Basic Pharmacology in Medicine

Fourth Edition

Basic Pharmacology in Medicine

Fourth Edition

Joseph R. DiPalma, M.D., D.Sc. (Hon.)
Professor Emeritus of Pharmacology and Medicine

G. John DiGregorio, M.D., Ph.D.
Professor of Pharmacology and Medicine

Edward J. Barbieri, Ph.D.
Associate Professor of Pharmacology

Andrew P. Ferko, Ph.D.
Associate Professor of Pharmacology

Department of Pharmacology
Division of Toxicology
Medical College of Pennsylvania and Hahnemann University
Philadelphia, Pennsylvania

Medical Surveillance Inc.
West Chester

Basic Pharmacology in Medicine

Fourth Edition

ISBN 0-942447-04-2

Printed in the United States of America

Printing: 1 2 3 4 5 6

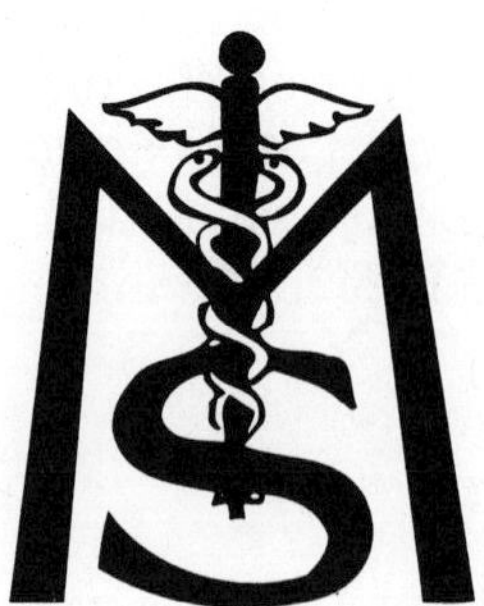

CONTENTS

Contributors xi

Preface xv

PART I

MODERN APPROACHES TO PHARMACOLOGY

Section Editor Joseph R. DiPalma

1 Introduction to Pharmacology 3
Joseph R. DiPalma

2 The Drug-Receptor Interaction 16
Richard R. Neubig

3 Receptors and Intracellular Signals 28
Stephen P. Halenda

4 Pharmacokinetics 42
Edward J. Barbieri

5 Biotransformation 65
William J. Cooke

6 Clinical Pharmacology 76
Anthony J. Piraino and Jay Roberts

PART II

THE AUTONOMIC NERVOUS SYSTEM

Section Editor Edward J. Barbieri

7 Introduction to the Autonomic Nervous System 99
Domenic A. DeBias

8 Adrenergic Drugs *113*
Terriann Crisp

9 Adrenergic Blocking and Neuronal Blocking Drugs *130*
Andrew P. Ferko and G. John DiGregorio

10 Cholinomimetics Drugs *147*
Frank J. Dowd

11 Antimuscarinic Drugs and Ganglionic Blocking Agents *163*
Edward J. Barbieri

12 Skeletal Muscle Relaxants *173*
Edward J. Barbieri

PART III

LOCAL CONTROL SUBSTANCES

Section Editor Edward J. Barbieri

13 Histamine, Histamine Receptor Antagonists, 5-Hydroxytryptamine, and Its Congeners *185*
Edward J. Barbieri and Andrew P. Ferko

14 Prostaglandins and Related Eicosanoids *205*
J. Bryan Smith

PART IV

CENTRAL NERVOUS SYSTEM DRUGS

Section Editor G. John DiGregorio

15 General Anesthetics *219*
Jan C. Horrow and Ruby M. Padolina

16 Sedatives and Hypnotics *233*
Laurence A. Carr

17 Antianxiety Drugs *244*
Lynn Wecker

18 Ethanol and Related Alcohols *253*
Andrew P. Ferko

19 Psychotomimetic Drugs *262*
Alan S. Bloom

20 Antipsychotic Drugs and Lithium *275*
Martin D. Schechter

21 Antidepressant Drugs *289*
Beth Hoskins

22 Antiepileptic and Antiparkinsonian Drugs *303*
Arthur Raines

23 Opioid Analgesics *319*
Anthony J. Triolo

24 Nonsteroidal Anti-Inflammatory Drugs and Drugs Used in the Treatment of Gout *345*
Joan Y. Summy-Long

25 Local Anesthetics *365*
Jonathan T. Abrams and Jerry D. Levitt

26 Drug Dependence *375*
Charles P. O'Brien

PART V

THE CARDIOVASCULAR AND RENAL AND RESPIRATORY SYSTEMS

Section Editor Joseph R. DiPalma

27 Congestive Heart Failure: Cardiac Glycosides and Other Inotropic Agents and Vasodilator Therapy *387*
Joseph R. DiPalma

28 Drugs for Tachyarrhythmias *400*
Joanne I. Moore

29 Antianginal Drugs *425*
Joanne I. Moore

30 Agents Used in Hyperlipoproteinemia *439*
Evangelos T. Angelakos and G. John DiGregorio

31 Diuretics *455*
Charles T. Stier, Jr.

32 Antihypertensive Drugs *468*
Cathy A. Bruner

33 Drugs for Chronic Obstructive Pulmonary Diseases *485*
Bruce R. Pitt and William J. Calhoun

PART VI

THE HEMATOPOIETIC SYSTEM

Section Editor Andrew P. Ferko

34 Antianemia Agents *503*
David L. Topolsky and Sigmund B. Kahn

35 Anticoagulant and Procoagulant Drugs *520*
Carl Barsigian and José Martinez

PART VII

THE GASTROINTESTINAL SYSTEM

Section Editor Joseph R. DiPalma

36 Vitamins *539*
David R. Schneider

37 Gastrointestinal Drugs *560*
Joan S. DiPalma

PART VIII

ENDOCRINES

Section Editor Andrew P. Ferko

38 Thyroid and Parathyroid Drugs *583*
Jeffrey L. Miller and Leslie I. Rose

39 Insulins and Oral Hypoglycemic Agents 596
Norman Altszuler

40 Female Sex Hormones, Oral Contraceptives, and Fertility Agents 611
Ira Weinstein

41 Androgens, Anabolic Steroids, and Inhibitors 630
Gerald H. Sterling

42 Corticotropin and Corticosteroids 638
Jeffrey L. Miller and Leslie I. Rose

PART IX

ANTINEOPLASTIC AGENTS

Section Editor Joseph R. DiPalma

43 Cancer Chemotherapy 653
Pamela A. Crilley and Michael J. Styler

44 Immunopharmacologic Drugs 676
Eric M. Scholar

PART X

ANTI-INFECTIVE AGENTS

Section Editor G. John DiGregorio

45 Antimicrobials I: General Concepts, Beta-Lactam Antibiotics, and Glycopeptides 691
Abdolghader Molavi

46 Antimicrobials II: Aminoglycosides and Quinolones 719
Abdolghader Molavi

47 Antimicrobials III: Macrolides, Clindamycin, Metronidazole, Sulfonamides, Trimethoprim, Chloramphenicol, and Tetracyclines 729
Abdolghader Molavi

48 Antimicrobials IV: Antimycobacterial Drugs 747
Abdolghader Molavi

49 Antifungal and Antiviral Drugs *757*
Henry W. Hitner

50 Drugs Used in Protozoan Infections *771*
Joseph R. DiPalma

51 Chemotherapy of Helminthiases *787*
Benjamin Z. Ngwenya

PART XI

TOXICOLOGY

Section Editor Joseph R. DiPalma

52 Toxicology *803*
Thomas L. Pazdernik

53 Non-Metallic Toxicants *810*
Thomas L. Pazdernik

54 Heavy Metals and Antagonists *821*
Thomas L. Pazdernik

Index *835*

C O N T R I B U T O R S

Jonathan T. Abrams, M.D.
Assistant Professor of Anesthesiology
Department of Anesthesiology
Medical College of Pennsylvania
and Hahnemann University
Philadelphia, Pennsylvania

Norman Altszuler, Ph.D.
Professor
Department of Pharmacology
New York University Medical Center
New York, New York

Evangelos T. Angelakos, M.D., Ph.D.
Professor
Department of Pharmacology
Medical College of Pennsylvania
and Hahnemann University
Philadelphia, Pennsylvania

Edward J. Barbieri, Ph.D.
Associate Professor
Department of Pharmacology
Medical College of Pennsylvania
and Hahnemann University
Philadelphia, Pennsylvania

Carl Barsigian, Ph.D.
Assistant Professor of Medicine
and Pharmacology
Cardeza Foundation for Hematologic Research
Department of Medicine
Jefferson Medical College
of Thomas Jefferson University
Philadelphia, Pennsylvania

Alan S. Bloom, Ph.D.
Professor
Department of Pharmacology and Toxicology
Medical College of Wisconsin
Milwaukee, Wisconsin

Cathy A. Bruner, Ph.D.
Associate Professor
Department of Pharmacology and Toxicology
Albany Medical College
Albany, New York

William J. Calhoun, M.D.
Associate Professor
Department of Medicine
University of Pittsburgh School of Medicine
Pittsburgh, Pennsylvania

Laurence A. Carr, Ph.D.
Professor
Department of Pharmacology and Toxicology
University of Louisville
Louisville, Kentucky

William J. Cooke, Ph.D.
Professor and Chairman
Department of Pharmacology
Eastern Virginia Medical School
Norfolk, Virginia

Pamela A. Crilley, D.O.
Assistant Professor
Department of Medicine
Medical College of Pennsylvania
and Hahnemann University
Philadelphia, Pennsylvania

Terriann Crisp, Ph.D.
Associate Professor
Department of Pharmacology
Northeastern Ohio Universities
Rootstown, Ohio

Domenic A. DeBias, Ph.D.
Professor and Chairman
Department of Physiology and Pharmacology
Philadelphia College of Osteopathic Medicine
Philadelphia, Pennsylvania

G. John DiGregorio, M.D., Ph.D.
Professor
Department of Pharmacology
Medical College of Pennsylvania
and Hahnemann University
Philadelphia, Pennsylvania

Joan S. DiPalma, M.D.
Associate Professor
Department of Pediatrics
Georgetown University, School of Medicine
Washington, D.C.

Joseph R. DiPalma, M.D.
Professor Emeritus
Departments of Pharmacology and Medicine
Medical College of Pennsylvania
and Hahnemann University
Philadelphia, Pennsylvania

Frank J. Dowd, D.D.S., Ph.D.
Professor and Chairman
Department of Pharmacology
Creighton University
Omaha, Nebraska

Andrew P. Ferko, Ph.D.
Associate Professor
Department of Pharmacology
Medical College of Pennsylvania
and Hahnemann University
Philadelphia, Pennsylvania

Stephen P. Halenda, Ph.D.
Associate Professor
Department of Pharmacology
University of Missouri
Columbia, Missouri

Henry W. Hitner, Ph.D.
Professor
Department of Physiology and Pharmacology
Philadelphia College of Osteopathic Medicine
Philadelphia, Pennsylvania

Jan C. Horrow, M.D.
Professor
Department of Anesthesiology
Medical College of Pennsylvania
and Hahnemann University
Philadelphia, Pennsylvania

Beth Hoskins, Ph.D.
Professor
Department of Pharmacology and Toxicology
University of Mississippi Medical Center
Jackson, Mississippi

Sigmund B. Kahn, M.D.
Professor
Department of Medicine
Medical College of Pennsylvania
and Hahnemann University
Philadelphia, Pennsylvania

Jerry D. Levitt, M.D.
Associate Professor of Anesthesiology
Department of Anesthesiology
Medical College of Pennsylvania
and Hahnemann University
Philadelphia, Pennsylvania

José Martinez, M.D.
Professor of Medicine
Cardeza Foundation for Hematologic Research
Department of Medicine
Jefferson Medical College
of Thomas Jefferson University
Philadelphia, Pennsylvania

Jeffrey L. Miller, M.D.
Associate Professor of Medicine
Department of Medicine
Medical College of Pennsylvania
and Hahnemann University
Philadelphia, Pennsylvania

Abdolghader Molavi, M.D.
Professor
Director, Division of Infectious Diseases
Department of Medicine
Medical College of Pennsylvania
and Hahnemann University
Philadelphia, Pennsylvania

Joanne I. Moore, Ph.D.
Professor and Head
Department of Pharmacology
University of Oklahoma
College of Medicine and Dentistry
Oklahoma City, Oklahoma

Richard R. Neubig, Ph.D.
Associate Professor of Pharmacology
Department of Pharmacology
University of Michigan Medical School
Ann Arbor, Michigan

Benjamin Z. Ngwenya, Ph.D.
Associate Professor
Department of Microbiology and Immunology
Medical College of Pennsylvania
and Hahnemann University
Philadelphia, Pennsylvania

Charles P. O'Brien, M.D., Ph.D.
Professor and Vice Chairman
Department of Psychiatry
University of Pennsylvania
Philadelphia, Pennsylvania

Ruby M. Padolina, M.D.
Associate Professor of Clinical Anesthesiology
Department of Anesthesiology
Medical College of Pennsylvania
and Hahnemann University
Philadelphia, Pennsylvania

Thomas L. Pazdernik, Ph.D.
Professor
Department of Pharmacology, Toxicology
and Therapeutics
University of Kansas Medical Center
Kansas City, Kansas

Anthony J. Piraino, M.D., Ph.D.
Professor
Departments of Medicine and Pharmacology
Medical College of Pennsylvania
and Hahnemann University
Philadelphia, Pennsylvania

Bruce R. Pitt, Ph.D.
Professor
Department of Pharmacology
University of Pittsburgh School of Medicine
Pittsburgh, Pennsylvania

Arthur Raines, Ph.D.
Professor
Department of Pharmacology
Georgetown University School of Medicine
Washington, D.C.

Jay Roberts, Ph.D.
Professor and Chairman
Department of Pharmacology
Medical College of Pennsylvania
and Hahnemann University
Philadelphia, Pennsylvania

Leslie I. Rose, M.D.
Professor of Medicine
Director, Division of Endocrinology
Department of Medicine
Medical College of Pennsylvania
and Hahnemann University
Philadelphia, Pennsylvania

Martin D. Schechter, Ph.D.
Professor and Chairman
Department of Pharmacology
Northeastern Ohio University College of Medicine
Rootstown, Ohio

David R. Schneider, Ph.D.
Professor
Department of Pharmacology
Wayne State University School of Medicine
Detroit, Michigan

Eric M. Scholar, Ph.D.
Associate Professor
Department of Pharmacology
University of Nebraska Medical Center
Omaha, Nebraska

J. Bryan Smith, Ph.D.
Professor and Chairman
Department of Pharmacology
Temple University, School of Medicine
Philadelphia, Pennsylvania

Gerald H. Sterling, Ph.D.
Associate Professor
Department of Pharmacology
Temple University, School of Medicine
Philadelphia, Pennsylvania

Charles T. Stier, Jr., Ph.D.
Associate Professor
Department of Pharmacology
New York Medical College
Valhalla, New York

Michael J. Styler, M.D.
Senior Instructor
Department of Medicine
Medical College of Pennsylvania
and Hahnemann University
Philadelphia, Pennsylvania

Joan Y. Summy-Long, Ph.D.
Professor
Department of Pharmacology
Milton S. Hershey Medical Center
Hershey, Pennsylvania

David L. Topolsky, M.D.
Assistant Professor
Department of Medicine
Medical College of Pennsylvania
and Hahnemann University
Philadelphia, Pennsylvania

Anthony J. Triolo, Ph.D.
Professor
Department of Pharmacology
Jefferson Medical College
of Thomas Jefferson University
Philadelphia, Pennsylvania

Lynn Wecker, Ph.D.
Professor and Chairman
Department of Pharmacology
University of Florida College of Medicine
Tampa, Florida

Ira Weinstein, Ph.D.
Professor
Department of Pharmacology
University of Tennessee, College of Medicine
Memphis, Tennessee

PREFACE

The fourth edition of Basic Pharmacology in Medicine continues its tradition of providing a teaching text which is authentic, is up to date, and is written in enough depth to provide a sound foundation, yet is brief enough to be digestible. Because of its emphasis on Clinical Pharmacology, students will find that this text effectively bridges the gap between basic facts and clinical applications.

A new publisher, Medical Surveillance, has offered the opportunity to the editors to recast the book to better serve its purpose. The value of a multi-authored book ultimately must rest upon the selection of contributors who are knowledgeable, write well, and have extensive experience in their subject. To this end, 28 new contributors have been selected to revise and improve existing text. Most of these individuals are pharmacology medical school course directors and hence in a position to have judgement about the latest pertinent information. Other major changes include an introductory chapter which orients the discovery of new pharmacological agents to the advances in medicine's control of disease. Nutritional agents are now recognized to be important risk factors in many diseases. This subject is addressed in a new chapter in vitamins. Important attention is now devoted to the environment and its influence on disease processes. To address this subject the toxicology section has been expanded to three chapters. Gastrointestinal disease, always a mainstay of medical practice, now has a separate chapter on drugs which are effective in the treatment of peptic ulcer, inflammatory bowel disease and other entities. This has caused some expansion, partially compensated by elimination of redundant material such as preparations and doses, which second year medical students are not required to know and which need to be looked up in a prescribing manual.

The editors are deeply grateful to their many collaborators. The entire book is now on computer files and our secretarial help, Linda Bush and Elizabeth Ju, have shown extraordinary cooperation and patience. Thomas Nicosia of Medical Surveillance has been especially generous and stimulating. Emil Bobyock, Robert McMichael, and Eileen Ruch have been of enormous help in the publication of this text.

Joseph R. DiPalma
G. John DiGregorio
Edward J. Barbieri
Andrew P. Ferko

PART I

Modern Approaches to Pharmacology

SECTION EDITOR

Joseph R. DiPalma

CHAPTER 1

Introduction to Pharmacology

Joseph R. DiPalma

Since the beginning of recorded civilization humans have sought substances which would give them an advantage in the alleviation of disease, in the search for food, and for defense. One of the earliest documents, the Egyptian papyri of Ebers (1550 BC) lists many therapeutic preparations, including digitalis and opium which are still used today in modified and refined forms. Since ancient times the natives of the upper Amazon and the Orinoco rivers perfected a very effective arrow poison (curare) extracted from the vines of *Chondodendron tomentosum* and *Strychnos lethalis*. The active alkaloid of curare, tubocurarine, is still used today as a neuromuscular blocking agent during surgery. As recently as 1992, a very powerful (and toxic) chemical which has remarkable analgesic properties has been synthesized from an extract of the glands of a frog *Epipedobates tricolor*. It has been reported that Ecuadorian indians have been using this venom as an arrow poison for generations. The active ingredient of this material is epibatidine which has a chemical structure different from any known analgesic agent; it has a specific receptor because only one enantiomer is active. Nature still provides more diversity of chemical structure than can be synthesized by the chemical industry.

These two arrow poisons found empirically by more primitive cultures illustrate the powerful advance in technology of the 20th century. Curare took over 50 years to develop to its present useful drug form; epibatidine is projected to be a useful analgesic drug in 3 or 4 years, if its toxicity can be controlled.

Advances in pharmacological information developed painfully and slowly over the centuries. As shown in Table 1-1 each step was vital to the next until accumulated knowledge arrived at a critical point about 1900. Until this time there were no university chairs of Pharmacology except for that of Rudolph Buchheim (1820 - 1879) at Dorpat (Tartu). His pupil, Oswald Schmiedeberg (1838 - 1921) held the Chair of Pharmacology at Strasbourg. John Jacob Abel one of his fellows, held the first Chair of Pharmacology in the United States at the University of Michigan Medical School (1892). Mostly all medical schools in the U.S. now have separate departments of pharmacology. The amazing development of drug therapy since 1900 is summarized in Table 1-2. The great majority of useful drugs have been discovered by observing the effects of large numbers of chemical compounds in animal test systems, hoping to find chemical entities with worthwhile pharmacologic activity and minimal toxicity. With the powerful new technology exemplified in Table 1-2, it is almost certain that most novel, effective drugs will be designed, rather than found empirically.

An excellent illustration is the development of captopril, an angiotensin converting enzyme (ACE) inhibitor, and a very useful drug for the treatment of hypertension and congestive heart failure. In 1975, it was known that angiotensin II was an important factor in human hypertension. It was also understood that a converting enzyme was needed to produce active angiotensin II from a precursor. If the converting enzyme could be inhibited by a drug, then a useful antihypertensive agent might be found. Unfortunately, the exact structure of the converting enzyme was not known at that time. However, the conformation of a closely related enzyme was known and using this information it was found that a modified and substituted proline derivative was suitably active in blocking ACE: the resulting drug was captopril. Using this information, investigators designed other modifications of proline resulting in other useful ACE inhibitors, e.g., enalapril and lisinopril.

Many of the advances presented in Table 1-2 are actually discoveries in other basic sciences, for

TABLE 1-1 Some significant events in the development of pharmacology from ancient times to 1900

Author	Date(s)	Discovery	Significance
Ebers papyri	1550 BC	Remedies used in ancient times.	One of the first authentic documents describing the use of substances for the cure of disease.
Theophrastus	370 - 286 BC	Botanical descriptions.	Rudimentary beginnings of pharmacognosy.
Dioscorides	100 AD	Classified materia medica by substances rather than by disease syndromes.	Forerunner of modern pharmacopeias.
Galen	200 AD	Extended the work of Dioscorides. Perfected many remedies. Invented tincture of opium.	Works preserved and followed for centuries during the middle ages.
Avicenna	980 - 1037	Added new remedies of natural sources.	Preserved knowledge during the dark ages.
Paracelsus	1493 - 1541	An alchemist who popularized the use of salts of potassium, iron, and arsenic. Developed tinctures.	Broke away from the classical doctrines of Galen. Established a chemical basis for drug action.
Serturner	1806	Isolated morphine from opium.	Important step in identifying active ingredients from natural substances.
Magendie, F.	1783 - 1855	A physiologist who published the first medical formulary of purified chemical agents.	Among the drugs now identified were quinine, emetine, and strychnine.
Ehrlich, P.	1854 - 1915	Established the "lock and key" theory of drug action. Also, famous for the discovery of the cure for syphilis.	Basis of drug-receptor interaction. A fundamental beginning of immunology.
Fischer, E.	1852 - 1919	Synthesis of barbital, the first barbiturate.	The industrial revolution gave rise to a chemical industry which could synthesize new agents.

example, physiology, biochemistry, and microbiology. Pharmacology combines these innovations into a logical body of information which aims to integrate knowledge into a pattern which makes it possible to use chemicals effectively and safely as drugs for the therapy of disease. In this effort there is close integration with clinical medicine, especially with internal medicine and anesthesiology, but actually with all clinical subspecialities. Certainly, the amazing surgical feats of today, such as organ transplantation, would not be possible without the use of drugs.

TABLE 1-2 Some of the main drug and theoretical discoveries since 1900.

Date	Drug and discoveries	Comments
1900 to 1920	Autonomic Nervous System Epinephrine Acetylcholine Anesthesia Local anesthetics (cocaine and procaine) Central Nervous System Barbital Phenobarbital Chemotherapy Arsphenamine Lock and Key Theory Histamine Ergot Cardiology Digitalis Heparin Vitamins A, D, B_1, and niacin Aspirin and other Salicylates	Autonomic nervous system concepts are refined and the primary neurohumors are identified. Development of local anesthetics advanced for anesthesia. Barbiturates replace older drugs for sedation and hypnosis. Treatment of syphilis is greatly advanced by the development of arsphenamine. Erhlich's lock and key theory of drug action reinforces the receptor concept. Histamine's role in the body advances the concept of allergic reactions. The discovery of ergot derivatives introduce the concept of autonomic blockade. Drugs are used in the treatment of migraine headaches. Digitalis is rediscovered as a very useful cardiac drug. Heparin becomes the first clinically-effective anticoagulant. Importance of vitamins in the therapy of deficiency diseases come into prominence. Salicylates are considered the best therapy for arthritis and rheumatic heart disease.
1921 to 1940	Hormones Insulin Estrogen Testosterone Progesterone Anterior Pituitary Hormone Chemotherapy Sulfonamides Anesthetics Thiopental Cyclopropane Nitrous oxide Cardiology Quinidine Gastroenterology Antacids Antispasmodics Vitamins Ascorbic Acid Liver Extract Beginnings of Biochemical Pharmacology	Diabetics now could be controlled with insulin. Pernicious anemia, a uniformly fatal disease, could now be controlled by a liver extract. Introduction of the sex hormones open up therapy of many sexual aberrations. Anterior pituitary hormone is mainly of scientific interest at this time. Discovery of sulfonamides are of major importance in the therapy of infections; these drugs open up the whole field of chemotherapy. Thiopental, an ultra-short acting barbiturate, makes short-term anesthesia possible. Cyclopropane, a gas, becomes an important addition to diethyl ether and chloroform. Nitrous oxide is also widely used. Quinidine, the sole antiarrhythmic drug, receives much attention. Antacids are more widely used for gastric ulcer. Atropine-like compounds (antispasmodics) become the main therapy for gastrointestinal complaints. Ascorbic acid is synthesized and its role is more firmly established. Adenosine triphosphate (ATP) is synthesized. Metabolism of drugs begin to be studied; this forms an early basis of pharmacokinetics.

TABLE 1-2 (continued) Some of the main drug and theoretical discoveries since 1900.

Date	Drug and discoveries	Comments
1941 to 1960	Antibiotics Penicillins Cephalosporins Streptomycin Chloramphenicol Tetracyclines Vancomycin Central Nervous System Antipsychotics Chlorpromazine Haloperidol Lithium Antidepressants Tricyclics MAO inhibitors Antianxiety Agents Benzodiazepines Antiepileptic Drugs Phenytoin Ethosuximide Valproic acid Antiparkinsonian Drugs Levodopa Opioid Antagonists Naloxone Naltrexone Synthetic Opioids Methadone Meperidine Cardiovascular Drugs Antihypertensives Reserpine Methyldopa Clonidine Hydralazine Antiarrhythmics Procainamide Lidocaine Diuretics Mecurials Thiazides Oral Anticoagulants Warfarin, others	The introduction of penicillin start a world-wide search for antibiotics from fungi and other organisms. Drug resistance becomes a problem, but almost every infectious disease can now be treated with antibiotics. The introduction of phenothiazines for schizophrenia start a flood of central nervous system (CNS) drugs. CNS neurotransmitters, norepinephrine, serotonin, γ-aminobutyric acid (GABA), and glutamate are identified as CNS neurohumors, which open up avenues for new drug development. Effective drugs for epilepsy and Parkinson's disease become available. Antagonists to opioids are developed. A number of synthetic opioids extend the use of these drugs. Addiction to opioids increases and methadone therapy is established. Enkephalins are discovered. The introduction of antihypertensive drugs revolutionize the therapy of this condition. For the first time, blood pressure can be safely returned to normal and thus life span is prolonged and the incidence of morbidity is decreased. Open heart surgery becomes possible because of more effective anesthesia, antibiotics, and the development of pulmonary by-pass. Many antiarrhythmic drugs become available. The use of effective, non-explosive anesthetics like halothane is started. An increased use of curariform agents, e.g., tubocurarine and succinylcholine, make many types of surgery safer. Organic mercurial diuretics, which had to be given parenterally are soon replaced by the oral thiazide diuretics. This makes the therapy of congestive heart failure much more pleasant and effective. Nitroglycerin and other nitrates are still widely used. No more effective therapy for angina is available. The oral anticoagulants extend the use of heparin in conditions of hypercoagulation of blood.

TABLE 1-2 (continued) Some of the main drug and theoretical discoveries since 1900.

Date	Drug and discoveries	Comments
1941 to 1960	Blood Vitamin K Vitamin B_{12} Folic Acid Diabetes Oral Hypoglycemics Newer insulins Hormones Newer estrogens Newer progestins Gonadotropins Cortisone Adrenocorticotropic Hormone (ACTH) Prednisone, others Cancer Chemotherapy Antimetabolites Alkylating Agents Steroid Hormones Antibiotics Plant Alkaloids Theoretical discoveries: Separation of α- and β-adrenergic receptors in the autonomic nervous system Use of radioactive isotopes in drug research Testing of drugs in man; placebo effect Structure of DNA elucidated Teratogenic effects of drugs Field of Clinical Pharmacology developed	The discovery of vitamin K makes liver surgery and other types of bowel surgery much safer. At last, the mystery of the effectiveness of liver extract in pernicious anemia is solved with the discovery of vitamin B_{12}. Folic acid metabolism and its relationship to blood production is elucidated. The role of intrinsic factor is classified. The development of tolbutamide and related oral hypoglycemic agents make therapy for non-insulin dependent diabetics much more effective. The newer, long acting insulins simplify therapy of insulin-dependent diabetics. Estrogens are now widely used for menopausal symptoms. There is great use of diethylstilbestrol, an inexpensive synthetic drug. Progesterone is widely used for functional uterine bleeding, amenorrhea and infertility. The advent of the synthesis of cortisone and its more useful congener, prednisone, make the therapy of a wide variety of diseases possible; prominent among these is rheumatoid arthritis and lupus erythematosus. Addison's Disease can now be cured. Remarkable advances in drugs that inhibit cell growth permit more effective therapy of cancer. Drugs like methotrexate and 6-mercaptopurine are much more effective than prior drugs. The alkylating agents, particularly the polyfunctional ones, prove to be especially useful. The use of steroids as adjuncts increase overall "cure" rates. Use of multiple agents improve the kill ratio and tend to inhibit the development of resistance. The finding that there are different receptors in the autonomic neurons system is a great stimulus to the development of new autonomic drugs. Receptor concepts are strengthen and amplified. The structure of the nicotine receptor is anticipated. Radioactively-tagged drugs enable metabolic studies, not possible before, to be conducted. Drug levels too low to be measured can now be detected. The structure of DNA is defined. This makes possible the study of the action of drugs on this most vital cellular structure. This is the early beginning of the molecular biology movement and genetic technology. The field of Biochemical Pharmacology becomes more important with the flood of new drugs. The discovery of the placebo effect enforces the testing of new drugs by blind and double-blind techniques in humans. The thalidomide episode awakens the public and the FDA to the importance of drug effectiveness and safety.

TABLE 1-2 (continued) Some of the main drug and theoretical discoveries since 1900.

Date	Drug and discoveries	Comments
1961 to 1980	Autonomic Nervous System Adrenergic Agonists: Norepinephrine Dopamine β-Adrenergic Receptor Blockers α-Adrenergic Receptor Blockers Nicotinic receptor subtypes Central Nervous System Benzodiazepines Psychotomimetics Antidepressants Opioids Bromocriptine General Anesthetics Enflurane Ketamine Cardiovascular Drugs Antiarrhythmics Tocainide Mexiletine Bretylium Antihypertensives ACE Inhibitors New β-Adrenergic Blockers Verapamil Congestive Heart Failure Sodium Nitroprusside Digoxin Antihyperlipemic Drugs Clofibrate Nicotinic Acid Cholestyramine Colestipol Prostaglandins Nonsteroidal Antiinflammatory Drugs (NSAIDs) Ibuprofen Naproxen Indomethacin Gastrointestinal Drugs H_2-Receptor Blockers Cimetidine	Autonomic receptors are more clearly defined. Greater use of adrenergic agents in shock occurs. β-Adrenergic blockers begin to be used in a wide variety of diseases. α-Adrenergic blockers become useful as antihypertensives. Surgery to block the autonomics is no longer necessary (due to chemical sympathectomy). Benzodiazepines find wide use as sedatives, antianxiety agents, short-term anesthetic agents, and anticonvulsants; all involving a major inhibitory system of the brain — the GABA receptor. The use of LSD gives rise to the psychedelic experience. Increased abuse of amphetamines and phencyclidine occurs; cocaine abuse increases greatly. Bromocriptine, a dopamine receptor agonist which acted centrally, augmented the knowledge of the function of dopamine in the brain. The development of newer, non-explosive halogenated volatile general anesthetics (e.g., enflurane), and IV drugs (e.g., ketamine) make surgical anesthesia safer and more effective. A greater interest in antiarrhythmic drugs begins. The use of some of the older antihypertensive drugs ceases; β-adrenergic blockers and diuretics dominate therapy. In severe heart failure, the use of vasodilators become a useful therapeutic modality. Digoxin becomes the primary digitalis glycoside in clinical use. Blood cholesterol becomes a major risk factor in coronary artery disease and stroke. Antihyperlipemic drugs are more widely used. β-Adrenergic blockers are shown to lessen the incidence of mortality after a myocardial infarction. Discovery of the mechanism of action of aspirin (i.e., inhibition of the synthesis of prostaglandins) leads to the development of many nonsteroidal anti-inflammatory drugs (NSAIDs) which have wide uses as analgesics and antiinflammatory agents. Some may be superior to aspirin. Prostaglandins are used as drugs in neonates with patent ductus arteriosus and in pregnant women as abortifacients. New histamine receptors (H_2) are discovered. Cimetidine, an H_2-receptor antagonist, becomes a best selling drug, replacing antacids as a main therapy for peptic ulcers and reflux esophagitis.

TABLE 1-2 (continued) Some of the main drug and theoretical discoveries since 1900.

Date	Drug and discoveries	Comments
1961 to 1980	Hormones Human insulin Oral Contraceptives Anabolic Steroids Tamoxifen Clomiphene Antibacterials New penicillins New cephalosporins Antiviral Drugs Amantadine Vidarabine Idoxuridine Acyclovir Antifungal Agents Griseofulvin Ketoconazole Antituberculosis Drugs Isoniazid Rifampin Ethambutol Immunosuppressive Drugs Azathioprine Theoretical Developments Pharmacokinetics Epidemiological study of drugs Orphan Drugs Environmental effects of chemicals	Human insulin, produced by recombinant DNA technology, results in the use of a non-allergic insulin. Oral contraceptives become widely used. The illicit use of anabolic steroids to enhance athletic performance occurs; extensive abuse results. Tamoxifen, a competitive antagonist of estradiol, is found to be effective against breast cancer. The antiestrogen, clomiphene, improves fertility of some women and causes multiple births. Many new antibacterial penicillins and second- and third-generation cephalosporins are synthesized that have a wider spectrum of activity. Antiviral drugs become fairly effective in eye infections Antifungal drugs are effective in a number of infections. Tuberculosis, which had been virtually wiped out in the 60's and 70's, increases in incidence due to the emergence of resistant strains of *M. tuberculosis*. Azathioprine enables the transplantation of organs such as heart and kidney to occur. Pharmacokinetics develops with the precise determinations of drug disposition. This makes it possible to study congeners of drugs for superior properties and makes precise dosing more feasible. Epidemiological studies help to uncover effects of drugs on populations as a whole and the long-term environmental effects of chemicals. For example, DDT was found to persist for long periods of time and may cause birth defects and cancer. The establishment of "orphan drugs" (sponsoring by the government with tax breaks and special grants) make it possible to develop useful drugs for rare diseases that are not commercially feasible. Recombinant DNA technology is developed so as to be practically able to synthesize any substance. Insulin is one of the first major examples.

TABLE 1-2 (continued) Some of the main drug and theoretical discoveries since 1900.

Date	Drug and discoveries	Comments
1981 into the 90's	Autonomic Nervous System M_1, M_2 receptors Dopamine receptors Adenylate cyclase G Proteins Central Nervous System GABA receptors New Antidepressants Fluoxetine Sertraline Paroxetine New Antipsychotics Clozapine New Anesthetics Midazolam Propofol Anticonvulsants Carbamazepine Cardiovascular System Antiarrhythmics Flecainide Propafenone Amiodarone Moricizine Sotalol Antihypertensives ACE inhibitors Calcium Channel Blockers Verapamil Diltiazem Nifedipine Congestive Heart Failure ACE inhibitors Amrinone Milrinone Antihyperlipemic Drugs Lovastatin Myocardial Infarction Aspirin Alteplase Anistreplase Streptokinase Nonsteroidal Antiinflammatory Drugs (NSAIDs) Ketorolac Flurbiprofen Oxaprozin Nabumetone	Autonomic receptors continue to be defined. Mechanisms of signal transduction are described, including the important role of G proteins and second messengers such as calcium. The role of adenylate cyclase is clarified. Greater understanding of the role of GABA occurs. Many new benzodiazepines are developed with a variety of uses such as anticonvulsants, sedatives, hypnotics, and anesthetics. New blockers of serotonin reuptake (e.g., fluoxetine, sertraline, and paroxetine) open a new series of antidepressant drugs. Tricyclics antidepressants are still widely, used as are monoamine oxidase inhibitors. Lithium is more widely used as an agent for bipolar disease. The development of clozapine allows for improvement in some psychotic patients who have not responded to the classical antipsychotic agents. Newer agents for IV anesthesia (e.g., midazolam and propofol) are found to be very useful for short operations and procedures. Carbamazepine competes with phenytoin as a primary antiepileptic drug. Sudden death from an arrhythmia is declared an epidemic and, as a result, many new antiarrhythmics are developed. The value of some drugs are later seriously questioned and restricted in use. ACE inhibitors now become dominant antihypertensives. Monotherapy is emphasized; there is less use of thiazide diuretics. Calcium channel blockers also become important as antihypertensive and antianginal drugs. ACE inhibitors are found to be an effective therapy for congestive heart failure. Digoxin is still useful. Other new inotropes are developed, but are not very effective. The development of lovastatin becomes a superior therapy for hyperlipidemia. Other HMG-CoA inhibitors follow and become widely used to lower blood cholesterol. Aspirin inhibition of platelet aggregation reduces the risk of myocardial infarction. The use of thrombolytic agents becomes effective as therapy for acute myocardial infarction. NSAIDs are now the most widely used drugs for osteoarthritis, rheumatoid arthritis, and pain. Ketorolac becomes available in a parenteral form.

TABLE 1-2 (continued) Some of the main drug and theoretical discoveries since 1900.

Date	Drug and discoveries	Comments
1981 into the 90's	Gastrointestinal Drugs Ranitidine Famotidine Nizatidine Omeprazole Misoprostol Metoclopramide Cisapride Antibacterial Drugs New cephalosporins Imipenem Fluoroquinolones Ciprofloxacin Enoxacin Norfloxacin Antiviral Drugs Zidovudine Ribavirin Amantadine Foscarnet Didanosine Antifungal Drugs Flucytosine Miconazole Antimalarial Drugs Mefloquine Halofantrine Antiprotozoal Drugs Pentamidine Metronidazole Trimethoprim Sulfamethoxazole Eflornithine	H_2-receptor blockers become very popular for the therapy of peptic ulcer and reflux esophagitis. Newer compounds compete with cimetidine. Omeprazole, a proton pump inhibitor becomes an important new agent for refractory cases of peptic ulcer and reflux esophagitis. Misoprostol, a prostaglandin analog, is developed to protect the stomach against the ulcerogenic activity of NSAIDs. Metoclopramide, a dopamine receptor antagonist, increases gastric emptying. It is also an effective antiemetic. Cisapride is also effective. New antibacterial drugs are developed which have a broader spectrum of activity and pharmacokinetic advantages. The development of clavulanic acid as a beta-lactamase inhibitor increases the activity of certain compounds. The unique chemical structure of imipenem resists beta-lactamases. The fluoroquinolones become a new group of antibacterial drugs and are found to be active against some previously resistant bacteria. The discovery of human immunodeficiency viruses and the acquired immunodeficiency disease syndrome (AIDS) epidemic increases the search for new antiviral drugs. Zidovudine is partially effective, as is didanosine. Other antiviral agents are found to be useful in retinitis, cystic fibrosis, and respiratory infections. Newer antifungal drugs make therapy of fungal infections more amenable, especially in immunocompromised patients. The incidence of tuberculosis continues to rise due to resistance and to AIDS. New drugs are investigated. Malaria becomes an increasing problem worldwide. New drugs for resistant *P. falciparum* are needed. Two new antimalarial agents, mefloquine and halofantrine, are a partial answer to the problem. Protozoal diseases increase due to AIDS. Metronidazole, an antibacterial compound, becomes an important antiprotozoal agent. *Plasmodium carinii* infections respond to pentamidine and the sulfamethoxazole-trimethoprim combination in AIDS patients. Eflornithine becomes an important new drug for the treatment of trypanosomiasis; it is also effective in the treatment of *P. carinii* infections.

TABLE 1-2 (continued) Some of the main drug and theoretical discoveries since 1900.

Date	Drug and discoveries	Comments
1981 Into the 90's	Skeletal Muscle Blockers Atracurium Vecuronium Mivacurium Doxacurium Immunosuppressives and Immunomodulators Cyclosporine Muromonab-CD3 Interferons Interleukins Cancer Chemotherapy Carmustine Cisplatin Etoposide Flutamide Ifosfamide Paclitaxel (Taxol) Hormones GnRH Agonists Gonadorelin Leuprolide Nafarelin Growth hormone Blood Modifiers Epoetin alfa Ticlodipine Alteplase Antihemophilic factor Factor IX complex Theoretical Developments Receptors Cell cycle Synthesis of peptides Structure of enzymes Computer technology Ethical considerations Gene therapy Epidemiology Environmental factors Cost considerations	There is a renewed interest in neuromuscular blocking agents and the development of new curariform compounds. Cyclosporine greatly improves the transplantation of heart, liver, kidney, and other organs by suppressing the immune system. Muromonab-CD3 becomes useful in renal transplants. Interferons and interleukins are found to be useful as immunomodulator drugs in certain cancers. Many new cancer chemotherapeutic agents are developed. Combination of agents continues to overcome the development of resistance to therapy and insures a more complete cell kill. The incidence of "cure" improves, but cancers are still increasing. The availability of the GnRH agonists makes possible tests of pituitary function. Leuprolide is useful in prostatic cancer. The availability of synthetic growth hormone leads to human experiments on aging and increase in stature. Recombinant human erythropoietin (epoetin alfa) stimulates blood production in renal insufficiency and other debilitating diseases. Ticlodipine is developed as a new agent for inhibition of platelet aggregation and is used to prevent stroke. Thrombolytic agents become the first-line therapy for acute myocardial infarction. Treatment of hemophilia is improved by the greater availability of antihemophilic factors. There is an amazing development of the knowledge of receptors. The structure and function of most receptors become known. The cell cycle and the factors that influence it are elucidated. The ability to synthesize peptides and proteins makes a large number of new drugs available, which were not possible previously. Computer technology begins to solve the problems of the fit of agonists and antagonists with receptors. Drugs can be designed purely on computer modelling and theoretical grounds. Use of certain processes, such as gene therapy and fertility technology raises serious ethical questions. Drug therapies may affect worldwide populations and the environment; there is enhanced interest in epidemiological studies. The cost of drugs has risen much faster than the general rate of inflation. This has caused great concern in view of the high cost of present-day medical care.

A text in pharmacology aims to provide medical students and students in the allied health professions (e.g., pharmacists, nurses, physician assistants, respiratory therapists) with information which will make it possible to understand how drugs act, what effects they produce in the body, how the body disposes of these foreign compounds, and what are their therapeutic uses. Organization of pharmacological information into district categories makes it possible to retain and use large bodies of this acquired knowledge. The following are the categories of information concerning most drugs: names, chemistry, mechanism of action, effects on organ systems, pharmacokinetics, therapeutic uses, adverse reactions, and preparations and dosages.

Drug Names

One confusing aspect of pharmacology is the naming of drugs. Each drug has at least 3 names: the *chemical name*, the *generic name* and the *proprietary* or *trade name*. Thus the chemical name of aspirin is 2-(acetyloxy benzoic acid or acetylsalicylic acid); the generic name is aspirin and it has at least 50 trade names depending on the manufacturer and country of origin. Incidentally, the name aspirin was originally a trade name of Bayer, one of the largest manufacturers of the drug. Common usage has established the aspirin name as generic.

Today there is nothing haphazard about drug names. The chemical name generally follows Chemical Abstracts Service (CAS). The generic name is set by a committee of scientists, pharmacists, and physicians called United States Adapted Names (USAN). Trade names are invented by manufacturers and are designed to be easy to pronounce and suggestive of therapeutic effect. For example, the tranquilizer chlordiazepoxide is named *Librium* by one manufacturer. The generic name is the proper name for usage by scientists, physicians, and pharmacists. However in actual practice, the trade name is more commonly used and stressed in drug advertisements.

For the student, there is a distinct advantage in knowing the generic name, as it often indicates the chemical and functional classification of the drug. With a few exceptions, all drugs whose generic name ends in *-olol* are β-adrenergic receptor blocking agents. Some concept of the chemistry is immediately deduced from knowing the chemical structure of propranolol, the first of this class of drugs, i.e., the *prototype*. The rest of the drugs in the series of β-adrenergic blocking agents are called congeners. They have chemical similarities, although their pharmacological actions may differ quantitatively and qualitatively particularly in regard to absorption, distribution, and elimination.

Chemistry

A sound knowledge of organic chemistry is essential in pharmacology. The student does well to have a visual memory of the chemical structures of drugs. Drug action depends upon a close fit of the chemical structure of the drug to a portion of the receptor. Slight alterations in structure sometimes change an agonist into an antagonist. In addition changes in structure can profoundly affect the absorption, distribution, and elimination of a drug, thus changing the time sequence during which a drug may act. This field of chemical manipulation is known as structure-activity relationships. Derivatives of the prototype, which vary slightly from the original structure, may have superior attributes — or they may not.

Mechanism of Action

Physicians and other health personnel have an intimate knowledge of how a particular drug exerts its effect on the body. Armed with this information, they are better able to made expert clinical judgements.

There is a vast array of knowledge concerning the intimate mechanism of action of most drugs at a molecular level. For example, it now can be stated that digoxin inhibits Na^+,K^+-ATPase; aspirin inhibits the synthesis of prostaglandins; nitroglycerin achieves its effects by being converted to an endogenous vasodilator, nitric oxide, which is equivalent to endothelial-derived relaxant factor (EDRF); morphine binds to specific cellular receptors mimicking the action of endogenous opiate-like substances.

The technology for the synthesis of complex peptides is far advanced. This makes it possible to manufacture synthetic insulin and other peptide hormones. Altering the structure of these peptides allows one to deduce the mechanism of action at a molecular level which were not anticipated before. Furthermore, it is possible to make computer models of receptor proteins allowing a study of the exact chemical configuration. Thus smaller molecules may be designed to either block or stimulate the receptor. It is anticipated that this will lead to the discovery of many new and effective drugs for diseases hitherto resistant to present therapeutics.

Pharmacodynamics

This body of knowledge relates to the effect of drugs on the physiological functions of the individual and it also includes the mechanism of action. Pharmacodynamics describes which tissues and organ systems of the body are affected by a particular drug and, for this reason, is often referred to as "Effect on Organ Systems". Some examples are the effects of the administered drug on the central nervous system, autonomic nervous system, and cardiovascular system. Thus anesthetics, sedatives, autonomic drugs, gastrointestinal drugs, hormonal agents, etc. affecting practically every organ system in the body. Drugs are also classified by mechanism of action although they may affect the same organ system. The cardiovascular system drugs include calcium channel blockers, angiotensin converting enzyme inhibitors, and inotropics such as digitalis and vasodilators. Thus, mechanisms of action are intimately related to pharmacodynamics.

Pharmacokinetics

This subject concerns the movement of drugs in body. Fortunately, modern technology allows the measurement of drug concentrations in all body fluids. Also in most cases, at equilibrium the blood level of a drug relates directly with the drug concentration at a receptor site. This permits a precision of dosage which aims at a maximum therapeutic action with a minimum of toxicity. Pharmacokinetics is so important that two chapters are devoted to it.

Therapeutic Uses

There would be little interest in drugs if they did not relieve symptoms or correct conditions which might lead to increased morbidity and mortality. Clinical medicine depends heavily on drugs. The average hospitalized patient receives an average 7 to 10 drugs. Even surgery would, in many cases, be impossible without anticoagulants, anesthetics, antibiotics, and analgesics. The objective of pharmacology is, in the final analysis, to be related to the clinical sciences.

Adverse Reactions

Drugs are beneficial in their desired effects; unfortunately they also have unwanted or noxious actions. These may be only an overextension of the beneficial effect, such as dizziness caused by lowering blood pressure in a hypertensive individual or lethargy in a patient receiving a sedative. Such responses are known as, "side effects" since they occur at therapeutic doses. Many drugs have additional toxic effects which may affect the liver, kidneys, brain, and other organs and usually occur at higher dosages. These are known as the more severe adverse effects. Occasionally a drug may have a bizarre and unexpected toxic effect which is termed "idiosyncratic", usually as a result of a genetic abnormality in the individual. There may also be allergic responses to drugs which are a result of the genetic constitution.

The use of more than one drug in the same patient at the same time is now a common practice. The possibility that drugs may interact or interfere with each other is a real consideration. This subject is known as *Drug Interactions* and comprises an important segment of iatrogenic disease. Drugs also may interact with foods. This subject is discussed fully in Chapter 6.

The toxicity of drugs assumes great significance in relation to the disease to be treated and the status of the patient. Drugs are generally more toxic to the very young and the aged. A greater risk of toxicity may be tolerated in a serious and deadly disease such as cancer. In contrast, a sedative should have practically no toxicity. This concept is now generally known as the *benefit to risk ratio*.

Preparations and Doses

Drugs would not be useful unless they were available in proper and convenient dosage forms. They must also be in the suitable dosage forms for the particular schedule of dosage. In this edition of the text, the preparations and dosage forms as well as specific dosages of drugs have been eliminated. In a basic text, it is impossible to do justice to the many preparations now available to the clinician or to the doses that should be used in patients of all ages. Reference must be made to texts on this subject, such as the Physicians' Desk Reference (PDR), Drug Evaluations Annual, or Facts and Comparisons. In any event, the package insert should be read before prescribing any drug for the first time.

Pharmacology is a rapidly changing subject. Each year, approximately 20 new drugs are marketed in the United States, and new concepts as to how older drugs are to be better utilized are constantly being proposed. Large scale clinical investigations are in progress such as the optimum use of thrombolytic agents in the therapy of acute myocardial infarction. The student must develop the habit of continually educating himself or herself in the newer medical knowledge and one of the best ways of doing this is by reading quality medical journals. The references name some of the best journals in pharmacology. It is hoped that the student will become acquainted with these to supplement basic knowledge of this subject.

BIBLIOGRAPHY

Historical

Bradley, D.: "Frog Venom Cocktail Yields A One-handed Pain Killer," *Science* **261**: 1117 (1993).

Bugg, C.E., W.M. Carson, and J.A. Montgomery: "Drugs by Design," *Scientific American* **269**: 92-98 (1993).

Krantz, J.C.: *Historical Medical Classics Involving New Drugs*, Williams & Wilkins, Baltimore, 1974.

Lyons, A.S., and R.J. Petrucelli: *Medicine, An Illustrative History*, Harry N. Abrams, Inc., New York, 1978.

Journals

Clinical Pharmacology and Therapeutics, Mosby-Year Book, Inc. Official journal of the American Society for Pharmacology and Experimental Therapeutics.

The Journal of Clinical Pharmacology, J.B. Lippincott, Hagerstown, MD. Official publication of the American College of Clinical Pharmacology.

Journal of Pharmaceutical Sciences, American Pharmaceutical Association, Washington, D.C.

Journal of Pharmacology and Experimental Therapeutics, Williams & Wilkins, Baltimore, MD. A publication of the American Society for Pharmacology and Experimental Therapeutics.

Journal of Pharmacy and Pharmacology, Royal Pharmaceutical Society of Great Britain.

European Journal of Pharmacology, Elsevier Science Publishers, B.V., New York.

Pharmacological Reviews, Williams & Wilkins, Baltimore, MD. A journal of the American Society for Pharmacology and Experimental Therapeutics.

Prescribing Books

Drug Evaluations Annual 1993, American Medical Association.

Facts and Comparisons, Olin, B.R. (ed.). Facts and Comparisons Inc., St. Louis, MO. Loose leaf monthly and annual volume.P

Physicians' Desk Reference (PDR), Medical Economics Company Inc., Montvale, N.J. Published annually.

CHAPTER 2

The Drug-Receptor Interaction

Richard R. Neubig

Modern textbooks define pharmacology broadly as "the effects of chemicals upon living systems." Medical pharmacology focuses on those chemicals, called drugs, that influence the course of disease or maintain well-being. It follows that any substance, usually a chemical of relatively small molecular size, that is found to have utility in the therapy or prevention of disease is defined as a drug. Improved biotechnology has expanded the range of drugs to include macromolecules such as proteins or DNA.

Recent advances in molecular pharmacology have also provided the means of understanding the mechanisms of drug action that make possible the more accurate control of disease and indeed the development of new and superior drugs. It is permissible now to think of pharmacology as related mainly to *the action of chemicals on receptors in a living system*. What a receptor is and what the consequences of a drug-receptor interaction are will occupy the second and third chapters of this text.

Of all the controllable variables in the investigation of drug action, the *dose* is of crucial importance. In all instances the response of the drug-receptor interaction is dependent on the dose. Therefore, a logical approach to the understanding of the drug-receptor interaction would be to study the terminology and methods used to measure responses in relationship to dose. Later, methods and theoretical implications of dealing with receptor quality and quantity may be defined.

DOSE-RESPONSE RELATIONSHIPS

The principle that the magnitude of the drug effect is related to the dose administered is, though self evident, one of the most important in the science of pharmacology. Four variables enter into this relationship: time, biologic unit, dose of drug administered (or, with *in vitro* experiments, the drug concentration in the bath fluid), and the effect produced by the given quantity of drug. To make effects easier to visualize, we arbitrarily select two variables and represent their functional relationship graphically, keeping other variables constant. Two choices of variables are in common use. First, the *graded* dose-response plot presents the magnitude of the response as the dose varies, keeping the time and the biologic unit constant by using the same biologic object (e.g., animal or human subject) throughout the experiment and making measurements at the time when the system has come to steady state, i.e., when the effect has become constant as long as the drug concentration does not change. Second, the *quantal* dose-response curve represents the relationship between the dose of a drug and the proportion of biologic objects manifesting a specified pharmacologic effect. Here the dose and the number of subjects vary, and the magnitude of the response and the time are constant.

Graded Dose-Response Curve

Graded dose-response curves generally look like that shown in Fig. 2-1. When the dose of a drug is gradually increased and the first noticeable effect is observed, the dose that produced this effect is called the *threshold* dose. Increments of drug administration result in larger effects; the curve obtained from the experiment is found to be a hyperbola and as such asymptomatically approaches the *ceiling* effect, where further increments of drug administration no longer change the response. The ceiling effect thus reveals the *intrinsic activity* of the drug. However, representing the results on an arithmetic scale, as shown in

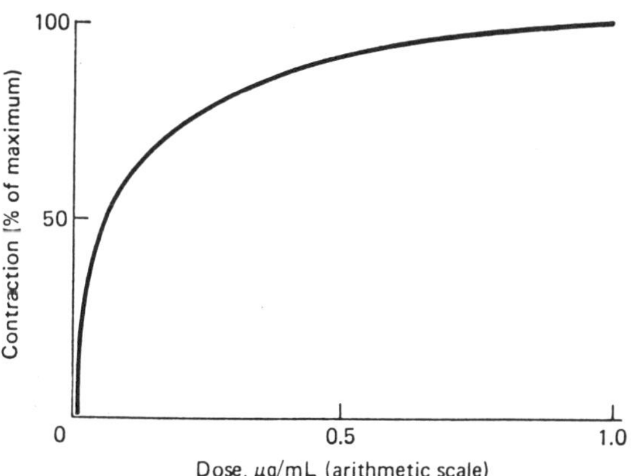

FIGURE 2-1 *A graded response curve for increasing concentrations of a drug in a perfusion bath of a perfused isolated intestine. Plotted on an arithmetic scale, the contraction response is hyperbolic as the concentration of the drug is increased until a ceiling effect is achieved.*

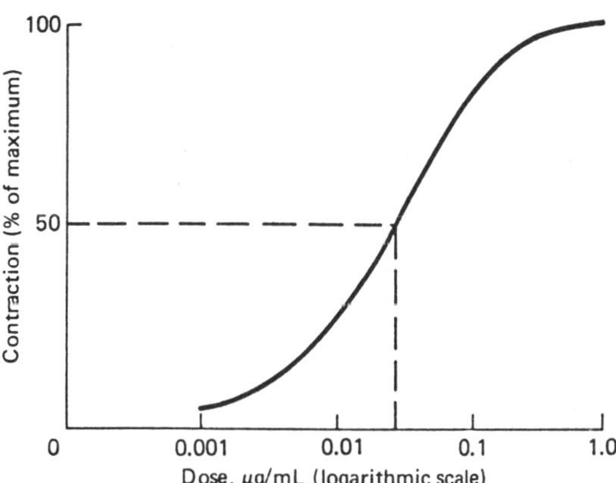

FIGURE 2-2 *The same data as in Fig. 2-1 except that the dose is now plotted as a negative logarithm. The curve now becomes sigmoid in shape with a nearly linear central portion. This is far more convenient to interpret and has the advantage that the 50 percent maximal response may be easily determined. For these reasons, the log-concentration curve has become the standard dose-response curve.*

Fig. 2-1, has its disadvantages; the data in the beginning of the curve are so crowded that drug doses responsible for different effects cannot be discerned. It is customary, therefore, to plot the effect not against the dose of the drug (or its concentration) but against the logarithm of the dose (Fig. 2-2). Such a *logarithmic* representation of the data results in a sigmoid (S-shaped) curve; it expands the lower part of the hyperbola (where the effect changes greatly with increasing drug dose) and compresses its upper part (where there is little change in effect). In addition, it has the advantage that the middle part of the sigmoid curve is very nearly a straight line.

Quantal Dose-Response Curve

Quantal (or all-or-none) dose-response curves, in which the time and the magnitude of the effect are constant and the variables are the drug dose and the number of individuals responding with the specified effect, are actually a statement on the population statistics of drug response. They show the proportion of a human or animal population, or of a population of isolated tissues, that displays a specified response to a given drug dose. As a consequence of biologic variability, in a population of sufficient size there are always some few individuals so drug-sensitive that they respond to rather small doses, equally few so drug-insensitive that they require substantial doses, and the largest number responsive to a middle dose, with gradual transitions from the middle to the extremes. Hence a *Gaussian*, or *normal distribution*, *curve* (Fig. 2-3) will best represent the population statistics of drug response. In such a curve the drug dose is plotted on the abscissa and the frequency of response, i.e., the percentage of the population responding to each drug, on the ordinate. The curve is seen to be symmetric; therefore, the *mean* (or average) dose, the *median* dose (which bisects the total population into two equal parts), and the *mode* (the dose which draws the most frequent response) are all identical. Also, all the points on the curve deviate from the mean as much to the right (in a positive direction in the coordinate system) as to the left (in a negative direction), so that the sum of the deviations is zero; but, the sum of their squares is a positive number. The *variance* is obtained by dividing the sum of squares by the number of individual values that have been squared, and the *standard deviation* is the square root of the variance. This is an important parameter, which describes the width of the curve, i.e., the scatter of individual points about the mean due to biologic variation. (The standard deviation is to be distinguished from the *standard error*, which is a measure of scatter of

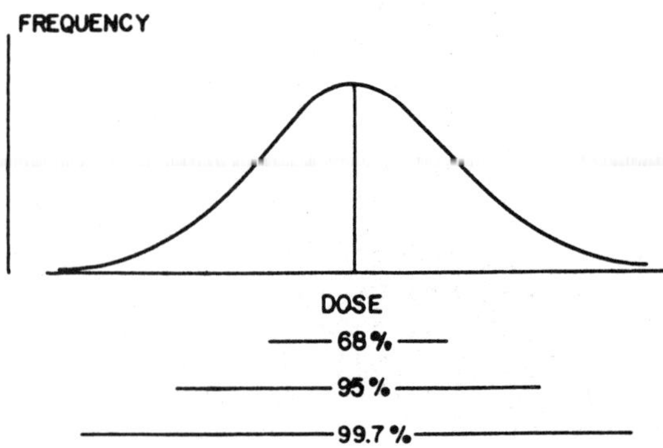

FIGURE 2-3 *A graphic expression of the theoretical normal distribution of doses needed to elicit a quantal response in subjects from a large sample. The horizontal bars delineate the borders of plus or minus one, two, and three standard deviations from the mean dose, which is shown by the vertical bar. The proportion of subjects requiring doses within the boundaries is indicated as a percentage of the sample. The dose units are unspecified.*

individual measurements due to experimental inaccuracy.) In the Gaussian curve, one unit of standard deviation encompasses 34 percent of the total population, two units 47.5 percent, three units 49 percent, and so on.

In practice, distribution curves are seldom perfect because the sample may be too small for serviceable statistics, or the curve is *truncated* (one or the other end of the distribution curve is experimentally not available), or some extraneous influence or other experimental limitation opposes or modifies the drug action observed. In such cases the mean, the mode, and the median dose may differ. The situation can be improved by trying to eliminate disturbing influences, and, most importantly, by increasing the size of the population studied. But only an infinite population guarantees perfect results. Therefore all actual statistical findings have limited reliability, expressed as the *confidence limit*, a figure arrived at by known mathematical rules, which states the probability of some measured value being the true value. The statement that a particular value is, for example, 0.63 to 0.65 with a confidence limit of 0.95 means that in 95 out of 100 experiments, the value can be expected to be found between 0.63 and 0.65.

As in the case of graded dose-response curves, efforts have been made to convert the bell-shaped quantal dose-response curve to a form that is at least partially linear. To this end one may plot the results cumulatively, that is, instead of the number of individuals responding to some particular drug dose and not to lower ones, one records the total number of individuals who have responded up to that dose, as a percentage of the total population studied. This procedure transforms the bell-shaped Gaussian curve into a sigmoid one with a linear midsection (Fig. 2-4).

Therapeutic Index

The data provided by quantal dose-response plots can be utilized for a statement on the safety of a drug. Consider Fig. 2-4. It reports experiments conducted on a population of laboratory mice with a hypnotic drug, both parts of the figure showing two curves, sleep as the specified therapeutic effect in one curve and death—the ultimate toxic effect—in the other. Obviously, the farther apart the two curves are, the safer the drug. Numerically, the safety of the drug can be expressed as the *therapeutic index* TI_{50}, defined as the ratio of the median toxic dose TD_{50}, or the median lethal dose LD_{50}, to the median effective dose ED_{50}. But this information is insufficient; the TI_{50} is only a statement about the distance between the median effective and the median toxic dose in the plot. It

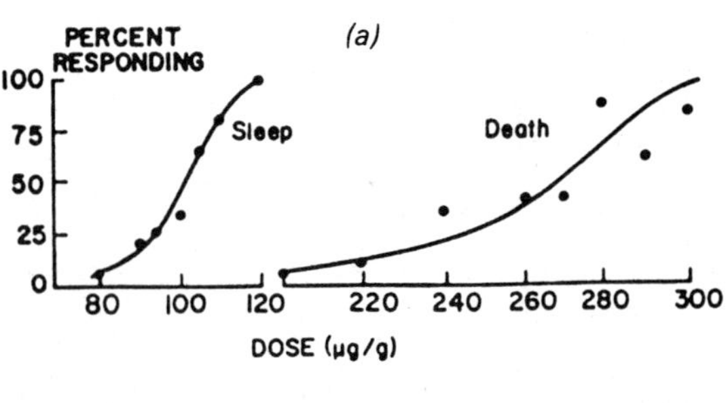

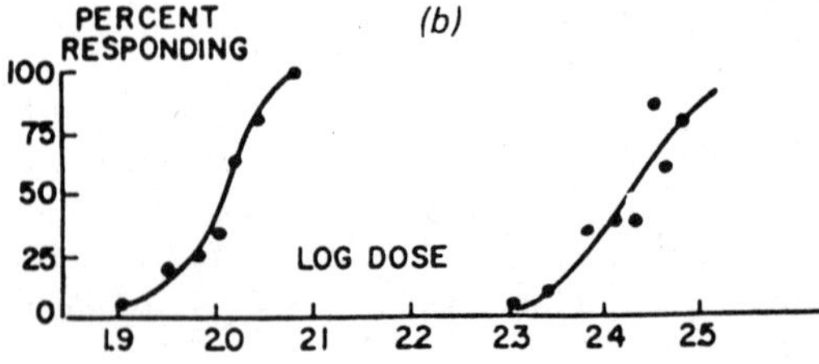

FIGURE 2-4 *Cumulative quantal dose-response curves. Percent responding (a) against the drug dose and (b) against the logarithm of the dose.*

says nothing about the standard deviations, i.e., the width of the two Gaussian curves, and hence nothing about whether the lower end of the toxicity curve overlaps the upper end of the effect curve. If such an overlap occurs, then a dose of the drug, which is just the threshold dose for some individuals, is toxic and may even be lethal to others. (This is not a hypothetical problem: beverage alcohol is such a dangerous drug.) It is therefore customary to supplement the information given by the therapeutic index with the *standard safety margin* (see Table 2-1), which indicates the relative positions of the upper end of the effect curve and the lower end of the toxicity curve by a number which states by what percentage the ED_{99}, the drug dose effective in 99 percent of the population, must be increased in order to equal the TD_1, the dose that causes toxicity in 1 percent of the same population. (Instead of 99 percent and 1 percent, one may use, for example, 99.9 percent and 0.1 percent, or other values).

TABLE 2-1 Safety margin or therapeutic index calculated from the data in Fig. 2-4

Therapeutic index and symbol	Value of index
Median therapeutic index	2.62
$\dfrac{TD_{50}}{ED_{50}} = \dfrac{262\text{ mg}}{100\text{ mg}}$	
Standard safety margin	67%
$\left[\dfrac{TD_1}{ED_{99}} - 1\right] \times 100$	
Standard safety margin	8%
$\left[\dfrac{TD_{0.1}}{ED_{99.9}} - 1\right] \times 100$	

Time-Action Curves

It was noted earlier that in choosing the two variables on which the graded and quantal dose-response curves are based one keeps the time variable constant by stipulating that observations are to be made when steady state has been attained, i.e., a constant effect at constant drug dose. It may be desirable, however, to record the time course of the appearance of the effect as well, both as a tool in the analysis of the mechanism of action of the drug and as information for scheduling drug administration to patients. Fig. 2-5 illustrates the three important phases of *time-action curves:* the time of onset (time interval from the moment of drug administration to the moment when the drug effect is first perceived), the time to peak effect (when the drug has reached all cells of the responsive tissue and has induced the maximum effect in all responsive cells, yet the physiologic factors antagonizing drug action have not yet diminished it perceptibly), and the duration of action (time from the onset to the disappearance of the effect). In some cases there are also residual effects, perceived only as increased potency of the same drug on re-administration or as a modification in the activity of a different drug with which the first drug interacts positively or negatively.

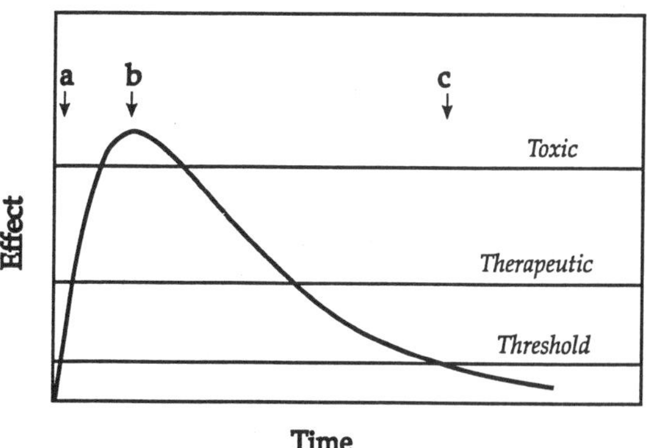

FIGURE 2-5 *The intensity of effect related to the time after administration of a single dose of a drug. The effect first reaches the threshold of detection at the time marked "a". It rises to a peak at time "b", which in this case produces some toxic effects. The effect has fully disappeared at time "c". The duration of detectable drug action is "c - a" but the duration of the therapeutic effect would be somewhat less.*

The major determinant of the time course of drug action *in vivo* is, in most cases, the *pharmacokinetics* of the drug (see Chapter 4). That is, the absorption of drug from the site of administration, distribution to the site of action, and the clearance from the body are slow relative to the action of the drug at the receptor. Thus the drug effect follows the time course of drug concentration at the site of action. In some cases, there is a substantial lag time between binding of the drug to the receptor and the perceived biological effect (e.g., with the metabolic effects of steroid hormones). Also, for drugs which bind irreversibly to their receptors, the drug effect may last longer than the time the drug is detectable in the body. When the drug effect does not precisely parallel drug concentration in time, the term *pharmacodynamics* is used to refer to the time course of drug effect, as contrasted to the pharmacokinetics which is the time course of drug concentrations.

RECEPTORS

The extreme specificity and potency of drugs (with effects occurring at picomolar (10^{-12} M) to nanomolar (10^{-9} M) concentrations) indicated to early workers in pharmacology such as Ehrlich and Langley (see Chapter 3) that such drugs worked by binding to special components of cells which they termed *receptors*. The classical definition of receptors includes specialized proteins which, having bound to ligands, trigger a physiologic response. It is appropriate now, with many important drugs working by inhibition of enzymes, to expand the definition of receptor to include any molecule (usually protein or DNA) to which a drug binds in a specific manner and which is responsible for the action of the drug. The binding is made possible by a close structural complementarity between the receptor and the ligand. (The analogy with a lock-and-key relationship is often used.) In the case of classical receptors, if a drug can stimulate the receptor to trigger a response, then the drug is termed an *agonist*. On the other hand, an *antagonist* drug complexes with the receptor without evoking a response and removes the receptor from the pool available to the endogenous ligand or to an agonist, thus blocking the receptor response.

Another important characteristic of receptors is that they are present in very small numbers, yet they can cause actions on a large scale, such as muscle contraction or substantial amounts of glucose uptake and metabolism. The ability of femtomole (10^{-15} mole) quantities of receptors to cause these actions depends on a large degree of signal amplification. An extreme example of this is the ability of the eye to detect a single photon of light. The photon activates a receptor in the retina called rhodopsin. As discussed in Chapter 3, rhodopsin is very similar to many classical drug receptors (e.g., adrenergic receptors) and both rhodopsin and many drug receptors transmit their signals via guanine nucleotide binding proteins. The details of this and several other signal amplification mechanisms are described in Chapter 3.

Receptors and Acceptors

It should be noted that many binding agents in the body, such as blood proteins, particularly serum albumin, can bind numerous compounds, including drugs. However, this binding does not result in drug action and the binding agent is an *acceptor* rather than a receptor. The binding of drugs by acceptors may modify their pharmacological effect, as the amount of free drug available to the true receptor is decreased but the acceptor generally does not contribute to the response.

Experimental Study of Receptors

There are three major methods to study receptors: functional measurements, binding measurements, and direct purification and biochemical characterization. The dose-response curve, discussed above, is the primary tool for functional studies of receptors. Binding methods use a radioactively-labelled agonist or antagonist ligands. Such methods have been very useful in directly proving the existence of receptors, in rapidly screening chemicals for potential activity at receptors, and for the purification and isolation of the very small quantities of receptors present in tissues. A number of receptors have been isolated, taking advantage of the powerful technique of affinity chromatography in which a ligand is attached to a solid support and the receptor isolated by binding it specifically to the ligand, then eluting the purified receptor with the same ligand in solution. This can enrich and purify the receptors 200,000-fold in a single step. The receptors may then be identified as proteins and their structure elucidated by standard methods of amino acid sequencing. As discussed in Chapter 3 this has resulted in an explosion of information about the structure and mechanism of many different types of receptors.

Many receptors are located in cell membranes, held in place by the compatibility of the cell membrane with an accumulation of hydrophobic amino acid side chains on the outside of that part of the receptor-protein helix which is in contact with the membrane, while hydrophilic portions of the helix protrude both into the extracellular fluid and into the cytosol. The outside hydrophilic portion contains the actual receptor site, a grouping of amino acids serving as the lock which the ligand fits as the key. The stimulation of the receptor by the ligand is then passed on by a complex transduction system to a second messenger (e.g., cyclic AMP or calcium ions) inside the cell. In the next chapter there are schematic pictures of such receptors whose structure has been established. Other receptors, particularly those which respond to corticosteroid hormones and to thyroxin, are located in the cytosol or nucleus rather than in the cell membrane.

As discussed above, it is reasonable to consider the active sites of the enzymes as drug receptors. If there is medical reason to depress the activity of such an enzyme, this can be done by means of a drug which functions as an inhibitor of the enzyme. Such a procedure is particularly important in inhibiting the enzymes involved in the metabolism or the reproductive function of harmful cells, such as those of microbial invaders or of malignant cells of the organism. Other enzymes that function as drug receptors are prostaglandin synthase and hydroxymethylglutaryl-CoA (HMG-CoA) reductase. The former is inhibited by aspirin and related drugs, which prevent prostaglandin effects such as pain, fever, and inflammation. The latter enzyme is required for cholesterol synthesis and can be blocked to reduce the amount of cholesterol in the blood.

The Drug-Receptor Association

The forces involved in the drug-receptor interaction are determined by the protein nature of most receptors and by the fact that drug-receptor association is usually reversible. Chemical agents can also attach themselves irreversibly to receptors by covalent bonds, but except for rare cases, such as nitrogen mustards (see Chapter 43) or organophosphorus insecticides (see Chapter 10), it is not usually desirable to inflict irreversible changes on the organism. Thus, the forces causing drug and receptor to associate are usually ionic, hydrophobic, or hydrogen bonds, all of which have energies low enough to be easily broken under physiologic conditions. Hydrogen bonds and hydrophobic bonds are too weak and fall off too fast with increasing distance to cause significant binding unless there are many of them and unless the bonded parts of drug and receptor molecules come in very close contact. Hence the distribution of charges and of potential hydrogen-bonding and hydrophobic-binding groups in a receptor specifies structural features in a drug. In order to be able to attach itself to the receptor, the drug must have charges and hydrogen-bonding and hydrophilic-binding groups so arranged that they fit corresponding groups in the receptor closely.

This is the lock-and-key relationship mentioned earlier. Therefore, certain structural characteristics must be present in all drugs capable of interacting with the same receptor, much as they must be present in all substrates capable of interacting with the same enzymatic active site. (It will be noted later that receptors are in many ways similar to enzymes.)

By similar reasoning, when a drug molecule is asymmetric, only one of its enantiomers will fit the receptor accurately; therefore drug-receptor interactions are often *stereospecific*. Examples illustrating this conclusion are found in drugs capable of interacting with receptors for epinephrine and norepinephrine (Chapter 8), for acetylcholine (Chapter 10), and for opioids (Chapter 23). Drugs acting on adrenergic receptors are, like the natural adrenergic agents epinephrine and norepinephrine, derivatives of phenylethylamine; and those among them which are asymmetric show stereospecificity. Thus the natural (−)-epinephrine is 1000 times more potent than (+)-epinephrine. The effect of the alkaloid (−)-muscarine, a potent cholinergic agent, is 700 times greater than that of (+)-muscarine. As another example, morphine and all other opioid drugs are derivatives of γ-phenylpiperidine; and while the natural (−)-morphine is a powerful drug, the biologic activity of its (+)-enantiomer is minimal.

Thus the nature of the forces involved in the drug-receptor interaction leads to the realization that, when drug action is based on receptors, a given pharmacologic activity hinges on a specific molecular structure of the drug. Conversely, when it is observed that some particular pharmacologic action is contingent on some particular chemical structure, this is evidence that the effect is mediated by receptors. The important principle of *structure-activity relationship* will be often illustrated in later chapters of this book.

THE PHYSICAL CHEMISTRY OF DRUG-RECEPTOR ASSOCIATION

If the association of a drug D with its receptor R is reversible,

$$D + R \rightleftharpoons DR$$

then the law of mass action is applicable to the interaction:

$$\frac{[D][R]}{[DR]} = K \qquad (1)$$

where K is the *equilibrium dissociation constant* with units of concentration (moles/liter). Noting that the total receptor concentration $[R]_t$, is the sum of the concentrations of free receptor [R] and drug-occupied receptor [DR],

$$[R]_t = [R] + [DR]$$

one may substitute $[R]_t$ − [DR] for [R] in Equation (1):

$$\frac{[D]([R]_t - [DR])}{[DR]} = K \qquad (2)$$

which can be rearranged to

$$[DR] = \frac{[R]_t}{(K[D]) + 1} \qquad (3)$$

This is an important equation because it shows how the concentration of the drug-receptor complex [DR] depends on the amount of receptor present $[R]_t$, the binding constant, K, and the concentration of drug [D]. The magnitude of the drug effect E depends on the concentration of the drug-receptor complex [DR], so if we assume that this functional dependence is a simple proportion with the proportionality constant α then

$$E = \alpha[DR] = \frac{\alpha[R]_t}{(K/[D]) + 1} \qquad (4)$$

The technical term for α is *intrinsic activity*. Drugs with a greater intrinsic activity produce larger responses at saturating drug concentrations. This equation is formally similar to a fundamental equation of enzyme kinetics: substitute V for E, k_{cat} for α, K_m for K, enzyme for receptor, and substrate for drug; and Equation (4) becomes the Michaelis-Menten equation. This is so because both Equation (4) and the Michaelis-Menten equation are derived from the application of the law of mass action to the reversible association of two molecules followed by an observable consequence of the association. Like the Michaelis-Menten equation, Equation (4) contains two variables, [D] and E, both of which are measurable in favorable cases. Even though $\alpha[R]_t$, and K may not be known, it is enough to know that they are constants in order to make the statement (which follows from elementary algebra) that the effect depends hyperbolically on the drug concentration and that a plot of E versus log[D] is the sigmoid curve discussed above, as indeed experiments shows that it is (Fig. 2-6).

By directly measuring binding of a drug to its receptor, it is possible to find the values of $[R]_t$, and K. It is possible to determine [DR] by measuring total drug binding, then subtracting the lower affinity acceptor or non-specific binding. The biologic material under study is incubated with a solution of a radioactive drug known to be a specific ligand for the receptor, and the total amount bound is established by measuring the

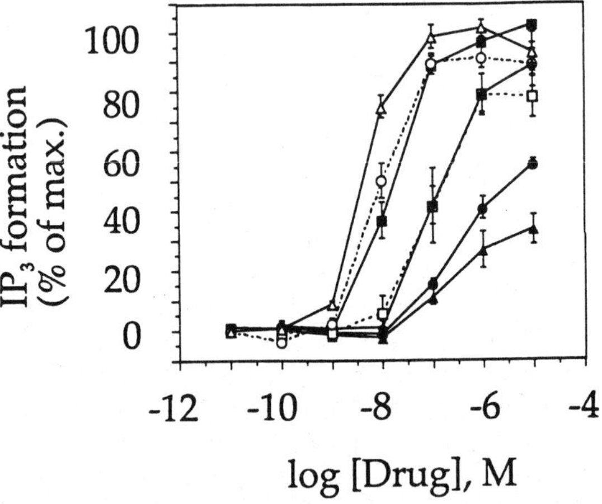

FIGURE 2-6 *Dose-response curves for serotonin analogs activating a biochemical response. Cells transfected with the 5-HT_{2f} subtype of the serotonin receptor were stimulated with the indicated concentrations of serotonin (filled squares) and several serotonin analogs. Release of the second messenger inositol trisphosphate (IP_3) was measured. Most analogs are full agonists, producing the same maximum response as serotonin, but the filled circles and filled triangles show partial agonist responses in which the maximum is less than that of serotonin. [Modified from Wainscott, D.B., et. al., Mol. Pharmacol. **43**: 419-426 (1993).]*

radioactivity of the biologic material after the incubation. Drug will bind both to receptors and to the much more numerous, but lower affinity, acceptors. The experiment is then repeated, but this time in the presence of an excess of nonradioactive drug. The relatively few receptors will be saturated by nonradioactive drug, and the modest amount of radioactivity found at the end of the experiment can be attributed to an equally small fraction of acceptor binding. The difference between the results of the two experiments therefore represents the receptor-bound radioactivity which, knowing the radioactivity of the drug, can be recalculated as [DR]. Equation (2) can be rearranged, not only to Equation (3), but also to

$$\frac{[DR]}{[D]} = \frac{1[R]_t}{K} - \frac{1[DR]}{K} \qquad (5)$$

This linear equation is very useful in binding studies for determining the number and affinity of receptors in a tissue or membrane preparation. A plot of [DR]/[D] against [DR] (Scatchard plot) yields a slope of $-1/K$ and an x-intercept of $[R]_t$. Hence, one can determine $[R]_t$ and K from the Scatchard plot (Fig. 2-7). Knowing the number of cells, one can calculate from such results that a typical cell bears 10,000 to 100,000 receptors.

The dissociation constant K is an important parameter of drug action in that its reciprocal, the *affinity constant* 1/K, is a measure of the affinity of the drug for its receptor. The other important parameter in determining receptor responses is the intrinsic activity, α. Between these two parameters the magnitude of the drug effect can be calculated, as clearly shown by Equation (4). A drug with high intrinsic activity and high affinity will have a large effect, but drugs with either low affinity or low intrinsic activity will have a smaller effect, the former because relatively few drug molecules will be attached to receptors, the latter because, even though many receptors are occupied, they are not fully stimulated by the drug's low intrinsic activity.

The simple assumption that E is proportional to [DR] is called the *occupancy theory* of drug action. While a number of conclusions may be derived from this assumption about drug-receptor interactions, recognition of the remarkable properties of signal amplification described in Chapter 3 have lead to the *efficacy theory* of Stephenson. The reader who wishes to find a full presentation of these theories and their algebraic derivations is referred to the excellent text *Pharmacologic Analysis of Drug-Receptor Interaction* by Kenakin.

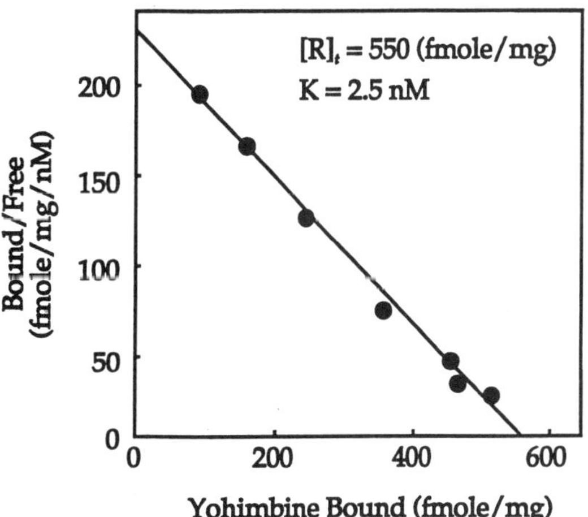

FIGURE 2-7 *Scatchard plot of the binding of radiolabelled yohimbine, an α_2-adrenergic receptor antagonist. Human platelet membranes were incubated with increasing concentrations of ^{3}H-labelled yohimbine. Non-specific binding determined in the presence of excess yohimbine was subtracted to calculate specific, receptor-associated binding. Data were converted to a Scatchard plot and the total receptor content $[R]_t$ and binding constant K were calculated from the intercept and slope, respectively. [Modified from Neubig, R.R., R.D. Gantzos, and R.S. Brasier: Mol. Pharmacol. 28: 475-486 (1985).]*

SIMULTANEOUS ACTION OF TWO DRUGS AND ITS THEORETICAL INTERPRETATION

Agonist and Antagonist

Equation (4) describes the relation between the effect E with the concentration [D] of an agonist. This relation hinges on the magnitudes of the parameters K and α. If a drug has affinity for a receptor without having a measurable intrinsic activity (i.e., α = 0), then from Equation (4) it follows that this drug is an antagonist. It will diminish the effect of an agonist present at the same time. This is analogous to the situation in enzyme kinetics of a competitive inhibitor and such a drug is called a *competitive antagonist*. The theory predicts that, just as in the parallel situation in enzyme kinetics, when an agonist acts in the presence of a competitive antagonist, a higher concentration of agonist will be required to obtain any particular level of response; the log dose-response curve of the agonist is displaced in a parallel fashion to the right. Figure 2-8 illustrates an experimental example complying with these predictions. It is seen that, even in the presence of the antagonist, a sufficiently large drug dose can overcome the antagonism, resulting in the same maximum effect. The antagonist, in effect, reversibly occupies part of the receptor pool, but a sufficient agonist concentration can take it back. That is the meaning of competition. From the algebra of competitive antagonism, it follows that when the concentration of the antagonist is equal to its equilibrium dissociation constant K_A, the amount of agonist needed to produce a given response doubles. Indeed, the ratio of agonist concentrations D′/D needed to produce the same response increases linearly with antagonist concentration:

$$D'/D = 1 + A/K_A$$

where D′ and D are the agonist concentrations needed to produce a response in the presence and absence of antagonist, respectively, and A is the antagonist concentration.

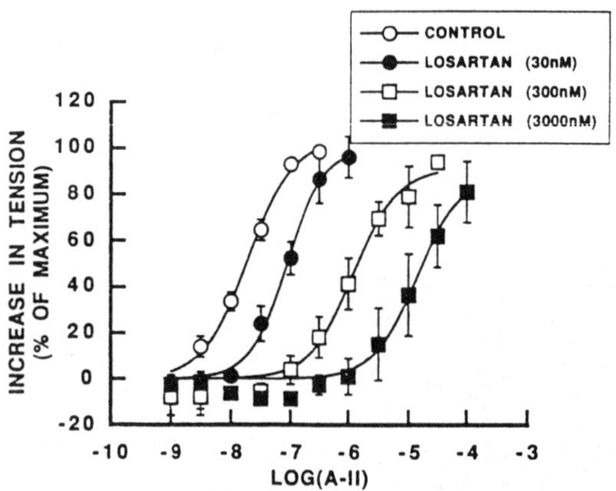

FIGURE 2-8 *Competitive inhibition of angiotensin II by losartan. The effect of angiotensin II (A-II) to enhance nerve activity in the rabbit vas deferens was measured in vitro (control curve). The angiotensin II receptor antagonist losartan was incubated with the vas deferens preparation at the three indicated concentrations (30, 300, and 3000 nM) while A-II dose-response curves were determined. The competitive antagonist caused a concentration-dependent parallel right-ward shift of the dose-response curves as expected. [From Hegde, S.S., and D.E. Clarke: J. Pharmacol. Exp. Ther.* ***265****: 601 (1993)].*

Competitive antagonism is not the only way to diminish receptor responses. There are at least five other types of antagonism: *irreversible, noncompetitive, physiological* and *chemical*, as well as a phenomenon called *desensitization*.

Irreversible antagonists generally bind to the same site as the agonist but by means of a covalent or very slowly dissociating non-covalent interaction. Examples of irreversible antagonists include the cancer chemotherapeutic agents known as nitrogen mustards (Chapter 43) and the α-adrenergic receptor blocker phenoxybenzamine (Chapter 9). These drugs will not come off of the receptor binding site even when there is a large amount of agonist competing for that binding site. Thus the result is that the available number of receptors $[R]_t$ is decreased and the maximum response to the agonist is decreased.

An antagonist is *noncompetitive* when it does not associate with the same site on the receptor as the agonist does, but lowers the intrinsic activity of the agonist. Although the mechanism is different, the result is usually the same as that of an irreversible antagonist, i.e., a lower maximum effect (Fig. 2-9).

The phenomenon of two drugs acting on the same organ through independent receptors, but in opposite directions, is known as *physiologic antagonism*. An example is the drug pair epinephrine and carbamylcholine. Both are agonists on the heart, but epinephrine accelerates the pulse by stimulating β-adrenergic receptors in the heart, while carbamoylcholine stimulates muscarinic cholinergic receptors and slows the heartbeat.

Chemical antagonism occurs when one compound interferes chemically with another. An example is a chelating agent used to sequester harmful metal ions, such as ethylenediaminetetraacetic acid or dimercaprol in lead poisoning (see Chapter 53).

Finally, with many drugs it is observed that on repeated administration their effect decreases. This phenomenon, to be discussed in some of the later chapters, has various names, such as *desensitization, drug resistance, tolerance,* and *tachyphylaxis*. It also has various causes, such as fatigue (i.e., depletion of endogenous substances required for manifestation of the drug effect) and increased rate of biotransformation of the drug. What interests us in the present context is desensitization, interpreted as a change in the ability of the receptor to transmit its signal to downstream components of the transduction cascade. In

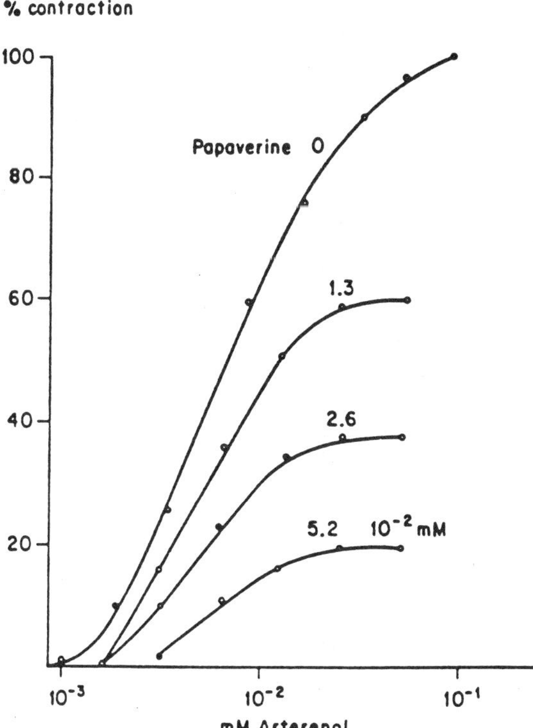

FIGURE 2-9 *Experimental dose-response curves demonstrating noncompetitive antagonism of norepinephrine (arterenol) by papaverine.*

recent years evidence has accumulated of several mechanisms which underlie receptor desensitization. The receptor can become uncoupled from the signal transduction system but remain in the surface or plasma membrane, the receptor can be internalized into the intracellular membranes and later returned to the plasma membrane, and finally it can undergo *down-regulation* in which some of the receptor is destroyed and the total number of receptors in the cell is decreased. Similarly *up-regulation* can occur by increased synthesis of receptors. In this instance the phenomenon is called sensitization.

From the point of view of therapy, competitive and physiologic antagonism are probably the most important mechanisms of drug interaction (Fig. 2-10). Atropine, a competitive antagonist of acetylcholine, is widely used to block such parasympathetic actions as nasal and bronchial secretions and bradycardia (Chapter 11); naloxone, a competitive antagonist of morphine, is the standard antidote in cases of morphine poisoning (Chapter 23); and antihistamines are utilized to block allergic conditions caused by the release of histamine from body stores (Chapter 13). However, while histamine is also one of the causative agents of asthma, an acute asthmatic attack is better treated with the physiological antagonist isoproterenol, which dilates bronchioles by stimulating β-adrenergic receptors, while histamine constricts bronchioles by stimulating histamine receptors (Chapter 33).

Synergism and Potentiation

When two agonist drugs act on the same target organ through different receptors (i.e., a functional interaction), the effect produced by the two drugs may greater than the sum of the separate effects of the component drugs, a phenomenon known as *synergism*. This is in contrast to *additivity*, where the total effect is equal to the sum of the separate effects. When two drugs act on the same receptor, it is also possible to observe sub-additive effects when a high concentration of one drug has already saturated most of the receptors and the second drug can not increase the response any further.

The term *potentiation* is sometimes used as a synonym of synergism. More correctly, it applies to that special case of synergism where one of the two drugs has zero intrinsic activity, that is, where an inactive drug enhances the activity of the other. For example, the analgesic effect of morphine is enhanced by the simultaneous administration of phenothiazine derivatives, which, by themselves, are not analgesic.

Nonspecific Drugs

Finally, drugs must be mentioned that do not act by way of receptors, but rather by physical alteration of some essential part of the organism, for instance, cell membranes in the central nervous system. A number of drugs are soluble in the lipid cell membrane and, when so dissolved, inhibit the function of the membrane which is to carry messages by the mechanism known as *conduction*. The drugs that perform in this manner (e.g., general anesthetics and certain cardiac muscle depressant drugs, display no clear structure-activity relationship. What they have in common is the physical characteristic of solubility in cell membranes, and it has been found that their depressant potency is reasonably well correlated with the

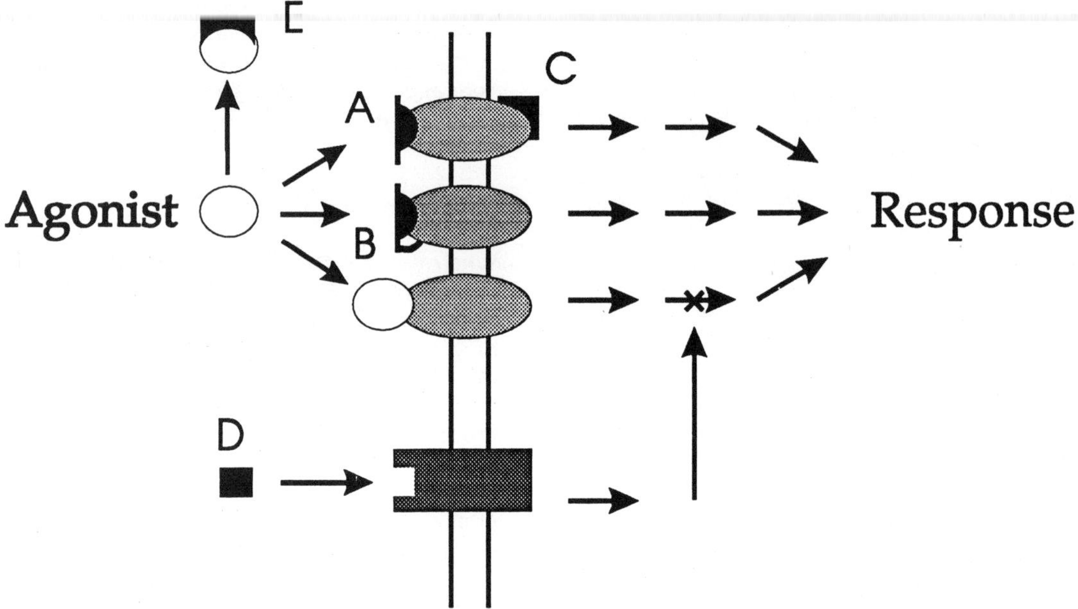

FIGURE 2-10 *Mechanisms and locations of antagonist action. A membrane bound receptor (gray oval) is activated by an agonist (white oval). The signal is transmitted intracellularly via several amplification steps before the response is produced. Antagonists (black shapes) can block competitively (A) or irreversibly (B) at the agonist binding site. They can block non-competitively (C) at a distinct site on the receptor, possibly inside the cell. They can interfere as a physiological antagonist (D) with the downstream signals by activating a distinct receptor (gray rectangular shape). Finally, they can interfere chemically (E) by binding to the agonist itself.*

thermodynamic concentration c/c_s, where c is the actual concentration of the drug and c_s, its saturation concentration (Ferguson's principle). The validity of this correlation is such that often when a series of drugs has equal potency at equal c/c_s, this has been considered evidence that the action of those drugs is *nonspecific*, i.e., not mediated by receptors.

While the concept of nonspecific drug action is a useful and valid one, it must be admitted that in some instances a drug which was considered to be nonspecific, as a result of new discoveries turns out to have a very specific receptor. An example is local anesthetics, which were considered to act nonspecifically on membranes but now are definitely known to interact with the sodium channels in membranes (Chapter 25). There is also the possibility that lipids may themselves act as receptors.

Regarding the cell membrane as a receptor, there is a hypothesis that general anesthetics act by increasing *fluidity* of the membrane, in other words, a transition of the lipid bilayer from a gel to a liquid-crystal form. While there is much indirect evidence of the validity of this hypothesis, including pressure reversal of anesthesia, it cannot be considered to be definitely proven.

BIBLIOGRAPHY

Cuatrecasas, P.: "Affinity Chromatography of Macromolecules," *Adv. Enzymol.* **36**: 29-89 (1972).

Kenakin, T.P.: *Pharmacologic Analysis of Drug-Receptor Interaction, 2nd Ed.*, Raven Press, New York, 1993.

Caron, M.G., and R.J. Lefkowitz: "Catecholamine Receptors: Structure, Function, and Regulation," *Recent Prog. Horm. Res.* **48**: 277-290 (1993).

Hegde, S.S., and D.E. Clarke: "Characterization of Angiotensin Receptors Mediating the Neuromodulatory Effects of Angiotensin in the Vas Deferens of the Rabbit ," *J. Pharmacol. Exp. Ther.* **265**: 601-608 (1993).

Neubig, R.R., R.D. Gantzos, and R.S. Brasier: "Agonist and Antagonist Binding to α_2-Adrenergic Receptors in Purified Membranes from Human Platelets. Implications of Receptor-Inhibitory Nucleotide-Binding Protein Stoichiometry," *Mol. Pharmacol.* **28**: 475-486 (1985).

Pratt, W.B., P. Taylor: *Principles of Drug Action: The Basis of Pharmacology, 3rd Ed.*, Churchill Livingstone, New York, 1990.

Wainscott, D.B., M.L. Cohen, K.W. Schenck, J.E. Audia, J.S. Nissen, M. Baez, J.D. Kursar, V.L. Lucaites, and D.L. Nelson: "Pharmacological Characterization of the Newly Cloned Rat 5-Hydroxytryptamine$_{2F}$ Receptor," *Mol. Pharmacol.* **43**: 419-426 (1993).

CHAPTER 3

Receptors and Intracellular Signals

Stephen P. Halenda

The actions of many of our most important drugs are mediated by physiological receptors and their associated cellular signaling pathways. These pathways serve an essential function in the transmission of signals by hormones, neurotransmitters, and other biological mediators. Receptors provide the means by which information arriving from outside of the cell, in the form of a hormone or transmitter molecule, is translated into a functional response within the cell. Consider, as an example, the mechanism by which the neurotransmitter norepinephrine causes contraction of vascular smooth muscle. Upon its release from adrenergic nerve endings, norepinephrine binds to and activates α_1-adrenergic receptors at the surface of the smooth muscle cell. Within a few seconds, a number of additional events occur within the target cell as a result of receptor activation; these include the production of the second messenger inositol-1,4,5-trisphosphate and the consequent rise in the cytosolic concentration of calcium ions. These initial steps in the signaling pathway culminate in the activation of the actin/myosin system and muscle contraction. Of course, the muscle cell also possesses many types of receptors in addition to α_1-adrenergic receptors. Some are also coupled to stimulation of contraction, others inhibit contraction, and some receptors may have other functions (such as regulation of cell growth and differentiation) that are entirely unrelated to contraction. At any moment, the functional state of the smooth muscle cell is determined by the integrated effects of a network of receptor-coupled signaling pathways. The same generalization can be made for essentially all cells in the organism. Clearly, the administration of drugs that bind to physiological receptors may have profound effects on cell function.

For the purposes of this discussion, a physiological receptor is defined as a cellular macromolecule (nearly always a protein or complex of protein molecules) to which an endogenous mediator binds, producing a conformational change in the receptor that results in its activation. In the activated conformation, the receptor is capable of initiating intracellular biochemical changes that eventually result in an end response such as action potential generation, muscle contraction, secretion, enhanced production of fuel molecules, increased synthesis of certain proteins, or cell growth. On the other hand, some receptors are coupled to inhibitory signaling pathways that block these responses. The endogenous mediators include hormones, neurotransmitters, and locally acting hormone-like substances such as cytokines, prostaglandins, and bradykinin. In signal transduction parlance, these mediators collectively are considered *first messengers* because they originate from a source external to the target cell and, by binding to and activating their specific receptors, they constitute the first step in their respective signaling pathways. In many cases, the initial receptor activation leads to production of additional intracellular molecules that transmit the signal within the cell, i.e., *second messengers*. Well known examples of second messengers are cyclic AMP, cyclic GMP, inositol-1,4,5-trisphosphate, and 1,2-diacylglycerol. The cell's response to receptor activation depends on the type of signaling pathway that is called into play by that receptor. Furthermore, the same hormone or neurotransmitter may have very different effects in other cell types due to cell-specific differences in the receptors to which the ligand binds or the response pathways to which the receptors are coupled.

A large number of drugs produce their therapeutic (and sometimes toxic) effects by binding to physiological receptors at the same site utilized by the endogenous mediator. Thus, the drug may function as an *agonist*, mimicking the effect of the endogenous mediator. The analgesic agent morphine, obtained from the opium poppy, is an agonist at opioid receptors that are normally activated by endogenous opioid peptides. An *antagonist* is a drug with no agonist activity of its own, but with sufficient affinity for the receptor that it blocks the action of endogenous or exogenous agonists. Naloxone, an antagonist at opioid receptors, dramatically reverses the effects of morphine overdosage. Certain drugs act upon physiological receptors at a site distinct from the natural agonist binding site, thereby causing allosteric regulation of receptor activity. An example of such a drug is the sedative-hypnotic phenobarbital that enhances the effect of the inhibitory neurotransmitter γ-aminobutyric acid (GABA) at $GABA_A$ receptors (see below). Finally, a drug might affect receptor coupled signaling pathways at steps downstream from the receptor, for example, by inhibiting the degradation of a second messenger and, consequently, prolonging its action. High concentrations of caffeine, a familiar central nervous system stimulant, can inhibit the phosphodiesterases that inactivate cyclic AMP (although this drug is actually more potent as an adenosine receptor antagonist). Many drugs produce their effects by binding molecules other than physiological receptors. In this regard, ion channels, enzymes, and carrier proteins are targets for drugs that act as inhibitors or competitive substrates. These additional sites of drug action will be encountered frequently in later chapters.

Advances in molecular cloning and gene expression techniques, allied with more traditional protein purification methodology, have led to the identification of several hundred receptors or receptor candidates. Fortunately, most of these molecules fall into distinct families based on structural similarities, as will be discussed in the following paragraphs. The intracellular pathways that transduce receptor-generated signals have proven to be more difficult to elucidate than the receptors themselves, despite the purification and cloning of many of the proteins involved. In fact, there are few examples of entirely defined pathways from receptor to the ultimate cellular response. In contrast to the situation with receptors, it appears that the number of discrete signaling pathways may be limited to a dozen or fewer. Therefore, a large number of receptors can exert their effects by evoking one or more of only a handful of signaling pathways. Clearly, much remains to be learned about the means by which specificity of signaling is attained at the cellular level.

MAJOR RECEPTOR CLASSES

An exciting aspect of the recent discoveries of new receptor candidates, by cloning and sequence analysis, is that by knowing the amino acid sequence of the molecule, accurate predictions can be made as to its function. Receptors have traditionally been categorized into general classes based on the molecular mechanisms by which the receptors transduce signals (Fig. 3-1). At least four distinct classes of receptors are identified on this basis: (1) ion channel receptors, (2) receptors that interact with guanine nucleotide binding proteins (G proteins), (3) receptors with intrinsic tyrosine kinase activity, and (4) nuclear receptors. The first three types of receptors transduce information delivered extracellularly at the plasma membrane into ionic or biochemical signals within the cell, whereas the last receptor type is associated with the nuclear matrix and is activated by lipophilic ligands (e.g., steroids) that easily diffuse across membrane barriers. Within each class of signal transduction mechanism, individual receptor proteins conform to specific structural motifs. It is relevant to point out that the classification of membrane receptors is not necessarily based on the primary structure of the receptor proteins, but rather on their higher order structure. In other words, members of the same receptor class, as defined above, all have an essentially identical predicted configuration within the membrane (Fig. 3-1).

Ion Channel Receptors

The mechanism of action of several hormones and neurotransmitters is attributed directly to enhanced movement of ions across the plasma membrane. In some cases the hormone or neurotransmitter receptor is itself an ion channel. These systems are referred to as *ligand-gated* ion channels or ion channel receptors. Included in this superfamily of receptors are the nicotinic acetylcholine receptor (nAChR), the $GABA_A$ receptor ($GABA_AR$), the glycine receptor (GlyR), and certain of the receptors for glutamate (GluR) and serotonin (5-HT) (Table 3-1). By and large these signaling systems are confined to excitable tissue of the central nervous system, the autonomic ganglia, and the neuromuscular junction. The ion channel

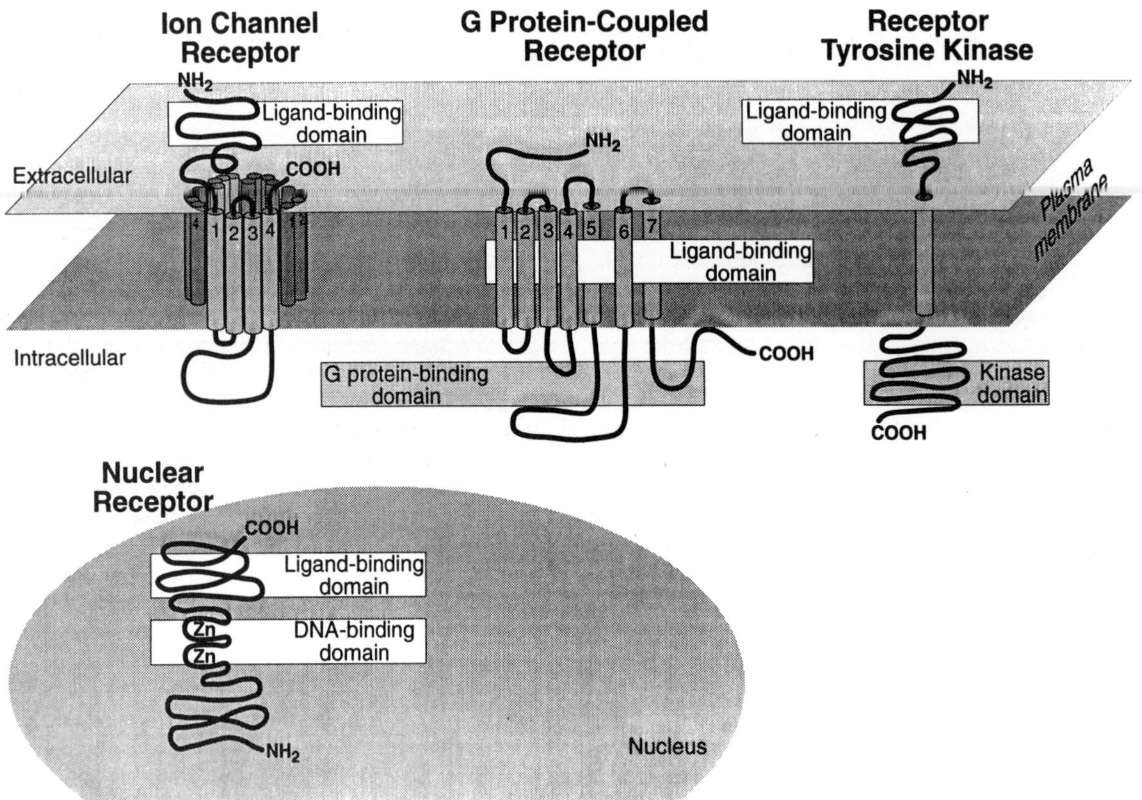

FIGURE 3-1 *Schematic models of the major classes of physiological receptors. Membrane-spanning domains are depicted as cylinders. For clarity, the N- and C-terminal tails and connecting loops are shown for only one of the five subunits of the ion channel receptor. The transmembrane regions of a G protein-coupled receptor are probably arranged in a cluster, forming a ligand binding pocket within the membrane.*

receptors are activated by agonists on a millisecond time scale, and the resultant ion movements serve either to increase (depolarize) or decrease (hyperpolarize) the electrical potential across the membranes of postsynaptic neurons and muscle cells. As a class, these receptor systems are involved in the rapid propagation of electric impulses and the transfer of information across synapses throughout the nervous system. Other types of ion channels are regulated by membrane potential (e.g., *voltage-gated* sodium and potassium channels) or are regulated by physically distinct receptors through the action of intermediary transducer proteins or second messengers. These latter classes of ion channels can also be modulated by certain drugs. For example, local anesthetics block ion flux through voltage-gated sodium channels and therefore prevent action potential propagation.

At the molecular level the ion channel receptors show remarkable similarity. All are multimeric proteins arranged across the membrane to contain an anion- or cation-selective channel whose conductivity is controlled by agonist binding to specific extracellular sites. These receptors have a molecular mass of 250 to 300 kDa and are composed of several nonidentical subunits of 50 to 60 kDa (approximately 450 to 500 amino acid residues). The overall structure of the ion channel receptors, based on electron microscopy of the nAChR, indicates that the subunits are arranged in a rosette around a central core of low election density that forms the ion channel through the membrane (Fig. 3-1).

To date, the primary structures of more than 80 distinct subunits of the ion channel receptor superfamily have been determined from complimentary DNA sequences obtained from many

TABLE 3-1 Examples of ion channel receptors

Receptor	Ion selectivity
Nicotinic acetylcholine	Na^+, K^+
$GABA_A$	Cl^-
Glycine	Cl^-
Glutamate	
NMDA	Na^+, K^+, Ca^{2+}
AMPA	Na^+, K^+
Kainate	Na^+, K^+
Serotonin	
$5\text{-}HT_{1A}$	K^+
$5\text{-}HT_3$	cations

different species. The complete subunit sequences of the nAChR, the $GABA_AR$, and the GlyR have been determined, and all show a striking homology. This homology suggests that there are important structural features necessary to accommodate the function of a ligand-gated ion channel. The similarities among the gene sequences encoding the receptor subunits also indicate a common evolutionary origin and substantiate the identification of ion channel receptors as a superfamily of proteins.

The deduced amino acid sequence of each of the protein subunits includes a large extracellular N-terminal domain, four hydrophobic, α-helical domains (M1 to M4), each of which is predicted to span the plasma membrane, and a long intracellular loop between the M3 and M4 transmembrane domains. Common features of the extracellular domain of each subunit are its length, accounting for approximately 50 percent of the entire polypeptide, the existence of multiple N-glycosylation sites, and the presence of two conserved cysteine residues that may form a disulfide bond to produce a loop structure. This loop contains invariant amino acid residues and a conserved glycosylation site. The function of this highly conserved structural region is unknown, although it has been hypothesized to be involved in some stereotypical way, either in the binding of agonist or in the intramolecular transduction of that signal. A second conserved structural feature among this class of receptors is the series of four hydrophobic segments (M1 to M4) common to all receptor subunits. Each segment is 19 to 27 amino acid residues long and is thought to adopt an energetically favorable α helix that spans the thickness of the membrane. These segments orient with each other and with segments from the other subunits to form the ion channel through the membrane, somewhat like the staves of a barrel. The M2 segments are amphipathic; the hydrophobic side aligns with other hydrophobic segments, and the hydrophilic side lines the central channel rendering it conducive to ion flow. Despite these findings, the precise molecular workings of the ion channel receptors are not known. According to current models, agonist binding causes the subunits to undergo either an "all-or-none twist" or a "bloom", as with the petals of a flower, such that the diameter of the central pore is altered and ions are allowed to pass.

Nicotinic Acetylcholine Receptor

The best understood of the ion channel receptors is the nicotinic acetylcholine receptor (nAChR). Different isoforms of this receptor mediate the action of acetylcholine at excitable synapses in ganglia (both sympathetic and parasympathetic), at the neuromuscular junction, and at sites in the central nervous system. A separate class of cholinergic receptor, the muscarinic receptor, mediates the effects of acetylcholine at the effector organs. The muscarinic cholinergic receptor is a member of the G protein-associated receptor family (see below).

Activation of the nAChR depolarizes excitable membranes by increasing the permeability of the ion channel to sodium primarily, although the channel is also permeable to potassium and calcium ions. The ganglionic and neuromuscular nAChRs differ in their pharmacology, indicating that they are distinct proteins. For example, nondepolarizing neuromuscular blocking drugs have variable effects in producing ganglionic blockade. Tubocurarine will block at both sites but acts predominantly as a true acetylcholine antagonist at the muscle nicotinic receptor and largely by noncompetitive channel blockade in the mammalian ganglia. Furthermore, α-bungarotoxin blocks the muscle receptor nearly irreversibly, whereas most neuronal receptors are unaffected.

Isolation of the nicotinic acetylcholine receptor was aided greatly by the availability of excellent pharmacological tools, i.e., α-bungarotoxin and other snake venom toxins, that bind selectively and with high affinity to the receptor. Equally important was the use of the receptor-rich electric organs of the electric fish *Torpedo californica* and the electric eel *Electrophorus electricus* as starting materials for receptor purification. The electrocytes of these electric organs are derived ontogenetically from muscle cells, and it is not surprising, therefore, that the *T. californica* nAChR very much resembles that of the mammalian neuromuscular junction. The purified receptor has a pentameric structure composed of 4 distinct subunits (denoted α, β, γ, δ) with a stoichiometry of 2:1:1:1, respectively. Reconstitution studies in lipid vesicles and planar lipid bilayers show that agonist-controlled ion channel activity is wholly contained in this purified multimeric receptor complex. Furthermore, injection of *Xenopus* oocytes with mRNA coding for the four receptor subunits results in expression of functional nAChR. The subunits are of molecular masses ranging from 50 to 58 kDa and are arranged in the membrane in a quasi-fivefold symmetry surrounding a central channel. The receptor contains, mainly within its α subunits, two acetylcholine binding sites that are important in both regulation of ion conduction and fast desensitization in response to agonist. Desensitization is a process by which receptor responsiveness decreases in the continued presence of agonist. Fast desensitization in the nAChR is unique in that it appears to be an intrinsic property of the receptor complex that can occur even after reconstitution of the purified protein.

Comparison of the *T. californica* receptor genes with those encoding the acetylcholine receptor of the neuromuscular junction in several different animal species shows that these proteins are highly conserved. At least 90 percent amino acid sequence identity is seen for a particular subunit compared to its homologue in other species. In fact, greater sequence differences are seen between the receptors of the skeletal muscle end plate and of the postsynaptic neurons of autonomic ganglia in the same species. As indicated above, these receptors show pharmacologic differences as well.

Recombinant DNA studies support the existence of a diverse family of mammalian nAChR proteins. Muscle cells make both fetal and adult forms of the receptor, which differ in structure and in channel conductance. In the adult muscle nAChR, a distinct ϵ subunit substitutes for the γ subunit present in the fetal receptor. The ganglionic nAChR differs from the muscle cell types and also from forms identified in the brain. In contrast to the nAChR from muscle, neuronal nAChRs are composed of only two different subunit classes, α and β, with a proposed stoichiometry of two α and three β subunits in the functional pentameric receptor.

GABA$_A$ Receptor

γ-Aminobutyric acid (GABA) is the main inhibitory neurotransmitter in the mammalian brain. GABA-mediated neuronal hyperpolarization results from increased membrane chloride conductance and is attributed to the activation of an integral chloride channel. This chloride channel contains a specific GABA binding site and is classified as the GABA$_A$ receptor (GABA$_A$R). Less well characterized GABA$_B$ receptors, that have a pharmacology distinct from the GABA$_A$R, are probably members of the G protein-associated receptor family. GABA$_A$Rs have binding sites for several pharmacologic agents that act *allosterically* to modulate chloride ion conduction, i.e., they bind in regions other that the neurotransmitter binding site. Benzodiazepines such as diazepam bind with high affinity to the receptor complex and increase the GABA-stimulated ion current by increasing the frequency of channel opening. There is evidence that the benzodiazepine site itself might interact with substances normally present in the brain ("endogenous benzodiazepines"), raising the possibility that this chloride channel is subject to coordinate regulation by multiple ligands *in vivo*. Barbiturates like phenobarbital bind to a different site on the receptor and increase the mean open time of the chloride channel. The potentiation of GABA-mediated neuronal hyperpolarization by these drugs offers a compelling molecular explanation for their anxiolytic and depressant activities. This intriguing receptor is thus a site of action of many sedative-hypnotic agents; it is also thought that general anesthetics, alcohol, and other drugs may exert some of their depressant actions by affecting GABA$_A$R function. Of further interest is the observation that certain experimental drugs that bind to the benzodiazepine site can actually *inhibit* GABA-stimulated chloride flux and therefore produce central nervous system excitation. These substances are known as *inverse agonists* because they produce an effect that is opposite to the typical benzodiazepine agonist effect.

The GABA$_A$R conforms to the superfamily of ligand-gated ion channels. Molecular cloning studies have revealed the existence of six α, four β, three γ, one δ, and two ρ subunits of the receptor. Although the exact subunit composition of any native GABA$_A$R is unknown, it is generally thought that five subunits associate to form the ion channel in a topology similar to the nAChR. As different brain regions express distinct patterns of $GABA_AR$ subunits, it is likely that numerous isoforms of the receptor are present. These may be composed of different α and β subunits, alone, or in combination with members of the other classes of subunits, providing for a great diversity of structural (and presumably functional) characteristics.

Each of the $GABA_AR$ subunits contains the four stretches of hydrophobic amino acids (putative membrane-spanning regions) that are the hallmark of all ion channel receptors. The $GABA_AR$ is distinctive in that there is a clustering of positively charged, basic amino acids at both ends of the membrane-spanning helices. In contrast, these sites in the nAChR are either negatively charged or uncharged. It is likely that these charged regions are involved in the anion and cation selectivity of the respective channels.

Glycine Receptor

Glycine is the principal inhibitory neurotransmitter in the mammalian spinal cord and brain stem. Like GABA, glycine inhibits neuronal firing by activating a chloride ion conductance which effectively hyperpolarizes excitable membranes. A glycine receptor (GlyR) has been affinity-purified, and when reconstituted in planar lipid bilayers, glycine-dependent ion conductances are observed. The convulsant alkaloid strychnine has been particularly useful in characterizing the pharmacology and molecular biology of the GlyR and its subunits. Strychnine acts as a competitive antagonist of glycine binding and inhibits glycine-mediated, but not GABA-mediated chloride conductances. Strychnine binding to synaptic membranes is antagonized by glycine and other GlyR agonists including the amino acids β-alanine and taurine.

The GlyR conforms to the superfamily of ion channel receptors. The affinity-purified GlyR is a pentamer of homologous, glycosylated 48 kDa and 58 kDa subunits that constitute the glycine-regulated chloride channel. A 93 kDa subunit is a peripheral protein that is associated with the cytoplasmic portion of the GlyR and the role of this subunit is not clear. Strychnine photoaffinity labels the 48 kDa subunit, and to a lesser extent the 58 kDa subunit. The cloned and sequenced cDNA of the 48 kDa strychnine-binding subunit of the GlyR bears significant similarity to the subunit cDNAs of the nACh and $GABA_A$ receptors.

Glutamate Receptors

The glutamate receptors, i.e., the excitatory amino acid receptors, which are ionotropic are divided into three subtypes based on pharmacologic agonist selectivity: the N-methyl-D-aspartate (NMDA) receptor, the D,L-α-amino-3-hydroxy-5-methyl-4-isoxalone propionic acid (AMPA) receptor (previously called the quisqualate receptor), and the kainate receptor. The AMPA and kainate receptors mediate conventional sodium ion and potassium ion depolarizing conductances and are responsible for most fast excitatory postsynaptic potentials in the brain and spinal cord. In this way the AMPA and kainate receptors resemble the nAChRs; receptor activation allows rapid ion flow, immediate depolarization, and summate to give an all-or-none activation of the postsynaptic cell. On the other hand, the NMDA receptor mediates not only monovalent cation but also calcium ion conductances, and these responses require both agonist binding and concurrent membrane depolarization. Depolarization is required because the ion channel is blocked under resting conditions in a voltage-dependent manner by magnesium. A strychnine-insensitive, modulatory glycine binding site is present on the NMDA receptor; this site must be occupied by glycine in order for receptor activation to occur. NMDA receptors are therefore not directly involved in fast synaptic transmission but in the modulation of postsynaptic neuronal activity. These properties of NMDA receptors support their proposed role in the complex phenomena of neuronal plasticity, long-term potentiation, and learning.

Little is known about the molecular structures of glutamate receptors except that separate genes and mRNAs encode the receptor subtypes. The purification, sequencing, and expression of the encoding mRNAs should indicate whether any or all of the glutamate receptors conform to the superfamily of ion channel receptors.

RECEPTOR-G PROTEIN-EFFECTOR SYSTEM

A second major pattern of signal transduction involves receptors that produce their cellular effects indirectly. In this system, the receptors interact with transducer molecules within the plane of the plasma membrane; the transducers in this case are heterotrimeric guanine nucleotide binding proteins known as *G proteins*. The G proteins in turn transmit the receptor-generated signal to a downstream *effector* that functions as either an enzyme or an ion channel. In many cases, effector enzymes trigger a cascade of cellular events involving the generation of second messengers, activation of additional enzymes, and changes in ion levels. Although the initial receptor-G protein-effector interactions occur at the plasma membrane, downstream events may take place in the cytosol or intracellular organelles due to the involvement of diffusible messengers. The added complexity of this signaling system, by comparison with the ion channel receptors, means that cell responses usually occur on a time scale of seconds to minutes rather than milliseconds. A few examples of the receptor-G protein-effector system are given in Table 3-2.

Receptors Coupled to G Proteins

Most of the pharmacologically important hormone and neurotransmitter receptors are known to interact with G proteins. Included among these receptors are the adrenergic, muscarinic acetylcholine, serotonergic, and dopaminergic receptors as well as a multitude of peptide receptors. The genomic and deduced amino acid sequences of many of these receptors are now known. The receptors are all monomeric proteins. The most striking feature of these receptors is the conservation of seven stretches of 20 to 28 hydrophobic amino acids that likely represent membrane-spanning regions. Electron optical analysis of the related protein, bacteriorhodopsin, confirms the existence of the membrane-spanning regions; they are arrayed as a bundle of α helices within the membrane. Many additional studies, both biophysical and biochemical in nature, also support the model of a "serpentine" structure for G protein-coupled receptors, as depicted in Fig. 3-1. It is likely that all the receptors in this class have a similar topology. With an extracellular amino terminus and an odd number of transmembrane segments, this arrangement dictates that there are three extracellular connecting loops (EI to EIII), three cytosolic connecting loops (CI to CIII), and an intracellular carboxyl terminus (Fig. 3-1).

The ligand binding site in the G protein-coupled receptors, surprisingly, appears to be buried deep within the membrane-spanning regions rather than in the extracellular N-terminal tail. The photoreceptor protein rhodopsin in the mammalian retina is a well-established prototype of this family of receptors. In rhodopsin, the chromophore 11-*cis* retinal is covalently bound to a lysine residue midway down the seventh transmembrane do-

TABLE 3-2 Some representative receptor-G protein-effector systems

Receptor	G-protein	Effector	Tissue	Response
β_1-Adrenergic	G_s	Increased adenylate cyclase activity	Heart	Increased rate, increased contractility
β_2-Adrenergic	G_s	Increased adenylate cyclase activity	Bronchioles	Bronchodilation
α_1-Adrenergic	G_q	Increased phosphoinositide-specific phospholipase C activity	Blood vessels	Contraction
α_2-Adrenergic	G_i	Decreased adenylate cyclase activity	Adipocytes	Decreased lipolysis
M_2 Cholinergic	G_i	Increased K^+ channel opening	Heart	Decreased rate, Decreased contractility
Rhodopsin	G_t	Increased cyclic GMP phosphodiesterase activity	Retinal rods	Hyperpolarization
Glucagon	G_s	Increased adenylate cyclase activity	Liver	Glycogenolysis

main. Interactions between retinal and amino acids in other transmembrane helices are critical for light-stimulated signal transmission by rhodopsin, suggesting that the membrane-spanning regions form a binding pocket for retinal. There is considerable evidence that other receptors bind their respective ligands in a similar configuration, although the interaction is usually noncovalent. Absorption of a photon by retinal, or binding of agonist by other G protein-coupled receptors, is thought to induce a conformational change in the receptor that facilitates its interaction with a G protein.

Receptor mutants, synthetic peptides corresponding to specific receptor regions, and sequence-specific antibodies have been utilized to map the possible sites of interaction between the receptor and its G protein. Based on these studies, portions of the cytoplasmic surface of the receptor contained within the CII and CIII loops and the C-terminal tail are implicated in receptor-G protein association. The amino acid composition of these regions is an important determinant of G protein binding specificity as well as the ability of the receptor to activate the G protein. One form of retinitis pigmentosa is associated with an amino acid substitution in the CII loop of rhodopsin that prevents the interaction of this receptor with its G protein, transducin.

Sequences of the C-terminal segments are highly enriched in serines and threonines. These residues are potential sites for phosphorylation. Strong evidence exists for a β-adrenergic receptor desensitization system involving phosphorylation of the receptor by a specific kinase followed by binding of an intracellular protein known as β-arrestin. A very similar system had previously been established for rhodopsin. It remains to be seen whether this same basic mechanism of desensitization is conserved among all G protein-coupled receptors.

A fascinating variation on the G protein-coupled receptor theme is a receptor for thrombin that is present on blood platelets and other cell types. It has recently been demonstrated that thrombin, a protease generated during blood coagulation, activates its receptor by cleaving off a segment of the N-terminus, thereby creating a new N-terminus. The new N-terminus is thought to function as a "tethered ligand", interacting with a binding site within the receptor. Synthetic peptides based on the new N-terminus are in fact full agonists at the uncleaved thrombin receptor, although, as is the case for most agonists at other receptors, their action is reversible.

G proteins

G proteins are a family of homologous guanine nucleotide binding proteins that function as intermediaries in signal transduction between receptors and effectors (Fig. 3-2). The G proteins are on the cytoplasmic face of the plasma membrane, thus facilitating interaction with both membrane-bound proteins and cytosolic components (i.e., guanine nucleotides). The G proteins are heterotrimeric, consisting of α subunits (40 to 46 kDa), β subunits (37 kDa), and γ subunits (7 to 9 kDa). The α subunits bind guanine nucleotides and, in most cases, determine the specificity of receptor-effector coupling. The α subunits display by far the greatest structural diversity of the three types of subunits, constituting a family of more than 20 proteins. The β and γ subunits form a tightly associated, highly hydrophobic complex. The $\beta\gamma$ subunit complex is required for receptor-induced activation of the G protein, and may serve to anchor the α subunits to the plasma membrane. The $\beta\gamma$ subunits appear to be functionally interchangeable among different α subunits.

The action of G protein involves a cycle of guanine nucleotide binding and hydrolysis. At rest, the G protein has guanosine diphosphate (GDP) bound to the nucleotide binding site of the α subunit. The agonist-occupied hormone receptor interacts with the G protein, stimulating it to release GDP and subsequently bind guanosine triphosphate (GTP). The receptor-G protein complex dissociates at this point, releasing the $\beta\gamma$ complex and a free α subunit with its bound GTP. Free α-GTP directly activates effector systems until a GTPase activity, intrinsic to the α subunit, hydrolyzes bound GTP to GDP. The α-GDP unit reassociates with the $\beta\gamma$ complex, and the G protein complex is then available for another receptor-stimulated activation cycle. Since GTP hydrolysis by the α subunit is slow, a single ligand-activated receptor can activate a number of G proteins in a catalytic fashion, thereby amplifying the signal. Recent evidence suggests that the $\beta\gamma$ complex may also play a role in the activation of certain effector molecules. A highly simplified depiction of the receptor-G protein-effector system is presented in Fig. 3-2.

G proteins were initially identified by their functional interactions: transducin (G_t), which couples rhodopsin activation to cyclic GMP phosphodiesterase in retinal rods, and the G proteins (G_s and G_i), which mediate stimulation and inhibition of adenylate cyclase, respectively. Subsequently, a distinct, "other" G protein (G_o) of

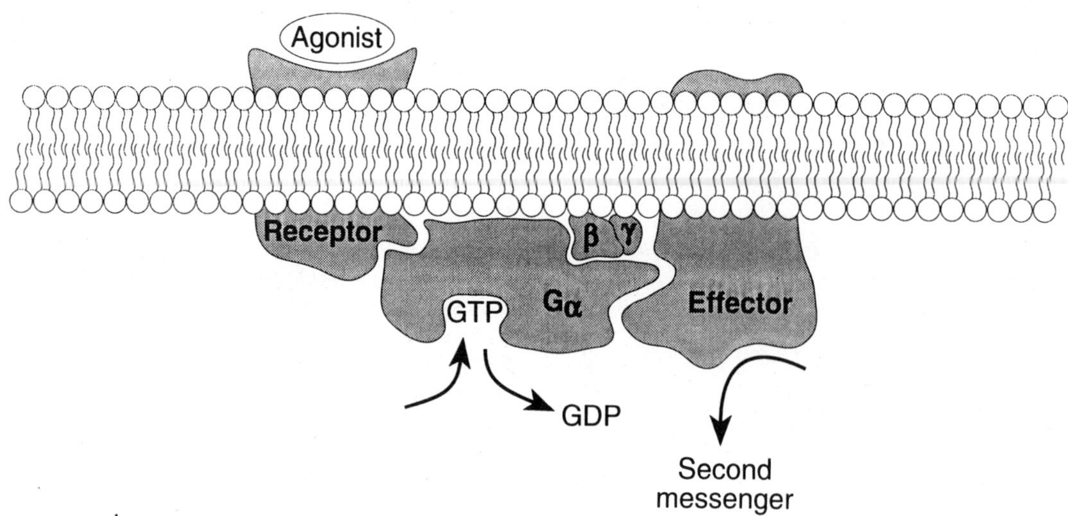

Figure 3-2 *Illustration depicting the receptor-G protein-effector system at the plasma membrane. The receptor is of the seven-transmembrane-domain class, as shown in Fig. 3-1. Occupation of the receptor by agonist causes receptor-G protein association, release of guanosine diphosphate (GDP) and subsequent binding of guanosine triphosphate (GTP) by the G protein α subunit, and then activation of the effector by free α-GTP or perhaps by free $\beta\gamma$ subunits. Hydrolysis of GTP by the α subunit terminates effector activation and allows reassociation of α-GDP with $\beta\gamma$. Some known effectors are adenylate cyclase, phospholipase C, and calcium channels.*

unknown function was isolated from brain, and additional G proteins that couple to effector systems other than adenylate cyclase have recently been identified. In not all cases have G proteins been unambiguously assigned to specific receptors and effectors. The fact that the receptors, G proteins, and effectors are separate molecules provides for a high degree of potential versatility in cell signal transduction. Signals initiated by more than one type of receptor often converge on a common pool of G proteins. Alternatively, one receptor might be capable of activating more that one type of G protein. And in some instances, it appears that a single G protein may couple to multiple effector systems, some systems being more potently activated than others.

A property of some G protein α subunits is their susceptibility to covalent modification by certain bacterial toxins. Cholera toxin catalyzes the ADP-ribosylation of an arginine residue of G_s α, resulting in the inhibition of intrinsic GTPase activity and in the persistent activation of adenylate cyclase. Transducin is similarly activated by cholera toxin. Pertussis toxin catalyzes the ADP-ribosylation of a cysteine residue located in the carboxy terminus of α_i, α_o, and α_t. ADP-ribosylation by pertussis toxin blocks interactions between receptors and G proteins, thus inhibiting effector activities linked to these systems. This suggests that the C-terminal domain of G proteins is involved in receptor contact. Support for this idea is obtained from the *unc* mutant of the mouse S49 lymphoma cell line in which G_s cannot be activated by hormone receptors. The *unc* mutation encodes a variant α_s with a single amino acid change six residues from the carboxy terminus. It has also been observed that antibodies specific for the carboxy termini of α_i, α_s, and α_t block the interaction of these proteins with their respective receptors, whereas antibodies to other regions in the α subunits do not affect receptor binding.

Effector Systems

G proteins are coupled to effector systems that in turn regulate membrane potential or the cellular levels of various second messengers. The best studied G protein effector systems are regulation of adenylate cyclase activity in many tissues, and visual signal transduction in the retina. In the past few years, it has become clear that cellular phospholipases are also subject to control by G proteins.

In retinal rod cells, light-activated rhodopsin associates with transducin (G_t) and elicits the production of free α_t-GTP. The activated α subunit stimulates a cyclic GMP phosphodiesterase, resulting in a *decreased* cytosolic level of the second messenger, cyclic GMP. The drop in cyclic GMP results in hyperpolarization of the rod cell due to closure of sodium channels that are controlled by this second messenger. Hyperpolarization causes decreased neurotransmitter release by the rod cell. A similar system operates in retinal cone cells, in this case mediated by forms of opsin and transducin that are specifically expressed in cone cells.

Adenylate cyclases are enzymes that convert adenosine triphosphate (ATP) to cyclic AMP, a ubiquitous second messenger. β-adrenergic receptors are but one type of receptor that stimulates adenylate cyclase via the G protein, G_s. Free α_s-GTP binds to and activates adenylate cyclase to produce a rise in cytosolic levels of cyclic AMP. The consequent activation of cyclic AMP-dependent protein kinase typically leads to a signal-amplifying cascade of additional kinase steps that determine the eventual functional response in the cell, such as the activation of glycogenolysis in liver or relaxation of vascular smooth muscle. In addition to adenylate cyclase, G_s is coupled to activation of calcium channels and inhibition of sodium channels.

It has been known for some time that α_2-adrenergic receptors and other receptors coupled to G_i can evoke an inhibition of adenylate cyclase, although the exact mechanism and physiological significance of this phenomenon remain uncertain. Depending on the particular isoform of adenylate cyclase and experimental conditions, α_i-GTP usually inhibits the cyclase, while $\beta\gamma$ subunits can be inhibitory, stimulatory, or have no effect at all. G_i may have a more important role in regulation of effectors other than adenylate cyclase, such as certain cation channels and phospholipases. For example, it has been proposed the pertussis toxin-sensitive activation of phospholipase C, observed in some systems, may be mediated by $\beta\gamma$ complexes released from G_i.

A separate series of G proteins that are not substrates for cholera or pertussis toxins have been discovered. G proteins of the G_q family, present in virtually all tissues, are coupled to activation of phosphoinositide-specific phospholipase C (specifically, phospholipase C-β). Phosphatidylinositol-4,5-bisphosphate is a minor membrane phospholipid that is, in essence, two second messengers covalently linked in an inactive form. Its hydrolysis by phospholipase C releases 1,2-diacylglycerol, a hydrophobic neutral lipid that remains in the membrane, and inositol-1,4,5-trisphosphate (IP_3), a hydrophilic molecule that is now free to diffuse through the cytosol. Diacylglycerol activates a multifunctional protein kinase known as protein kinase C. IP_3 binds to a receptor located on the endoplasmic reticulum, an intracellular organelle that is packed with calcium ions. It may come as no surprise that the IP_3 receptor is a ligand-gated ion channel, similar in many respects to the plasma membrane channels discussed earlier. Binding of IP_3 to its receptor induces the release of calcium into the cytosol, where it activates calcium-dependent protein kinases, contractile proteins, and additional phospholipases. In response to the binding of calcium, a cytosolic phospholipase A_2 translocates to membranes and cleaves arachidonic acid away from phospholipids. The free arachidonic acid is then converted into a series of products known as eicosanoids (including prostaglandins, leukotrienes, and lipoxins). Eicosanoids diffuse out of the cell to play the role of "local hormones"; they bind to receptors on other cells in the vicinity. Eicosanoid receptors themselves are coupled to G proteins that activate adenylate cyclase or phospholipase C. It should be apparent at this point that the phospholipase C pathway constitutes an effector system of astounding complexity and versatility.

RECEPTOR TYROSINE KINASES

In comparison with the first two major classes of receptors, whose ligands are usually small molecules, the receptor tyrosine kinase family is distinctive in its specificity for large polypeptide ligands such as insulin, epidermal growth factor (EGF), platelet-derived growth factor (PDGF), macrophage colony stimulating factor (CSF-1), insulin-like growth factor (IGF-1), and many other growth factors (Table 3-3). Activation of the receptor tyrosine kinases leads to cell-specific changes in proliferation, differentiation, and metabolic activity. The common structural features of these receptors are an N-terminal extracellular domain that contains the ligand binding site, a single transmembrane segment, and an intracellular protein kinase domain (Fig. 3-1). Binding of the ligand extracellularly causes activation of the cytosol-facing kinase domain, thereby transmitting a signal across the membrane.

TABLE 3-3 Examples of receptor tyrosine kinases

Subclass	Receptor and molar mass	Characteristics
I	EGF (170 kDa)	Single polypeptide chain (monomeric) Two extracellular cysteine-rich regions Uninterrupted tyrosine kinase domain
II	Insulin (α, β: 135 kDa, 90 kDa) IGF-1 (α, β: 135 kDa, 90 kDa)	Heterotetrameric structure ($\alpha_2\beta_2$) One extracellular cysteine-rich region Uninterrupted tyrosine kinase domain
III	PDGF (180 kDa) CSF-1 (165 kDa)	Single polypeptide chain (monomeric) No cysteine clusters 70 to 100 amino acid insertion in tyrosine kinase domain

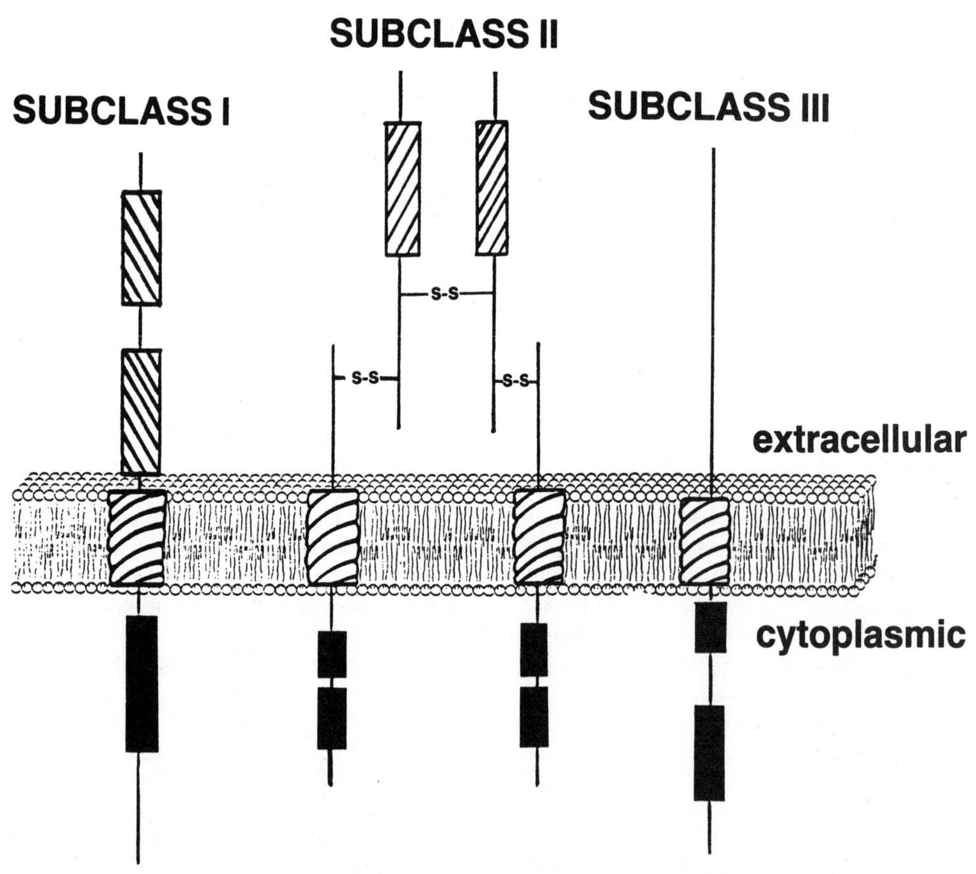

FIGURE 3-3 *Schematic models of the structural subclasses of the receptor tyrosine kinase superfamily. Extracellular cysteine-rich domains are indicated by hatched areas. Tyrosine kinase domains are indicated by blackened boxed regions.*

The receptors for EGF, PDGF, and CSF-1 are monomeric proteins, as depicted in Fig. 3-3. In contrast, the insulin and IGF-1 receptors are disulfide-linked multimeric proteins, consisting of two extracellular α chains that bind the ligand, and two β chains that span the membrane and possess the tyrosine kinase regions. Since the insulin and CSF-1 receptors consist of dual ligand-binding, membrane-spanning, and kinase domains, they may be thought of functionally as receptor dimers. Binding of EGF and PDGF to their monomeric receptors in fact induces these receptors to dimerize. It is thought that dimerization is a molecular mechanism by which ligand binding can result in a kinase-activating conformational change in the intracellular portion of the receptor.

Receptor tyrosine kinases play a critical role in the control of cell function. The activation of receptor tyrosine kinases induces a pleiotropic cellular response consisting of both early and late events (on a time scale of a few minutes to many hours, respectively). Upon agonist binding, the tyrosine kinase domain becomes activated and the receptor undergoes autophosphorylation on specific tyrosine residues. Short sequences of amino acids that contain the phosphorylated tyrosines serve as highly selective recognition sites for other signaling molecules within the cell. These molecules often include phosphatidylinositol-3-kinase, phospholipase C-γ, and GTPase-activating protein. The interaction between the phosphorylated receptor and other proteins is specified by sequences of amino acids known as *src* homology-2 (SH2) domains that are contained in these proteins. Each type of SH2 domain binds a particular phosphotyrosine-containing sequence. The SH2-containing proteins that associate with the activated receptor are also substrates for tyrosine phosphorylation catalyzed by the receptor tyrosine kinase. The resultant activation of the multiple SH2-containing proteins provides a means for generation of many intracellular signals downstream from the receptor.

The signaling pathways coupled to the receptor tyrosine kinases are just beginning to be elucidated. It appears that a complex series of protein-protein interactions, involving linker/adapter molecules, tyrosine kinases, serine/threonine kinases, monomeric GTP-binding proteins, protein phosphatases, and other enzymes, occurs following the initial receptor activation. Ultimately, specific changes in gene expression and cell phenotype take place. The importance of this receptor family to normal growth and development is indicated by the large number of retroviral oncogenes that code for similar proteins. Invariably, the viral analogs are lacking in normal regulation. An example is the v-*erbB* oncogene that codes for a truncated form of the EGF receptor. The v-*erbB* product has no ligand-binding domain, but retains a functional tyrosine kinase that is constitutively active, transmitting a continual signal for cell proliferation. Thus, selective inhibitors of tyrosine kinases might have important applications in the treatment of neoplastic disease.

NUCLEAR RECEPTORS

A number of pharmacologically important hormones and drugs bind to receptors that are capable of direct interaction with DNA, thereby altering the rate of synthesis of key cellular proteins. The ligands for these *nuclear receptors* include steroid hormones (glucocorticoids, mineralocorticoids, sex steroids), thyroid hormones, and retinoids; these are all small, lipophilic molecules whose movement is not blocked by cell membranes. The lipophilic hormones are important in the regulation of diverse developmental and homeostatic processes. These hormonal effects require increases or decreases in gene transcription and protein synthesis that take place on a time scale of hours to days. The thyroid hormone triiodothyronine (T_3) binds to a cytoplasmic binder or directly enters the nucleus and attaches to its receptor; this complex then binds to DNA. The mechanism of action of steroid hormones is attributable to their penetration into cells and their high affinity binding to soluble, intracellular receptors. Agonist binding induces a structural change in the receptor that facilitates its association with specific chromatin regions in the nucleus. These nuclear acceptor sites, known as hormone response elements, lie within the promoter regions of inducible genes. Thus, the interaction of the ligand-occupied receptor with its hormone response element affects the binding of RNA polymerase and the expression of regulated genes. By comparison, cell surface receptors can also be linked to changes in gene expression through the action of intermediary messenger molecules. However, only the nuclear receptors produce their effects by direct binding to DNA, and are therefore classified as ligand-responsive transcription factors.

As with the other receptor superfamilies, nuclear receptors all possess certain characteristic structural features (Fig. 3-1). Notably absent is a transmembrane domain, consistent with the fact that these proteins are not associated with membranes. Nuclear receptors are single polypeptides ranging from 427 to 984 amino acids in length. The most highly conserved structural region of the nuclear receptors is a sequence of 66 to 68 amino acids that constitutes the DNA binding domain. In the native receptor, this domain complexes two atoms of zinc in a conformation similar to the DNA-binding "zinc fingers" found in other transcription factors. Ligand binding takes place in a much larger carboxy-terminal domain that shows some degree of amino acid sequence similarity among the different receptors. Additional regions, located throughout the polypeptide chain, are important for various receptor functions: transcriptional activation, receptor dimerization, nuclear localization, and interaction with heat shock proteins.

In the ligand-free state, steroid hormone receptors are tightly associated with the 90 and 70 kDa heat shock proteins. The heat shock proteins function as masking proteins, preventing receptor interaction with DNA. Binding of steroid agonist to the ligand binding site causes release of the heat shock proteins, whereupon the free receptors combine to form homodimers. The dimeric receptor complex is then capable of binding its hormone response element. Retinoid and thyroid hormone receptors, on the other hand, do not associate with heat shock proteins; these receptors are able to bind DNA even in the absence of ligand, although ligand binding is required to initiate transcriptional activity. Nuclear receptors are thought to undergo protein/protein interactions with other transcription factors to form a stable initiation complex, resulting in transcriptional activation. The mechanisms by which nuclear receptors cause *repression* of transcription are less well understood, but may involve a competition between receptor and other transcription factors for binding to DNA.

OTHER RECEPTOR TYPES

The above discussion has far from exhausted the possible mechanisms of transmembrane signaling and potential sites of action for drugs. Entirely new classes of receptors continue to be discovered; some will be briefly mentioned here. For example, receptor tyrosine kinases are not the only family of ligand-regulated enzymes: atrial natriuretic peptide has been shown to bind to a plasma membrane-spanning receptor that has intrinsic guanylate cyclase activity. Activation of this receptor leads to a rise in the second messenger, cyclic GMP. The endothelium-derived relaxing factor, nitric oxide, directly activates a cytosolic form of guanylate cyclase. This is the site of action of a number of clinically important nitrate vasodilator drugs. Other cell surface receptor classes whose signal transduction mechanisms are not as well understood include the cytokine receptor family (e.g., the receptors for interleukin-3 and granulocyte/macrophage colony-stimulating factor) that consist of two different subunits, as well as the multicomponent T-cell antigen receptor complex. Neither of these receptors has intrinsic ion channel or enzymatic activity, nor do they appear to interact with G proteins. Instead, the activation of intracellular tyrosine kinases is thought to be essential for their biological activity. Finally, integrins and other classes of cell surface proteins have an established role in cell adhesion to extracellular matrix proteins such as fibronectin, vitronectin, and laminin. In addition to their adhesive function, evidence is accumulating that these membrane proteins may serve as physiological receptors, transmitting intracellular signals upon binding their extracellular ligand.

SUMMARY AND PERSPECTIVE

Receptors and their cellular signaling pathways are essential for controlling and coordinating the complex functions of multicellular organisms. One might then predict that defects in any element of a signaling pathway could lead to disease. In particular, those pathways concerned with regulation of cell growth and differentiation are strong candidates for involvement in neoplasia. Many oncogenes code for signaling proteins that have lost their normal mechanisms of activation or signal termination. The example of the *erbB* tyrosine kinase was given above. The product of the *ras* oncogene is a GTP-binding protein that lacks the ability to hydrolyze GTP and is therefore continually in the "on" state, much like the effect of cholera toxin on G_s discussed previously. Some forms of cancer are associated with amplification of genes that code for growth factors or their receptors. The rational design of antineoplastic therapies that act selectively at the level of signal transduction holds great promise. One example of such an approach is the use of retinoids, agonists at nuclear receptors, to induce tumor cells to undergo terminal differentiation and cease proliferation. Much remains to be learned of the function of signaling systems in health and disease.

Cloning and expression techniques offer the

means of developing selective new pharmaceuticals. Specific *in vitro*-synthesized mRNA encoding receptors can be injected into *Xenopus laevis* oocytes or other expression systems. Receptor subtypes identified from cDNA clones can be expressed individually, and pharmaceuticals can be screened for their specificity at that subtype. This approach offers the advantage of not only being able to express individual receptor subunits but also allowing the functional effects on signal transduction to be determined. G protein coupling, activation of second messenger systems, and electrophysiologic events can all be assessed in this system.

A second powerful approach to drug design is through structural analysis of the receptor site. It is now possible to think about the design of a drug molecule which will bind specifically to the active site as either an agonist or antagonist. The database of structural information on a wide range of biologically active molecules enables us to begin to develop drugs on a rational basis, in terms of models of intermolecular interaction. The physical chemistry of drug-receptor recognition includes an analysis of hydrogen bonding, electrostatic interactions, van der Waals contact distances, solvent effects, and hydrophobic interactions. With the aid of computers, this information will yield predictions of the appropriate molecular shapes that effective agonists or antagonists must adopt. These approaches should enable chemists to tailor ligands so as to recognize specific subtypes of receptors, leading to the development of more selective and effective therapeutic agents.

BIBLIOGRAPHY

Burgen, A., and E.A. Barnard (eds.): *Receptor Subunits and Complexes*. Cambridge University Press, 1992.

Dohlman, H.G., J. Thorner, M.G. Caron, and R.J. Lefkowitz: "Model Systems for the Study of Seven-transmembrane-segment Receptors," *Annu. Rev. Biochem.* **60**: 653-688 (1992).

Fantl, W.J., D.E. Johnson, and L.T. Williams: "Signalling by Receptor Tyrosine Kinases," *Annu. Rev. Biochem.* **63**: 453-482 (1993).

Parker, M.G. (ed.): *Nuclear Hormone Receptors: Molecular Mechanisms, Cellular Functions, Clinical Abnormalities*, Academic Press, 1991.

Spiegel, A.M., A. Shenker, and L.S. Weinstein: "Receptor-Effector Coupling by G Proteins: Implications for Normal and Abnormal Signal Transduction," *Endocrine Rev.* **13**: 536-565 (1992).

Various authors: *Trends in Biochemical Sciences, vol. 17*, pp. 367-443, October 1992. (The entire issue is devoted to reviews on receptors and signal transduction mechanisms.)

CHAPTER 4

Pharmacokinetics

Edward J. Barbieri

It is known that the intensity of the biologic response produced by a drug is related to the concentration of the drug at its site of action. As discussed in the previous chapter, an important factor in determining the magnitude of the response is the dose of drug administered; however, this dictates only the maximum amount of drug that can reach the site of action. The fraction of the dose that actually is attained at the active site(s) in the body is dependent on a multitude of factors, including the route of drug administration and the dosage form. It is advantageous to be able to select a route of administration, dose, and dosage form that place a drug at its site of action in a suitable concentration and maintain this concentration for a desired time. This goal can be attained for a considerable number of therapeutic agents if we understand the physiologic processes that influence drug concentrations throughout the body and the physical and chemical properties of drugs that determine their interactions with these processes.

Some of the physiologic factors that influence the concentration of a drug at its site of action (Fig. 4-1) are as follows: (1) absorption, i.e., the ability of a drug to enter the bloodstream; (2) distribution, i.e., the movement of a drug throughout the body to various tissue sites; (3) biotransformation, i.e., the alteration of the chemical structure of a drug; and (4) excretion, i.e., the ability of the living system to remove a drug and its biotransformation products from its internal environment. These vital biologic processes constitute *pharmacokinetics*, a subspecialty of pharmacology which describes the movement of drugs through the body, but not their actions or effects. In a more restricted sense, the word *pharmacokinetics* refers to the mathematical analysis of drug absorption, distribution, biotransformation, and excretion and, therefore, is a detailed study of these processes in a quantitative and temporal fashion.

Pharmacodynamics is the study of mechanisms of action, the therapeutic and toxicologic effects of drugs, chemical structure-activity relationships, and many other drug-organism interactions. This discipline relies on and builds upon the subjects of biochemistry, physiology, microbiology, immunology, molecular biology, and pathology to both describe and quantify drug actions and effects.

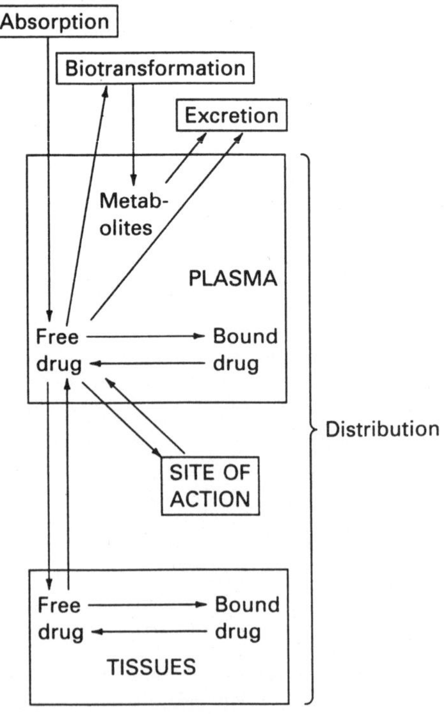

FIGURE 4-1 *Factors affecting the concentration of a drug at its site of action.*

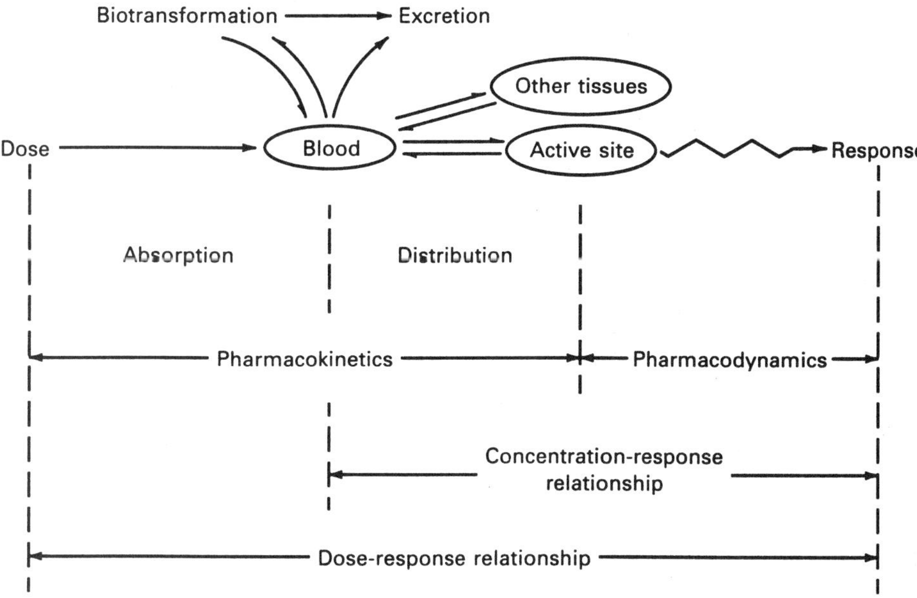

FIGURE 4-2 *Interconnections among the dose-response relationship, the concentration-response relationship, pharmacokinetics and pharmacodynamics.*

As shown in Fig. 4-2, the dose-response relationship, which was developed and explained in Chapter 2, can be divided into two parts, pharmacokinetics and pharmacodynamics. Both of these fields have been greatly aided by the development of technologies capable of measuring accurately even very minute quantities of drugs and their metabolites in body fluids and tissues. However, the measurement of drug concentrations in the plasma remains the most useful method of directly assessing pharmacokinetics and forecasting pharmacodynamics. For most drugs, changes in plasma concentrations are indicative of changes that occur at other tissues (including the active site) throughout the body. Analogous to the time-action curve, the time-plasma drug concentration curve (Fig. 4-3) is a useful device for monitoring the pharmacokinetics of a drug in relation to the therapeutic response of the patient. The goals in utilizing pharmacokinetics are to maximize the time that plasma drug concentrations are within the therapeutic range, to minimize the time the drug concentrations are within the ineffective range, and to avoid toxic concentrations. A thorough understanding of the principles of pharmacokinetics provides for greater insight into the action of drugs and leads to more knowledgeable and rational drug selection and prescribing. Furthermore, many important drug-body and drug-drug interactions have been discovered by the application of these principles. This chapter provides the necessary information for a working knowledge of pharmacokinetics.

ABSORPTION

Absorption is the process by which a drug enters the bloodstream without being chemically altered. Various factors influence the rate of absorption, including types of transport, the physicochemical properties of the drug (e.g., lipid solubility, ionization), protein binding, the routes of administration, dosage forms, circulation at the site of absorption, and the concentration of the drug.

An important physiologic factor that determines the absorption of a drug, as well as its distribution and elimination, is the membranes that separate the biologic compartments. Electron microscopic studies of tissues suggest that all body membranes are composed of a fundamental structure called the *unit membrane,* or *plasma membrane*. This boundary, which is approximately 8 to 10 nm thick, surrounds single cells such as the erythrocyte, epithelial cell, and neuron, and also subcellular structures such as the mitochondrion and nucleus.

Cellular membranes appear to be composed of

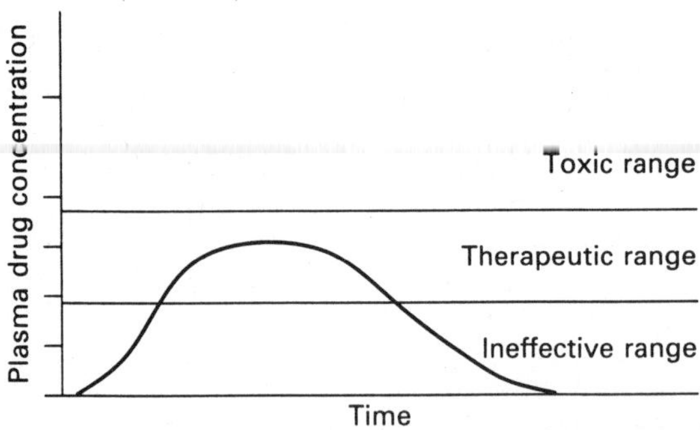

FIGURE 4-3 *The time-plasma drug concentration curve showing the ineffective range, therapeutic range, and toxic range for a drug. These ranges are spaced according to arbitrary units of drug concentration for the purpose of illustration.*

a bimolecular layer of phospholipids, with the hydrophilic heads facing the outer surfaces and the hydrocarbon chains pointing toward the interior and creating a continuous hydrophobic band within the membrane. *Integral proteins* (also called *intrinsic proteins)* of varying size appear to be interspersed, either singularly or as composites, in the lipoid matrix. The position of these within the membrane is determined by the distribution of hydrophilic and hydrophobic regions of the protein. Such proteins are found to extend through the entire lipid bilayer and are called *transmembrane proteins.* Other proteins are confined to either surface of the membrane and do not interact with the hydrophobic core of the membrane; these are known as *peripheral proteins* or *extrinsic proteins.*

The unit membrane is considered to be a constantly changing, dynamic structure. Phospholipids in the bilayer have lateral and rotational mobility, which allows the membrane to be flexible, pliable, and readily deformed (termed *fluidity*) while retaining relative impermeability to highly water-soluble compounds. Intrinsic proteins can function as drug receptors, ionophores, enzymes, and regulatory substances. In addition these proteins may act in transporting drugs across the membrane. Extrinsic proteins appear to function largely as structural components of the membrane, although when associated with intrinsic proteins they may assist these molecules in their specific function.

While lipid-soluble substances penetrate the membrane by dissolving in the lipoid phase, many water-soluble molecules enter only if they are small enough to pass through small aqueous channels or pores. The cell membranes also possess specialized transport processes, and certain large water-soluble molecules, such as sugars and amino acids, can penetrate cells readily by these routes. The diverse ways in which drugs move across membranes can be grouped under two general headings: passive and specialized transport. The major difference between these is that specialized transport involves membrane-associated protein carriers for drugs and passive transport does not.

Passive Transport

Two main types of passive transport are recognized: filtration and simple diffusion. Neither of these processes is saturable, nor can they be inhibited by drugs.

Filtration is the process by which compounds cross membranes by hydrodynamic flow. In this passive process, when a hydrostatic or osmotic pressure difference exists across a membrane, water flows, in bulk, through the membrane pores, carrying with it any solute molecules whose dimensions are less than those of the pores. Solutes with molecular weights greater than 100 to 200 generally do not pass through membrane pores. Since most drugs often exceed this size limitation, they cannot filter through *cell* membranes. Furthermore, the filtration of highly ionized substances may be limited because of attraction to, or repulsion from, ionic charges which are carried on membrane surfaces or within the pores.

Filtration of drugs (by dissolving in the fluid that flows through *intercellular pores*) is the predominant process by which drugs cross most capillary endothelial membranes. With the exception of blood vessels in the central nervous system, where tight cellular junctions are numerous, capillary (and some epithelial) intercellular pores are large enough to permit the passage of most drugs. For example, the water that filters through the relatively large pores of the renal glomerular membrane is accompanied by all the solutes of plasma except the protein molecules.

Most drugs penetrate body membranes by *simple diffusion*; that is, their rate of transfer is directly proportional to their concentration gradient across the membrane. Some of the substances transverse the membrane as though it were a layer of lipoid material, the relative speed of passage being determined by the lipid solubility or, more precisely, the lipid-to-water partition coefficient of the substances. The higher the lipid-to-water partition coefficient, the greater the rate of transfer across the membrane. In contrast, a number of water-soluble (relatively lipid-insoluble) compounds of low molecular weight diffuse across the membrane as though it were a sieve made up of small aqueous channels, the smaller molecules crossing more rapidly than the larger ones. With water-soluble ions, however, the speed of transfer may be determined more by the ionic charge than by the molecular size; for example, in the red blood cell, anions penetrate much more rapidly than cations.

In considering the diffusion of drugs across membranes, it is necessary to take into account that most drugs are weak acids or weak bases which exist in solution as a mixture of the ionized and nonionized forms. This complicates the problem of describing the passage of drugs across a lipoid membrane. Usually only the nonionized species of the compound is sufficiently lipid-soluble to diffuse across cell membranes and the ionized form of the molecule is too large to pass readily through the membrane channels. Accordingly, the nonionized component of a drug penetrates many cellular membranes at a rate related to its lipid-to-water partition coefficient and its concentration gradient across the membrane, whereas the ionized form penetrates at a very slow rate. This process is sometimes called *nonionic diffusion*.

The proportion of a drug in the nonionized form depends on the dissociation constant of the drug on the pH of the medium in which it is dissolved, a relationship shown by the Henderson-Hasselbalch equation. Thus for a weak acid:

$$pK_a = pH + \log \frac{\text{conc. of nonionized acid}}{\text{conc. of ionized acid}}$$

For a weak base:

$$pK_a = pH + \log \frac{\text{conc. of ionized base}}{\text{conc. of nonionized base}}$$

In these equations, the dissociation constant of both acids and bases is expressed as a pK_a, which is the negative logarithm of the acidic dissociation constant. From the equations, it can be determined that phenobarbital, a weak acid with a pK_a of 7.4, is approximately 91 percent ionized at pH 8.4, 50 percent ionized at pH 7.4, and 9 percent ionized at pH 6.4. Quinine, a weak base with a pK_a of 8.4, is about 91 percent ionized at pH 7.4, 50 percent ionized at pH 8.4, and 9 percent ionized at pH 9.4. While most drugs have pK_a values between 3 and 11 and are therefore partly ionized and partly nonionized over the range of physiologic pH values, some compounds are at the extreme ends of the scale. For example, acetanilide, a weak base with a pK_a of 0.3, is almost completely nonionized at all body pH values. Sulfonic acids, with a pK_a below 1, are almost completely ionized at all pH values. Neutral molecules, e.g., ethanol, are always in the nonionized state, and quaternary compounds such as acetylcholine exist only as cations regardless of pH.

Drugs that penetrate a biologic membrane by simple diffusion become distributed across the membrane according to their degree of ionization, the charge of their ionized form, and the extent to which they are bound to proteins or other macromolecules in the solutions bathing the membrane. A difference in pH on the two sides of a membrane affects the distribution of a partly ionized substance because of the preferential permeability of membranes to the lipid-soluble, nonionized form of the compound. This is illustrated in Fig. 4-4, which shows the distribution of a weak acid (pK_a = 6) between solutions of pH 7 and 5; the solutions are separated by a membrane permeable only to the nonionized form of the compound. At equilibrium, the concentration of the nonionized solute is the same in both solutions, but the concentrations of the ionized form are unequal because of the difference in pH of the two fluids. Accordingly, the total concentration of solute (ionized plus nonionized) on both sides of the membrane is a function of the pH of the two fluids and the pK_a of the solute.

Specialized Transport

Although passive transfer across a lipoid boundary adequately describes the penetration of body membranes by most drugs and other foreign organic compounds, it does not explain the rapid penetration and peculiar kinetic behavior of certain large, lipid-insoluble molecules and ions. For example, glucose and a number of other monosaccharides are readily absorbed from the small intestine and renal tubule and penetrate most cells at a rapid rate; moreover, the same is true of the highly ionized amino acids. In addition, a number of sulfonic acid anions and quaternary cations are rapidly transported across cell membranes of the liver, renal tubule, and choroid plexus. Not only

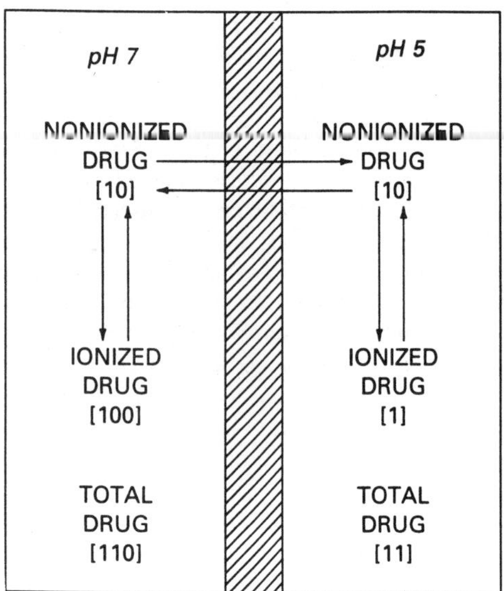

FIGURE 4-4 *Distribution of a weak acid (pK_a = 6) between aqueous solutions of pH 7 and pH 5. The solutions are separated by a membrane that is permeable only to the nonionized form of the weak acid. Concentrations at equilibrium are shown in brackets.*

are the rates of transport rapid, but in most cases the substances can move across membranes in an "uphill" direction, that is, from a solution of low concentration into one of higher concentration. The concept of membrane *carriers* offers an explanation for the unique permeability of membranes to these substances.

Membrane carriers are viewed as proteinaceous components of the unit membrane, which are capable of combining with a solute at one surface of the membrane. The carrier-solute complex moves across the membrane, the solute is released, and the carrier then returns to the original surface where it can combine with another molecule of solute.

Two main types of carrier-mediated transport are recognized: *active transport* and *facilitated diffusion*. Active transport signifies a process in which (1) the solute crosses the membrane against a concentration gradient, or, if the solute is an ion, it crosses against an electrochemical potential gradient; (2) the transport mechanism becomes saturated at high solute concentrations and thus shows a *transport maximum*; (3) the process is selective for certain ionic or structural configurations; (4) if two compounds are transported by the same mechanism, one will competitively inhibit the transport of the other; (5) the transport process can be inhibited noncompetitively by substances which interfere with cell metabolism. The term *facilitated diffusion* denotes a transport process that shows all the above characteristics except that the solute is *not* transferred against a concentration or electrochemical potential gradient and does *not* require energy.

Proteins and other macromolecules are transported across most membranes slowly, as compared with the rates of transfer of smaller lipid-soluble drugs and carrier-transported substances. A specialized transport process by which these large molecules (usually greater than 1000 daltons) can be transported to the interior of cells is by *pinocytosis*. In this complex process, the cell invaginates a small portion of the cellular membrane and engulfs a droplet of extracellular fluid containing the compound. The droplet becomes completely surrounded by a portion of the membrane, and the resulting vesicle buds off and moves into the cell cytoplasm where the transported compound is released. In many cases pinocytosis is initiated by complexation of the drug to a membrane receptor; it appears that the size and charge of the drug macromolecule are important factors in determining its degree of uptake.

SITES OF ABSORPTION, ROUTES OF ADMINISTRATION, AND DOSAGE FORMS

Alimentary Canal

The alimentary tract is by far the most common site of administration when a drug is intended for systemic action. The dosage forms include tablets, capsules, caplets, specially formulated tablets or capsules for prolonged or repeated action, powders, various flavored or unflavored liquids (syrups, solutions, suspensions, elixirs, emulsions, tinctures, fluid extracts), and rectal suppositories.

Gastrointestinal Tract The passage of drugs and other foreign compounds across the epithelial lining of the oral cavity, stomach, small intestine, colon, and rectum is explainable, for the most part, in terms of simple diffusion across a lipoid membrane. Drugs in true solution are readily absorbed in their lipid-soluble nonionized forms; the relative rates of absorption are directly related to the lipid-to-water partition coefficients of the molecules.

The stomach is a significant site of absorption for many acidic and neutral compounds but not for basic compounds. For example, acidic drugs like the salicylates and barbiturates, which exist as nonionized lipid-soluble molecules in the acid gastric contents, are readily absorbed, whereas basic drugs like the plant alkaloids, which exist largely as ions, are hardly absorbed at all. In other portions of the alimentary tract where the intraluminal pH is closer to neutrality, many weak acids and bases are, to a considerable extent, nonionized and are absorbed at rates related their lipid-to-water partition ratios. At all levels of the tract, slowest rates of absorption are found with completely ionized drugs, such as the quaternary ammonium compounds and sulfonic acids, and with lipid-insoluble neutral molecules, such as sulfaguanidine and mannitol. Certain quaternary amines may be absorbed in part in the form of chemical complexes.

The rate of absorption of most drugs is directly proportional to drug concentration in accordance with the process of simple diffusion. If the intraluminal concentration is raised threefold, 3 times as much drug will be absorbed per unit of time, the percentage absorption remaining constant.

The absorption of drugs is increased by changes in pH which increase the fraction of drug in the lipid-soluble nonionized form. For example, raising the gastric pH to 8 with sodium bicarbonate results in a markedly increased rate of absorption for many basic drugs; conversely, the gastric absorption of most acidic compounds is decreased at the elevated pH value. A similar relationship between pH and absorption rate occurs in the mouth, small and large intestines, and rectum.

In the small intestine, weak acids and bases become distributed between intestinal fluid of pH 6.6 and plasma of pH 7.4 (see Fig. 4-4) as though the intestinal pH were 5.3. Thus the pH at the absorption surface appears to be lower than that of the intestinal contents, and it is this lower pH value that may determine the degree of ionization and hence the rate of absorption of weak electrolytes. The colonic and rectal mucosae also show an apparent surface pH somewhat lower than that of the luminal contents.

While most drugs cross the intestinal boundary by a process of simple diffusion, a drug can be absorbed by specialized active transport if its chemical structure is similar enough to that of a substrate which is naturally transported; for example, the antitumor compound 5-fluorouracil is actively transported across the intestine by the process which transports the natural pyrimidines uracil and thymine. Macromolecules are absorbed from the small intestine in trace quantities. Examples include enzymes, food proteins, and bacterial toxins, and the absorption of these occurs via pinocytosis or diffusion through imperfections in the epithelium.

The oral route of administration is the safest, most convenient, and most economical. However, it has a number of disadvantages: (1) irritation to the gastric mucosa with resultant nausea or vomiting; (2) destruction of some drugs by gastric acid or digestive enzymes; (3) precipitation or insolubility of some drugs in gastrointestinal fluids; (4) formation of nonabsorbable complexes between drugs and food materials; (5) variable rates of absorption due to physiologic factors such as gastric emptying time, gastrointestinal motility, and mixing; (6) too slow an absorption rate for effectiveness in an emergency situation; (7) inability to use the oral route in an unconscious patient; and (8) the unpleasant taste of some drugs.

Some of the disadvantages of the oral route can be overcome in various ways. Gastric irritation, as well as the destruction, precipitation, or complexing of drugs in the stomach, can be avoided by using an enteric coated tablet or capsule which resists gastric acid but dissolves in the higher pH range of the intestine or in the presence of intestinal enzymes. In some cases, gastric irritation can be minimized or avoided simply by administering a drug at mealtime or immediately after a meal.

Conversely, for rapid and more complete absorption, some drugs should be taken with the stomach empty; a glass of water should accompany a solid dosage form to dissolve the drug and wash it into the intestine.

Prolonged-action dosage forms for oral administration have been developed with the idea of supplying in one capsule, tablet or caplet, all the drug that will be needed over a period of many hours. For a particular drug, the objective might be to produce quickly a desired plasma concentration of drug and then supply additional drug to maintain this concentration for a number of hours. Or the objective might be to release various doses of one or more drugs at widely spaced intervals. Many names are used to describe these preparations, including *sustained-release*, *timed-release*, *extended-release*, *repeat action*, and *long-acting*. A major obstacle to the use of these dosage forms is the high variability of physiologic factors in patients.

An important point to be emphasized in considering absorption after oral administration is that a drug must be dissolved before it can be absorbed. The drug administered in solid form will be absorbed at a rate limited by the rate at which it dissolves in the gastrointestinal fluids. Many factors influence the dissolution rate; these include (1) solubility, particle size, crystalline form, and salt form of the drug; (2) the rate of disintegration of the solid-dosage form in the gastrointestinal lumina; and (3) gastrointestinal pH, motility, and food content.

Oral bioavailability is the measure of the rate and extent of drug absorption through the oral route. A drug is considered to be bioavailable once it reaches the systemic circulation. Therefore, oral bioavailability is decreased by a low rate and extent of absorption through the gastrointestinal mucosa and by biotransformation of the drug during its first passage through the portal circulation of the liver (the so-called *first pass effect* or *presystemic biotransformation*). Bioavailability is discussed in greater detail in the last section of this chapter.

Oral Mucosa Due to the extensive vascularity and relatively thin mucosal surfaces, many drugs are readily absorbed from the oral cavity. The *sublingual* route, in which a small tablet is placed under the tongue and allowed to dissolve, offers a simple, convenient method of administration. Drugs may also be given by the *buccal* route, in which a tablet is placed between the cheek and gingiva. Advantages of these routes include (1) delayed degradation of the drug by avoiding early passage through the liver and (2) avoidance of many of the disadvantages of oral administration. Disadvantages of the sublingual and buccal routes include the unpleasant taste and the local irritating effects of some drugs.

Rectal Mucosa Drugs can be administered rectally, for either local or systemic effect, in the form of suppositories which melt at body temperature. The rectal route is useful when unconsciousness or vomiting preclude use of the oral route. Approximately 50 to 60 percent of a drug dose, administered rectally, is absorbed directly into the general circulation (via the inferior and middle hemorrhoidal veins), avoiding the portal circulation and presystemic biotransformation. Local irritation to the rectal mucosa and inconvenience are major disadvantages of rectal administration; furthermore, as compared to other avenues of drug use, drug absorption from the rectum is slow and often erratic.

Injection Routes

The term *parenteral* literally means "by some other route than through the intestine" (the *enteral* route) and includes drug administration by injection, through the respiratory tract, and topical application to the skin, conjunctiva, urethra, and vagina. However, through common usage parenteral administration usually refers to the injection of drug by the subcutaneous, intramuscular, intravenous, intra-arterial, and intrathecal routes. In the following discussion parenteral will be used in this more limited context. Each of the injection routes has its own merits and pitfalls, but a number of features are shared by all. Generally, parenteral administration produces a more prompt response than that obtained after oral administration, and more accurate dosage is usually attained. Injection routes are valuable when vomiting or unconsciousness preclude the use of the oral route.

Parenteral administration has several drawbacks. Because of the generally rapid rate of absorption, there often is not much time to combat adverse drug reactions and accidental overdoses. Moreover, parenteral administration requires sterile dosage forms and aseptic procedures; it may be painful; it is relatively expensive; and patients cannot readily administer the drug to themselves.

Subcutaneous Route Absorption of drugs from aqueous solutions injected at a subcutaneous site is rapid, occurs by simple diffusion, and depends mainly on the ease of penetration of the capillary wall, the area over which the solution has spread, and the rate of blood flow through the area. Accordingly, the rate of absorption can be influenced by a number of procedures. Absorption can be hastened by massage or application of heat to the injected area, or it can be slowed by reducing circulation to the injected area, for example, by local cooling or by inclusion of a vasoconstrictor, e.g., epinephrine, in the drug solution.

To obtain a slow, continuous rate of absorption from a subcutaneous site, drugs may be injected as a suspension of poorly soluble crystals (e.g., some insulin preparations) or implanted under the skin in the form of a compressed pellet (e.g., some sex hormones).

Irritating drugs should not be injected subcutaneously. They can produce severe pain, local necrosis and sloughing.

Intramuscular Route Drugs injected into skeletal muscle in the form of aqueous solutions are absorbed rapidly. As with the subcutaneous route, the rate of absorption is determined mainly by the speed of penetration of the capillary wall, the area of solution exposed to the circulation, and the rate of blood flow. For many drugs, the rates of absorption from muscle and subcutaneous sites are comparable.

The intramuscular route is often used for depot forms of drugs, for example, aqueous or oil suspensions of poorly soluble salts. In addition, some irritating medicinals that cannot be administered subcutaneously may be injected intramuscularly.

Intravenous Route Injection of drugs directly into the bloodstream avoids all delays and variables of absorption. Penetration to the site of drug action is usually very rapid, and this is advantageous in emergency situations and in the continuous control of the degree of pharmacologic action, e.g., during general anesthesia, because the drug can be given slowly and the rate of administration varied as necessary. Other advantages of the intravenous route include (1) the greatest accuracy in drug dosage, (2) the ability to give large volumes of solutions over a long period of time, and (3) the ability to administer irritating, hypertonic, acidic, or alkaline solutions, since these become diluted in the large volume of circulating fluid when given slowly. However, it is important to avoid extravasation of these solutions into tissue surrounding the vein, which may result in pain and tissue necrosis.

The intravenous route is the most dangerous of all avenues of drug administration because of the speed of onset of pharmacologic action. An overdosage cannot be withdrawn, nor can its absorption be retarded. If a safe dose is given too rapidly, toxicity can result from the undesirable high drug concentration which initially perfuses reactive tissue sites.

Drugs which precipitate readily at the pH of blood and drugs suspended or dissolved in oily liquids should not be given intravenously because of the danger of embolism.

Intrathecal Route Injection of drugs into the spinal subarachnoid space is used for producing spinal anesthesia with local anesthetic agents. It is also used for treating infections or tumors of brain and spinal tissues with drugs that do not penetrate well into the central nervous system from the blood.

Respiratory Tract

Due to the large surface area, many drugs and other chemicals are rapidly absorbed through the membranes and pulmonary epithelium of the respiratory tract. Drugs may be administered as gases, sprays, aerosols, or powders. With the exception of oxygen and anesthetic gases, this route of absorption for systemic drug administration has had rather limited use in therapeutics. A major problem is the difficulty of administration and retention of exact quantities of drug. Physiologic variables may include respiratory tract infections and other pathologic states, ciliary action, and the mucous coating of the tract.

An *aerosol* is an air suspension of liquid or solid particles so small that they do not readily settle out under the force of gravity. Particles with a diameter greater than 10 μm become deposited mainly in the nasal passages, whereas particles smaller than 2 μm in diameter penetrate deeper into the respiratory tract before deposition occurs. For significant penetration into the alveolar ducts and sacs, it is probably necessary to have particles smaller than 1 μm in diameter.

Pulmonary administration of drugs for localized activity on the respiratory tree is a valuable dosing method. Certain sympathomimetics, for example, applied directly to the nasal mucosa are used as nasal decongestants; bronchodilators and other antiasthmatic compounds are inhaled as aerosols through the mouth for their effect in the lower portion of the respiratory tract.

Skin

For local effects on the skin, drugs are often applied in the form of ointments, creams, gels, lotions, liniments, and pastes. Drugs penetrate the skin much more slowly than through most other body membranes due to the relatively thick epithelial barrier and the reduced and less consistent blood perfusion. Lipid-soluble drugs are absorbed at greater rates than water-soluble compounds, and absorption can be enhanced by dissolving a drug in oil, an ointment base, or other organic solvents and rubbing it into the skin, a procedure known as *inunction*.

Although the skin is not ordinarily employed as a site for the systemic absorption of drugs, it has some useful applications. Nitroglycerin is slowly absorbed from ointments and is used in this form for the prophylaxis of nocturnal angina pectoris. In addition, drugs are commonly administered to the skin for systemic absorption via the *transdermal patch*. This is a unique bandagelike therapeutic system which provides for the continuous controlled release of the drug from a reservoir through a semipermeable membrane. The active compound gains access to the systemic circulation prior to any biotransformation in the liver, and a more consistent therapeutic plasma level is attained. However, systemic drug absorption through the skin is highly dependent on the site (due to thickness and vascularity) and its condition, i.e., intact versus broken and inflamed skin.

Other Routes of Administration

Drugs can be absorbed from sites other than those described above, for example, the conjunctiva, urethra, and vagina. Although medicinals are applied at these sites, the purpose is almost always for local action.

DISTRIBUTION

Once a drug enters the vascular space, its distribution to other tissues is assured; every tissue which has a blood supply eventually comes into equilibrium with the plasma concentration of the drug. The distribution of drugs will depend on the physicochemical properties of the drug (e.g., the lipid-to-water partition coefficient), cardiac output, blood flow to and capillary permeability in various tissues, binding to plasma proteins and other macromolecules, lipid content of the tissues, and tissue binding. Most drugs traverse the capillary wall by a combination of two processes, diffusion and filtration (hydrodynamic flow). In addition, most drugs, whether lipid-soluble or not, cross the capillary wall at rates which are extremely rapid in comparison with their rates of passage across other body membranes. Thus, the supply of drugs to the various tissues may be limited more by the blood flow than by the restraint imposed by the capillary endothelium.

The passage of drugs into and out of the central nervous system involves transfer between three compartments: brain, cerebrospinal fluid (CSF), and blood. The boundary between blood and brain consists of several membranes: those of the capillary wall, the glial cells closely surrounding the capillary, and the neuron. The *blood-brain barrier*, which provides the main hindrance to the diffusion of drugs, is located at the capillary wall-glial cell region. After a drug penetrates this barrier and enters the extracellular fluid of the brain, it must then cross the neuronal cell membrane to enter nervous tissue. The *blood-CSF barrier* consists mainly of the epithelium of the choroid plexuses located within the cerebral ventricles.

Drugs pass from blood into brain and CSF at rates related to the lipid-to-water partition coefficient and degrees of ionization of the compounds. Lipid-soluble, nonionized substances penetrate readily, whereas water-soluble molecules and ions penetrate with great difficulty. For example, a highly lipid-soluble compound such as thiopental passes from blood into CSF thousands of times more rapidly than do certain quaternary ammonium compounds or sulfonic acids.

Although most drugs that enter the central nervous system do so by simple diffusion through the blood-brain barrier, specific carrier-mediated and receptor-mediated transport systems have been described (Table 4-1). Carrier-mediated systems appear to be involved predominantly in the transport of a variety of nutrients through the blood-brain barrier; however, the thyroid hormone, triiodothyronine, can also enter the brain via carrier-mediated transport. Moreover, drugs such as levodopa and methyldopa, which are structural derivatives of phenylalanine, cross the blood-brain barrier by the neutral amino acid transport system. Receptor-mediated transport (also known as *receptor-mediated transcytosis*) functions to allow certain peptides, e.g., insulin, to gain access to the brain. The awareness of these specialized transport systems in the blood-brain barrier has stimulated interest in using selected lipid-soluble prodrugs (i.e., inactive nutrient-drug complexes that can be transported into the brain and then split to release the active drug moiety) as a novel approach to drug delivery into the central nervous system.

The exit of drugs from the central nervous system involves more pathways than the entrance. Drugs can diffuse across the blood-brain barrier and the blood-CSF barrier in the reverse direction at rates determined by their lipid solubility and degree of ionization. Moreover, all drugs, whether lipid-soluble or not, pass from CSF into blood at similar rates as CSF drains into the dural blood sinuses by flowing through the wide channels of

TABLE 4-1 Carrier-mediated and receptor-mediated transport systems of the blood-brain barrier

Transport System	Representative Substrate
Carrier-mediated	
Hexose	Glucose
Amine	Choline
Basic amino acid	Arginine
Neutral amino acid	Phenylalanine
Monocarboxylic acid	Lactic acid
Purine	Adenine
Nucleoside	Adenosine
Thyroid hormone	Triiodothyronine
Receptor-mediated	
Insulin	Insulin
Transferrin	Transferrin
Growth factors	Insulin-like growth factors 1 and 2

the arachnoid villi. In addition, certain organic anions and cations are rapidly transferred from CSF to blood by active transport across the choroid plexuses; anions such as penicillin are transported by one process, and cations such as choline by another. Because of the ready removal of certain poorly lipid-soluble drugs from the CSF by active transport as well as by the CSF drainage mechanism, many of these substances never attain a concentration in CSF equal to that in plasma.

The ocular fluid is similar to CSF in regard to the entry and exit of drugs. Thus the blood-ocular fluid boundary, which consists mainly of the ciliary-body epithelium and the capillary walls and surrounding connective tissue of the iris, behaves as a lipoid barrier to most organic compounds.

Drugs applied to the corneal surface of the eye penetrate into the aqueous humor at rates related to the lipid-to-water partition coefficient of their nonionized form. Drug penetration increases when there is injury to the epithelium.

Protein and Macromolecule Binding

Binding of drugs to proteins and other macromolecules is known to occur in almost every tissue of the body. It has been demonstrated with albumin, mucopolysaccharides, nucleoproteins, and other substances.

Binding is generally a reversible process and, therefore, arrives at an equilibrium in which only the unbound (free) fraction of the drug is available to act and to be biotransformed and excreted, while the bound fraction functions as a depot from which the drug is released as the equilibrium is reestablished after removal of the free fraction. The forces responsible for the binding are weak bonds of the van der Waals, hydrogen, and ionic types. The position of the equilibrium and the rate at which the free fraction of the drug is removed by biotransformation and excretion determines the biologic half-life of the drug, which can vary widely.

Thus, the reversible binding of drugs to various intracellular and extracellular substances is important in determining how long a drug remains in the body. Without these storage pools, many drugs would be biotransformed and excreted so rapidly that they would hardly have time to exert their pharmacologic action.

Binding to Plasma Proteins

Most drugs show some degree of protein binding in plasma; usually this is due to binding with plasma albumin for acidic drugs and α_1-acid glycoprotein for basic drugs. The extent to which drugs bind to plasma proteins is determined by the drug concentration, its affinity for and the number of available binding sites on plasma proteins. Plasma protein binding of drugs is usually expressed as the percent of total drug that is bound and simple mass-action relationships are used to describe the free and bound concentrations of drug. (Since both low and high drug concentrations can result in great variability in the amount of drug binding to plasma proteins, the percentages listed throughout this text refer only to the plasma protein binding within the therapeutic concentration range for each drug.) Examples of highly bound compounds include phenylbutazone, warfarin, imipramine, and thiopental (80 to 98 percent bound); compounds with moderate degrees of binding include caffeine, phenobarbital, and terbutaline (20 to 50 percent bound). Drugs such as barbital, lithium, and tobramycin exhibit a low degree of plasma binding

(1 to 8 percent).

Because albumin, α_1-acid glycoprotein, and other plasma proteins possess a limited number of binding sites and these sites are rather nonselective with respect to the drugs that will bind, two drugs with an affinity for the same site will compete with one another for binding. Furthermore, if one of the drugs is administered after the other has established an equilibrium between its free and protein-bound moieties, the second drug will displace a portion of the first from the binding sites, and there may be a marked increased in plasma concentration of pharmacologically active compound. With a drug that is normally highly bound, the usual therapeutic dose may be toxic when followed by administration of a drug that displaces it from its storage sites.

Competition between drugs for binding sites can also bring about significant changes in the distribution of drugs between plasma and tissues. For example, one drug that has a high percentage binding to plasma proteins may displace another highly bound drug from plasma albumin; as a result, the free fraction of the latter drug diffuses into tissues, thereby causing the (total) plasma concentration to decline.

The influence of protein binding on the passive transfer of drugs across membranes has already been mentioned. When binding to plasma proteins creates an equilibrium mixture of free and protein-bound drug, only the free fraction can diffuse across membranes. It is true that, as free drug is removed, more is liberated as the equilibrium is reestablished, but when the equilibrium is strongly influenced by binding, only a very small portion of the total drug may leave the blood on a single passage of the blood through an organ. This situation is modified when a drug is actively transported across a membrane or crosses by some other form of specialized transport. As an example, penicillin is tightly bound in plasma, but is actively transported into the urine by the renal tubular epithelium and is almost completely cleared from the plasma in one passage through the kidney. The speed of reversibility of the drug-protein interaction is apparently great enough to keep pace with the rapid removal of free drug from plasma by the membrane carriers.

Binding to Tissues

The binding of drugs to components of various tissues (other than plasma proteins) is difficult to measure quantitatively. Certain drugs show a much greater affinity for tissues than for plasma proteins, and in some instances, the affinity for one tissue is considerably greater than for another. As examples, tetracycline has a high affinity for bone, guanethidine for cardiac muscle, and digoxin for skeletal muscle.

Redistribution

The pattern of distribution of drugs is governed by two factors: (1) the affinity of the drug for the various tissues, i.e., the equilibrium between the blood and each tissue, and (2) the rate of blood flow to each tissue. As mentioned previously, those tissues with the greatest blood flow come into equilibrium with the blood almost immediately; those with the poorest blood flow equilibrate very slowly. As a result, the tissues with good blood supply initially accumulate an inordinately high proportion of the total drug present, which is then gradually redistributed in the body as other tissues also come into equilibrium with the blood. The final situation, where all tissues are in equilibrium with each other by the intermediary of the blood which supplies them, may take many hours.

Thiopental, a highly lipid-soluble drug that penetrates all cells readily and has an especially high affinity for body fat, does not initially become localized in adipose tissue. Rather, after intravenous administration, it first reaches high concentrations in brain, liver, kidney, and other tissues that have high rates of blood flow (see Fig. 4-5). The concentration of the drug in muscle rises slowly because of the slower rate of delivery to that tissue, and the concentration in the adipose rises even more slowly for the same reason. As thiopental is taken up by the large muscle mass of the body as well as by fat, the plasma concentration declines, and the drug begins to redistribute by diffusing out of the brain and other early sites of deposition.

ELIMINATION

Elimination includes all processes that terminate the presence of a drug in the body. The major processes are biotransformation, renal excretion, and biliary excretion. Other elimination processes occur via saliva, sweat, milk, tears, feces, and exhaled air. Although these routes of elimination are of minor importance for many drugs, they may play a significant role in the elimination of others. For example, the lung is the major route of elimina-

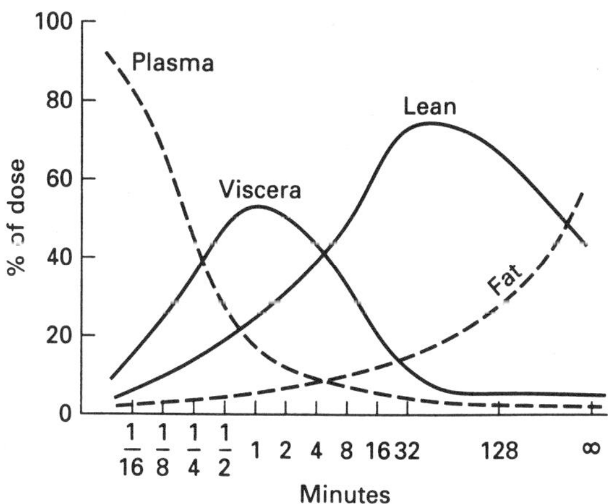

FIGURE 4-5 *Distribution of thiopental in different body tissues at various times after intravenous injection. Time scale (in minutes) progresses geometrically. Final values are at infinity.*

tion of gaseous substances, such as the inhalational general anesthetics.

Biotransformation

Biotransformation is the process by which drugs or endogenous substances are altered chemically. It occurs mainly in the liver, but may occur in plasma or other tissues such as the lung or kidney. This subject is discussed at length in Chapter 5; however, in the interest of continuity a brief discussion follows here.

There are four major biotransformation reactions that occur within the body; they are oxidation, reduction, hydrolysis, and conjugation. Drugs which undergo oxidative, reductive, or hydrolytic reactions may or may not be converted to a pharmacologically inactive product. Alternatively, some drugs are taken as pharmacologically inactive compounds that are biotransformed to an active product by oxidation, reduction, or hydrolysis; these compounds are known as *prodrugs*. Once a drug has been conjugated as a result of the addition of another molecule (such as sulfate or glucuronic acid) to itself or its metabolite, the drug tends to be pharmacologically inert. In general, conjugation reactions follow oxidation, reduction, or hydrolytic reactions. A conjugated drug is generally more polar and therefore more water-soluble; this greatly enhances renal excretion of the compound.

Renal Excretion

The kidney serves as the major route of excretion of unchanged and biotransformed drugs. There are two major renal routes of excretion: filtration and secretion. Filtered drugs are generally polar and water-soluble. They pass into Bowman's capsule and traverse the tubular lumen, and most reach the collecting duct without significant reabsorption. Drugs can be actively secreted into the tubular lumen by proximal tubular carrier-mediated mechanisms that transport naturally-occurring organic acids or organic bases. These systems are nonselective and organic acids (e.g., penicillin, aspirin, and diuretics) or organic bases (e.g., quinine) compete for transport. In addition, these carrier systems can function in a bidirectional manner, i.e., a compound can be both actively secreted into the lumen and actively reabsorbed from the lumen.

Following its passage into the renal tubule, if a drug is nonionized, or becomes nonionized due to the acidic pH of the tubular filtrate, and has an appropriate molecular size, then passive reabsorption of the drug into the bloodstream at both the proximal and distal portions of the nephron may occur. As the renal tubular fluid becomes more concentrated, nonionized drug molecules are reabsorbed by diffusion across the tubular epithelium at rates related to their lipid-to-water partition coefficients. Accordingly, compounds of low lipid solubility, which are poorly reabsorbed, are excreted in the urine more readily than are compounds of high lipid solubility.

In accordance with the principles governing the distribution of weak electrolytes across a lipoid membrane, when the tubular urine is made alkaline, weak bases become less concentrated in the urine than in plasma and, as a result, are excreted more slowly; when the urine is made acidic, weak bases concentrate in the urine and are excreted more rapidly. Conversely, weak acids are excreted more readily in an alkaline urine and more slowly in an acidic urine.

Biliary Excretion

The hepatic parenchymal cell is readily penetrated by most drugs. In addition to the rapid penetration of many nonionized compounds, which pass through lipoid areas as well as pores in the cell membrane, a wide variety of organic anions and cations are readily taken up by liver parenchymal cells by carrier-type transport processes.

The liver has at least three active transport processes for the biliary excretion. One process excretes a variety of poorly lipid-soluble organic anions including sulfonic acid dyes, bile acids, bilirubin, penicillins, and many drug biotransformation products such as glucuronides and other acidic conjugation substances. A second process is responsible for the biliary excretion of organic cations, including certain quaternary ammonium compounds and tertiary amines. A third process excretes a number of steroids and related compounds, e.g., cardioactive glycosides. In each of these processes, compounds are transported from plasma into bile against a large concentration gradient, the excretion mechanism becomes saturated at high plasma levels of the compound, the carrier systems are nonselective and substances that are excreted by the same process inhibit the transport of one another in a competitive manner.

In contrast, most lipid-soluble, nonionized drugs do not appear in the bile in high concentrations. During their passage through the bile duct, reabsorption may occur whereby these molecules can diffuse readily across the bile duct epithelium and thus remain in equilibrium with the drug concentration in plasma.

After a drug has been excreted into the intestine via the bile, it may be partly reabsorbed and partly excreted in the feces. Glucuronides or other conjugated forms of drugs may be split within the intestinal lumina to release free, lipid-soluble drug molecules. Obviously the free drug is readily reabsorbed in the intestine, reconjugated in the liver, and again excreted into bile. This enterohepatic cycle can delay considerably the elimination of a drug from the body. Some drugs which undergo enterohepatic recirculation are morphine, glutethimide, digitoxin, and indomethacin.

Other Elimination Processes

Drugs and their biotransformation products can be secreted into saliva, sweat, tears, nasal excretions and mammary secretions. Although most compounds that are eliminated from the body by way of any of these media are water-soluble, it is important to remember that they pass into these fluids by simple diffusion and that only the free form of the drug or its metabolites can pass across the particular organs and their membranes. The amount of compound excreted by any of these routes represents only a small fraction of the of the total amount of drug eliminated from the body.

Of particular importance are mammary secretions in a nursing mother. Since the pH of milk is usually about 0.7 unit below that of plasma, basic drugs appear in milk in a concentration greater than that in plasma, and acidic drugs in a concentration less than that in plasma. Completely neutral substances, e.g., ethanol, become distributed equally between the two fluids. Breast-fed infants will thus become exposed to drugs ingested by the mother with consequent pharmacologic effects. Therefore, it is a good general rule to advise drug abstinence by the mother if she is breast-feeding her child.

FUNDAMENTAL MATHEMATICAL PRINCIPLES OF PHARMACOKINETICS

In order to simplify the discussion of the mathematical relationships in pharmacokinetics, it is necessary to assume that the factors which influence drug absorption, distribution, and elimination in a single individual remain constant over a period of time. This assumption is made with the full realization that drug-drug interactions and changes in the function of the cardiovascular system, the liver, and the kidney may alter the pharmacokinetic pattern of a compound.

Pharmacokinetic Models and Compartments

As mentioned previously, the use of time-plasma drug concentration curves, as exemplified in Fig. 4-3, has become a useful standard device with which to monitor pharmacokinetics. Drugs are absorbed, distributed, biotransformed, and excreted at different rates. Since a variety of biologic and physicochemical processes influence how a particular drug is handled by the body, it would appear that a mathematical description of drug pharmacokinetics would be very complex and would vary for each drug. In contrast, due to the equilibrium nature of drug disposition in the body, certain patterns, which tend to simplify pharmacokinetic analyses, emerge from using time-plasma drug concentration curves. These patterns, conceptualized into *pharmacokinetic models*, or *compartment models*, help to explain human pharmacokinetic data.

The simplest pharmacokinetic model, the *one-compartment model* (Fig. 4-6), assumes that, after administration, drugs are rapidly and homogeneously distributed throughout all body fluids.

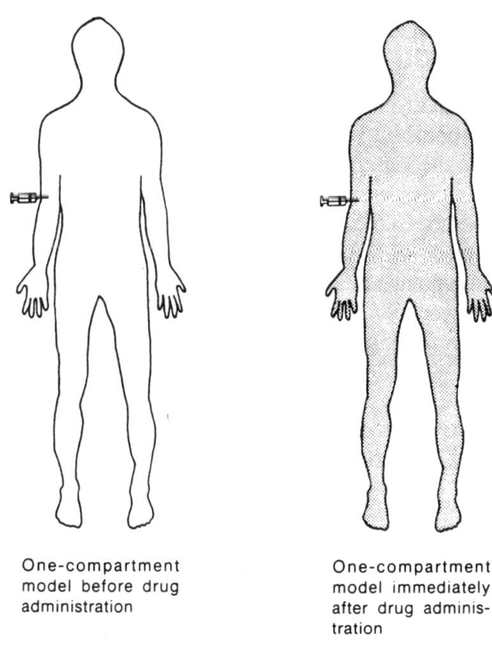

One-compartment model before drug administration
One-compartment model immediately after drug administration

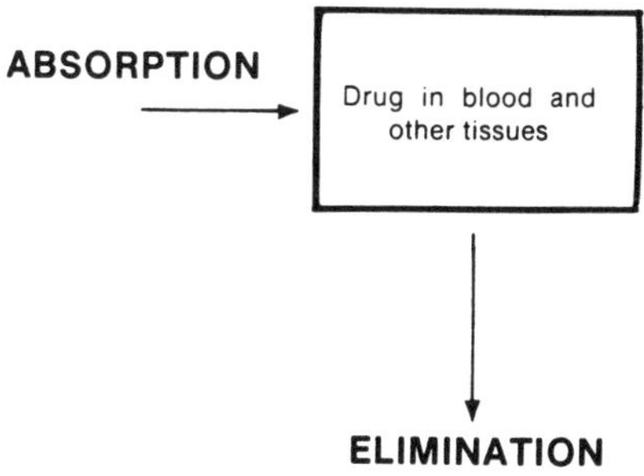

FIGURE 4-6 *The one-compartment model before and after intravenous drug administration. [Modified from Dvorchik, B.H., and E.S. Vesell: Clin. Chem. 22: 868 (1976).]*

This does not necessarily mean that the concentration of drug in plasma and other tissues is equal, rather, that the entire system is at equilibrium and changes in plasma drug concentrations quantitatively reflect changes in drug concentrations occurring in other fluids and tissues. Many drugs equilibrate between plasma and other tissues very rapidly. Furthermore, at the usual plasma sampling times, the one-compartment pharmacokinetic model adequately describes the data of time-plasma drug concentration curves (see Fig. 4-10). Therefore, this model, although the most elementary, is often the most appropriate pharmacokinetic model for many drugs.

The *two-compartment model* (Fig. 4-7) considers the fact that drugs distribute to different tissues at rates related to the blood flow in each tissue, and therefore, divides tissues primarily upon vascularization. For example, tissues with high blood flow, i.e., adrenals, kidneys, heart, brain, and the blood vessels, may compose the "central compartment" and receive drugs rapidly. All other tissues (with lower blood flow) constitute the "peripheral compartment" and, therefore, exchange drugs at a slower rate. If drug distribution throughout the body is relatively slow or if plasma sampling is performed frequently and quickly following drug administration, "two-phase" time-plasma drug concentration data can be seen (see Fig. 4-12). In this case, the two-compartment model describes drug disposition in the body. Three- and four-compartment models have been described but are rarely used. It is important to realize that these "compartments" have no real physiologic meaning; they vary in extent depending on the particular drug under consideration.

Kinetics

Kinetics is the study of rates of reactions. In general, drug absorption, distribution, and elimination (i.e., biotransformation and excretion) processes follow *first-order kinetics*. A first-order kinetic process is one in which a constant *fraction*, or *percentage*, of a drug is handled per unit of time. This is true for both passive processes (e.g., glomerular filtration) and active processes (e.g., renal tubular secretion) where drug concentrations do not saturate the enzyme or carrier system. In selected instances, drug concentrations may saturate the metabolic or transport system. When the capacity of those systems is exceeded, a constant *amount* of drug is handled per unit of time. This is known as *zero-order kinetics*.

First-Order Rate Equations With first-order kinetics, the rate of an absorption, a biotransformation, a distribution, or an excretion process is directly proportional to the concentration of the substance remaining to be handled by the system at any given time. For example, if drug A is absorbed through the intestinal mucosa into the blood, then the rate of transfer of drug A from the intestinal lumen is proportional to the concentration of drug A in the intestine. The following

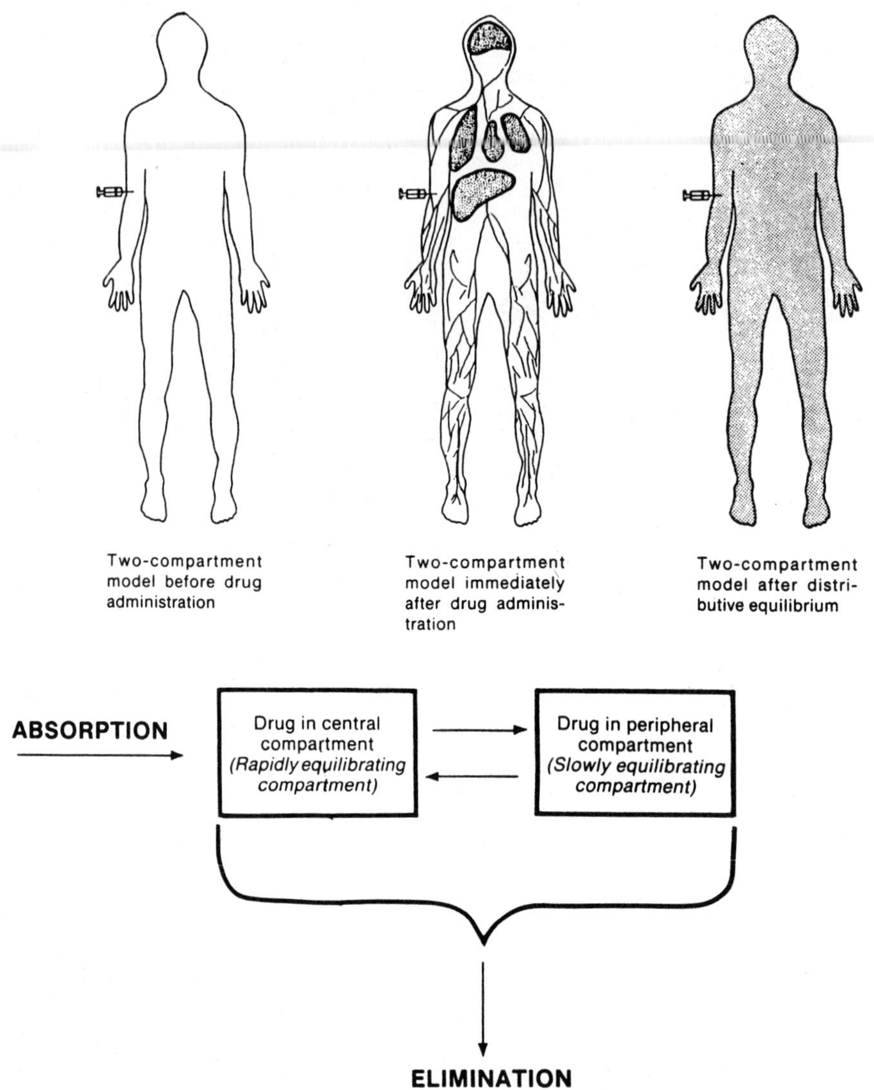

FIGURE 4-7 *The two-compartment model before and after intravenous drug administration. [Modified from Dvorchik, B.H., and E.S. Vesell: Clin. Chem. 22: 868 (1976).]*

relationships are applicable:

$$\text{Rate of transfer} \propto [A] \text{ in the intestine}$$

or

$$\text{Rate} = k[A]$$

where k is the proportionality constant or rate constant for the process. This is one form of the first-order rate equation.

For a biotransformation reaction where drug A is converted to its metabolite, drug B, the rate of reaction is also equal to k[A]. The rate of this reaction is the increase in the concentration of B with respect to time, $d[B]/dt$; therefore,

$$Rate = \frac{d[B]}{dt} = k[A]$$

The rate of the formation of B is equal to the rate

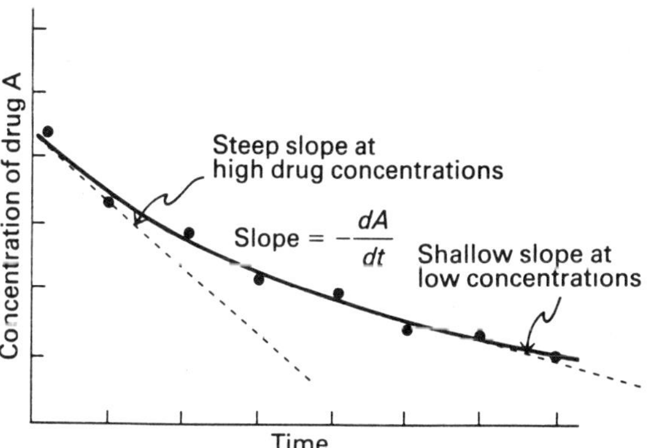

FIGURE 4-8 *Arithmetic plot of drug concentration versus time for a first-order process.*

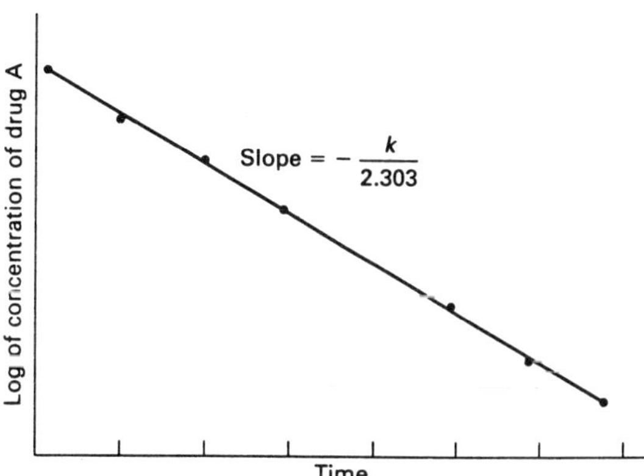

FIGURE 4-9 *Logarithmic plot of drug concentration versus time for a first-order process.*

of the biotransformation of A, or

$$\frac{d[B]}{dt} = \frac{-d[A]}{dt}$$

where the minus sign denotes that [A] is decreasing with time. This provides another form of the first-order rate equation:

$$Rate = \frac{-d[A]}{dt} = k[A]$$

which is plotted in Fig. 4-8. Note that the slope of the line reflects the rate of the reaction; at high [A], the rate is high (steep slope), and as the [A] decreases, so does the rate of the process (shallower slope). The same relationship holds for the gain or loss of a drug from a tissue or organ site, e.g., from gastric juice, plasma, or cerebrospinal fluid.

If it is of interest to determine the rate constant k for absorption or elimination of a drug, the first-order rate equation as expressed graphically in Fig. 4-8 is difficult to analyze and leads to a considerable error in the estimate of k because of the constantly changing slope of the line. This equation can be converted mathematically (through rearrangement and integration) to

$$\ln[A] = \ln[A_o] - kt$$

where $\ln[A_0]$ is the natural logarithm of concentration of drug A before the process begins, or at time = 0, and ln[A] is the natural logarithm of the concentration of drug A at any subsequent time t. This equation, which is in a linear format, can also be written using common logarithms:

$$\log[A] = \log[A_o] - \frac{k}{2.303}t$$

$$y = a + b\ x$$

The relationship between the log-concentration of drug A and time is shown in Fig. 4-9.

Sample Problem 1

The aminoglycoside amikacin was cleared from the plasma of one patient with a rate constant of 0.277/h. If the initial concentration of amikacin in the plasma was 30 μg/mL, how long would it be before the plasma concentration was reduced to 12 μg/mL?

$$2.303 \log \frac{\text{initial drug concentration}}{\text{final drug concentration}} = kt$$

$$2.303 \log \frac{30\ \mu g/mL}{12\ \mu g/mL} = \frac{0.277}{h}t$$

$$t = 3.3\ h$$

The half-life ($t_{1/2}$) of a first-order process is the time necessary for the drug concentration to decrease to one-half of its original value or the time required for the process to be half completed. At the half-life, $[A] = \frac{1}{2}[A_o]$; therefore

$$\log \tfrac{1}{2}[A_o] - \log[A_o] = -\frac{k}{2.303}t_{1/2}$$

and

$$2.303 \log \frac{[A_o]}{\tfrac{1}{2}[A_o]} = kt_{1/2}$$

The left side of the equation equals 2.303 log 2, or 0.693. Therefore

$$t_{1/2} = \frac{0.693}{k}$$

which shows that the half-life for a first-order process is dependent only on k and is independent of the initial concentration of the drug. In addition, if the half-life is known, k can easily be calculated (see Fig. 4-10).

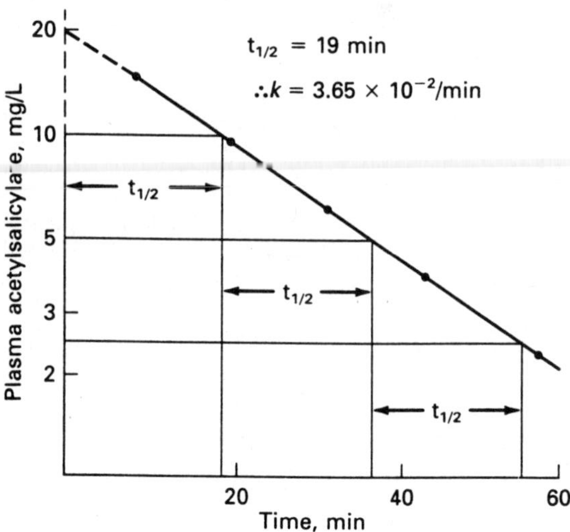

FIGURE 4-10 *Logarithmic plot showing the rate of removal of acetylsalicylate from human plasma in vivo and the estimation of half-life ($t_{1/2}$). [Modified from Lamont-Havers, R.M., and B.M. Wagner (eds.): Proceedings of the Conference on Effects of Chronic Salicylate Administration, New York, June 13-14, 1966; U.S. Department of Health, Education and Welfare.]*

Sample Problem 2

Calculate the elimination half-life of the opioid analgesic codeine in a patient if the elimination rate constant was 0.173/h.

$$t_{1/2} = \frac{0.693}{k}$$

$$t_{1/2} = \frac{0.693}{0.173/h}$$

$$t_{1/2} = 4.0 \text{ h}$$

It is important to remember that k for any first-order pharmacokinetic process does not have a definitive value. It is a variable that depends on the individual patient's ability to handle a particular drug. Furthermore, when two or more first-order processes are involved in drug kinetics, the rate constants of each are additive. For example, in drug elimination which encompasses both hepatic biotransformation and renal excretion, the *systemic elimination rate constant* k_e is a composite of the rate constants for biotransformation and excretion. It follows that the *systemic half-life* of a drug equals $0.693/k_e$. It is the systemic half-life that is most useful clinically.

The Zero-Order Rate Equation Most enzyme-catalyzed processes in the body, such as facilitated diffusion, active transport, and biotransformation reactions, are saturable. That is, the drug in *too great a concentration* will overwhelm the capacity of the enzyme or carrier. In such a case, the rate of the process becomes independent of the drug concentration and dependent on only the rate constant k of the process. If the concentration of a drug (not the log) is plotted versus time, a linear plot results with the slope equal to $-k$. In zero-order kinetics a constant *amount* of drug is handled per unit of time; the clearance of ethanol from the plasma provides an excellent example of zero-order kinetics (see Figure 4-11).

Apparent Volume of Distribution Every drug has a characteristic distribution pattern which depends on the physicochemical properties of the drug as well as the inherent biologic variability of the organism.

For the one-compartment model, distribution of a drug is considered to be relatively rapid.

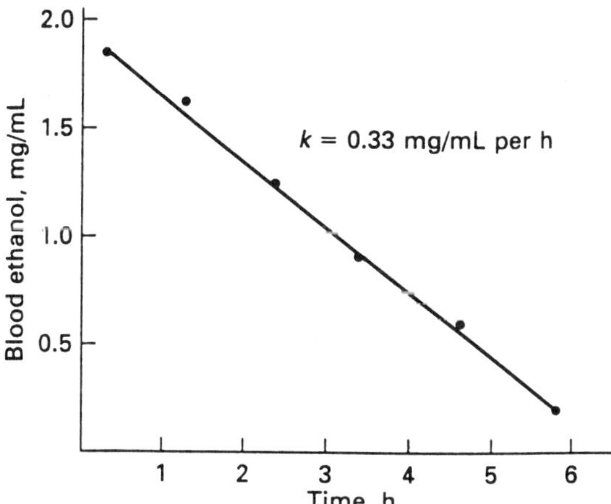

FIGURE 4-11 *Arithmetic plot of the changes in blood ethanol concentrations with respect to time following intraperitoneal injection of ethanol to rats. [Modified from Ferko, A.P., and Bobyock, E.: Toxicol. Appl. Pharmacol.* ***46:*** *235-248 (1978).]*

Regardless of the rate at which distribution occurs, the extent of distribution varies widely among drugs. Some drugs are highly distributed throughout the body, others are largely confined to the plasma and therefore do not distribute well. The *apparent volume of distribution* V_d was developed as an index to compare the extent of drug distribution. V_d is defined as the volume of fluid into which a drug appears to distribute, with a concentration equal to that of plasma. Mathematically this is expressed as

$$V_d = \frac{\textit{total amount of drug in the body}}{\textit{concentration of drug in the plasma}}$$

An important questions to consider is: How long after drug administration should the plasma concentration of that drug be measured? Time-plasma concentration curves vary for every drug in every patient, depending on the rates and extent of absorption, distribution, and elimination. Therefore, by convention, elimination data are used, i.e., plasma levels taken at various times following administration, and extrapolated back to the drug concentration of time = 0. For example, using data shown in Fig. 4-10, plasma acetylsalicylate concentrations were taken at various times following IV administration of 200 mg of the drug. Extrapolation of the linear elimination data to time = 0 gives the acetylsalicylate concentration of 20 mg/L. This would be the plasma concentration if absorption and distribution of the drug were rapid enough to be essentially instantaneous. In this example, V_d = (200 mg)/(20 mg/L), or 10 L.

If drug data appear to follow a two-compartment model, the distribution phase is ignored in estimating the plasma concentration at time = 0 for calculating V_d. This is because V_d describes drug distribution after *equilibrium has occurred,* which is not until the elimination phase is observed. Using the data in Fig. 4-12 for calculating V_d, the plasma concentration of morphine at time = 0 would be approximately 60 ng/mL.

V_d is a theoretical concept that provides some indication of the extent of drug distribution; it is generally a characteristic of the drug rather than the biologic system (however, biologic variability affects patient V_d values to some extent). Most drugs have a V_d between 0.1 and 6 L/kg. Often V_d is expressed in liters per 70 kg or simply liters (which assumes a 70-kg weight). A low V_d indicates that the drug remains largely within the plasma and does not readily distribute to other tissues. This may be due to a high degree of drug binding to plasma proteins or a very low lipid-to-water partition coefficient and low penetrability

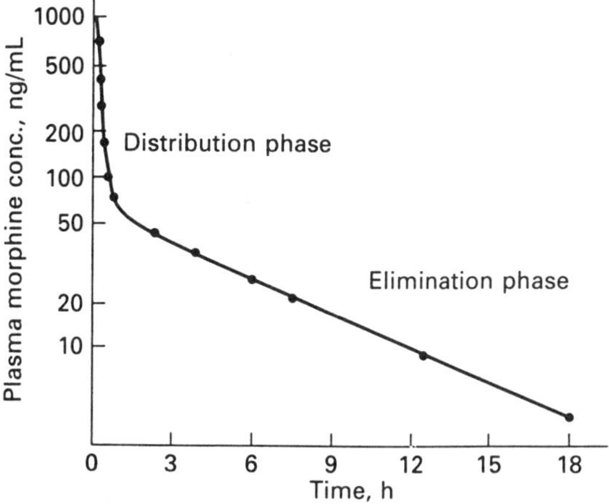

FIGURE 4-12 *Logarithmic plot of plasma morphine concentrations following intravenous administration of morphine to a patient. Note that the first phase of the curve (the distribution phase, or the α phase) shows a rapid decline. This is due to prompt distribution into the slowly equilibrating tissues. After the phase, the concentration of drug in the body is at equilibrium and the elimination phase (or the β phase) proceeds more slowly. [Modified from Stanski, D.R., et al.: Clin. Pharmacol. Ther.* ***24:*** *52-59 (1978).]*

through membranes and storage in adipose tissue. A high V_d is indicative of significant uptake by many tissues and widespread distribution of the compound. In addition to providing insight into the distribution of a drug, V_d is useful for estimating the plasma concentration after a dose of the drug or in calculating the total amount of drug in the body when the plasma concentration is known.

Sample Problem 3

The pharmacokinetics of 2 benzodiazepines (diazepam and clonazepam) were being compared in a clinical study. A 70 kg subject received 10 mg of diazepam IV and, on a separate occasion, 2 mg of clonazepam IV. The plasma concentrations (extrapolated to time = 0) were: diazepam = 120 ng/mL; clonazepam = 11 ng/mL. Calculate the V_d for each drug. Which drug has the greater distribution throughout the body?

1 The V_d for diazepam:

$$V_d = \frac{10 \text{ mg per } 70 \text{ kg}}{120 \text{ ng/mL}} = \frac{0.143 \text{ mg/kg}}{0.12 \text{ mg/L}}$$

$$V_d = 1.2 \text{ L/kg (or 83 L per 70 kg)}$$

2 The V_d for clonazepam:

$$V_d = \frac{2 \text{ mg per } 70 \text{ kg}}{11 \text{ ng/mL}} = \frac{0.029 \text{ mg/kg}}{0.011 \text{ mg/L}}$$

$$V_d = 2.6 \text{ L/kg (or 182 L per 70 kg)}$$

3 Clonazepam has the greater distribution (approximately twice that of diazepam).

Clearance Clearance is defined as the apparent volume of a biologic fluid from which a drug is removed by elimination processes per unit of time. Clearance is *not* a measure of the quantity of drug being eliminated; it provides an indication of the *volume of fluid* from which the drug is eliminated. For example, if drug A is biotransformed in the liver to metabolite B and has a hepatic clearance of 1 mL/min/kg (or 70 mL/min), this means that as blood flows through the liver containing drug A, every minute 70 mL of blood leaves the organ containing only drug B (i.e., completely cleared of drug A).

Organ clearance CL_{organ} is dependent on (1) the blood flow Q through the organ and (2) the maximum ability of the organ to remove the free drug from the circulation (known as the *intrinsic clearance*, or the *extraction efficiency E*. Therefore

$$CL_{organ} = Q \times E$$

The extraction efficiency is determined by the difference between the arterial drug concentrations C_A and venous drug concentrations C_V divided by the arterial drug concentration, or

$$E = \frac{C_A - C_V}{C_A}$$

Therefore, after substitution

$$CL_{organ} = Q \times E = Q \times \frac{C_A - C_V}{C_A}$$

One generally discusses clearance of a drug from the plasma (or blood) by elimination processes that affect the whole body. Total body clearance CL_{total} is the rate of removal of a drug from the body and represents the sum total of clearance of all the organs that eliminate a drug, i.e.,

$$CL_{total} = CL_{liver} + CL_{kidney} + CL_{lung} + \ldots..$$

Total body clearance is influenced by the apparent volume of distribution V_d and the elimination rate constant k_e. Kinetically,

$$CL_{total} = V_d \times k_e = \frac{0.693 \times V_d}{t_{1/2}}$$

or expressed in terms of half-life,

$$t_{1/2} = \frac{0.693 \times V_d}{CL_{total}}$$

Therefore, the elimination half-life of a drug is dependent on how widely a drug is distributed throughout the body and its rate of clearance.

Sample Problem 4

A 70 kg patient was given aminophylline, 5 mg/kg IV, resulting in a plasma concentration of 10 μg/mL. The elimination half-life of the drug in this patient was estimated to be 6 hours. What was the total body clearance of aminophylline in this patient?

$$CL_{total} = \frac{0.693 \times V_d}{t_{1/2}}$$

1 Calculate the V_d

$$V_d = \frac{5\text{ mg/kg} \times 70\text{ kg}}{10\ \mu\text{g/mL}} = 35\text{ L per }70\text{ kg}$$

2 Calculate the CL_{total}

$$CL_{total} = \frac{0.693 \times V_d}{t_{1/2}} = \frac{0.693 \times 35\text{ L}}{6\text{ h}}$$

$$CL_{total} = 4\text{ L/h or }67\text{ mL/min}$$

DOSAGE REGIMENS AND PHARMACOKINETIC PROFILES

Single Doses

Intravenous Administration After intravenous injection of a drug as a bolus, the compound mixes with and becomes diluted by circulating blood. Although distribution within the circulation and to other tissues begins to occur rapidly, uniform systemic distribution usually is not established for several minutes after drug administration. As distribution equilibrates, plasma concentrations of the drug decrease rapidly; following this distribution phase, drug elimination from the plasma takes the form of a first-order process.

If plasma concentrations of the drug are measured quickly enough following intravenous bolus administration and at various times thereafter, time-plasma drug concentration data will resemble those shown in Fig. 4-12 and will appear to follow a two-compartment model. If, on the other hand, the rate of drug distribution is more rapid than the ability to quantitate the initial plasma concentrations, then the data for the distribution phase will be lost, only the elimination phase will be observed (see Fig. 4-10), and the data will appear to follow a one-compartment model.

Oral Administration Oral dosing of a substance introduces absorption as a significant variable factor. In addition to the inherent biologic variations in rates of drug absorption, differences in dosage forms, formulations of a dosage form, or salts of a drug may dramatically alter the pharmacokinetic pattern of a compound. These problems relate to bioavailability of drugs and bioequivalence of drug products.

As discussed previously, due to the ability of drugs to traverse membranes, once within the systemic circulation, they become *available* to the tissues of the body. The term used to describe the amount of drug that is delivered the general circulation and the rate at which this occurs is *bioavailability*. If a drug is injected by the intravenous route, it is at once completely bioavailable. All other avenues of drug administration usually result in incomplete bioavailability due to (1) incomplete absorption, (2) biotransformation of some of the drug prior to reaching the systemic circulation, or (3) both. Therefore, bioavailability *F* is a measure of the fraction of an administered dose that reaches the general circulation.

The area under the time-plasma drug concentration curve, or simply the *area under the curve* (AUC), for any drug represents the total amount of that drug delivered to the circulation (during the time period of measurement) following administration. Using IV dosing as the basis of comparison and assuming no changes in drug distribution or elimination, the bioavailability of a drug (given by any route) can be calculated by the AUCs according to the following:

$$F = \frac{AUC \times dose_{IV}}{AUC_{IV} \times dose}$$

If the doses are equal, the relationship simplifies to the ratio of AUC values only. In this context, the bioavailability of a drug by any route is the *absolute bioavailability*. Usually oral bioavailability of drugs is of most interest, since the oral route is the most common method of drug administration. As an example, the antimicrobial drug penicillin G has an oral bioavailability of approximately 20 percent, i.e., only about 20 percent of an oral dose reaches the systemic circulation. A compound with similar antimicrobial activity and potency, penicillin V, has an oral bioavailability of over 80 percent and would be preferred to penicillin G for oral use since more drug would reach the bloodstream at equivalent oral doses.

When bioavailability comparisons are made between two different dosage forms of a drug, e.g., capsules versus tablets, or between two different manufacturers of the same type of dosage form and the dose and route of administration are the same, the AUC ratio refers to the *relative bioavailability*.

Multiple Doses

It is rare that a drug will be used in a single-dose regimen; in most therapeutic situations including the treatment of acute illnesses, drugs are usually given in multiple doses. Regardless of the route of administration, if these doses are spaced far enough apart, complete elimination of the first dose may occur prior to the administration of the second dose; the second dose will be completely eliminated prior to the third dose, etc.; the time-plasma drug concentration curves resulting from this schedule of drug administration will resemble individual single doses, separated by the dosing interval (Fig. 4-13). Pharmacokinetic data may be calculated for each dose using the concepts and equations developed previously in this chapter.

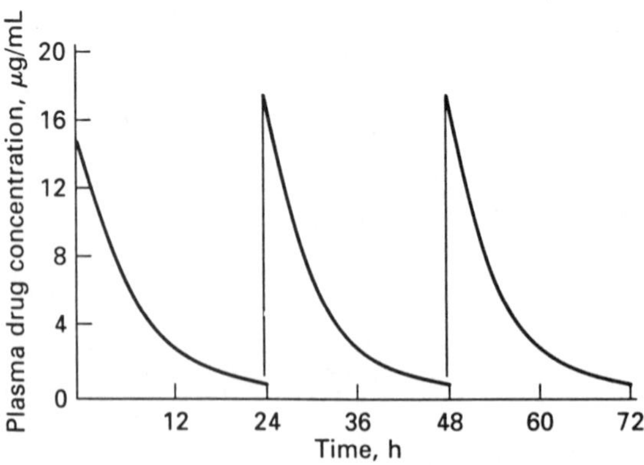

FIGURE 4-13 *Arithmetic plot of plasma drug concentration versus time following multiple intravenous bolus injections given every 24 h. There is no accumulation of the drug since the doses are widely separated and each dose is almost completely eliminated prior to the next injection.*

Repeated administration of a drug at intervals selected so that complete elimination of the compound has not occurred, will result in drug accumulation. Plasma concentration will fluctuate in response to the inherent pharmacokinetics of the drug and in proportion to the dosage interval selected. Accumulation of the compound within the body will continue to occur until the amount of drug eliminated per dosing interval equals the amount of drug absorbed per dose. When this condition is attained, the plasma level will be at the *plateau* or *steady state*.

Multiple Intravenous Administration Figure 4-13 shows the time-plasma drug concentration curve of a drug with a 4-h half-life given by IV injection every 24 h. If this drug were administered at more closely spaced intervals, e.g., once every half-life (4 h), the data would appear as shown in Fig. 4-14. The plasma drug concentration will continue to increase until the steady state is attained, at which time the drug concentration will fluctuate between a minimum C_{min} and maximum C_{max} during each dosing interval.

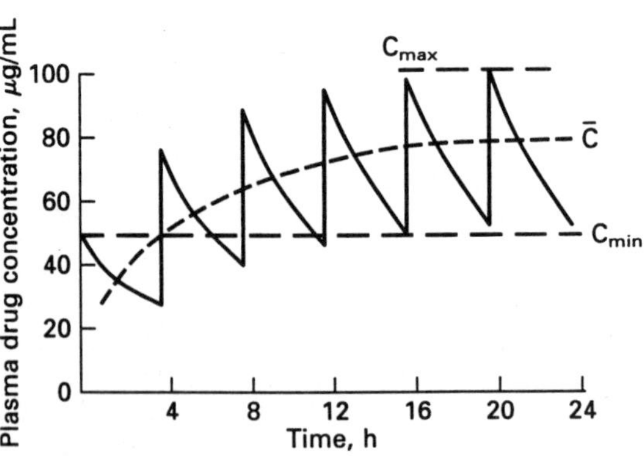

FIGURE 4-14 *Arithmetic plot of plasma drug concentration versus time following multiple intravenous bolus injections given every 4 h. Since the drug is not completely eliminated prior to each succeeding dose, drug accumulation will occur. Eventually, plasma drug concentrations will attain the steady state, fluctuating between the maximum (C_{max}) and minimum (C_{min}) drug concentrations at the beginning and end of each dosing interval, respectively.*

The average plasma concentration at the steady state $\bar{C}$ during multiple IV administration can be calculated by

$$\bar{C} = \frac{D}{V_d \times k_e \times T} = \frac{D}{CL_{total} \times T}$$

where D is the dose, V_d the apparent volume of distribution, k_e the elimination rate constant, CL_{total} the total body clearance, and T the dosing interval. Therefore, given some pharmacokinetic data following a single dose of a drug, one can estimate the plasma concentration at the steady state with a variety of dosage regimens.

Sample Problem 5

The inotropic drug digoxin was administered to a 75 kg, 60 year old man with normal renal function at a dose of 0.125 mg IV every 4 hours. Assuming a V_d of 8 L/kg and a $t_{½}$ of 24 hours for digoxin, what would be the average plasma concentration of the drug in this patient at the steady state?

1 Calculate the k_e

$$k_e = \frac{0.693}{24\text{ h}} = 0.0289/\text{h}$$

2 Calculate $\bar{C}$

$$\bar{C} = \frac{D}{V_d \times k_e \times T}$$

$$\bar{C} = \frac{0.125\text{ mg}}{8\text{ L/kg} \times 0.0289/\text{h} \times 4\text{ h}}$$

$$\bar{C} = \frac{0.125\text{ mg}}{0.924\text{ L/kg} \times 75\text{ kg}}$$

$$\bar{C} = 0.0018\text{ mg/L or } 1.8\text{ ng/mL}$$

Continuous Intravenous Infusion This can be considered a variation of multiple IV injections where the dosing interval is infinitely small. Instead of many small single IV doses, a suitable constant rate of drug infusion and duration of infusion is chosen. If the infusion is continued indefinitely, the plasma concentration will increase until the rate of elimination (which increases as drug concentration increases) becomes equal to the rate of infusion. At this point a steady-state plasma concentration will be achieved (Fig. 4-15). With this form of drug administration, the infusion rate = dose/T, and therefore

$$\bar{C} = \frac{\textit{infusion rate}}{CL_{total}}$$

Multiple Oral Dosing Similar to the case of multiple IV injections, with multiple oral dosing, the average plasma concentration $\bar{C}$ is related to the dose, dosage interval, and clearance of the compound, but is complicated by the inclusion of a first-order absorption step. Therefore the dose administered is reduced by the oral bioavailability F, and the equation for calculating C becomes

$$\bar{C} = \frac{F \times D}{V_d \times k_e \times T} = \frac{F \times D}{CL_{total} \times T}$$

Using this relationship, a uniform maintenance dose and dosage interval can be selected for any drug in order to achieve any average steady-state plasma concentration that is desired. This works

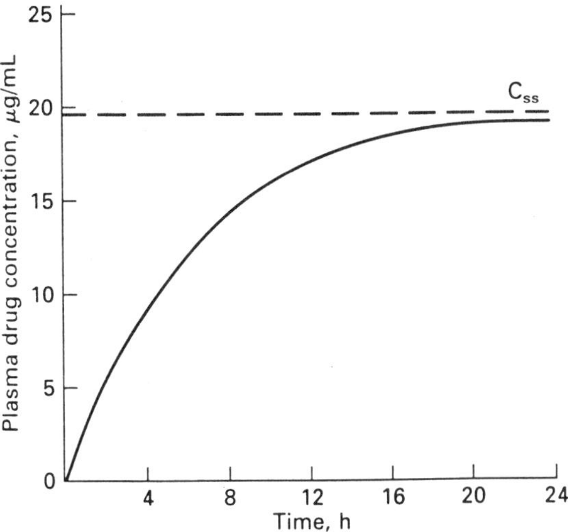

FIGURE 4-15 *Arithmetic plot of plasma drug concentration versus time following continuous intravenous infusion. The plasma drug concentration will, in time, reach the steady-state (C_{ss}) concentration.*

well when patients are instructed to take medication with a uniform dosing interval, for example, four times a day around the clock, i.e., every 6 h. Unfortunately, in practice uniform dosing regimens such as this are seldom used and rarely adhered to by the patient. Thus drug plasma levels often tend to fluctuate more than desired, leading to ineffective therapy, and/or unwanted adverse drug effects.

BIBLIOGRAPHY

Azarnoff, D.L., and D.H. Huffman: "Therapeutic Implications of Bioavailability," *Annu. Rev. Pharmacol. Toxicol.* ***16:*** 53-66 (1976).

Bend, J.R., C.J. Serabjit-Singh, and R.M. Philpot: "The Pulmonary Uptake, Accumulation and Metabolism of Xenobiotics," *Annu. Rev. Pharmacol. Toxicol.* ***25:*** 97-125 (1985).

Benet, L.Z., N. Massoud, and L.G. Gambertoglio: *Pharmacokinetic Basis for Drug Treatment*, Raven, New York, 1984.

Bochner, F., G. Carrothers, J. Kampmann, and J. Steiner: *Handbook of Clinical Pharmacology*, Little, Brown, Boston, 1983.

Bourne, D.W.A., E.J. Triggs, and M.J. Eadie: *Pharmacokinetics for the Non-mathematical*, MTP Press Limited, Lancaster, 1986.

Creasey, W.A.: *Drug Disposition in Humans*, Oxford, London, 1979.

Gladtke, E., and H.M. von Hattingberg: *Pharmacokinetics, An Introduction*, Springer-Verlag, New York, 1979.

Greenblatt, D.J., and R.I. Shader: *Pharmacokinetics in Clinical Practice*, Saunders, Philadelphia, 1985.

Ladua, B.N., H.G. Mandel, and E.L. Way (eds.): *Fundamentals of Drug Metabolism and Drug Disposition*, Williams and Wilkins, Baltimore, 1971.

Levine, R.R.: *Pharmacology: Drug Actions and Reactions,* 3rd ed., Little, Brown, Boston, 1983.

Partridge, W.M.: "Recent Advances in Blood-Brain Barrier Transport," *Annu. Rev. Pharmacol. Toxicol.* **28**: 25-39 (1988).

Rowland, M., and T.N. Tozer: *Clinical Pharmacokinetics: Concepts and Applications, Second Edition*, Lea & Febiger, Philadelphia, 1989.

Ther, L., and D. Winner: "Drug Absorption," *Annu. Rev. Pharmacol.* **11**: 57-70 (1971).

Williams, R.L.: "Pharmacokinetics," in R.L. Williams, D.C. Brater, and J. Mordenti (eds.), *Rational Therapeutics*, Marcel Dekker, Inc., New York, 1990, pp. 1-18.

CHAPTER 5

Biotransformation

William J. Cooke

The chemical changes undergone by a drug within the body are referred to as *drug biotransformation*. The majority of these chemical alterations result from the interaction of drugs with endogenous enzyme systems, although nonenzymatic reactions are also involved for particular compounds. Many of the enzymes exhibit broad substrate specificity and thus catalyze reactions involving a wide range of foreign chemicals referred to as xenobiotics. Pharmacologic agents, or drugs, represent a particular type of xenobiotic.

The liver is the major organ responsible for the biotransformation of drugs and other xenobiotics. The smooth endoplasmic reticulum, a subcellular membrane system rich in enzymes for xenobiotic metabolism, is especially prominent in hepatic tissue. When liver is homogenized the endoplasmic reticulum forms small membrane vesicles which can then be isolated by differential centrifugation, and are known as *microsomes*. Thus, the group of enzymes associated with the smooth endoplasmic reticulum, and obtained by the technique indicated, is often termed the *drug-metabolizing microsomal system* (DMMS). Extrahepatic metabolism, involving similar enzymes, can also be important for many drugs and occurs mainly in kidney, lung, and intestine.

TYPES OF BIOTRANSFORMATION REACTIONS

Lipid-soluble xenobiotics introduced into the body are usually not excreted until they undergo chemical changes that result in an increase in polarity. Since many drugs are lipophilic, biotransformation increases their water solubility. This solubility change restricts further penetration of the drug through cellular membranes, reduces systemic distribution, and promotes elimination through excretory systems such as the kidney. Therefore, biotransformation of a drug usually limits its pharmacologic activity by altering the compound's structure as well as its solubility.

Traditionally, drug biotransformation reactions have been regarded as occurring in two separate phases. Phase I reactions consist of oxidations, reductions, and hydrolyses which introduce new functional groups to the parent drug molecule. Phase I reactions often alter the chemical reactivity of a drug and increase its aqueous solubility. Phase II reactions consist of conjugation (synthetic) reactions in which an endogenous substrate, such as glucuronic acid, sulfate, or glutathione, is coupled to the drug molecule. Conjugation reactions generally involve the new chemical groups introduced during phase I reactions. Phase II reactions further increase the water solubility of the drug molecule, thus promoting its elimination.

Phase I and phase II reactions may occur either sequentially or simultaneously and often involve multiple functional groups on the drug molecule. Phase I reactions usually precede phase II reactions, but in some cases phase II reactions occur prior to those of phase I. Alternatively, a given drug may undergo only phase II reactions. The pattern of drug biotransformation reactions, as well as the pattern of metabolites formed, is determined by the chemical structure and reactivity of each particular drug in addition to the particular enzymes available in the body.

It is important to recognize that biotransformation can result in conversion of (1) a pharmacologically active drug to an inactive metabolite, (2) a pharmacologically active drug to a pharmacologically active metabolite, or (3) an inactive agent to a pharmacologically active metabolite.

As an example of the first case, phase I biotransformation of phenytoin (an anticonvulsant agent) by hydroxylation leads to its inactivation, or loss of pharmacological activity:

Phenytoin [active] ⟶ hydroxyphenytoin [inactive]

In the second case, a metabolite of a drug retains pharmacologic activity similar to the parent drug. An important example is provided by the phase I dealkylation of diazepam (an antianxiety agent):

Diazepam [active] ⟶ desmethyldiazepam [active]

When an inactive precursor is metabolized to a pharmacologically active drug, the parent compound is known as a *prodrug*. An example is:

Sulindac (sulfoxide) [inactive] ⟶ sulindac sulfide [active]

A corollary to the above is that a metabolite can exhibit greater toxicity than its precursor. This may be especially important with respect to carcinogenesis, for example, where a xenobiotic is converted to a more reactive metabolite (e.g., an electrophile) capable of inducing a modification in the genome (DNA). An example of this is the metabolism of benzo[a]pyrene to a highly reactive epoxide:

Benzo[a]pyrene ⟶ benzo[a]pyrene epoxide

Phase I and phase II biotransformation reactions are mediated by enzymes located in various subcellular compartments, such as cytoplasm, mitochondria, lysosomes, and microsomes. In general, highly lipid-soluble foreign chemicals that do not resemble endogenous metabolic intermediates tend to be metabolized through the microsomal enzyme systems. On the other hand, drugs that are structural analogs of endogenous compounds compete with the latter and thus may be metabolized by microsomal and nonmicrosomal enzymes.

STRUCTURE AND FUNCTION OF MICROSOMAL CYTOCHROMES P-450

The most important and widespread enzyme system active in biotransformation reactions is that of microsomal cytochromes P-450. These electron transfer proteins contain a prosthetic group having a single iron atom coordinated to protoporphyrin IX. The prosthetic group, termed *heme*, undergoes reduction and oxidation during the catalytic cycle of the enzyme. The noncovalent binding of the heme prosthetic group with the apoprotein forms an enzyme active in oxidation-reduction reactions known as a *cytochrome*. It functions to activate molecular oxygen to a form capable of insertion into various types of chemical bonds on organic substrates. Because it is an oxygen-binding hemoprotein, cytochrome P-450 is inhibited by carbon monoxide (CO), an electronic analog of molecular oxygen. The name *P-450* derives from the spectral position of the distinctive absorbance maximum observed when the reduced enzyme is mixed with CO. Under such conditions, a maximum, or peak, is seen at 450 nm.

Cytochrome P-450 is now known to be a group of closely related proteins, rather than a single protein, which catalyze a diverse number of oxidative reactions involved in metabolism of drugs and other xenobiotics. Cytochromes P-450 and other enzymes of the drug-metabolizing microsomal system are encoded by a supergene cluster on mammalian nuclear DNA. Several distinct isoenzymes (isozymes) of cytochrome P-450 exist within the microsomal membrane. These exhibit broad and partially overlapping substrate specificities but are unique by immunologic criteria. The mix of particular cytochrome P-450 isozymes present within the microsomal membrane is subject to complex genetic and environmental regulatory influences. Effectors operate at the level of transcription through both induction and repression mechanisms, leading to marked alterations in membrane enzyme composition.

From a practical view, this means that metabolism of a given drug can be influenced by factors such as nutrition, age, presence of disease, or prior exposure to structurally related drugs. For example, such physiologic and environmental factors may cause microsomal enzyme induction resulting in more rapid metabolism of the drug. Consequently, the duration and intensity of pharmacologic action may be curtailed.

MICROSOMAL OXIDATION REACTIONS IN DRUG BIOTRANSFORMATION

Many of the reactions catalyzed by the microsomal drug metabolizing enzyme system may be classified as oxidations. These include oxygenation or hydroxylation reactions, dealkylation reactions at both carbon and nitrogen atoms, as well as a number of other types of reactions (Table 5-1). Microsomal enzymes act on a broad spectrum of

TABLE 5-1 Types of microsomal cytochrome P-450-dependent oxidation reactions

Reaction type	Chemical change	Examples
Aliphatic hydroxylation	$R \longrightarrow R{-}OH$	Pentobarbital Phenylbutazone
Aromatic hydroxylation	$Ar \longrightarrow Ar{-}OH$	Phenytoin
Epoxidation	$R_1{-}CH{=}CH{-}R_2 \longrightarrow R_1{-}\overset{O}{\widehat{CH{-}CH}}{-}R_2$	Benzo[a]pyrene Aflatoxin
N-Dealkylation	$R_1{-}\underset{\mid \atop CH_3}{N}{-}R_2 \longrightarrow R_1{-}\underset{\mid \atop H}{N}{-}R_2$	Diazepam Prazepam Methadone
O-Dealkylation	$R{-}O{-}CH_3 \longrightarrow R{-}OH$	Codeine
S-Dealkylation	$R{-}S{-}CH_3 \longrightarrow R{-}SH$	Methylthiopurine
N-Hydroxylation	$R_1{-}\underset{\mid \atop H}{N}{-}R_2 \longrightarrow R_1{-}\underset{\mid \atop OH}{N}{-}R_2$	2-Acetylaminofluorene
Sulfoxidation	$R_1{-}S{-}R_2 \longrightarrow R_1{-}\overset{O \atop \parallel}{S}{-}R_2$	Chlorpromazine
Desulfuration	$R_1{-}\overset{S \atop \parallel}{P}{-}R_2 \longrightarrow R_1{-}\overset{O \atop \parallel}{P}{-}R_2$	Parathion
Dehalogenation	$R_1{-}\overset{H \atop \mid}{\underset{\mid \atop X}{C}}{-}R_2 \longrightarrow R_1{-}\overset{H \atop \mid}{\underset{\mid \atop OH}{C}}{-}R_2 + XH$	Halothane

Note R, R_1,R_2, etc. can be alkyl, aryl, or hydrogen groups for most reaction types. Additional oxidation reactions, such as oxidative deamination, are catalyzed by FAD-containing monooxygenase.

aliphatic and aromatic structures. These diverse oxidations are catalyzed by cytochromes P-450, which activate molecular oxygen using reducing equivalents derived from NADPH. The reducing equivalents are transferred to a cytochrome P-450 through a flavoprotein known as NADPH-cytochrome P-450 reductase. These proteins are embedded within a lipid membrane which is relatively fluid, thus permitting the enzymes and lipophilic substrates to interact by diffusion.

In microsomal monooxygenase or "mixed-function oxidase" (MFO) reactions, reducing equivalents from NADPH are utilized to activate molecular oxygen, which is then incorporated into the drug substrate (e.g., as a hydroxyl group). The general stoichiometry for cytochrome P-450-linked monooxygenase reactions is

$$RH + NADPH + O_2 + H^+ \longrightarrow ROH + NADP^+ + H_2O$$

The catalytic cycle for activation of molecular oxygen by cytochrome P-450 includes several steps and is simplistically outlined in Fig. 5-1. Reducing equivalents are delivered in two separate

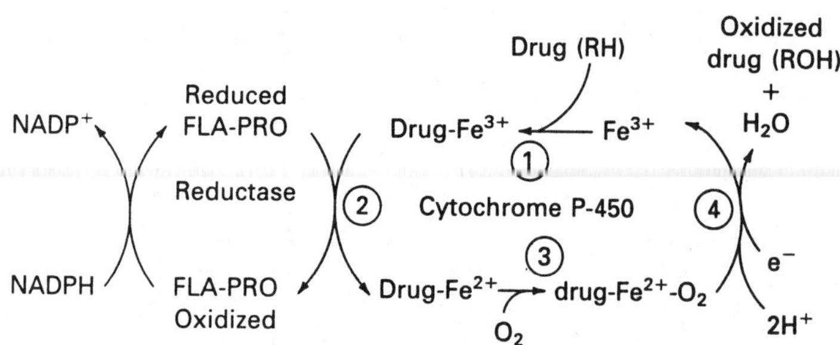

FIGURE 5-1 *Catalytic cycle for cytochrome P-450-dependent monooxygenase reactions. The sequence of steps in the hydroxylation of a drug substrate (RH) is illustrated (flavoproteins = FLA-PRO). (1) Drug binds to the oxidized heme of the enzyme; (2) the first electron from NADPH-cytochrome P-450 reductase reduces the drug-enzyme complex; (3) oxygen binds to the reduced enzyme-drug complex; (4) an intramolecular oxidation-reduction reaction forms "activated oxygen" concomitant with entry of the second electron from the reductase. This activated oxygen is inserted into the drug substrate, and the hydroxylated product (ROH) is released, regenerating the oxidized enzyme. [Adapted from White, R.E., and M.J. Coon: Annu. Rev. Biochem.* ***49****: 315-356 (1980).]*

one-electron transfer reactions from NADPH-cytochrome P-450 reductase. An enzyme-bound activated species of oxygen, possibly a free radical, is an intermediate in the cycle.

An alternative branch of the microsomal electron transport system consists of a distinct NADH-cytochrome b_5 flavoprotein reductase and cytochrome b_5. This branch of the microsomal electron transport system normally functions in fatty acid desaturation, the synthesis of long-chain unsaturated fatty acids from saturated precursors. Fatty acid desaturation requires oxygen. It can be inhibited by cyanide, but not by CO, indicating that it proceeds independently of cytochromes P-450. With certain xenobiotic substrates, however, the second electron required in the P-450 catalytic cycle can be provided by NADH, rather than NADPH, through the NADH-cytochrome b_5 reductase/cytochrome b_5 system.

The hepatic microsomal electron transport system also contains a third distinct flavoprotein known as FAD-containing monooxygenase. This enzyme, formerly known as amine oxidase, catalyzes the oxidative deamination of substituted amines, such as amphetamine, to the corresponding ketones plus ammonia. Microsomal FAD-containing monooxygenase requires oxygen and NADPH but acts independently of cytochromes P-450. It is not inhibited by CO. This enzyme also functions as a sulfur oxidase, converting thioethers to sulfoxides and sulfones. The flow of reducing equivalents through the microsomal electron transport system is shown in Fig. 5-2.

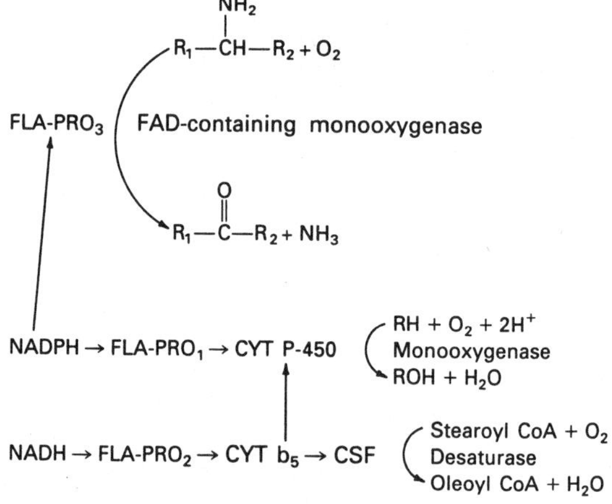

FIGURE 5-2 *Pathways for microsomal electron transport. Flow of reducing equivalents (electrons) through branches of the microsomal electron transport chain is indicated by the arrows. The various microsomal flavoproteins are designated by the abbreviation FLA-PRO. FLA-PRO_1 = NADPH-cytochrome P-450 reductase; FLA-PRO_2 = NADH-cytochrome b_5 reductase; FLA-PRO_3 = FAD-containing monooxygenase (amine oxidase); CSF = cyanide-sensitive factor of the fatty acid desaturase complex. With some cytochrome (CYT) P-450-dependent substrates, the second electron of the catalytic cycle (Fig. 5-1) can be derived from NADH, rather than NADPH, by way of cytochrome b_5.*

The utilization of oxygen by the drug-metabolizing microsomal system outlined above is mechanistically different from that of mitochondria. Microsomal electron transport results in conversion of molecular oxygen to a chemically more reactive form that is capable of condensing with an organic substrate. In mitochondrial respiration, reducing equivalents (hydrogen atoms) from substrates such as glutamate or succinate are transferred through sequential oxidation-reduction reactions to molecular oxygen, which is then reduced to water. The stepwise transfer of reducing equivalents through the mitochondrial respiratory chain catalyzed by hydrogen and electron carriers (e.g., cytochromes) is coupled to the synthesis of adenosine triphosphate (ATP) by means of an intermediate transmembrane electrochemical proton gradient. In this way, the energy of substrate oxidation is conserved as ATP. By contrast, microsomal electron transport is not coupled to ATP synthesis and thus does not conserve energy.

NONMICROSOMAL OXIDATION REACTIONS IN DRUG BIOTRANSFORMATION

Enzymes localized in subcellular compartments other than the endoplasmic reticulum also play a role in drug biotransformation. For the most part, these enzymes tend to have broad substrate specificities (Table 5-2).

1. *Alcohol oxidation* The oxidation of primary and secondary alcohols to the corresponding aldehydes is catalyzed by NAD-linked alcohol dehydrogenase. This enzyme is localized in the cytoplasm and is found predominantly in liver, with lesser amounts in kidney and lung. Hepatic alcohol dehydrogenase is responsible for the bulk of ethanol metabolism following consumption of alcoholic beverages. The enzyme exhibits reactivity with a variety of alcohols. Retinol has been suggested to be its natural endogenous substrate.
2. *Aldehyde oxidation* The oxidation of aliphatic aldehydes to carboxylic acids is catalyzed by NAD-linked aldehyde dehydrogenase. Several isozymes with different substrate preferences exist. An intra-mitochondrial isozyme having a high affinity for acetaldehyde is primarily involved in metabolism of ethanol-derived acetaldehyde, while a low affinity cytoplasmic isozyme is active in catabolism of aldehydes derived from xenobiotics and biogenic amines.
3. *Monoamine and diamine oxidation* Monoamine oxidase (MAO), a flavoprotein localized on the outer mitochondrial membrane, oxidatively deaminates short-chain monoamines (e.g., catecholamines and tyramine) to aldehydes. Short-chain amines having a methyl group on the adjacent carbon, such as amphetamine, are not substrates for MAO and are oxidized instead by the microsomal enzyme system. A distinct diamine oxidase acts on short-chain unsubstituted diamines such as histamine.
4. *Purine oxidation* Xanthine oxidase, a flavoprotein found in the cytosol, catalyzes the oxidation of xanthine to uric acid. It is also active with a number of purine derivatives, including theophylline and caffeine.

REDUCTION REACTIONS IN DRUG BIOTRANSFORMATION

Reductions are less common in biotransformation than are oxidations. Table 5-3 provides a few pharmacologically important examples. Reductions of nitro and azo groups are involved in the biotransformation of drugs such as chloramphenicol and prontosil, respectively. Microsomal cytochromes P-450-linked reductions can occur under conditions of low oxygen tension. Reductive dehalogenation reactions catalyzed by cytochrome P-450 are implicated in the toxicities of carbon tetrachloride, the pesticide DDT and the general anesthetic halothane.

The most important microsomal reduction reactions involve NADPH-cytochrome P-450 reductase. Many quinone-containing drugs can function as electron acceptors with this flavoprotein. These drugs become reduced by a single electron to give unstable semiquinone species. The latter autooxidize with molecular oxygen, forming free radicals which can potentially initiate pathologic processes, and regenerate the parent drug. Such a sequence of enzymatic reduction followed by autooxidation provides a mechanism for catalytic amplification of oxygen radical production by the drug itself. This process is referred to as redox cycling (Fig. 5-3). Cytotoxicity of the anticancer agents doxorubicin and mitomycin C

TABLE 5-2 Nonmicrosomal oxidative reactions in biotransformation

Reaction type	Chemical change	Examples
Alcohol oxidation	$RCH_2OH + NAD^+ \longrightarrow RCHO + NADH$	Ethanol Retinol
Aldehyde oxidation	$RCHO + NAD^+ \longrightarrow RCOOH + NADH$	Acetaldehyde
Monoamine oxidation	$RCH_2NH_2 + O_2 \longrightarrow RCHO + NH_3$	Tyramine Epinephrine Norephinephrine Dopamine Serotonin
Diamine oxidation	$NH_2RCH_2NH_2 + O_2 \longrightarrow NH_2RCHO + NH_3$	Histamine
Purine oxidation	$Ar(N) \longrightarrow Ar(O)$	Xanthine Theophylline

TABLE 5-3 Reduction reactions in biotransformation

Reaction type	Chemical change	Examples
	Microsomal	
Nitro reduction	$Ar—NO_2 \longrightarrow Ar—NH_2$	Chloramphenicol Clonazepam
Azo reduction	$Ar_1—N{=}N—Ar_2 \longrightarrow Ar_1NH_2 + Ar_2NH_2$	Prontosil
Reductive dehalogenation	$RCCl_3 \longrightarrow RCHCl_2$	Carbon tetrachloride DDT
	Nonmicrosomal	
Aldehyde reduction	$RCHO + NADH \longrightarrow RCH_2OH + NAD^+$	Chloral hydrate
Ketone reduction	$R_1—C(=O)—R_2 + NADPH \longrightarrow R_1—CH(OH)—R_2 + NADP^+$	Naloxone
Quinone reduction	$Q + NADPH \longrightarrow QH_2 + NADP^+$	Menadione

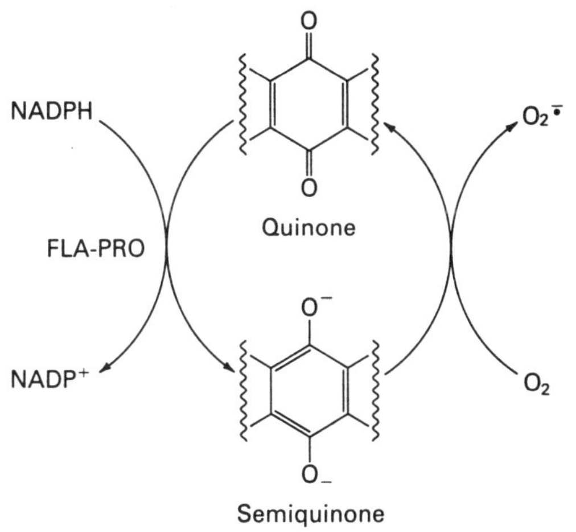

FIGURE 5-3 *Redox cycling by a quinone-containing drug. Enzymatic one-electron reduction of a quinone-containing xenobiotic catalyzed by a flavoprotein (FLA-PRO), such as NADPH-cytochrome P-450 reductase, forms an unstable semiquinone. The semiquinone undergoes autooxidation with molecular oxygen in a spontaneous nonenzymatic reaction, forming an oxygen radical (superoxide anion O_2^-) and regenerating the parent quinone. The quinone thus acts catalytically to promote the formation of oxygen free radicals which are potentially toxic. A quinone can also undergo two-electron reduction to a hydroquinone, which is often more stable than the corresponding semiquinone species. The relative formation of semiquinone and hydroquinone species is dependent on both the oxidation-reduction chemistry of the quinone itself and the catalytic mechanism of the flavoenzyme catalyzing the reduction. Redox cycling mechanisms have been demonstrated in vitro with the anticancer drug doxorubicin and the xenobiotic paraquat.*

may involve such a sequence of reactions.

Alcohol dehydrogenase, a reversible enzyme, can catalyze the reduction of chloral hydrate to trichloroethanol. Quinone reductase, a flavoprotein found in the cytoplasm of hepatocytes and formerly known as diaphorase, catalyzes the NADPH-dependent two-electron reduction of menadione (vitamin K_3) and several quinone-containing xenobiotics. Other carbonyl reductase catalyze reduction of certain aldehydic sugars (aldoses) and prostaglandins.

HYDROLYSIS REACTIONS IN DRUG BIOTRANSFORMATION

Esterases and amidases hydrolyze ester and amide groups, respectively, producing carboxylic acids (Table 5-4). These enzymes typically exhibit low substrate selectivity. They are widely distributed throughout mammalian cells and in the plasma. Recent studies have indicated that both types of hydrolytic activities are often catalyzed by the same enzyme. In most cases, amides are hydrolyzed at a slower rate than the corresponding esters.

CONJUGATION REACTIONS IN PHASE II BIOTRANSFORMATION

The coupling of endogenous small molecules with polar functional groups on a xenobiotic is termed *conjugation*. In humans, the synthesis of glucuronides is the most prevalent type of conjugation in drug biotransformation. Glucose-1-phosphate is first activated by condensation with uridine triphosphate (UTP) to form uridine diphosphoglucose (UDPG), a normal intermediate in the synthesis of glycogen. UDPG is subsequently oxidized to uridine diphosphoglucuronic acid (UDPGA) in an NAD-dependent reaction catalyzed by a specific dehydrogenase. Both of these reactions are accomplished by cytoplasmic enzymes. A microsomal glucuronyl transferase then catalyzes transfer of the glucuronic acid moiety to a polar group (often hydroxyl or carboxyl) on the drug molecule (ROH). These reactions can be described as:

$$\text{Glucose-1-P} + \text{UTP} \longrightarrow \text{UDPG} + \text{PP}_i$$

$$\text{UDPG} + 2\text{NAD}^+ \longrightarrow \text{UDPGA} + 2\text{NADH}$$

$$\text{UDPGA} + \text{ROH} \longrightarrow \text{RO-glucuronide} + \text{UDP}$$

The polar nature of the glucuronic acid residue in addition to the increased molecular weight makes the conjugated molecule to be more readily excreted than the parent drug. Glucuronyl transferase, like other microsomal enzymes, is inducible by various drugs or xenobiotics which cause proliferation of endoplasmic reticulum.

Other important, but less frequent, routes of phase II biotransformation in humans include sulfate ester synthesis, methylation, acylation, and conjugation with glutathione (Table 5-5). These reactions are catalyzed mainly by nonmicrosomal enzymes. Sulfate groups are transferred by means

TABLE 5-4 Hydrolysis reaction in biotransformation

Reaction type	Chemical change	Examples
Ester hydrolysis	$R_1\text{—}\overset{O}{\overset{\parallel}{C}}\text{—}OR_2 + H_2O \longrightarrow R_1\text{—}\overset{O}{\overset{\parallel}{C}}\text{—}OH + R_2OH$	Acetylcholine Succinylcholine Aspirin Procaine
Amide hydrolysis	$R_1\text{—}\overset{O}{\overset{\parallel}{C}}\text{—}NH\text{—}R_2 + H_2O \longrightarrow R_1\text{—}\overset{O}{\overset{\parallel}{C}}\text{—}OH + R_2NH_2$	Procainamide Lidocaine Indomethacin
Peptide hydrolysis	$-R_1\text{—}\overset{O}{\overset{\parallel}{C}}\text{—}NH\text{—}R_2\text{—} + H_2O \longrightarrow -R_1\text{—}\overset{O}{\overset{\parallel}{C}}\text{—}OH + -R_2NH_2$	Proinsulin

of an activated intermediate form, 3′-phosphoadenosine-5′-phosphosulfate, synthesized by an ATP-dependent enzyme. Sulfate is typically conjugated to hydroxyl groups on a drug molecule by a cytoplasmic sulfotransferase. Sulfation is less common than glucuronide formation in biotransformation owing to the limited availability of inorganic sulfate.

Methyl groups are transferred in the form of S-adenosyl methionine to various functional groups on xenobiotics. Nonspecific N-, O-, and S-methyl transferase enzymes, found mainly in the cytosol, are responsible for these conjugations. By contrast with other phase II reactions, methylation tends to decrease the polarity of the xenobiotic molecule.

Acylation reactions utilize coenzyme A (CoA) esters as acyl donors and commonly result in transfer of the acyl group to compounds containing amino, hydroxyl, or sulfhydryl groups. This reaction is catalyzed by various acyl transferase enzymes. Drug-acyl CoA derivatives are subsequently conjugated with amino acids such as glycine or glutamic acid prior to excretion, regenerating free coenzyme A in the process.

Coupling of glutathione, the principal sulfhydryl buffer of mammalian cells, with a drug functional group leads to the formation of thioether compounds. This reaction is catalyzed by broad-specificity glutathione-S-transferases present in liver and, to a less extent, in other tissues. The glutathione conjugates are subsequently hydrolyzed to cysteine derivatives by enzymes in the kidney. The latter are then acetylated to form N-acetylcysteine conjugates, known as mercapturic acids, which are readily excreted into the urine. Mercapturic acid formation is a frequent route for detoxication of electrophilic metabolites of xenobiotics. For example, it is the depletion of glutathione that contributes to the toxicity of acetaminophen (a widely used analgesic) following high doses. Conjugation reactions with glutathione are also involved in the synthesis of leukotrienes from endogenous arachidonic acid.

TABLE 5-5 Conjugation reactions in biotransformation

Reaction type	Enzyme	Examples
Glucuronidation	UDP-glucuronyl transferase	Bilirubin, chloramphenicol, diazepam
Sulfation	Sulfotransferases	Estrone, androsterone, acetaminophen
Acetylation	Acyl CoA transferases	Isoniazid, sulfonamides
Methylation	Methyl transferases	Norepinephrine, thiouracil
Glutathione conjugation	GSH transferases	Ethacrynic acid

RATE OF DRUG BIOTRANSFORMATION

The biotransformation of most drugs is not enzyme limited, but is proportional to the plasma concentration, a phenomenon referred to as *first-order kinetics*. Thus, an increase in plasma concentration will result in a proportional increase in the rate of drug biotransformation. However, there are notable exceptions: alcohol dehydrogenase becomes saturated at modest plasma concentrations of ethanol resulting in a constant amount of ethanol being biotranformed per unit time, rather than a constant percentage. This is referred to *zero-order kinetics*. The anticonvulsant phenytoin also demonstrates zero-order kinetics at plasma concentrations that are not markedly above therapeutic concentrations. The consequence is that small increases in exposure to the drugs can result in significant increase in plasma concentration and subsequently to an increased incidence of adverse effects.

DRUGS WITH LIMITED BIOTRANSFORMATION

Highly polar and charged compounds, such as moderately strong acids and bases, have restricted permeability through lipid membranes and consequently are not metabolized to a significant extent. Hexamethonium, a quaternary ammonium compound, is an example of a polar compound that is not biotransformed prior to excretion. Likewise, nonpolar compounds which are relatively inert and chemically unreactive are not biotransformed to a significant extent. Examples are some gaseous anesthetics such as isoflurane and halothane. These anesthetic agents are mainly excreted unchanged via the lungs, although minor amounts are metabolized through the hepatic microsomal system.

INDUCTION OF THE DRUG-METABOLIZING MICROSOMAL SYSTEM

The level of activity of the drug-metabolizing microsomal system determines the duration and intensity of pharmacologic action of many drugs due to its predominance in biotransformation reactions. One of the most important aspects of the microsomal enzyme system is its ability to be induced, or increase in activity, in response to various physiologic, pharmacologic, and environmental factors. Molecular biology has begun to unravel the mechanisms responsible for this phenomenon. As mentioned earlier, cytochrome P-450 is now known to be a group of closely related hemeproteins with overlapping substrate specificities. At least 12 species of cytochrome P-450 have been identified on the basis of DNA coding sequences as well as by immunologic and enzymatic criteria. Unique cytochrome P-450 species are involved in reactions with several aliphatic and aromatic hydrocarbons, steroids, fatty acids, ethanol, and a variety of drugs and xenobiotics.

The two most thoroughly studied inducers of microsomal drug-metabolizing enzymes are phenobarbital and 3-methylcholanthrene. These are representative of barbiturates and polycyclic aromatic hydrocarbons, respectively. Administration of phenobarbital causes proliferation of the liver endoplasmic reticulum, associated with an increase in the microsomal content (nanomoles per milligram of protein) of cytochromes P-450, and enhancement of the metabolism of a variety of xenobiotic substrates. Methylcholanthrene induces a distinct isozyme of cytochrome P-450 and elicits a different pattern of enhancement of microsomal enzyme activities compared to phenobarbital. Chronic ethanol consumption likewise induces a unique form of cytochrome P-450 which is involved in ethanol metabolism (microsomal ethanol oxidizing system, MEOS).

The molecular mechanism by which activity is induced is thought to involve binding of an inducer, commonly the substrate or drug, to a specific receptor molecule in the cytoplasm of the hepatocyte. The receptor-inducer complex is subsequently translocated into the nucleus whereupon it activates transcription of specific genes through an interaction with DNA. The mRNA transcribed from DNA is translated, leading to synthesis and incorporation of new cytochrome P-450 species into the membrane of the smooth endoplasmic reticulum. In addition, a regulatory control site, termed the A_h *locus*, is present on the DNA. This site controls transcription of several genes for related microsomal enzymes, particularly NADPH-cytochrome P-450 reductase and UDP-glucuronyl transferase, as well as the cytochrome P-450 genes themselves. Thus the induction sequence involves interaction of the receptor-inducer complex with the A_h *locus* and leads to increased amounts of the complement of microsomal enzymes. For this reason, factors such as sex (hormonal status), age, nutrition, and prior exposure to related xenobiotics can alter metabolism of a drug by changing the amount and/or relative composition of the enzymes present in the smooth endoplasmic reticulum membrane. However, the most important factor is prior exposure to the drug itself. This exposure often results in induction of the microsomal enzymes responsible for its biotransformation, thus altering its pharmacokinetics. When the enzymes responsible for biotransformation of a drug are induced, the administered drug will be metabolized more rapidly. Consequently, a normally effective dose may be completely ineffective.

ROLE OF METABOLIC EFFECTS IN DRUG-DRUG INTERACTIONS

The overlapping substrate specificities of the cytochrome P-450 enzymes and the phenomenon of enzyme induction play roles in drug-drug interactions. Exposure to one drug sometimes alters the pharmacokinetics and pharmacodynamics of a second, often structurally unrelated, drug. Induction of the microsomal drug-metabolizing system provides a molecular mechanism which can account for such a situation. That is, alteration of the content of enzymes involved in biotransformation of the second drug as a consequence of enzyme induction caused by the first drug will modify the pharmacokinetics of the second drug. A clinically important example of this concerns the action of barbiturates in alcoholics. Chronic alcohol abusers, in the absence of ethanol, show a reduced sedative effect following administration of barbiturates, due in part to an enhanced rate of barbiturate metabolism through the cytochrome P-450 system. On the other hand, nonalcoholics who become acutely intoxicated by the concomitant use of both ethanol and barbiturates show enhanced central nervous system depression. This arises from an additive sedative effect plus decreased biotransformation of the barbiturate. In this case, competition between ethanol and the barbiturate for metabolism through the microsomal system, as well as competition for reducing equivalents, slows the inactivation and elimination of both agents. There are clinically important examples of pharmacological agents whose mechanism of action is attributable to their ability to influence a biotransformation pathway: disulfiram inhibits aldehyde dehydrogenase, resulting in a very unpleasant experience in an individual who consumes ethanol; allopurinol inhibits xanthine oxidase, causing a reduced rate of uric acid synthesis and subsequently a decreased incidence of gout attacks in susceptible individuals.

ENVIRONMENTAL FACTORS IN REGULATION OF BIOTRANSFORMATION

The commonality of the enzymatic pathways involved in biotransformation of drugs and other xenobiotics may account for many drug-drug interactions observed clinically. Both direct effects, such as two agents acting as substrates for the same enzyme, and indirect effects, such as enzyme induction, can be important factors. In addition to drugs, many chemicals present in the environment are known to stimulate the activity of the hepatic microsomal system. Polychlorinated biphenyls (PCBs), a group of chemicals formally widely employed in manufacturing and electrical industries, are potent inducers of the microsomal drug-metabolizing system. Likewise, may pesticides and herbicides used in agriculture in addition to and many organic solvents used in industry are metabolized via the microsomal enzyme systems. These can function as both inducers and inhibitors of microsomal enzyme activities.

Tobacco smoke, which contains a complex mixture of hydrocarbons, including benzo-[a]-pyrene, and gases such as CO, also affect microsomal enzyme activities. For this reason, smokers may exhibit markedly different pharmacokinetic profiles as compared to nonsmokers with respect to drugs biotransformed via microsomal enzymes. Most often, smokers demonstrate enhanced rates of drug biotransformation owing to preinduction of the microsomal enzymes.

PHYSIOLOGIC FACTORS IN REGULATION OF BIOTRANSFORMATION

Physiologic factors are also clinically important for modulating drug actions. For example, newborns have low levels of drug-metabolizing enzymes and thus may be more sensitive to drugs. Likewise, liver damage makes individuals more sensitive to a variety of drugs. Obstructive jaundice, hepatitis, and cirrhosis impair the formation of glucuronide and sulfate conjugates. Thus caution should be taken in prescribing drugs for such patients.

PHARMACOGENETIC VARIANTS IN BIOTRANSFORMATION

Many enzymes involved in biotransformation exhibit substantial variation in activity levels between individuals. This phenomenon was first identified with respect to acylation reactions involved in metabolism of the antitubercular drug isoniazid. Measurements of the rate of acylation of isoniazid in various populations have demonstrated a distinct bimodal distribution of "slow" and "fast" acetylators. Genetic polymorphism has also been found for cytochrome P-450-dependent hydroxylation of debrisoquine and related drugs.

The existence of pharmacogenetic variants can account for markedly different pharmacokinetic profiles between individuals. For example, the prolonged duration of action of the normally short acting neuromuscular blocking agent succinylcholine in individuals with an atypical plasma cholinesterase. Such genetic differences illustrate the central role of biotransformation in governing pharmacologic activity. Likewise, genetic differences may result in altered metabolite profiles between individuals. Pharmacogenetic variations may also underlie, at least in part, idiosyncratic drug toxicities. For example, the trait of rapid acetylation of procainamide has been associated with the development of systemic lupus erythematosus-like conditions in some patients.

In summary, an awareness of the basic metabolic patterns involved in drug biotransformation allows the physician to employ the full spectrum of modern pharmaceutical agents to greater advantage in treatment of disease.

BIBLIOGRAPHY

Creasey, W.A.: *Drug Disposition in Humans*, Oxford, Oxford, England, 1979.

Gibson, G.C. and P. Skett: *Introduction to Drug Metabolism*, Chapman and Hall, London, 1986.

Gram, T.E., L.K. Okine, and R.A. Gram: "The Metabolism of Xenobiotics by Certain Extrahepatic Organs and Its Relation to Toxicity," *Annu. Rev. Pharmacol. Toxicol.* **26**: 259-291 (1986).

Greenblatt, D. and R.I. Shader: *Pharmacokinetics in Clinical Practice*, Saunders, Philadelphia, 1985.

Hodgson, E.: "Metabolism of Toxicants: Phase I Reactions," In E. Hodgson and P.E. Levi (eds.), *Introduction to Biochemical Toxicology, 2nd Ed.*, Appleton and Lange, Norwalk, Connecticut, 1994, pp. 75-112.

Kappus, H.: "Overview of Enzyme System Involved in Bioreduction of Drugs and in Redox Cycling," *Biochem. Pharmacol.* **35**: 1-6 (1986).

Kupfer, A.: "Genetic Differences in Drug Metabolism in Man: Polymorphic Drug Oxidation," In G. Siest (ed.), *Drug Metabolism: Molecular Approaches and Pharmacological Implications*, Pergamon, Oxford, England, 1985, pp. 25-33.

Mulder, G.J.: "Glucuronidation and Its Role in Regulation of Biological Activity of Drugs", *Annu. Rev. Pharmacol. Toxicol.* **32**: 25-49 (1992).

Nebert, D.W., and F.J. Gonzalez: "P450 Genes: Structure, Evolution, and Regulation," *Annu. Rev. Biochem.* **56**: 945-993 (1987).

Sipes, I.G. and A.J. Gandolfi: "Biotransformation of Toxicants," In Amdur, M.O., J. Doull, and C.D. Klaassen (eds.): *Casarett and Doull's Toxicology, 4th Ed.*, Pergamon Press, New York, 1991, pp 88-126.

Waterman, M.R. and R.W. Estabrook: "The Induction of Microsomal Electron Transport Enzymes," *Molec. Cell Biochem.* **53/54**: 267-278 (1983).

White, R.E. and M.J. Coon: "Oxygen Activation by Cytochrome P-450," *Annu. Rev. Biochem.* **49**: 315-356 (1980).

Whitlock, J.P.: "The Regulation of Cytochrome P-450 Gene Expression," *Annu. Rev. Pharmacol. Toxicol.* **26**: 333-369 (1986).

Zieglar, D.M.: "Recent Studies on the Structure and Function of Multisubstrate Flavin-containing Monooxygenases," *Annu. Rev. Pharmacol. Toxicol.* **33**: 179-199 (1993).

CHAPTER 6

Clinical Pharmacology

Anthony J. Piraino and Jay Roberts

Clinical pharmacology is that branch of the medical sciences which is most concerned with the rational development, the effective and safe use, and the proper evaluation of drugs in humans for the diagnosis, prevention, alleviation, and cure of disease and disease syndromes. It also involves the exploration of chemical entities other than drugs. Clinical pharmacology occupies a continuum which spans the gap between animal studies of a drug's safety (toxicology), the evaluation of its efficacy and disposition in humans, and the medical discipline of therapeutics. In a broader sense, clinical pharmacology has been identified in many contexts: as a component of preclinical and clinical drug investigations, as the initial phase of new drug development and as the entire spectrum of drug use in human subjects or patients, as well as the field of clinical pharmacy. Even veterinary medicine has some claim to the tenets of clinical pharmacology in the therapy of animal disease. While no consensus exists regarding the definition of clinical pharmacology, the importance of applying clinical pharmacological principles to achieving a rational use of drugs in both clinical and preclinical situations cannot be over-emphasized.

This chapter is devoted to those areas in pharmacology which are the special province of clinical pharmacology and therapeutics. Briefly discussed are a review of some pharmacokinetic and pharmacodynamic concepts, factors affected drug dosage in patients, and information concerning how new drugs are discovered and developed for therapeutic use.

All physicians who elect to prescribe drugs should know and apply the principles of clinical pharmacology. For this reason a modern text of medical pharmacology is also a text of clinical pharmacology. Most medical school curricula now include formal clinical pharmacology instruction in the third and fourth years of study.

ROLE OF CLINICAL PHARMACOLOGY IN THE ACHIEVEMENT OF THERAPEUTIC OBJECTIVES

The exercise of prescribing a drug to a patient implies the physician's expectation of one or more of the spectrum of effects attributable to that agent. Among the possible outcomes, the preferred outcome is a therapeutic response which often represents the most important step in achieving the desired medical objectives for that patient. Clinical pharmacology provides a rational approach to therapeutics in that, by properly applying its principles, the prescriber can improve the probability of using the right drug in the correct dosage to achieve the desired biological response in a well-defined (properly diagnosed) and well-understood disease.

Clinical pharmacology also provides a framework within which to distinguish and predict the beneficial and undesirable effects a drug may produce. Drug effects which are not among the prescriber's therapeutic goals are frequently called *side effects*. These can be unexpected or anticipated effects which are outside of the physician's main therapeutic objectives. Whether these effects are desirable or undesirable depends upon the perspective of the patient, the physician, and the extent to which they contribute to or detract from the overall goals of the therapy. For example, the antihistamine diphenhydramine is frequently used to ameliorate symptoms of seasonal allergies and the common cold. The main action of diphenhydramine is blockade of binding of histamine to receptors whose activation by histamine causes the rhinorrhea, sneezing, and upper airway irritation typical of cold and allergies. The side effects of diphenhydramine include sedation. This effect is clearly undesirable in many clinical circumstances and could interfere with a patient's ability to operate a car or perform other tasks which require alertness and quick reaction to changing conditions. However, drowsiness might be desirable for the patient experiencing cold, flu, or allergy symptoms at night which interfere with sleep. In fact, many over-the-counter sleep aids intended for the self-treatment of mild insomnia, incorporate antihistamines like diphenhydramine to take advantage of this "side effect".

A more clear cut distinction can be made between those side effects which can be beneficial and therapeutic and those which can result in toxicity. The opioid analgesic, morphine, can produce significant respiratory depression. At higher doses this effect may be life threatening. Side effects which have toxic consequences are also called *adverse reactions* or adverse experiences. Adverse reactions are most often extensions of a drug's primary pharmacologic action. Sometimes these effects are attributable to a drug's biotransformation products and are predictable on that basis. On the other hand, adverse reactions may be attributable to a patient's genetic constitution and be manifest as a hypersensitivity or drug allergy. Such *idiosyncratic* adverse drug reactions are not easily predictable under most circumstances although genetic testing and a more complete understanding of pathophysiology may help explain some of these reactions which typify the inter-individual variations in the response to a drug (see Pharmacogenetics below).

Adverse reactions which are manifest before the appearance of the drug's therapeutic response or which become the predominate effect which a patient experiences following the use of a drug usually preclude further use of that agent in that individual. Some drugs are specifically toxic to certain tissues, and this effect extends beyond their pharmacologic actions. Thus the antifungal agent amphotericin B may cause renal damage, and the antibiotic tetracycline may cause staining of the teeth when given to young children. Unfortunately, not all toxic effects can be predicted by *in vitro* or animal studies. However, it is quite certain that if a toxicity occurs in two animal species such as rats and dogs it is very likely to occur also in humans. It follows that the same general rules apply to the prediction of beneficial actions.

PHARMACOKINETICS AND PHARMACODYNAMICS

Among the topics encompassed by clinical pharmacology, *pharmacokinetics* occupies a place of particular importance. Many clinical trials are performed to enhance our knowledge of a drug's pharmacokinetics, i.e., its absorption, distribution, biotransformation, and elimination.

Pharmacodynamics, the study of a drug's mechanism(s) of action at biochemical and physiological levels, is also the topic of many important clinical investigations. A knowledge of both pharmacokinetics and pharmacodynamics is essential to the rational use of existing therapeutic agents and the design and discovery of new and better drugs.

BIOAVAILABILITY AND BIOEQUIVALENCE

Among pharmacokinetic parameters, drug absorption is frequently studied because it can vary significantly depending upon the product formulation used and the route of administration, among other things. The extent to which a drug administered by a route, other than intravenously, achieves a particular concentration in the blood is a measure of its efficiency of absorption or its *bioavailability*. A variety of factors specific to the drug's physical form (called the dosage form) including solubility, particle size, and the presence of excipients, wetting agents, etc., can influence its bioavailability. Local factors such as the time during which the drug has contact with the absorptive site are also very important. In the intestine, for example, this parameter is influenced by the tremendous surface area and by the gastrointestinal transit time. The extent to which an orally administered drug is biotransformed as it passes through the liver prior to establishing its initial presence in the blood (the so-called "first pass effect") can also influence the efficiency of absorption as measured by its bioavailability.

When a particular dosage form of a drug is produced by different processes (for example, at different manufacturing sites, or using different manufacturing or production techniques), and contain the same amount of active ingredient and are to be used for the same therapeutic purpose, the extent to which the bioavailability of one dosage form differs from that of another of the same drug must be evaluated. In the body, these dosage forms should produce similar blood, plasma, or serum concentration-time curves. The comparison of the bioavailability of two such dosage forms is called *bioequivalence*.

To determine the bioequivalence of different

preparations, three parameters are assessed: (1) the peak height concentration achieved by the drug in the dosage form, (2) the time to reach the peak concentration of the drug, and (3) the area under the concentration-time curve. Fig. 6-1 shows the three parameters used to measure bioequivalence.

In addition, the ascending limb of the curve is considered to be a general reflection of the rate of drug absorption from the dosage form. The descending limb of the concentration-time curve is a general indication of the rate of elimination of the drug from the body.

DRUG INTERACTIONS

In the United States more than 1.5 billion outpatient prescriptions are filled annually. In fact, about two-thirds of all physician visits lead to a prescription. Hospitalized patients receive, on average, fifteen drug administrations per day. It is quite common for a patient to receive two or more drugs concurrently for a variety of reasons, among them the presence of several concurrent diseases or conditions and the advantages offered by combination drug therapy in the treatment of some conditions. As the number of concomitantly administered drugs increases, the probability of an interaction increases as well. Most drug interactions probably are mild and escape notice by patient or clinicians; but there still are many which seriously affect the effectiveness and safety of the therapy, and some are even fatal. Clinical pharmacology provides a framework within which the interaction between or among drugs can be evaluated in a systematic way.

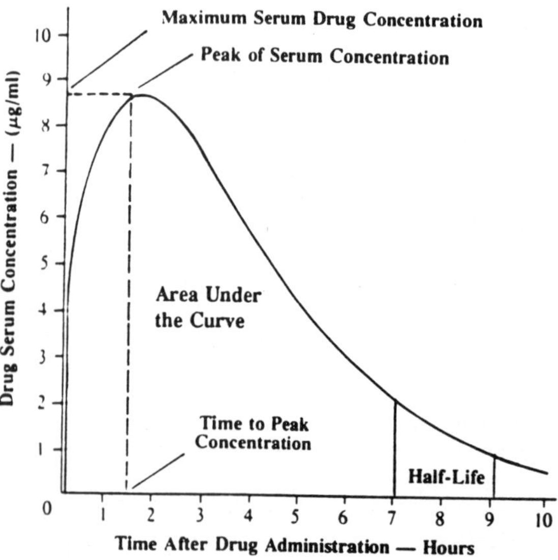

FIGURE 6-1. *Serum concentration-time curve after the oral administration of a single dose of a hypothetical drug. Shown are the 3 parameters that are measured in a study of bioequivalence: the peak serum concentration, the time to peak concentration, and the area under the concentration-time curve. [Modified from Koch-Weser, J.: N. Engl. J. Med.* ***291:*** *234 (1974).]*

The mechanisms of drug interactions are complex and varied. Although any classification suffers from oversimplification, drug-drug interactions can generally be divided into two main categories: those attributable to changes in pharmacokinetic parameters and those which are pharmacodynamic in nature. Most interactions stem from changes in pharmacokinetic modalities such as the effect of one drug upon a second with respect to its absorption, plasma protein binding, increased or decreased drug biotransformation, and factors affecting excretion such as urinary pH. In a pharmacodynamic sense, drugs may also have synergistic or additive effects which exaggerate responses or they may antagonize each other by various mechanisms involving either the same or different receptors. The best approach to understanding and predicting drug interactions is to have a working knowledge of the major mechanisms and to realize which drugs are likely to be involved. Table 6-1 summarizes the pharmacokinetic drug-drug interactions and provides several examples of each type.

Pharmacokinetic Drug Interactions

Drug Absorption Some drug interactions can advance the physician's therapeutic objectives. For example, co-administration of the vasoconstrictor, epinephrine, can limit the systemic absorption of the local anesthetic, procaine, producing a beneficial and synergistic therapeutic effect. Other drug interactions may have a negative effect upon absorption. Insoluble complexes may be formed when two drugs are given simultaneously, for example, a calcium-containing antacid which chelates with tetracycline and prevents its absorption. Antacids may also prevent the absorption of drugs which depend on an acidic pH in the stomach for absorption. Drugs such as anticholinergics and metoclopramide affect gastrointestinal motility and transit time, which may increase absorption or decrease absorption, respectively, depending upon

TABLE 6-1 Classification and examples of drug interactions involving pharmacokinetics[a]

Pharmacokinetic Parameter	Response	Example	Comment
Rate of absorption	↑	Metoclopramide and acetaminophen	Metoclopramide hastens gastric emptying
	↓	Epinephrine and procaine	Epinephrine reduces blood flow to subcutaneous and intramuscular sites of administration
Oral bioavailability	↑	Cimetidine and metoprolol	Cimetidine inhibits the metabolism of metoprolol, expressed as a reduced first-pass effect
	↓	Calcium and tetracycline	Calcium forms an insoluble, non-absorbable complex with tetracycline
Volume of distribution	↑	Aspirin and phenylbutazone	Competitive displacement from plasma (and tissue) binding sites
	↓	Quinidine and digoxin	Quinidine displaces digoxin from tissue binding sites
Hepatic clearance	↑	Phenobarbital and warfarin	Phenobarbital induces microsomal enzymes
	↓	Erythromycin and theophylline	Erythromycin inhibits the metabolism of theophylline
Renal clearance	↑	Bicarbonate and salicylates	Elevated urinary pH by bicarbonate reduces the tubular reabsorption of salicylates
	↓	Probenecid and penicillins	Probenecid inhibits the active secretion of penicillins

[a] Modified from Rowland, M., and T.N. Tozer: *Clinical Pharmacokinetics - Concepts and Applications, Second Edition*, Lea & Febiger, Philadelphia, 1989, p. 258.

the drugs. Phenytoin may inhibit the activity of specific enzymes, which may prevent the conversion of folic acid to an absorbable form, eventually causing megaloblastic anemia. Other interaction mechanisms may involve changes in intestinal flora and inhibition of vitamin K synthesis or absorption, thus influencing the production of vitamin K-dependent blood clotting factors and, consequently, anticoagulant therapy.

Protein Binding Drugs in body fluids exist in a dynamic equilibrium between the free form and that which is bound by protein components of plasma or other tissues (Fig. 6-2).

A drug bound to plasma proteins or other pharmacologically inactive tissue components is generally not available to cross membranes or exert its effect(s). In the plasma there are two primary binding proteins: albumin and alpha$_1$ acid glycoprotein. In general, acidic drugs bind to albumin; basic drugs bind to alpha$_1$ acid glycoprotein and, to a lesser extent, to lipoprotein.

These blood proteins bind nearly all drugs to varying degrees, and this binding provides the opportunity for another type of drug interaction. A second drug, which has a greater affinity for

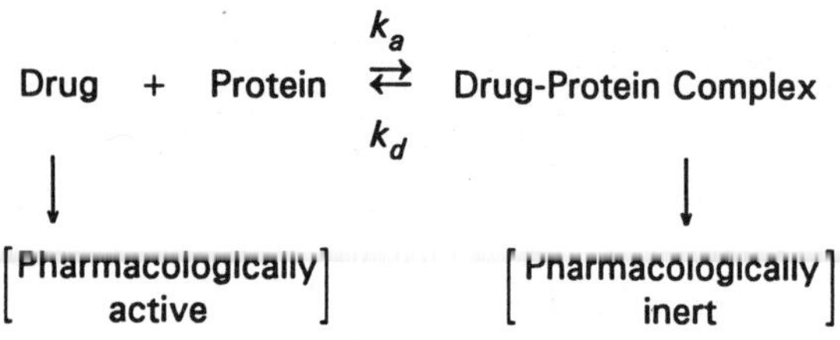

FIGURE 6-2 *The equilibrium between free and protein-bound drug, where k_a is the affinity constant and k_d is the dissociation constant.*

binding to plasma proteins, may displace the first drug. Also, because of competition for a limited number of binding sites, both drugs experience lower protein binding than that which would have been expected if each were administered individually. Consequently the free drug concentration of each agent is higher, potentially leading to a greater effect than might be expected from a particular dose of either drug (or, in some cases, increased clearance resulting in a loss of effect). An example might be displacement of the oral anticoagulant warfarin by the calcium channel blocking agent nifedipine, leading to enhanced antiprothrombin effect and perhaps bleeding tendencies. Another example is the displacement of the anticancer agent methotrexate from plasma proteins by salicylates. This has caused increased methotrexate toxicity.

Biotransformation Historically, the term *drug interaction* arose from studies which implicated the potential of one drug to influence greatly the biotransformation of another through an intermediary mechanism.

It is now known that many drugs and chemicals are capable of causing a proliferation (both in activity and quantity) of certain enzyme systems. For example, barbiturates induce the hepatic drug-metabolizing microsomal system; this may result in an accelerated biotransformation of the barbiturate itself or other drugs which are handled by this system. Consider the circumstance in which a cardiac patient is receiving both a barbiturate for sedation and an anticoagulant such as warfarin to prevent thromboembolic accidents. The dose of anticoagulant must be controlled carefully and is monitored by the prothrombin time. The addition of the barbiturate causes enzyme proliferation and activity, resulting in increased biotransformation of the anticoagulant. This in turn requires that a higher dose of anticoagulant be administered to maintain the prothrombin time within the therapeutic range. If the anticoagulant therapy continues but the barbiturate is withdrawn, the biotransformation of the anticoagulant returns to the lower, baseline level which elevates the anticoagulant concentration in the blood and its effect. If the dose of the anticoagulant is not promptly lowered, it might cause excessive and even fatal bleeding episodes. (See Chapter 5 for a discussion of the drug-metabolizing microsomal system).

It is also well known that drugs may inhibit or impede the usual functions of an enzyme or enzyme system. Cimetidine, an anti-ulcer medication, inhibits the biotransformation of a variety of drugs including theophylline, a bronchodilator used in the therapy of asthma. This interaction increases theophylline blood levels, in some cases to toxic concentrations.

Excretion *Renal Tubular Transport* In some instances a drug may inhibit the excretion of a second drug at the renal tubular level. One of the classic drug interactions is that of probenecid and its blockade of penicillin secretion. This is an example of a drug interaction which may be used to achieve a useful purpose, specifically, to increase and prolong the therapeutic blood level of an antibiotic. On the other hand, there are instances in which probenecid has produced toxic effects by causing the accumulation of a second drug. For example, indomethacin secretion is blocked by probenecid.

There are many other drugs which act on the renal tubule. It should be mentioned that dicumarol, phenylbutazone, and salicylates inhibit the excretion of oral hypoglycemic drugs, causing an excessive hypoglycemic effect.

The excretion or clearance of drugs which takes place both in the liver (via the bile) and the kidneys is another pharmacokinetic process which can present an opportunity for drug interactions.

Urinary pH and Drug Excretion Altering the pH of the urine has a profound effect on the rate of excretion of many drugs. Creation of an alkaline urine by diet or drug therapy will cause an increased excretion of phenobarbital, salicylic acid, and some sulfonamides. In fact, the excretion of most drugs that are weak acids will be increased; conversely, in acidic urine their excretion will be decreased. On the other hand, many weak bases will demonstrate an increased excretion in acidic urine and decreased excretion in alkaline urine. Examples of these drugs are amphetamine, meperidine, and quinidine.

TABLE 6-2 Examples of drug interactions involving pharmacodynamics[a]

Response	Example	Comment
↑	Chlorothiazide and digoxin	By inducing hypokalemia, chlorothiazide enhances the cardiotoxicity of digoxin
↑	Diphenhydramine and alcohol	Additive sedative effects
↓	Chlorpromazine and guanethidine	Chlorpromazine blocks the uptake of guanethidine into postganglionic sympathetic neurons
↓	Warfarin and vitamin K	Vitamin K antagonizes the anticoagulant activity of warfarin

[a] Modified from Rowland, M., and T.N. Tozer: *Clinical Pharmacokinetics - Concepts and Applications, Second Edition*, Lea & Febiger, Philadelphia, 1989, p. 258.

Pharmacodynamic Drug Interactions

Some pharmacodynamic drug interactions result from additive effects of two drugs (for example, excessive sedation caused by the administration of an antihistamine like diphenhydramine with alcohol) or antagonistic activity of compounds with opposing effects (e.g., warfarin and vitamin K). In addition, many drug interactions result from an interaction with transmitter systems. Table 6-2 shows a few examples of pharmacodynamic drug interactions.

Transmitter Mechanisms Transmitter systems consist of several elements including synthesis, storage, release, uptake, metabolism, receptor stimulation by the transmitter, and post-receptor events leading to the response. As a result there are many processes and sites where drugs can interact.

Adrenergic Mechanisms The neurotransmitter norepinephrine (NE) can participate in several possible drug interactions. There are a number of drugs which modify the metabolism of NE, i.e., monamine oxidase (MAO) inhibitors, and which are used as antidepressants. As a result of inhibition of MAO, the action of substances such as tyramine (which causes the release of NE) found in wine and cheese or the use of medications which are metabolized by MAO (e.g., phenylephrine), will be prolonged and their action potentiated. There are other drugs like tricyclic antidepressants which prevent neuronal reuptake of NE. This reuptake represents the principal means by which the action of NE is terminated at the neuroeffector junction and its inhibition prolongs the duration of action of the neurotransmitter. Using such drugs, in combination with an MAO inhibitor would markedly increase the local concentration and the effect of the neurotransmitter. It should also be noted that cocaine, which also blocks the reuptake of the neurotransmitter results in increased NE effect. Cocaine could also increase the effect of sympathomimetic amines like epinephrine which are also taken up by the adrenergic nerve terminal.

Blockers of neuronal reuptake also prevent the access of indirect acting sympathomimetic agents like tyramine (see above) or any substance that requires access into the nerve terminal to produce its effect. The effect of these agents would be decreased or abolished in these circumstances. It should be noted that the action of drugs like clonidine which is an antihypertensive agent and acts by reducing sympathetic nerve outflow, also has an independent action on the blood vessels to cause constriction. Increased circulating catecholamines, induced by the effect of tyramine, could add to the activity of clonidine resulting in a reduction of its antihypertensive effect.

Cholinergic Mechanisms When cholinergic transmission is considered, the same principles as mentioned for NE with respect to the release, storage, and receptor mechanisms are operative. However, in this case the enzymes known as the cholinesterases represent the main route of terminating the action of the cholinergic transmitter, acetylcholine (ACh). The duration of action of the neurotransmitter will be affected by agents which inhibit these enzymes. Cholinesterase inhibitors which block the degradation of ACh, are found in some pesticides and, as such, these substances may gain access to the body by penetration through the skin, by inhalation, or by oral ingestion. Cholinesterase inhibitors may cause neuromuscular paralysis and may potentiate the actions of the cholinergic neurotransmitter at other sites, e.g., in the gastrointestinal tract, heart, and glands. In addition, cholinergic toxicity is seen with the ingestion of certain varieties of mushroom in which one of the components of the mushroom (muscarine) can increase the effect of the cholinergic neurotransmitter.

Anticholinergic (or antimuscarinic) activity, i.e., antagonism of the effect of ACh, is exhibited by many drugs, e.g., meperidine, tricyclic antidepressants, diphenhydramine, and phenothiazines. Such drugs, when given in conjunction with conventional anticholinergics like atropine can produce excessive anticholinergic effects, e.g., confusion and/or urinary retention.

Neuromuscular Junction The neuromuscular junction is another example of a cholinergic transmission system where drug interactions may occur. For example, the antibiotic gentamicin may exert a blocking effect at the neuromuscular junction and, when used with inhalation anesthetics, such as halothane, may cause excessive muscle paralysis. Cholinesterase inhibitors may prolong the duration of action of the neuromuscular blocking agent, succinylcholine, because cholinesterase enzymes are needed to hydrolyze this substance and terminate its effect.

Other Neurotransmitters Drug interactions at other transmitter systems, for example the serotonergic and dopaminergic systems, also have to be taken into account since many drugs affect these. Drugs which affect dopaminergic transmission may cause an imbalance in the central nervous system, for example in the extrapyramidal system and could result in Parkinsonian symptoms and/or abnormal muscular movements, i.e., tardive dyskinesia. Certain antipsychotic drugs like the phenothiazines may produce these effects.

There are other mechanisms of drug interactions which are mentioned throughout this text. The above cited examples are some of the most frequently encountered. Fortunately, there are now many sources of drug interaction information (see Bibliography).

FACTORS AFFECTING DRUG DOSAGE

Once a particular drug is selected for a disease or disease syndrome, the determination of the dosage regimen is the next important consideration. Most dosage ranges given in standard texts are for average adults. The vast majority of all patients are well served by such ranges, but there are important modifications in particular cases that are, for the most part, dictated by factors of age, sex, pregnancy, lactation, and renal and hepatic disease.

Infancy and Childhood

Recommended doses such as those in the *United States Pharmacopoeia Dispensing Information* (USPDI) are generally intended for an adult who weighs in the neighborhood of 70 kg. It follows that a dose for an infant or child should be smaller. If weight alone is to be considered, one can easily calculate that a 3-month old infant weighing 9.5 kg should receive only 13.5 percent of the adult dose. Unfortunately, weight is not the only factor. Rate of biotransformation is higher in the young, and it is more closely related to surface area than to weight. In young patients there is also active growth and proliferation of tissues, as well as different hormonal balances. The very young are more easily dehydrated and lose electrolytes faster than the adult. Some enzyme systems are not developed until 6 months or even a year of life. Fortunately, exact doses on a milligram per kilogram basis are available for most drugs used in pediatrics, and the physician very rarely has to estimate dosage. Formulas which were developed for the adjustment of pediatric dosages relative to adult dosages are generally not reliable, and it is better to rely on specific information about the proper doses of particular drugs in children.

Elderly Patients

It is now well known that in the elderly the response to drugs may be different than those in younger groups. As exemplified in Table 6-3, the response may be due to pharmacodynamic or

TABLE 6-3 Cardiovascular drugs having an increased risk of adverse effects in the elderly[a]

Drug	Mechanism of increased risk	Pharmacokinetic changes	Pharmacodynamic changes
Antihypertensives	Pharmacodynamic	—[b]	Increased risk of postural hypotension
Digoxin	Pharmacokinetic	Decreased volume of distribution Decreased renal elimination	None
Disopyramide	Pharmacodynamic	—	Increased risk of urinary retention and glaucoma due to anticholinergic effects
Diuretics	Pharmacodynamic	—	Increased risk of hypokalemia, hyperglycemia, postural hypotension, urinary retention, or incontinence
Heparin	Pharmacodynamic [possible]	—	Increased risk of bleeding complications
Lidocaine	Pharmacokinetic Pharmacodynamic	Increased volume of distribution Increased half-life Decreased clearance	Increased sensitivity to adverse effects
Propranolol	Pharmacokinetic Pharmacodynamic[c]	Decreased hepatic elimination	Decreased response to a given IV dose of drug Greater prevalence of disease aggravated by β-blockade
Quinidine	Pharmacokinetic	Decreased renal elimination	None
Warfarin	Pharmacodynamic	None	Increased sensitivity to anticoagulant effects, possibly due to decreased vitamin K absorption

[a] Modified from Roberts, J., and N. Tumer: "Pharmacodynamic Basis for Altered Drug Action in the Elderly," *Clin. Ger. Med.* **4**: 127-149 (1988).

[b] No data available.

[c] Mechanism of lesser importance.

pharmacokinetic changes. Pharmacodynamic changes suggest that at a given site of drug action, drug-receptor interactions produce responses which may be qualitatively or quantitatively different in the elderly when compared with young individuals. A pharmacokinetic alteration may result from changes in drug disposition in older people which result in different concentrations at the site of action than in younger individuals. Such changes may result in higher concentration of drugs at the site of action and result in increased end organ response.

There are clearly major changes in distribution, metabolism, and excretion of drugs in the elderly which result in part or in whole from alteration of drug action with age. Many of these changes are associated with diseases and may not be related to the aging process. For example, a reduction in cardiac output that is observed in elderly subjects is due to latent cardiovascular disease rather than an aging effect per se. On the other hand, the diminution of kidney function seems to be more related to age than disease. Nevertheless, it is important to ascertain whether, in the elderly person, the systems that are responsible for pharmacokinetic handling of a drug have changed regardless of whether the change is the result of age or disease or some combination of the two. Changes in absorption from the gastrointestinal tract, distribution (in the elderly there is a relative increase in weight attributable to fatty tissue relative to the lean mass), hepatic metabolism, renal excretion of drugs, and in the extent of protein binding, all play a major role in determining the dose of a drug in the elderly. Information is available on the doses of a particular drug to be used in the elderly, and the reader is encouraged to consult these sources, e.g., the USPDI.

In addition to pharmacokinetic changes, major pharmacodynamic changes occur in the elderly which most often become manifested at age 70 or 75. Studies of middle age or late middle age subjects may not reveal such changes. To determine if alteration in drug action on an effector organ is due to pharmacodynamic changes it is necessary to determine whether pharmacokinetic parameters have changed. For example, recovery from succinylcholine-induced paralysis is longer in the elderly than in a young person. Because of an age-related decline in plasma cholinesterase levels, succinylcholine is biotransformed in the elderly at a slower rate (pharmacokinetics). The dose-response relationship in elderly patients, however, was found to be comparable to that observed in the younger groups (pharmacodynamics). Consequently, the alteration in drug action is due to pharmacokinetic changes. However, there are other agents such as antihypertensive drugs, barbiturates, digoxin, and morphine which show increased responsiveness in the elderly due to pharmacodynamic changes.

Gender

Gender is a factor to consider in the determination of doses of some drugs. On a weight basis alone (milligram per kilogram) there would appear to be no reason to administer drugs differently to a female than to a male. Certainly a frail 40-kg female should not receive the same dose as a robust 80-kg male. Formerly, clinical trials to determine the safety and the pharmacokinetics of drugs were performed only on healthy males. Recently the restriction on inclusion of women in these trials has been lifted and the Food and Drug Administration (FDA) is actively encouraging the inclusion of females, minorities, and elderly subjects in early drug development trials.

Gender also has an effect on drug responses, particularly with regard to pharmacokinetic changes. It is known that the male and female sex hormones affect the liver's microsomal enzymes (i.e., testosterone induces, while estrogen inhibits these drug-metabolizing enzymes). This would influence the metabolism of such drugs as barbiturates and anticoagulants. Consequently, excessive or deficient levels of sex hormones can modify a drug's effects by altering its metabolism. Alterations in the sex hormone milieu does occur with aging in both females and males.

Pregnancy and Lactation

In pregnancy there is the consideration that any drug administered to the mother is also administered to the developing fetus because many drugs cross the placental barrier. Most drugs now carry the warning "not recommended in pregnant females." Since the thalidomide episode of 1962, all drugs are suspected of being capable of causing birth defects. This is of particular importance in the first trimester of pregnancy, as it is now recognized that many drugs, including hormones and cancer chemotherapeutic agents, are definitely teratogenic. It is extremely difficult to prove that any drug is completely safe in the first trimester of pregnancy, and drug manufacturers, encouraged by the FDA, always label their drugs as contraindicated in pregnancy, especially in the first trimester. Few would dare to argue with this dictum, but on occasion, e.g., in problems of cancer chemotherapy and other serious disease syndromes, the physician must wrestle with the problem of treating the mother with obvious risk to the fetus. Certainly, there is more latitude in deciding whether or not to prescribe therapy for symptomatic relief, for example, antinausea or sedative agents, in the first trimester of pregnancy.

During lactation, most drugs will be secreted in the milk. The risk here is that treatment of the mother will also result in the drug reaching the nursing child. For example, morphine easily enters the milk supply, and an addicted mother will have an addicted nursing child. The safest rule is that any mother who needs continuing drug therapy of any type, but especially lithium or tricyclic antidepressants, should stop nursing her child. Aspirin, barbiturates, and antibiotics may be prescribed to the nursing mother in modest doses for limited periods of time without much danger. However, if serious antipsychotic therapy is to be undertaken, it would be wiser to stop the nursing.

Renal Disease, Uremia

Impairment of renal function profoundly affects the dosage used to achieve a therapeutic effect while avoiding toxicity. The interplay of altered pharmacokinetics and pharmacodynamics influences the relationship between dosage and therapeutic effect and toxicity. Obviously, the most important factor is diminished glomerular filtration and tubular secretion of unchanged drug and active biotransformation products. However, the delayed absorption, altered protein binding, impaired biotransformation, and abnormalities of distribution of drugs in the body which are characteristic of renal insufficiency all play a role in the increased incidence of adverse drug reactions observed to occur in uremic states. Many ingenious approaches to this problem have been advanced. The most practical of these relates the dosage adjustment to the estimated decrease of excretion of the unchanged drug in the impaired kidney as compared with the normal kidney. The degree of impairment of the diseased kidney is calculated from the reduction of creatinine clearance (normally 120 mL/min). This may be calculated from serum creatinine levels using available nomograms. Tables of dosage adjustments of common drugs necessary in various degrees of renal failure as measured by serum creatinine levels are also available. Package inserts also carry this information where pertinent. It is also evident that the uremic patient can benefit from more frequent measurement of serum drug levels. This is especially true for drugs which have a high risk/benefit ratio such as digitalis or aminoglycosides.

Considerations of potential toxicity require that special care be taken regarding dosage with particular drugs. In uremia, for example, anticoagulants are especially prone to cause bleeding tendencies, salicylates and other analgesics have an increased incidence of gastric ulceration, and drugs which affect potassium homeostasis, such as spironolactone, may cause hyperkalemia. Such drugs as gold, aminoglycosides, and amphotericin B, among others, are apt to be more toxic even in smaller doses.

The treatment of chronic renal failure patients using hemodialysis presents other therapeutic challenges. Drugs with low lipid solubility are easily removed by the dialysis process and require more frequent dosing to remain effective. Highly lipid soluble drugs are often not dialyzable and remain in the organism for a prolonged time after dosing. For these drugs, hemodialysis is ineffective in reversing toxicity when an overdose occurs.

Hepatic Disease

It appears reasonable to assume that a loss of liver parenchyma would lead to a decrease in the capacity of this organ to biotransform drugs. This is true only in certain instances, and it turns out in practice that such factors as protein binding and changes in distribution may be more important. The influence of liver disease on various drugs is shown in Table 6-4.

It turns out that the rate of blood flow through the liver becomes of crucial importance for drugs which experience first-pass biotransformation (see Chapter 4). Thus in heart failure or advanced cirrhosis of the liver, where blood flow through this organ is markedly impaired, drugs such as meperidine, propranolol, propoxyphene, and lidocaine may have a markedly reduced clearance. On the other hand, drugs with a much lower extraction ratio, such as warfarin and phenytoin, may not be affected very much. One of the problems which remains to be solved is an accurate measure of liver function comparable to creatinine clearance in the kidney. Unfortunately,

TABLE 6-4 Serum half-life of some drugs as affected by parenchymal liver disease

Prolonged half-life	Unchanged half-life
Erythromycin	Gentamicin
Chloramphenicol	Penicillin G
Diazepam	Digoxin
Lidocaine	Tubocurarine
Meperidine	
Prednisone	

the liver-function tests generally available in the practice of medicine correlate poorly with impairment of drug-biotransformation capacity. Unless the liver is markedly impaired, drug-biotransformation capacity does not seem to be decreased. Even so, a modest decrease in biotransformation capacity may not show any distinct changes clinically.

It is also important to consider that many drugs are inherently toxic to the liver, such as ethanol, tetracycline, and isoniazid. These drugs as well as those drugs which cause hypersensitivity like reactions in the liver, such as halothane, long-acting sulfonamides, phenytoin, and phenylbutazone, should be avoided wherever possible when impaired liver function is present.

It appears most practical to measure serum or blood levels of drugs in advanced liver disease in an attempt to avoid overt toxicity. The correlation of the clinical effect(s) with the blood level is most important as a means to adjust the dose to a satisfactory level.

Pharmacogenetics

There are hereditary factors which influence the dosage of drugs. In fact the explanation of idiosyncratic and hypersensitivity reactions resides in the different genetic constitution of individuals. Often the difference lies in an altered rate of biotransformation because of the lack of, or excess amount of, a certain critical enzyme. Some of the classical genetic defects which change drug biotransformation are listed in Table 6-5.

DRUG INVESTIGATION AND NEW DRUG DEVELOPMENT

The process through which new drugs are discovered and developed as prescription medicines is complex, expensive, and time consuming. It is estimated that for every 4000 new chemical entities which are discovered, only 7 will successfully complete preclinical testing to be studied in man. Of those 7 drugs which are evaluated in clinical trials, only 1 will become a marketed drug. The time which is typically required to get from discovery to the market is estimated to be about 12 years; the cost is estimated at $200 to $300 million. A large portion of this time and these resources are expended in performing the clinical trials which confirm the safety and efficacy of a new drug in humans.

Properly designed, properly conducted clinical trials, as will be described later, are essential to the successful development of new pharmaceuticals and many research protocols are performed in the pursuit of this objective each year. Many other clinical trials are conducted with the goal of expanding our knowledge of how new and existing drugs interact with organs, organ systems and the organism *in toto* in their therapeutic application.

Statistics

A mandatory feature of the design of any protocol for drug investigation is the assurance of the statistical validity of the results. This starts with insistence on *random selection* of subjects and the enrollment of appropriate number of individuals based on the estimated probability of securing a statistically valid result. In an all-or-none situation (cure of a bacterial infection which is ordinarily incurable) a small number of subjects would suffice. In the study of an analgesic which relieves pain in only 20 percent of patients, many hundreds of subjects might be needed to prove efficacy. In epidemiologic studies of a drug to prevent coronary thrombosis, thousands of subjects and years of study would be required to secure conclusive results. Large and complex studies, as a consequence, require that a statistician be part of the research team.

Clinical drug development trials are designed to evaluate, in an unbiased way, the safety, tolerability, and efficacy of new pharmaceutical agents. As a general rule, the subject is administered two different treatments, one of which is the test substance, the other of which is an inert dosage form or placebo (see below). These two dosage forms are typically administered to each subject in separate identical visits. The placebo which usually consists of lactose powder is prepared in a dosage form (e.g., capsule, tablet, elixir) exactly matched to the test material. To preserve the objectivity of the subjects participating in reporting their responses in these trials and the objectivity of the investigator evaluating them, clinical trials are often performed using a *single blind* or a *double blind* design. In a single blind clinical trial, the subject is not informed by the investigator as to the sequence of administration of the test substance and placebo. In a double blind design, neither the test subject or the investigator know the order of administration. Blinding the subject to the order in which the test medication and placebo are administered makes it less

TABLE 6-5 Some examples of genetic defects which modify drug biotransformations

Enzymatic reaction	Examples of drugs involved	Effect
Glucose-6-phosphate dehydrogenase deficiency in erythrocytes	Acetylsalicylic acid Nitrofurans Para-aminosalicylic acid Primaquine 8-Aminoquinolines Quinidine Sulfonamides	Acute hemolytic anemia
Glucuronyl transferase deficiency (found in Crigler-Najjar syndrome and newborn infants)	Chloral hydrate Codeine Chloramphenicol Indomethacin Morphine Nicotinic acid Probenecid	Exaggerated drug toxicity
δ-Aminolevulinic acid (ALA) synthetase stimulation	Barbiturates Chloroquine Estrogens Griseofulvin Sulfonamides	Acute intermittent porphyria
Pseudocholinesterase abnormality or deficiency	Succinylcholine	Prolonged apnea
Acetylase deficiency	Isoniazid	Peripheral neuropathy
Methemoglobin reductase deficiency	Chloroquine Dapsone Primaquine	Methemoglobinemia

likely for spurious subjective reactions to be attributed to the study drug.

A particularly valuable technique to ensure reliability of results is the *crossover design*. Here the experimental and the control groups are exchanged once a therapeutic endpoint has been obtained. Thus each subject serves as his or her own control in addition to a comparison with the whole group.

The use of a placebo as a comparator for these crossover design drug studies helps to delineate those effects which are more likely the consequence of dosing with the study medication. However, this is not to say that a placebo is without its own measurable pharmacologic effects.

Placebo Effect

Early in this century it was realized that certain drugs which had been used for years for specific conditions actually had no pharmacologic effect when studied objectively. *Placebo* is a Latin verb meaning "I shall please". The *placebo effect* may or may not occur and is defined as the psychological or physiologic effect of a therapeutic drug or procedure which is not related to its specific pharmacologic activity. Many observers believe that the placebo effect can be explained by a psychological mechanism. Experienced clinicians are well aware that many therapeutic effects are the results of a good sales talk and a pat on the back.

More recently, however, the elucidation of receptor theory and its association with therapeutic analgesia has demonstrated that, at least in pain management, the placebo response **is** a pharmacologic effect produced by the interaction of endogenous analgesic substances with a specific receptor, the same receptor with which morphine interacts to produce pain relief. The production, release, and receptor binding of these endogenous substances can be initiated by a variety of neural stimuli. For example, electrical stimulation of discretely distributed loci in the brain elicits analgesia which lasts for several hours. Three groups of endogenous analgesics have been identified: enkephalins, dynorphins and ß-endorphin. These substances each have their own anatomic distribution within the central nervous system. Neurons containing enkephalins and dynorphins frequently terminate in synapses which contain opioid (morphine) receptors. It is also interesting to note that in some clinical studies, administration of an antagonist of opioid analgesics, naltrexone for example, was able to block the pain relief which resulted from release of these endogenous analgesic substances just as it antagonizes the effect of morphine. Other possible placebo effects may exist and the responses which placebos produce are often highly variable among individual patients.

In any population some individuals are more susceptible to placebos than others. It must also be pointed out that while a greater number respond to a placebo with positive effects there are a minority who react negatively. Double blind and single blind studies help to identify placebo effects because the patient does not know when he or she is receiving the active ingredient or the placebo.

NEW DRUG DEVELOPMENT

Once a new chemical entity or an older established drug with a new indication has been studied in a variety of animal species and a distinctly favorable benefit/risk ratio is anticipated with the expectancy of low toxicity, it is desirable to study the compound in humans. How to do this safely has been the subject of much investigation. Furthermore, the study of new drugs in humans must be performed in a meaningful and statistically valid manner. Some standard techniques (e.g., single and double blind studies) have been adopted which lessen the risk and make the probability of useful results more likely.

Animal versus Human Dose

One of the main problems in the initial human trials of a new drug is to extrapolate the first dose to be used from the data obtained in animal studies. These data predict the quantitative and qualitative effects that may be expected from a compound. The basis of extrapolation is a comparison of animal species with regard to their body weights, metabolic rates, and rates of drug metabolism. One current conversion technique employs body surface area to establish comparable dosages between animal species. A conservative approach in determining the first dose to be administered to humans is recommended because of possible unexpected reactions. These include idiosyncrasy, hypersensitivity, effects on specific brain centers, blood and bone marrow disturbances, and unusual metabolic actions. Usually, based on the data from acute animal toxicity studies, logarithmically increasing doses of the agent are administered to the selected animal to obtain the minimum effective dose. From these data are made estimates of the therapeutic index and therapeutic range. For example, perhaps a parasympathomimetic agent is studied in a group of animals; the dose-response relationship is as follows:

mg/kg dose	Pharmacologic response
2.5	No effect
5.0	Mild diarrhea
10.0	Bradycardia
20.0	Hyperpyrexia and achromodacryorrhea

The initial single human dose would be a fraction of the minimum effective dose, which in this example is 5.0 mg/kg. If the rat were the test animal, a safe arbitrary suggestion might be 1/200 of this dose as the total single initial dose for an average-size (70 kg) human, using the same route of administration. If the dog were the test animal, then 1/10 of this minimum effective dose might be used.

Although mice, rats, rabbits, cats, and dogs are the animal species generally used, it is highly desirable to study nonhuman (monkey) and subhuman (orangutan or baboon) primates because of their physiologic similarity to humans. Here, one-half the minimum effective dose might be used in the initial human studies.

If an atropine-like agent is studied in certain rodents, a much smaller fraction of the minimum effective dose would be used in humans, since the rodent is resistant to compounds having atropine-like structures, and consequently, humans can be expected to be more sensitive. Such preclinical evaluations are important considerations.

Single-Dose Methodology

When there is no detectable response in the human to the initial dose (based on the estimated dose suggested by the preceding considerations), the dose is slowly increased until a response appears. The response may or may not be the anticipated one, but all subjective and objective reactions are recorded. A second subject is given the same dose, and the reactions are again observed and recorded. When there is no response to these initial human trials using the estimated dosage, the dose is slowly increased until drug activity is manifested. Once this minimum effective dose has been determined, the dose is further increased to establish the maximum tolerated dose, or the dose which does not elicit undesirable effects. No individual should be exposed to more than a single dose in a short period of time. Usually, a rest period of at least 1 week between subsequent doses is allowed to prevent cumulative effects.

Single Blind and Double Blind Format

When evaluation of drug efficacy involves personal judgment, either subjective on the part of the patient or objective on the part of the investigator, further controls are necessary to prevent bias. This is particularly true for such drugs as analgesics, sedatives, antianginals, or tranquilizers, which are usually evaluated by their subjective effects. Even in diseases with such objective signs as hypertension, patient reassurance alone may produce a therapeutic effect and thereby mask the effect of the test substance. Because of psychological influences, proper control is often difficult to achieve. Transference and counter transference between the enthusiastic investigator and subject or patient may lead to a variety of results. To avoid these bias factors, statistical techniques are employed and blinding as described above becomes necessary. When a completely dispassionate evaluation is needed, a double blind trial is performed. In blinded trials all material is coded, including the test substance and a placebo and, if possible, an already known active substance therapeutically similar to the one being tested (standard reference or positive control). Occasionally, negative controls are used to duplicate certain side effects to prevent identification of the test substance. For example, quinine may be used to mimic the taste of a bitter substance. Obviously, the physical appearance and manner of handling the materials should render them indistinguishable.

THE ROLE OF THE FOOD AND DRUG ADMINISTRATION IN NEW DRUG DEVELOPMENT

In the United States, the Food and Drug Administration (FDA) is the federal agency responsible for regulating investigational drug studies in humans and for determining the adequacy of pharmacologic, animal-toxicologic, and manufacturing-control information for new pharmaceuticals before and during clinical trials. The FDA also determines whether the drug development plan for a new compound is adequate and whether the design of specific clinical trials in that plan is appropriate in relation to the objectives listed and questions asked in the studies.

A pharmaceutical company, as the sponsor, who intends to conduct clinical trials on a new drug, or a new dosage form of an already marketed drug, will request an *Investigational New Drug Application* (IND) from the FDA. The agency reviews this application, which consists of all the preclinical data on the proposed new drug, over the 30 day period after it is submitted. If the sponsor receives no response from the FDA within this review period, the proposed clinical research program may begin. It is not the function of the FDA to approve an IND, but after review, the agency may elect to disapprove the application for cause. The primary focus of this review process is to confirm the safety of the compound and to ensure that subjects of the clinical trials testing are not exposed to undue risks.

In an effort to shorten and streamline the drug approval process the FDA, in March 1987, introduced new regulations known as the *IND rewrite* which defined the four phases of clinical investigation (see below) used to study new drugs. These phases overlap each other and are designed to progressively reveal the drug's beneficial and adverse properties. In addition, the rewrite more clearly defined the clinical investigator's responsibilities during the investigational phase of drug development and strengthened communication between the FDA and the pharmaceutical sponsors of clinical trials.

Upon completion of the first three phases of clinical investigations for a new drug, the sponsor submits the results to the FDA in order to receive approval to market that agent as a prescription drug in the United States. The package submitted by the sponsor is embodied in a *New Drug Application* (NDA). The NDA package, which frequently consists of many volumes of clinical trial data, is carefully reviewed by the FDA. The review process typically involves FDA scientists and professionals including physicians, pharmacologists, chemists, pharmacokineticists, biometricians, and where applicable, microbiologists. In important or difficult cases, the NDA may be presented to an advisory committee of extramural experts. These experts may or may not approve the drug for marketing, or they may suggest additional studies to be done.

The protocol for the study of a new drug in humans differs depending on the compound and its purported pharmacologic activity. For example, Phase I studies which customarily involve healthy males could not be used in the development of oncology drugs due to the potential toxicity of the investigational agent. In this instance a population of selected cancer patients would be studied. In general, however, four phases of clinical investigations are conducted.

Phase I

In this phase, small numbers (20 to 80) of human volunteers, usually healthy with no disease syndrome, are given single doses of the drug. In 1993 the Food and Drug Administration lifted its 1977 policy of excluding women of child-bearing potential from participating in early-phase clinical trials. The FDA maintains that women are underrepresented in the approval process of many new drugs where there might be specific gender differences in the indications for use, the use of concomitant medications, pharmacodynamic data, or pharmacokinetic data. Carefully selected patients may also be used in Phase I studies. This is typically the case in the evaluation of drugs for treatment of life-threatening illnesses like cancer or acquired immunodeficiency syndrome (AIDS) but otherwise this is the exception, not the rule. Careful pharmacodynamic and pharmacokinetic studies are done in Phase I. The aim is to establish a minimum effective dose to achieve activity without significant adverse reactions. Often, Phase I studies also seek to identify the maximum tolerated doses of drugs. If the drug being developed is likely to be used chronically, then after single-dose parameters have been established, it may be given chronically to simulate the therapy of a disease situation and thus to determine its feasibility for chronic usage. If after these studies the drug shows promise and no serious or unexpected adverse reactions become evident in the anticipated dosage range, then with the approval of the FDA the development plan may proceed to phase II.

Phase II

In phase II, small numbers of patients are selected with the symptoms or diseases for which the drug is purported to be effective. A clinical trial design is established which aims to conclusively demonstrate efficacy in relation to safety. Again, the design may follow a single blind or a double blind format or indeed any rational approach indicated for a particular drug or disease. As new data accumulate from human trials, ongoing chronic toxicity studies in animals are also conducted. Additional metabolic and pharmacokinetic studies may also be performed. If the drug is to be used for long periods of time in females, special studies of its effects on reproduction and fertility are necessary to rule out teratogenic effects. Usually there will be a stage late in phase II at which findings are finalized and any additional observations are performed which are believed to be important.

Phase III

If the drug survives phase II, then, with the approval of the FDA, phase III may be initiated. This is actually a program of broad clinical trials each employing a large sample of specified patients. Here the attempt is to prove efficacy in the patients for whom the drug would be indicated. The investigation is usually performed by a number of different clinicians in different medical centers or even under actual medical practice conditions. Phase III clinical trials are designed to be rather restrictive about the test conditions in order to control variability. Dosage forms, methods, and routes of administration are clearly defined. As in all preceding phases, the phase III clinical development plan must be approved by the FDA, and any toxicity must be immediately reported. The battery of clinical trials which constitute Phase III usually require from 1 to 3 years to complete.

Following the collection and documentation of all data in humans which culminate in the filing of the NDA, the FDA may allow the drug to be marketed for specified therapeutic purposes and applications. In most instances, clear proof must be advanced that the new drug is superior to an established product of the same therapeutic class.

Phase IV

Phase IV clinical studies are initiated following the FDA's approval of the NDA. It is through this mechanism that pharmaceutical companies and the FDA are able to obtain new information about recently approved, newly marketed drugs. Unlike earlier clinical trials, post-approval testing is not usually required by the FDA, but is initiated by the sponsor to gain more data on the safety and effectiveness of the drug. There are, however, specific instances when the FDA will request Phase IV clinical studies. For example, when pharmaceutical companies manufacture drugs approved as part of the accelerated development program to treat life-threatening and seriously debilitating conditions, post-marketing studies to delineate additional information about the drug's benefits, risks and optimal use may be requested. In 1987 the FDA changed the regulations to make available promising new drugs to patients who are desperately ill where no satisfactory alternative therapy exists. The initiation of the *Treatment IND* allows these patients the benefit of therapy while clinical development and agency review proceeds.

Table 6-6 is a flow chart which summarizes the phases of new drug development. It is estimated that up to 12 years is required to introduce a new drug for use in humans. The length of time required to develop and approve new pharmaceuticals in the United States has given rise to criticism that there is a drug lag in the United States as compared with other countries because of the more stringent requirements of the FDA in this country. In the case of drugs being developed for life-threatening illnesses (like AIDS), where no satisfactory alternative treatment exists, drug development has been accelerated by the use of parallel track clinical trials and a variety of treatment protocols. Whether the benefits of expediting the investigation and development of such new pharmaceuticals outweighs the risks to the patients participating in these trials is yet to be determined. In general, however, despite the high cost and long time frame required to develop new drugs, it is not likely that there will be a lessening of vigilance in the introduction of new drugs in the United States.

ETHICS OF DRUG INVESTIGATION IN HUMANS

In view of the inevitable toxicity of drugs, it might well be asked, "What are the moral and humanistic aspects of human investigation?" Obviously, when the only object of administering a drug is an attempt to alter a course of a usually or uniformly fatal disease, considerable toxicity may be justified, for example, in cancer chemotherapy or in the treatment of AIDS. However, systematic medical research may not have as its sole or even major aim the cure of immediate disease but the explanation of mechanisms which may later lead to beneficial therapeutic agents. Under what conditions may an individual then serve as a subject in a clinical trial? The code laid down in 1947 by the judges of the Nuremberg Military Tribunals for War Criminals following the atrocities of World War II still stands as a classic document. It clearly states the principles which are still followed today:

1. The voluntary consent of the human subject is absolutely essential.

   This means that the person involved should have legal capacity to give consent; should be so situated as to be able to exercise free power of choice, without the intervention of any element of force, fraud, deceit, duress, over reaching, or other ulterior form and constraint or coercion; and should have sufficient knowledge and comprehension of the elements of the subject matter involved to enable him to make an understanding and enlightened decision. The latter element requires that before the acceptance of an affirmative decision by the experimental subject, there should be made known to the subject the nature, duration, and purpose of the experiment; the method and means by which it is to be conducted; all inconveniences and hazards reasonably to be expected; and the effects upon his/her health or person which may possibly come from his/her participation in the experiment.

TABLE 6-6 The controlled clinical trial as a means of developing a new drug in humans

Start

2 to 3 years

Phase I.

Cautious administration to human volunteers, and in specific cases patients, to determine pharmacologic activity and pharmacokinetics. Usually done by clinical pharmacologists in a research setting.

1 to 2 years — Phase II.

1. Early: Selection of few patients with appropriate disease syndrome. Determination of potential usefulness and dosage ranges. Review of finding by experts. Performance of additional studies in animals as indicated by findings. Special toxicity studies if indicated.
2. Late: Larger number of clinical patients. Further determination of activity and toxicity. Longer periods of therapy. Review of data by experts.

1 to 2 years

Phase III.

Clinical trial in selected centers. May have to be set up as blind or double blind with randomized selection of patients and controls, depending on the nature of the drug. Determination of safety and efficacy under various clinical situations. This phase is usually performed by physicians who are experts in their selected field.

1 to 3 years — Phase IV.

1. Approval of NDA by the FDA for marketing. Efficacy and safety of the drug still has to be followed carefully by the manufacturer, who reports periodically to the FDA. Drug may be withdrawn if unexpected undue toxicity becomes evident.
2. Conditional approval. The drug may be released only for limited use in selected patients under strict post-market surveillance by physicians agreeing to participate in the study.

Review of findings and decision to continue marketing.

The duty and responsibility for ascertaining the quality of the consent rests upon each individual who initiates, directs, or engages in the experiment. It is a personal duty and responsibility which may not be delegated to another with impunity.

2. The experiment should be such as to yield fruitful results for the good of society, unprocurable by other methods or means of study, and not random and unnecessary in nature.

3. The experiment should be so designed and based on the results of animal experimentation and a knowledge of the natural history of the disease or other problem under study that the anticipated results will justify the performance of the experiment.

4. The experiment should be so conducted as to avoid all unnecessary physical and mental suffering and injury.

5. No experiment should be conducted where there is *a priori* reason to believe that death or disability injury will occur.

6. The degree of risk to be taken should never exceed that determined by the humanitarian importance of the problem solved by the experiment.

7. Proper preparations should be made and adequate facilities provided to protect the experimental subject against even remote possibilities of injury, disability, or death.

8. The experiment should be conducted only by scientifically qualified persons. The highest degree of skill and care should be required through all stages of the experiment of those who conduct or engage in the experiment.

9. During the course of the experiment the human subject should be at liberty to bring the experiment to an end if he has reached the physical or mental state where continuation of the experiment seems to him to be impossible.

10. During the course of the experiment the scientist in charge must be prepared to terminate the experiment at any stage, if he/she has probable cause to believe, in the exercise of the good faith, superior skill, and careful judgement required of him/her that a continuation of the experiment is likely to result in injury, disability, or death to the experimental subject.

Since this code was promulgated, other declarations have been published. The American Medical Association affirmed the concepts of consent, competence, and care. The British Medical Association, the Medical Research Council, and the World Medical Association have issued guidelines for conduct of experimentation not essentially different in principle. The World Medical Association approved the Declaration of Helsinki in 1964, which established a code of ethics for guiding physicians in biomedical research that involves human subjects:

> "In the field of clinical research, a fundamental distinction must be recognized between clinical research in which the aim is essentially therapeutic for a patient, and clinical research, the essential object of which is purely scientific and without scientific value to the person subjected to the research."

The declaration asserts that where research is combined with professional care:

> "If at all possible, consistent with patient psychology, the doctor should obtain the patient's freely given consent after the patient has been given a full explanation."

The Helsinki declaration is the current *vade mecum* to guide us through the ethical maze.

In addition, there are the elements of informed consent in the FDA regulations (Title 21 of the Code of Federal Regulations Part 50.25). This regulation states that investigators must inform any human being used in the tests or controls that the agent is being used for investigational purposes; it also states that investigators will obtain the informed consent of such individuals or their representatives.

In all human drug studies performed under a government contract or grant (for example, the National Institutes of Health), and in order to comply with the more recent regulations of the FDA, there is the additional requirement that the study be approved by a human research review committee often called Institutional Review Board (IRB). Such a committee must be composed of at least 5 members with varying backgrounds, i.e., impartial scientists, clinicians, and lay people from the community. Individuals of different, non-medical vocations, for example, lawyers, members of the clergy, or homemakers would be among those who could serve in this capacity. Full disclosure of the drug's chemical and biologic background to the IRB is required. The risks to the human subjects relative to the benefits, both to the individual and society, of participating in a trial are estimated, responsibility for the conduct of the investigation is established, and it is determined that the facilities available for the investigation are adequate and ensure safety. The use of consultants to the IRB is sometimes necessary in cases where the research under consideration is outside the expertise of the IRB's regular membership. Disclosure of the risk involved to the volunteer is mandatory as part of the process of obtaining the informed consent of each participant. The informed consent process which must be performed by the investigator or his/her designee may be witnessed and supervised by the IRB if deemed appropriate or necessary. The IRB carefully reviews the protocol of the proposed investigation. The IRB is also empowered to perform surveillance of the conduct of the investigation and the facility in which it is performed to ensure that both are satisfactory. Investigators must periodically report the progress and/or results of the approved investigation for the IRB's review. Of course any toxicity observed by the investigator or that which becomes known to the investigator from the work of others must be immediately reported to the committee. The work of IRBs becomes more difficult as ethical questions arise which in the past were not even considered. For example, who pays for therapies and diagnostics which are clearly experimental? Is it ethical to have a washout period in testing a new antiarrhythmic agent when the standard drug is effective and the arrhythmia might be lethal? What is the appropriate pay for volunteer subjects to fairly compensate them for their time and cooperation but not to encourage them unduly to submit to participate in a research project? When a tissue is obtained from a donor, who owns it? This is especially important when the tissue is put to a profitable use, the development of a new drug or therapy, for example.

These and other issues challenge the discipline of clinical investigation. With the rising cost of health care the public seriously questions the increasing cost of developing new drugs and therapies. In addition, litigation over drug toxicity is growing. It is estimated that approximately 20 percent of all hospital admissions are attributable to adverse drug reactions and that up to 15 percent of all hospitalized patients experience an adverse reaction to drug(s) they received while hospitalized. Thus the societal function of clinical pharmacology is not only the development of new and better drugs but also to contain their cost and most of all to ensure their safety.

FATE OF MARKETED DRUGS

Results of the experimental and clinical evaluation of new drugs often become well publicized and may have a tremendous influence on a drug's use and its sales. The clinical results obtained by practicing physicians using a new drug after its approval for marketing may or may not match those obtained under experimental conditions. In order to be widely prescribed and hence successful in the marketplace, a new drug must offer a therapeutic advantage over drug already available, otherwise physicians may become reluctant to use the new product and third party payers (health insurance/maintenance organizations) may disallow its use by their policy holders. Keen competition among over 1000 manufacturers in the pharmaceutical industry ensures that research programs will be constantly initiated and intensified to develop innovative products which fill unmet medical needs, but newer pharmaceuticals are more expensive to develop than their predecessors and the higher costs of these prescription medicines to the consumer has been cited as a significant factor in the rising cost of health care. However, within the overall context of medicine, new drugs, even if expensive, are a good value because their use makes it possible, in many cases, to avoid even more expensive medical intervention like invasive procedures, surgery, and hospitalization. For these reasons and others, using drugs remains one of the most cost effective modalities available in health care.

BIBLIOGRAPHY

Drug Evaluations Annual 1993, prepared by the Department of Drugs, Division of Drugs and Toxicology, American Medical Association, Milwaukee, 1993.

Bennett, W.M., and S.K. Swan: in E. Rubenstein and D.D. Federman (eds.), *Drug Therapy in Renal Disease in Scientific American Medicine,* Appendix A, Scientific American, New York, 1992.

Blaschke, T.F.: in E. Rubenstein and D.D. Federman (eds.), *Pharmacokinetics and Pharmacoepidemiology in Scientific American Medicine*, Appendix A, Scientific American, New York, 1986.

Branch, R.A., and R. Johnston: "Therapeutic Advisory Program: An Opportunity for Clinical Pharmacology," *Clin. Pharmacol. Ther.* **43**: 223-227 (1988).

Code of Federal Regulations, Title 45, Public Welfare. Department of Health and Human Services National Institutes of Health, Office for Protection from Research Risks, Part 46-Protection of Human Subjects, Revised June 18, 1991, Appendix 4.

DiGregorio, G.J., E.J. Barbieri, A.P. Ferko, G.H. Sterling, J.F. Camp, and M.F. Prout.: *Handbook of Pain Management, Fourth Edition*, 1994, pp. 9-13.

Dollery, C.T.: "The Future of Clinical Pharmacology and Therapeutics," *Clin. Pharmacol. Ther.* **41**: 1-2 (1987).

Eighteenth World Medical Assembly Helsinki, Finland, June 1964.

Kaitin, K.I., N.R. Bryant, and L. Lasagna: "The Role of the Research-Based Pharmaceutical Industry in Medical Progress in the United States," *J. Clin. Pharmacol.* **33**: 412-417 (1993).

Kaitin, K.I., B.W. Richard, and L. Lasagna: "Trends in Drug Development: The 1985-86 New Drug Approvals," *J. Clin. Pharmacol.* **27**: 542-548 (1987).

Koch-Weser, J.: "Drug Therapy: Bioavailability of Drugs," *N. Engl. J. Med.* **291**: 233-237 (1974).

Lind, S.E.: "Can Patients Be Asked to Pay for Experimental Treatment?," *Clin. Res.* **32**: 393-398 (1984).

Martin, E.W.: *Hazards of Medication, Second Edition*, J.B. Lippincott Company, Philadelphia, p. 371 (1978).

McMahon, G.F.: "Does Your Institutional Review Board Review Advertising for Recruits?", *Clin. Pharmacol. Ther.* **43**: 1-3 (1988).

Merkatz, R.B., R. Temple, S. Sobel, and D.A. Kessler: "Women in Clinical Trials of New Drugs: A Change in FDA Policy," *New Engl. J. Med.* **329**: 292-96 (1993).

Niebyl, J.R.: *Drug Use in Pregnancy, Second Edition*, Lea & Febiger, Philadelphia, 1988.

Nierenberg, D.W., and K.L. Melmon: "Introduction to Clinical Pharmacology," *Clinical Pharmacology - Basic Principles in Therapeutics, Third Edition*, in K.L. Melmon, et al., editors, New York, 1992, pp. 1-51.

Piraino, A.J.: "Why New Drugs Are So Expensive," *Philadelphia Medicine* **86**: 322-326, (1990).

Riedenberg, M.M.: "The Discipline of Clinical Pharmacology," *Clin. Pharmacol. Ther.* **38**: 2-5 (1985).

Roberts, J., and N. Tumer: "Age and Diet Effects on Drug Action," *Pharmacol. Ther.* **37**: 111-149 (1988).

Roberts, J., and N. Tumer: "Pharmacodynamic Basis for Altered Drug Action in the Elderly," *Clin. Ger. Med.* **4**: 127-149 (1988).

Rowland, M. and T.N. Tozer: "Interacting Drugs," *Clinical Pharmacokinetics - Concepts and Applications, Second Edition*, Lea & Febiger, Philadelphia, 1989, pp. 255-275.

Spector, R., G.D. Park, G.F. Johnston, and E.S. Vessell: "Therapeutic Drug Monitoring," *Clin. Pharmacol. Ther.* **48**: 345-353 (1988).

Speight, T.M.: "Principles and Practice of Clinical Pharmacology and Therapeutics," *Avery's Drug Treatment, Third Edition*, Williams and Williams, Baltimore, 1987.

Trials of War Criminals before the Nuremberg Military Tribunals under Control Council Law No. 10, Vol. 2, U.S. Government Printing Office, Washington, D.C., 1949. pp. 181-182,

Tsujimoto, G., K. Hashimoto, and B.B. Hoffman: "Pharmacokinetic and Pharmacodynamic Principles of Drug Therapy in Old Age. Part 2," *Int. J. Clin. Pharm., Ther., and Tox.* **27**: 102-116 (1989).

Tumer N., P. . Scarpace, and D.T. Lowenthal.: "Geriatric Pharmacology: Basic and Clinical Considerations," *Annu. Rev. Pharmacol. Toxicol.* **32**: 271-302 (1992).

Vesell, E.S.: "Clinical Pharmacology: A Personal Perspective," *Clin. Pharmacol. Ther.* **38**: 603-612 (1985).

Weinshilbaum, R.M.: "The Therapeutic Revolution," *Clin. Pharmacol. Ther.* **42**: 481-484 (1987).

PART II

The Autonomic Nervous System

SECTION EDITOR

Edward J. Barbieri

CHAPTER 7

Introduction to the Autonomic Nervous System

Domenic A. DeBias

GENERAL CONSIDERATIONS

The autonomic nervous system provides an important means whereby major visceral functions are regulated so that the limits for survival are not surpassed. The system is organized into two specialized subsystems, the parasympathetic and the sympathetic. In controlling bodily function under normal physiologic conditions, such as rest and/or restoration, the parasympathetic nervous system usually predominates; the sympathetic nervous system generally directs the response of the organism to various environmental stresses. When mammals are confronted with danger, the heart beats more rapidly and more forcefully, the pupils dilate to permit more light to reach the retina, blood flow through skeletal muscles is enhanced, blood sugar is elevated, the sphincters of the alimentary tract close, and the mind becomes more alert. Each of these responses is achieved by activation of the sympathetic nervous system through various somatic and visceral afferent (sensory) fibers. The autonomic nervous system consists of spinal and supraspinal peripheral components. Excitation of many autonomic reflexes can occur at the spinal level, whereas integration of several autonomic activities occurs at supraspinal levels.

ANATOMIC CONSIDERATIONS

The efferent pathways of each of the two major subdivisions of the autonomic nervous system consist of two neurons (Fig. 7-1). The cell body of the first is found in the brain or spinal cord, and its neural endings synapse with the cell body of the second outside the central nervous system (CNS), either in discrete ganglia or within the innervated organ. With few exceptions, the preganglionic fibers are myelinated, and the postganglionic fibers are nonmyelinated.

The *parasympathetic division* of the autonomic nervous system, with its preganglionic cell bodies in the brain stem (tectobulbar) and the sacral cord, is also called the *craniosacral division* (or tectobulbosacral division). The cells of the postganglionic fibers are near, on, or within the innervated organ. The cranial division of the parasympathetic nervous system distributes fibers through the oculomotor (III), facial (VII), glossopharyngeal (IX), and vagal (X) nerves to terminal ganglia. Fibers from these innervate structures of the head, neck, thorax, and abdominal viscera; exceptions are the descending colon and the pelvic viscera, which are innervated by the sacral division. The sacral division arises from the sacral cord (S2-S4) and forms the pelvic nerve *(nervus erigens)*, which synapses in terminal ganglia near, on, or within the innervated organs. Only in the head are there discrete parasympathetic ganglia separated from the innervated structure.

The *sympathetic division* of the autonomic nervous system, with its preganglionic cell bodies in the intermediomedial or intermediolateral column of the thoracic and upper lumbar (T1-L2 or L3) spinal cord, is called the *thoracolumbar division*. Sympathetic preganglionic fibers pass out of the spinal cord with the ventral root and into the chain ganglia through the *white rami communicantes*. The cells of origin of the postganglionic sympathetic nerves are in autonomic ganglia of three types: (1) chain, or paravertebral; (2) collateral, or prevertebral; (3) terminal, or peripheral. The synapses of sympathetic nerves occur in the first two ganglia, but occasionally sympathetic nerves synapse in terminal ganglia.

Autonomic ganglia consist of small preganglionic nerve terminals, the ganglionic cells and their associated dendritic processes, and satellite or

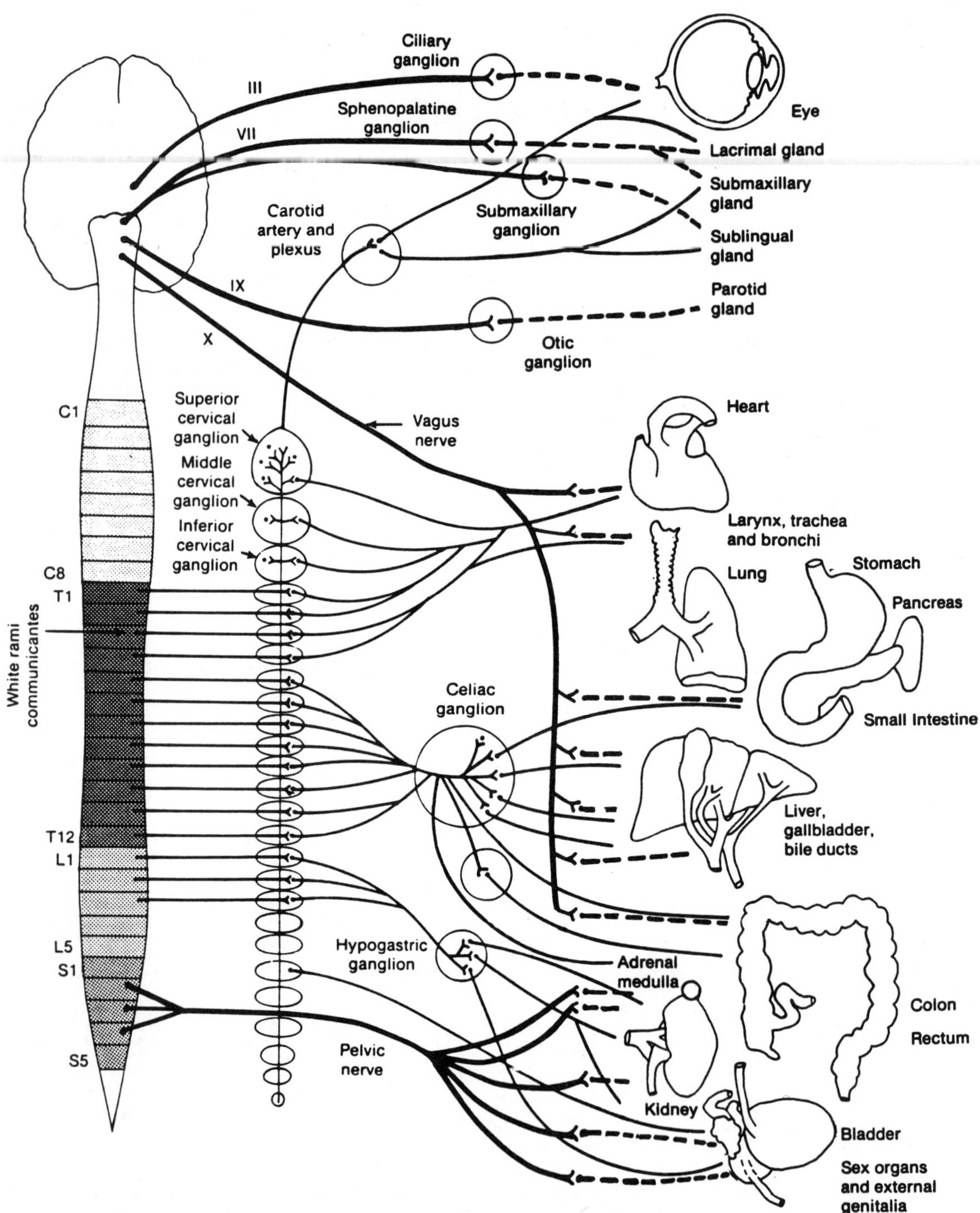

FIGURE 7-1 *Schematic representation of the autonomic nervous system. Innervation to various effector organs is shown for both the parasympathetic nervous system (———<— — —) and the sympathetic nervous system (———<———). The parasympathetic nervous system distributes fibers from cranial nerves (III, VII, IX, and X) and from the sacral cord (▒); sympathetic fibers originate from the thoracic (■) and lumbar (░) spinal cord through the white rami communicantes. Autonomic fibers do not originate from the cervical (░) spinal cord.*

glial cells. In mammalian sympathetic ganglia, the ratio of preganglionic to postganglionic fibers is of the order of 1:20; mammalian parasympathetic ganglia usually have a ratio of 1:1 or 1:2 (e.g., ciliary ganglion). The differences between sympathetic and parasympathetic ganglia, together with the widespread distribution of postganglionic sympathetic fibers, as compared with localized postganglionic parasympathetic fibers, is often regarded as the anatomic basis for the different physiologic characteristics of the two divisions of the autonomic nervous system. While activation of the sympathetic division results in a generalized response of many organ systems, activation of the parasympathetic division results in a more localized and discrete response. The organization of parasympathetic innervation by the vagus nerve is a notable exception to this generalization. The ratio of preganglionic vagal fibers to postganglionic fibers in the plexuses of Auerbach and Meissner is about 1:8000.

PHYSIOLOGIC CONSIDERATIONS

The actions of the various autonomic nerves on effector cells are summarized in Table 7-1 and require little additional comment. Many organs receive both sympathetic and parasympathetic fibers and are influenced in opposite ways by the two divisions of the autonomic nervous system. In some instances, e.g., heart and intestine, the organs are endowed with intrinsic activity and require dual innervation with opposing actions in order to elevate or suppress this inherent activity when appropriate. In other instances, control of function is regulated by opposing actions on different effector cells. For example, pupillary constriction occurs following the activation of parasympathetic nerves to the circular muscles of the iris or following the inactivation of sympathetic nerves to the radial muscles of the iris. Conversely, pupillary dilation occurs following activation of sympathetic fibers to the radial muscles or the inactivation of parasympathetic fibers of the circular muscles. Stated in other terms, the circular muscles of the iris are under the control of parasympathetic nerves and the radial muscles are under sympathetic control, with pupil size determined by the interplay between the sympathetic and parasympathetic nerves. Parallel action of sympathetic and parasympathetic innervation to effector cells is illustrated by the increase in conduction velocity in atrial fibers following either sympathetic or vagal stimulation. However, the increase in atrial conduction by vagal stimulation is not a constant finding.

It follows from these considerations that the activity of most organ systems reflects a balance of modulating influences between the sympathetic and parasympathetic nervous systems. Blockade of the sympathetic nervous system by drugs can be expected to result in an exaggeration of parasympathetic activity. Conversely, blockade of parasympathetic activity results in the exaggeration of sympathetic activity. When both pathways are blocked, the effect on the organ system depends on its inherent activity and on the pathway that normally dominates the organ system.

SYNAPTIC TRANSMISSION

The release of neurotransmitter substances from the small, unmyelinated neuronal endings is initiated by nerve action potentials (Figs. 7-2 and 7-3). Obviously, drugs or procedures modifying conduction of impulses in neuronal terminals can be expected to produce corresponding changes in the release of the synaptic transmitter.

Vesicular organelles, which contain transmitter substances, are present in synaptic neuronal terminals and move toward the terminal membrane to discharge their contents into the junctional cleft during nervous activity. Release of transmitter occurs when an action potential, propagated down the axon by activation of voltage-sensitive sodium channels, terminates at the nerve ending. As the membrane depolarizes, voltage-sensitive calcium channels in the membrane open, allowing an influx of ionic calcium. The increase in intracellular calcium facilitates fusion of the vesicular membrane with the neuronal membrane resulting in exocytotic release of neurotransmitter into the junctional cleft.

The neurotransmitter diffuses through the synaptic cleft and attaches reversibly with the receptors on the postsynaptic membrane at a rapid rate, causing changes in membrane activity. At many junctions, the dissociation of the transmitter and receptor must occur at a rapid rate for synaptic activity to remain responsive to succeeding incoming impulses. Equally important, mechanisms must be available for the elimination of the transmitter from the junctional region in order to prevent the accumulation within the synapse of concentrations of transmitter, which may interfere with further synaptic activity. Termination of transmitter activity can occur by a variety of means. After dissociation of the transmitter from

TABLE 7-1 Major effector responses to autonomic nervous system activity

	Sympathetic		Parasympathetic	
Effector	Receptor	Response	Receptor	Response
Eye				
Iris				
Radial muscle	α_1	Contraction	—[a]	—
Sphincter muscle	—	—	M	Contraction
Ciliary muscle	β_2	Relaxation	M	Contraction
Glands				
Sweat	α_1/M	Secretion[b]	M	Secretion
Salivary	α_1	Potassium and water secretion	M	Potassium and water secretion
	β_2	Amylase secretion		
Lacrimal	—	—	M	Secretion
Nasopharyngeal	—	—	M	Secretion
Gastrointestinal tract	—	—	M	Secretion
Skin				
Pilomotor muscles	α_1	Contraction	—	—
Lung				
Tracheal muscle	β_2	Relaxation	M	Contraction
Bronchial muscle	β_2	Relaxation	M	Contraction
Heart				
SA node	β_1	Increase in rate	M	Decrease in rate
Atria	β_1	Increase in contractility and conduction velocity	M	Decrease in contractility; usual: increased conduction velocity
AV node	β_1	Increase in conduction velocity	M	Decrease in conduction velocity
His-Purkinje system	β_1	Increase in conduction velocity	—	—
Ventricles	β_1	Increase in contractility and conduction velocity	—	—
Arterioles				
Coronary	α_1	Constriction[c]	—	—
Skin and mucosa	α_1	Constriction	—	—
Skeletal muscle	β_2	Dilation[d]	—	—
Pulmonary	α_1	Constriction[c]	—	—
Abdominal viscera	α_1	Constriction	—	—
	D_1	Dilation		
Salivary glands	α_1	Constriction	M	Dilation
Renal	α_1	Constriction	—	—
	D_1	Dilation		
Veins (systemic)	α_1	Constriction	—	—
	β_2	Dilation		

TABLE 7-1 (continued) Major effector responses to autonomic nervous system activity

	Sympathetic		Parasympathetic	
Effector	**Receptor**	**Response**	**Receptor**	**Response**
Gastrointestinal tract				
Longitudinal muscle (tone and motility)	α_2/β_2	Decrease	M	Increase
Sphincters	α_1	Contraction	M	Relaxation
Urinary bladder				
Detrusor	β_2	Relaxation	M	Contraction
Trigone & sphincter		Contraction	M	Relaxation
Adrenal medulla	N_N	Secretion[e]	—	—
Uterus				
Nonpregnant	β_2	Relaxation	M	Variable[f]
Pregnant	α_1	Contraction	M	Variable[f]
	β_2	Relaxation		
Male sex organs	α_1	Ejaculation	M	Erection
Spleen capsule	α_1	Contraction	—	—
Liver	α/β_2[g]	Glycogenolysis and gluconeogenesis		
Pancreas				
Acini	α_1	Decreased secretion	M	Secretion
Islets (β cells)	α_2	Decreased secretion	—	—
	β_2	Increased secretion		
Fat cells	β_3	Lipolysis	—	—
Pineal gland	β_3	Melatonin synthesis	—	—
Anterior pituitary	D_1/D_2	Inhibition of prolactin release	—	—

[a] No known functional innervation
[b] Thermoregulatory sweat (cholinergic); apocrine [stress] activation sweat (adrenergic).
[c] β_2-Receptor-mediated dilation observed *in situ* (autoregulatory phenomenon).
[d] Predominant effect over α receptor-mediated constriction.
[e] Secretion of epinephrine and norepinephrine in response to sympathetic preganglionic cholinergic fibers.
[f] Depends on the phase of the ovulatory cycle and amounts of estrogen and progesterone circulating.
[g] Species-dependent.

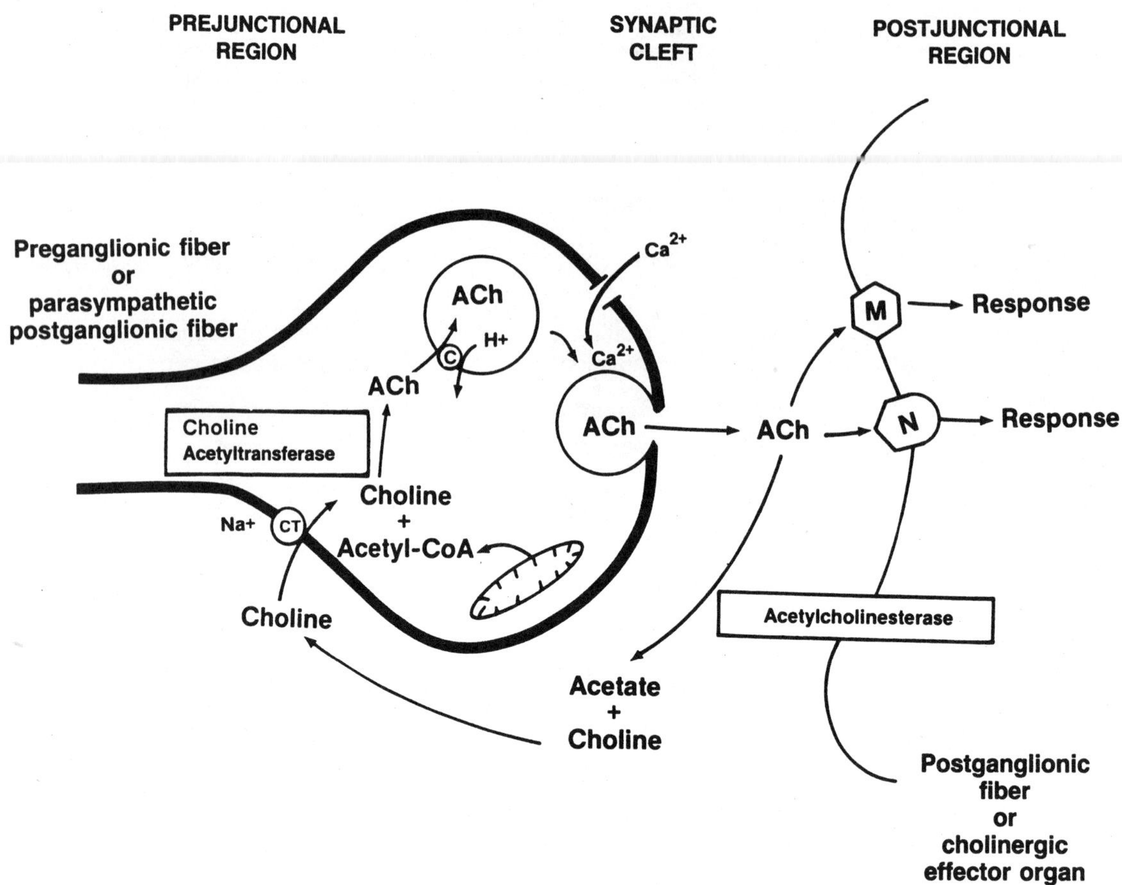

FIGURE 7-2 *Schematic representation of neurohumoral transmission at cholinergic nerve endings. Choline is taken up into the neuron by a Na^+-dependent carrier transport (CT) and is combined with acetyl CoA, released by mitochondria, to form acetylcholine (ACh). Synthesized ACh is transported into storage vesicles by a carrier which utilizes effluxing protons as a source of energy. Influx of ionic calcium (Ca^{2+}) through Ca^{2+} channels causes fusion of the vesicular and neuronal membranes and liberation of ACh into the synaptic cleft. ACh will interact with muscarinic (M) and/or nicotinic (N) receptors on the postjunctional tissue and can be hydrolyzed by acetylcholinesterase to acetate and choline.*

the postsynaptic receptor, the transmitter may (1) diffuse away from the synapse, (2) be converted to inactive degradation products by metabolic means, or (3) be taken up (reuptake) into neuronal terminals from the extracellular space. At cholinergic junctions, a significant portion of the neurotransmitter is terminated by enzymatic means; at adrenergic junctions, re-uptake of the transmitter by nerve endings is the major route of inactivation.

Cholinergic Transmission

The transmission of impulses at preganglionic, nerve endings, postganglionic parasympathetic and some postganglionic sympathetic nerve endings, as well as somatic nerve endings, occurs by means of acetylcholine (ACh) that is synthesized in the axonal terminal and is liberated from storage vesicles within the nerve terminals (Fig. 7-2).

The chemical processes involved in the formation of ACh within the nerves are complex; however, the major step in the biosynthetic process is the acetylation of choline catalytically by choline acetyltransferase. This reaction requires the presence of acetyl coenzyme A (CoA) and choline. Acetyl CoA is formed by and released from mitochondria, found in large numbers in

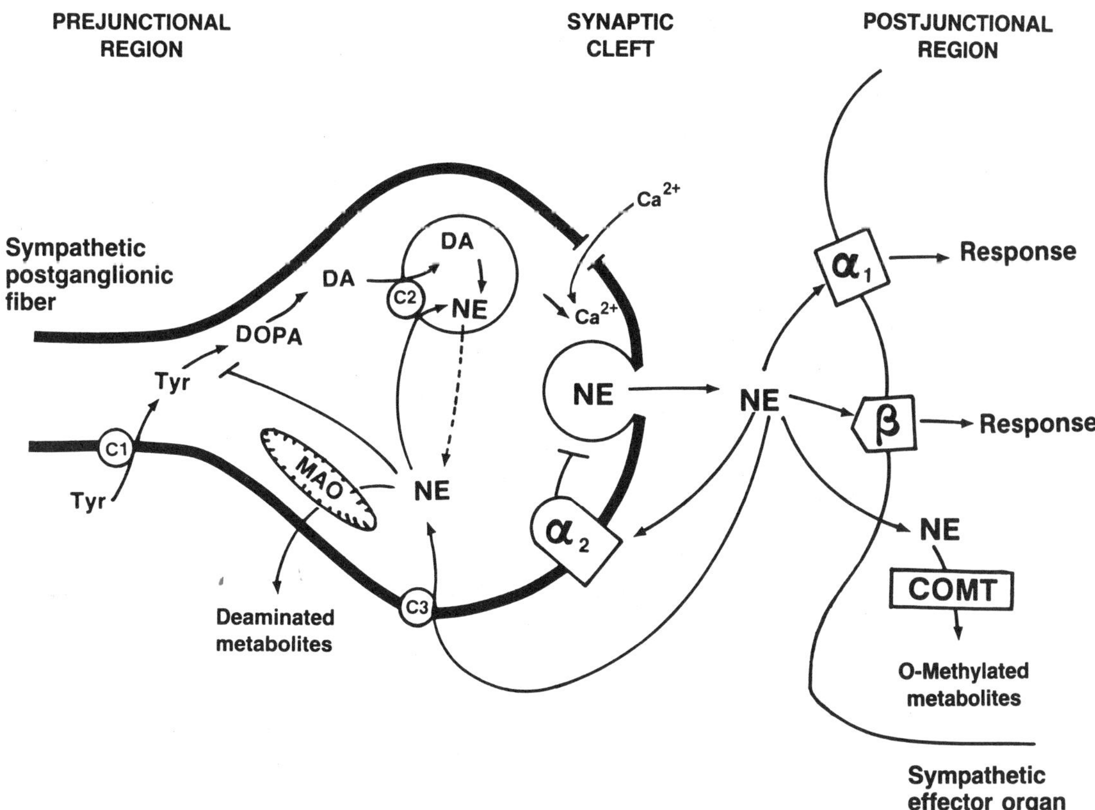

FIGURE 7-3 *Schematic representation of neurohumoral transmission at adrenergic nerve endings. Tyrosine (Tyr) enters sympathetic postganglionic neurons by an active carrier transport (C1) system. Dopamine (DA), formed from DOPA in the cytoplasm is transported into the storage vesicle by another active transport mechanism (C2); norepinephrine (NE) is synthesized from DA with the vesicles and stored for release. Influx of ionic calcium (Ca^{2+}) through Ca^{2+} channels causes fusion of the vesicular and neuronal membranes and liberation of NE into the synaptic cleft. NE will (1) complex with postjunctional α_1- and β-adrenergic receptors and initiate a physiologic tissue response, (2) bind to neuronal α_2-adrenergic receptors and inhibit further NE release from neurons, and (3) be inactivated by carrier transport (C3) mediated re-uptake into the neuron (uptake 1) and effector tissue (uptake 2). Cytoplasmic NE will (1) be transported back into the storage vesicle, by the same active transport mechanism (C2) transports DA, (2) be metabolized by mitochondrial monoamine oxidase (MAO), and (3) inhibit the formation of DOPA. NE that is accumulated in effector tissues will be metabolized by catechol-O-methyl transferase (COMT).*

axonal terminals. Choline is taken up into the axoplasm from the extracellular fluid by active transport, a process which is Na^+-dependent and can be inhibited by hemicholinium (a congener of choline).

$$\text{Acetyl CoA} + \text{choline} \xrightarrow{\text{choline acetyltransferase}} \text{ACh} + \text{CoA}$$

Following its formation in the cytoplasm, ACh is stored in vesicles that accumulate at neuronal endings and range in diameter from 20 to 40 nm. Among the inorganic ions present in nerve tissue, calcium plays a prominent role in the release mechanism. As previously mentioned, depolarization of the axonal terminal results in calcium ion influx through voltage-sensitive calcium channels. Ionic calcium binds to negative charges on the internal surface of the neuronal membrane, an interaction which promotes fusion of the neuronal and vesicular membranes, resulting in ACh release into the synaptic cleft. In addition to the marked hyperirritability of neural structures associated with calcium deficiency, there is a profound reduction in the output of ACh from cholinergic nerves resulting in the failure of transmission. Conversely, an elevation in the concentration of calcium ions bathing the nerve terminals enhances the output of the neurotransmitter.

Acetylcholine is subjected to a number of inactivation processes following its release from the nerve endings. These include diffusion from the site of release, dilution in extracellular fluids, binding to nonspecific sites, and enzymatic destruction. For most cholinergic junctions, the most important inactivation process is the enzymatic hydrolysis of ACh to acetate and choline. This reaction is catalyzed by the enzyme acetylcholinesterase and occurs at a rate sufficiently rapid to prevent the accumulation of ACh in the synaptic cleft.

Acetylcholinesterase is one of a family of enzymes which catalyze the hydrolysis of ester linkages. It differs from other members of the family in being almost completely specific for ACh, which it hydrolyzes with great efficiency. For this reason it is also termed *true*, or *specific, cholinesterase*. Apart from neural structures, it also occurs in red blood cells, in the placenta, and in the motor end plate of skeletal muscle. Another member of this family of enzymes is butyrylcholinesterase (also called *nonspecific cholinesterase*, or *pseudocholinesterase*), which is not specific for ACh but hydrolyzes a great variety of esters in addition to acetylcholine. This enzyme is found in the plasma in the liver, and in glial and other cells associated with nerve tissues.

Adrenergic Transmission

The transmission of impulses at adrenergic nerve endings occurs by means of norepinephrine liberated from storage granules within the nerve terminals (Fig. 7-3). Norepinephrine is one of several naturally occurring biogenic catecholamines; other important catecholamines are epinephrine, which is found in high concentrations in the adrenal medulla and other chromaffin cells, and dopamine, a precursor of both norepinephrine and epinephrine found in adrenergic nerve endings and in some areas of the CNS.

The synthetic pathway for norepinephrine in adrenergic neurons, appropriate cells of the CNS, and chromaffin tissue involves a complex series of enzymatic steps (Fig. 7-4). At adrenergic nerve endings the amino acid tyrosine is transported from the extracellular fluid to the intraneuronal cytoplasm by metabolically dependent processes. In the first step of the enzymatic series, tyrosine undergoes hydroxylation to form dopa. This cytoplasmic reaction is catalyzed by the enzyme tyrosine hydroxylase and requires tetrahydrobiopterin as a cofactor. When compared with other enzymes involved in the formation of catecholamines, the activity of tyrosine hydroxylase is the lowest. Therefore, the hydroxylation of tyrosine is the primary rate-limiting step in the series of reactions. Inhibition of tyrosine hydroxylase by analogs of tyrosine results in a depletion of catecholamine stores in the brain and adrenergic nerves and is the most effective mechanism for impairing the synthetic pathway for catecholamines. In addition, this step is subject to end-product (norepinephrine) feedback inhibition. The second step in the pathway results in the conversion of dopa to dopamine by a decarboxylation reaction catalyzed by dopa decarboxylase (aromatic L-amino acid decarboxylase) with the cofactor pyridoxal phosphate. The enzyme is not specific for dopa and will bring about the decarboxylation of histidine, tyrosine, and 5-hydroxytryptophan. In addition, the enzyme is present in many nonnervous tissues. Dopamine is actively transported into vesicles; the transport system requires Mg^{2+} and is driven by pH and potential gradients through an ATP-dependent proton translocase. In the vesicle the hydroxylation of the β carbon of dopamine to form norepinephrine takes place under the control of the enzyme dopamine-β-oxidase. This enzyme has been isolated from the chromaffin granules of the adrenal medulla and the synaptic vesicles of adrenergic nerves. The vesicles also contain relatively high concentrations of ATP (in a ratio of ATP to norepinephrine of 1:4), proteins known as chromogranins, certain peptides (e.g., enkephalin precursors), and ascorbic acid (a cofactor for dopamine-β-oxidase). These electron-dense vesicles range in size from 40 to 130 nm and have the capacity to concentrate norepinephrine from the cytoplasm. The formation of epinephrine from norepinephrine is confined primarily to the adrenal medulla (and similar tissues), and the enzyme catalyzing the conversion, phenylethanolamine-N-methyltransferase, is localized in those tissues.

Similar to cholinergic neurons, calcium ions appear to be the required link between membrane excitation and the release of catecholamines from adrenergic neurons and adrenal medullary cells. At both sites calcium deprivation causes a failure of the release mechanisms, and at both sites there is

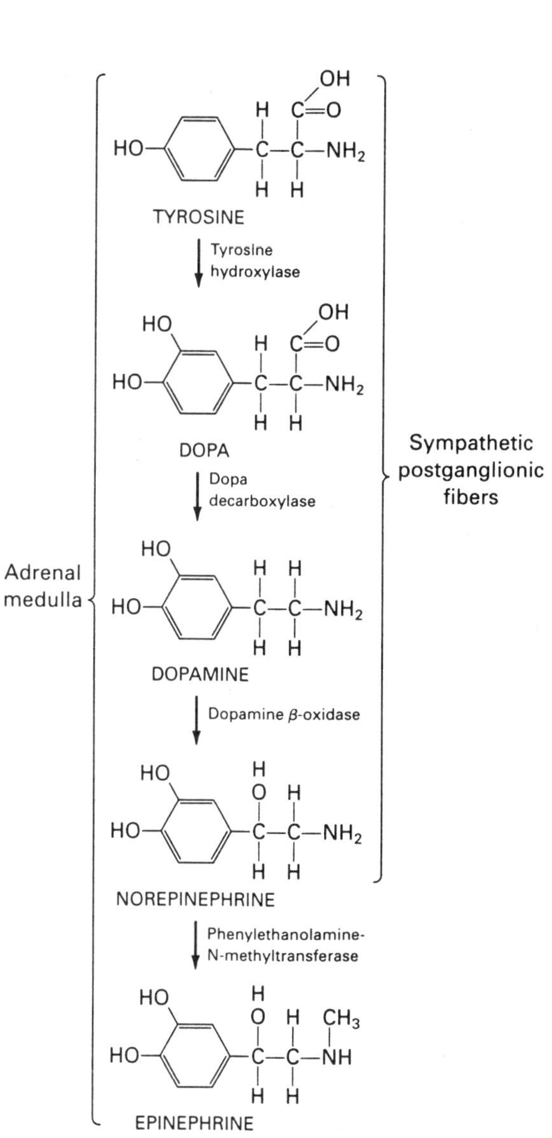

TYROSINE

Tyrosine hydroxylase

DOPA

Dopa decarboxylase

DOPAMINE

Dopamine β-oxidase

NOREPINEPHRINE

Phenylethanolamine-N-methyltransferase

EPINEPHRINE

Adrenal medulla

Sympathetic postganglionic fibers

FIGURE 7-4 *Metabolic syntheses of norepinephrine and epinephrine from tyrosine. Since postganglionic sympathetic neurons do not contain significant amounts of the enzyme phenylethanolamine-N-methyltransferase (PNMT), the synthetic pathway terminates with production of norepinephrine. PNMT is present in the adrenal medulla and continues the synthetic pathway to the biosynthesis of epinephrine. For this reason the adrenal medulla secretes both epinephrine and norepinephrine directly into the blood, whereas adrenergic resources secrete only norepinephrine into the synaptic cleft.*

an influx of calcium ions during the release of the catecholamines. The mechanism whereby calcium brings about the release of norepinephrine is exocytosis. The vesicular membrane fuses with the neuronal membrane, and the entire contents of the vesicle (including norepinephrine, dopamine, dopamine-β-oxidase, ATP, etc.) are discharged into the synaptic cleft.

By comparing the depletion of catecholamine stores produced by nerve stimulation and chemical agents such as tyramine and reserpine, it is apparent that the intraneuronal distribution, binding, and release of catecholamines are heterogeneous. As determined by isotopically labeled norepinephrine, there are two major neuronal compartments for the storage of catecholamines. The first compartment (pool I) contains norepinephrine, which undergoes rapid turnover (half-life of approximately 2 h). The second compartment (pool II) contains a storage form of norepinephrine with a slower turnover rate (half-life of about 24 h) and may represent a neuronal transmitter reserve. Norepinephrine released into the synaptic cleft from the first compartment is metabolized by the enzyme catechol-O-methyltransferase (COMT). The norepinephrine released into the neuronal cytoplasm from the second compartment is metabolized by monoamine oxidase (MAO).

The activity of norepinephrine released from adrenergic neurons can be terminated by (1) re-uptake into the neuron (uptake 1), (2) enzymatic inactivation, and (3) diffusion away from the synapse and uptake at extraneuronal sites (uptake 2). Re-uptake (both uptake 1 and uptake 2) is the most important method of terminating neuronally released norepinephrine as well as circulating norepinephrine and epinephrine, i.e., catecholamines present in the blood as a consequence of sympathetic nerve activity, release from the adrenal medulla, and/or release from chromaffin tissues. *Neuronal re-uptake* is a Na^+-dependent active process which transports catecholamines from the junctional extracellular fluid, across the neuronal membrane, into the cytoplasm. *Vesicular transport* involves the transfer of the compound from the cytoplasm, across the membrane of the vesicle, into the storage vesicle and appears identical to the active transport of dopamine into the vesicle during norepinephrine synthesis.

There are two major enzyme systems involved in the transformation of the catecholamines to inactive degradation products (Fig. 7-5). Oxidative deamination of epinephrine and norepinephrine is catalyzed by MAO. Adrenergic nerve endings contain large quantities of the enzyme, which is

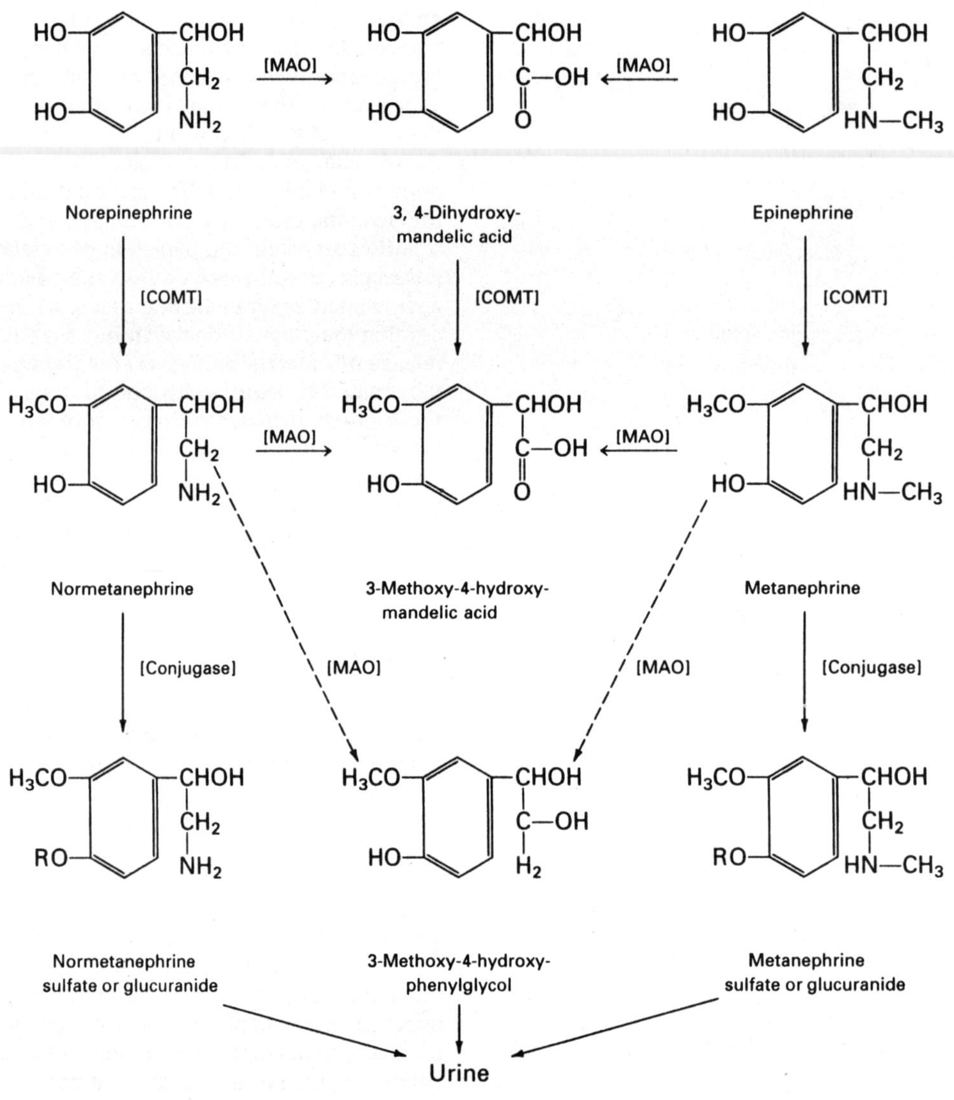

Norepinephrine [MAO] → 3, 4-Dihydroxy-mandelic acid ← [MAO] Epinephrine

[COMT] [COMT] [COMT]

Normetanephrine [MAO] → 3-Methoxy-4-hydroxy-mandelic acid ← [MAO] Metanephrine

[Conjugase] [MAO] [MAO] [Conjugase]

Normetanephrine sulfate or glucuranide

3-Methoxy-4-hydroxy-phenylglycol

Metanephrine sulfate or glucuranide

Urine

FIGURE 7-5 *Metabolic pathways showing the inactivation of norepinephrine and epinephrine by various enzyme systems.*

localized on the outer surface of mitochondrial membranes. Apparently, because of its intraneuronal localization, MAO plays more of a role in the regulation of the intraneuronal disposition of catecholamines than the destruction of circulating biogenic amines, which takes place in the liver. Inhibition of MAO leads to an increase in the tissue concentration of the catecholamines but has no appreciable effect on the responses to injected epinephrine or norepinephrine.

The second major enzyme involved in the metabolism of the catecholamines is COMT. This enzyme is responsible for the inactivation of circulating catecholamines. Although the enzyme is widely distributed, highest concentrations are found in the liver and kidneys; lesser amounts are localized in the neuroeffector junction, especially in the tissues served by the adrenergic nerves. Sympathetic nerves contain very little COMT activity. The metabolic conversion by 0-methyltransferase of the catecholamines to inactive forms is due to the transfer of a methyl group from "activated" methionine to the 3-hydroxyl group of the phenyl ring. Part of the norepinephrine released from adrenergic nerves during nerve stimulation as well as circulating catecholamines, is taken up by the effector cells (uptake 2) and acted upon by COMT.

NEURONAL COTRANSMITTERS

Although junctional transmission is currently conceived as involving a single transmitter from each neuron, there is evidence that more than one transmitter is released from a single neuron. Enkephalins can be demonstrated to be present in preganglionic neurons, postganglionic sympathetic neurons, and adrenal medullary cells. Vasoactive intestinal polypeptide (VIP) can also be found in peripheral cholinergic nerves to exocrine glands. Stimulation of the preganglionic sympathetic nerve to the adrenal medulla results in a release of substance P along with acetylcholine. The vesicles in autonomic nerve terminals contain ATP which is also released with the neurotransmitter. Therefore there appears to be an association of neuropeptides with the more familiar cholinergic and adrenergic neurotransmitters. Although specific receptors and antagonists are readily discernible for many of the neuropeptides, data to substantiate their roles as neurotransmitters are not presently conclusive.

RECEPTORS

Virtually all hormones and drugs initiate their physiologic or pharmacologic actions by binding to specific cellular sites referred to as *receptors*. Receptor binding initiates alterations of cellular metabolic events such as enzyme activities, ion fluxes, glandular secretions, muscle contractions, and other activities characteristically expressed as physiologic or pharmacologic.

Exogenously administered drugs, such as epinephrine and acetylcholine, mimic the effects of autonomic nervous activity and produce their characteristic effects on suitably denervated structures; thus, these drugs react directly with specific receptors on the effector cell rather than on the nerve endings.

In effector cells innervated by sympathetic and/or parasympathetic fibers, the responses to the neurotransmitter upon activation of the nerve fiber or to the administered mimetic agent are similar. It is therefore postulated that responding cells possess receptors for acetylcholine and other receptors for norepinephrine. These two general classes of receptors are often referred to as *cholinergic receptors* and *adrenergic receptors*, respectively (Table 7-2). Additionally, it should be noted that specific dopamine receptors are found in certain renal and mesenteric blood vessels.

The receptor concept is based on the presence of distinct cellular macromolecules which are capable of binding with the biologically active agonists or their functionally inert antagonists. The molecular structure of the ligand-binding site determines the specificity of the physiologic or pharmacologic action characteristic of the tissue. The specific binding of an agonist with the receptor must therefore activate a biologic process which terminates in a response such as glandular secretion, muscle contraction, ion channel regulation, and other such actions. Receptor-effector coupling mechanisms are discussed in detail in Chapter 3.

Cholinergic Receptors

There are many peripheral efferent nerves which are cholinergic. It is convenient and empirically useful to group them into three categories: (1) preganglionic fibers of the autonomic nervous system, (2) postganglionic fibers of the parasympathetic division and some postganglionic fibers of the sympathetic division, and (3) somatic motor nerves (Fig. 7-6). Although each of these nerves transmits to a cell which contains receptors for ACh (cholinergic receptors, cholinoceptive sites) and each of these cells responds to properly applied exogenous ACh, the pharmacologic characteristics of the receptors at the three sites are different in significant ways. Drugs that strongly mimic the effects of ACh at one cholinergic junction may have a markedly reduced effect at another. Similarly, drugs that block cholinergic transmission at one site may have no effect on cholinergic transmission at another site.

All three groups of cholinergic receptors respond to ACh; the differences among the receptors have been determined by using drugs which act like ACh (cholinomimetic) or which antagonize the effects of ACh (anticholinergic). The cholinergic effects of *muscarine* and *nicotine* have long been known and form the basis for classifying the cholinergic receptors. The alkaloid muscarine produces all the effects of postganglionic parasympathetic nerve stimulation and also induces sweating (a response produced by cholinergic sympathetic postganglionic fibers). The effects of muscarine are readily suppressed by atropine, as

TABLE 7-2 Autonomic receptors

Designation	Typical locations
CHOLINERGIC RECEPTORS	
Muscarinic (M)	
M_1	Parasympathetic effector cells (e.g., gastric mucosa), neurons (e.g., cerebral cortex, ganglia)
M_2	Parasympathetic effector cells (e.g., intestinal smooth muscle, cardiac muscle, exocrine glands), central nervous system
M_3	Central nervous system, exocrine glands, smooth muscle
Nicotinic (N)	
N_N	Autonomic ganglia, central nervous system
N_M	Skeletal muscle end plate
ADRENERGIC RECEPTORS	
Alpha (α)	
α_1	Postsynaptic effector cells (e.g., vascular smooth muscle)
α_2	Adrenergic nerve terminals (presynaptic) and smooth muscle (postsynaptic); also nonsynaptic sites (e.g., platelets, lipocytes)
Beta (β)	
β_1	Postsynaptic effect cells (especially heart and kidney); also non synaptic sites (e.g., lipocytes)
β_2	Postsynaptic effector cells (e.g., smooth muscle)
β_3	Postsynaptic effector cells (e.g., lipocytes)
DOPAMINERGIC RECEPTORS	
D_1	Brain (e.g., presynaptic receptors on nerve terminals) and vascular smooth muscle of the abdominal viscera and renal beds
D_2	Brain and peripheral receptors on nerve terminals

are those of ACh on these same responses. On this basis, the receptors for ACh on effector cells innervated by postganglionic cholinergic fibers (all parasympathetic and certain sympathetic postganglionic fibers) may be called *muscarinic receptors* or *atropine-sensitive receptors*. Drugs with the same pattern of activity as muscarine have been termed *muscarinic agents* or *parasympathomimetic drugs*. Muscarinic cholinoceptive sites are also found in some tissues that are not innervated; most arterioles do not receive parasympathetic innervation but are extremely sensitive to the actions of muscarine and muscarine-like drugs.

Based on the selectivity of specific agonists and antagonists, muscarinic receptors are subdivided into M_1, M_2 and M_3 types. Current nomenclature is presented in Table 7-2. All of these receptors are found in the CNS. M_1 receptors are found in the autonomic ganglia and both M_2 and M_3 receptors are found on effector organs, especially smooth muscle. M_2 receptors are found on the sinoatrial node and cardiac muscles while M_3

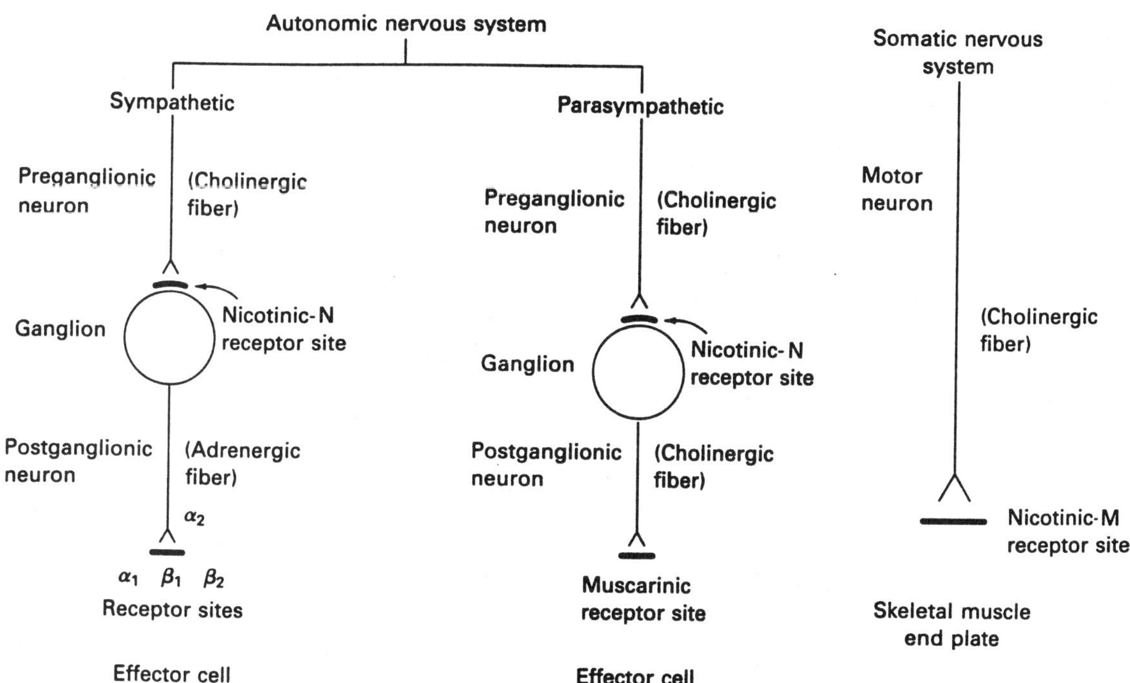

FIGURE 7-6 *Diagrammatic representation of the distribution of cholinoceptive and adrenoceptive sites in the autonomic nervous system and the somatic nervous system.*

receptors are found on exocrine glands. Muscarine is the specific agonist for all of these receptors, and atropine is the specific antagonist.

The cholinergic receptors in autonomic ganglia and at the neuromuscular junction are responsive to low concentrations of nicotine and to ACh applied in adequate concentrations by an appropriate route of administration. The responses to ACh at these sites are called *nicotinic effects*, and the respective cholinoceptive sites *nicotinic receptors*. The nicotinic receptors for ACh are further subdivided into two groups: N_N (found mainly in autonomic ganglia and the CNS); and N_M (located at the skeletal muscle end plate). Although genes have been cloned for other receptor subtypes, they have not been functionally identified. There are drugs which selectively interfere with transmission in autonomic ganglia (*ganglionic blocking agents*) and others that selectively interfere with neuromuscular transmission (*neuromuscular blocking drugs*). It is important to remember that cholinergic fibers to skeletal muscle and the nicotinic receptors associated with the muscle end plate are part of the somatic nervous system, not the autonomic nervous system.

Adrenergic Receptors

The organs innervated by adrenergic nerves respond to exogenous epinephrine or norepinephrine in a manner which qualitatively mimics the effects of sympathetic nerve stimulation; drugs which act in this manner are termed *sympathomimetic agents*. The primary reaction between norepinephrine or epinephrine and the effector cell is mediated by *adrenergic receptors* (*adrenoceptive sites*).

A careful study of the relative potencies of several sympathomimetic amines for producing the characteristic sympathetic response in several tissues has suggested that adrenergic receptors could be grouped into two major classes: alpha (*α*) and beta (*β*) receptors (Table 7-2). The synthesis of selective blocking agents has allowed a further subdivision of β-adrenergic receptors into β_1 (chiefly at cardiac and renal sites) and β_2 (most other sites). More recently, α-adrenergic receptors have been subdivided into α_1 (found mainly on effector organs) and α_2 (located on adrenergic neurons at presynaptic sites and to a lesser extent on effector tissues). Receptor subtypes for dopamine (D_1 and D_2) have been described in the CNS and in certain peripheral vascular beds.

Although there are exceptions, activation of α_1 receptors generally results in an excitatory response; activation of β_2-adrenergic receptors generally results in tissue relaxation or an inhibitory response. Activation of β_1-adrenergic receptors results in a stimulatory effect on the heart and kidney, and activation of *presynaptic* α_2-adrenergic receptors appears to constitute a mechanism for presynaptic feedback inhibition of neuronal release of norepinephrine, while stimulation of *postsynaptic* α_2 receptors, similar to α_1 receptors, mediates tissue excitation.

Effector organ response to epinephrine and/or norepinephrine is primarily determined by the type of adrenoceptor as well as the proportion of α-adrenergic and β-adrenergic receptors. The radial muscle of the eye will contract in response to epinephrine and norepinephrine because the receptor mediating this effect is α_1; since both epinephrine and norepinephrine are capable of activating α_1-adrenoceptors, mydriasis will be a consistent response. Blood vessels of striated muscle have both α_1- and β_2-adrenergic receptors, but β_2 receptors predominate; in response to circulating epinephrine these blood vessels dilate as β_2-adrenergic receptors are activated; norepinephrine resulting from sympathetic discharge has little effect on these blood vessels because of the low density of α_1-adrenoceptors. Conversely, cutaneous blood vessels contain predominantly α_1 receptors and will respond to both epinephrine and norepinephrine with vasoconstriction.

The catecholamines cause striking changes in the metabolism of most organs. An increase in oxygen consumption, a breakdown of glycogen, an increase in the formation of lactic acid, and an increase in the mobilization of free fatty acids represent the major metabolic effects. In mammals, the metabolic effects of epinephrine include hyperglycemia, the release of free fatty acids, and an increase in plasma lactic acid. These effects are produced by the action of epinephrine on β-adrenergic receptors and the subsequent increase in the formation of cyclic AMP by the adenylate cyclase enzyme system (see Chapter 3).

PHYSIOLOGIC REGULATION OF RECEPTORS

A diminution of responsiveness to pharmacologic action with time is a fundamental mechanism of cellular adaptation which is known as *desensitization* (tolerance, tachyphylaxis, refractoriness). Desensitization markedly limits the therapeutic efficacy of drugs, including parasympathomimetic and sympathomimetic agents; the refractoriness to bronchodilators administered to asthma patients is a classic example. Detailed information concerning desensitization phenomena is given in Chapter 2.

BIBLIOGRAPHY

Bylund, D.B.: "Subtypes of Alpha1 and Alpha2 Adrenergic Subtypes," *FASEB J.* **6**: 832-840 (1992).

Fernandes, L.B., A.D. Fryer, and C.A. Hirshman: "M2 Muscarinic Receptors Inhibit Isoproterenol-Induced Relaxation of Canine Airway Smooth Muscle," *J. Pharmacol. Exp. Ther.* **262**: 119-126 (1992).

Hoffman, B.B., and R.J. Lefkowitz: "Radioligand Binding Studies of Adrenergic Receptors: New Insights Into Molecular and Physiological Regulation," *Annu. Rev. Pharmacol. Toxicol.* **20**: 581-608 (1980).

Hoffman, B.B., and R.J. Lefkowitz: "Alpha-adrenergic Receptor Subtypes," *N. Engl. J. Med.* **302**: 1390-1396 (1980).

Lefkowitz, R.J., M.G. Caron, and G. L. Stiles: "Mechanisms of Membrane-Receptor Regulation," *N. Engl. J. Med.* **310**: 1570-1579 (1984).

Levitzki, A.: "β-Adrenergic Receptors and Their Mode of Coupling to Adenylate Cyclase," *Physiol. Rev.* **66**: 819-854 (1986).

Moreland, R.S., and D.F. Bohr: "Adrenergic Control of Coronary Arteries," *Fed. Proc.* **43**: 2858-2861 (1984).

Ruffolo, R.R.: "Interactions of Agonists with Peripheral α-Adrenergic Receptors," *Fed. Proc.* **43**: 2910-2916 (1984).

Ruffolo, R.R., A.J. Nichols, J.M. Stadel, and J.P. Hieble: "Structure and Function of Adrenceptors," *Pharmacol. Rev.* **43**: 475-505 (1991).

Whiting, P.J., R. Schoeffer, W.G. Conroy, M.J. Gore, K.T. Keyser, S. Shimasaki, F. Esch, and J.M. Lindstrom: "Expression of Nicotinic Acetylcholine Receptor Subtypes in Brain and Retina," *Brain Res.* **10**: 61-70 (1991).

CHAPTER 8

Adrenergic Drugs

Terriann Crisp

Adrenergic drugs and *sympathomimetic amines* are conventional terms used in reference to a class of chemicals that evoke responses in the living organism which simulate the functional consequences of sympathetic nerve activation or the hormonal secretion of epinephrine by the adrenal glands. Both naturally occurring and synthetic compounds make up this diverse group of substances. Indeed, three *endogenous catecholamines* — epinephrine, norepinephrine, and dopamine — are clinically useful as sympathomimetic drugs.

Norepinephrine and dopamine are released from neurons in the brain and periphery; their physiologic roles as neurotransmitter molecules have been extensively studied. Norepinephrine is considered to be the principal neurotransmitter of the sympathetic division of the autonomic nervous system. Epinephrine is recognized as a hormonal substance synthesized and released into the systemic circulation from chromaffin cells of the adrenal medulla during the defensive "fight or flight" reaction. Relatively small amounts of epinephrine also occur in some regions of the brain, where it apparently functions as a neurotransmitter or neuromodulator.

Sympathetic neurons exert a prominent regulatory influence on the heart and vasculature. Thus, many therapeutic uses of sympathomimetic drugs are based on their ability to alter the cardiovascular status of the organism.

Some typical and important pharmacologic actions of the wide variety of adrenergic drugs include the following:

Cardiac stimulation Increased heart rate and myocardial contractile force (also known as positive chronotropic and inotropic effects, respectively)

Vasomotor changes Vasoconstriction and/or vasodilation

Bronchodilation and a "decongestant" action on mucous membranes

Ocular effects Mydriasis and a reduction of intraocular pressure

Regulation of endocrine status Modulation of insulin, renin, and pituitary hormones

Regulation of metabolic status Enhanced glycogenolysis in liver and muscle and liberation of free fatty acids from adipose tissue

Behavioral changes Complex stimulatory or "alerting" effects in the central nervous system

The spectrum of cardiovascular, respiratory, hormonal, metabolic, and neuropsychic responses that may be elicited by adrenergic drugs in general clearly resembles many of the systemic adaptive reactions to increased physical activity and psychic stress. Both pharmacodynamic and pharmacokinetic distinctions among the drugs included in this broad classification scheme provide the rationale for their specific therapeutic applications. Considered individually, adrenergic drugs exhibit notable quantitative and qualitative differences with respect to their potencies and most prominent actions. The variation in responses to subclasses of adrenergic drugs is largely based on their relative selectivity of interaction with populations of receptor molecules that are differentially distributed in effector structures (heart, vasculature, lungs, brain, peripheral nerves, etc.) throughout the body.

SITES AND MODE OF ACTION

Conceptually, sympathomimetic drugs induce their effect by:

1. Binding directly to and thereby activating adrenergic receptors on the cell membranes of target tissues. The term *direct-acting agonist* is descriptively used for such drugs (Figure 8-1). Examples include epinephrine, phenylephrine, and isoproterenol.
2. Evoking the neuronal release of stored catecholamines, which then bind to and activate adrenergic receptors. The sympathomimetic activity of the drug is therefore dependent on the presence of endogenous catecholamines. The phrase *indirect-acting agent* is used with reference to this mode of action (Figure 8-1). Tyramine, a compound used as an experimental tool, is an example of an indirect-acting sympathomimetic.
3. A combination of direct adrenergic receptor activation and indirect catecholamine-releasing actions. Drugs with this duality of action are referred to as *mixed-acting* and are exemplified by ephedrine, amphetamine, and dopamine.

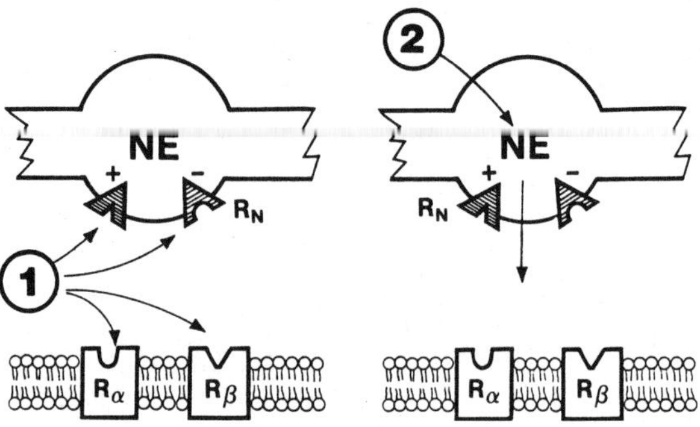

FIGURE 8-1 *Diagrammatic illustration of direct and indirect actions of sympathomimetic drugs. (1)* ***Direct-acting agonists*** *activate adrenergic receptors (R_α, R_β) on the target cell membrane (i.e., postsynaptic site) and on presynaptic neuronal receptors (R_N) located on the neurilemma. Presynaptic "autoregulatory" receptors modulate [enhance (+) or reduce (−)] release of the endogenous neurotransmitter [norepinephrine (NE)]; presynaptic receptors can be inhibitory (α_2-adrenergic) or excitatory (β-adrenergic). Examples of direct-acting drugs: phenylephrine (selective for α_1 receptors) and isoproterenol (selective for β receptors. (2)* ***Indirect-acting compounds*** *promote the release of the neurotransmitter (NE) from sympathetic neurons. An example of an indirect-acting drug is tyramine.* ***Note:*** *the distinction between actions 1 and 2 is not necessarily absolute; many* ***mixed-acting adrenergic drugs*** *combine both actions, e.g., dopamine, ephedrine, and amphetamines.*

Figure 8-1 depicts direct and indirect-acting modes of action of sympathomimetic agents. Examples of direct-acting adrenergic receptor agonists, indirect-acting agents, and mixed-acting adrenergic drugs are listed in Table 8-1.

Adrenergic receptors (adrenoceptors) exist throughout the body — in the brain, peripheral nerves, and non-neural cells (muscles, glands, blood cells). From a molecular perspective, the binding of an adrenergic agonist drug to a complementary receptor on the cell membrane regulates a cascade of biochemical reactions within the cell ultimately to alter its intrinsic metabolic status. The drug (or an endogenous neurotransmitter or hormone) thus provides an informational message which is transduced into the cell interior and subsequently amplified (see Chapter 3). From a macroscopic perspective, altered cellular activity elicits a measurable effect at the tissue or organ level. Two major classes of adrenergic drug-binding receptor proteins have been historically designated as *alpha (α)* and *beta (β)*. Several subtypes of these two classes have been characterized on the basis of anatomic, pharmacologic, biochemical, and molecular criteria. Currently, four subtypes are widely recognized and designated as α_1, α_2, β_1, and β_2. This classification of adrenergic receptor subtypes may yield to modified schemes as detailed structural and functional characterization is accomplished. For example, recently some adrenergic receptors in fat cells have been designated as β_3.

Drugs such as epinephrine, norepinephrine, and isoproterenol are nonselective agonists, i.e., they stimulate all subtypes of α- and/or β-adrenergic receptors. Several examples serve to illustrate the variation in pharmacologic effects of drugs that *selectively* activate subpopulations of adrenergic receptors.

The activation of α-adrenergic receptors in vascular smooth muscle elicits vasoconstriction. Consequently, drugs with α-adrenergic agonist activity increase vascular resistance and thereby elevate arterial blood pressure. Phenylephrine is a

TABLE 8-1 Examples of direct-acting, indirect-acting, and mixed-acting adrenergic agents

DIRECT-ACTING AGONISTS	
Catecholamines	**Non-catecholamines**
α_1-Adrenoceptor Agonists	
dopamine norepinephrine epinephrine	phenylephrine metaraminol methoxamine
α_2-Adrenoceptor Agonists	
dopamine norepinephrine epinephrine	clonidine guanabenz guanfacine
β_1-Adrenoceptor Agonists	
dopamine norepinephrine epinephrine isoproterenol dobutamine	prenalterol
β_2-Adrenoceptor Agonists	
epinephrine isoproterenol isoetharine	salmeterol terbutaline albuterol metaproterenol bitolterol pirbuterol ritodrine
INDIRECT-ACTING SYMPATHOMIMETICS	
tyramine	
MIXED-ACTING SYMPATHOMIMETICS	
Catecholamines	**Non-catecholamines**
dopamine	ephedrine amphetamines methylphenidate

representative vasopressor drug with highly selective α_1-adrenergic agonist activity. The term *vasopressor* refers to the ability of sympathomimetic drugs to elicit a rise in arterial blood pressure.

The activation of *presynaptic* α_2 "autoreceptors" located on peripheral postganglionic sympathetic neurons causes a reduced amount of norepinephrine to be released in response to electrical stimulation of the nerve. *Postsynaptic* α_2-adrenergic receptors also exist in target tissues such as blood vessels, where their activation results in vasoconstriction. When α_2-adrenergic receptors located on blood platelets are activated, enhanced platelet aggregation occurs. α_2-Adrenoceptors in the brain stem modulate sympathetic neural outflow to peripheral organs. Clonidine, guanabenz and guanfacine are centrally active α_2-adrenergic agonists which lower systemic blood pressure and heart rate.

β_1-Adrenergic receptors in the heart regulate myocardial contractility, heart rate, and the electrophysiologic characteristics of cardiac cells. β_2-Adrenergic receptors in the trachea and bronchi of the lungs modulate the contractile state of airway smooth muscle. Isoproterenol, a potent selective agonist on β-adrenergic receptors, is a powerful myocardial stimulant (β_1-adrenergic receptors) and bronchodilator (β_2-adrenergic receptors). Sympathomimetic drugs that can activate pulmonary β_2 receptors in preference to cardiac β_1 receptors, e.g., salmeterol, terbutaline, albuterol, metaproterenol, and isoetharine, are widely used as bronchodilators to treat bronchospastic disorders.

The terms *desensitization* and *down-regulation* are used to describe certain biochemical phenomena, associated with reduced functional responsiveness, which have been noted when target tissues are continually exposed to drugs that activate adrenoceptors. Desensitization refers to cellular events possibly following relatively brief periods of tissue exposure to adrenergic drugs, such as redistribution of receptors on the cell membrane, uncoupling of the receptor from distal regulatory components, internalization of receptors within the cell cytosol, and possibly, receptor phosphorylation. Down-regulation refers to a reduction in number of adrenoceptors, i.e., lowered receptor density, following longer periods of contact with adrenergic drugs. Such phenomena have been more thoroughly documented for β-adrenergic receptors than for α-adrenoceptors. They offer several plausible mechanistic explanations for observations — variously described as refractoriness, tolerance, and tachyphylaxis — of diminished effectiveness of an adrenergic drug during prolonged, continuous, or repeated administration. The possible relevance of these dynamic aspects of adrenergic receptor proteins to clinical pathologic states is under investigation.

CHEMISTRY and STRUCTURE-ACTIVITY RELATIONSHIPS

Figure 8-2 shows some key structural features of several representative adrenergic drugs. The physiologic catecholamines (which have —OH groups substituted on the 3 and 4 positions of the aromatic ring) and most synthetic sympathomimetic drugs are viewed as substituted phenylethylamines. It is noteworthy that substituted imidazolines and some aliphatic amines also have sympathomimetic activity. The sympathomimetic characteristics of substituted phenylethylamines are, to some extent, predictable from an inspection of their structural differences. Several general statements can be made about such correlations between molecular structure and biologic activity (refer to Figure 8-2):

1. Sympathomimetic activity is maximal when two carbon atoms separate the aromatic ring from the amino group.
2. The lesser the degree of substitution on the amino group, the greater is the selectivity for activating α-adrenergic receptors. Conversely, increasing the bulk of substituents on the primary amino group confers greater selectivity for β-adrenergic receptors.
3. Maximal activity at α- and β-adrenoceptors depends on the presence of hydroxyl groups at positions 3 and 4 on the aromatic ring, i.e., the catecholamines.
4. Compounds with large amino subsitituents and hydroxy groups at positions 3 and 5 and show greater selectivity for β_2-adrenergic receptor sites.
5. Noncatecholamines elicit more prominent central nervous system stimulatory effects than catecholamines.
6. Substitution on the α carbon atom blocks oxidative inactivation of the molecule by monoamine oxidase (MAO) and thus greatly prolongs the duration of activity. α-Carbon substitution also enhances the ability of the molecule to release endogenous catecholamines from neuronal storage sites.
7. Compounds with only a 3-hydroxy substitution on the aromatic ring (e.g., phenylephrine) yield a high ratio of direct/indirect agonist activity.
8. Compounds with only a 4-hydroxy substitution on the aromatic ring yield a high ratio of indirect/direct activity, as exemplified by tyramine.

DIRECT-ACTING AGONISTS

Epinephrine

This endogenous catecholamine is also known by its official British name *adrenaline*. Epinephrine is a potent agonist on both α- and β-adrenergic receptors. Its actions are complex, being dependent not only on the relative distribution of adrenergic receptor sites in various tissues and organs but also on the conditions of dosage and route of administration. Although prominent pharmacologic actions are exerted on the cardiovascular and respiratory systems, the full profile of its effects throughout the body reflects its physiologic importance as a systemic neurohormone involved in "defense activation". Since it can represent the prototype of many adrenergic drugs reviewed in this chapter, the pharmacodynamic characteristics of epinephrine on several organ systems are presented below in some detail.

Pharmacodynamics

Cardiovascular System The typical cardiovascular response to an intravenous injection or infusion of epinephrine is an immediate rise in systemic arterial blood pressure. Systolic pressure is usually elevated to a greater degree than diastolic pressure; thus, pulse pressure is increased (Fig. 8-3). This pressor response to epinephrine is due to the combined actions of (1) vasoconstriction in many, but not all, vascular beds and (2) myocardial stimulation, i.e., increased contractile force and heart rate.

Significant differences in reactivity to epinephrine are observed among the regional vascular networks of the body. Such variations in response have been shown to be related to the distribution of adrenergic receptor types in different blood vessels. The vasoconstrictive action of epinephrine results from activation of α-adrenergic receptors and is principally exerted on small arterioles and precapillary sphincters (i.e., resistance vessels) and also on veins (i.e., capacitance vessels). Vascular constriction is particularly marked in blood vessels supplying the skin and mucous membranes, in the splanchnic circulation and in the kidneys. Although *vasopressor amine* is an appropriate reference to the vasoconstrictor action, small doses of epinephrine can sometimes evoke a fall in diastolic blood pressure. This *vasodepressor* component is a consequence of regional vasodilation in blood vessels supplying

Many adrenergic drugs can be considered as substituted derivatives of phenylethylamine

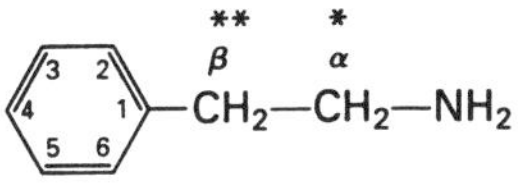

$$\text{C}_6\text{H}_5\text{—}\overset{**}{\underset{\beta}{\text{CH}_2}}\text{—}\overset{*}{\underset{\alpha}{\text{CH}_2}}\text{—NH}_2$$

(ring positions numbered 1–6)

* Designates the *alpha* carbon atom of the molecule.
** Designates the *beta* carbon atom of the molecule.

REPRESENTATIVE CATECHOLAMINES

Norepinephrine

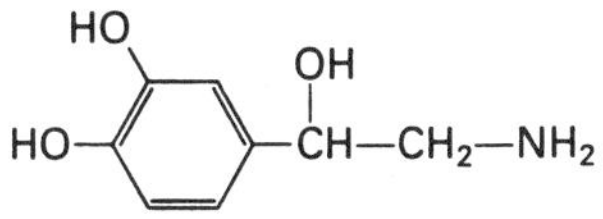

$(HO)_2C_6H_3\text{—}CH(OH)\text{—}CH_2\text{—}NH_2$

Epinephrine

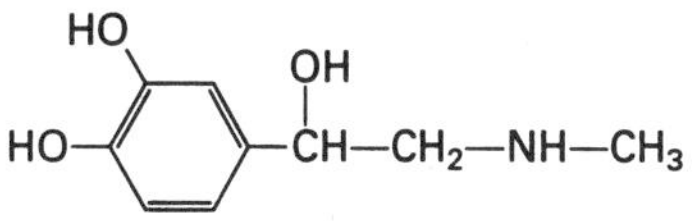

$(HO)_2C_6H_3\text{—}CH(OH)\text{—}CH_2\text{—}NH\text{—}CH_3$

Isoproterenol

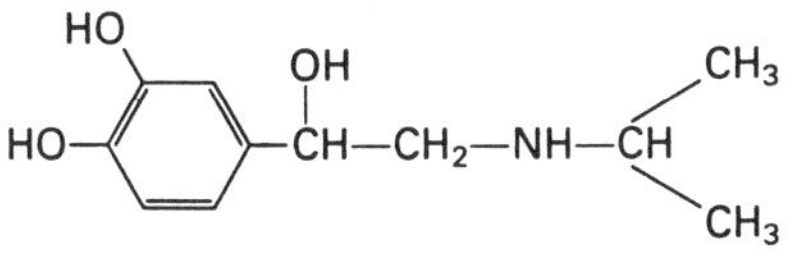

$(HO)_2C_6H_3\text{—}CH(OH)\text{—}CH_2\text{—}NH\text{—}CH(CH_3)_2$

Dobutamine

$(HO)_2C_6H_3\text{—}CH_2\text{—}CH_2\text{—}NH\text{—}CH(CH_3)\text{—}CH_2\text{—}CH_2\text{—}C_6H_4\text{—}OH$

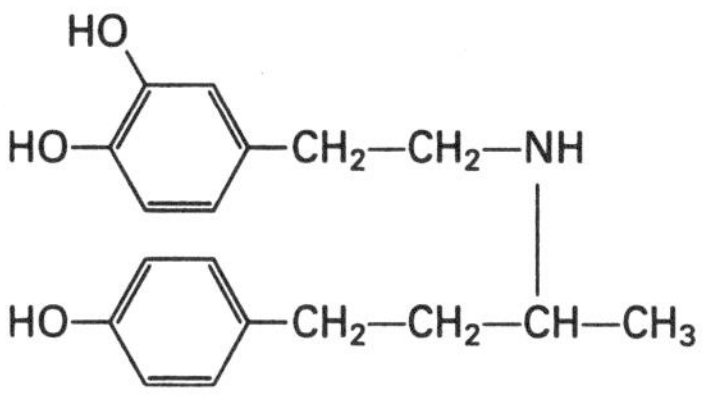

REPRESENTATIVE NONCATECHOLAMINES

Phenylephrine

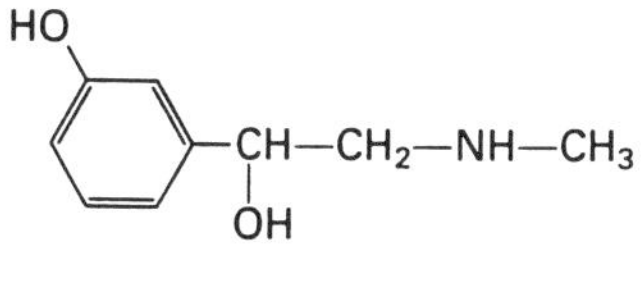

$HO\text{—}C_6H_4\text{—}CH(OH)\text{—}CH_2\text{—}NH\text{—}CH_3$

Phenylpropanolamine

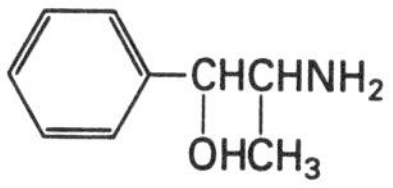

$C_6H_5\text{—}CH(OH)CH(CH_3)NH_2$

Amphetamine

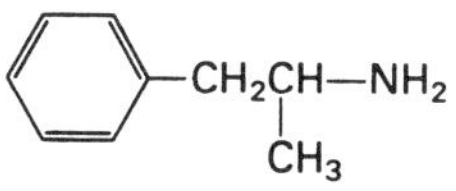

$C_6H_5\text{—}CH_2CH(CH_3)\text{—}NH_2$

Ephedrine

$C_6H_5\text{—}CH(OH)CH(CH_3)NH\text{—}CH_3$

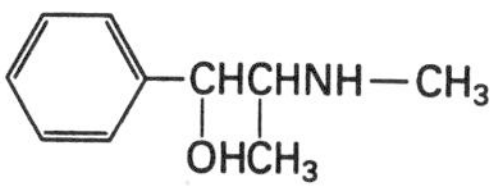

Tetrahydrozoline
(an imidazoline derivative)

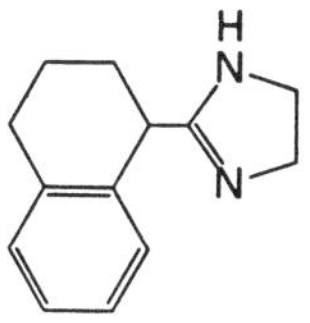

Albuterol

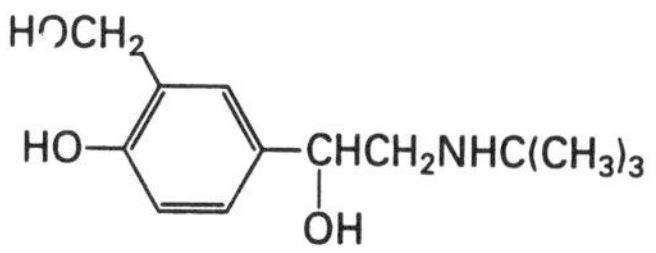

$HOCH_2(HO)C_6H_3\text{—}CH(OH)CH_2NHC(CH_3)_3$

FIGURE 8-2 *Structural aspects of adrenergic drugs.*

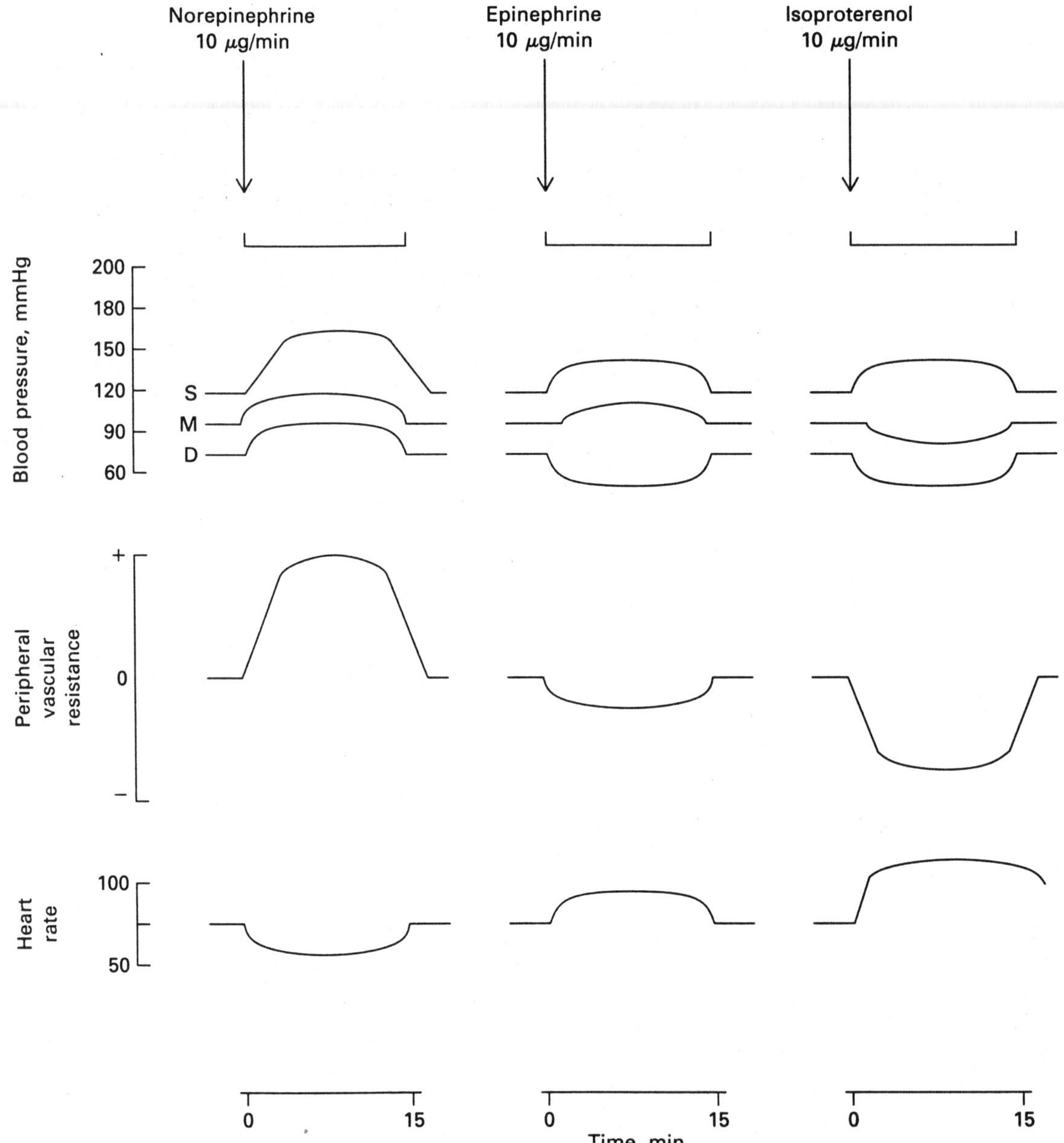

FIGURE 8-3 *The cardiovascular effects of IV administration of norepinephrine, epinephrine, and isoproterenol. Under blood pressure: S = systolic pressure; M = mean blood pressure; D = diastolic pressure. [Modified from Allwood, M.J., et al., Br. Med. Bull.* ***19****: 132-136 (1963)].*

skeletal muscle because of the activation by epinephrine of vascular β_2-adrenergic receptors which subserve vasodilation. Depending on dose and route of administration, the total peripheral vascular resistance may be increased, decreased, or relatively unchanged, as determined by the net combined vasoconstrictive (α-adrenergic) and vasodilatory (β_2-adrenergic receptor) regional vascular responses.

Cardiostimulation is primarily mediated via the

activation of β_1-adrenergic receptors, and is coupled to an elevated intracellular concentration of cyclic AMP and augmented influx of calcium into cardiac cells. Epinephrine alters both the mechanical (contractile) and electrophysiologic (rhythmic) properties of the heart. The increase in myocardial contractility is referred to as a positive inotropic action. Myocardial work, cardiac output, coronary blood flow, and myocardial oxygen consumption are increased by epinephrine.

Epinephrine elevates heart rate (a positive chronotropic action) by increasing the rate of depolarization of pacemaker cells in the sinoatrial node. However, depending on the dosing conditions *in vivo*, baroreceptor reflexes triggered by a rapidly elevated arterial blood pressure may elicit vagal discharge, and thus avert any significant appearance of tachycardia, or result in reflex bradycardia. Blockade of this vagal cholinergic effect by the administration of atropine unmasks the direct cardioaccelerating effect of epinephrine. Large doses of epinephrine can activate latent, i.e., abnormal, pacemaker cells, induce complex changes in impulse formation and conduction characteristics, and thereby precipitate various cardiac arrhythmias such as premature ventricular systoles, ventricular tachycardia, and fibrillation. Accidental intravenous and even conventional subcutaneous doses of epinephrine have the potential to cause lethal arrhythmias.

Respiratory System β_2-Adrenergic receptors which mediate relaxation are found in the smooth muscle of the bronchi. Epinephrine and other sympathomimetic drugs with β_2-adrenergic agonist properties are thus capable of relaxing bronchial muscle and evoking bronchodilation. This therapeutically important action is most pronounced in circumstances when the bronchial muscle is abnormally constricted. Examples of such conditions include bronchial asthma, the administration of bronchoconstrictive drugs, and the release of autacoids (e.g., histamine) during an allergic reaction. Additionally, the α-adrenergic agonist activity of epinephrine produces a respiratory mucosal decongestant effect. The combined bronchodilatation and relief of airway congestion result in an improved vital capacity in bronchospastic states. These effects of epinephrine are attainable when the drug is given systemically by subcutaneous injection, or by inhalation in the form of an aerosolized solution. The respiratory actions of epinephrine are rapid in onset and rather brief in duration and may be accompanied by adverse cardiovascular reactions and other sympathomimetic side effects.

Although epinephrine is clearly valuable in acute bronchospastic states, the use of this catecholamine as a primary medication in the chronic treatment of asthma has waned as longer acting and safer β_2-selective adrenergic agonists have been developed (e.g., salmeterol, albuterol, bitolterol, terbutaline and pirbuterol). Members of this subgroup of adrenergic agonists are discussed in a later section of this chapter.

Ocular Effects Epinephrine and other α-adrenergic agonists (e.g., phenylephrine) contract the radial muscle of the iris to produce mydriasis. The mydriatic effect of topically applied epinephrine is weaker than that of the more selective α-adrenergic agonists. Of greater therapeutic importance is the reduction of intraocular pressure that occurs upon local administration of epinephrine in patients with open-angle glaucoma. The precise mechanism by which epinephrine evokes ocular hypotension is not fully understood but is probably caused by facilitating the outflow of aqueous humor through the ocular drainage network (the trabecular meshwork and Schlemm's canal). Instillation of epinephrine into the eyes can reduce intraocular tension for 12 to 24 h. Dipivefrine (dipivalyl epinephrine), a lipophilic analog of epinephrine, penetrates the tissues of the eye more readily. Dipivefrine, a prodrug, is hydrolyzed into active epinephrine by esterase enzymes in ocular tissues. It is employed for its ocular hypotensive action in chronic glaucomas.

Gastrointestinal System Smooth muscle of the gastrointestinal tract contains α- and β-adrenergic receptors, both of which subserve relaxation. Thus epinephrine and other sympathomimetic drugs may reduce gastric and intestinal contractions, but the magnitude of this inhibitory action depends on the preexisting tone of the muscle. There is also evidence that sympathomimetic agents activate inhibitory presynaptic adrenergic receptors located on cholinergic neurons in the gastrointestinal tract to suppress the release of acetylcholine. These inhibitory effects of sympathomimetic amines on gastrointestinal function are considered to be of minor therapeutic importance.

Genitourinary System Epinephrine and other sympathomimetics relax the urinary bladder detrusor muscle (mediated by β-adrenergic receptors), constrict the trigone and urethral sphincter (mediated by α-adrenergic receptors), and thus promote bladder continence. The reactivity of uterine smooth muscle to adrenergic drugs is influenced by several factors: species, stage of the estrus cycle, and pregnancy. In pregnant women, uterine relaxation occurs upon activation of myometrial β_2-adrenergic receptors. This effect provides the basis for the use of selective β_2-receptor agonists (e.g., ritodrine and terbutaline) in the prevention of premature delivery. In males, sympathetic control of ejaculation is accomplished via α-adrenergic receptors. Inhibition of ejaculation is a relatively common side effect of drugs with α-adrenergic antagonist activity.

Metabolic Effects Epinephrine has prominent and complex actions on several key aspects of intermediary metabolism. Following injections of epinephrine, glycogenolysis in liver and skeletal muscle is enhanced, and lipolysis in adipose tissue is accelerated. Elevated plasma concentrations of glucose (hyperglycemia), lactate (hyperlactacidemia), and free fatty acids (hyperlipidemia) occur. For the most part, these metabolic stimulatory effects of epinephrine result from activation of β-adrenergic receptors with the associated increase in intracellular cyclic AMP. Epinephrine inhibits the pancreatic secretion of insulin and augments glucagon secretion, which facilitates the catabolism of stored hepatic glycogen. Liberation of potassium from the liver leads to a transient hyperkalemia, which is followed by a more prolonged hypokalemia as potassium is taken up by muscle cells. A calorigenic action of epinephrine is manifested by an increase in oxygen consumption and elevated body temperature. These metabolic actions of epinephrine represent an integrated mobilization of energy reserves. In contrast, norepinephrine is significantly less potent in evoking these metabolic alterations.

Central Nervous System Following their peripheral systemic administration, the polar nature of catecholamines, such as epinephrine, greatly limits their access into the central nervous system. Nevertheless, in some patients epinephrine may provoke reactions such as headache, anxiety, restlessness, confusion, and skeletal muscle tremor. Many of these untoward reactions may be secondary to the marked peripheral cardiovascular, respiratory and metabolic actions of epinephrine. The more lipid-soluble noncatecholamines, particularly amphetamine and its congeners (e.g., methamphetamine and benzphetamine), are capable of inducing much more pronounced central stimulatory effects.

Pharmacokinetics

Parenteral administration is required to elicit the systemic effects of epinephrine and other catecholamines; little or no actions are observable if these drugs are given orally. Several factors accounting for this lack of oral activity include: (1) inactivation by digestive secretions, (2) poor absorption due to a low lipid-to-water partition coefficient, (3) local vasoconstriction which diminishes blood flow and absorptive ability of mucous membranes, and (4) rapid enzymatic inactivation in the intestines and liver. The usual routes of parenteral administration of epinephrine are by subcutaneous or intramuscular injection. Intravenous infusion is uncommon in the clinical setting and potentially hazardous.

Solutions of epinephrine may be topically applied to mucous membranes for control of capillary bleeding. Epinephrine and other vasoconstrictive sympathomimetics may be combined with local anesthetics to reduce systemic absorption of the local anesthetic from the injection site.

In bronchial asthma, epinephrine solution is aerosolized in a suitable nebulizer, and the fine mist is inhaled through the mouth. Adverse reactions due to systemic absorption may occur; the risk of toxicity is higher in geriatric patients and in patients with longstanding chronic lung disease.

The metabolism of catecholamines is based on an interplay of several biochemical reactions, including oxidative deamination, methylation, and conjugation. Only a minute fraction of circulating epinephrine and norepinephrine are excreted unchanged. Two key enzyme systems — monoamine oxidase (MAO) and catechol-*O*-methyltransferase (COMT) — participate in the degradation of catecholamines, and the group of metabolic products resulting from the actions of both enzymes is excreted in the urine. An estimate of catecholamine turnover can be obtained from analysis of the urinary concentrations of these metabolites.

The biotransformation of these compounds, as well as important tissue re-uptake processes which are involved in terminating the activity of neurally released catecholamines are discussed in Chapter 7.

Adverse Reactions

Many untoward reactions from epinephrine and related catecholamines are predictable extensions of their sympathomimetic effects resulting from α-

and β-adrenoceptor activation. Due to the transient duration of activity of the catecholamines, palpitations, mild tachycardia, hypertension, anxiety, headache, and tremor may not represent serious complications. However, increased cardiac work with an attendant increase in myocardial oxygen requirement may precipitate angina pectoris or myocardial infarction. Excessive or inappropriate dosing with catecholamines can promote convulsive seizures, extremely high arterial pressure resulting in cerebrovascular hemorrhage, and life-threatening ventricular arrhythmias. The halogenated volatile general anesthetics, e.g., halothane, are well known to sensitize the myocardium to the arrhythmogenic actions of the catecholamines.

General contraindications to the use of epinephrine include hypertension, hyperthyroidism, ischemic heart disease, cerebrovascular insufficiency, organic brain damage, and predisposition to narrow angle glaucoma. Because of cardiac stimulation and vasoconstriction, pulmonary hypertension leading to pulmonary edema may be a cause of fatality.

Several important drug interactions are possible with epinephrine. The cardiovascular effects of epinephrine may be potentiated to a dangerous degree in patients receiving monoamine oxidase inhibitors, tricyclic antidepressants, thyroxine, or other sympathomimetic agents (e.g., vasoconstrictors and nasal decongestants). Propranolol and other β-adrenergic blockers antagonize the cardiostimulatory and bronchodilator effects, and intensify the pressor effect of epinephrine. Dosage adjustments of insulin or oral hypoglycemic drugs may be necessitated because of the hyperglycemic effect of epinephrine. Fatal cardiac arrhythmias can occur in digitalized patients receiving epinephrine.

Therapeutic Uses

Epinephrine (given by subcutaneous injection) can be lifesaving and is the drug of choice in the treatment of anaphylactic shock and related acute hypersensitivity reactions. By its combined cardiorespiratory actions on α-, β_1-, and β_2-adrenergic receptors, it is able to reverse the syndrome of cardiovascular collapse, bronchospasm, airway congestion, and angioedema.

The use of epinephrine by aerosol as a bronchodilator and pulmonary decongestant in the treatment of bronchial asthma has been previously described, as was its value in lowering intraocular tension in the treatment of simple, wide-angle glaucoma. Other ophthalmic indications are based on its decongestant (vasoconstrictive) and mydriatic actions in the eye. Similarly, the use of epinephrine as a topical hemostatic to control superficial bleeding and its combination with local anesthetics to prolong their action are based on a local vasoconstrictive effect. Epinephrine and other cardiostimulatory catecholamines have been used in the emergency treatment of complete heart block and cardiac arrest.

Norepinephrine

Norepinephrine, the principal neurotransmitter produced and released by adrenergic neurons, is also known as *(−)-noradrenaline* and *levarterenol*. This vasopressor catecholamine constricts both resistance and capacitance blood vessels (by stimulating α-adrenergic receptors) and has direct cardiostimulatory actions on the heart (mediated through β_1-adrenergic receptor activation). Norepinephrine has significantly weaker effects than epinephrine on vascular β_2-adrenergic receptors mediating vasodilation. The typical response to intravenous infusion of this drug consists of a rise in both systolic and diastolic arterial blood pressure resulting from an increased peripheral vascular resistance, accompanied by bradycardia. Thus, the direct chronotropic action on the heart is overshadowed by vagal reflexes. Norepinephrine may be used by intravenous infusion in acute hypotensive states when a potent vasoconstrictor is needed to maintain tissue perfusion. It can cause ischemic tissue necrosis at the infusion site. In contrast to epinephrine, norepinephrine has little or no stimulatory effect on carbohydrate and lipid metabolism.

Isoproterenol

This synthetic catecholamine is representative of a sympathomimetic drug with high selectivity for β-adrenergic receptors. Substitution of a bulky alkyl group on the amino nitrogen atom of the phenylethylamine skeleton confers greater affinity for β-adrenergic receptor sites than for α-adrenergic sites (Fig. 8-2). Thus, isoproterenol lacks significant α-adrenergic agonist actions.

The activation by isoproterenol of β_1-adrenergic receptors in the heart evokes positive chronotropic and inotropic actions. Peripheral vascular resistance is reduced via β_2-adrenergic-mediated vasodilation, principally in skeletal muscle but also in the renal and mesenteric circulations. These combined cardiostimulatory and vasodilatory effects result in a marked increase in stroke volume and cardiac output. Since the drug does not activate α-adrenergic receptors, isoproterenol lacks a vasoconstrictive action and does not elevate systemic arterial blood pressure as do norepinephrine and epinephrine. Arterial pulse pressure increases as a consequence of increased stroke volume in the face of reduced peripheral vascular resistance. Large doses of isoproterenol can produce a significant fall in systemic blood pressure. Figure 8-3 illustrates the differential profiles of three representative sympathomimetic catecholamines exhibiting relatively selective α-adrenergic agonist (norepinephrine), β-adrenergic agonist (isoproterenol), or both α- and β-adrenergic agonist (epinephrine) actions on the cardiovascular system.

Bronchodilation is another prominent action of isoproterenol, resulting from activation of pulmonary β_2-adrenergic receptors. Inhalation of a mist of isoproterenol can prevent and relieve bronchoconstriction in asthmatics but may be accompanied by cardiac stimulation. The use of isoproterenol as a bronchodilator has decreased as newer β_2-selective adrenergic agonists have become available (see Table 8-1). When compared to isoproterenol, this latter group of drugs has an advantage of causing fewer cardiac side effects (palpitations, tachycardia, arrhythmias) at doses that are equally bronchodilatory.

Phenylephrine

This synthetic drug is a noncatecholamine but is related both in chemical structure (see Fig. 8-2) and pharmacologic activity to norepinephrine. The characteristic feature of phenylephrine is its marked selectivity for α-adrenergic receptors (specifically, α_1). Thus, phenylephrine evokes vasoconstriction but little or no cardiostimulation. Parenteral administration results in elevated arterial blood pressure, accompanied by reflex bradycardia. Blood vessels in mucous membranes are constricted. Topical application to the nasal mucosa of patients with infectious or allergic rhinitis promotes a local decongestant effect by reducing blood flow to engorged, edematous tissue. Instillation to the eye results in mydriasis as well as a decongestant effect on ocular tissues. Central stimulatory effects are minimal with this drug.

Other Sympathomimetic Decongestants

Phenylephrine and *phenylpropanolamine* (see below) are among the most popular sympathomimetic drugs used for their mucosal decongestant action. Drugs such as *naphazoline*, *oxymetazoline*, *tetrahydrozoline*, and *xylometazoline* are chemically related imidazolines (see Fig. 8-2) used topically as mucosal decongestants. These are α-adrenergic agonists which cause a "drying" effect when applied to congested membranes by constricting nasal mucosal blood vessels. The onset of effects is less than 10 min, and duration of action may be longer than 5 h; oxymetazoline is somewhat longer acting than the others. Phenylephrine, naphazoline and tetrahydrozoline are used also as ocular decongestants (vasoconstriction of conjunctival blood vessels) for the relief of redness of the eye due to minor eye irritations.

Continued use of topical decongestant drugs can result in rebound congestion. As the drug effect wanes, the congestion returns with increased severity and encourages further use of the medication. Prolonged use over several days may lead to rhinitis medicamentosa, a disorder characterized by chronic swelling and a red, boggy edematous appearance of the mucosa.

Clonidine

As previously mentioned, this drug is a selective α_2-adrenergic agonist. Clonidine, methyldopa, guanabenz and guanfacine lower systemic blood pressure and heart rate by stimulating α_2-adrenergic receptors in certain areas of the central nervous system and are used primarily as antihypertensive drugs. The pharmacology of these drugs is discussed in Chapter 32.

Dobutamine

The increased myocardial contractility produced by intravenous infusion of dobutamine has been attributed to selective activation of cardiac β_1-adrenergic receptors. However, the mechanism of action of this compound is more complex since dobutamine can also activate α_1-adrenoceptors in the myocardium and vascular β_2-adrenoceptors. In moderate doses, dobutamine increases cardiac output without greatly increasing heart rate and tends to lower peripheral vascular resistance. Higher doses elevate blood pressure and increase heart rate.

The onset of action of dobutamine occurs within 2 min of intravenous infusion; peak activity usually occurs within 10 min. Dobutamine is a synthetic catecholamine which is not effective by the oral route. The plasma half-life of a single intravenous injection is 2 min. Biotransformation of this compound is primarily via methylation of the catechol group and subsequent conjugation (see Fig. 8-2). Conjugates of 3-*O*-methyl dobutamine, an inactive biotransformation product, and the parent compound are the major urinary excretion products.

Dobutamine is used when parenteral therapy is necessary to improve myocardial function in the short-term treatment of patients with severe refractory cardiac failure and to provide inotropic support following cardiac surgery. A greater improvement in cardiac performance may be attained when dobutamine is used in combination with intravenously administered vasodilators such as nitroprusside and nitroglycerin.

Hypertension, tachycardia, and ventricular arrhythmias are the most commonly encountered adverse effects. More rarely, nausea, headache, anginal pain, palpitations, and shortness of breath may occur. Dobutamine may also accelerate AV conduction. Untoward cardiovascular reactions to this drug can usually be controlled by reducing the dose.

Terbutaline

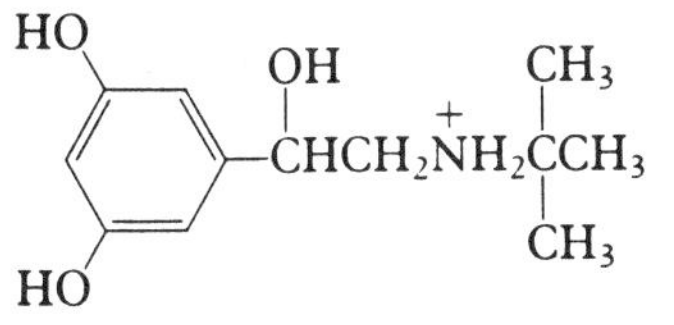

HO
OH CH₃
CHCH₂N⁺H₂CCH₃
CH₃
HO

Terbutaline, a synthetic noncatecholamine sympathomimetic amine, is a direct-acting β-adrenergic receptor agonist. In therapeutic doses, terbutaline selectively stimulates the β_2-adrenoceptors found in bronchial smooth muscle with relatively little activity on the cardiac β_1-adrenergic receptors (Table 8-1). Although this drug is one of the more selective β_2-adrenergic receptor stimulants, the degree of selectivity of terbutaline and similar agents will vary with dose, and cardiovascular effects have been reported.

Terbutaline can be administered orally, by inhalation or by subcutaneous injection. Since it is not a catecholamine, terbutaline is not susceptible to enzymatic inactivation by COMT nor is it a substrate for the cellular uptake processes for catecholamines. Thus, its duration of action is considerably longer than that of isoproterenol and epinephrine. By the oral route the onset is within 30 min and the duration of effect up to 8 h; by inhalation the duration of the drug is somewhat shorter.

Terbutaline is used in the treatment of bronchial spasm such as occurs in chronic obstructive pulmonary diseases (e.g., bronchitis and emphysema) and as a bronchodilator in asthma.

Adverse reactions produced by terbutaline are those commonly associated with other sympathomimetic amines, and include tremors, nervousness, and more rarely headache, tachycardia, palpitations, sweating, drowsiness, nausea, and vomiting. Tolerance appears to develop to these untoward effects as therapy with terbutaline continues.

Albuterol

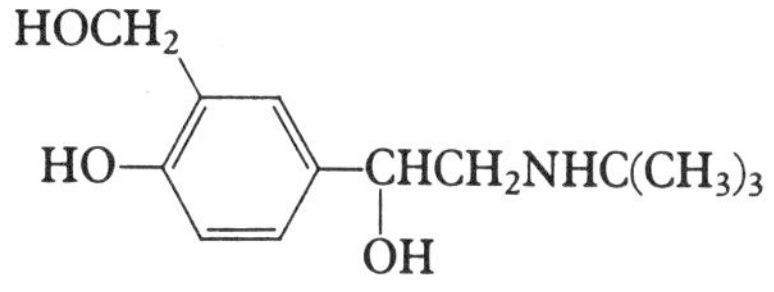

HOCH₂
HO— —CHCH₂NHC(CH₃)₃
OH

Albuterol is another noncatecholamine selective β_2-adrenergic sympathomimetic with pharmacologic characteristics similar to terbutaline and several other adrenergic bronchodilators. It is widely used in acute and chronic bronchial asthma, bronchitis, and other chronic obstructive pulmonary diseases. When administered by the inhalation route, significant bronchodilation occurs within 15 min and lasts for 3 to 4 h. Following oral administration, albuterol is conjugated in the intestinal mucosa and liver; urinary excretion of both the unchanged drug and sulfate conjugates occurs. Greater separation of β_2 effects (bronchodilation) from β_1 effects (cardiostimulation) can be achieved when the drug is used by inhalation than by systemic administration.

Similar to other selective β_2 agonists, a common side effect of albuterol is skeletal muscle tremor, more frequently encountered during oral dosing regimens. Fine finger tremors may interfere with manual activities. Disturbances in cardiac rate and rhythm may also occur but are less problematic than with epinephrine or isoproterenol. Excessive use may lead to a state of tolerance and refractoriness to the bronchodilatory effect.

Salmeterol

Salmeterol is a long-acting, selective β_2-adrenergic receptor agonist that is structurally-related to albuterol. It differs in that it contains a long, lipophilic, N-substituted side chain that binds irreversibly to a site adjacent to the active site of the β-adrenergic receptor (called an "exo-site"). The long side chain and the lipophilicity of the compound are believed to be responsible for the prolonged effects of the drug. *In vitro* studies have shown that salmeterol is the most selective β_2-adrenergic receptor stimulant of all of the drugs available for clinical use. At present, salmeterol is only available for use by inhalation.

The onset of action of salmeterol is dose-related and ranges from 10 to 20 min; peak activity occurs in 3 to 4 h. The duration of the bronchodilation after inhalation is at least 12 h; however, some pulmonary effects have been observed for up to 30 h after dosing. Approximately 96 percent of salmeterol found in the circulation is bound to plasma proteins. The drug is extensively biotransformed and eliminated primarily in the feces.

Salmeterol is generally well tolerated with adverse effects similar to other β_2-adrenergic receptor agonists. The drug is indicated for use in the treatment of patients with bronchial asthma and the prevention of bronchospasm in those with reversible obstructive airway disease (see Chapter 33).

Pirbuterol

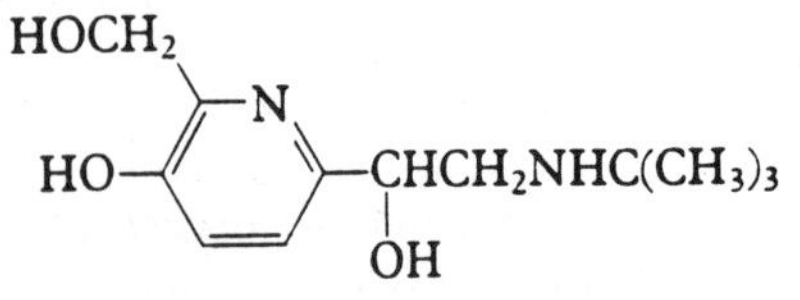

HOCH$_2$ N HO CHCH$_2$NHC(CH$_3$)$_3$ OH

Pirbuterol is structurally related to albuterol, stimulates β_2-adrenoceptors, and produces similar bronchodilatory and cardiovascular effects. Although pirbuterol is less potent on a weight basis, when administered by inhalation, the onset of action, time to peak effect, and duration of action are similar to albuterol. The drug is used to treat patients with reversible bronchospasm and asthma. As with other sympathomimetics, pirbuterol should be used with caution in patients with cardiovascular disease (e.g., hypertension, ischemia and arrhythmias).

Bitolterol

Bitolterol is a bronchodilatory β_2-adrenoceptor agonist; it is a prodrug that is slowly hydrolyzed by blood and tissue esterases to its active form, colterol. Used by inhalation, the onset of action of bitolterol is rapid (3 to 4 min) and its duration of action is between 5 and 8 h. The drug is used to treat bronchial asthma and reversible bronchospasm.

Metaproterenol

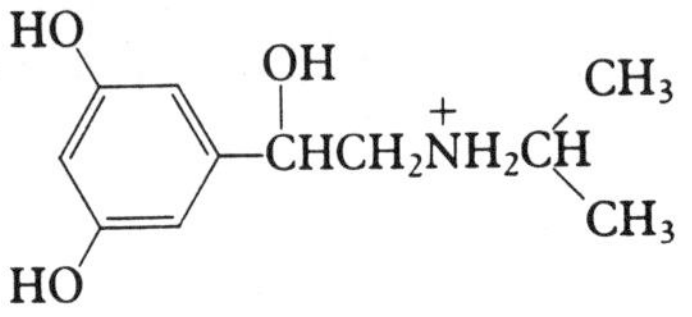

HO OH CH$_3$ CHCH$_2\overset{+}{N}$H$_2$CH CH$_3$ HO

Metaproterenol is less selective than terbutaline, albuterol, pirbuterol and bitolterol as a β_2-adrenergic stimulant, but the drug is still useful in the treatment of chronic obstructive airway diseases. It can be administered by either the oral or inhalational route. It is not biotransformed by COMT as is the case with the catecholamines but is excreted primarily as glucuronide conjugates via the kidney. Duration of action is approximately 4 h following a single dose. Adverse reactions are similar to the other aforementioned drugs.

Isoetharine

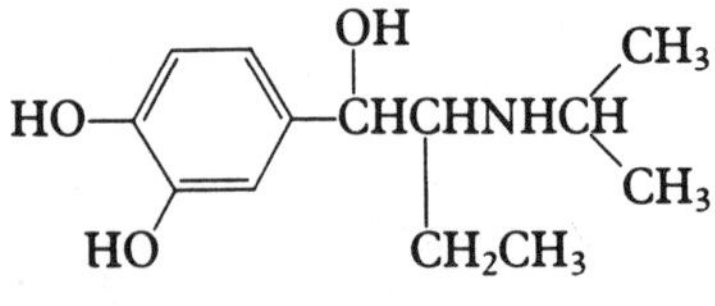

OH CH$_3$ HO CHCHNHCH CH$_3$ HO CH$_2$CH$_3$

Isoetharine is a direct-acting sympathomimetic with relatively low selectivity for β_2-adrenergic receptor sites. However, this drug produces more rapid relief of bronchial spasms than the more selective bronchodilator agonists. Isoetharine is a catecholamine, metabolized by COMT to an inactive compound. As such, isoetharine is not active following oral administration, rather it is effective only by inhalation. As with other sympathomimetic amines administered by inhalation, tolerance may develop with prolonged continuous use of isoetharine.

Ritodrine

This selective β_2-adrenergic agonist is approved for use both intravenously and orally in carefully selected patients as a uterine relaxant for the prevention of premature labor (terbutaline and albuterol have been used to arrest premature labor but are as yet unapproved for this use in the United States). Intravenous therapy with ritodrine is initiated when contraindications have been ruled out; if successful, oral maintenance dosing is then instituted. Cardiovascular and metabolic reactions, i.e., hypokalemia and diabetogenic effects, have been noted in both mother and fetus, especially during intravenous infusion of this drug. Ritodrine therapy has largely replaced the previous use of intravenous alcohol to inhibit premature labor.

INDIRECT-ACTING AGENTS

The only indirect-acting compound that will be mentioned here is tyramine, which exerts its sympathomimetic effect by causing the release of endogenous norepinephrine from storage vesicles in the adrenergic neuron. Tyramine has no other action, and because its effectiveness is limited by the extent of neuronal norepinephrine stores and it is rapidly inactivated by intraneuronal MAO, it is of no clinical value. Tyramine is, however, important as an experimental laboratory tool and has toxicologic importance with some types of antidepressant drugs (see Chapter 21).

MIXED-ACTING AGENTS

The mixed-acting sympathomimetic drugs discussed below all possess, to some extent, a tyramine-like indirect action in addition to direct adrenergic receptor activation.

Dopamine

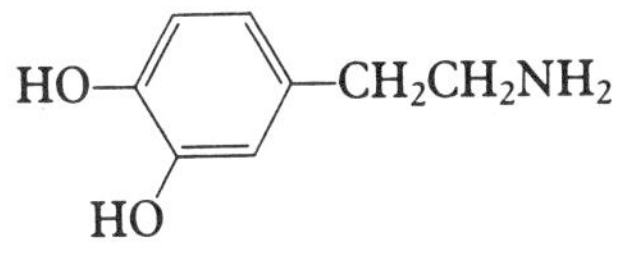

HO— (benzene ring) —$CH_2CH_2NH_2$

HO

Dopamine is one of the intermediate products in the synthesis of norepinephrine and is formed by the decarboxylation of DOPA. Dopamine has been found in all sympathetic neurons and ganglia, and in the CNS.

As a drug, dopamine stimulates both α- and β_1-adrenoceptors in addition to dopaminergic receptors; it has little activity on β_2-adrenergic receptors. Dopamine can also release norepinephrine from storage sites in neuronal tissues. Although dopamine has activity at central dopamine receptors, exogenously-administered drug does not cross the blood-brain barrier to any significant extent and only the administration of the prodrug levodopa will elicit a central response (see "Antiparkinsonian Agents" in Chapter 22).

Dopamine exerts its major effects on the cardiovascular system and on renal and mesenteric vasculature. Intravenous infusion of this endogenous catecholamine evokes a unique complex of hemodynamic actions which is dependent on the dose administered. Small doses produce increases in renal and mesenteric blood flow by activating dopaminergic receptors which mediate vasodilation in these areas. Somewhat greater doses additionally stimulate the heart via β_1-adrenergic receptor activation; cardiac output is increased without markedly increasing heart rate or blood pressure and with less oxygen consumption than occurs with the catecholamines. Larger doses of dopamine evoke vasoconstriction (an α-adrenergic receptor-mediated effect) resulting in elevated systolic and diastolic blood pressure.

Dopamine is commonly used as a temporary adjunct in treating hypotension and circulatory shock caused by myocardial infarction, trauma, renal failure, and endotoxic septicemia. Because of its renal vasodilatory action, it may be more beneficial than other sympathomimetic amines (e.g., norepinephrine, metaraminol) in patients with impaired renal function. However, excessive doses can decrease renal blood flow and urine output. Dopamine is a more potent vasopressor agent than dobutamine.

The most common adverse reactions to dopamine include nausea, vomiting, CNS disturbances, and a variety of cardiovascular manifestations: tachyarrhythmias, palpitations, hypotension, vasoconstriction, and anginal pain. An improvement in hemodynamic status may be accompanied by increased myocardial oxygen demand. Large doses or long infusion periods have resulted in peripheral ischemia and gangrene. Since dopamine is metabolized by monoamine oxidase, a tenfold reduction in dosage is warranted if the drug is administered to patients receiving monoamine oxidase inhibitors.

Ephedrine

Ephedrine, an alkaloid which occurs in certain species of the plant genus *Ephedra*, is now produced synthetically (see Fig. 8-2). Ephedrine is a "mixed-acting" noncatecholamine sympathomimetic agent that, lacking the catechol moiety, is distinguished from epinephrine and norepinephrine by its oral efficacy, longer duration of effect, more pronounced actions on the CNS, and significantly lower potency. The drug directly stimulates both α- and β-adrenergic receptors and also causes the release of norepinephrine from sympathetic neurons. Two principal uses of ephedrine as a mucosal decongestant and bronchodilator are consequences of activating α- and β-adrenoceptors, respectively. *Pseudoephedrine* is a stereoisomer with pharmacologic actions only subtly different from ephedrine; it is used orally as a decongestant.

Pharmacodynamics

Cardiovascular System If given intravenously, ephedrine produces cardiovascular effects similar to those of epinephrine. Systemic arterial blood pressure rises (both systolic and diastolic) and reflexly-mediated cardiac slowing occurs. If vagal reflexes are blocked, heart rate is seen to increase. The hypertensive response is due to a combination increased vascular resistance resulting from vasoconstriction and an increase in cardiac output resulting from cardiac stimulation. In comparison with epinephrine, the pressor response to ephedrine is slower in onset, lasts considerably longer, and requires a much higher dose to obtain an equivalent pressure elevation. If a second identical intravenous dose of ephedrine is administered shortly thereafter, the ensuing pressor response proves weaker than that following the first dose. This phenomenon, known as *tachyphylaxis* (i.e., "rapid tolerance"), is a characteristic of sympathomimetic amines with an indirect-acting component that liberate norepinephrine from storage sites in the body. Tachyphylaxis is not observed with norepinephrine, epinephrine, and other direct-acting sympathomimetic amines. One explanation which has been given for this phenomenon is neuronal depletion of the neurotransmitter following repetitive exposure to the indirect-acting compound.

Respiratory System The smooth muscle of the bronchial tree is relaxed by ephedrine as a result of activating bronchopulmonary β_2-adrenergic receptors. Compared to epinephrine, the bronchodilation produced by ephedrine is significantly weaker and is slower in onset but more sustained.

Other Smooth Muscles and Glands In general, ephedrine has effects on smooth muscle and glands that are qualitatively similar to epinephrine. Inhibition of the intact gastrointestinal musculature and contraction of the splenic capsule and of pilomotor muscles may be produced.

Central Nervous System Ephedrine passes the blood-brain barrier and is a corticomedullary stimulant, as are other sympathomimetic amines with structural features of an unsubstituted phenyl ring and a methyl group on the alpha carbon. The mental "alerting" activity of ephedrine is less pronounced than that of central nervous system stimulants such as amphetamine and methamphetamine. Depending on the dose, ephedrine can produce insomnia, restlessness, anxiety, agitation, and tremor.

Pharmacokinetics

Ephedrine is readily and completely absorbed after oral administration. If given subcutaneously or intramuscularly, local vasoconstriction at the injection site is not significant enough to prevent systemic absorption. Ephedrine resists oxidative deamination by MAO, but deamination and conjugation do occur to some extent via the hepatic microsomal system. Up to 40 percent of an administered dose of the drug may be secreted unchanged in the urine. The pharmacologic activity of a single dose persists for several hours.

Ephedrine is usually administered orally in tablet, capsule, or liquid forms. Sterile solutions can be given by the subcutaneous, intramuscular, and intravenous routes, but the parenteral use of the drug is relatively uncommon. For local decongestion of the nasal mucosa, ephedrine solutions are applied directly by drops or as a spray.

Therapeutic Uses

Ephedrine is an orally effective, long-acting sympathomimetic drug. Its clinical applications include allergic disorders, nasal congestion, and bronchial asthma. The drug is not useful for severe attacks of bronchial asthma because of its limited potency, but it is employed in several oral medications as a mild bronchodilator. Unfortunately, tolerance develops during prolonged administration. Both ephedrine and pseudoephedrine are popular ingredients of many proprietary decongestants and cough and cold formulations. Ephedrine can also be used as a pressor agent in spinal anesthesia, and occasionally as a CNS stimulant.

Adverse Reactions

Untoward reactions from ephedrine such as nervousness, insomnia, nausea, vertigo, and tremor are related to its actions on the central nervous system. Cardiovascular complications are similar to those with epinephrine. Many nonprescription drug products for the symptomatic relief of allergies and upper respiratory infections contain ephedrine, pseudoephedrine, or related sympathomimetic drugs such as phenylpropanolamine. Patients with hypertension, cardiac problems, hyperthyroidism, and diabetes mellitus should be warned of the potential risks entailed by injudicious use of these products. Prolonged and continuous use of ephedrine can result in tolerance.

Phenylpropanolamine

The pharmacologic actions of phenylpropanolamine are similar to those of ephedrine. This sympathomimetic agent can cause transient elevations of blood pressure and is used for its nasal decongestant activity. A weak central stimulant, phenylpropanolamine has anorexigenic properties similar to but weaker than those of the amphetamines. It is currently available in nonprescription drug products promoted for (1) use as an upper respiratory decongestant in colds and allergies, and (2) short-term use as an adjunctive drug in weight control programs. The appetite suppressant effect of phenylpropanolamine is probably mediated at adrenergic neurotransmission sites in the brain stem.

Adverse effects can include both cardiovascular and CNS reactions such as hypertension, stroke, nausea, nervousness, insomnia, and neuropsychiatric problems. The incidence of such adverse reactions is relatively low when used at recommended oral therapeutic doses, but there appear to be individuals who are highly sensitive to the drug. Contraindications to the use of phenylpropanolamine are the same as those of epinephrine.

Amphetamines

This term is commonly used in reference to racemic amphetamine, dextroamphetamine, and methamphetamine. As mixed-acting drugs, the amphetamines activate adrenergic receptors, central dopaminergic receptors, and also release endogenous catecholamines (norepinephrine and dopamine) from neurons in the brain and periphery. Their peripheral sympathomimetic properties closely resemble ephedrine. Oral administration raises systolic and diastolic blood pressure often with reflex cardiac slowing, but bronchodilation is a less prominent effect. The most distinguishing characteristic of the amphetamines relates to their psychic stimulatory activity. Both methamphetamine and dextroamphetamine (the (+) isomer of racemic amphetamine), are more potent than the (−) isomer in evoking CNS excitatory effects. The stimulatory actions of amphetamines result in increased alertness, elevated mood states, insomnia, irritability, and dizziness. Large doses can induce hallucinations, violent behavior, and a psychotic state that resembles paranoid schizophrenia.

Amphetamines are biotransformed by oxidative deamination in the drug-metabolizing microsomal system, and their metabolic fate may be affected by agents which alter the response of this system.

Amphetamines were the first drugs widely prescribed for appetite suppression in treating obesity. They are no longer recommended for use as anorexiants because of their striking psychic and physical dependence liability. Tolerance to the anoretic effect (and euphoric "high") can develop quite rapidly, and progressively larger doses must be taken to obtain the desired psychic response. Based on its central actions, dextroamphetamine has been used in treating narcolepsy, urinary incontinence, and attention deficit disorder in children. Prolonged use in children can impair linear growth and reduce weight gain.

Several substituted phenylethylamines have anorexiant and CNS stimulant properties similar to those of amphetamine, although they differ in potency and other actions. *Diethylpropion, phendimetrazine* and *phenteramine* are representative of this group.

The use of an amphetamine or an amphetamine-like sympathomimetic drug is contraindicated in patients with cardiovascular disease, hypertension, hyperthyroidism, glaucoma, and pregnancy. Persons with a history of emotional disorders or drug abuse should not receive these agents.

Metaraminol

Metaraminol is a sympathomimetic amine that has both direct and indirect actions and has hemodynamic characteristics similar to those of norepinephrine. Because of its prominent α-adrenergic agonist activity it may be useful parenterally as a vasoconstrictor, e.g., in treating acute hypotensive states during spinal anesthesia.

SUMMARIZED USES OF ADRENERGIC DRUGS

Cardiovascular Uses

The positive inotropic effect of adrenergic agents with β-adrenoceptor agonist properties provides a basis for their use in conditions in which myocardial stimulation and increased cardiac output are desired. Cardiostimulatory sympathomimetics have been used in circulatory and cardiogenic shock, for the short-term therapy of severe congestive heart failure, and in the emergency management of complete heart block and cardiac arrest.

Vasoconstrictor agents (e.g., phenylephrine) may convert episodes of paroxysmal atrial tachycardia to a sinus rhythm by elevating arterial blood pressure and thereby activating vagal cholinergic reflexes. Regional vasoconstriction may be desirable to control hemorrhage in surgical procedures and to reduce diffusion of local anesthetics from their site of injection. Vasoconstriction in mucous membranes forms the basis of use of sympathomimetics as nasal, bronchopulmonary, and ocular decongestants.

Bronchopulmonary Uses

β-Adrenergic agonists, and in particular the selective β_2-receptor agonists, are an important class of drugs used in both acute and chronic therapy of bronchial asthma and certain other obstructive respiratory diseases. Their efficacy is primarily based on their ability to reverse bronchoconstriction, but evidence also exists that they can inhibit the release of chemical mediators of inflammation and increase the rate of mucociliary clearance. Other classes of drugs used in bronchial disorders are described in Chapter 33.

Central Nervous System Uses

Sympathomimetic drugs with central stimulatory actions, i.e., the amphetamines, have been used as anorexiants in obesity, in the treatment of narcolepsy, and in children diagnosed with attention deficit disorder (ADD). The clinical efficacy of amphetamines in many of these neuropsychiatric applications is not well proven and controversial. Physical dependence and addiction to amphetamines severely limits their therapeutic value. The illicit sale of amphetamine-like stimulants and their widespread abuse for "antifatigue" and euphoric effects is a major social problem. Their legitimate use in medicine for trivial purposes is unwarranted.

Methylphenidate is a mild CNS stimulant, similar to amphetamine, which is primarily used to treat hyperkinesis in children with ADD. The prescribed dose of methylphenidate is usually dependent on behavioral severity. This agent has been found to improve the concentration and learning ability of children with ADD. Some of the more common side effects of methylphenidate include insomnia, anorexia, elevated heart rate and irritability. Side effects can be diminished by reducing the dosage. Methylphenidate also has a high abuse potential.

Pemoline is a CNS stimulant that is structurally dissimilar to the amphetamines. Pemoline is used to treat ADD, but the exact site and mechanism of its pharmacological action is unknown. As with methylphenidate, pemoline is most effective when used as an adjunct to educational and psychological therapy for treating hyperactive patients.

Other Uses

Ophthalmic uses of sympathomimetics are based on their mydriatic and decongestant properties and their ability to reduce intraocular pressure in open-angle glaucoma. The use of β_2-adrenergic agonists (specifically ritodrine) for their uterine relaxant activity has replaced older therapies in suppressing premature labor.

BIBLIOGRAPHY

Allwood, M.J., A.F. Cobbold, and J. Ginsburg: "Peripheral Vascular Effects of Noradrenaline, Isopropylnoradrenaline and Dopamine," *Br. Med. Bull.* **19**: 132-136 (1963).

Axclrod, J., and T. Reisine: "Stress Hormones: Their Interaction and Regulation," *Science*, **224**: 452-459 (1984).

Barach, E.M., R.M. Nowak, G.L. Tennyson, and M. C. Tomlanovich: "Epinephrine for Treatment of Anaphylactic Shock," *Am. Med. Assoc.* **251**: 2118-2122 (1984).

Barnes, P.J.: "A New Approach to the Treatment of Asthma," *N. Engl. J. Med.*, **321**: 1517-1527 (1989).

Bilezikian, J.P.: "Defining the Role of Adrenergic Receptors in Human Physiology," in P.A. Insel (ed.), *Adrenergic Receptors in Man*, Marcel Dekker, New York, 1987, pp. 37-68.

Bravo, E.L.: "Phenylpropanolamine and Other Over-the-Counter Vasoactive Compounds," *Hypertension* **Mar 11 (3 Pt 2):II** 7-10 (1988).

Bulbring, E., and T. Tomita: "Catecholamine Action on Smooth Muscle," *Pharmacol. Rev.* **39**: 49-96 (1987).

Dohlman, H.G., M.G. Caron, and R.J. Lefkowitz: "A Family of Receptors Coupled to Guanine Nucleotide Regtilatory Proteins," *Biochemisity* **26**: 2657-2664 (1987).

Drug Evaluations Annual 1991, prepared by the Department of Drugs, Division of Drugs and Toxicology, American Medical Association, Milwaukee, 1991.

Dwyer, J.M.: "Pharmacologic Approach to Management of Asthma," *Ration. Drug Ther.* **18**: 1-8 (1984).

Feldman, R., and L.E. Limbird: "Biochemical Characterization of Human Adrenergic Receptors, in P. A. Insel (ed.), *Adrenergic Receptors in Man*, Marcel Dekker, New York, 1987, pp. 161-200.

Goldberg, L.I.: "Dopamine: Clinical Uses of an Endogenous Catecholamine," *N. Engl. J. Med.* **291**: 707-710 (1974).

Kesten, S., and A.S. Rebuck,: "Management of Chronic Obstructive Pulmonary Disease," *Drugs* **38**: 160-174 (1989).

Kopin, I.J.: "Catecholamine Metabolism: Basic Aspects and Clinical Significance," *Pharmacol. Rev.* **37**: 333-364 (1985).

Lefkowitz, R.J., and M.C. Caron: "Molecular and Regulatory Properties of Adrenergic Receptors," *Recent Prog. Horm. Res.* **43**: 469-487 (1987).

Mefford, I.N.: "Epinephrine in Mammalian Brain," *Prog. Neuro-Psychopharmacol. & Biol. Psychiat.* **12**: 365-388 (1988).

Minneman, K.P.: "α-Adrenergic Receptor Subtypes, Inositol Phosphates, and Sources of Cell Ca^{2+}" *Pharmacol. Rev.* **40**: 87-119 (1988).

Ruffolo, R.R., Jr.: "The Pharmacology of Dobutamine," *Am. Med. Sci.* **294**: 244-248 (1987).

Sarnoff, S.J., S.K. Brockman, J.P. Gilmore, R.J. Linden, and J.H. Mitchell: "Regulation of Ventricular Contraction. Influence of Cardiac Sympathetic and Vagal Nerve Stimulation on Atrial and Ventricular Dynamics," *Circ. Res.* **8**: 1108-1122 (1960).

Sonneblick, E.H.: "Implications of Muscle Mechanics in the Heart," *Fed. Proc.* **21**: 975-990 (1962).

Strader, C.D., I.S. Sigal, and R.A.F. Dixon,: "Structural Basis of β-Adrenergic Receptor Function," *FASEB J.* **3**: 1825-1832 (1989).

Whitehouse, A.M., and J.M. Duncan: "Ephedrine Psychosis Rediscovered," *Br. J. Psychiatry* **150**: 258-261 (February 1987).

CHAPTER 9

Adrenergic Blocking and Neuronal Blocking Drugs

Andrew P. Ferko and G. John DiGregorio

Adrenergic blocking drugs have been used for a number of years in therapy. These drugs are employed in a wide variety of diseases and symptoms in which the adrenergic nervous system has a pathogenic role. The main organ system that is the target for the therapeutic intervention of adrenergic blockade is the cardiovascular system. The earlier drugs that were developed showed nonselective inhibition of all alpha (α)- or beta (β)-adrenergic receptors. With the knowledge that there were subgroups of these receptors, newer compounds were introduced that exhibited selective blockade for the individual subgroups of α- or β-adrenergic receptors at therapeutic doses.

Adrenergic blockade refers to the capacity of a drug to antagonize the effects elicited by either sympathetic nerve stimulation or the administration of adrenergic drugs. The drugs in this chapter are classified into three general groups: *β-adrenergic blocking agents*, *α-adrenergic blocking agents*, and *adrenergic neuronal blocking drugs*.

The first group, drugs which block β-adrenergic receptor sites, is divided into nonselective and selective blockers. The nonselective β-adrenergic blocking agents have affinity for all β-adrenergic receptor sites (i.e., β_1, β_2, and β_3), although for the purposes of this discussion only the first two are important. Drugs such as propranolol, carteolol, labetalol, nadolol, penbutolol, pindolol, sotalol and timolol are in this category. The selective β-adrenergic blocking agents preferentially attach to β_1-adrenergic receptor sites at therapeutic doses. Drugs with selectivity for these receptors are acebutolol, atenolol, betaxolol, bisoprolol, esmolol, and metoprolol. To date there are no therapeutically useful selective β_2- or β_3-adrenergic receptor blockers, although a number of experimental compounds exist.

The second group of drugs block α-adrenergic receptors. These agents are also divided into nonselective and selective blockers. The nonselective α-adrenergic blocking agents bind to both α_1- and α_2-adrenergic receptors. Examples of drugs in this classification include phentolamine and phenoxybenzamine. The selective α-adrenergic blocking agents exhibit, at therapeutic doses, a high degree of affinity for either the α_1-adrenergic site (e.g., prazosin, terazosin, and doxazosin) or the α_2-adrenergic site (e.g., yohimbine).

The final group of adrenergic blocking drugs include those which act primarily in the nerve terminal to impair biogenic amine (norepinephrine, dopamine, or 5-hydroxytryptamine (serotonin)) synthesis, storage, or release. These drugs are termed *adrenergic neuronal blocking agents*. Examples of drugs in this group are reserpine, guanadrel, guanethidine, and metyrosine. Figure 9-1 illustrates the sites of action of the various adrenergic blocking drugs.

β-ADRENERGIC BLOCKING DRUGS

The introduction of the β-adrenergic blocking drugs has been one of the major advances in cardiovascular pharmacology. Initially these drugs had been utilized only in the treatment of essential hypertension; presently they are used in a wide variety of clinical situations such as angina pectoris, supraventricular and ventricular arrhythmias, migraine headaches, glaucoma, and the hyperactive phase of myocardial infarction. Their effectiveness in many diseases is based primarily on the competitive blockade of the β-adrenergic receptors within the autonomic nervous system that occurs with all of these drugs. Included in this large group of compounds are acebutolol, atenolol, betaxolol, bisoprolol, carteolol, esmolol, labetalol, metoprolol, nadolol, penbutolol, pindolol, propranolol, sotalol, and timolol.

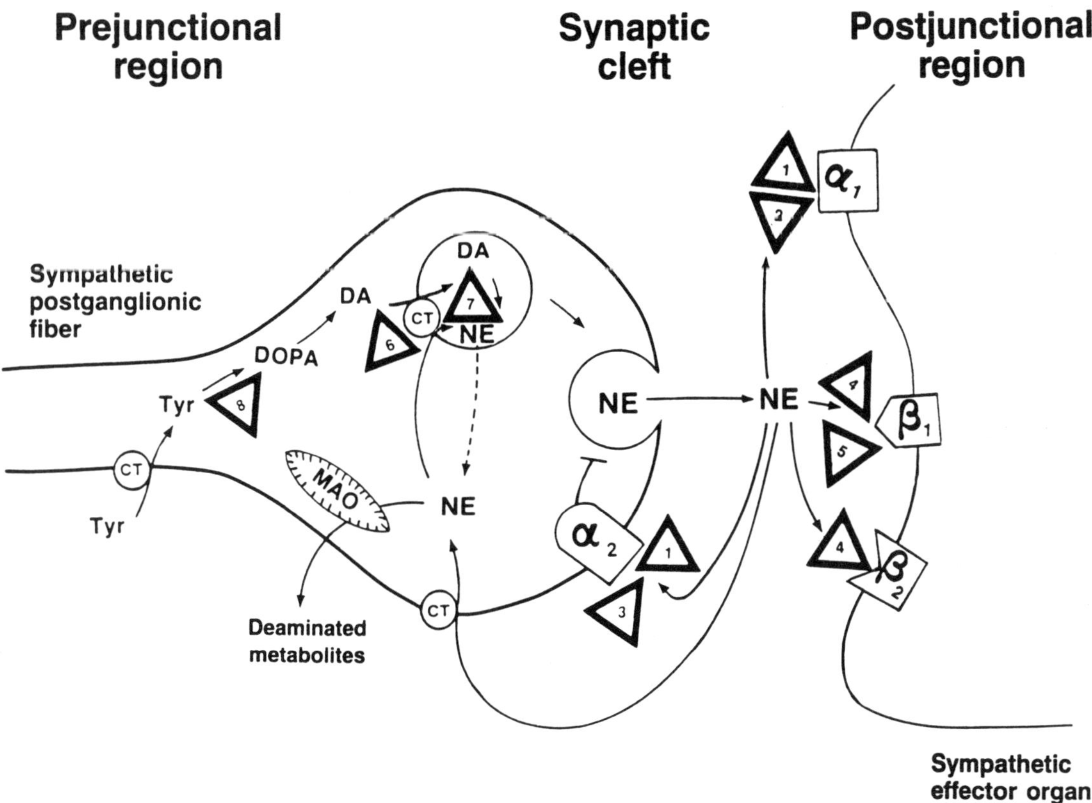

FIGURE 9-1 *Sites of action of adrenergic blocking drugs and adrenergic neuronal blockers. The diagram illustrates an adrenergic synapse, which shows the synthesis of norepinephrine, its storage in intraneuronal vesicles or granules, and its release into the synaptic cleft. The primary location of α_1-, α_2-, β_1-, and β_2-adrenergic receptors is shown. Numbered triangles represent the blocking drugs: [1] phentolamine and phenoxybenzamine; [2] prazosin, terazosin, and doxazosin; [3] yohimbine; [4] nonselective β-adrenergic blockers; [5] selective β-adrenergic blockers; [6] reserpine; [7] guanethidine and guanadrel; and [8] metyrosine. Abbreviations: Tyr = tyrosine; DOPA = dihydroxyphenylalanine; DA = dopamine; NE = norepinephrine; MAO = monoamine oxidase; and CT = catecholamine transport (uptake).*

Chemistry

The chemical structures of some β-adrenergic blockers are shown in Fig. 9-2. There are several structural features that are common to these drugs: (1) a substituted or unsubstituted aromatic or heterocyclic group, (2) a methoxy linkage ($-OCH_2-$), and (3) a substituted ethanolamine side chain [$-CH(OH)-CH_2-NH-$] with either a tertiary butyl group (as in nadolol and timolol) or an isopropyl group on the terminal nitrogen. The substituted ethanolamine group is similar to that found in many compounds with β-adrenergic receptor agonist activity (e.g., isoproterenol and albuterol, see Fig. 8-2), and believed to be responsible for the high affinity of these blocking agents for binding to β-adrenergic receptors. The levorotatory stereoisomers of these drugs are much more potent with respect to their β-adrenoceptor blocking activity than the dextrorotatory isomers; however, all of these compounds are marketed as racemic mixtures.

Mechanism of Action

These drugs attach reversibly to β-adrenergic receptor sites and competitively prevent the activation of these receptors by catecholamines released by the sympathetic nervous system or by

Acebutolol

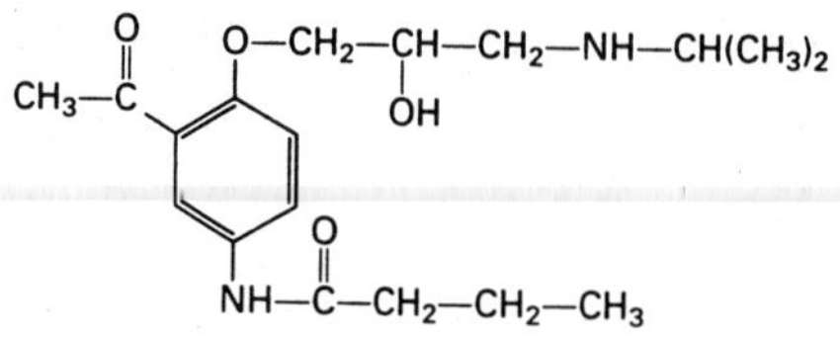

Atenolol

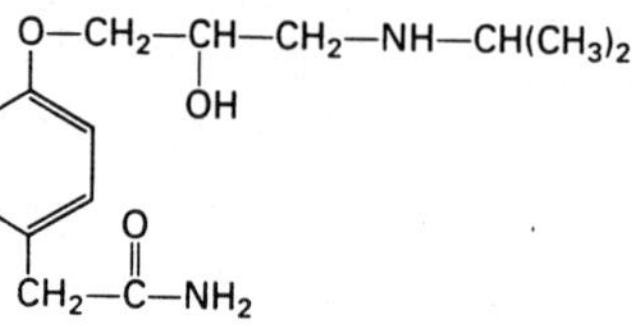

Esmolol

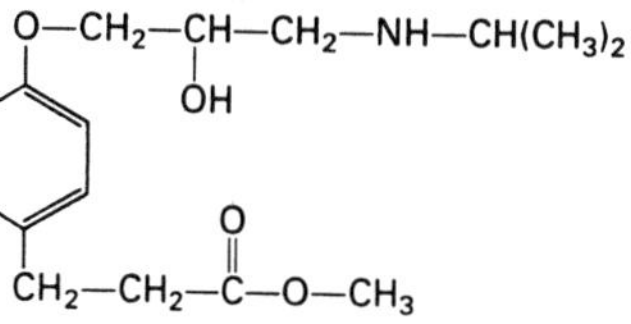

Metoprolol

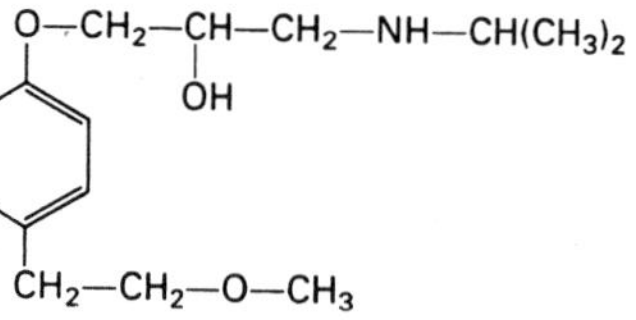

Nadolol

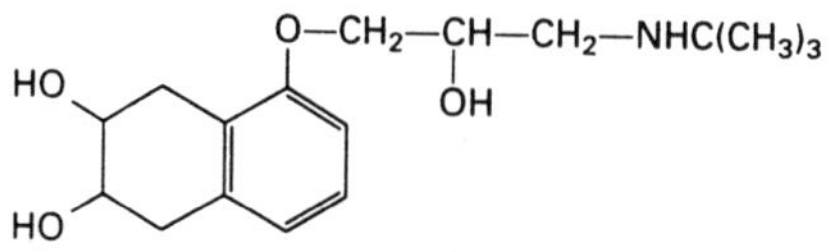

Pindolol

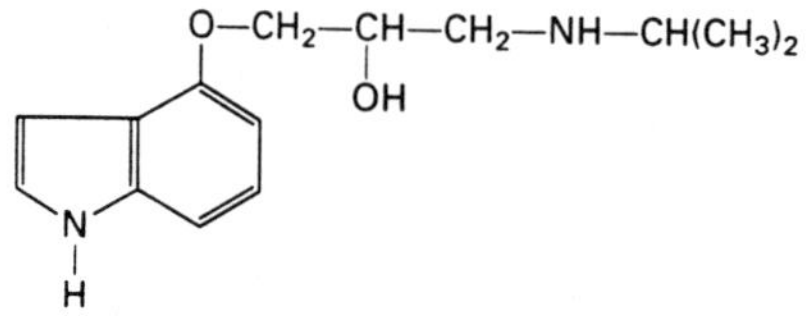

Propranolol

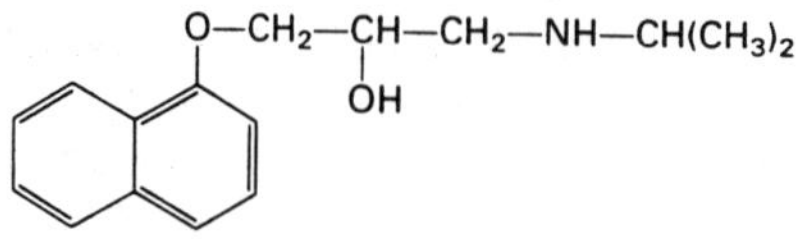

Timolol

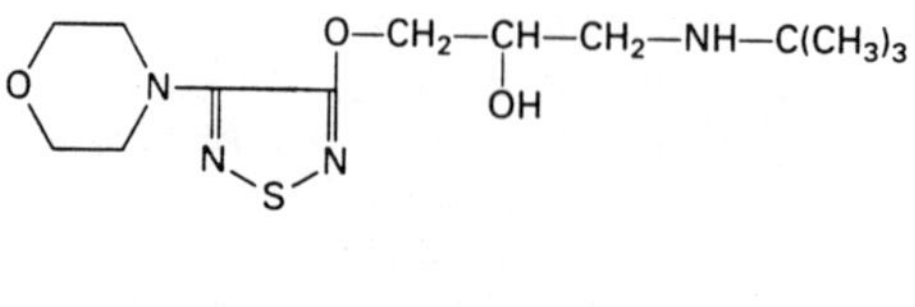

FIGURE 9-2 *Chemical structures of some β-adrenergic receptor blocking drugs.*

exogenously administered sympathomimetics (Fig. 9-1). β-Adrenergic receptors are divided into β_1 receptors (located mainly in cardiac tissue), β_2 receptors (located mainly in bronchial and vascular musculature), and β_3 receptors (found in adipose tissue and the pineal gland) (see Chapter 7 for more details). The β-adrenergic blocking drugs may be classified according to their selectivity toward β_1 and β_2 receptors. Those drugs that have approximately equal affinity for both β_1- and β_2-adrenoceptors, independent of dose, are referred to as *nonselective* blocking agents and include carteolol, labetalol, nadolol, penbutolol, pindolol, propranolol, sotalol, and timolol. Those agents that have a higher affinity for the β_1 receptors than the β_2 receptors (at therapeutic doses), e.g., acebutolol, atenolol, betaxolol, bisoprolol, esmolol, and metoprolol, are classified as *selective* (or *cardioselective*) β-adrenergic blockers. It is important to remember, however, that this receptor selectivity is not absolute; rather, it is dose-dependent, i.e., the selective blocking agents, administered at high therapeutic doses, will loose their selectivity and inhibit both of these β-adrenergic receptor subtypes equally. Presently no compounds are available for clinical use that selectively block β_2- or β_3-adrenergic receptors.

In addition to blocking β-adrenoceptors, these drugs have other properties which result in certain cardiovascular effects (Table 9-1). Propranolol, acebutolol, betaxolol, metoprolol, and pindolol have a nonspecific myocardial depressant effect (also known as a *quinidine-like effect* or *membrane stabilizing activity (MSA)*), which usually occurs at higher dosage regimens and has been suggested as being partly responsible for the antiarrhythmic properties of certain β-adrenergic blockers. There are, however, β-adrenoceptor blocking drugs which lack this property but still possess certain antiarrhythmic activities (e.g., esmolol).

Pindolol and, to a lesser extent, acebutolol, carteolol, and penbutolol have partial agonist activity, also known as *intrinsic sympathomimetic activity (ISA)* (Table 9-1). ISA is most often manifested at the β_1-adrenergic receptor site resulting in less of a depression of heart rate and cardiac output than drugs lacking this property.

Propranolol

Propranolol is the oldest of the clinically useful β-adrenergic blocking agents. It is considered the prototypical drug in this category and will be discussed in greater detail than the other drugs.

Effects on Organ Systems *The Cardiovascular System* Propranolol is a cardiac depressant which can affect the mechanical and electrophysiologic properties of the myocardium. It can block atrioventricular (AV) conduction and automaticity of cardiac pacemaker potentials and the adrenergic stimulation induced by catecholamines; therefore, the drug lowers myocardial contractility, heart rate, blood pressure, cardiac work, and myocardial oxygen demand. Because of these effects, propranolol and some other β-adrenergic blockers are useful as antiarrhythmic agents (see Chapter 28) and as antianginal drugs (see Chapter 29).

Propranolol reduces the blood pressure of most patients with essential hypertension without causing orthostatic hypotension. The antihypertensive effect of propranolol may be the result of a number of proposed mechanisms:

1 *Reduced cardiac output.* As mentioned, the blockade of adrenergic stimulation to the heart, reduces heart rate and cardiac output. These effects are more pronounced during exercise and are a potential problem in active individuals.

2 *Inhibition of renin release.* By decreasing the release of renin from the juxtaglomerular cells in the kidney, a reduction in serum angiotensin II (a potent vasoconstrictor) occurs.

3 *Decreased sympathetic outflow from the central nervous system.* This mechanism effectively lowers sympathetic tone to the heart, kidney, and vasculature.

4 *Inhibition of norepinephrine release from sympathetic postganglionic neurons.* In addition to blocking postsynaptic β-adrenergic receptors, it has been suggested that presynaptic β-adrenoceptors enhance neurotransmitter release from sympathetic neurons; blockade of these receptors would reduce sympathetic activity to the heart and vascular smooth muscle.

None of these mechanisms, however, adequately explains the antihypertensive activity of propranolol and the other β-adrenergic blocking drugs. For example, some of these drugs (e.g., nadolol and atenolol) do not enter the central nervous system (CNS) very readily, yet these are no less effective as antihypertensive drugs than propranolol.

A mild increase in peripheral vascular resistance is associated with propranolol and the other

TABLE 9-1 Comparison of some pharmacodynamic properties of β-adrenergic blocking drugs

Drug	β_1-Adrenoceptor selectivity[a]	Intrinsic sympathomimetic activity (ISA)	Membrane stabilizing activity (MSA)
Acebutolol	Yes	+	+
Atenolol	Yes	−	−
Betaxolol	Yes	−	+
Bisoprolol	Yes	−	−
Carteolol	No	+	−
Esmolol	Yes	−	−
Labetalol	No	−	+
Metoprolol	Yes	−	+
Nadolol	No	−	−
Penbutolol	No	+	−
Pindolol	No	+ +	+
Propranolol	No	−	+ +
Sotalol	No	−	−
Timolol	No	−	−

[a] At therapeutic dosage

nonselective β-adrenergic blockers. This is due to inhibition of peripheral β_2 receptors, resulting in an α-adrenergic receptor effect (i.e., vasoconstriction) which will be unopposed by reduced β-adrenergic receptor-mediated vasodilatation. During chronic administration of these drugs, the antihypertensive effect predominates and the increased peripheral vascular resistance returns to the pretreatment level and does not significantly affect systemic blood pressure.

Respiratory System Due to β_2-adrenergic receptor blockade throughout the pulmonary system, the resting bronchiolar smooth muscles become hypersensitive to agents which increase airway resistance and induce bronchoconstriction. This is of little or no consequence in patients with normal respiratory function; however, in susceptible individuals an asthmatic attack can be precipitated. Bronchoconstriction is less evident with the selective β_1-adrenergic blocking agents.

Metabolic Effects Propranolol has effects on carbohydrate and fat metabolism which are a result of the blocking activity of these drugs on catecholamine-induced β-adrenergic receptor-mediated responses.

The effects of propranolol and the other β-adrenergic blockers on carbohydrate metabolism is complicated. Glycogenolysis can be inhibited in the heart and skeletal muscle resulting in the depression of blood glucose levels. Hypoglycemia is not common, however, but may present difficulty should it occur in a diabetic patient since propranolol may mask some of the premonitory signs of acute hypoglycemia, e.g., tachycardia. In addition, propranolol may delay the recovery of blood glucose to normal levels following insulin-induced hypoglycemia in a diabetic patient.

Propranolol will also inhibit the rise in plasma free fatty acids induced by sympathomimetic agents such as epinephrine and will subsequently inhibit the lipolytic action of the sympathetic nervous system. Serum triglyceride levels generally increase with β-receptor blockade; however, these drugs generally do not significantly alter serum cholesterol levels. In some specific cases, some β-blockers may decrease high-density lipoproteins (HDL) slightly, whereas other drugs may increase this serum lipoprotein. Low-density lipoprotein (LDL) levels may be raised modestly, or no effect may be observed.

Pharmacokinetics Propranolol is well absorbed after oral administration, but the systemic bioavailability is low due to high first pass biotransformation (Table 9-2). Of all the β-adrenergic blockers, propranolol has the highest lipid solubility, which results in the greatest penetration into the CNS. In addition, this drug has a high degree of binding to plasma proteins, mainly albumin and α_1-acid glycoprotein.

Propranolol is converted by the hepatic mixed-function oxidase system to 4-hydroxypropranolol, an active metabolite; the half-life of the 4-hydroxy derivative is short (approximately 2 h) and does not account for the major effects of propranolol during chronic oral therapy. Propranolol can also be biotransformed to a number of inactive products; these and the small amounts of the parent compound are all excreted in the urine.

The pharmacokinetic profile of propranolol is complex and depends to a great extent on the route of administration. β-Adrenergic blockade usually develops within 30 min following oral ingestion and is maintained for approximately 3 to 8 h. The duration is about 12 to 24 h following a single oral dose. When administered by the intravenous route, the onset of action occurs within 2 min and reaches a peak effect in 3 to 5 min; the duration of effect is 2 to 4 h. The elimination half-life has been estimated at 3 h after intravenous use and 4 to 6 h following oral administration. Plasma levels of propranolol and many other drugs in this group are not closely correlated with therapeutic responses.

There are certain factors, such as genetics,

TABLE 9-2 Physicochemical and pharmacokinetic properties of β-adrenergic blockers

Drug	Lipid solubility	Plasma protein binding, %	Elim. half-life, h	Percent excreted unchanged	Major metabolic process	Active metabolites
Acebutolol	Low	25	3 to 7	20	Acetylation	N-acetyl acebutolol (diacetolol)
Atenolol	Low	5 to 15	6 to 7	100	None	None
Betaxolol	Low	50	14 to 22	15	Oxidation	None
Bisoprolol	Moderate	30	9 to 12	50		None
Carteolol	Low	23 to 30	6	50 to 70	Oxidation	8-hydroxycarteolol
Esmolol	Low	55	0.16	1	Hydrolysis	None
Labetalol	Moderate	50	5 to 8	20	Conjugation	None
Metoprolol	Moderate	10	3 to 4	5	Oxidation	None
Nadolol	Low	30	20 to 24	100	None	None
Penbutolol	High	80 to 98	5	17	Oxidation	4-hydroxypenbutolol
Pindolol	Moderate	50 to 70	3 to 4	40	Oxidation & conjugation	None
Propranolol	High	90 to 95	3 to 4	1	Oxidation	4-hydroxypropranolol
Sotalol	Low	0	12	100	None	None
Timolol	Low	25 to 60	3 to 5	20	Oxidation	None

age, and various disease states, that can influence the pharmacokinetics of propranolol and other β-adrenergic blockers. The biotransformation of the drugs may be influenced by genetic differences in oxidation or by disease. Hence patients having gene characteristics which result in poor oxidative metabolism, or individuals with liver disease, may acquire higher plasma concentrations of β-adrenergic blockers, which may lead to drug toxicity. In the neonate and the elderly patient, the renal excretion of the drugs may be delayed due to decreased renal function.

Therapeutic Uses Propranolol is indicated in the management of hypertension, angina pectoris, supraventricular and ventricular arrhythmias, prophylaxis of migraine headache, hypertrophic subaortic stenosis, essential tremors, and pheochromocytoma. It is also indicated to reduce cardiovascular mortality in the post-acute phase of myocardial infarction. Additional information concerning the use of propranolol in arrhythmias, angina, and essential hypertension is found in Chapters 28, 29, and 32, respectively.

Adverse Reactions Propranolol produces mild and transient side effects that rarely require cessation of therapy. Some of these include nausea, vomiting, anorexia, gastric pain, flatulence, dizziness, vertigo, fatigue, insomnia, depression, hallucinations, visual disturbances, mild diarrhea or constipation, and cutaneous eruptions such as rash and pruritus. Agranulocytosis and thrombocytopenic purpura are very rare, as is the development of antinuclear antibodies.

Serious adverse effects resulting from the pharmacologic action of β-adrenergic blockade include severe hypotension, bradycardia, atrioventricular conduction delay (which may lead to heart block), and congestive heart failure especially in patients that require an active sympathetic nervous system for their myocardial drive. Other adverse effects associated with β-receptor blockade include decrease in exercise tolerance, bronchoconstriction, and the induction of Raynaud's phenomenon. Following abrupt cessation of propranolol, as well as the other β-adrenergic blocking drugs, episodes of angina and myocardial infarction have occurred. This effect is probably related to the increase in the β-adrenoceptor population after chronic β-adrenergic blocker use, i.e., up-regulation of receptor sites. When administration of the antagonist is suddenly stopped, there is an overabundance of β-adrenoceptors available to interact with endogenous catecholamines causing increased cardiac activity.

Since propranolol may precipitate an acute, severe crisis in asthmatic patients and since these patients may respond poorly to β-adrenergic bronchodilators, propranolol is contraindicated in the presence of bronchial asthma. This drug must also be given with extreme caution to patients with borderline cardiac reserve or frank congestive heart failure, unless the failure is due to an arrhythmia that may be controlled by propranolol.

The drug should also be used with caution in diabetics and patients subject to hypoglycemia, since propranolol may mask some of the symptoms of acute hypoglycemia reactions, e.g., tachycardia.

Drug Interactions Since β-adrenergic blockers are widely administrated with other drugs, the occurrence of drug interactions is not uncommon. Table 9-3 lists some of the important drug interactions and the possible mechanisms. The most important drug interactions are those that occur between the β-blockers and other drugs associated with the myocardium. For example, both digoxin and verapamil will decrease heart rate and de-

TABLE 9-3 Some drug interactions of β-adrenergic blockers

Drug	Response with the β-adrenergic blocker
Antacids	Decreases absorption of the β-blocker
Cardiac glycosides	Increased bradycardia
Lidocaine	Increased lidocaine blood levels
Phenytoin	Additive cardiac depression
Quinidine	Additive cardiac depression
Tricyclic antidepressants	Inhibits negative inotropic and chronotropic effects of the β-blocker
Tubocurarine	Enhanced neuromuscular blockade
Verapamil	Potentiation of bradycardia and myocardial depression

crease conduction across the AV node; if administered with propranolol, a serious bradycardia may occur.

Metoprolol

Metoprolol was the first cardioselective β-adrenergic receptor blocking agent available and will be mentioned as the protoptype of this subgroup. Unlike propranolol, which blocks both β_1- and β_2-adrenergic receptors, metoprolol has a cardioselective action, i.e., in therapeutic doses metoprolol will block β_1-adrenoceptors with little effect on β_2-adrenergic receptors (Table 9-1). Metoprolol is *less likely* to induce bronchoconstriction and does not compromise bronchodilation provided by isoproterenol, albuterol, or other such agents. The drug has no ISA and only weak MSA.

Metoprolol is rapidly and completely absorbed from the gastrointestinal tract following oral administration; however, like propranolol, its systemic bioavailability is reduced significantly (about 50 percent) due to high first pass biotransformation (Table 9-2). Only about 10 percent of metoprolol is bound to plasma proteins, resulting in a relatively high apparent volume of distribution (4.2 L/kg); the elimination half-life is 3 to 4 h. The drug is biotransformed to a small extent to an active oxidation product (which has no clinical significance) and to inactive products, all of which are eliminated in the urine.

Metoprolol is indicated for essential hypertension and angina pectoris and appears comparable to propranolol in these diseases. It is also indicated for use in the post-myocardial infarcted patient. The adverse reactions of this drug are similar to propranolol.

Other β-Adrenergic Receptor Blockers

The other β-adrenergic blocking agents are very similar to propranolol and metoprolol in their pharmacology. The nonselective blocking agents like propranolol are carteolol, labetalol, nadolol, penbutolol, pindolol, sotalol, and timolol; those agents that have a higher affinity for the β_1-adrenoceptors than the β_2-adrenergic receptors, the cardioselective β-adrenergic blockers, are acebutolol, atenolol, betaxolol, bisoprolol, esmolol, and metoprolol (Table 9-1). The cardioselective β-adrenergic blockers exhibit selective affinity for the β_1-adrenergic receptor at therapeutic doses. When the dosage is increased above the recommended dosage, these drugs may lose their selectivity and bind to both β_1- and β_2-adrenergic receptor sites. Therefore, the minimum effective dose should be used to maintain the cardioselective property.

The major difference with respect to these drugs resides in their pharmacokinetics, and some of these properties are outlined in Table 9-2. With the exception of esmolol, all of these compounds are absorbed from the gastrointestinal tract; nadolol and atenolol are absorbed to the extent of 30 and 50 percent, respectively, while all the others are absorbed greater than 80 percent. Once absorbed, acebutolol and timolol, like propranolol, undergo a high first pass metabolism within the liver. Pindolol, betaxolol, bisoprolol, carteolol, penbutolol, atenolol, nadolol and sotalol have a high systemic bioavailability because they escape this initial hepatic inactivation; in fact, atenolol, sotalol, and nadolol are not biotransformed and are excreted in the urine unchanged. The remaining β-adrenergic blockers are metabolized in the liver to either active or inactive metabolites. All the resulting metabolites and parent compounds are excreted primarily in the urine. The elimination half-lives of these drugs ranges from 3 to 24 h. Plasma protein binding to both albumin and α_1-acid glycoprotein ranges from 5 to 98 percent.

With respect to pharmacokinetics, esmolol is unique. It is an ester that is metabolized rapidly by hydrolysis of the ester linkage, chiefly by esterases in the cytosol of erythrocytes (not by plasma cholinesterase or red cell membrane acetylcholinesterase) to an inactive product, resulting in a compound with an elimination half-life of approximately 10 min. Less than 2 percent of the drug is excreted unchanged in the urine.

These drugs are used for a wide variety of clinical conditions. Each drug or preparation has a specific Food and Drug Administration (FDA)-approved indication. Acebutolol is indicated for the treatment of essential hypertension and ventricular arrhythmias (premature ventricular contractions, PVCs). Atenolol, metoprolol, and nadolol are indicated for the treatment of hypertension and long-term management of patients with angina pectoris. Esmolol is indicated for the rapid control of ventricular rate in patients with atrial fibrillation or atrial flutter in preoperative, postoperative, or other emergency circumstances where short-term control of ventricular rate is necessary. Pindolol, betaxolol, bisoprolol, carteolol, and penbutolol are indicated only for the management of hypertension. Timolol is indicated for the treatment of hypertension, prophylaxis in migraines, and to reduce the cardiovascular mortality and the risk of re-infarction after an acute phase of a myocardial infarction. Sotalol is used in severe ventricular arrhythmias such as ventricular tachycardia that is life-threatening.

Timolol and betaxolol administered topically to the eye, are used in the treatment chronic open-angle glaucoma and in secondary glaucoma. A summary of uses is presented in Table 9-4.

Labetalol

Chemically, labetalol differs somewhat from other β-adrenergic blockers in that it is a substituted phenylpropylamino salicylamide derivative.

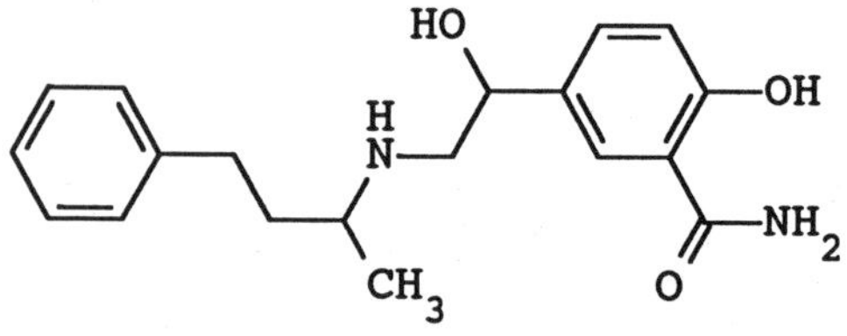

HO, H, N, OH, NH_2, CH_3, O

Labetalol also differs in its pharmacologic properties; it is a competitive blocker of both α- and β-adrenergic receptors. The drug will selectively block α_1-adrenergic receptors and β_1- and β_2-adrenergic receptors in a nonselective fashion; the potency ratios for α:β blockade is 1:3 for the oral route and 1:7 following intravenous administration; therefore it has greater blocking activity at β-adrenergic than α-adrenergic receptors.

Labetalol will block cardiac β_1-adrenoceptor sites resulting in a decreased heart rate. There appears to be little or no effect on intraventricular conduction or QRS duration; a mild prolongation of the AV conduction time has been observed in some patients. Peripheral vascular resistance will decrease slightly due to both α- and β-adrenergic blocking action, and both of these actions of labetalol contribute to the decrease in blood pressure in hypertensive patients. Because of the α-adrenergic blocking activity, blood pressure is decreased more in the standing than in the supine position, and symptoms of postural hypotension can occur. Labetalol lowers blood pressure without significant reflex tachycardia. As with the other β-adrenergic blockers, abrupt withdrawal of the drug may lead to an exacerbation of angina and, in some cases, myocardial infarction.

Following oral administration, labetalol is subjected to a high first pass effect resulting in an oral bioavailability of only 25 percent. Plasma protein binding is approximately 50 percent. The elimination half-life of the drug is about 5.5 h after intravenous use and 6 to 8 h following oral administration. Total body clearance is estimated at

TABLE 9-4 Some indications of β-adrenergic blockers

Therapeutic Use	Drugs
Angina	Atenolol, metoprolol, nadolol, and propranolol
Arrhythmias	Acebutolol, esmolol, propranolol, and sotalol
Glaucoma	Betaxolol and timolol
Hypertension	Acebutolol, atenolol, betaxolol, bisoprolol, carteolol, labetalol, metoprolol, nadolol, penbutolol, pindolol, propranolol, and timolol
Migraine Headaches (Prophylactic)	Propranolol and timolol
Myocardial Infarction	Atenolol, metoprolol, propranolol, and timolol

about 33 mL/min/kg. Metabolism of labetalol is by the drug-metabolizing microsomal system with the production of glucuronide conjugates. Approximately 55 to 60 percent of the dose appears in the urine as conjugates or unchanged drug within the first 24 h of dosing. In patients with hepatic dysfunction, labetalol should be used cautiously.

Labetalol is usually well-tolerated. The most common adverse reactions include dizziness, fatigue, nausea, vomiting, nasal stuffiness, impotence, and edema.

The indication for labetalol is in the treatment of essential hypertension.

NONSELECTIVE α-ADRENERGIC BLOCKING AGENTS

These adrenergic blocking drugs include a structurally heterogeneous group of compounds which possess varied pharmacologic effects. All of these drugs have one common property: the ability to block α_1- and α_2-adrenergic receptors.

Phentolamine

Chemistry Phentolamine is an imidazoline derivative which has α-adrenergic blocking, direct smooth muscle relaxant, cholinomimetic, histaminic, and sympathomimetic activity. The drug is one of a group of substituted imidazolines which share these properties. Structural changes make some actions more prominent. For example, tolazoline, a structural congener of phentolamine, has greater smooth muscle relaxant and histaminic effects than phentolamine, but less α-adrenergic receptor blocking activity.

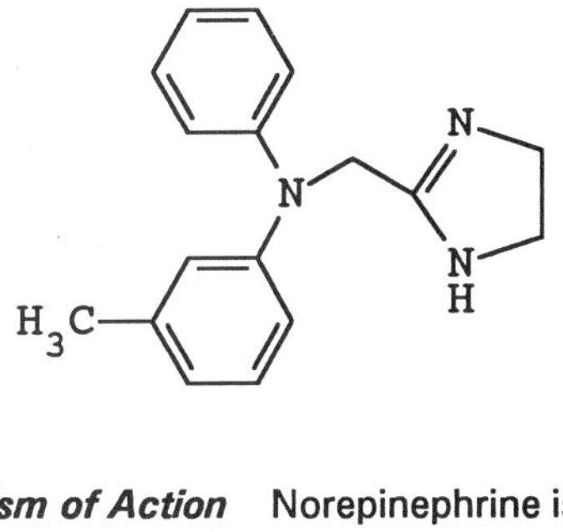

N
N
N
H
H_3C

Mechanism of Action Norepinephrine is released from sympathetic nerve terminals during neuronal activity; it diffuses across the synaptic space, binds to adrenergic receptors on the effector cells of smooth muscle, cardiac muscle, or exocrine glands, and a response occurs. Circulating catecholamines elicit similar responses by stimulating the same effectors.

Phentolamine exerts its action by competing for α-adrenergic receptors and therefore is termed a *competitive blocking agent*, which has high affinity for, but little intrinsic activity at, these receptor sites. Such drug-receptor combinations reduce the availability of the α-adrenergic receptors for reaction with sympathomimetic amines and therefore reduce the magnitude of the response elicited either from endogenous or administered amines. The duration of the blockade of the α-adrenergic receptor by phentolamine is relatively short when compared with phenoxybenzamine (see below).

Effects Phentolamine produces a moderately effective, transient, competitive α-adrenergic blockade; in addition, it has a direct relaxant (musculotropic spasmolytic) effect on vascular smooth muscle. The vasodilatation and reduced blood pressure which occur are due to the direct relaxant effect on the vasculature (in low doses) and to α-adrenergic blockade (at higher, therapeutic doses).

The physiologic responses of the heart to epinephrine and norepinephrine are not effectively blocked by phentolamine or by other α-adrenergic blocking agents, since the cardiac response to these drugs is mediated by β_1-adrenergic receptors, and therefore α-adrenergic blockers have little effect on arrhythmias induced by adrenergic stimuli. Tachycardia and increased cardiac output may result as reflex responses to the decreased blood pressure induced by phentolamine. In addition, phentolamine has a sympathomimetic action on the heart, which appears to be the result of increased endogenous norepinephrine release due to blockade of presynaptic α_2-adrenergic receptors and a reduction in negative feedback inhibition of neurotransmitter release (see Fig. 9-3). Therefore, cardiac stimulation resulting from therapeutic doses of the drug is more than just a reflex response to the vasodilatation and hypotension.

In addition to the ability of phentolamine to antagonize α-adrenergic receptors, this compound has activity at other receptor sites. Phentolamine can block the effects of 5-hydroxytryptamine (serotonin). At the H_1 and H_2 histamine receptor sites, phentolamine has both affinity and intrinsic activity. This is observed as a histamine-like effect on the stomach, causing secretion of both acid and pepsin. Phentolamine increases the motility of the intestine by a cholinomimetic

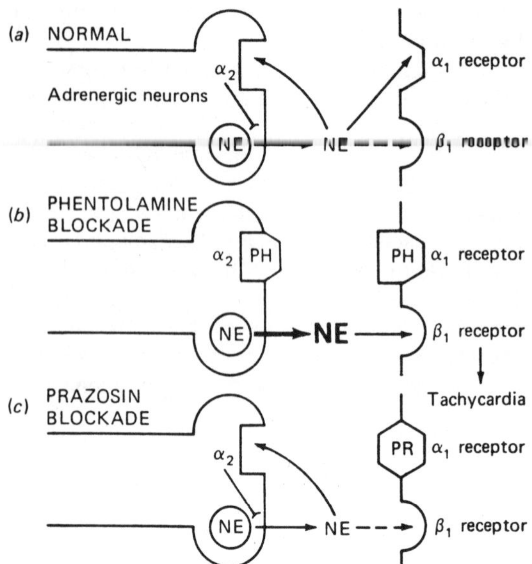

FIGURE 9-3 *Diagrammatic representation of the mechanism of action of certain α-adrenergic receptor blocking agents. (a) Normal autoregulation of norepinephrine (NE) release from adrenergic neurons via α_2-adrenergic receptor stimulation. (b) Blockade of α_1- and α_2-adrenoceptors by classic α-adrenergic blocking drugs, e.g. phentolamine (PH), leads to a reduction in the negative feedback inhibition of NE release. Greater NE release from the sympathetic neurons in the heart allows for greater cardiac β-receptor activation and greater tachycardia. (c) Selective α_1-adrenergic blockade by prazosin (PR) does not significantly effect α_2-adrenergic receptors; NE release is controlled, and tachycardia is minimal.*

action, which is the result of a direct effect on muscarinic receptors and unrelated to its α-adrenergic blockade.

Pharmacokinetics Phentolamine has low bioavailability when it is given by the oral route. Upon intravenous administration, the compound has a half-life of 19 min, and approximately 10 percent of an injected dose is found in the urine unchanged. The actual biotransformation reactions that phentolamine undergoes in the body are unknown.

Adverse Reactions Adverse effects are common with phentolamine and are attributable to cardiac and gastrointestinal stimulation. Tachycardia, anginal pain, cardiac arrhythmias, and episodes of hypotension may occur, especially after parenteral administration. Gastrointestinal stimulation may produce nausea, vomiting, abdominal pain, diarrhea, and exacerbation of peptic ulceration.

Clinical Uses Although the drug causes hypotension, phentolamine is not useful in the treatment of essential hypertension because of the frequency of adverse reactions and the development of tolerance. However, phentolamine is of use in controlling severe acute hypertensive crises due to an excess in circulating catecholamines from pheochromocytoma or drug interactions involving monoamine oxidase inhibitors. Its use is based on the fact that the α-adrenergic receptor-mediated effects of circulating catecholamines, e.g., vasoconstriction, are readily blocked by phentolamine. In pheochromocytoma, phentolamine is indicated both preoperatively and during surgical removal of the tumor to prevent or control excessive elevation of blood pressure.

This α-adrenergic receptor blocking agent is also indicated in the diagnosis of pheochromocytoma. In patients with this tumor, the administration of phentolamine may cause a reduction in the sustained or paroxysmal hypertension that is present. However, many false-positive responses can occur with this test; therefore, measurement of urinary concentrations of catecholamine metabolites (e.g., vanillymandelic acid, VMA) is a more reliable diagnostic procedure.

In addition, during the treatment of arteriolar hypotension and shock with intravenous norepinephrine, small doses of phentolamine have been added to the infusion to prevent local tissue necrosis following extravasation of the catecholamine.

Phenoxybenzamine

Chemistry Phenoxybenzamine is a haloalkylamine that is structurally related to the nitrogen mustard alkylating agents used in cancer chemotherapy. The chemical mechanism responsible for the long-lasting α-adrenergic receptor blockade appears to be related to alkylation of these receptors.

O CH_3 N CH_2Cl

Mechanism of Action Phenoxybenzamine produces a persistent ("irreversible") α-adrenergic receptor blockade. Chemically it appears that the terminal N-C-C moiety cyclizes at the alkaline pH of body fluids to form an ethylenimonium intermediate (Fig. 9-4). The drug, as a highly reactive carbonium ion, produced when the unstable cyclic structure opens, forms a stable covalent bond with the receptor. This antagonist-receptor complex cannot be affected by even large concentrations of α-adrenergic receptor agonists. Therefore the blockade is referred to as *nonequilibrium receptor blockade.*

In addition to the blockade of α-adrenergic receptors, high doses of phenoxybenzamine can inhibit responses to 5-hydroxytryptamine, acetylcholine, and histamine.

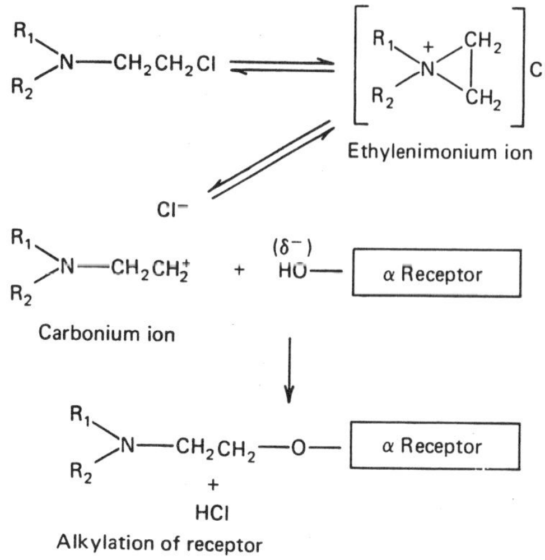

Effects Most actions of phenoxybenzamine, as well as other α-adrenergic blockers, are dependent on the normal level of adrenergic tone, i.e., the greater the sympathetic tone the greater the observed effect of the drug that is due to receptor blockade. For example, phenoxybenzamine has little effect on blood pressure in normal, recumbent subjects. However, hypotension may result in any situation involving compensatory sympathetic vasoconstriction, such as an upright posture. Therefore, *postural (orthostatic) hypotension* is a prominent effect of α-adrenergic receptor blockade of the vascular system. As a reflex response to the hypotension produced by phenoxybenzamine and blockade of presynaptic α_2-adrenergic receptors on sympathetic neurons (as with phentolamine), tachycardia is generally observed.

In addition to blocking the vascular effects of endogenous norepinephrine, small doses of phenoxybenzamine will diminish the pressor responses to exogenously administered epinephrine, norepinephrine, and other adrenergic drugs. Large doses of phenoxybenzamine "reverse" the pressor action of epinephrine, so that a depressor response is the prominent effect (Fig. 9-5). These larger doses antagonize the pressor responses to injected norepinephrine or sympathetic vasoconstrictor nerve stimulation but do not reverse them. *Epinephrine vasomotor reversal,* as it is commonly called, is best understood by remembering that epinephrine has pronounced β_2-adrenergic receptor stimulant activity, notably in skeletal muscle vasculature, which is not blocked by α-adrenergic blocking agents. As would be expected, α-adrenergic blocking agents have no effect on the vasodepressor action of isoproterenol, since this drug is predominantly a potent stimulant of β-adrenergic receptor-mediated responses.

$R_1R_2N{-}CH_2CH_2Cl \rightleftharpoons [R_1R_2N^+(CH_2)_2]\,Cl^-$

Ethylenimonium ion

Cl^-

$R_1R_2N{-}CH_2CH_2^+$ + (δ^-) HO— α Receptor

Carbonium ion

$R_1R_2N{-}CH_2CH_2{-}O{-}$ α Receptor + HCl

Alkylation of receptor

FIGURE 9-4 *Schematic representation of the mechanism by which α-adrenergic receptors are alkylated by phenoxybenzamine.*

Phenoxybenzamine has a negligible effect on the gastrointestinal tract. The drug can affect the CNS and cause nausea, vomiting, and drowsiness.

Pharmacokinetics Although phenoxybenzamine has a low bioavailability, the drug is sufficiently absorbed from the gastrointestinal tract to provide a therapeutic effect. Little information is known about its biotransformation and excretion from the body.

Adverse Reactions The use of this drug is generally limited by the frequent occurrence of adverse reactions; nasal congestion, miosis, inhibition of ejaculation, and severe hypotension with reflex tachycardia may occur. These adverse reactions are manifestations of adrenergic blockade and vary according to the degree of blockade.

Therapeutic Uses Phenoxybenzamine is effective in the treatment of pheochromocytoma. The drug is indicated preoperatively or chronically in patients with inoperable tumors of pheochromocytoma. The drug has also been employed in vasospastic peripheral vascular diseases associated with increased α-adrenergic activity, e.g., Raynaud's syndrome, and in cases of endotoxin-induced shock where the vasoconstrictor effect of

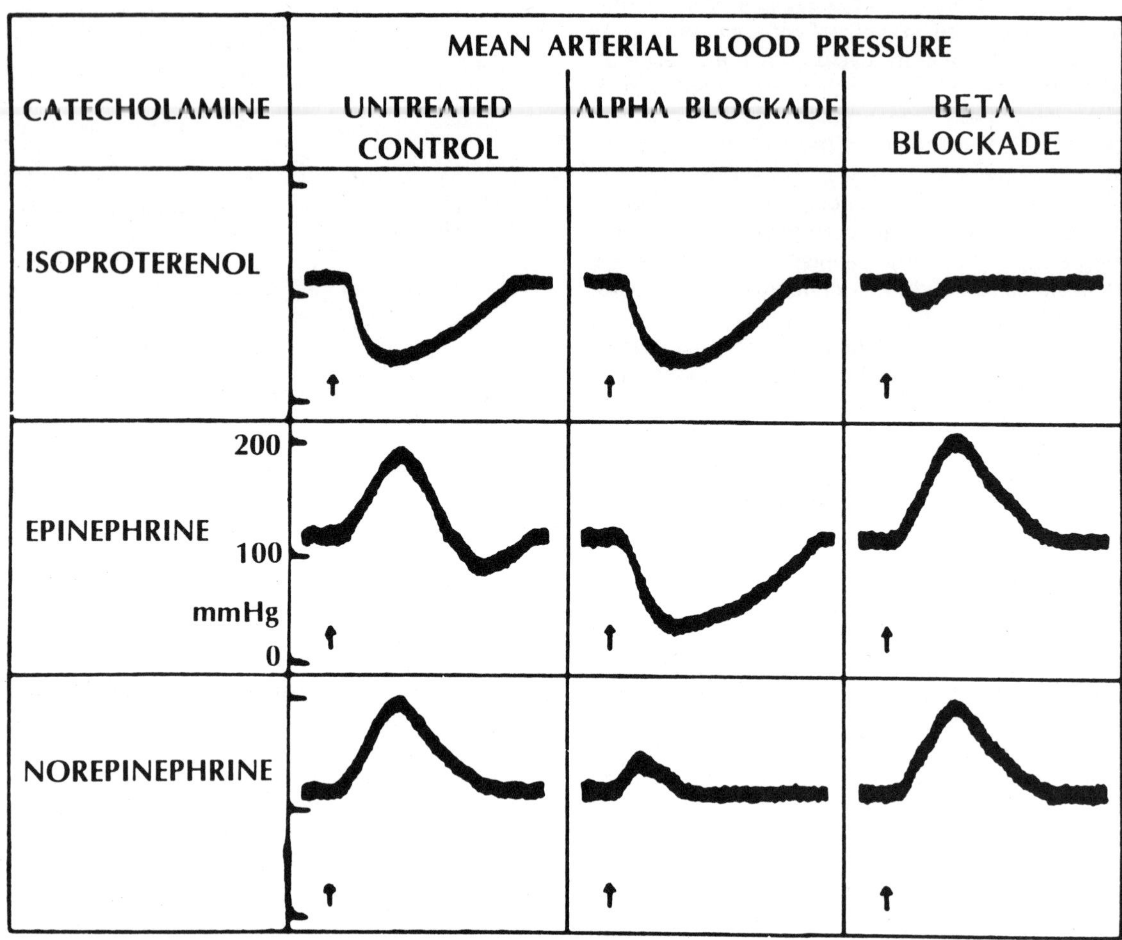

FIGURE 9-5 *The influence of α- and β-adrenergic blocking agents on the idealized responses of the mean arterial pressure to intravenous injections of three catecholamines. The direction of the blood pressure response is largely determined by the influence the amines exert on total peripheral resistance. In the first column the responses in untreated animals are presented. Isoproterenol, which is predominantly an evoker of β-adrenergic responses, dilates the arterioles and pressure falls. Epinephrine, which is a potent stimulant of both α- and β-adrenoceptor responses, tends to constrict and dilate simultaneously. The algebraic summation of these opposing effects on peripheral vascular resistance frequently yields a biphasic effect on blood pressure. Pressure is first greatly increased, then falls somewhat below control level before recovering. Norepinephrine, which predominantly evokes α-adrenergic responses, constricts the resistance vessels, and only a pressor response is observed.*

In the presence of an effective dose of an α-adrenergic receptor blocking agent, catecholamine-induced vasoconstriction is inhibited. Isoproterenol exerts its full depressor activity, epinephrine is purely depressor, and norepinephrine exerts only slight or no pressor effect. In the presence of an effective dose of a β-adrenergic blocking agent, catecholamine-induced vasodilation is inhibited. Isoproterenol has only slight or no depressor activity. Epinephrine is purely pressor, and the magnitude of the response is increased. Norepinephrine retains its usual pressor effect.

Arrows indicate time at which the catecholamine is injected intravenously (abscissa is time).

endotoxin is mediated by release of epinephrine and norepinephrine. Phenoxybenzamine has found some usefulness in patients with urinary retention caused by a spastic detrusor.

SELECTIVE α-ADRENERGIC BLOCKING AGENTS

Prazosin, Terazosin, and Doxazosin

These drugs are peripheral vasodilators which have been found to possess significant α-adrenergic receptor blocking activity. Prazosin, terazosin, and doxazosin differ from the aforementioned α-adrenergic blocking drugs in their selectivity for α-adrenergic receptors at therapeutic doses.

Prazosin, terazosin, and doxazosin, unlike phentolamine and phenoxybenzamine, appear to selectively block postsynaptic α_1-adrenergic receptors with little affinity for presynaptic α_2-adrenergic receptors. It has been shown that norepinephrine regulates its own release from adrenergic neuronal terminals via a negative feedback mechanism mediated by α_2-adrenergic receptors located on the presynaptic membrane. Since prazosin, terazosin, and doxazosin do not block α_2-adrenergic receptor sites at therapeutic doses, feedback inhibition of norepinephrine release is not greatly affected, which may account for the low degree of tachycardia with these drugs (Fig. 9-3). Prazosin, terazosin, and doxazosin are used for the treatment of hypertension.

In addition, terazosin is indicated in the treatment of benign prostatic hyperplasia with its associated urinary symptoms such as interrupted or slow urine flow, need for frequent urination, and the sensation that the bladder has retained urine in it. Terazosin appears to relax muscle in the prostate gland and decreases the urinary symptoms due to benign prostatic hyperplasia. A more complete discussion of these selective α-adrenergic receptor blockers is presented in the chapter on antihypertensive drugs (Chapter 32).

Yohimbine

Yohimbine is a selective α_2-adrenergic antagonist. Chemically this compound resembles the alkaloid reserpine in that it is an indolealkylamine. Since yohimbine can block α_2-adrenergic receptor sites on the nerve terminal, it can attenuate the negative feedback mechanism on the release of the neurotransmitter, norepinephrine.

There is evidence that this drug has some sympathomimetic effects. In addition, other studies indicate that yohimbine can promote a sympatholytic effect, which can result in an enhanced parasympathetic activity. In clinical studies yohimbine has been used to treat and diagnose certain types of male erectile impotence. It also is a mydriatic and sympathicolytic agent.

ADRENERGIC NEURONAL BLOCKING DRUGS

The adrenergic neuronal blocking agents cause a depletion of biogenic amines in neuronal terminals. These drugs may interfere with the synthesis, storage, or release of norepinephrine, dopamine, and serotonin.

Reserpine

Reserpine is the principal alkaloid found in the roots of *Rauwolfia serpentina* and is presently isolated from the plant for medical purposes. Other *Rauwolfia* alkaloids related structurally and pharmacologically to reserpine (deserpidine, rescinnamine, and alseroxylon) have largely been abandoned for therapeutic use. In the following discussion, reserpine is used as the prototype compound of the *Rauwolfia* alkaloids. The structure of reserpine is

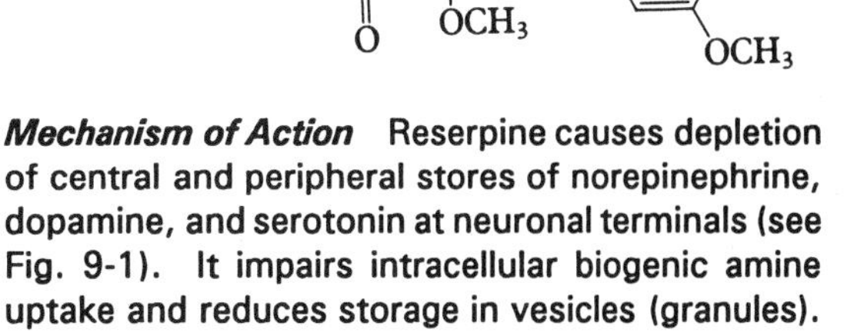

CH_3O N N H H H H OCH_3 O CH_3OC O OCH_3 OC OCH_3 OCH_3

Mechanism of Action Reserpine causes depletion of central and peripheral stores of norepinephrine, dopamine, and serotonin at neuronal terminals (see Fig. 9-1). It impairs intracellular biogenic amine uptake and reduces storage in vesicles (granules). Reserpine appears to act on the membranes of vesicles to irreversibly inhibit the Mg^{2+}-ATP-dependent transport process that is responsible for uptake of biogenic amines into intraneuronal vesicles. Catecholamine depletion results in decreased sympathetic predominance. A reduction in intraneuronal 5-hydroxytryptamine and dopamine produces an attenuation of serotonergic and dopaminergic activity, respectively.

Effects Reserpine acts in the CNS to produce sedation and tranquilization. It is believed that these effects are due to depletion of stores of catecholamines and 5-hydroxytryptamine centrally. Large doses cause hypothermia and respiratory depression.

The cardiovascular effects of reserpine include hypotension and reduced heart rate and cardiac output. The hypotensive response to the drug is due to impairment of adrenergic transmission both centrally (inhibition of the vasomotor center of the hypothalamus) and peripherally (arteriolar dilatation, decreased peripheral resistance). Reflex tachycardia is effectively blocked.

Adverse Reactions The use of reserpine has been limited, largely because of the adverse reactions which commonly occur.

Central nervous system effects include drowsiness, lethargy, depression, and nightmares. The most serious adverse effect is depression, which may require hospitalization and may persist for several months after the drug has been discontinued. Therefore, the drug should be used with extreme caution in patients with a history of depressive episodes. On occasion parkinsonian and other extrapyramidal reactions may be observed.

Parasympathetic predominance due to reduced sympathetic function may occur, and results in nasal congestion, bradycardia, salivation, and diarrhea. Increased gastric secretion with aggravation of peptic ulcer frequently occurs.

Endocrinologic disturbances have been reported. Reserpine inhibits ovulation and menstruation, probably through an action on the hypothalamus which alters the secretion of regulatory hormones. Gynecomastia in males has also been observed.

In addition, reserpine has been reported to cause angina pectoris, thrombocytopenia purpura, decreased libido, and cardiac arrhythmias.

Therapeutic Uses Reserpine is employed in the treatment of hypertension because of its cardiovascular effects. It is not a drug of choice, principally because of the high incidence of adverse reactions, but it may be combined with more effective, less toxic antihypertensive drugs such as diuretic agents. Reserpine has been used in the chronic treatment of Raynaud's disease.

Guanethidine

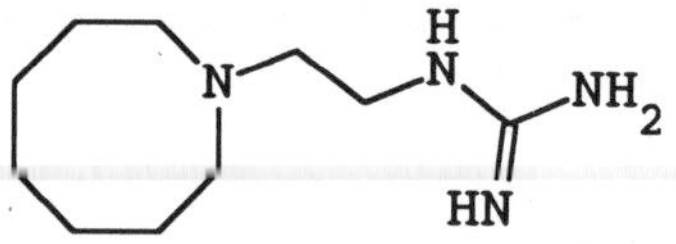

H
N NH$_2$ N
HN

Mechanism of Action The terminal and varicosities of the sympathetic neurons are filled with vesicles that contain norepinephrine. In these vesicles, norepinephrine appears to be bound to adenosine triphosphate (ATP) in a ratio of 4 molecules of norepinephrine to 1 molecule of ATP. Upon nerve stimulation, the vesicular membrane fuses with the presynaptic neuronal membrane and releases the adrenergic neurotransmitter. The released norepinephrine impinges on the effector cells, which are adjacent to the nerve ending.

Guanethidine does not act on the effector cells, as do adrenergic blocking agents. It acts on the terminal ramifications of the peripheral sympathetic nerve fibers. Guanethidine enters into the neuron by the same reuptake mechanism that returns norepinephrine to the terminal portion of the neuron from the synaptic area (see Fig. 9-1). Inside the neuron guanethidine is actively transported into the adrenergic storage vesicles where it accumulates. Guanethidine and norepinephrine compete for the same storage sites in the vesicles. As guanethidine increases in concentration, norepinephrine is displaced and there is a decrease in the neurotransmitter available for release. Guanethidine itself may be released by nerve stimulation but is ineffective as an adrenergic receptor stimulant. In addition to depletion of catecholamine stores from adrenergic nerve endings, it readily acts on catecholamine stores in organs such as the heart, spleen, and aorta. Guanethidine does not affect central sympathetic neurons, since the drug does not readily cross the blood-brain barrier.

Effects Guanethidine may produce an initial pressor response that is followed by decreased mean blood pressure as a result of decreased peripheral vascular resistance, bradycardia, and decreased cardiac output. The initial pressor response is due to displacement of large amounts of norepinephrine; this effect is generally observed after intravenous administration of the drug. The drug has considerably greater hypotensive effects when patients are in the standing position than when patients are supine. Such postural hypotension is a characteristic response to agents which block the sympathetic nervous system. The hypotension is presumably due to a reduction in the capacity of vasoconstrictor fibers to bring about the usual reflex compensations upon standing.

Pharmacokinetics Guanethidine is incompletely but predictably absorbed from the gastrointestinal tract. Approximately 40 percent of an oral dose is biotransformed to several inactive metabolites. The parent compound and its metabolites are excreted into the urine via glomerular filtration and tubular secretion.

Adverse Reactions Orthostatic hypotension can occur frequently. Additionally, dizziness, weakness, lassitude, syncope, bradycardia, diarrhea, inhibition of ejaculation, fluid retention, and edema are common side effects. Severe organ toxicity is very rare with this drug. Unlike reserpine, guanethidine does not produce any central adverse reactions.

Therapeutic Uses Guanethidine is indicated in the treatment of severe hypertension in which other more commonly used therapeutic agents have not been successful in patients. This drug reduces elevated arterial pressure in short-term therapy and is also effective in long-term management of hypertension. In addition, guanethidine may be useful in the treatment of Raynaud's disease, a vasospastic disorder.

Guanethidine is a very potent and long-lasting antihypertensive agent with a slow onset of activity. It primarily causes postural hypotension. The antihypertensive effect of guanethidine is usually delayed for 2 or 3 days following oral administration of an effective dose. The ensuing pressure reduction is sustained for several days. Because of its long duration of action, the drug can be administered effectively in a single daily dose or a dose every other day.

Guanadrel

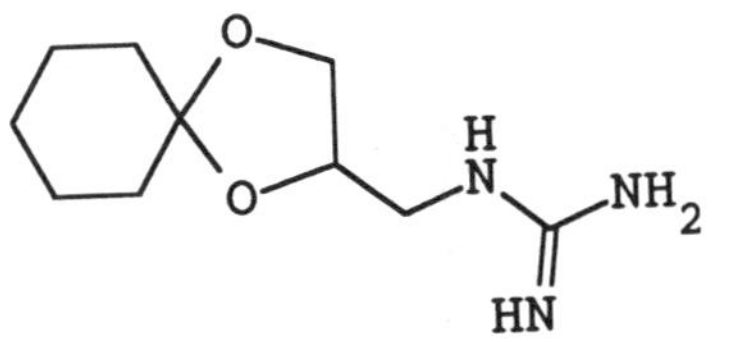

O O H N NH_2 HN

Guanadrel is an adrenergic neuronal blocking agent that is used in the treatment of essential hypertension. Its mechanism of action and adverse reactions are similar to those of guanethidine. The drug is well absorbed from the gastrointestinal tract but does not readily enter the CNS. Guanadrel appears to be somewhat more useful than guanethidine in the treatment of essential hypertension and may produce less of an incidence of diarrhea, morning orthostatic hypotension on arising, and impaired ejaculation.

Metyrosine

Metyrosine is the α-methylated derivative of tyrosine. This drug competitively inhibits the activity of tyrosine hydroxylase and thus decreases the endogenous formation of epinephrine and norepinephrine (see Fig. 9-1). Metyrosine is used in patients with pheochromocytoma who produce excessive quantities of these catecholamines, which results in hypertension. The drug is not recommended for the control of essential hypertension.

Metyrosine is well absorbed from the gastrointestinal tract. Approximately 30 percent of an oral dose is biotransformed to methyldopa, methyldopamine, and methylnorepinephrine; the remainder is excreted unchanged in the urine.

Adverse reactions include sedation, extrapyramidal symptoms, anxiety, depression, nausea, vomiting, diarrhea, abdominal pain, and nasal stuffiness. Crystalluria and transient dysuria have been observed in a few patients.

BIBLIOGRAPHY

Bravo, E.L., and R.W, Gifford, Jr.: "Pheochromocytoma: Diagnosis, Localization and Management," *N. Engl. J. Med.* **311**: 1298-1303 (1984).

Flaker, G.C., and V.N. Singh: "Prevention of Myocardial Reinfarction. Recommendations Based on Results of Drug Trials," *Postgrad. Med.* **94**: 94-98, 102-104 (1993).

Frishman, W.H.: "β-Adrenergic Blockers," *Medical Clin. North Am.* **72**: 37-81 (1988).

Hoffmann, B.B., and R.J. Lefkowitz: "Alpha-Adrenergic Receptor Subtypes," *N. Engl. J. Med.* **302**: 1390-1396 (1980).

Lewis, R.V., and C. Lofthouse: "Adverse Reactions with Beta-Adrenoceptor Blocking Drugs. An Update", *Drug Safety* **9**: 272-279 (1993).

Kincaid-Smith, P.S.: "Alpha Blockade. An Overview of Efficacy Data," *Am. J. Med.* **82**: 21-25 (1987).

McDevitt, D.G.: "Pharmacological Characteristics of β-Blockers and Their Role in Clinical Practice," *J. Cardiovasc. Pharmacol.* **8 (Suppl. 6)**: S5-S11 (1986).

McNeil, J.J., O.H. Drummer, E.L. Conway, B.S. Workman, and W.J. Louis: "Effect of Age on Pharmacokinetics of and Blood Pressure Responses to Prazosin and Terazosin," *J. Cardiovasc. Pharmacol.* **10**: 168-175 (1987).

Prichard, B.N.C.: "Pharmacologic Aspects of Intrinsic Sympathomimetic Activity in Beta-Blocking Drugs," *Am. J. Cardiol.* **59**: 13F-17F (1987).

Riddell, J.G., D.W.G. Harron, and R.G. Shanks: "Clinical Pharmacokinetics of β-Adrenoreceptor Antagonists," *Clin. Pharmacokinet.* **12**: 305-320 (1987).

Singh, B., and A.R. Laddu: "Esmolol: A Novel Ultra-short Acting, β-Adrenoreceptor Blocking Agent," *Rational Drug Therapy*, **20**: 1-7 (1986).

Titmarsh, S.: "Terazosin. A Review of Its Pharmacodynamics and Pharmacokinetic Properties and Therapeutic Efficacy in Essential Hypertension," *Drugs* **33**: 461-477 (1987).

Wong, Y.W., and T.M. Ludden: "Determination of Betaxolol and its Metabolites in Blood and Urine by High-Performance Liquid Chromatography with Fluorimetric Detection," *J. Chromatogr.* **534**: 161-172 (1990).

CHAPTER 10

Cholinomimetic Drugs

Frank J. Dowd

Cholinomimetic agents are drugs which evoke responses similar to both those produced by acetylcholine and those which result from activation of all ganglia and the parasympathetic nervous system. These drugs mimic the actions of acetylcholine released endogenously. Those drugs that act primarily on muscarinic receptors and mimic stimulation of the parasympathetic nervous system are called *parasympathomimetics*. Cholinomimetic agents produce their effects through two mechanisms: (1) direct stimulation of cholinergic receptors and (2) indirectly, through inhibition of acetylcholinesterase, the enzyme responsible for the chemical destruction of acetylcholine at its site of action. The primary mechanism of action of each drug can be used to classify the agents.

DIRECT ACTING CHOLINOMIMETIC DRUGS

The direct-acting cholinomimetic agents are those drugs which act by direct stimulation of cholinergic receptors. The drugs can be subdivided based on their selectivity in stimulating muscarinic or nicotinic receptors. A description of these receptors including their location and major effects elicited by receptor activation is found in Chapter 7. Those drugs whose effectiveness is based primarily on their stimulation of muscarinic receptors include (1) choline esters consisting of acetylcholine and structural analogs and (2) the naturally occurring alkaloids, muscarine and pilocarpine. (Although some of these compounds can activate nicotinic receptors, their most prominent effects are mediated through stimulation of muscarinic receptor sites). Drugs whose actions are based primarily on their stimulation of nicotinic receptors include nicotine and lobeline.

Choline Esters

Drugs in this class consist of acetylcholine and its structural analogs, methacholine, bethanechol, and carbachol (carbamylcholine) (Fig. 10-1). Although these compounds have the ability to directly stimulate all cholinergic receptors, their therapeutic effectiveness is due to their action on muscarinic receptors (e.g., subtypes M_1, M_2 and M_3). The compounds differ only in the duration of their effects and, to some degree, in their selectivity for receptors. Acetylcholine is the prototype for the group. No agonist, selective for a muscarinic receptor subtype, is currently available for therapeutic use. A detailed description of muscarinic receptors is found in Chapter 3.

Acetylcholine

Acetylcholine is composed of a molecule of choline with an acetyl functional group connected by an ester linkage (Fig. 10-1). Due to its highly polar, positively charged ammonium group, acetylcholine does not readily cross lipid membranes. For that reason, the exogenously administered drug is confined to extracellular spaces of the body and does not cross the blood-brain barrier. To obtain systemic effects, acetylcholine must be administered intravenously; oral bioavailability is extremely low. Moreover, being an ester, this compound is readily hydrolyzed and inactivated by acetyl- and plasma cholinesterases. Even large intravenous doses would produce effects with a very brief duration.

Pharmacodynamics *Cardiovascular system* The cardiovascular system is affected more profoundly than any other organ system following intravenous administration. At low doses, acetylcholine

$CH_3{-}COOCH_2{-}CH_2{-}\overset{+}{N}(CH_3)_3$ Acetylcholine

$CH_3{-}COOCH(CH_3){-}CH_2{-}\overset{+}{N}(CH_3)_3$ Methacholine

$NH_2{-}COOCH_2{-}CH_2{-}\overset{+}{N}(CH_3)_3$ Carbachol

$NH_2{-}COOCH(CH_3){-}CH_2{-}\overset{+}{N}(CH_3)_3$ Bethanechol

FIGURE 10-1 *Structures of choline esters.*

produces vasodilatation in essentially all vascular beds, including cutaneous, cerebral, pulmonary, and coronary vessels. Although these blood vessels are not innervated by cholinergic vasodilator fibers, they do contain cholinergic (muscarinic) receptors which can be stimulated by exogenously administered drugs. Vasodilatation from acetylcholine is an indirect effect. Stimulation of muscarinic receptors located on endothelial cells leads to the release of nitric oxide (NO), originally called endothelium-derived relaxing factor. NO stimulates guanylate cyclase and the production of cyclic-GMP in vascular smooth muscle, leading to muscle relaxation. The vasodilatation may be accompanied by reflex tachycardia; this would partially be masked by direct actions on cardiac tissue. At higher doses, bradycardia may accompany the vasodilatation.

Acetylcholine has prominent direct actions on cardiac rhythm, conduction processes of the heart, and the atrial myocardium; these actions parallel almost exactly those produced by stimulation of the vagus nerve. Acetylcholine reduces heart rate by slowing the rate of firing of the sinoatrial node, an effect which is associated with hyperpolarization of the pacemaker membrane. Acetylcholine also slows conduction velocity across the AV node. The His bundle and Purkinje system appear to be relatively resistant to these effects of the compound. Atrial fibers are also inhibited by acetylcholine, causing a decrease in the force of contraction of atrial muscle. Ventricular fibers, which are not innervated by cholinergic neurons, are resistant to stimulation by the vagus. However, exogenously administered acetylcholine will slightly reduce the force of contraction of ventricular muscle fibers due to the presence of some muscarinic receptors.

In addition to the changes in cardiac activity, the local application of acetylcholine can also induce atrial fibrillation. The fibrillation is not due to an increase in the sinus rate but appears to be due to a phenomenon called *reexcitation by reentry*. This phenomenon results from the circular movement of excitation and the reexcitation of fibers which have already passed through their refractory periods. It is favored by (1) a restriction of normal pathways as a result of local block, (2) a reduced refractory period, and (3) reduced conduction velocity. In addition to producing various degrees of blockade, both vagal stimulation and acetylcholine reduce the refractory period of atrial fibers by shortening the duration of the action potentials. Thus, two of the conditions which predispose the atrium to fibrillation are produced by acetylcholine and stimulation of the vagus nerve. All the direct effects of this drug on the heart are reversed by atropine, a muscarinic antagonist, and enhanced by cholinesterase inhibitors.

Smooth muscle cells In contrast with vascular smooth muscle cells, those of most other organs respond to acetylcholine with an increase in tone. By direct stimulation of muscarinic receptors, acetylcholine causes contraction of smooth muscle cells of the (1) bronchioles causing bronchoconstriction, (2) gastrointestinal tract increasing motility, (3) bladder and ureters increasing the frequency of urination, (4) uterus, and (5) iris sphincter and ciliary muscle of the eye, causing miosis and accommodation for near vision, respectively. The contraction of smooth muscle is antagonized by atropine and enhanced by cholinesterase inhibitors.

Glands All glands which are innervated by cholinergic neurons are stimulated by exogenous administration of acetylcholine. This causes increased salivation, lacrimation, and sweating, in addition to increases in gastrointestinal, pancreatic, and bronchial secretions. These are also muscarinic effects, antagonized by atropine.

Neuromuscular junction Although acetylcholine is the primary neurotransmitter at the neuromuscular junction, the exogenous administration of this drug causes little contraction of skeletal muscle. This is because acetylcholine, a quaternary compound, cannot readily get to its site of action, which is surrounded by lipoid membranes. Higher doses, however, will cause some contraction of skeletal muscle. Intravenously administered acetylcholine also does not penetrate very well to the autonomic ganglia. The effects of acetylcholine at the ganglia and neuromuscular junction are due to stimulation of nicotinic receptors, and these would not be antagonized by the administration of atropine.

Therapeutic Use Acetylcholine has no therapeutic effectiveness by intravenous administration. This is due to its diffuse action and rapid inactivation by cholinesterases. It is, however, used as a sterile solution for intraocular administration to produce miosis during cataract surgery. Its short duration of action is advantageous, allowing rapid recovery postoperatively.

Adverse Reactions Administered locally in the eye, acetylcholine only rarely produces systemic side effects. Reactions may include hypotension, bradycardia, flushing, sweating, and dyspnea. No local toxic reactions have been reported.

Methacholine

As shown in Fig. 10-1 this compound differs from acetylcholine only by the addition of a methyl group to the β carbon of choline. This structural change results in two important alterations in the pharmacologic properties of the molecule (Table 10-1). Unlike acetylcholine, methacholine is hydrolyzed only by acetylcholinesterase, and the rate of hydrolysis of methacholine is considerably slower than that of acetylcholine. Thus the actions of methacholine are more persistent than those of acetylcholine. The introduction of the methyl group to the β carbon also endows the compound with more selectivity. Methacholine acts primarily on muscarinic receptors in smooth muscle, glands, and the heart and has very little activity on nicotinic receptors at the autonomic ganglia and skeletal muscle. These two features, duration of response and improved selectivity, represent the primary differences between the pharmacologic actions of methacholine and acetylcholine.

The actions of methacholine on the cardiovascular system are the same qualitatively as those described above for acetylcholine. Its clinical use in selected cases of atrial tachycardia not responding to other forms of therapy has been replaced by other modalities. Methacholine is currently used in the diagnosis of bronchial hyperreactivity in patients who do not have clinically apparent asthma.

Carbachol (Carbamylcholine)

In contrast to acetylcholine and methacholine, carbachol contains a carbamic rather than esteratic functional group (Fig. 10-1). The carbamate group is not readily susceptible to hydrolysis by cholinesterases. Although enzymatic destruction has been demonstrated *in vitro*, the rate of hydrolysis is too slow to be of any practical significance.

Carbachol is a potent choline ester, stimulating both muscarinic and nicotinic receptors. It therefore possesses all the pharmacodynamic properties of acetylcholine. In addition to producing vasodilatation, reduced heart rate, increased tone and contraction of smooth muscle and stimulation of salivary, lacrimal, and sweat glands, carbachol also stimulates autonomic ganglia and skeletal muscle.

Carbachol is more selective in stimulating muscarinic receptors in the gastrointestinal tract, urinary bladder and eye, compared to the cardiovascular system. Nevertheless, its lack of overall cholinergic selectivity (muscarinic vs nicotinic) limits its therapeutic usefulness. At present, the principal use of carbachol is in ophthalmology as a miotic agent. The drug is applied topically to the conjunctiva, producing prolonged miosis during ocular surgery.

Bethanechol

Bethanechol combines the structural features of methacholine and carbachol, containing both β-methyl and carbamate functional groups (Fig. 10-1), and therefore has pharmacologic properties of both drugs. Bethanechol, like carbachol, is resistant to hydrolysis by acetyl- and plasma cholinesterases. Similar to methacholine, bethanechol has very little action at nicotinic receptors of autonomic ganglia or neuromuscular junctions.

Bethanechol has a more selective action at muscarinic receptors of the gastrointestinal tract and urinary bladder than do the other choline esters. Its therapeutic application is based on these actions; the primary use of bethanechol is in treatment of postoperative nonobstructive urinary retention and neurogenic atony of the bladder. It was also used in the past for treatment of gastro-

TABLE 10-1 Comparison of the pharmacologic properties of choline esters

	Susceptibility to cholinesterases	Muscarinic effects	Nicotinic effects	Therapeutic use
Acetylcholine	+4	+3	+3	Miotic
Methacholine	+1	+4	+1	Diagnosis of bronchial hyperreactivity
Carbachol	0	+2	+3	Miotic
Bethanechol	0	+2[b]	0	Nonobstructive urinary retention

[a] 0 to +4 indicates increasing activity, where 0 is no effect and +4 is the greatest effect.
[b] Bethanechol has more selectivity for muscarinic receptors of the gastrointestinal tract and urinary bladder than do other choline esters.

intestinal disorders including postoperative abdominal distention, but this has been largely replaced by other agents. Bethanechol has also been used with very limited success in the treatment of Alzheimer's disease.

Bethanechol is available for both oral and subcutaneous administration; it is readily absorbed from either route. Following oral administration, onset of action is approximately 30 min with peak effects in 1 to 1.5 h; its duration is about 2 to 2.5 h. Subcutaneous administration provides a more rapid onset (15 to 30 min) with a duration of about 2 h.

Adverse effects of bethanechol are due to overstimulation of the parasympathetic nervous system and include gastrointestinal distress, abdominal cramping, sweating, flushing, hypotension, and bronchoconstriction. Reactions are less likely to occur following oral administration than after dosing by the subcutaneous route. Bethanechol is contraindicated in patients with peptic ulcer, bronchial asthma, pronounced bradycardia, hyperthyroidism, coronary artery disease and parkinsonism (although very little crosses the blood-brain barrier).

Naturally Occurring Muscarinic Alkaloids

Muscarine

Muscarine (Fig. 10-2) is an alkaloid present in various wild mushrooms with wide geographic distribution (Europe, Asia, North and South America, and South Africa). *Amanita muscaria*, in which muscarine was first identified, contains low

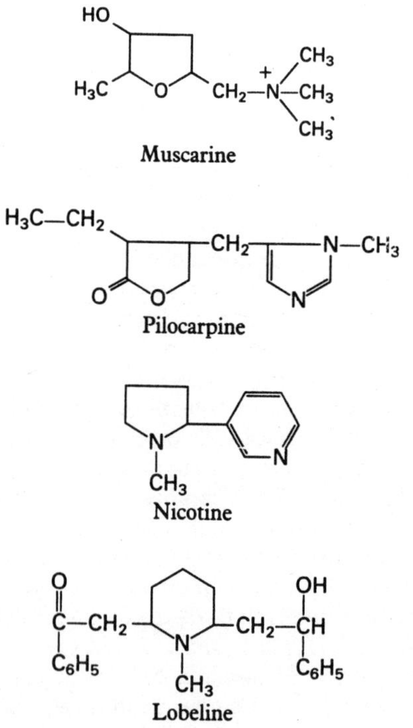

Muscarine

Pilocarpine

Nicotine

Lobeline

FIGURE 10-2 *Structures of naturally occurring alkaloids and a synthetic analog.*

concentrations of the compound; much higher levels are found in *Clitocybe inocybe*. Although it is not useful as a therapeutic agent, muscarine is of interest because of its toxic properties and because historically it was one of the first cholinomimetic drugs to be systematically studied. The compound has provided the basis for classification of cholinergic muscarinic receptors. The actions of muscarine are similar to those of acetylcholine on peripheral autonomic effector organs and are antagonized by atropine. Unlike acetylcholine, muscarine has no effects on nicotinic receptors.

Mushroom poisoning is still fairly common and may constitute a serious medical emergency, requiring intensive supportive therapy. Muscarine is well absorbed from the gastrointestinal tract, and therefore ingestion can lead to accidental intoxication. It is much more potent than acetylcholine, probably as a result of its greater stability; not being an ester, muscarine is resistant to hydrolysis by cholinesterases. It is important that a physician be able to differentiate the symptoms of muscarine intoxication (overstimulation of the parasympathetic nervous system) from that of other toxins found in mushrooms so that proper treatment can be started. Muscarine poisoning is treated with atropine, a muscarinic receptor antagonist.

Pilocarpine

Pilocarpine is an alkaloid obtained from the leaf of the tropical American shrub *Pilocarpus jaborandi*. Its actions are primarily due to stimulation of muscarinic receptor sites and, therefore, given systemically are similar to acetylcholine. The compound differs from acetylcholine in that it does not have any effects on nicotinic receptors, and since it is a tertiary amine (Fig. 10-2), it can produce central nervous system stimulation. All these effects are blocked by atropine.

The primary therapeutic use of pilocarpine is in ophthalmology as a miotic. Pilocarpine is an important drug for initial and long-term treatment of various types of glaucoma, i.e., primary open-angle glaucoma, other chronic glaucomas, and emergency therapy of acute angle closure glaucoma. Topical administration produces miosis by contracting the circular muscle of the iris. It also causes contraction of the ciliary muscle, leading to an increased opening of the trabecular space and hence an increase in the outflow of aqueous humor, which reduces intraocular pressure. The drug has an onset of action of 15 to 30 min and a duration of 4 to 8 h. It can be used alone or in combination with other agents such as epinephrine or physostigmine. Pilocarpine is available for treatment of chronic glaucoma in a specialized drug delivery system (Ocusert); this is placed directly in the conjunctival sac, allowing for continuous release of the drug. Pilocarpine, 5 mg orally, is being evaluated in the treatment of xerostomia (dry mouth).

Although pilocarpine is generally well tolerated, it can produce local burning and irritation. Systemic cholinergic effects following topical administration are uncommon.

Naturally Occurring Nicotinic Alkaloids

Nicotine

Nicotine has been extensively studied for several reasons. First, the chemical was used experimentally to characterize cholinergic nicotinic receptors and to simulate or block the autonomic ganglia. Second, the inherent toxicity of nicotine has been applied in the control of insects and is of concern because of the possibility of accidental poisoning. Today, nicotine is also important owing to its presence in tobacco products and the link of habitual cigarette smoking to cancer of the lung, mouth, larynx, and esophagus. Chronic bronchitis and emphysema are common in smokers. Nicotine is also a risk factor for coronary artery disease, arteriosclerosis, and hypertension.

Source and Chemistry Nicotine (Fig. 10-2) is an alkaloid found in the dried leaves of *Nicotiana tabacum* and *N. rustica* to the extent of 2 to 8 percent. The nicotine content varies from about 2 percent in the average cigarette to about 1 percent in so-called denicotinized preparations.

Mechanism of Action Nicotine acts by interacting with the peripheral cholinergic nicotinic receptors at the postsynaptic membrane in the autonomic ganglion (N_N) and neuromuscular junction (N_M) as well as nicotinic receptors in the central nervous system. At low doses (such as obtained in cigarette smoking) or initially at high doses, nicotine stimulates the receptors causing depolarization of the membrane and influx of sodium and calcium. If large doses are used, the stimulation is followed by a prolonged blockade of repolarization. This makes the receptor refractory to subsequent stimulation by acetylcholine released from the preganglionic cholinergic fibers and, therefore, there is a block of transmission. This is referred to as a *depolarizing ganglionic blockade*, in which the actions of all nicotinic agonists, including the endogenous neurotransmitter, acetylcholine, is blocked.

Pharmacodynamics *Central nervous system* The effects of nicotine on the CNS are both stimulatory and depressive. Nicotine causes excitation of the motor cortex leading to tremors and even convulsions at toxic doses. The tremors are also due to peripheral stimulation of the neuromuscular junction. Nicotine stimulates release of antidiuretic hormone, possibly causing a temporary antidiuresis following cigarette smoking. Nausea and vomiting are frequent effects on first exposure to nicotine due to stimulation of the chemoreceptor trigger zone in the area postrema as well as vagal and spinal afferent nerves. Respiration can be stimulated or depressed. Tolerance develops fairly rapidly to these effects.

Autonomic nervous system Actions of nicotine extend to all autonomic ganglia, both sympathetic and parasympathetic. These manifestations are further complicated by actions of nicotine outside the autonomic ganglia, namely, the release of epinephrine from the adrenal medulla, and activation of visceral receptors with resulting reflex actions. The combined picture is an increase in sympathetic activity of some organs (heart, blood vessels, pupil) and in parasympathetic activity of others (salivary glands, gastrointestinal tract).

Respiratory system Nicotine initially stimulates respiration; with increasing doses the stimulation is followed by respiratory depression. The initial increase in rate and depth of respiration from small doses is due to stimulation of chemoreceptors in the carotid body and aortic arch. Larger doses cause direct stimulation of the medullary pontine respiratory center. At toxic levels, respiratory depression is caused by (1) depression of the respiratory center and (2) blockade of nicotinic receptors in skeletal muscles (i.e., intercostals and diaphragm).

An intravenous injection of nicotine would elicit respiratory stimulation, but this is often preceded by a brief period of apnea, which arises from stimulation of receptors in the lungs. From the toxicologic standpoint, the reflex apnea is not so important as the paralysis of respiratory muscles brought about by a direct action of nicotine on the neuromuscular junction.

Cardiovascular system The effects of nicotine on the cardiovascular system are complex and a summation of its actions at multiple sites: sympathetic and parasympathetic ganglia and the adrenal medulla. Chronic smokers (as well as occasional smokers) show an increase in pulse rate from a few to over 50 beats per minute. Nicotine-induced increases in heart rate may be accompanied by a rise in cardiac output and an increase in total peripheral resistance, both contributing to an increase in blood pressure. These effects can exacerbate cardiovascular disease and hypertension.

Pharmacokinetics Nicotine is highly lipid-soluble and is readily absorbed through all mucosal membranes and also via the intact skin. When administered by mouth, nicotine is absorbed through the buccal mucosa, the stomach, and the intestine. Nicotine is rapidly distributed throughout the body, readily crossing the blood-brain barrier, placenta, and also accumulating in breast milk. Approximately 80 to 90 percent of the drug is oxidized in the liver, lung, and kidney to the inactive products cotinine and nicotine-N-oxide, which are excreted in the urine.

Therapeutic Use The only therapeutic use of nicotine is as a temporary aid to an individual attempting to quit smoking. Nicotine is available as a chewing gum, bound to an ion exchange resin. The drug has proven effective but should only be used for periods shorter than 3 months. Though abuse potential is considered minimal, nicotine gum does maintain the patient's addiction and should be withdrawn gradually. Nicotine is also available in a transdermal preparation for smoking cessation. The preparation consists of a multilayered skin patch which, depending on the preparation, can provide up to a 24 hour release of the drug upon contact with the skin. As with nicotine gum, patch therapy should be limited in duration (4 to 8 weeks) and withdrawal should be preceded by gradual reduction in drug dosage.

Adverse Reactions The adverse reactions associated with the use of nicotine are generally mild. Gastrointestinal distress, nausea, and vomiting are most common. Headache, dizziness, insomnia, and irritability occur in 1 to 2 percent of patients. Nicotine induced hiccoughs have also been reported. The use of nicotine gum is associated with an increased incidence of nausea and vomiting, indigestion, hiccoughs, and excessive salivation. Erythema, local edema and contact dermatitis have been reported with the transdermal preparations. Contact dermatitis may be followed by a more serious allergic reaction following a second challenge with nicotine.

Poisoning may occur from the accidental exposure to large doses of this compound, e.g., the accidental ingestion of tobacco products in children, the exposure of tobacco workers to wet tobacco leaves, or the extensive contact with an insecticide containing nicotine. The symptoms of nicotine poisoning which appear immediately include salivation, nausea or vomiting, abdominal pain and diarrhea, mental confusion, and marked weakness. The pupils become constricted and later dilated; pulse rate is at first slow and then rapid; blood pressure rises and then falls. Respiration becomes irregular when convulsions appear. Death results from respiratory paralysis followed by cardiovascular collapse. Therapy for acute poisoning should include vomiting induced by syrup of ipecac or gastric lavage with activated charcoal. Respiratory and cardiovascular support may be necessary. There is no specific antidote for nicotine.

Chronic toxicity to nicotine is a major problem owing to the large number of people exposed through smoking of cigarettes, cigars, and pipes. There is a causal connection between chronic smoking and cardiovascular disease and lung cancer. Cardiovascular diseases associated with tobacco smoking include peripheral vascular disease, cerebrovascular disease, and coronary artery disease. These are due not only to nicotine but also to other constituents of tobacco smoke.

Tolerance and Dependence Tolerance does develop to some of the effects of nicotine following chronic smoking. The dizziness, nausea, and vomiting experienced by first-time smokers usually are not observed in the chronic smoker. However tolerance does not appear to develop to the hand tremor, increase in blood pressure and pulse rate, and increased secretion of certain hormones. The mechanism for tolerance appears to be pharmacodynamic, although chronic smokers also biotransform nicotine more rapidly than nonsmokers owing to the induction of the drug-metabolizing microsomal system.

An abstinence syndrome may occur on cessation of chronic smoking. Symptoms may include irritability, restlessness, anxiety, headache, insomnia, gastrointestinal upset, increased appetite, and a craving to start smoking again. Symptoms may begin within 24 h, with some persisting for several weeks or months.

Lobeline

Lobeline (α-lobeline; L-lobeline; inflatine) is the principal alkaloid of the dried leaves and tops of *Lobelia inflata*. The actions of lobeline are in many respects similar to those of nicotine, but lobeline has a lower mg potency. Like nicotine, lobeline is a primary stimulant and secondary depressant to the sympathetic ganglia, parasympathetic ganglia, adrenal medulla, central medullary centers (especially the emetic centers), neuromuscular junction, and chemoreceptors in the carotid body and aortic arch. Lobeline is used therapeutically as a smoking deterrent to aid an individual to give up cigarette smoking. It is not to be used for longer than 6 weeks. Adverse reactions including nausea, vomiting, heartburn, belching, epigastric pain, and dizziness.

INDIRECT ACTING CHOLINOMIMETIC DRUGS

As a class, the cholinesterase inhibitors (or anticholinesterases) are very important members of the cholinomimetic family of drugs. In addition to their importance therapeutically, some compounds are widely used as agricultural pesticides and others are extremely toxic chemical warfare agents. All uses of these compounds are based on the changes which occur following inactivation of cholinesterases, i.e., the effects observed are due to the accumulation and action of acetylcholine at the neuronal-effector junctions. Before discussing the pharmacologic effects of individual agents, some of the characteristics of the cholinesterases and the inhibitors will be considered.

Acetylcholinesterase is depicted schematically as shown in Fig. 10-3. Acetylcholine binds to the enzyme, orienting the molecule for enzymatic hydrolysis of the ester linkage. The choline portion of the molecule binds to a hydrophobic site which is in close proximity to anionic sites to which the charged nitrogen is attracted. The carbonyl group of the acetyl portion of the substrate forms a covalent bond at the esteratic site. This substrate-enzyme complex results in acetylation of the enzyme, destruction of the ester linkage, and removal of the choline. The acetylated enzyme then reacts with water to form acetate and a regenerated enzyme. Acetylcholine is cleaved within 100 to 150 μs. Plasma cholinesterase (or pseudocholinesterase) acts in a similar manner to hydrolyze acetylcholine. It is, however, less specific for acetylcholine and biotransforms other aliphatic and aromatic esters as well.

The cholinesterase inhibitors can inhibit both cholinesterases. They are divided based either on their chemical structure or their chemical interaction with the enzyme which determines their time course of action. There are three broad chemical classes of cholinesterase inhibitors (Fig. 10-4): (1) mono-carbamates, e.g., physostigmine, neostigmine, pyridostigmine, and several insecticides represented by carbaryl; (2) other quaternary amines, e.g., edrophonium, ambenonium, and demecarium; and (3) organophosphates, e.g., isofluorophate, echothiophate, insecticides represented by malathion and parathion, and toxins represented by soman. In addition, an acridine derivative, tacrine, was recently made available for the treatment of Alzheimer's disease. Based on differences in their time course of inhibition, cholinesterase inhibitors can also be classified as reversible and irreversible inhibitors. The reversible inhibitors comprise the mono-carbamates, the quaternary amines, and tacrine; organophosphates are irreversible inhibitors of the cholinesterases.

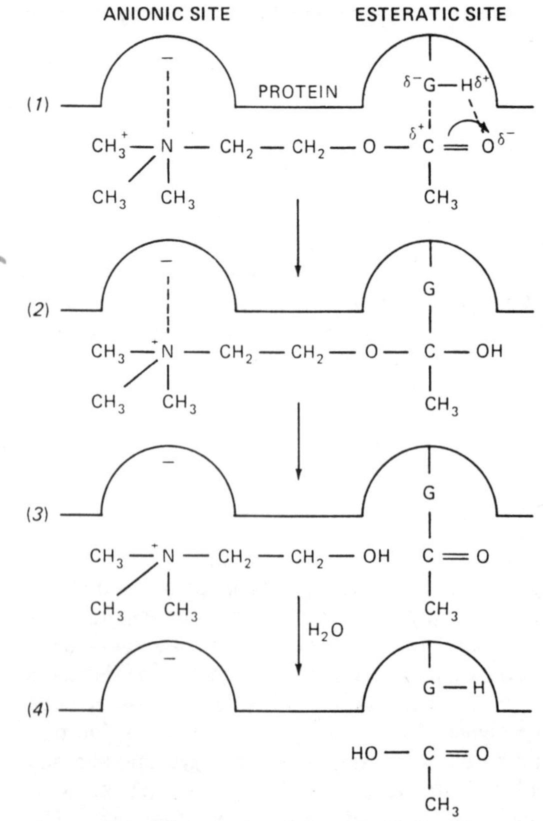

FIGURE 10-3 *Steps in the acetylcholinesterase-catalyzed hydrolysis of acetylcholine (ACh): (1) Attachment of ACh to the anionic site (–) and esteratic site (G–H) of the enzyme. (2) Formation of a covalent bond to the esteratic site, with loss of the resonance energy of the C=O group. (3) Cleavage of the ACh-enzyme complex into choline and acetylated enzyme. (4) Very rapid hydrolysis of the acetylated enzyme and regeneration of the acetylcholinesterase.*

Reversible Cholinesterase Inhibitors

As the name implies, the reversible cholinesterase inhibitors form a transient complex with the enzyme, in much the same way as does acetylcholine. These compounds compete with acetylcholine for binding at the active site of the enzyme. The chemical structure of the classic reversible inhibitors physostigmine and neostigmine suggests a similarity to acetylcholine like the carbonyl moiety of acetylcholine, the carbonyl group of physostigmine and neostigmine attaches to the esteratic site of the enzyme. In addition, neostigmine also forms an ionic bond between its quaternary nitrogen and the anionic site of the enzyme, thus forming a two-point attachment to the enzyme. Edrophonium, also a potent reversible inhibitor (but not a carbamate), binds primarily to the anionic site, with hydrogen bonding to the esteratic site. While these compounds have high affinity for the enzyme, the inhibition of the enzyme is reversible. These inhibitors differ from acetylcholine in that they are not readily degraded by the enzyme; the enzyme is reactivated much more slowly than following hydrolysis of acetylcholine. Therefore, the pharmacologic effects produced by these drugs are reversible.

Physostigmine

Physostigmine is an alkaloid extracted from the calabar bean, the dried ripe seed of a wood vine *Physostigma venenosum* that grows in tropical West Africa. Unlike most other reversible cholinesterase inhibitors, physostigmine is a tertiary amine (Fig. 10-4); thus physostigmine is readily absorbed from the gastrointestinal tract and from other mucous membranes, but it is not used by the oral route. It is available for topical and parenteral administration. Once physostigmine enters the bloodstream, the drug is widely distributed throughout the organism, readily crossing the

MONO-CARBAMATES

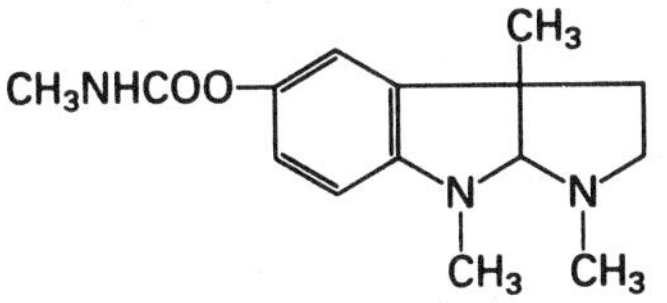

Physostigmine

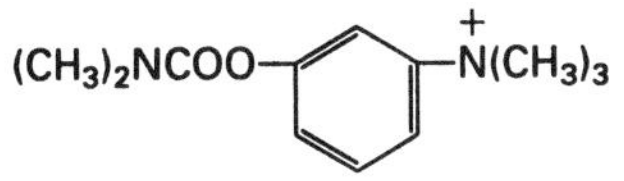

Neostigmine

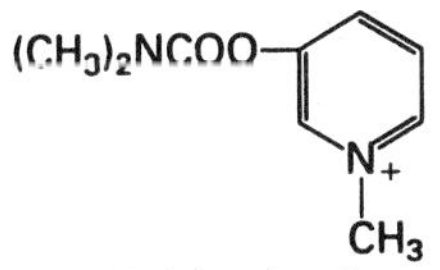

Pyridostigmine

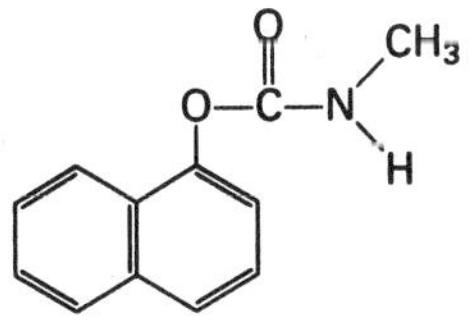

Carbaryl

QUATERNARY COMPOUNDS

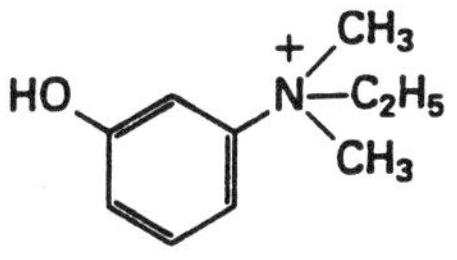

Edrophonium

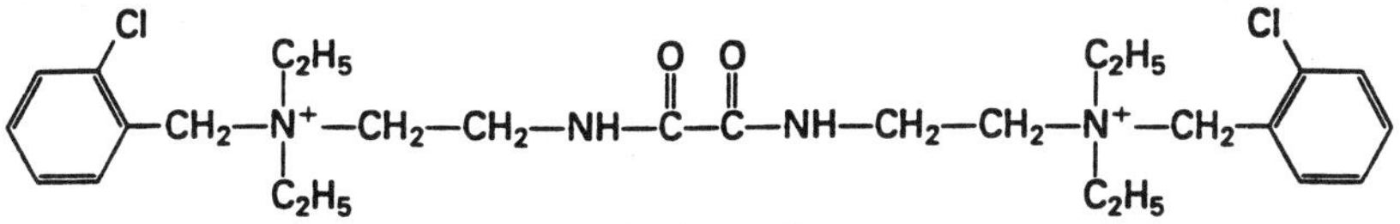

Ambenonium

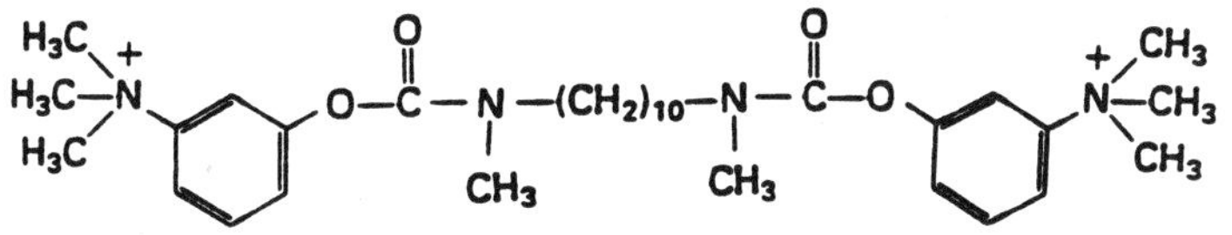

Demecarium

ORGANOPHOSPHATES

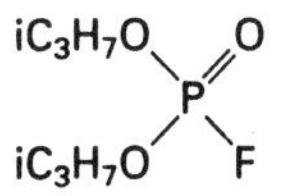

Isoflurophate (DFP)

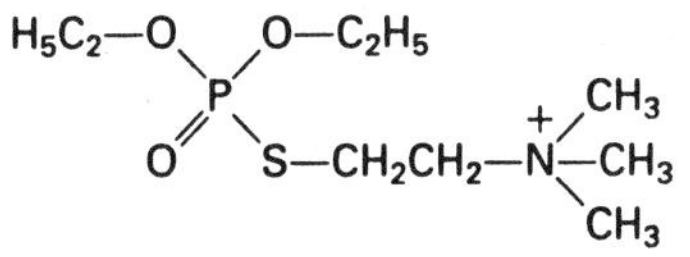

Echothiophate

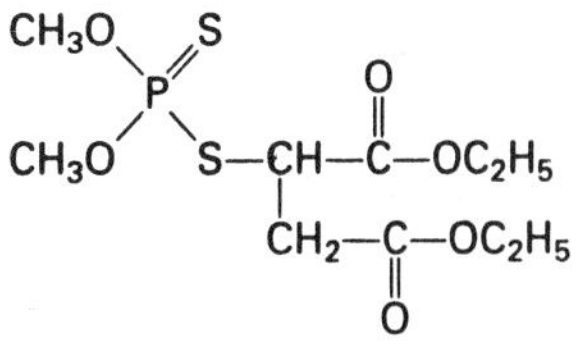

Malathion

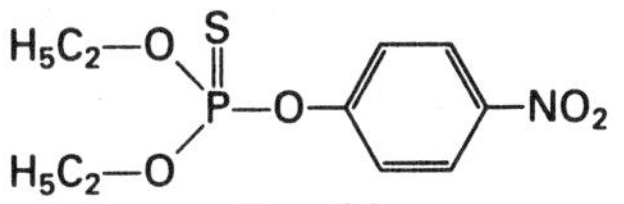

Parathion

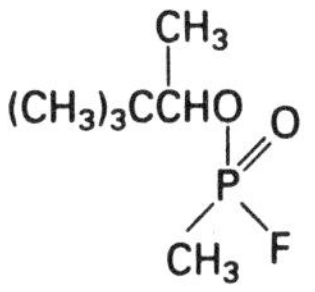

Soman

FIGURE 10-4 *Structures of representative cholinesterase inhibitors.*

blood-brain barrier. The drug is inactivated by plasma cholinesterases. Renal impairment has noeffect on drug elimination. Following intravenous administration, the duration of action is approximately 0.5 to 2 h, depending on the dose.

All those systems which normally produce and respond to acetylcholine are affected by physostigmine. At each of these sites, following the administration of adequate amounts, the resultant accumulation of acetylcholine gives rise to marked cholinergic stimulation. Physostigmine has minimal direct effects on cholinergic receptors. Since the responses to physostigmine are essentially the same as mentioned for acetylcholine and those described in Table 10-2, they will not be described here except as they relate to the therapeutic uses of physostigmine. In ophthalmology, physostigmine is useful topically in the treatment of glaucoma. It lowers intraocular pressure by increasing the outflow of aqueous humor. As mentioned before, it can be used in conjunction with pilocarpine.

One of the most striking aspects of the pharmacologic actions of physostigmine is its effect on transmission at the neuromuscular junction. When administered systemically, physostigmine produces fasciculations and, with large doses, paralysis of striated muscle. As stated earlier, these responses are due to the inhibition of acetylcholinesterase and the resulting accumulation of acetylcholine in the neuromuscular junction. It is by this mechanism that physostigmine antagonizes the blockade of neuromuscular transmission produced by tubocurarine and other competitive neuromuscular blockers. Since tubocurarine blocks transmission by competing with acetylcholine for nicotinic receptor sites on the skeletal muscle end plate, the accumulation of acetylcholine which occurs following the inhibition of acetylcholinesterase shifts the competition in favor of the neurotransmitter and mediates the anticurare action of physostigmine. This is a useful tool for anesthesiologists. However, the use of physostigmine for this purpose has largely been replaced by pyridostigmine, neostigmine, and edrophonium since they have no central nervous system effects.

Because of the ability of physostigmine to penetrate into the central nervous system, the drug is useful to antagonize toxic concentrations of drugs with anticholinergic properties, such as atropine, antihistamines, phenothiazines, and tricyclic antidepressants. For emergency treatment, the drug must be given intravenously. Physostigmine has also been used, with limited success, in the treatment of Alzheimer's disease, which is characterized, in part, by serious reduction in acetylcholine levels in cerebral cortex and hippocampus.

The severity of adverse reactions associated with the drug depends on the route of administration. Topically in the eye, physostigmine often causes hyperemia of the conjunctiva and iris. Systemically, adverse reactions are the result of overstimulation of cholinergic effectors. Physostigmine can exacerbate peptic ulceration and bronchial asthma. It can also produce a reduction in heart rate and even bradyarrhythmias. Since it crosses the blood-brain barrier, physostigmine can worsen the symptoms of parkinsonism by further disrupting the balance of acetylcholine and dopamine.

Neostigmine

Neostigmine is a synthetic cholinesterase inhibitor which differs from physostigmine in that it contains a quaternary nitrogen (Fig. 10-4). As a consequence, neostigmine has a limited pattern of distribution in the organism. Neostigmine is poorly and irregularly absorbed from the gastrointestinal tract although it is used by the oral route. In addition, it poorly penetrates other lipoidal barriers and membranes. Thus, it is difficult to regulate plasma levels of neostigmine when the drug is given orally. On the other hand, the poor penetration by the drug of the blood-brain barrier tends to minimize any occurrence of toxicity due to the inhibition of cholinesterases of the brain.

The presence of a quaternary nitrogen in the molecule introduces another important difference between physostigmine and neostigmine. The latter compound, in addition to inhibiting the cholinesterases, also has a direct stimulatory action on the skeletal muscle. Apart from these important differences, the general actions of neostigmine are like those of physostigmine and comparable to hyperactivity of cholinergic nerves.

Like other reversible cholinesterase inhibitors, neostigmine possesses a powerful anticurare action. This probably occurs by a combination of two mechanisms: (1) preservation of released acetylcholine by inhibiting acetylcholinesterase and (2) a direct stimulation of nicotinic (N_M) receptors on the skeletal muscle end plate. Use of this effect of neostigmine is made in anesthesiology to overcome the paralysis of skeletal muscles produced by curariform drugs.

The neuromuscular actions of neostigmine,

TABLE 10-2 Signs and symptoms produced in humans by anticholinesterase drugs

Site of action	Signs and symptoms
	Following local exposure
Pupils	Miosis, marked, usually maximal (pinpoint), sometimes unequal
Ciliary body	Frontal headache, eye pain on focusing, slight dimness of vision, occasional nausea and vomiting
Conjunctiva	Hyperemia
Nasal mucous membranes	Rhinorrhea, hyperemia
Bronchial tree	Tightness in chest, sometimes with prolonged wheezing expiration suggestive of bronchoconstriction or increased secretion, cough
Sweat glands	Sweating at site of exposure to liquid
Striated muscle	Fasciculation at site of exposure to liquid
	Following systemic absorption
Bronchial tree	Tightness in chest, with prolonged wheezing expiration suggestive of bronchoconstriction or increased secretion, dyspnea, slight pain in chest, increased bronchial secretion, cough
Gastrointestinal system	Anorexia, nausea, vomiting, abdominal cramps, epigastric and substernal tightness (cardiospasm?) with "heartburn" and eructation, diarrhea, tenesmus, involuntary defecation
Sweat glands	Increased sweating
Salivary glands	Increased salivation
Lacrimal glands	Increased lacrimation
Heart	Slight bradycardia
Pupils	Slight miosis, occasionally unequal, later more marked miosis
Ciliary body	Blurring of vision
Urinary bladder	Frequency, involuntary micturition
Striated muscle	Easy fatigue, mild weakness, muscular twitching, fasciculations, cramps, generalized weakness, including muscles of respiration, with dyspnea and cyanosis
Sympathetic ganglia	Pallor, occasional elevation of blood pressure
Central nervous system	Giddiness; tension; anxiety; jitteriness; restlessness; emotional lability; excessive dreaming; insomnia; nightmares; headache; tremor; apathy; withdrawal and depression; bursts of slow waves of elevated voltage in EEG, especially on overventilation; drowsiness; difficulty in concentrating, slowness of recall, confusion; slurred speech; ataxia; generalized weakness; coma, with absence of reflexes; Cheyne-Stokes respiration; convulsions; depression of respiratory and circulatory centers with dyspnea, cyanosis, and fall in blood pressure

more than those of physostigmine, have also been beneficial in the treatment of myasthenia gravis. For many years neostigmine was the most commonly used drug for this disorder. Although it is still used at present for this purpose, it has been displaced to some extent by newer cholinesterase inhibitors, such as pyridostigmine, which are better tolerated because of less intense side effects at therapeutic doses and have a longer duration of action.

There are some difficulties attending the use of neostigmine (and other cholinesterase inhibitors) for the treatment of myasthenia gravis. First, the dosage of neostigmine is difficult to regulate. With an overdose, the accumulation of acetylcholine at the end plate may be excessive and paralysis of transmission may occur. This situation due to excessive drug administration is termed *cholinergic crisis*. In the absence of prior knowledge of drug administration, it then becomes necessary to distinguish between the muscle weakness of the undertreated patient, i.e., *myasthenic crisis*, and the paralysis caused by an overdose of the anticholinesterase agent. The differential diagnosis is aided by the use of an ultra-short-acting anticholinesterase agent, edrophonium, which is described below. A second difficulty with neostigmine is the maintenance of a stable level of strength. Since neostigmine is a reversible cholinesterase inhibitor, its actions are relatively short-lived (mean half-life less than 1 h). Accordingly, muscle strength waxes and wanes as the drug effect takes place and then diminishes. This necessitates repeated administration of the drug and incurs the risk of cumulation. For some patients, it may also be necessary to interrupt their sleep for drug administration. The third problem is the ever-present one of side effects. For the cholinesterase inhibitors, these include excessive salivation, perspiration, abdominal distress, nausea, and vomiting. The side effects can be controlled by giving the drug in conjunction with atropine. However, these effects are the indicators of cumulation and overdose of the anticholinesterase agent, and their blockade by atropine may mask an impending cholinergic crisis.

In addition to its use in myasthenia, neostigmine has also been used for the treatment of postoperative abdominal distension and urinary retention.

Pyridostigmine

Qualitatively, the pharmacologic properties of pyridostigmine are the same as those of neostigmine. Pyridostigmine, although useful by the oral route, is poorly absorbed from the gastrointestinal tract. Pyridostigmine is also slowly inactivated by plasma cholinesterases; the parent compound and metabolite are primarily excreted in the urine. The drug directly stimulates both muscarinic and nicotinic cholinergic receptors, in addition to its inhibition of cholinesterase. Pyridostigmine, however, is less potent than neostigmine.

Pyridostigmine is principally used for its nicotinic effects. It is the drug of choice for the treatment of myasthenia gravis. The improvement of muscle strength is more sustained than that produced by neostigmine. Accordingly, less frequent administration is required. Other advantages of pyridostigmine, compared to neostigmine, are (1) less danger of overdosage and (2) reduced frequency and severity of muscarinic side effects. Pyridostigmine is also used by anesthesiologists, to reverse the skeletal muscle blockade produced by curare-like drugs.

Adverse reactions associated with pyridostigmine include muscarinic (nausea, vomiting, diarrhea, miosis, increased bronchial secretions) and nicotinic (muscle cramps, fasciculation, and weakness) manifestations. Atropine may be used to reduce muscarinic side effects, but as mentioned can inadvertently mask cholinergic crisis.

Edrophonium

Edrophonium is similar structurally to neostigmine, with two exceptions: (1) edrophonium has an ethyl group on the nitrogen and (2) it lacks an ester functional group (Fig. 10-4).

The pharmacologic properties of the compound qualitatively resemble those of neostigmine. However, the structural changes give edrophonium more selective direct receptor activity. In addition to inhibiting cholinesterases, edrophonium stimulates nicotinic receptors at the neuromuscular junction at lower doses than that which stimulate other cholinergic receptors. Therefore, edrophonium will enhance neuromuscular transmission at doses that do not stimulate the heart, smooth muscle cells, and glands. Two additional features distinguish the actions of edrophonium from those of neostigmine and pyridostigmine: (1) its onset of action is more rapid than either drug, and (2) its duration of action is considerably shorter, 10 to 15 min, compared with 0.5 to 2 h for neostigmine and 4 to 6 h for pyridostigmine. These characteristics are more consistent with a direct acting drug than with one that exerts its effect only by inhibiting an enzyme.

The brief duration of action of edrophonium compared with the longer-acting anticholinesterase drugs is, for some purposes, a distinct advantage. It minimizes the problem of managing overdosage and reduces the possibility of cumulation of the drug.

Edrophonium plays a prominent role in establishing the diagnosis of myasthenia gravis and in making a differential diagnosis between myasthenic weakness and cholinergic crisis. In these situations, use is made of the transient actions of the drug. For the diagnosis of myasthenia, edrophonium is injected intravenously in divided doses. The brief duration of its effect requires that measurements of muscle strength be made quickly. The improvement in strength, if it occurs, will last for less than 5 min. The test can be repeated several times on the same day. For the differentiation between myasthenic and cholinergic crises, edrophonium is also given intravenously. If the crises is due to inadequate anticholinesterase therapy, edrophonium will result in an improvement of muscle strength. Conversely, edrophonium will further decrease muscle strength if the weakness if due to an overdose of the anticholinesterase agent. In the case of cholinergic crisis, the short-lived actions of edrophonium will not substantially prolong the crisis, and other measures, such as maintenance of airways and artificial ventilation, can be instituted.

A second important therapeutic use of edrophonium is based on its ability to antagonize curariform drugs, It is unlikely that the anticurare action is due to the inhibition of acetylcholinesterase, since doses of edrophonium which effectively antagonize the blockade of neuromuscular transmission have no effect on the sensitivity of the end plate to injected acetylcholine.

Ambenonium

Ambenonium is a cholinesterase inhibitor with pharmacologic properties similar to those of neostigmine and pyridostigmine (see Fig. 10-4 for structure). The pharmacologic actions of ambenonium are brought about primarily through the reversible inactivation of the cholinesterases.

The principal therapeutic use of ambenonium is in the management of myasthenia gravis. It is however considered a secondary drug to pyridostigmine. Though ambenonium appears to have a slightly more sustained action, it has a higher incidence of muscarinic side effects and consequently has been less used.

Demecarium

Demecarium is a bisymmetric compound containing two quaternary ammonium and two carbamate functional groups (Fig. 10-4). The compound is a reversible cholinesterase inhibitor, but with a duration of action longer than that of other reversible inhibitors. Demecarium has higher affinity for acetylcholinesterase than for plasma cholinesterase.

Demecarium is used in the management of glaucoma; when instilled topically into the eye, it lowers intraocular pressure. A single instillation into the conjunctival sac of normal subjects produces miosis, which is apparent within 1 h, attains a maximum within 4 h, and persists for 3 to 10 days. The miosis is accompanied by spasm of the intraocular muscles of accommodation.

Adverse reactions include local burning and itching. Systemic signs of cholinesterase inhibition can occur from prolonged administration.

Tacrine

Tacrine is an acridine derivative that is classified as a reversible cholinesterase inhibitor; this drug is indicated in the treatment of Alzheimer's disease. In some patients with mild-to-moderate symptoms, tacrine appears to improve cognitive functions such as memory, attention, language and common task.

It is proposed that tacrine acts as a noncompetitive inhibitor of acetylcholinesterase in the CNS and thereby increases the acetylcholine concentration in the cholinergic synaptic space. It also acts as a partial agonist at muscarinic receptors and may alter the concentrations of neurotransmitters such as dopamine and norepinephrine.

Upon oral administration, peak plasma concentration of the drug occur within 2 hours. The presence of food in the stomach decreases absorption. The drug readily crosses the blood-brain barrier. The site of biotransformation of tacrine is the liver and only small amounts of the parent compound are excreted in the urine. The elimination half-life of tacrine in elderly patients with Alzheimer's disease is about 3.5 hours, while in young adults it is approximately 2 hours.

Some adverse reactions reported for tacrine include nausea, vomiting, diarrhea, anorexia and ataxia. Elevation of serum transaminase can occur and there are reports of some cases of liver dysfunction.

Irreversible Cholinesterase Inhibitors

The second class of cholinesterase inhibitors is a group of organophosphorus compounds. They all have the same general formula:

$$\begin{matrix} R_1O & & O \text{ (or S)} \\ & P & \\ R_2O & & X \end{matrix}$$

where R_1 and R_2 are alkyl functional groups and the X is a halogen or other functional group. Structures of individual compounds are shown in Fig. 10-4.

The organophosphates act by complexing to the serine hydroxyl group at the esteratic site of the cholinesterase enzymes; the phosphorous atom covalently bonds with this site. A schematic representation of the phosphorylated enzyme is illustrated in Fig. 10-5. In contrast with the rapid hydrolysis of acetylcholine from the enzyme and slower hydrolysis of carbamates, the phosphorylated enzyme reacts very slowly with water, leading to essentially irreversible inhibition. For most of the organophosphorus compounds, de novo synthesis of the enzyme must take place for the cholinesterase activity of tissue to return. For others, a limited amount of spontaneous reactivation of the enzyme occurs. Although this type of inhibition is generally regarded as irreversible, chemical agents such as oximes can reactivate the enzyme. However, the phosphorylated enzyme can undergo a process called *aging*, in which the organophosphate loses an alkyl group, forming a tighter irreversible bond to the enzyme — this renders the enzyme insensitive to reactivation by oximes.

The signs and symptoms of acute toxicity which occur following the administration of an organophosphorus anticholinesterase agent can be readily predicted and are attributable to hyperactivity of the parasympathetic nervous system, neuromuscular junction, autonomic ganglia, and cholinergic nerves of the CNS. These signs and symptoms are listed in Table 10-2. Death is due primarily to depression of respiration caused by depression of the CNS, paralysis of the diaphragm and intercostal muscles, bronchospasm, and the accumulation of bronchosecretions. Each is due to the accumulation of excessive amounts of acetylcholine.

Some organophosphates are useful therapeutically, others are used as insecticides and potential chemical warfare agents based on their extreme toxicity. The pharmacology of representative individual agents is discussed below.

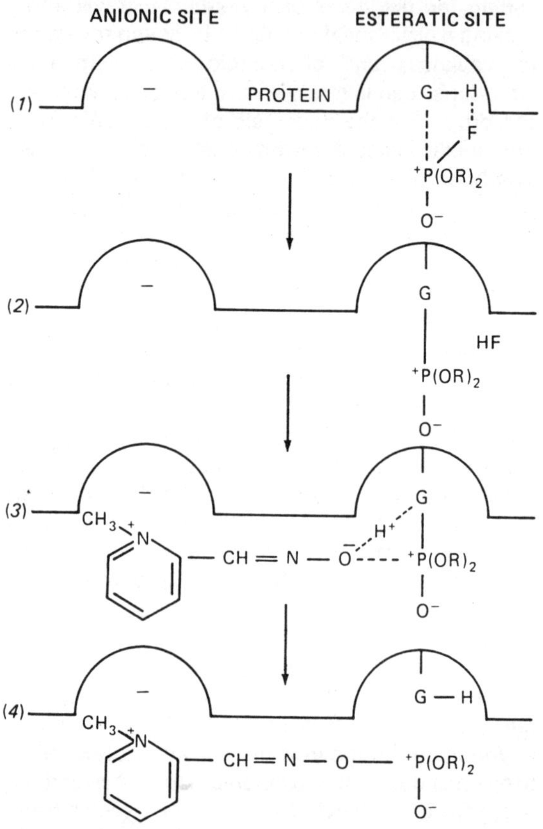

FIGURE 10-5 *Steps in the inactivation of acetylcholinesterase by isoflurophate (DFP) and its regeneration by pralidoxime (2-PAM): (1) Attachment of DFP to the esteratic site. (2) Formation of a phosphoryl enzyme which, in contrast to the acetylated cholinesterase, is hydrolyzed extremely slowly, making the enzyme unavailable for hydrolysis of ACh. (3) Attachment of 2-PAM to the anionic site of the enzyme and to the phosphorylated esteratic site by virtue of the pronounced acidity of the oxime: the anionic (nucleophilic) O^- is attracted to the positively charged P atom, and the proton of the oxime to site G. (4) The complex formed in the preceding step breaks up into phosphorylated 2-PAM and regenerated enzyme.*

Isoflurophate (DFP)

The primary difference between isoflurophate and agents such as physostigmine lies in the persistency of action. By the mechanism described above for the organophosphorus cholinesterase inhibitors isoflurophate produces an irreversible inactivation of the cholinesterases. Both acetylcholinesterase and "nonspecific" plasma cholinesterase are inactivated by isoflurophate; however, isoflurophate has a greater affinity for the latter enzyme.

Isoflurophate is used in the treatment of certain types of glaucoma, when short-acting miotics are inadequate. The compound has also been used in certain types of strabismus. Maximal reduction in intraocular pressure occurs within one day of a single dose. Effects can persist for several days. The intensity and duration of action are much greater for isoflurophate than for pilocarpine or physostigmine and approximately the same as demecarium. Since isoflurophate is highly lipid-soluble, it must be administered in peanut oil, which is very irritating to the eye.

Echothiophate

Echothiophate is a phosphorylthiocholine (see Fig. 10-4). It is a long-acting cholinesterase inhibitor with pharmacologic actions on the peripheral nervous system similar to those of isoflurophate. Spontaneous regeneration of the phosphorylated enzyme occurs more rapidly with echothiophate than with isoflurophate.

Echothiophate is used in ophthalmology for the treatment of glaucoma and other disorders of the eye amenable to therapy with cholinesterase inhibitors. In this regard, the water-soluble property of echothiophate affords one practical advantage over the lipid-soluble irreversible inhibitor. Lacrimation evoked by the irritation produced by solvents such as peanut oil may result in the removal of the anticholinesterase drug from the conjunctiva. Usually this does not occur with echothiophate. The use of echothiophate for ocular diseases is governed by the same precautions and limitations as are the other long-acting anticholinesterase agents. Long-term administration is limited due to the development of cataracts.

Other Organophosphorus Cholinesterase Inhibitors

Several organophosphate compounds are available for use as household and agricultural insecticides. Most are highly lipid-soluble compounds, which are rapidly and completely absorbed by practically all routes, including the skin and the respiratory and gastrointestinal tracts. Some commonly used compounds include malathion and parathion.

Most organophosphates are biotransformed by hydrolysis and are excreted in the urine. Malathion, widely used in the home and garden, has low toxicity in humans because it is readily hydrolyzed and detoxified by plasma esterases acting on the carboxyl ester bond of the insecticide. This rapid inactivation does not occur in insects. Other organophosphates (e.g., parathion and chlorpyrifos) are not readily detoxified and are responsible for many cases of accidental toxicity every year.

Still other organophosphates, first synthesized in Germany during World War II, are some of the most toxic compounds known and are potential chemical warfare agents. These include soman, sarin, and tabun. What makes these compounds so toxic is the fact that they induce very rapid "aging" of the enzyme, making the enzyme insensitive to reactivation by oximes. Hence there is no adequate therapy for intoxication with these compounds.

Management of Organophosphate Poisoning

Treatment of acute organophosphate intoxication includes (1) artificial respiration; (2) atropine sulfate, a muscarinic receptor antagonist; and (3) pralidoxime, a cholinesterase reactivator. The pharmacology of atropine is covered in Chapter 11. The properties of pralidoxime are discussed below. In addition to acute toxicity, the organophosphates can induce a neuropathy upon chronic exposure. This is characterized by neuronal degeneration and demyelination. The toxic mechanism apparently involves inhibition of neurotoxic esterase, which is distinct from cholinesterases.

Pralidoxime Chloride

Studies of the reactivity of organophosphorus compounds and of the mechanism by which they inhibit the activity of acetylcholinesterase and other cholinesterases has resulted in the discovery of agents which are capable of reactivating the inhibited enzymes. These reactivators also possess considerable antidotal effect. The present compound of choice in this country is pralidoxime chloride (2-pyridine aldoxime methylchloride or 2-PAM chloride).

This drug is used as an adjunct to atropine in the treatment of organophosphate pesticide intoxication. It is not effective against carbamate cholinesterase inhibitors. Standard treatment of toxicity by soman and related compounds with atropine and pralidoxime (or other oximes) is not of practical value due to the rapid aging of these compounds to the enzyme.

Pralidoxime is a strong nucleophilic compound. It reactivates the phosphorylated enzyme in a two-step reaction (Fig. 10-5). First a complex forms between the oximate ion and the phosphorylated enzyme; this is followed by liberation of the phosphorylated oxime and regeneration of enzyme activity.

The high reactivating potency of pralidoxime has been attributed to its ability to combine with a negatively charged group on the enzyme surface and to a high degree of molecular fit between oxime and phosphorylated cholinesterase. The rate of the reactivation is very much dependent on the type of the phosphorylated enzyme and on other factors in addition to oxime concentration. In summary, it appears that the oximes *in vitro* and *in vivo*, (1) react directly with the inhibitor, converting it to a harmless compound and (2) reactivate the inhibited enzyme, both in blood and tissues. At high concentrations, the oximes can act as mild cholinesterase inhibitors, a factor which does not appear to be of other than academic importance.

Pralidoxime is given by intravenous administration for severe organophosphate poisoning or by the oral route for mild poisoning. Being a quaternary compound, pralidoxime does not cross the blood-brain barrier and, therefore, will not reverse the central nervous system toxicities of organophosphates. Pralidoxime is largely metabolized in the liver, with its products excreted in the urine.

Pralidoxime may produce several adverse reactions including headache, dizziness, drowsiness, nausea, tachycardia, increased blood pressure, and muscle weakness when administered parenterally. There are no significant toxic effects following oral administration.

BIBLIOGRAPHY

-------- "Parasympathetic Neuroeffector Mechanisms in the Heart" (Symposium), *Fed. Proc.* **43**: 2597-2623 (1984).

-------- "Tacrine for Alzheimer's Disease," *The Medical Letter* **35**: 87-88 (1993).

Aquilonius, S-M., and P-G. Gillberg (eds): "Cholinergic Neurotransmission: Functional and Clinical Aspects," *Prog. Brain Res.*, **vol. 84** (1990).

Dowdall, M. (ed.): *Cellular and Molecular Basis of Cholinergic Function*, Plenum, New York, 1988.

Drachman, D.B. (ed.): "Myasthenia Gravis: Biology and Treatment," *Ann. N.Y. Acad. Sci.* **vol. 505** (1987).

Hosey, M.M.: "Diversity of Structure, Signalling and Regulation Within the Family of Muscarinic Cholinergic Receptors," *FASEB J.* **6**: 845-852 (1992).

Hucho, F., J. Jarv, and C. Weise: "Substrate-Binding Sites in Acetylcholinesterase," *Trends Pharmacol. Sci.* **12**: 422-426 (1991).

Hulme, E.C., N.J.M. Birdsell, and J.J. Buckley: "Muscarinic Receptor Subtypes," *Annu. Rev. Pharmacol. Toxicol.* **30**: 675-706 (1990).

Johnson, M.K.: "The Target for Initiation of Delayed Neurotoxicity by Organophosphorus Esters," in E. Hodgson, E. Band, and R.M. Philpot (eds.), *Reviews in Biochemical Toxicology*, Elsevier, New York, 1982, vol. **4**, pp. 141-272.

Karlin, H.: "Exploration of the Nicotinic Acetylcholine Receptor," *Harvey Lect.* **85**: 71-107 (1991).

Kaufman, P.L., T. Weidman, and J.R. Robinson: "Cholinergics," in M.L. Sears (ed.), *Pharmacology of the Eye. Handbook of Experimental Pharmacology*, Springer-Verlag, Berlin, 1984, **vol. 69**, pp. 149-192.

Moncada, S., M.W. Radomski, and R.M. Palmer: "Endothelium-Derived Relaxing Factor. Identification as Nitric Oxide and Role in the Control of Vascular Tone and Platelet Function," *Biochem. Pharmacol.* **37**: 2495-2501 (1988).

Pomponi, M., E. Giacobini, and E. Messamore: "Present State and Future Development of the Therapy of Alzheimer's Disease," *Aging* **2**: 125-153 (1990).

Soreq, H., A. Gnatt, Y. Loewenstein, and L.F. Neville: "Excavations into the Active-Site Gorge of Cholinesterases," *Trends Biochem. Sci.* **17**: 353-358 (1992).

Wesnes, K.A., P.M. Simpson, L. White, S. Pinker, G. Jertz, M. Murphy, and K. Siegfried: "Cholinesterase Inhibition in the Scopolamine Model of Dementia," *Ann. N.Y. Acad. Sci.* **640**: 268-271 (1991).

CHAPTER 11

Antimuscarinic Drugs and Ganglionic Blocking Agents

Edward J. Barbieri

As discussed in previous chapters, there are three major types of cholinergic receptors: muscarinic (M), neuronal type nicotinic (N_N), and muscle type nicotinic (N_M). Cholinergic receptor antagonists are classified based on their ability to selectively block one of these receptor types. *Antimuscarinic drugs* (muscarinic receptor blocking drugs) act at the muscarinic receptors of smooth muscle, cardiac tissues, and exocrine glands by blocking the actions of endogenous acetylcholine (ACh) released from cholinergic postganglionic autonomic neurons and the actions of cholinomimetic drugs administered exogenously. Antimuscarinic drugs also block M receptors in the central nervous system (CNS). *Ganglionic blocking agents* selectively interfere with neuronal transmission in autonomic ganglia mediated through N_N receptors. *Neuromuscular blocking drugs* act at N_M receptors of the skeletal muscle end plate.

The pharmacology of the antimuscarinic drugs and some features of the ganglionic blocking agents are discussed in this chapter. Information concerning neuromuscular blocking drugs is presented with the pharmacology of the skeletal muscle relaxants (Chapter 12).

ANTIMUSCARINIC DRUGS

The oldest drugs of the group are the various galenical (herbal) preparations of belladonna, hyoscyamus, and stramonium. All these are derived from plants of the potato family, the Solanaceae. The species used as drugs include *Atropa belladonna*, one of several plants known colloquially as "deadly nightshade"; *Hyoscyamus niger* (black henbane); and *Datura stramonium* (Jimson weed, Jamestown weed, or thorn apple). The active principle in all of these plants consist mostly of *l*-hyoscyamine, with smaller and variable amounts of *l*-scopolamine (hyoscine). *l*-Hyoscyamine is much more active as a muscarinic receptor blocking drug than *d*-hyoscyamine, both peripherally and on the CNS, but the racemic mixture *dl*-hyoscyamine, better known as *atropine*, is preferred for most medicinal purposes because it is more stable chemically and therefore more dependable for action. Scopolamine is found chiefly in *Hyoscyamus niger* and *Scopolia carniolica*.

Atropine and Scopolamine

Atropine and its congener scopolamine are two of the most important antimuscarinic drugs. As prototypes of the entire group, they will be discussed in greater detail than some of the other antimuscarinic drugs.

Chemistry

Atropine and scopolamine are esters of tropic acid with the organic bases tropine (tropanol) and scopine, respectively. Scopine differs from tropine only by the presence of the oxygen bridge between positions 6 and 7 (Fig. 11-1). The intact molecule is necessary for antimuscarinic activity; neither tropic acid nor the free bases show any appreciable antimuscarinic activity.

Mechanism of Action

Both atropine and scopolamine are competitive antagonists of ACh at all M receptors, i.e., they do not have selectivity in blocking any of the subtypes of M receptors (M_1, M_2, and M_3). Although the receptor blockade produced by atropine and

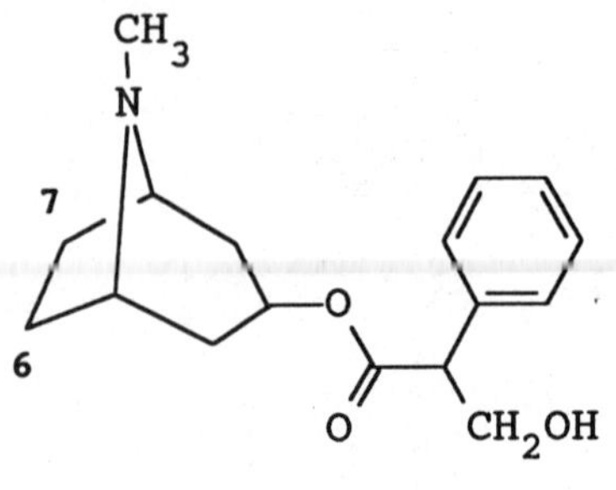

Atropine

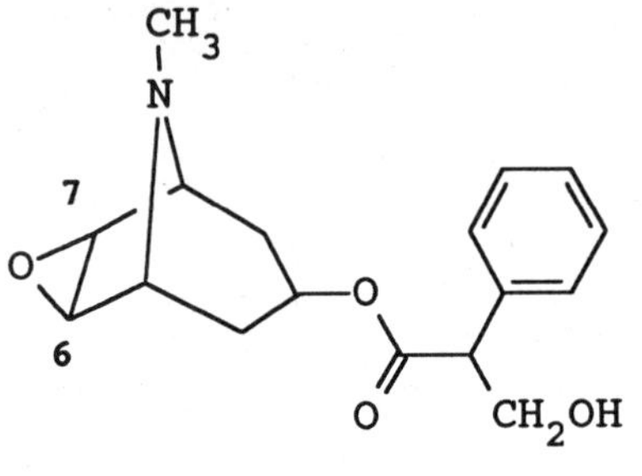

Scopolamine

FIGURE 11-1 *Structures of atropine and scopolamine.*

scopolamine is reversible, the dissociation constants with M receptors are several orders of magnitude lower than that of ACh. Therefore, their effects may persist for hours to days.

It has been observed repeatedly that atropine is more effective in blocking the effects of exogenously administered ACh or other parasympathomimetic agents than in blocking the effects following stimulation of parasympathetic, cholinergic nerve fibers. This is probably due to the fact that many postganglionic parasympathetic fibers release other neurotransmitters (e.g., adenosine triphosphate and vasoactive intestinal polypeptide), in addition to ACh, which are not blocked by atropine.

These drugs have other actions. In addition to their ability to block M receptors, these drugs can block nicotinic cholinergic receptors at autonomic ganglia and at the motor end plate of skeletal muscle, but only in doses far in excess of those employed clinically. The cutaneous flush that follows high doses of atropine is due to a direct vasodilator effect on arteriolar smooth muscle. Atropine is also a fairly potent local anesthetic and a histamine (H_1) receptor blocker in high doses.

Effects on Organ Systems

Atropine is somewhat more potent than scopolamine in its M receptor blocking actions on the heart, gastrointestinal tract, and bronchial muscle; the reverse is true for the iris sphincter, ciliary muscle, and exocrine glands.

Cardiovascular System *Heart* When atropine is administered orally or by subcutaneous, intramuscular, or intravenous injection, initially there is a temporary and moderate decrease in heart rate, which is followed by a more marked acceleration. The initial cardiac slowing is more prolonged following small doses, and is attributed to blockade of M_1 receptors on postganglionic parasympathetic neurons and a reduction in ACh-induced inhibition of neurotransmitter release. The tachycardia is due to blockade of M_2 receptors on the sinoatrial (SA) node and a reduction in the tonic vagal impulses to the heart, and is usually accompanied by an increase in cardiac output. The PR interval of the electrocardiogram is shortened by all doses of atropine. These effects are dose-related; therefore the acceleration of the heart rate occurs earlier, is more marked, and is more prolonged as the dose of atropine is increased.

With scopolamine, the reduction in heart rate is greater than with atropine. Tachycardia that occurs with higher doses is short-lived; heart rate usually returns to normal within 30 min.

Atropine will also prevent or reverse the decrease in refractory period, the lengthened PR interval, the slowing of atrioventricular (AV) conduction velocity, and the decrease in cardiac output and oxygen consumption produced by vagal stimulation or by cholinomimetic agents. The liberation of potassium from and the penetration of sodium into isolated atria produced by ACh are also reversed by atropine. Atropine will return the atrial fibrillation induced and maintained in animals by ACh or vagal stimulation to normal sinus rhythm.

Peripheral Circulation Normal doses of atropine (0.4 to 0.6 mg) have little effect on blood pressure. Larger doses (2 mg or more), although causing a marked increase in heart rate, usually decrease the systolic pressure by a few millimeters of mercury. This fall in blood pressure is more marked in warm environments and may be caused by decreased cardiac filling due to excessive heart rate.

When atropine sulfate is injected intravenously, into either conscious or anesthetized patients, the heart rate increases and the cardiac output rises, but the stroke volume, central venous pressure, and the total peripheral resistance decrease. The rise in the cardiac output is dependent on the degree of increase in heart rate and is accompanied by a rise in the arterial blood pressure; in anesthetized patients, the extent of these changes varies with the anesthetic used.

Atropine abolishes the vasodilation produced by ACh. On its own, it has a direct vasodilator effect on small blood vessels; this is not an anticholinergic phenomenon. Thus, a slight flushing of the skin may occur with small doses, and a pronounced reddening is a characteristic effect of toxic doses.

Central Nervous System On the CNS, atropine first causes stimulation and then depression, whereas scopolamine generally has a purely depressant effect. With the usual dose of atropine sulfate, effects on the CNS are not striking, except for the slowing of the heart, as mentioned above. Therapeutic doses of scopolamine, given by injection, have a profound sedative effect lasting 1 to 2 h. A similar dose given orally or topically (by a transdermal patch) has very little soporific effect, a fact that makes scopolamine useful by either of these routes as a therapy for motion sickness. Large doses of atropine produce drowsiness, hallucinations, disorientation, amnesia, and eventually coma. Similar toxic effects are produced by relatively smaller doses of scopolamine. On occasion, particularly in the presence of severe pain, scopolamine may be excitatory. For this reason, patients given scopolamine preoperatively should be kept under continual surveillance until taken to the operating room.

A normal clinical dose of atropine has no significant effect on respiration. Atropine is not considered effective in counteracting respiratory depression in poisoning by barbiturates or opioids. However, it is a specific antidote for the central respiratory depression (and peripheral bronchoconstriction and increased tracheobronchial secretion) occurring in poisoning with anticholinesterase agents.

Atropine decreases the muscle tremor and reduces the stiffness in parkinsonism. Scopolamine and many centrally-active synthetic anticholinergic drugs have a similar action. This is due to the restoration of the cholinergic-dopaminergic balance in the basal ganglia, since the primary defect in parkinsonism has been shown to be a deficiency of dopamine. This is discussed in greater detail in Chapter 22.

Secretions The exocrine sweat glands of the human skin are supplied by cholinergic fibers present in sympathetic nerves. Accordingly, sweating is diminished or abolished by small doses of atropine. This reduction or abolition of sweating may be responsible for the rise in body temperature that may follow moderate doses of atropine and is a regular consequence of toxic doses.

One of the most obvious effects of ordinary doses of atropine and scopolamine is dryness of the mouth (xerostomia). The copious watery flow of saliva induced by parasympathomimetic nerve stimulation is essentially abolished by atropine. In addition, nasal, pharyngeal, and bronchial secretions are all significantly reduced by these drugs.

Gastric secretion is under the influence of a number of nervous, hormonal, and local factors. Atropine does block increased gastric secretion induced by vagal stimulation, however, the effectiveness is variable and large doses may be required. Although there is some clinical use for atropine in this regard, the use of histamine H_2-receptor blocking drugs is a more practical therapeutic approach in most circumstances (see Chapter 13).

Atropine blocks the elaboration of pancreatic secretions caused by vagal stimulation or parasympathomimetic drugs, and this may be due to a blockade of the extrusion of zymogen granules. The drug has no effect on pancreatic secretion stimulated by secretin of pancreozymin.

Smooth Muscle *Alimentary Tract* In general, antimuscarinic drugs reduce the tone and decrease the amplitude and frequency of peristaltic contractions of the stomach, small intestine, and, to a lesser extent, the colon. The inhibitory effect of atropine on gastrointestinal motility is more pronounced and less variable than on gastric secretion. Normally motility is not appreciably altered by therapeutic doses of atropine, but hypermotility associated with peptic ulcer and certain other gastrointestinal disorders is usually reduced markedly.

Respiratory Tract The smooth muscles of the bronchioles are slightly relaxed by atropine blocking the constrictor effects of the vagus nerve. The result is a more open airway, which is useful in general anesthesia. Scopolamine has a longer bronchodilator effect than does atropine. When these drugs or their congeners (e.g., ipratropium) are given by inhalation, side effects on other systems are minimized (see Chapter 33).

Biliary Tract Atropine has little effect on the secretion of bile, but it exerts a mild antispasmodic effect on the gallbladder and the smooth muscle of the biliary tract, thus increasing bile flow through the duct. Consequently, even though its effect is slight, it is given with morphine for the relief of biliary colic.

Urinary Bladder Atropine decreases, but even in large doses does not abolish, the motor effect of the sacral cholinergic nerves supplying the urinary bladder. Therapeutic doses diminish the tone of the fundus of the bladder and increase the tone of the vesical sphincter. As a consequence, atropine may contribute to the retention of urine, which is often troublesome after surgical operations.

The Eye The circular smooth muscle of the iris, which constricts the pupil, is innervated by cholinergic fibers from the third cranial (oculomotor) nerve. Fibers from the same nerve cause contraction of the ciliary muscles, thus relaxing the suspensory ligament of the lens and allowing the lens to become more convex. In addition, this action may result in opening of the canal of Schlemm, improving drainage of aqueous humor from the anterior chamber and thereby decreasing intraocular pressure.

Atropine and scopolamine antagonize the binding of ACh to M receptors at the smooth muscle of the iris, causing mydriasis (dilation of the pupil). The pupillary dilation causes photophobia and abolition of the pupillary reflex constriction to light. These drug also block the action of the cholinergic neurotransmitter at the ciliary muscle, causing cycloplegia (paralysis of accommodation for near vision). Thus the lens becomes fixed for far vision and objects in the near field of vision become blurred. These effects can occur following systemic or local administration of atropine and scopolamine. However, systemic administration of atropine induces little ocular effect, while mydriasis and loss of accommodation may be significant following the systemic use of scopolamine.

Both the antimuscarinic compounds and the sympathomimetic drugs cause mydriasis (see Chapter 8); however, the antimuscarinic drugs also induce a loss of accommodation for near vision, an effect that does not occur with the sympathomimetic mydriatics.

Atropine-induced relaxation of the ciliary muscle tends to occlude the angle of attachment of the iris to the cornea, and dilatation of the pupil causes the iris to crowd the angular space and thus possibly obstruct the access of fluid to the venous sinus. The result is aggravation of the increased intraocular pressure of glaucoma, a disease characterized by increased intraocular pressure.

Narrow-angle glaucoma (angle-closure or closed-angle glaucoma) is a form of primary glaucoma in an eye characterized by a shallow anterior chamber and a narrow angle of attachment of the iris to the cornea, in which filtration of the aqueous humor is compromised as a result of the iris blocking the angle. Atropine and other cycloplegics and mydriatics should not be used in the eyes of patients with narrow-angle glaucoma or a predisposition to narrow-angle glaucoma since they will aggravate this condition. Open-angle glaucoma (wide-angle glaucoma) occur in a eye in which the angle of the anterior chamber remains open, but filtration is gradually diminished because of the tissues of the angle. Atropine has been used to treat ocular inflammation in patients with open-angle glaucoma.

Pharmacokinetics

Atropine and scopolamine are rapidly and almost completely absorbed from the gastrointestinal tract and from the conjunctiva; in addition, scopolamine can be absorbed across the skin (via transdermal administration). The peak serum concentration occurs about 1 h after oral administration of atropine and 15 to 20 min after intramuscular injection. The apparent volume of distribution is about 2 L/kg with plasma protein binding of 15 to 25 percent. Approximately 30 percent of atropine is hydrolyzed to tropic acid and tropine in the liver; atropine is also partly N-demethylated. The majority of the compound is excreted unchanged in the urine. The elimination of atropine appears to follow two-compartment first-order kinetics: the half-life of the distribution phase (α phase) is about 6 h, while the elimination half-life of the terminal β phase ranges from 13 to 38 h. The elimination kinetics of scopolamine are similar.

Adverse Reactions

Excessive dosage with atropine, one of the galenical preparation of belladonna, or one of the many drugs (e.g. H_1 receptor antagonists, tricyclic antidepressants, and phenothiazines) that have anticholinergic properties, gives rise to distinctive signs which include rapid pulse; dilated pupils; and dry, flushed skin. Patients may complain of thirst and difficulty in focusing their eyes, or may be restless, anxious, drowsy, garrulous, excited, disoriented, or even delirious. Nausea and vomiting, muscular weakness, and difficulty in swallowing may occur.

The classic description of atropine poisoning is: *red as a beet* (cutaneous vasodilation), *dry as a bone* (blockade of salivary secretion), *hot as a hare* (blockade of sweat secretion), *and mad as a hatter* (cortical stimulation). While these and the accompanying symptoms (tachycardia, mydriasis, blurred vision) can be frightening, they are rarely fatal, except in children. Although there is individual variation and sensitivity to atropine and its congeners, there is a wide margin of safety between therapeutic and lethal doses. If recovery ensues, there may be no recollection of the distressing episode. If the outcome is fatal, it usually follows a period of coma in which the respirations become rapid and shallow and finally cease. The toxic effects of scopolamine are similar to those of atropine except that stupor and delirium are more prominent and excitement is less so. Table 11-1 lists some of the dose-related effects that may be observed with toxicity to an antimuscarinic drug.

If the poisoning occurs by the oral route and the patient receives attention early, emesis should be initiated with syrup of ipecac or gastric lavage should be performed as soon as possible. A slurry of activated charcoal should be given in an attempt to adsorb and inactivate the portion of the drug remaining in the alimentary tract. Physostigmine, by slow intravenous injection, is useful to reverse the CNS, as well as the peripheral, anticholinergic effects of the poison. Respiratory failure is a common feature in the reported deaths from atropine and other anticholinergics so that artificial respiration should also be administered. Hyperthermia can be alleviated by keeping the skin wet with water until spontaneous sweating occurs.

TABLE 11-1 Dose-related adverse effects of antimuscarinic drugs

Dose	Effects
Low	Some dryness of the mouth; inhibition of sweating; slight reduction in heart rate
↓	Marked dryness of the mouth; thirst; increased heart rate; some pupillary dilation
↓	Pronounced dryness of the mouth; rapid heart rate; cardiac palpitations; widely dilated pupils; some blurring of near vision
↓	All of the above effects, and: restlessness; headache; fatigue; speech disturbances; difficulty in swallowing; muscular weakness; difficulty in urination; nausea and vomiting; reduced intestinal peristalsis; dry, hot skin
High	All of the above effects very marked, and: rapid, weak pulse; hot, dry, red and flushed skin; ataxia, restlessness and excitement; halucinations; stupor; delirium; shallow respiration; coma

Therapeutic Uses

Atropine is given frequently to patients in preparation for surgical anesthesia in order to minimize bronchial, nasal, and salivary secretions, which may accumulate and obstruct the respiratory passages. Scopolamine is preferred if additional sedative effect is desired.

Atropine is useful in treating patients when bradycardia is associated with a low cardiac output or ventricular irritability. The syndrome of bradycardia and falling arterial blood pressure is seen in patients with a hyperactive carotid sinus reflex, occasionally in patients with acute myocardial infarction, and during anesthesia when vagal stimulation is produced by intra-abdominal surgical traction. In such cases, atropine increases the heart rate and usually restores the blood pressure to a normal range. In addition, atropine can reduce the degree of AV block that may occur in patients taking a digitalis glycoside.

By relaxation of the detrusor muscle, atropine can allay the urgency and frequency of micturition, which often accompany urinary tract infections and cystitis. Atropine is effective in relieving biliary spasm, ureteral colic, pylorospasm, hypertonicity of the small intestine, and hypermotility of the colon. As mentioned previously, although effective in the treatment of peptic ulcers, the use of histamine H_2 receptor blocking drugs is presently a more acceptable therapeutic approach (see Chapter 37).

In parkinsonism, atropine is often effective in relieving the muscular rigidity and tremors which impair the speech, writing, and locomotion of patients with this disease. However, other antimuscarinic drugs (see below) are more commonly used.

Atropine, in conjunction with other measures, is indicated for the treatment of poisoning with cholinesterase inhibitors such as the organophosphate insecticides and nerve gases (see Chapter 10). In these case, atropine will block or reverse many of the toxic effects due to the abnormal concentrations of free ACh. If neuromuscular blockade is present, it will not be affected by atropine. It is important to remember that large doses of atropine may be necessary for the adequate treatment of these types of poisonings. Pralidoxime, a cholinesterase reactivator, should be given as an adjunct to atropine therapy.

In ophthalmology, atropine produces cycloplegia and mydriasis; it is used for diagnostic procedures such as ocular refraction, and in acute inflammatory conditions of the iris and uvea.

Scopolamine is used to treat nausea and vomiting associated with motion sickness. For this purpose, it is administered topically by application of an adhesive bandage-like device behind the ear. It is also used on occasion in obstetrics, in combination with an opioid analgesic, such as morphine or meperidine, to promote drowsiness with amnesia, or "twilight sleep". Like atropine, scopolamine is used topically in the eye as a cycloplegic-mydriatic for refraction, and in uveitis.

Synthetic Derivatives

The wide range of effects that occur following the systemic administration of atropine or scopolamine have encouraged attempts to develop synthetic antimuscarinic compounds with greater selectivity for particular tissues. Over the past several decades, a great number of compounds with antimuscarinic activity have been synthesized and tested. Most of these compounds proved unsatisfactory for clinical use. Until recently, the drugs that have been developed have not met the goal of being more selective muscarinic receptor antagonists with less adverse reactions.

Drugs that are considered as synthetic or semisynthetic substitutes for atropine and scopolamine are used in five major therapeutic areas: (1) for gastrointestinal disorders including peptic ulcer, pylorospasm, hypermotility of the gastrointestinal tract, and similar conditions; (2) for ophthalmology, i.e., for refraction and uveitis; (3) for parkinsonism; (4) for bronchospastic diseases such as chronic bronchitis, and (5) for urological disorders, e.g., dysuria and incontinence.

Drugs for Gastrointestinal Disorders

Most of these drug act by a variety of mechanisms including blockade of M receptors, direct depression of smooth muscle, and N_N receptor blockade at autonomic ganglia. All show some undesirable side effects at other cholinergically innervated sites. The list of drugs includes a number of quaternary ammonium derivatives (e.g., propantheline, methscopolamine, glycopyrrolate, mepenzolate, and clidinium) and a tertiary amine (dicyclomine). A short discussion of propantheline and dicyclomine will serve to describe the pharmacologic characteristics of all of these drugs.

Propantheline Bromide The pharmacologic effects of this compound are qualitatively similar to those of atropine. The quaternary nitrogen makes the drug more polar, and therefore it has less CNS effects than atropine. In contrast to atropine, propantheline has a high ratio of ganglionic blocking to antimuscarinic activity which may be attributed to the quaternary nitrogen and bulky rings and side chain. Propantheline inhibits gastrointestinal motility and gastric acid secretion.

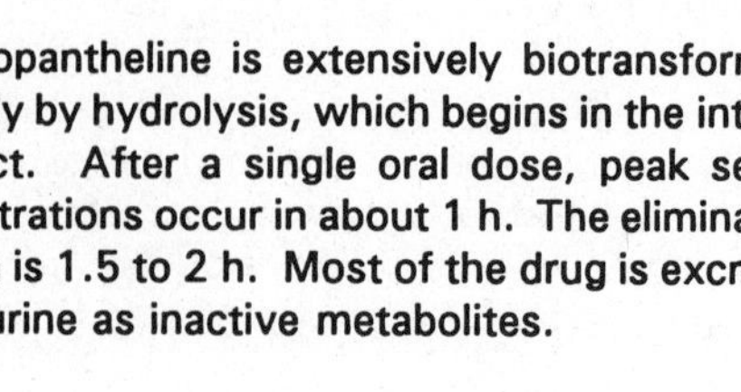

Propantheline is extensively biotransformed, primarily by hydrolysis, which begins in the intestinal tract. After a single oral dose, peak serum concentrations occur in about 1 h. The elimination half-life is 1.5 to 2 h. Most of the drug is excreted in the urine as inactive metabolites.

Adverse effects are similar to those of atropine and are antimuscarinic in nature as described above. Very high doses have been found to produce a neuromuscular blockade resembling curariform drugs. Therapy of severe toxicity requires the use of intravenous physostigmine, sodium thiopental, or diazepam to combat CNS agitation, and mechanical ventilation if progression of the curare-like paralysis of respiratory muscles occurs.

Propantheline is indicated as an adjunct in the treatment of peptic ulcer and is one of the more widely used drugs in this category.

Dicyclomine Dicyclomine is a tertiary amine that reduces gastrointestinal smooth muscle spasms by its antimuscarinic and musculotropic antispasmodic effects. On a milligram basis, it is about one-eighth as potent as atropine as a competitive M receptor antagonist.

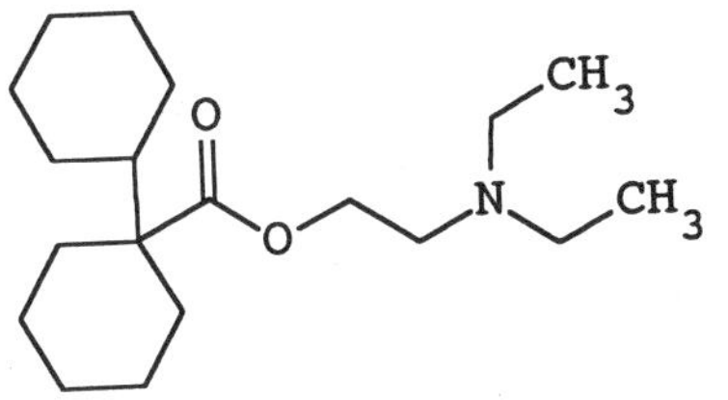

Dicyclomine is rapidly absorbed following oral administration; peak plasma levels occur in about 60 to 90 min. The drug has extensive distribution to other tissues (the volume of distribution is 3.7 L/kg) and the principal route of elimination is by the urine.

Adverse reactions are similar to atropine, with dry mouth, dizziness, and blurred vision being the most commonly observed. Because it is a tertiary amine, dicyclomine will induce a greater incidence of CNS adverse effects than propantheline, a quaternary amine. Dicyclomine is indicated for use in patients to treat the irritable bowel syndrome by the oral and intramuscular routes.

Selective M_1 Receptor Antagonists Pirenzepine and telenzepine are two complex tricyclic compounds that are relatively selective antagonists of ACh at M_1 receptors. They decrease both basal and stimulated gastric acid and pepsin secretion, but, because of their receptor selectivity, have less effect than other antimuscarinic drugs on gastric emptying and heart rate. They do not cross the blood-brain barrier; therefore, CNS effects are minimal. At present, these compounds are used in Europe to treat peptic ulcers, but are not yet available in the United States (see Chapter 37).

Drugs Used in Ophthalmology

In the refraction of children, a potent cycloplegic-mydriatic is generally used, e.g., atropine sulfate (1%) or scopolamine hydrobromide (0.5%). These drugs are also used in some diagnostic procedures and in the treatment of acute inflammatory conditions of the uveal tract when a potent, long-acting mydriatic is required.

Adults under the age of 40 to 50, in whom tension on the suspensory ligament of the lens is diminished, are generally refracted with short-acting, less potent cycloplegics such as homatropine hydrobromide (1%), cyclopentolate hydrochloride (0.5 to 2%), or tropicamide (0.5 to 1%). These less potent analogs, that produce mydriasis of brief duration with relatively little cycloplegia, are very useful in performing ophthalmoscopic examinations (Table 11-2). Sympathomimetic drug such as epinephrine and phenylephrine can also be used as adjuncts to produce mydriasis (see Chapter 8).

After the age of 50, the use of cycloplegics for routine refraction is generally omitted. The ciliary muscle exerts relatively little tone, and the danger of precipitating an attack of glaucoma by application of an antimuscarinic is present.

Drugs Used in Parkinsonism

The belladonna alkaloids and atropine were the first effective drugs introduced for the symptomatic treatment of parkinsonism. In contrast with the gastrointestinal antispasmodics, several synthetic compounds which cross the blood-brain barrier have proven to be more effective, with a lower incidence of adverse effects. The list of drugs includes biperiden, benztropine, orphenadrine, procyclidine, and trihexyphenidyl; diphenhydramine, an antihistamine with high anticholinergic activity, is also used occasionally.

While levodopa is now generally regarded to be the drug of choice in the treatment of parkinsonism, it has its limitations due to adverse effects and tolerance. Consequently, some physician prefer to initiate therapy with an antimuscarinic agent and continue with such until more effective therapy is required. In addition, the drugs in the foregoing list are effective in controlling the parkinson-like side effects that frequently occur during therapy with antipsychotics drugs (e.g., phenothiazines). The pharmacology of the antimuscarinic drugs used in parkinsonism is discussed in Chapter 22.

TABLE 11-2 Summary of peak and duration of mydriasis and cycloplegia with topical antimuscarinic drugs

Drug	Mydriasis		Cycloplegia	
	Peak, minutes	Recovery, days	Peak, minutes	Recovery, days
Atropine (1%)	30 to 40	7 to 12	60 to 180	6 to 12
Homatropine (1%)	40 to 60	1 to 3	30 to 60	1 to 3
Scopolamine (0.5%)	20 to 30	3 to 7	30 to 60	3 to 7
Cyclopentolate (0.5 to 2%)	30 to 60	1	25 to 75	0.25 to 1
Tropicamide (0.5 to 1%)	20 to 40	0.25	20 to 35	0.25

Drugs Used for Bronchospasm

Many years ago, *Datura stramonium* was available in cigarettes which were smoked by patients with bronchial asthma to relieve bronchoconstriction; the preparation was somewhat effective by virtue of its content of the belladonna alkaloids, atropine and scopolamine. Atropine itself (both by oral administration and aerosolized application to the respiratory tract) was used as a bronchodilator in patients with chronic obstructive pulmonary diseases (COPD), but was associated with numerous adverse effects due to its systemic antimuscarinic activity. Systemic adverse effects of antimuscarinic therapy can be minimized by the use of the quaternary ammonium derivative, ipratropium bromide.

Ipratropium bromide is poorly absorbed into the systemic circulation and does not freely cross the blood-brain. The drug is administered locally to the bronchioles by aerosol and is an effective bronchodilator in some patients with COPD. For additional information, see Chapter 33.

Drugs for Urological Disorders

Oxybutynin and **flavoxate** are two tertiary amine antimuscarinic drugs that exert direct antispasmodic activity on smooth muscle. Both compounds are less potent than atropine as M receptor antagonists (about one-fifth), but are more potent than atropine in relaxing smooth muscle (4 to 10 times). Neither drug has significant activity at nicotinic receptors.

Both oxybutynin and flavoxate are effective by the oral route. They are only used for the relief of symptoms assocated with urological disorders, e.g., urinary urgency, urinary frequency, urinary leakage, incontenence, and dysuria, that may occur due to bladder instability or inflammatory conditions of the urinary tract. These drugs are not indicated to treat urinary tract infections.

Adverse reactions to these compounds are similar to atropine with dry mouth, decreased sweating, and blurred vision being the most common. Since these drugs will cross the blood-brain barrier, CNS effects may occur.

GANGLIONIC BLOCKING DRUGS

During the 1950s and early 1960s, the ganglionic blocking agents were practically the only drugs available for the treatment of primary hypertension. They have now been almost totally replaced by more satisfactory antihypertensive drugs (see Chapter 32). Presently, the only two drugs that are available for clinical use in the United States are mecamylamine and trimethaphan. Although their clinical uses are few, they illustrate a number of important pharmacologic principles and are discussed briefly. In high doses, other drugs have ganglionic blocking activity. For example, nicotine toxicity is associated with ganglionic blockade (see Chapter 10) and tubocurarine has some antagonistic activity at ganglionic (neuronal type) nicotinic receptors (see Chapter 12).

Mechanism of Action

The primary event in sympathetic and parasympathetic ganglionic transmission is the release of acetylcholine (ACh) by presynaptic neuronal terminals. The neurotransmitter combines with neuronal type nicotinic (N_N) receptors on the postsynaptic neuronal membrane and, after a latent period of approximately 1 msec, results in the initial excitatory postsynaptic potential (EPSP); this in turn gives rise to action potentials in the postganglionic neuronal fibers. However, subsequent events modify this process. These events include:

1 *The inhibitory postsynaptic potential (IPSP)*, which occurs after a latency of approximately 35 msec and involves both muscarinic (M) receptors found on small neurons found within the synaptic cleft (called *SIF cells* because they are small, immunofluorescent cells) that release norepinephrine or dopamine which stimulate α-adrenergic receptors on the postganglionic neuronal membrane. M receptors on SIF cells are stimulated by ACh released in the synaptic cleft by the presynaptic neurons;

2 *The late EPSP*, which occurs at about 300 msec and results from activation of postganglionic M receptors; and

3 *The late slow EPSP*, which occur considerably later and may persist for several minutes. The late slow EPSP is produced by various peptides released along with ACh from the presynaptic terminals, e.g., enkephalins, vasoactive intestinal polypeptide, and substance P (see "Cotransmitters" in Chapter 7).

While the physiologic significance of these modulatory influences is still not defined, it is clear that ganglion cells contain M and N_N receptors, which accounts for cellular activation by muscarinic, as well as nicotinic agonists.

Ganglionic blocking agents can effectively reduce ganglionic transmission in both divisions of the autonomic nervous system by interacting with N_N receptors on the postsynaptic membrane. These drugs are classified into two groups: *depolarizing ganglionic blocking drugs* and *antidepolarizing blocking drugs*.

Depolarizing blocking drugs complex with and activate N_N receptors of the ganglia, producing depolarization of the postganglionic neuronal membrane (as does ACh), and then block transmission by causing persistent depolarization and blockade of membrane repolarization. Thus, these drugs have both a ganglionic stimulant and blocking action. Examples of drugs in this group are nicotine and lobeline. Since both of these compounds are used therapeutically for their agonist properties, their pharmacology is discussed in Chapter 10.

Antidepolarizing ganglionic blocking drugs act as competitive antagonists of ACh at N_N receptors. These compounds have a high affinity for the receptor site but lack intrinsic activity and, therefore, prevent the development of the initial EPSP; in this way they produce complete ganglionic blockade. Example of drugs in the group include mecamylamine and trimethaphan.

Effects on Organ Systems

Theoretically, ganglionic blocking agents can abolish all autonomic activity. The effects that occur following their administration reflect the predominance of sympathetic or parasympathetic tone on the tissue affected before they were given. For example, on vascular smooth muscle, sympathetic tone predominates. Accordingly, these drugs cause arteriolar vasodilatation with decreased peripheral resistance; venous dilatation leads to pooling of blood, diminished return to the heart, and decreased cardiac output. Both of these effects result in hypotension with relatively little compromise of peripheral blood flow, the desired therapeutic effect. At the same time they cause postural hypotension, an undesirable effect.

At most other autonomic effectors, parasympathetic tone normally predominates. Thus, many of the adverse effects of the ganglionic blocking agents are related to inhibition of parasympathetic tone on a variety of tissues and organs: the heart (tachycardia), iris (mydriasis), ciliary muscle (cycloplegia), gastrointestinal tract (reduced motility, constipation), urinary bladder (retention of urine), salivary glands (xerostomia), and sweat glands (anhydrosis).

In addition to the aforementioned side effects, the other limitations of the ganglionic blocking agents are their poor and irregular absorption from the gastrointestinal tract and the development of tolerance to their therapeutic effect in most patients.

The most surprising feature following the systemic use of a ganglionic blocking drug is the improvement in allocation or distribution of cardiac output in favor of the heart and brain. Observations in humans indicate that after the autonomic nervous is blocked, the local regulatory mechanisms (such as the metabolic control or cerebral and coronary vessels) and the local vascular (autoregulatory) factors in the kidney and splanchnic bed come into play. These mechanisms, which are independent of the autonomic nervous system, are active in normotensive and hypertensive individuals and account for the relative safety of the use of autonomic blocking agents in antihypertensive therapy. Without these mechanisms, cerebral and coronary insufficiency, manifested by fainting and cardiac arrhythmias, would be more frequently encountered.

Mecamylamine A secondary amine, mecamylamine, was introduced to overcome the problem of absorption following oral administration, common with most older quaternary amine ganglionic blocking drugs. Mecamylamine is almost completely absorbed from the gastrointestinal tract. However, its lipophilic structure also allows it to penetrate the blood-brain barrier so that it occasionally produces the additional side effects of malaise, choreiform movements, mania, and convulsions in some patients.

Mecamylamine has a slow onset of action (up to 2 h) and a prolonged duration (6 to 12 h or more). It is not biotransformed and is eliminated slowly into the urine. The rate of urinary excretion is marked influenced by urinary pH.

At the present time, mecamylamine is the only ganglionic blocking drug administered orally for the management of primary hypertension. It is only used in severe cases of hypertension that do not respond to other agents. Because of the development of tolerance and with the availability of many effective less toxic antihypertensive drugs (see Chapter 32), the routine use of mecamylamine is not necessary.

Trimethaphan Camsylate This compound differs from mecamylamine in its extremely brief duration of action. In addition to blocking N_N receptors, trimethaphan also exerts a direct peripheral vasodilator effect, and promotes the release of histamine from mast cells. By inducing vasodilation, the drug causes blood to pool in the dependent periphery and splanchnic system and reduces blood pressure. Since it is a charged compound, trimethaphan is not effective by the oral route and does not elicit significant CNS effects.

The onset of action following the initiation of intravenous infusion is almost immediate; the duration of action is short (10 to 30 min). Trimethaphan is used for the production of controlled hypotension during surgery when reduction of bleeding in the surgical field is required. It is also used in the emergency treatment of pulmonary edema from acute left ventricular failure, for reducing blood pressure in acute dissecting aortic aneurysm, and in the short-term control of blood pressure in hypertensive emergencies.

BIBLIOGRAPHY

Bonner, T.I., N.J. Buckley, A.C. Young and M.R. Brann: "Identification of a Family of Muscarinic Acetylcholine Receptor Genes," *Science* **237**: 527-532 (1987).

Gross, N.J.: "Ipratropium Bromide," *N. Engl. J. Med.* **319**: 486-494 (1988).

Higgins, S.T., R.J. Lamb, and J.E. Henningfield: "Dose-dependent Effects of Atropine on Behavioral and Physiologic Responses in Humans," *Pharmacol. Biochem. Behav.* **34**: 303 (1989).

Hinderling, P.H., U. Gundert-Remy, O. Schmidlin, and G. Heinzel: "Integrated Pharmacokinetics and Pharmacodynamics of Atropine in Healthy Humans, I. Pharmacokinetics," *J. Pharm. Sci.* **74**: 703-710 (1985).

Hinderling, P.H., U. Gundert-Remy, O. Schmidlin, and G. Heinzel: "Integrated Pharmacokinetics and Pharmacodynamics of Atropine in Healthy Humans, II. Pharmacodynamics," *J. Pharm. Sci.* **74**: 711-717 (1985).

North, R.V., and M.E. Kelly: "A Review of the Uses and Adverse Effects of Topical Administration of Atropine," *Ophthalmic Physiol. Opt.* **7**: 109-114 (1987).

Virtanen, R., J. Kanto, E. Iisalo, E.U. Iisalo, M. Salo, and S. Sjovall: "Pharmacokinetic Studies on Atropine with Special Reference to Age," *Acta Anaesthesiol. Scand.* **26**: 297-300 (1982).

Volle, R.L.: Nicotinic Ganglionic-Stimulating Agents," In Kharkevich, D.A. (ed.), *Pharmacology of Ganglionic Transmission*, Springer-Verlag, Berlin, 1980, pp. 281-312.

Wellstein, A., and H.F. Pitschner: "Complex Dose-response Curves of Atropine in Man Explained by Different Functions of M1- and M2-Cholinoceptors," *Naunyn Schmiedeberg Arch. Pharmacol.* **338**: 19-27 (1988).

Wilkinson, J.A.: "Side Effects of Transdermal Scopolamine," *J. Emerg. Med.* **5**: 389-392 (1987).

CHAPTER 12

Skeletal Muscle Relaxants

Edward J. Barbieri

The skeletal muscle relaxants are a diverse group of chemical compounds that share the capacity to interfere with the contraction of voluntary muscles. Some of these drugs are able to completely paralyze skeletal muscle; these compounds are used predominantly as adjuncts to anesthesia during surgical and orthopedic procedures in the controlled confines of the hospital environment. Other drugs in this broad category elicit a more modulatory effect on muscle contraction and do not completely block the activity of the skeletal musculature. These agents are useful in reducing muscle spasms and/or spasticity associated with myopathies and are commonly used in ambulatory patients.

Although the above separation of compounds is an appropriate therapeutic classification, the drugs discussed here are divided pharmacologically based on the site and mechanism of action. Three categories of drugs will be presented: (1) *neuromuscular blocking drugs*: peripherally acting muscle relaxants that act at the myoneural junction and impair the transmission of impulses from somatic neurons to skeletal muscle membranes; (2) a *direct-acting muscle relaxant*: one compound that acts directly on the muscle fiber by blocking the contractile process; and (3) *centrally acting drugs*: agents which depress the transmission of motor impulses at synapses within the central nervous system.

NEUROMUSCULAR BLOCKING DRUGS

These compounds block transmission from the motor nerve ending to skeletal muscle fibers. Conduction of impulses along somatic neurons is not impaired and the skeletal muscle is capable of contraction following direct stimulation. The effect of the neuromuscular blocking agents is usually transitory, and skeletal muscle function is completely restored after cessation of drug administration.

Chemistry

Curare is a generic term used to describe various resinous mixtures of paralyzing arrow poisons used by South American natives. The first neuromuscular blocking agent, *tubocurarine*, was an active alkaloid extracted from curare. Today, synthetic neuromuscular blocking agents are based upon certain structural features of tubocurarine and these compounds are known as *curariform drugs*. The structures of representative neuromuscular blocking agents are shown in Fig. 12-1. Although there are exceptions, tubocurarine and most other synthetic curariform agents are large, bulky molecules that contain two or more quaternary nitrogen groups (approximately 1.0 +/− 0.1 nm apart), which appear to be important to the ability of the drugs to bind to nicotinic receptors at the skeletal muscle end plate.

Mechanism of Action

By electron microscopy it has been estimated that the muscle-type nicotinic cholinergic receptor (N_M) density at the skeletal muscle end plate is approximately $10{,}000/\mu m^2$. Each nicotinic cholinergic receptor of the neuromuscular junction is envisioned to be an asymmetric complex of five proteins. This 250 to 300 kDa pentamer extends completely through the muscle membrane and is composed of four distinct subunits (two α, one each β, γ, and δ in embryonic muscle; the γ subunit is replaced by ϵ in adult tissue, which results in a receptor with slightly altered biophysical

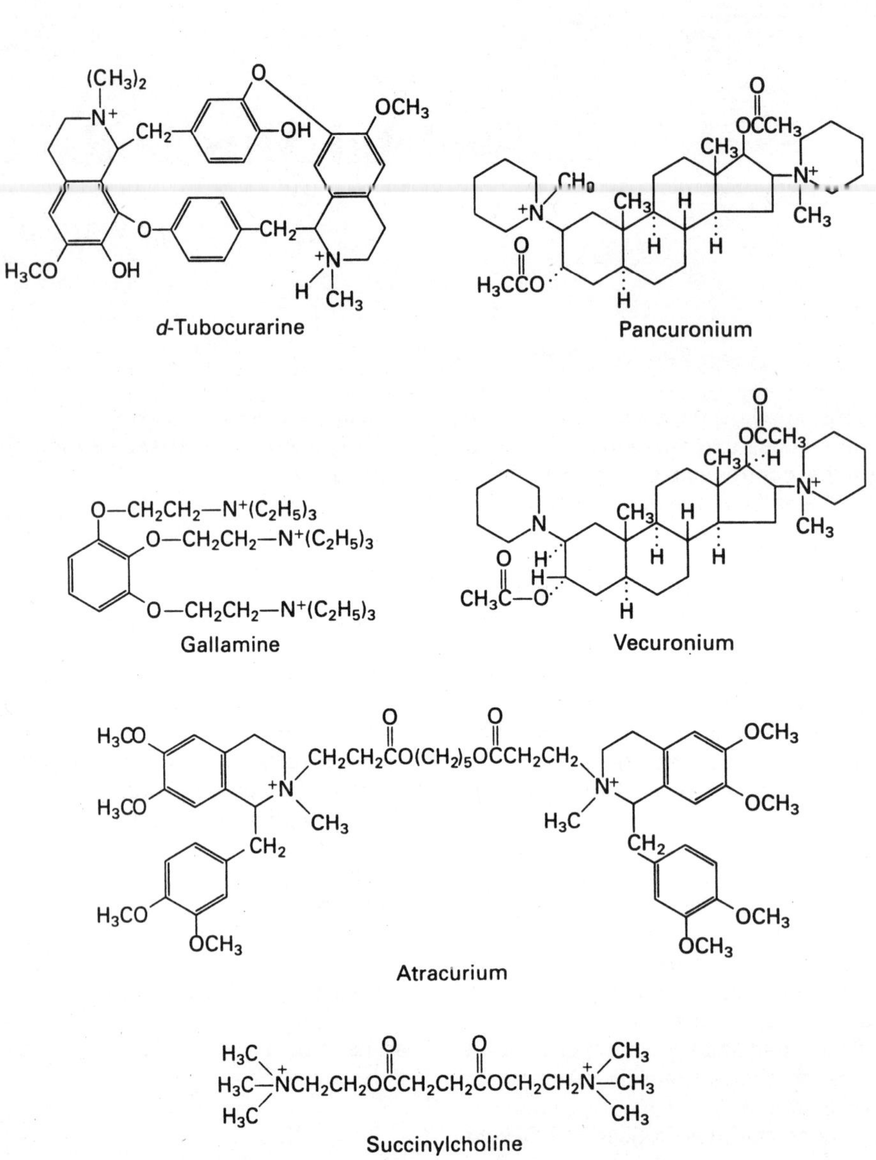

FIGURE 12-1 *Structures of some neuromuscular blocking drugs.*

properties) arranged around a single Na^+-K^+ ion channel as shown in Fig. 12-2. The α subunits contain the primary recognition sites for the endogenous neurotransmitter, acetylcholine, and these proteins are also the sites for binding of the antagonists that act as neuromuscular blocking drugs.

Following acetylcholine release from storage vesicles of activated motor neurons, the neurotransmitter diffuses across the synaptic cleft and binds to the α subunits of the N_M receptors. When one acetylcholine molecule binds to each α subunit, a conformational change occurs in the protein complex, opening the central ion channel (for about 1 msec) and making the muscle membrane permeable to the influx of Na^+ and the efflux of K^+. The ion flow induces a postjunctional end plate potential, which gives rise to a propagated muscle action potential. The muscle action potential spreads throughout the myofibril conduction system and the muscle contracts.

When the muscle relaxes, it is refractory to another stimulus until repolarization of the muscle end plate is complete. This requires dissociation

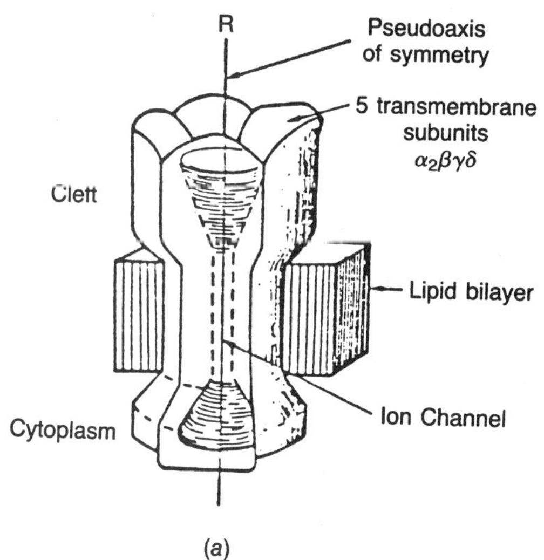

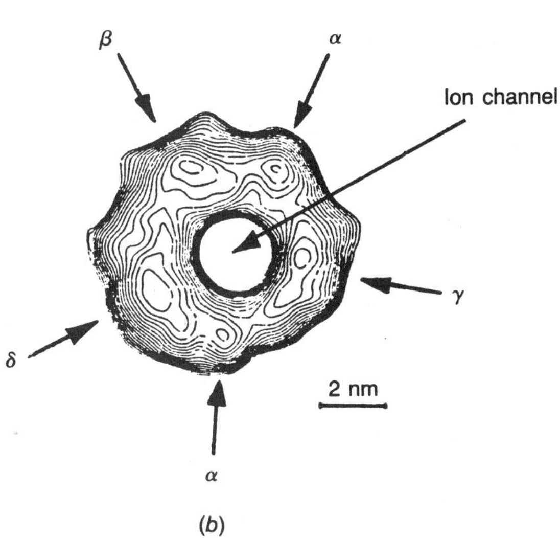

FIGURE 12-2 *Morphology of the muscle-type nicotinic (N_M) receptor. (a) Schematic model of the side view of the pentamer complex of the nicotinic receptor within the membrane of the neuromuscular junction. (b) Cross-sectional view of the asymmetric protein receptor complex showing the proposed positions of the α, β, γ, and δ subunits relative to the central ion channel. [From Changeux, J.-P., A. Devillers-Thiery, and P. Chemouilli: Science,* ***225****: 1335-1345 (1984).]*

of acetylcholine from the N_M receptor, re-establishment of the Na^+ and K^+ gradients across the membrane, and hydrolysis of acetylcholine by acetylcholinesterase located in the synaptic cleft. Neuromuscular blocking agents can depress skeletal muscle contraction either by (1) preventing acetylcholine-induced depolarization of the muscle end plate, i.e., the *nondepolarizing drugs*, or (2) blocking repolarization of the muscle end plate, i.e., the *depolarizing neuromuscular blocking agents*.

Nondepolarizing Drugs Compounds in this group, which are also referred to as *antidepolarizing* or *competitive blocking agents*, include tubocurarine, metocurine, gallamine, pancuronium, vecuronium, atracurium, pipecuronium, doxacurium, and mivacurium. The mechanism of action for all of these drugs is competition with acetylcholine for the postsynaptic N_M receptors. These drugs have affinity for, but no intrinsic activity on, the acetylcholine-binding sites on the α subunit of the N_M receptor complex. Since two molecules of an agonist are required to open the ionic channel, binding of one molecule of antagonist to the receptor will cause it to be nonfunctional. If a sufficient number of receptors are occupied by the antagonist, the number activated by acetylcholine will be too small to lead to the production of an end plate potential large enough to reach threshold for activation of the adjacent electrically excitable membrane. Thus transmission fails.

Depolarizing Drugs Succinylcholine is the only therapeutically useful neuromuscular blocker that acts as a *depolarizing agent* which blocks muscle repolarization. In contrast to the nondepolarizing agents, succinylcholine is not a competitive antagonist but rather a more stable agonist than acetylcholine: that is, as far as its action is concerned, succinylcholine differs from the neurotransmitter acetylcholine only in duration of action. Both agents act at the same receptor (N_M), and with both, channel opening and depolarization of the end-plate regions result. Succinylcholine is inactivated more slowly than acetylcholine and, since it lasts longer in the synapse, differs only from the neurotransmitter in that it produces a persistent depolarization.

The persistent depolarization of the end plate leads, by local circuit action, to a persistent depolarization of the adjacent electrically excitable membrane of the muscle. This brief period of repetitive excitation appears as an initial muscle fasciculation on administration of succinylcholine.

Since succinylcholine remains in the synaptic cleft for a relatively long period of time (in comparison to acetylcholine), the repolarization process is blocked and a flaccid paralysis results. This is *phase I* of the action of succinylcholine. Although stable depolarizing blocking agents can produce a depolarization which is quite prolonged compared with that produced by acetylcholine, they do not produce a depolarization of indefinite duration. Despite continued exposure to the depolarizing agent, the end plate does not stay depolarized to a constant extent and loses its responsiveness to the depolarizing agent, i.e., it becomes desensitized. Since the action of the neurotransmitter is identical to that of the more stable depolarizing agent, the neurotransmitter loses its effectiveness as well. A situation is reached, therefore, where the depolarizing drug may no longer be present but the neuromuscular block persists. This is called a *phase II block*, a *nondepolarization block*, or *desensitization block*.

Pharmacologic Effects

Neuromuscular Blockade When a neuromuscular blocking agent is administered, a flaccid paralysis of the voluntary musculature develops. The muscles which produce fine movements (for example, the extraocular muscles and muscles of the head, face, and neck) are most sensitive to these drugs and are blocked first. Muscles of the trunk, abdomen, and extremities are affected next; respiratory muscles are the most resistant to blockade with paralysis affecting the intercostal muscles prior to the diaphragm. Recovery of the musculature occurs in the reverse order following the cessation of drug administration.

When a depolarizing neuromuscular blocking agent (e.g., succinylcholine) is administered, the block is preceded by fasciculation, especially if the drug is given rapidly. Soon the fasciculation ceases, and the muscles become quiescent and superficially indistinguishable from those blocked by a competitive blocking agent.

The skeletal muscle relaxant activity of the competitive neuromuscular blocking agents is enhanced by certain inhalation general anesthetics, e.g., halothane, enflurane, and isoflurane; these drugs appear to stabilize the neuromuscular membrane. High doses of aminoglycoside antibiotics, such as streptomycin, neomycin, kanamycin, gentamicin, and tobramycin, inhibit acetylcholine release from cholinergic neurons and thus are reported to enhance neuromuscular blockade; due to widespread awareness, this interaction is now relatively rare. Tetracyclines, clindamycin, polymyxin B, and colistin also may increase the effect of curariform drugs by undetermined mechanisms. Enhanced neuromuscular blockade has occurred in antiarrhythmic therapy with quinidine and lidocaine. Fluid and electrolyte imbalances, such as acidosis, dehydration, and hypokalemia (produced by certain diuretics), may also enhance neuromuscular blockade. Postoperative respiratory depression due to neuromuscular blockade enhancement by quinine, magnesium, and lithium salts can occur. Patients with myasthenia gravis are extremely sensitive to nondepolarizing neuromuscular blocking agents.

The antagonism of neuromuscular blockade induced by the nondepolarizing blocking drugs is approached by the administration of a cholinesterase inhibitor so that acetylcholine released from the motor neurons will reach the end plate in higher concentrations and therefore will compete more effectively for the nicotinic receptor. Drugs such as neostigmine, pyridostigmine, and edrophonium are useful in this regard (see Chapter 10). The choice of dose is not too critical, the antagonism is distinct, and the effect is well maintained. These drugs also directly depolarize the nicotinic receptor. Therefore, the activity of these drugs is the result of inhibition of cholinesterases and a direct stimulation of the muscle end-plate.

Cholinesterase inhibitors should not be used in an attempt to reverse the action of the depolarizing blocker succinylcholine. Since succinylcholine is biotransformed via acetylcholinesterase at the neuromuscular junction, the use of a cholinesterase inhibitor would prolong the skeletal muscle relaxant effect of this drug.

Effect on Autonomic Ganglia Tubocurarine and metocurine are capable of producing ganglionic blockade at high therapeutic doses, which is, in part, responsible for the hypotension and tachycardia that may occur with these drugs. The activity of tubocurarine on ganglia is somewhat greater than that of metocurine. Because the potency of these drugs is still greater at the neuromuscular junction than at autonomic ganglia, in most cases a prominent effect on the ganglia during clinical use is rarely observed. None of the other drugs shows any significant ganglionic blocking activity. Succinylcholine can stimulate nicotinic receptors in ganglia of both divisions of the autonomic nervous system. Thus, succinylcholine drug may cause bradycardia (via stimulation of vagal ganglia), or hypertension and tachycardia (due to stimulation of sympathetic ganglia (see Table 12-1).

Histamine Release Tubocurarine is a potent liberator of histamine from mast cells, which can account quantitatively for an episode of hypotension during anesthesia. Histamine release can also produce bronchospasm or an increase in respiratory tract secretion and is occasionally seen following the administration of tubocurarine or metocurine. The other neuromuscular blocking agents do not act as potent histamine releasers, although some histamine release has been associated with the use of gallamine, atracurium, mivacurium, and succinylcholine, especially at high therapeutic doses (see Table 12-1).

Cardiovascular System As mentioned above, hypotensive reactions can be observed with tubocurarine and metocurine due to the ganglionic blocking activity associated with these drugs. Cardioacceleration, increased cardiac output, and mild hypertension may be seen with gallamine (Table 12-1). These effects seem to be the result of both an atropine-like antimuscarinic action and a tyramine-like effect of the drug, whereby norepinephrine is released from the sympathetic nerve endings supplying the vasculature and the pacemaker region of the heart. Pancuronium also causes increases in heart rate, cardiac output, and blood pressure. These changes are moderate and have been attributed to four distinct actions: (1) blockade of the negative chronotropic and inotropic actions of acetylcholine, (2) release of norepinephrine from postganglionic adrenergic fibers, (3) blockade of the re-uptake of catecholamines into adrenergic terminals, and (4) a mild ganglionic (N_N) stimulant effect.

Succinylcholine may occasionally elicit cardiovascular effects (e.g., bradycardia, tachycardia, increased blood pressure) due to activation of nicotinic receptors in autonomic ganglia. Although both tachycardia and bradycardia have been observed with the other neuromuscular blocking agents, these effects are not significant clinically.

Central Nervous System The cationic charge on all of these compounds makes permeation of the blood-brain barrier negligible, so that central nervous system effects are not observed in clinical practice.

Potassium Levels Succinylcholine can liberate potassium from skeletal muscles; continuous skeletal muscle depolarization can lead to an elevation of the plasma potassium concentration. This should be borne in mind when patients are encountered who will need prolonged administration of a neuromuscular blocking agent and whose electrolyte concentrations are already disturbed or who have congestive heart failure and are receiving digitalis or diuretics.

Eye Succinylcholine can cause a slight increase in intraocular pressure immediately after its injection and during the fasciculation phase. This is usually attributed to a sustained contraction of the extraocular muscles. This effect is transient, and the drug is not contraindicated in patients with glaucoma.

Pharmacokinetics

Since all of the neuromuscular blocking agents are charged, independent of pH, absorption from the gastrointestinal tract is very poor; therefore, all of these drugs must be administered intravenously. For the same reason these drugs are largely distributed to the extracellular space only. The apparent volume of distribution for these drugs is low (0.15 to 0.45 L/kg); plasma protein binding is variable, with pancuronium being the highest of the group at about 87 percent and metocurine one of the lowest at 35 percent. Elimination is predominantly via the urine and, to a lesser extent, through the bile. Since the molecular charge will prevent reabsorption across the tubular membrane in the kidney, all the drugs that cross the glomerular membrane will be excreted. The major differences with respect to the pharmacokinetics of these drugs is in their biotransformation and elimination half-lives. Accordingly, these drugs can be classified based upon their duration of action (Table 12-1).

A negligible fraction of tubocurarine is metabolized. This drug, as well as its methyl derivative metocurine, contains few unstable bonds, and the only reactive groups (the charged quaternary heads) are not susceptible to conjugation, oxidation, or reduction. The elimination half-life of tubocurarine is between 2 and 3 h; that of metocurine is about 3.5 h. Both drugs appear to be eliminated primarily via the kidney. Gallamine is also reasonably inert. Its ether linkages are stable, and so, like the aforementioned drugs, it is removed primarily by glomerular filtration. Such agents exert a prolonged action in patients with anuria. Doxacurium is not biotransformed; its major routes of elimination are through the bile and urine.

TABLE 12-1 Some pharmacodynamic and pharmacokinetic properties of the neuromuscular blocking agents

	Effect on Autonomic Ganglia	Effect on Histamine Release	Effect on Cardiac Muscarinic Receptors	Biotransformation and Active Product
Long-Acting (Duration of action: 1 - 2 hours)				
Tubocurarine	Blockade	High	None	Insignificant
Metocurine	Blockade	Moderate	None	Insignificant
Gallamine	None	Low	Blockade	Insignificant
Pancuronium	None	None	Blockade	Deacetylation: 3-hydroxy pancuronium
Pipecuronium	None	None	None	Deacetylation: 3-desacetyl pipecuronium
Doxacurium	None	None	None	Insignificant
Intermediate-Acting (Duration of action: 20 - 45 min)				
Vecuronium	None	None	None	Deacetylation: 3-desacetyl vecuronium
Atracurium	None	Low	None	Ester hydrolysis and spontaneous dissociation
Short-Acting (Duration of action: 5 - 15 min)				
Mivacurium	None	Low	None	Ester hydrolysis
Succinylcholine	Stimulation	Low	Stimulation	Ester hydrolysis: succinylmonocholine

Pancuronium, pipecuronium, and vecuronium are eliminated primarily unaltered by the kidneys, although up to 25 percent of these drugs may be deacetylated. Pancuronium is converted mainly to a 3-hydroxy derivative, but also to 17-hydroxy and 3,17-dihydroxy derivatives. Similarly, 3-deacetyl, 17-deacetyl, and 3,17-dideacetyl derivatives of pipecuronium and vecuronium have been identified. 3-Hydroxy pancuronium, 3-deacetyl pipecuronium, and 3-deacetyl vecuronium are about 50 percent as active as their parent compounds as neuromuscular blocking agents; the other metabolites are essentially inactive. Some of the unaltered drugs may undergo biliary excretion; for example, up to 50 percent of vecuronium may be eliminated by this route. The elimination half-lives of pancuronium and pipecuronium are between 1.5 and 2.5 h in patients with normal renal and hepatic function, whereas that of vecuronium is only about 1 h.

As shown in Fig. 12-1, atracurium is a complex molecule with two ester groups joined by a 5-carbon chain. The drug is inactivated in plasma by two nonoxidation pathways: (1) ester hydrolysis, catalyzed by nonspecific esterases, and (2) a spontaneous chemical reaction at physiologic pH in which the carbon bridge is split from the quaternary nitrogens (known as Hofmann elimination). The metabolites and any remaining atracurium are eliminated through both the urine and the bile. The elimination half-life of this drug is only approximately 20 min.

Mivacurium is a relatively short-acting mixture of three isomers (all esters) which do not interconvert *in vivo*. The two more potent isomers (that account for the majority of the mixture) are hydrolyzed by plasma cholinesterase. Mivacurium and its biotransformation products are eliminated through the urine and bile; the mean elimination half-life is estimated at under 10 minutes.

Succinylcholine is also biotransformed very rapidly. It contains two ester bonds and is an excellent substrate for plasma cholinesterase. The product of the hydrolysis is succinylmonocholine (an active product), which is also broken down by pseudocholinesterase to succinic acid and choline. Since the second stage is about 6 times slower than the first, appreciable quantities of the monocholine ester can accumulate, particularly during prolonged administration. The potency of the monocholine ester (about 5 percent that of succinylcholine itself) is great enough to contribute to the neuromuscular blockade. Succinylcholine also degrades spontaneously by alkaline hydrolysis at a slow rate, but fast enough to contribute to the biotransformation of the drug.

The rapid destruction of succinylcholine not only makes the action brief (half-life about 5 min) but also facilitates rapid onset. A larger dose can be given so that the effective concentration at the muscle end plate will be reached sooner, without prolonging unduly the overall duration of action. This feature has made succinylcholine popular for facilitation of endotracheal intubation during general anesthesia.

About one person in 3000 has atypical plasma cholinesterase which biotransforms some of these drugs less rapidly. If such a patient is given the usual dose of succinylcholine, for example, an overdose will result, and this will bring on prolonged apnea. The problem should be regarded as a form of overdosing as well as a situation in which the terminal phase of drug elimination is slowed.

Since the neuromuscular blocking agents are charged compounds, no marked transfer across the placenta would be expected. Some evidence of transfer has been reported for gallamine and tubocurarine, but it is negligible.

Therapeutic Uses

Anesthesia The purpose of anesthesia is not only to render the patient insensible to pain but also, where possible, to facilitate surgery. Normally the motor nerves carry a constant low level of traffic to the skeletal muscles. These signals induce a contraction of only a small fraction of the muscle fibers at any time, but the activity of these fibers place a slight tension on the muscle which prepares it for more intense activity at a moment's notice. This background state of light contraction is called *muscle tone*. Muscle tone can be a nuisance during surgery when the surgeon must struggle against it to reduce a fracture or when the tone in the flat muscles of the abdomen tends to expel the abdominal contents through an abdominal incision. Before the advent of neuromuscular blocking agents, larger doses of a general anesthetic, than were required simply to produce unconsciousness, had to be administered in order to stop the tonic outflow at the source. General anesthetics, however, have a rather low margin of safety; the concentrations required for muscle relaxation are too close to stage IV of anesthesia. It is therefore desirable to use a second agent to abolish muscle tone so that lower concentrations of the general anesthetic can be used. The neuromuscular blocking agents have proved to be a satisfactory group of agents for this role. They have subsequently found even wider use during induction of anesthesia when they are given to relax the laryngeal muscles and thereby facilitate endotracheal intubation.

Electroshock Therapy When electroshock therapy is used in the treatment of psychiatric disorders, muscular contraction can be intense enough to cause fractures. Since the therapeutic effect of the convulsion does not depend on the muscular response, prior administration of a neuromuscular blocking agent can be used to abolish the muscular component. The chief hazard that may be encountered is a synergism between the drug and a postictal depression of respiration. Preparations should be made to maintain the airway and assist respiration if necessary. Succinylcholine is the most popular agent for this purpose; its short duration of action apparently outweighs its propensity to produce fasciculations and the ensuing discomfort.

Mechanical Ventilation When a patient is unable to ventilate well enough to maintain normal arterial oxygen and carbon dioxide levels or is becoming exhausted in the attempts to do so, it is advantageous to assist or control respiration by means of a mechanical ventilator. This procedure is sometimes ineffective because the patient's attempts to breathe are not synchronous with the cycle of the respirator. Frequently sedation and depression of the respiratory center with opioids will improve the situation, but occasionally it is necessary to block all respiratory effort. Intravenous competitive blocking agents are most satisfactory. Often repeated administration is not needed, since the return of arterial blood-gas tensions to normal with the improved ventilation reduces the stimulus to increased respiration, and the patient no longer "fights" the respirator. Alert patients should be sedated while paralyzed.

Myasthenia Gravis Patients with myasthenia gravis are especially sensitive to the competitive neuromuscular blocking agents. Diagnosis of this disease can be facilitated in a borderline case by the use of a test dose of tubocurarine. However, tubocurarine is not used unless the more conventional tests with neostigmine or edrophonium have been inconclusive (see Chapter 10).

Adverse Reactions

The most important adverse reaction to the neuromuscular blocking agents is apnea, which may extend into the postoperative period and may require artificial respiration over long periods. This may result following overdosage or, in the case of succinylcholine, may be due to the patient's inability to adequately biotransform the drug. The nondepolarizing blockers, e.g., tubocurarine and pancuronium, can be antagonized by cholinesterase inhibitors.

Other mild and infrequent adverse reactions that have occurred with the nondepolarizing drugs include bradycardia, tachycardia, hypotension, hypertension, bronchospasm, excessive salivation, and rash. In addition to those reactions listed above, succinylcholine may cause hyperkalemia, postoperative muscle pain, and malignant hyperthermia.

DIRECT-ACTING SKELETAL MUSCLE RELAXANT

Dantrolene

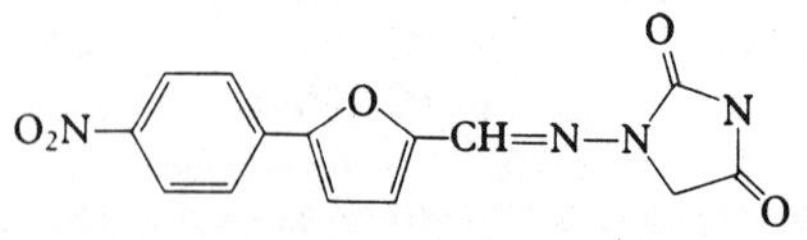

Dantrolene is a substituted hydantoin that relieves spasticity by an action on muscle. Unlike all other skeletal muscle relaxants, this agent acts directly on the contractile mechanism of skeletal muscle by interfering with the release of calcium from the sarcoplasmic reticulum. This results in uncoupling the excitation-contraction mechanism of skeletal muscles and is more pronounced in fast muscle fibers than in slow ones. Dantrolene will depress the CNS; however, its skeletal muscle relaxant effects do not appear to be mediated by actions on neurons.

The oral bioavailability of dantrolene is about 70 percent; oral absorption is slow but consistent. Peak plasma concentrations occur 4 to 6 h after a single oral dose. The mean biologic half-life is approximately 9 h after oral dosing and 4 to 8 h following IV administration. Dantrolene is slowly biotransformed to inactive hydroxy and acetamido derivatives, which, along with the parent drug, are excreted in the urine.

Dantrolene is used orally for controlling the manifestations of clinical spasticity resulting from serious chronic disorders such as injury, stroke, cerebral palsy, and multiple sclerosis. It is not recommended for the treatment for skeletal muscle spasms resulting from rheumatic disorders.

Because dantrolene interferes with the release of calcium from the sarcoplasmic reticulum to the myoplasma, it is also used in the therapy of life-threatening malignant hyperthermia caused by many inhalation general anesthetics and succinylcholine. For this purpose the drug is administered either orally or intravenously as soon as the malignant hyperthermia reaction is recognized. It can also be given preoperatively to prevent the development of this syndrome in patients who are judged to be susceptible to malignant hyperthermia.

The most frequent adverse effects of this drug are diarrhea, weakness, drowsiness, fatigue, dizziness, and general malaise. These are generally transient and disappear with continued drug use. The most serious adverse reaction is potentially fatal hepatocellular disease.

CENTRALLY ACTING SKELETAL MUSCLE RELAXANTS

Skeletal muscle paralysis achieved by curariform drugs is not useful in the large variety of common clinical spasticity states accompanying CNS lesions and local injury and inflammation. Neuromuscular blockade can relieve the spasm, but it also results in loss of voluntary skeletal muscle control. The aim in conditions of muscle spasticity is to find an agent that relieves the painful muscle spasm without loss of voluntary muscle function and without impairment of cerebral function.

Many CNS depressants cause skeletal muscle relaxation. Notable among these are the alcohols and the barbiturates, but these are ordinarily of no use since they also produce marked sedation and other untoward effects.

The search for selective CNS agents capable of achieving muscular relaxation has produced a number of interesting compounds, none of which has been completely successful. Nevertheless, centrally acting skeletal muscle relaxants are widely used in the treatment of sprains, arthritis, bursitis, and similar musculoskeletal disorders. This use is based on the assumption that spasms originating through spinal cord reflexes can be depressed by these muscle relaxants.

A number of heterogenous chemical compounds act within the spinal cord and depress monosynaptic and polysynaptic reflexes. Some of these are baclofen, cyclobenzaprine, carisoprodol, methocarbamol, chlorphenesin, chlorzoxazone, orphenadrine, and diazepam. The pharmacology of diazepam is presented in detail in Chapter 17. Baclofen and cyclobenzaprine are briefly discussed here as representative centrally acting skeletal muscle relaxants.

Baclofen

$$H_2NCH_2CH(C_6H_4Cl)CH_2C(=O)OH$$

An analog of the inhibitory neurotransmitter gamma aminobutyric acid (GABA), baclofen reduces transmission at monosynaptic extensor and polysynaptic flexor reflex pathways in the spinal cord; actions at supraspinal sites may also contribute to the effect of the drug. In the spinal cord the action of baclofen appears to occur presynaptically and involves the interaction with, and activation of, specific $GABA_B$ receptors, which leads to the inhibition of release of excitatory neurotransmitters.

Baclofen is well absorbed following oral administration. Peak blood concentration is reached in approximately 2 h. Plasma protein binding is only about 30 percent. Little of the compound is biotransformed; 70 to 85 percent of a dose is excreted unchanged by the kidney. The half-life of the drug is 3 to 4 h.

Baclofen is indicated for alleviating the signs and symptoms of muscle spasticity due to muscular sclerosis, clonus, and muscular rigidity. The drug may also be effective in patients with muscle spasms resulting from spinal cord injuries and other spinal diseases.

Drowsiness, dizziness, weakness, fatigue, confusion, headache, and insomnia are the most common adverse reactions observed with this compound. These are often transient and will disappear with continued therapy. Gastrointestinal complaints including nausea, anorexia, and constipation may occur; hypotension and increased urinary frequency have also been reported.

Cyclobenzaprine

$$=CHCH_2CH_2\overset{+}{N}H(CH_3)_2 \quad Cl^-$$

A compound which is structurally and pharmacologically related to the tricyclic antidepressants, cyclobenzaprine relieves muscle spasm associated with a variety of musculoskeletal conditions without interfering with skeletal muscle function. The drug acts primarily at the level of the brain stem, although it has some activity at spinal motor neurons, which may contribute to its overall skeletal muscle relaxant effects. The net response to cyclobenzaprine administration is a reduction in tonic somatic motor activity, influencing both descending alpha motor neurons and gamma motor neurons.

Cyclobenzaprine is generally well absorbed orally; however a significant first-pass effect occurs in some patients. Extensive hepatic biotransformation, primarily to inactive glucuronide conjugates, and renal excretion occur quite slowly and result in a half-life of 1 to 3 days. Because of the high plasma protein binding of the drug (93 percent), cyclobenzaprine is not long-acting, and administration three times daily is recommended for most patients.

The most frequent adverse reactions to this drug are drowsiness, xerostomia, and dizziness. Other adverse effects are similar in nature and incidence to those which are to be expected from a tricyclic compound (see Chapter 21).

BIBLIOGRAPHY

Argov, Z., and F.L. Mastaglia: "Disorders of Neuromuscular Transmission Caused by Drugs," *N. Engl. J. Med.* **301**: 409-413 (1979).

Burke, D., C.J. Andrews, and L. Knowles: "The Action of a GABA Derivative in Human Spasticity," *J. Neurolog. Sci.* **14**: 199-208 (1971).

Changeux, J.-P., A. Devillers-Thiery, and P. Chemouilli: "Acetylcholine Receptor: An Allosteric Protein," *Science* **225**: 1335-1345 (1984).

Colquhoun, D.: "Mechanisms of Drug Action at the Voluntary Muscle Endplate," *Annu. Rev. Pharmacol.* **15**: 307-326 (1975).

Elenbaas, J.K.: "Centrally Acting Oral Skeletal Muscle Relaxants," *Am. J. Hosp. Pharm.* **37**: 1313-1323 (1980).

Ellis, K.D.: "Mechanisms of Control of Skeletal Muscle Contraction by Dantrolene Sodium," *Arch. Phys. Med. Rehabil.* **55**: 362-369 (1974).

Feldman, S.: "Neuromuscular Blocking Drugs," in H.C. Churchill-Davidson and W. D. Wylie (eds.), *A Practice of Anaesthesia, 5th Ed.*, Year Book Medical, Chicago, 1984, pp. 722-734.

Galzi, J.-L., F. Revah, A. Bessis, and J.-P. Changeux: "Functional Architecture of the Nicotinic Acetylcholine Receptor: From Electric Organ to Brain," *Annu. Rev. Pharmacol.* **31**: 37-72 (1991).

Hubbard, J.I., and D.M.J. Quastel: "Micropharmacology of Vertebrate Neuromuscular Transmission," *Annu. Rev Pharmacol.* **13**: 199-216 (1973).

Hughes, R., and D.J. Chapple: "The Pharmacology of Atracurium: A New Competitive Neuromuscular Blocking Agent," *Br. J. Anaesth.* **53**: 31-44 (1981).

Lambert, J.J., N.N. Durant, and E.G. Henderson: "Drug-Induced Modification of Ionic Conductance at the Neuromuscular Junction," *Annu. Rev. Pharmacol. Toxicol.*, **23**: 505--539 (1983).

Reilly, C.S., and W.S. Nimmo: "New Intravenous Anaesthetics and Neuromuscular Blocking Drugs," *Drugs* **34**: 98-135 (1987).

Roizen, M.D., and T.W. Feeley: "Pancuronium Bromide," *Ann. Intern. Med.* **88**: 64-68 (1978).

Share, N.N., and C.S. McFarlane: "Cyclobenzaprine: A Novel Centrally Acting Skeletal Muscle Relaxant," *Neuropharmacology* **14**: 675-684 (1975).

Ward, A., M.O. Chaffman, and E.M. Sorkin: "Dantrolene," *Drugs* **32**: 130-168 (1986).

Young, R.R., and P.J. Delwaide: "Drug Therapy: Spasticity," *N. Engl. J. Med.* **304**: 28-33, 96-99 (1981).

PART III

Local Control Substances

SECTION EDITOR

Edward J. Barbieri

CHAPTER 13

Histamine, Histamine Receptor Antagonists, 5-Hydroxytryptamine, and Its Congeners

Edward J. Barbieri and Andrew P. Ferko

Both histamine and 5-hydroxytryptamine (5-HT, serotonin) are endogenous substances that have diverse physiological activities and participate in some pathological states. These substances have been called *autacoids* (from the Greek words *autos* ("self") and *akos* ("medicinal agent") because they have a brief duration of action and act locally near their sites of release. Other autacoids include the eicosanoids (see Chapter 14) and many peptides, including the cytokines and lymphokines (see Chapters 33 and 44). Primarily because there are drugs that can be used therapeutically or diagnostically to mimic the actions of histamine and 5-HT and there are a number of compounds available to antagonize their effects, this chapter will focus on the pharmacology of histamine, 5-HT, their congeners, and antagonists.

HISTAMINE

The discovery and synthesis of histamine more than 80 years ago was a landmark achievement in pharmacology, immunology, and medicine. This naturally occurring biogenic amine is widely distributed in tissues and is implicated in a variety of physiologic and pathophysiologic processes, including immediate hypersensitivity and allergic reactions, regulation of gastric acid secretion, and neurotransmission in the central nervous system.

The profound pharmacologic activity of histamine was first demonstrated in the early part of this century by investigations which established that similarities existed between pathophysiologic responses to histamine and to anaphylaxis. Both are characterized by smooth muscle contraction, signs of inflammation, vasodilation, and shock-like symptoms. These effects of histamine are known to be mediated through activation of specific histamine receptors (designated as H_1, H_2, and H_3). The first section of the chapter will focus on the physiological activity of histamine and drugs which have been found to inhibit its actions by blocking subtypes of histamine receptors selectively, i.e., H_1 receptor antagonists and H_2 receptor antagonists. Although several novel compounds have been synthesized that selectively block H_3 receptors, to date none are available for therapeutic use.

Synthesis, Distribution, Localization, and Binding

Histamine is synthesized in many tissues by the decarboxylation of the amino acid L-histidine. This reaction is catalyzed by the pyridoxal phosphate-dependent enzyme, L-histidine decarboxylase (Fig. 13-1). Unlike its less specific counterpart, aromatic L-amino acid decarboxylase, this enzyme is specific for L-histidine. Histamine may also be ingested from food or formed by bacteria in the gastrointestinal tract; however, these sources do not contribute significantly to the body's store of histamine, since absorbed amounts are catabolized readily in the intestinal mucosa or liver and eliminated in the urine.

Following its synthesis, histamine is distributed and stored. The primary histologic site is the mast cell (especially in perivascular tissues of most organs) in which preformed histamine is stored in localized secretory cytoplasmic granules as a heparin-protein complex along with other pharmacologically active substances, including eosinophil chemotactic factor of anaphylaxis (ECF-A), neutrophil chemotactic factor, and enzymes such as neutral proteases, β-glucuronidase, superoxide dismutase, and peroxidase (histamine constitutes approximately 10 percent of the weight of these granules). In the circulation the predominant site

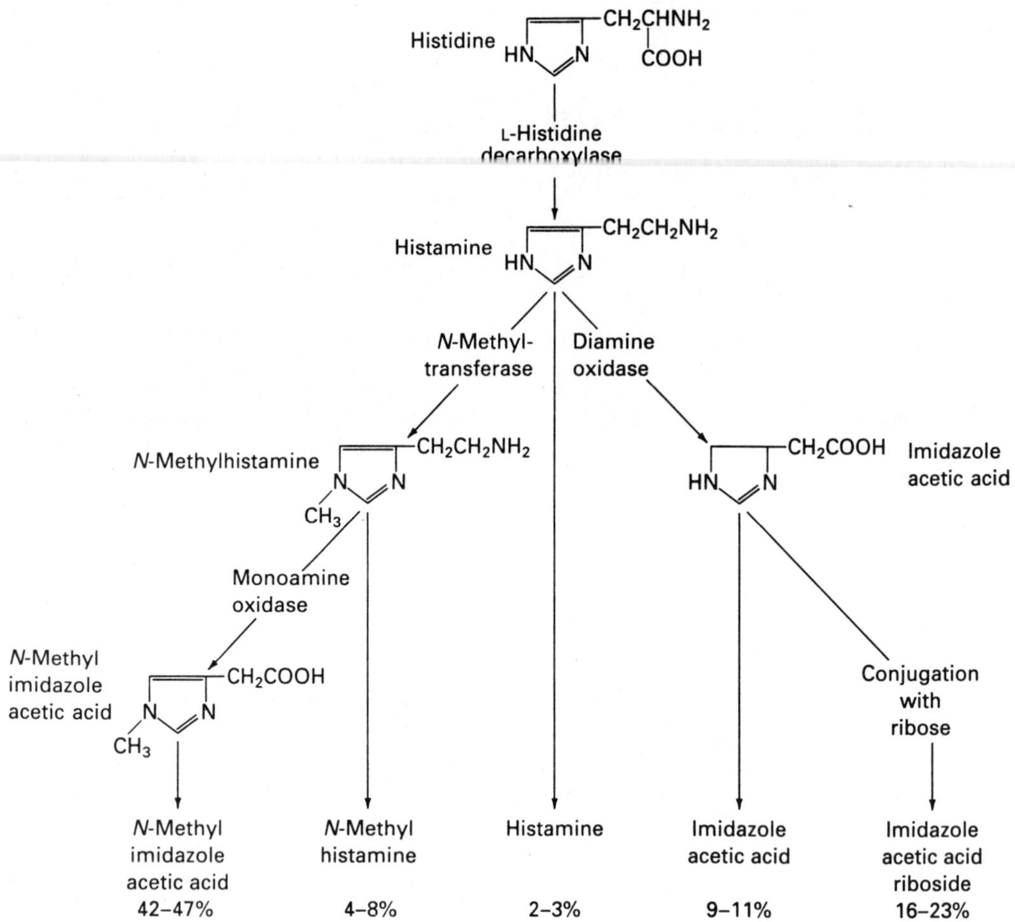

FIGURE 13-1 *Pathways of histamine synthesis and catabolism. Major urinary metabolites are listed at the bottom.*

of storage is the basophil (the cytologic counterpart of the tissue mast cell), in which histamine is bound to chondroitin sulfate. Generally, histamine becomes pharmacologically active only when released from storage sites. There is scarcely a tissue or organ which does not contain some histamine. Those especially rich in histamine include the gastrointestinal tract, lungs, and skin. Smaller amounts are found in the heart, liver, neural tissue, and reproductive mucosa. Furthermore, histamine has also been detected in bodily fluids, e.g., gastric juice, blood, urine, blister fluid, nasal washings, and pus.

Metabolism and Fate

There are two major enzymatic pathways for the metabolism of histamine (Fig. 13-1). Whereas only 2 to 3 percent of histamine is excreted unchanged in the urine, deamination with diamine oxidase (histaminase) and methylation via histamine N-methyltransferase account for the bulk of histamine biotransformation. Ring N-methylation transfers a methyl group from S-adenosylmethionine to histamine in the presence of N-methyltransferase (in the small intestine, liver, kidney, and monocytes). N-methylhistamine is either excreted in small amounts (4 to 8 percent) or is deaminated subsequently by monoamine oxidase to form N-methylimidazole acetic acid, which is the principal urinary metabolite of histamine in humans (42 to 47 percent). The other major catabolic pathway involves oxidative deamination of histamine by diamine oxidase (in the small intestinal mucosa, liver, skin, kidney, thymus, and leukocytes) to produce imidazole acetic acid, which is either excreted (9 to 11 percent) or conjugated with ribose and excreted in the urine as imidazole acetic acid riboside (16 to 23 percent). It is interesting that histamine is the only known compound to be metabolized by conjugation with ribose, although the relative importance of this step is unclear.

Release and Inhibitors of Release

The liberation of endogenous histamine and other autacoids can be stimulated by a wide variety of conditions. Perhaps the most important mechanism for the induction of mast cell and basophil granule extrusion (exocytosis) and subsequent histamine release is immunologic. During anaphylaxis and allergy, the specific interaction of an antigen with immunoglobulin E (IgE) antibody, attached to the surface of mast cells and basophils, triggers a cascade of biochemical events leading to mediator release without cell membrane disruption (Table 13-1). This "histamine hypothesis" of mediating immediate hypersensitivity reactions has achieved wide acceptance. The secretory behavior of histamine-containing cells is similar to that of exocrine and endocrine gland cells in which an increase in the concentration of intracellular calcium initiates stimulus-secretion coupling.

TABLE 13-1 Important biochemical events triggered by antigen-antibody interactions on mast cells and basophils

Activation of proteases
Influx of extracellular calcium ions via specific membrane channels
Activation of phospholipase A_2 and metabolism of arachidonic acid
Methylation of phospholipids
Altered levels of intracellular cyclic nucleotides
Phosphorylation of a specific protein
Release of histamine and other mediators from the cells

Individual sensitivity to this immunologic stimulus varies from species to species and among individuals. In sensitized persons, histamine will be produced along with a number of other key mediators of allergy and inflammation, e.g., leukotrienes C_4, D_4, and E_4 (constituents of slow-reacting substance of anaphylaxis, "SRS-A"); prostaglandin D_2; thromboxane A_2; bradykinin; ECF-A; neutrophil chemotactic factor; and platelet-activating factor. These mediators and certain enzymes, e.g., superoxide dismutase and neutral proteases, contribute directly or indirectly to the signs and symptoms of allergic disease.

There are many diverse classes of compounds which can liberate histamine without prior sensitization by affecting the integrity of the mast cell membrane so that the cell loses histamine from its granules. These include: enzymes (phospholipase A_2, chymotrypsin), venoms (cobra venom), organic bases (morphine, tubocurarine), and macromolecular polymers (dextran). Clinically, the actions of some of the above substances may account for unexpected anaphylactoid reactions. In addition, tissue injury may release histamine from storage sites, possibly through the action of released endogenous polypeptides, such as bradykinin.

Histamine release is blocked by various esterase inhibitors (e.g., isoflurophate), inhibitors of enzymes involved in energy production (e.g., fluoride ion), and other interfering agents (e.g., nicotinamide is a chymotrypsin inhibitor).

Cromolyn sodium is a drug which is presently employed as adjunct therapy in the management of allergic bronchial asthma. It is purported to behave as an inhibitor of mast cell degranulation, perhaps by stabilizing mast cell membranes and, therefore, is used prophylactically to prevent histamine release during allergic provocations; however, its clinical efficacy must also depend on other, as yet unknown, pharmacologic activities since a number of more effective and more potent mast cell stabilizers have failed clinically. The pharmacology of cromolyn sodium is discussed in depth in Chapter 33.

Histamine Receptors

The actions of histamine have been shown to be mediated through three separate and distinct membrane binding sites designated as H_1, H_2, and H_3 receptors (Table 13-2). The presence of more than one receptor was first suggested by the observation that the antihistamine mepyramine (pyrilamine) could block histamine-induced con-

TABLE 13-2 Differentiation of histamine receptor types

Receptor	Some Effects	Agonists[a]	Antagonists
H_1	Contraction of bronchial and intestinal smooth muscle Vasodilation and increased capillary permeability Pruritus Neurotransmission in the CNS	2-Methylhistamine 2-Thiazoylethylamine 2-Pyridylethylamine	Chlorpheniramine Diphenhydramine Pyrilamine
H_2	Gastric acid secretion Vasodilation Inhibition of neutrophil activation Inhibition of T cell cytotoxicity Neurotransmission in the CNS	4-Methylhistamine Dimaprit Impromidine	Cimetidine Ranitidine Famotidine Nizatidine
H_3	Neurotransmission in the CNS	(R) α-Methylhistamine	Thioperamide[a]

[a] All experimental compounds

tractions of the guinea pig ileum but not affect gastric acid secretions; subsequently the presence of H_2 receptors was confirmed, and the first H_2 receptor antagonists were discovered. Activation of H_1 receptors produces smooth muscle contraction and increases in microvascular permeability, which are blocked by "classical" antihistamines, e.g., pyrilamine, diphenhydramine, and chlorpheniramine. Stimulation of H_2 receptors mediates an increase in gastric acid secretion which is refractory to H_1 receptor antagonists but is sensitive to blockade by H_2 receptor antagonists, as exemplified by cimetidine, ranitidine, famotidine, and nizatidine. It appears that H_3 receptors only exist in the central nervous system.

There are some effects of histamine which are mediated by combined H_1 and H_2 receptor stimulation, including vasodilation, flushing, tachycardia, and headache. There are also species differences in the distribution of receptors, e.g., histamine contracts the uterus in most species (through H_1 receptors) but relaxes the uterus in the rat (an H_2 receptor effect). In addition, whereas the mouse and rat are highly resistant to the effects of histamine, the guinea pig and humans are extremely sensitive.

The availability and applicability of highly selective H_1 and H_2 receptor agonists and antagonists have provided the necessary tools to unravel the complex physiology and pathophysiology of histamine and to provide new pharmacotherapy for certain diseases.

Mechanism of Action

Molecular mechanisms underlying the actions of histamine on target cell responses have been the subject of intensive study. Although inhibition of adenylate cyclase has been suggested, the intracellular signaling mechanism associated with H_3 receptors has not been elucidated. The mechanism of action of histamine acting through H_1 and H_2 receptors is greatly dependent on the tissue and the type(s) of histamine receptor involved.

Altered ionic fluxes subsequent to an increase in cell membrane permeability can account for some stimulatory effects of histamine. For example, facilitation of ionic calcium entry down its electrochemical gradient or the mobilization of intracellular calcium stores may provide the link to histamine-induced smooth and cardiac muscle contraction. The positive inotropic effects in mammalian hearts, gastric acid secretion, and inhibition of basophil secretion are attributable to calcium ion influx and the elevation of intracellular cyclic AMP, effects which are blocked by H_2 receptor antagonists. Thus, intracellular levels of free calcium are a key to the regulation of contraction and secretion. Relaxation of smooth muscle is also associated with H_2 receptor activation and a rise in cyclic AMP, while contraction involves H_1 receptors and a rise in cyclic GMP.

H_1 receptors appear to be linked to phospholipase C; receptor activation results in an increase in intracellular formation of inositol-1,4,5-trisphosphate (IP_3), and 1,2-diacylglycerol. IP_3 binds to a receptor located on the endoplasmic reticulum, initiating the release of calcium into the cytosol, where it activates calcium-dependent protein kinases; diacylglycerol activates protein kinase C. H_2 receptors are associated with adenylate cyclase and stimulation of these receptors increases the cytosolic concentration of cyclic AMP and activation of cyclic AMP-dependent protein kinase.

Additionally, H_1 receptor stimulation may activate phospholipase A_2 and trigger the arachidonic acid cascade leading to prostaglandin production. Since different prostaglandins have variable effects on cyclic nucleotide accumulation, this complicates the measurement of any direct effect of histamine. Furthermore, in vascular smooth muscle, activation of H_1 receptors leads to the formation of endothelium-derived relaxing factor (EDRF), which in turn activates guanylate cyclase, increases cyclic GMP levels, activates cyclic GMP-dependent protein kinase, and reduces intracellular calcium ion concentrations. Thus vascular smooth muscle relaxation by histamine is believed to involve this pathway.

In bi-directional control systems found in a number of tissues, the signal transduction process that promotes a turnover of inositol phopholipids activates cellular functions, whereas the signal that raises cyclic AMP usually antagonizes such activation. Thus electrolyte, biochemical, and mechanical events are all linked in a complex process during stimulus-response coupling. See Chapter 3 for a more complete discussion of these intracellular signal transduction mechanisms.

Effects on Tissues

The most important pharmacologic actions of histamine are manifested principally on the cardiovascular system, extravascular smooth muscle, exocrine glands (especially the acid-secreting cells of the gastric mucosa), and neural processes.

Cardiovascular System The most prominent cardiovascular effects of histamine include an immediate fall in systemic blood pressure, flushing, and a lowering of peripheral resistance as a result of vasodilation of microcirculatory vessels (arterioles and capillaries). Histamine ranks among the most potent capillary vasodilators. This effect involves both H_1 and H_2 receptor activation and occurs diffusely throughout most vascular beds. H_1 receptors respond to low histamine concentrations in a rapid, short-lived fashion, whereas H_2 receptor activation leads to a slowly developing, yet more sustained, vasodilation. Thus, capillary vasodilator effects of histamine are completely blocked only by a combination of H_1 and H_2 receptor antagonists. Vasodilatation is most prominent in the skin and upper body as it produces heat, itching, and flushing ("blushing"). When cranial blood vessels dilate to histamine, abrupt and severe "cluster" headaches (also called *histamine headache* or *histamine cephalgia*) occur which are unilateral and involve the eye, temple, neck, and face.

Histamine also produces an increase in capillary permeability. Transudation of plasma and plasma macromolecules from vascular compartments to extracellular spaces in response to histamine occurs at postcapillary venules and is due to alterations in permeability manifested as increased hydrostatic pressure (venoconstriction) and enlarged endothelial intercellular spaces or gaps. This passage of fluid and proteins causes edema formation, a major component of the "triple response." This characteristic triad of reactions to intradermal histamine was described over 65 years ago and is composed of sequential localized vascular effects: (1) rapid reddening around the site of histamine injection ("erythema") resulting from direct local microcirculatory vasodilation, (2) bright red, diffusely shaped areas of hyperemia ("flare") around the initial erythema resulting from localized axonal reflex-induced arteriolar vasodilation, and (3) localized edema ("wheal") due to increased microvascular permeability. The triple response can also be induced by intradermal antigen in sensitized individuals, physical trauma, cold or thermal injury, or the injection of histamine liberators.

On the heart, histamine produces mechanical (positive inotropic and chronotropic) and electrophysiologic (slowed AV conduction) changes which are mediated by H_2 and H_1 receptors, respectively. Thus, cardiac pathophysiology due to either histamine or immediate hypersensitivity reactions should be effectively controlled by a combination of H_1 and H_2 receptor antagonists.

Smooth Muscle Nonvascular smooth muscle tone is generally stimulated in response to histamine (an H_1 receptor-mediated effect); however, depending on the species and the tissue studied, responses may vary greatly. Bronchial smooth muscle of humans is especially sensitive; indeed, even small amounts of histamine will provoke a marked bronchoconstriction in asthmatics and in patients with other hyperreactive airway diseases.

Although airway constriction involves direct H_1 receptor activation, histamine is also capable of triggering a localized reflex cholinergic discharge by stimulating afferent vagal nerve endings.

With regard to other smooth muscles, the human uterus responds poorly to histamine; smooth muscle of the urinary bladder, gallbladder, intestine, and iris are inconsistently and weakly stimulated by histamine.

Exocrine Glands Histamine is a potent stimulant of gastric acid and pepsin secretion, but a weak and relatively unimportant secretagogue for other exocrine glands, including salivary, bronchial, pancreatic, lacrimal, and intestinal mucosal glands. Its principal effect on gastric acid secretion results from a direct effect on parietal cell H_2 receptors. This can have important physiologic and pathophysiologic ramifications. As little as 0.025 mg injected subcutaneously will produce copious increases in acid secretion without evoking other histamine responses. Excessive production of acid induced by histamine (as in ulcers) is effectively reduced with H_2 receptor antagonists, e.g., ranitidine, which is discussed later in this chapter.

Peripheral Nerve Endings Histamine stimulates various sensory and autonomic nerve endings. The stimulation of sensory nerve endings is most conspicuous in the epidermis and dermis where itching and pain result. Together with its effect on capillaries (dilation and increased permeability), histamine-induced sensory nerve stimulation is responsible for the triple response (described previously) and for some indirect effects on the heart and lungs.

Stimulation of autonomic nerve endings in the adrenal medulla is probably responsible for histamine-induced release of the catecholamines epinephrine and norepinephrine into the bloodstream. Whereas this adrenal discharge is insufficient to block the direct vasodepressor response to the intravenous infusion of histamine in normal individuals, patients with functional pheochromocytoma respond with a rise in blood pressure following even a modest dose of histamine.

Central Nervous System The brain contains histamine, L-histidine decarboxylase, and diamine oxidase, and the thalamus, hypothalamus, cerebellum, and forebrain have high concentrations of H_1 receptors. Although little is known about the actual physiologic role of histamine in the central nervous system, it is believed that neurons containing the compound participate in temperature regulation, the perception of pain, the secretion of antidiuretic hormone, and the regulation of blood pressure. Histaminergic nerve terminal contain H_3 receptors, that are believed to play a role in the regulation of the neuronal synthesis and release of histamine.

Histamine does not penetrate the blood-brain barrier very well; however, when injected directly into the cerebral ventricles, histamine seems to stimulate both H_1 and H_2 receptors leading to a variety of effects, including changes in heart rate, blood pressure, body temperature, and state of arousal.

Tissue Growth and Repair Tissues which are undergoing rapid growth or repair, e.g., embryonic tissue, malignant growths, bone marrow, and wound and granulation tissue, have an extraordinarily high histamine-forming capacity to enhance growth. Newly formed ("nascent") histamine appears to function in a facilitative fashion in the anabolic processes to accelerate reparative growth, but its precise role is still unknown.

Immunoreactivity Histamine binds to T cells by specific receptor interactions, especially involving the H_2 receptor. As a result, intracellular levels of cyclic AMP are elevated and T cell-mediated cytotoxicity is blocked. In addition, H_2 receptor activation suppresses lymphocyte proliferation and the release of cytokines, inhibits E rosette formation, and stimulates T cells to release suppressor factors. Histamine also binds to H_1 receptors on T lymphocytes to inhibit suppressor cell function. With regard to other immunologic cells, histamine can reduce mast cell and basophil secretory capacity by increasing intracellular levels of cyclic AMP via H_2 receptor activation.

Diagnostic Uses

There are no therapeutic uses for histamine. It can be used in small doses (0.0275 mg/kg as the phosphate salt) by subcutaneous injection for the diagnosis of gastric function, i.e., to test the ability of the gastric mucosa to produce hydrochloric acid; however, it is not frequently used anymore. Rather, more selective H_2 receptor agonists, e.g., impromidine (available in Canada and the United Kingdom), may be used instead, and also pentagastrin is now more commonly used to test for achlorhydria. Pentagastrin is the C-terminal tetrapeptide of the natural gastrins, that act as the physiologic secretogogue for gastric acid.

Another application of histamine phosphate is as a provocative test for pheochromocytoma; however, it is indicated only for the occasional patient with paroxysmal signs of excessive catecholamine secretion.

Symptoms of Histamine Toxicity

The symptoms of histamine toxicity can be easily predicted on the basis of its pharmacologic activities. The primary finding is a precipitous fall in blood pressure accompanied by generalized vasodilation with a rise in skin temperature, headache, and visual disturbances. Smooth muscle stimulation leads to bronchoconstriction, dyspnea, and diarrhea. Additional effects noted are vomiting and a metallic taste. In severe cases, shock may supervene, and appropriate measures must be taken to treat this serious complication.

In general, non-shock cases can best be treated with epinephrine. Antihistamines (H_1 receptor antagonists) do not provide adequate therapy in cases of severe histamine toxicity because their effect develops too slowly to cope with life-threatening toxicity and also because many histamine actions, e.g., bronchoconstriction, are complicated by concomitant effects of other endogenous substances (e.g., prostaglandins, leukotrienes, kinins, ECF-A) which are released at the same time as histamine and are not antagonized by antihistamines.

H_1 RECEPTOR ANTAGONISTS

Prior to the elucidation of different types of histamine receptors in the 1970s, only one group of drugs were known to block the effects of histamine and these were commonly referred to as the *antihistamines*. Although the term *antihistamine* can refer to any compound that blocks H_1, H_2, or H_3 receptors, it has become commonplace to use this term when referring to the H_1 receptor antagonists.

Antihistamines were initially discovered in the late 1930s by investigators who reported that some amines with a phenolic ether substitution (1) afforded striking protection to guinea pigs from lethal doses of histamine, (2) lessened the symptoms of experimental anaphylactic shock, and (3) blocked histamine-induced contractions in a variety of smooth muscles *in vitro*. Although the original antihistamines were too toxic for clinical use, these compounds led to future successes with more acceptable derivatives, which were competitive and reversible antagonists, e.g., pyrilamine. Shortly thereafter, some highly effective histamine antagonists, diphenhydramine and tripelennamine, were developed, and by the 1950s there was a proliferation of these kinds of drugs.

Chemistry

Most conventional H_1 receptor antagonists resemble histamine structurally by sharing a substituted ethylamine side chain; however, they also have two aromatic moieties and are represented by the general formula shown in Table 13-3, where Ar_1 and Ar_2 are carbocyclic or heterocyclic aromatic rings, one or both of which may be separated from X by a carbon atom, where X is oxygen, carbon, or nitrogen connecting the ethylamine side chain to the rings. R_1 and R_2 represent alkyl substitutions, usually methyl groups. As an example, the structure of chlorpheniramine, one of the most widely used antihistamines, is shown below.

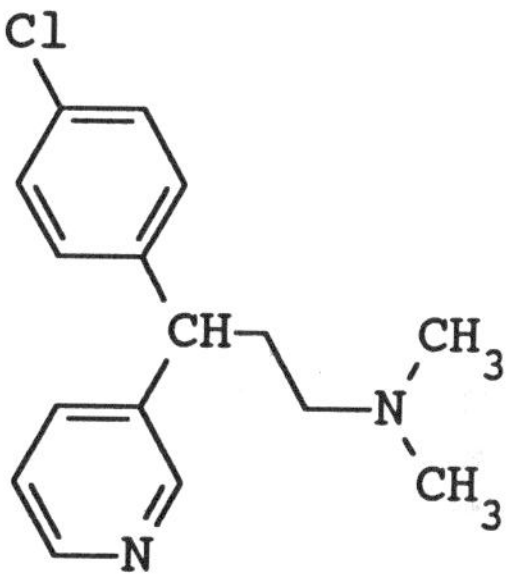

Cl

CH

CH_3

N

CH_3

N

Chlorpheniramine

Mechanism of Action

All of these compounds are competitive, reversible antagonists of histamine at H_1 receptors; they have no significant activity on H_2 receptors. Furthermore, these antihistamines only reduce or block the effects, not the synthesis, release, or metabolism of histamine. All the H_1 receptor antagonists block, to varying degrees, most effects of histamine on different organs and systems of the body and can afford protection against allergic and anaphylactic reactions. By themselves these agents exert little, if any, significant direct effects; by virtue of their affinity to H_1 receptors, they are therapeutically beneficial in antagonizing responses to histamine. Therefore,

TABLE 13-3 Structural classes and representative examples of H_1 receptor antagonists

$$\begin{matrix} Ar_1 & & & & & R_1 \\ & X & -C- & -C- & N & \\ Ar_2 & & & & & R_2 \end{matrix}$$

Structural classes	"X"	Examples
Ethylenediamines	$>N-$	Pyrilamine (mepyramine) Tripelennamine
Aminoalkylethers	$-O-$	Diphenhydramine Dimenhydrinate Clemastine
Alkylamines	$>CH-$	Chlorpheniramine Dexchlorpheniramine Brompheniramine Triprolidine
Piperazines	—N(piperazine ring)N— (Nitrogen in conjunction with a piperazine ring)	Meclizine Cyclizine Hydroxyzine
Phenothiazines	S, N— phenothiazine ring (Nitrogen in conjunction with a phenothiazine ring)	Promethazine Trimeprazine
Others	[contain different substitutions]	Cyproheptadine Terfenadine Astemizole Loratidine

antihistaminic effects are noted only in the presence of increased histamine activity. Although there are clearly differences in the relative potencies of these drugs when examined under different conditions, they do have comparable effects and therapeutic utility when considered as a group.

Effects

Smooth Muscle Most smooth muscle responses to histamine are blocked (or reduced) by H_1 receptor antagonists. For example, these compounds can inhibit histamine-induced constriction of intestinal and respiratory smooth muscle. The therapeutic utility of these classic antihistamines against anaphylactic bronchospasm in human asthma remains controversial. A variety of mediators (including histamine) are implicated in asthma and other chronic obstructive pulmonary diseases, e.g., leukotrienes, platelet-activating factor, ECF-A, and acetylcholine. To date, H_1 receptor antagonists have been remarkably ineffective or only of limited value in these more severe respiratory diseases.

With regard to vascular smooth muscle, the vasoconstrictor effects of histamine (H_1-mediated) can be blocked with these drugs, whereas a combination of H_1 and H_2 receptor antagonists are required for complete suppression of histamine-mediated vasodilation and hypotension.

Vascular Permeability The ability of systemic or local histamine, allergic cutaneous reactions, or anaphylaxis to produce vasodilation and increased capillary permeability, resulting in edema and wheal formation at the tissue site, can be prevented or antagonized by these antihistamines. Also, localized edema produced by various mechanical or chemical means and by inflammation can be reduced or blocked by these drugs, which may be acting directly on vascular and sensory nerve ending H_1 receptors or by actions against other mediators, e.g., acetylcholine and 5-hydroxytryptamine, or by a local anesthetic effect. For example, some compounds of the phenothiazine class (e.g., promethazine) as well as the piperidine derivative cyproheptadine (see below) have both histamine and 5-hydroxytryptamine receptor blocking activities, which may afford clinical advantages in the treatment of cutaneous allergies with itching.

Immediate Hypersensitivity Type I immediate hypersensitivity reactions, which include allergy and anaphylaxis, involve a number of autacoids, but the role of histamine as a primary mediator is universally accepted. Activated tissue-based mast cells and circulating basophils are the predominant cell sources which release histamine during type I immediate hypersensitivity reactions in quantities more than sufficient to account for much of the symptomatology of allergy and anaphylaxis. The relative importance of histamine versus other mediators can vary with the tissue and species examined, and therefore, the therapeutic benefit of H_1 receptor antagonists may also be variable. Whereas these drugs are valuable in treating edema formation, itching, rhinorrhea, and lacrimation, they are less effective in controlling hypotension and allergic bronchoconstriction.

Central Nervous System The effects of H_1 receptor antagonists on the central nervous system (CNS) are complex and dose-related. Depression of the CNS by therapeutic doses of most antihistamines will lead to varying degrees of diminished alertness, slowed reaction time, muscle weakness, mild sedation, and even somnolence. Some antagonists are more prone to produce these CNS manifestations than others, and patients seem to vary in susceptibility and responsiveness. The aminoalkyl ethers are especially liable to produce sedation; for example, diphenhydramine can produce drowsiness in 20 to 50 percent of the patients.

In some circumstances, physicians may take advantage of this sedative effect and prescribe the drug for patients with allergies who are also having problems sleeping. Most over-the-counter (OTC) preparation that aid in sleeping contain diphenhydramine. However, there are always dangers inherent in this type of self-medication in that the patient may neglect to seek a proper medical diagnosis.

Paradoxically, antihistamines may occasionally produce CNS stimulation even within a therapeutic dosage range, although stimulation occurs less frequently than sedation. This is manifested as restlessness, nervousness, hyperexcitability, and insomnia. Very small doses may provoke activation of the EEG, agitation, delirium, tremors, and epileptic seizures in some patients with focal CNS lesions. Infants may present with sensory and motor disturbances (convulsions) after poisoning with H_1 receptor antagonists, which is followed by depression or paralysis of the medullary-pontine cardiovascular and respiratory centers.

The specific mechanism by which these drugs produce CNS depression and excitation is unclear at present. They might be blocking responses to endogenously released histamine in the CNS, since these antagonists have been shown to be capable of high binding affinity to H_1 receptors in the brain. Alternatively, some compounds may replace α rhythms in the EEG with slow wave activity in the 3 to 4 per second range. Regardless, there does not appear to be a correlation between peripheral antihistaminic effectiveness and CNS activity.

The most important clinical advance in this field has been the development of "new generation" non-sedating antihistamines, which either do not enter the CNS or cross the blood-brain barrier only with great difficulty. Three of these newer antihistamines with reduced or minimal sedative liability are *terfenadine*, *astemizole*, and *loratadine*.

Terfenadine was the first of this new class of pharmacologically distinct, specific, peripherally acting H_1 receptor antagonists. It has no significant effect on α- or β-adrenergic receptors and is relatively free of 5-hydroxytryptamine and acetylcholine blocking activities and local anesthetic activity. Whereas antihistaminic activity is comparable to chlorpheniramine, terfenadine reportedly produces little, if any, characteristic depression of the EEG, behavioral effects, or impairment of motor function seen frequently with the older compounds. Although terfenadine may have equal affinity for peripheral and central H_1 receptors, it is thought to penetrate the blood-brain barrier poorly at effective therapeutic doses and, hence, produces a low incidence of CNS effects. Astemizole also has a high degree of H_1 receptor specificity, with little muscarinic, adrenergic, or other receptor activity. Loratadine may be less sedating because of either reduced ability to cross the blood-brain barrier or selective binding to peripheral rather than central H_1 receptors.

Diphenhydramine has been shown to have significant antitussive (cough suppressing) activity, probably mediated through an action on the cough center in the medulla. Whether this effect occurs through histaminic receptor blockade, an interaction with another receptor, or a sedative effect is unknown.

Another potentially useful CNS effect of some antihistamines is the ability to block emesis and motion sickness (car, sea, or air sickness). This activity is especially prominent with promethazine, diphenhydramine, dimenhydrinate (a salt of diphenhydramine), and meclizine. These drugs are helpful in alleviating most symptoms of disturbed equilibrium with minimal side effects. Perhaps promethazine owes its anti-motion sickness activity to the fact that it shows greater blockade of cholinergic muscarinic receptors than other antihistamines. The anticholinergic scopolamine is considered to be the most effective drug for the prophylaxis and treatment of motion sickness and other labyrinthine disturbances, such as Meniere's disease (see Chapter 11).

Anticholinergic Many H_1 receptor antagonists have some capacity to inhibit responses to cholinergic muscarinic and 5-hydroxytryptamine receptor activation, but these ancillary effects do not appear to be related to antihistamine activity or potency. The atropine-like actions are prominent enough to be useful clinically, such as in drying of excessive secretions in patients with allergic rhinitis. Among the classic antihistamines, diphenhydramine and promethazine have high anticholinergic activity; the one least with the least anticholinergic activity is pyrilamine.

Local Anesthesia Most of the known H_1 receptor antagonists exert some degree of local anesthetic action. Numerous clinical studies have been performed using ointments or solutions containing diphenhydramine, tripelennamine, promethazine, or pyrilamine; however, much higher concentrations are required for local anesthesia than for antagonizing responses to histamine. In fact, some of these drugs have been shown to be more potent than procaine in comparative tests, but are limited for use in minor surgical procedures by the incidence of mild-to-moderate irritation or the potential for local sensitization. They can be used locally for relief of itching and discomfort where the anesthetic component complements the antiallergic and antipruritic actions.

Pharmacokinetics

As a class, H_1 receptor antagonists are well absorbed from the gastrointestinal tract following oral administration. With most, effects begin within 30 min, peak within 1 to 2 h, and last approximately 3 to 6 h. Some drugs have a longer duration of action; for example, terfenadine and astemizole are effective for 12 to 24 hours. Extensive pharmacokinetic data are available on only a few of these drugs. For example, blood levels of diphenhydramine reach a maximum approximately 2 h after an oral dose and decrease exponentially with a plasma elimination half-life of 4 h. The drug is widely distributed through bodily tissues (including the CNS) and is biotransformed in the liver to inactive products, and these are excreted via the kidney within 24 h. Tripelennamine and other classical antihistamines have similar pharmacokinetic properties and are usually prescribed in doses which must be repeated every 4 h. These drugs are also capable of inducing liver microsomal enzymes which may facilitate their own metabolism.

Following oral administration, terfenadine undergoes extensive first pass biotransformation to two primary products: an inactive dealkylated metabolite and an active, acid metabolite (which has approximately 30 percent of the histamine receptor blocking activity of terfenadine). The oral bioavailability of terfenadine is low and in normal individuals plasma levels may be undetectable; therefore, a significant portion of the activity of the drug is dependent upon the accumulation of the active acid metabolite in the plasma. The plasma protein binding of the parent drug is 97 percent and that of the acid metabolite is 70 percent. Following biotransformation, 60 percent of an oral dose of terfenadine is eliminated in the feces, while 40 percent is excreted via the urine (mainly as metabolites in both cases). Terfenadine is longer lasting than most other antihistamines and is usually administered twice daily.

Loratadine is biotransformed to an active product (descarboethoxyloratadine) and astemizole is converted to active, hydroxylated derivatives (mainly desmethylastemizole). The plasma half-lives of loratadine, astemizole, and their active metabolites are 12 to 15 h and drug elimination occurs approximately equally through the feces and urine. Both loratadine and astemizole are used orally once a day.

Adverse Effects

The predominant central action of most H_1 receptor antagonists is sedation, but in children and some adults, agitation, nervousness, delirium, tremors, incoordination, hallucinations, and convulsions may occur. Sedation usually occurs within the therapeutic dose range for antihistaminic action and varies from diminished alertness and impaired ability to concentrate to muscle weakness and pronounced drowsiness. This effect interferes with daytime activities; patients are usually advised not to drive motor vehicles, operate heavy equipment and machinery, or imbibe alcohol or other CNS depressants, which would be additive or, perhaps, synergistic.

Lesser side effects may manifest on the digestive tract, i.e., anorexia, nausea, vomiting, diarrhea or constipation, and epigastric distress. These are reduced if the drug is given with meals. Other untoward effects include: dryness of the mouth, throat and airways; cardiac palpitations; hypotension; urinary retention; headache; faintness; tightness in the chest; and visual disturbances. (Many of these may be accounted for by atropine-like effects.) Because they can also release histamine or induce hypersensitivity of the skin, topical antihistamines can produce drug allergy (urticaria, dermatitis, photosensitization).

Laboratory animal teratogenesis has been observed with some piperazine derivatives (e.g., cyclizine and meclizine). Even though this has not been demonstrated in humans, administration of antihistamines to pregnant women is discouraged.

Rare cases of severe cardiovascular adverse effects, including prolongation of the QT interval, torsade de pointes, other ventricular arrhythmias, cardiac arrest, and death, have occurred in patients with high blood levels of terfenadine or astemizole. The use of these antihistamines is contraindicated in patients with hepatic dysfunction, in combination with other drugs known to prolong the QT interval (e.g., probucol, certain antiarrhythmics, tricyclic antidepressants, and calcium channel blockers), in combination with drugs other similar chemical structure (e.g., ketoconazole, itraconazole, and miconazole), or concomitant administration of macrolide antibiotics (e.g., erythromycin and clarithromycin).

In general, antihistamines possess a high therapeutic index such that it is rare to observe serious acute toxicity from their use. However, widespread use as self-medication or accidental overdose by children can lead to serious events as described earlier. Acute toxicity can culminate in coma, cardiorespiratory collapse, marked hyperthermia, and death within 2 to 15 h. Treatment is symptomatic and consists of supportive therapy with artificial ventilation.

Therapeutic Uses

Many physicians familiar with the advantages and disadvantages of each of the H_1 receptor antagonists prefer to have a working pool for selection and variation as indicated by individual patient needs in terms of efficacy and side effects. Few other classes of drugs possess such a depth in type and number for choice by the physician and acceptance by the patient.

Allergic diseases represent a complex series

of disorders with acute and chronic manifestations which may vary from mild urticaria or rhinitis to severe and possibly fatal anaphylaxis. It is estimated that approximately 10 percent of the population may suffer from some form of allergy. Therapy directed toward removal or avoidance of the offending allergen from the environment and specific patient desensitization is not always practical or successful. In a number of allergies, the causative allergen cannot be demonstrated; also, associated chronic infection and inflammation often complicate therapy. Therefore, symptomatic management with a variety of drugs has been exceptionally beneficial. H_1 receptor antagonists have earned their deserved, time-proven place, acceptance, and value in treating immediate hypersensitivity reactions, especially seasonal hay fever, allergic rhinitis, dermatoses, and conjunctivitis.

Allergic Rhinitis Antihistamines are especially effective in ameliorating the sneezing, rhinorrhea, and itching of the eyes, nose, and throat in most patients with seasonal allergic rhinitis and conjunctivitis (hay fever and pollinosis). They can be also used in combination with decongestants, e.g., phenylephrine or pseudoephedrine, and/or desensitization procedures. When exposure to the sensitizing allergen is prolonged or when nasal congestion is very prominent, these drugs become less effective. Similarly, they may only be of limited benefit in vasomotor rhinitis.

Dermatoses Both acute and chronic urticaria respond well to antihistamines, although the effect is more striking in acute disorders. The pruritus and wheals are usually resolved rapidly in a high percentage of patients. Angioedema (angioneurotic edema) also responds favorably, but when the larynx is involved, epinephrine must also be used as a life-saving measure. In patients with atopic dermatitis, contact dermatitis, insect bites, stings, and poison ivy, these drugs are particularly useful in treating the itch (local anesthetic properties may also be operative here), while topical corticosteroids treat the inflammation. The CNS depressant effects of most oral H_1 receptor antagonists may reduce the urge to scratch by decreasing the associated anxiety. Urticarial and edematous lesions of serum sickness also respond well to these drugs, but joint involvement and fever may require additional therapy. Caution should be exercised with individuals who may have a tendency to develop sensitization (allergic dermatitis) to topical application of these drugs.

Bronchial Asthma Although normal daily doses of classic antihistamines have been ineffective in treating bronchial asthma, higher doses may have been effective but could not be used because of limiting adverse side effects, such as sedation. This issue may finally be nearing resolution with the advent of the newer, long-lasting drugs, e.g., terfenadine, astemizole, and loratadine. Their effectiveness (or lack of same) in asthma is presently undergoing intensive worldwide clinical investigations to determine just how important histamine really is as a mediator of bronchial asthma. Until this issue is resolved, the utility of these compounds in asthma remains unproven.

Common Cold Antihistamines are generally considered as simple palliative therapy in treating the common cold. They will not cure the cold, which is of viral origin, but they will affect any concomitant allergic component (such as nasal discharge and sneezing). When combined with other traditional agents, antihistamines will provide some degree of symptomatic relief against the common cold, while producing only mild, if any, side effects.

Motion Sickness and Emesis Antihistamines have been used extensively in the prophylaxis of motion sickness to prevent nausea and vomiting. This effect cannot be correlated with antihistaminic potency and is probably due to a nonspecific central effect. The most effective antihistamines used in motion sickness include dimenhydrinate, cyclizine, meclizine, and promethazine. Their effectiveness as general antiemetic compounds is less than that of chlorpromazine and other phenothiazines, yet they are useful in vestibular disturbances such as Meniere's disease.

Miscellaneous Uses There are several other uses of the H_1 receptor antagonists. *Insomnia* can be treated using diphenhydramine as a mild hypnotic in OTC sleep-inducing medications. The tremors and muscular rigidity of *Parkinson's disease* can be modestly reduced through the use of an antihistamine with high anticholinergic activity on the CNS (e.g., diphenhydramine) as an adjunct to other therapy for this condition (see Chapter 22). Mild *Symptomatic relief of anxiety and tension associated with psychoneuroses* is an indication for hydroxyzine. *Antitussive activity (cough suppression)* is afforded by diphenhydramine. Most compounds can be used to reduce *adverse reactions to intravenous X-ray contrast media* which induce histamine release.

H_2 RECEPTOR ANTAGONISTS

While the conventional antihistamines block many histamine-induced effects that occur via H_1 receptors, they fail to antagonize H_2 receptor-mediated events, e.g., gastric acid secretion. In 1977, cimetidine was introduced in the United States as the first H_2 receptor antagonist approved for clinical use and it revolutionized the management of peptic ulcer disease. Several years later, ranitidine, a chemically different H_2 receptor antagonist, was developed and marketed. Because of the significant benefits associated with these agents, two other H_2 receptor antagonists, famotidine and nizatidine, with minor pharmacologic differences from ranitidine, entered clinical medicine.

Chemistry

The structure of cimetidine (Fig. 13-2) consists of a methylimidazole ring and a long side chain containing a sulfur atom and a cyanoguanidine group. It was thought that the imidazole moiety, as found in histamine, was required for H_2 receptor blocking activity; however, this proved untrue since ranitidine has a substituted furan ring and famotidine and nizatidine are thiazole derivatives and all are highly effective H_2 receptor antagonists. All four compounds have a substituted methyl thioethyl side chain ($-CH_2SCH_2CH_2-$), which may be important for potent H_2 receptor blockade.

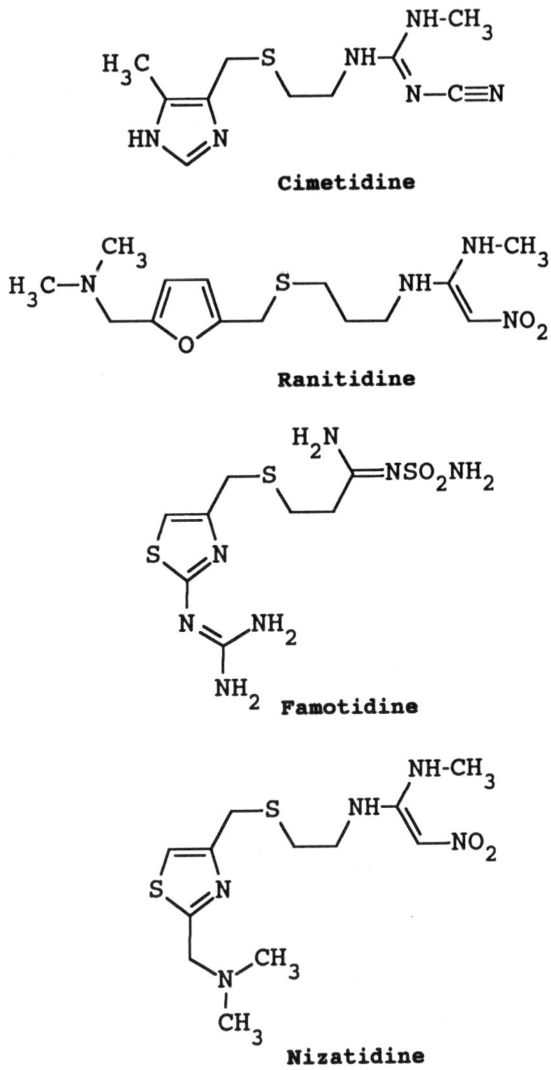

Cimetidine

Ranitidine

Famotidine

Nizatidine

FIGURE 13-2 *Structures of the H_2 receptor antagonists.*

Mechanism of Action

The H_2 receptor antagonists reversibly and competitively inhibit the actions of histamine on H_2 receptors in a dose-dependent fashion. They are pure antagonists, i.e., they have no agonistic activity. Numerous studies have lead to the conclusion that these drugs have no significant action at H_1 receptors, β-adrenergic receptors, or muscarinic receptors. Furthermore, neither the synthesis, release, or biotransformation of histamine is affected to any great extent by these compounds.

Effects

Although these drugs will block all H_2 receptor-mediated effects, the most important pharmacologic effect of these drugs is the ability to inhibit gastric acid secretion. All the drugs markedly reduce both daytime and nocturnal basal gastric secretory volume and acid output; gastric acid secretion induced by food, histamine, pentagastrin, insulin, and caffeine is also blocked. Pepsin secretion from the chief cells of gastric glands, which is mainly under cholinergic control, is reduced as the volume of gastric juice is lowered. These drugs do not appear to affect gastric motility or gastric emptying time, and alterations in gastric mucous secretion have not been observed.

Clinical data support the lack of significant pharmacodynamic differences between nizatidine 300 mg, cimetidine 800 mg, ranitidine 300 mg, and famotidine 40 mg (all administered orally at bedtime) in the acute therapy of peptic ulcer disease. On a weight basis, famotidine is more potent than the other drugs, but the efficacy of all four compounds in peptic ulcer disorders appears to be similar.

Pharmacokinetics

Table 13-4 summarizes some of the pharmacokinetic characteristics of cimetidine, ranitidine, famotidine, and nizatidine. Cimetidine and nizatidine are well absorbed from the gastrointestinal tract following oral administration; the oral absorption of ranitidine and famotidine are incomplete. Cimetidine undergoes extensive first pass biotransformation, while this is minimal with the other three compounds. Therefore, the oral bioavailability of nizatidine is greater than that of the other H_2 receptor antagonists. All drugs have a relatively low plasma protein binding, and their apparent volumes of distribution range from 1.0 to 1.9 L/kg. The elimination half-lives of these H_2 receptor antagonists are relatively short (from as short as 1.0 h for nizatidine to up to 3.5 h for famotidine).

The major biotransformation products of these drugs recovered in the urine are listed in Table 13-4. Approximately 50 percent of cimetidine is biotransformed (the sulfoxide is the major product); only a small percentage of the other drugs is metabolized. The only known active metabolite is monodesmethylnizatidine (which represents only 7 percent of the total nizatidine dose); it is 60 percent as active as the parent drug as an H_2 receptor antagonist.

For all these drugs the principal route of excretion is the urine. Renal elimination involves both glomerular filtration and tubular secretion. Precaution should be exercised when these compounds are administered to patients with renal insufficiency.

Adverse Reactions

In general, the H_2 receptor antagonists are remarkably safe agents, and side effects are usually moderate and reversible. These drugs infrequently produce headache, malaise, dizziness, constipation, diarrhea, skin rashes, and alterations of hepatic function. Various CNS disturbances, including somnolence, insomnia, confusion, and hallucinations, have been reported. Small elevations of plasma creatinine have occurred with cimetidine, and dosage adjustment for patients with impaired renal function is necessary.

Cimetidine and ranitidine may elevate serum prolactin concentrations, while famotidine and nizatidine have not shown this effect. Cimetidine binds to androgen receptors, an action which may be responsible for the sexual dysfunction (reduced libido and impotence) and gynecomastia which has been reported for this drug. These effects are only rarely, if ever, observed with the other drugs.

TABLE 13-4 Pharmacokinetic data for the H_2 receptor antagonists

Drug	Oral Bioavailability, %	Plasma protein binding, %	Half-life, h	Major metabolites	Renal clearance, mL/min
Cimetidine	60 to 70	20	1.8 to 2.0	Sulfoxide Hydroxymethyl	550
Ranitidine	50 to 60	15	2.0 to 3.0	N^2-oxide N^2-desmethyl S-oxide	600
Nizatidine	90 to 95	35	1.0 to 2.0	N^2-monodesmethyl N^2-oxide S-oxide	850
Famotidine	40 to 45	20	2.5 to 3.5	S-oxide	350

The frequency of these events appear greatest when cimetidine is administered in very high doses for the treatment of Zollinger-Ellison Syndrome.

Drug Interactions

Cimetidine reversibly inhibits the hepatic cytochrome P-450 system in either a competitive or noncompetitive manner, depending on the substrate, and therefore reduces phase I biotransformation reactions. This appears to be explained by the binding of the imidazole group to the heme portion of the enzyme, which is influenced by the lipophilicity of the molecule. Cimetidine does not inhibit phase II glucuronidation reactions. In contrast, ranitidine, famotidine, and nizatidine appear to have lower binding affinities to cytochrome P-450 and thus are only very weak inhibitors of drug metabolism. Therefore, cimetidine can interact with many drugs, thereby delaying their hepatic metabolism; for example, accumulation of the following drugs can occur: warfarin, phenytoin, theophylline, propranolol, diazepam, and phenobarbital. In contrast, none of the other three H_2 receptor antagonists affect P-450 drug metabolism to any significant extent.

By reducing gastric acid secretion, the absorption of drugs such as ketoconazole and clorazepate (enhanced at low stomach pH) is reduced by H_2 receptor blockers. In addition, antacids will reduce the bioavailability of cimetidine by 20 to 30 percent, and the administration of antacids and oral cimetidine should be separated by a 1 hour interval. Antacids may be given concomitantly with ranitidine, famotidine, and nizatidine.

Therapeutic Uses

The H_2 receptor antagonists are effective in the treatment of peptic acid disorders. They have proven to be invaluable in the treatment of duodenal ulcer disease because of their ability to lower basal and nocturnal gastric acid secretion. These agents also have proven to be effective therapy for the treatment of gastric ulcer, pathological hypersecretory conditions (e.g., Zollinger-Ellison Syndrome), and gastroesophageal reflux disease (GERD). All have been moderately effective in the prevention of duodenal ulcer recurrence.

All of these drugs can be administered orally and all except nizatidine are available for use by injection. Despite the relatively short elimination half-lives of these drugs, the duration of action is long, especially once plasma steady state conditions are attained, and once daily (often given at bedtime) or twice daily oral dosing regimens are commonly used.

5-HYDROXYTRYPTAMINE

Prior to 1950 it was known that a vasoconstrictor substance, named *serotonin*, was released into the serum when blood was allowed to clot. The compound was identified chemically as 5-hydroxytryptamine (5-HT), an indoleamine. 5-Hydroxytryptamine is widely distributed in the body including the intestines, the CNS, and platelets. This biogenic amine has been implicated in such physiological processes as temperature regulation, blood coagulation, transmission of pain, appetite, and sleep. With respect to pathophysiology, the compound is involved in such conditions as depression, migraine headaches, carcinoid tumors, vasospastic disorders, and (possibly) hypertension.

Synthesis, Storage, and Metabolism

The biosynthesis of 5-hydroxytryptamine occurs with the hydroxylation of tryptophan by the enzyme, tryptophan 5-monooxygenase (tryptophan hydroxylase) to form 5-hydroxytryptophan. This intermediate compound is decarboxylated by aromatic L-amino acid decarboxylase to 5-hydroxytryptamine (Fig. 13-3).

5-Hydroxytryptamine appears to function predominantly as an inhibitory neurotransmitter in the CNS, although some excitatory neural actions can occur. Following its synthesis in the cytoplasm of the neuron, the compound is stored within neuronal vesicles. After nerve stimulation and release of 5-hydroxytryptamine into the synaptic space, the actions of this biogenic amine are terminated by a reuptake mechanism in which the neurotransmitter is returned to the neuron. This mechanism is the same as the reuptake mechanism for norepinephrine (see Chapter 7). Reserpine, which causes the depletion of norepinephrine from adrenergic nerve terminals, also produces depletion of 5-hydroxytryptamine from its neurons.

The biotransformation of 5-hydroxytryptamine is mediated by the enzyme monoamine oxidase which involves an oxidative deamination reaction with the production of the inactive metabolite, 5-hydroxyindoleacetic acid (5-HIAA), which is excreted in the urine (Fig. 13-3).

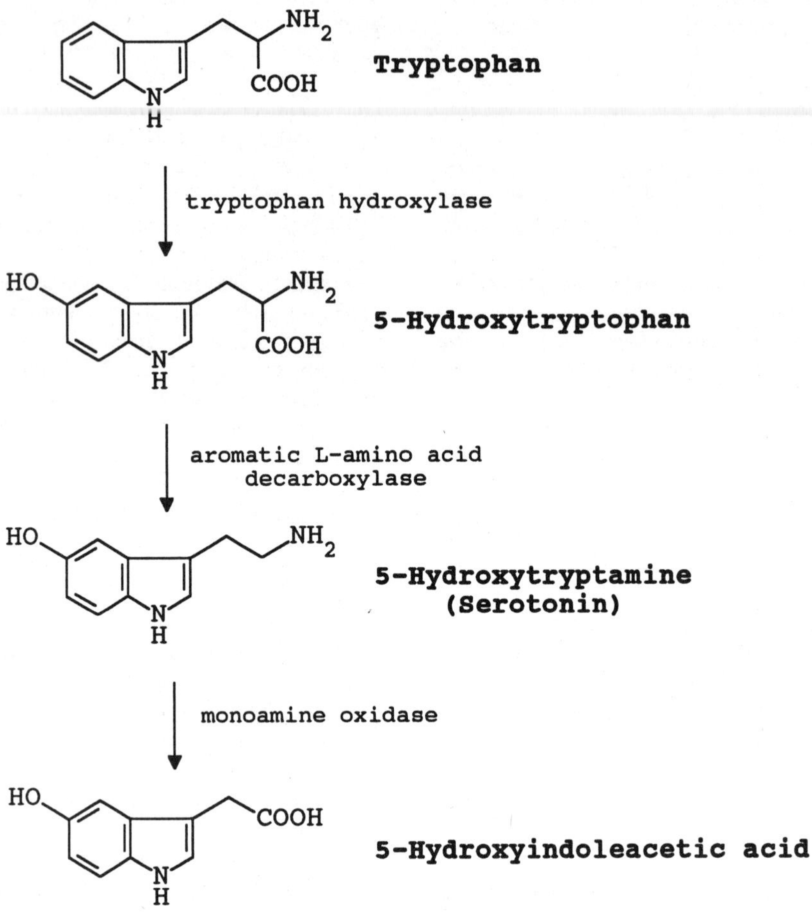

Tryptophan

tryptophan hydroxylase

5-Hydroxytryptophan

aromatic L-amino acid decarboxylase

5-Hydroxytryptamine (Serotonin)

monoamine oxidase

5-Hydroxyindoleacetic acid

FIGURE 13-3 *The biosynthesis of 5-hydroxytryptamine (serotonin) and its biotransformation.*

The compound, p-chlorophenylalanine, is an inhibitor of the synthesis of 5-hydroxytryptamine by blocking tryptophan hydroxylase which catalyzes the rate-limiting step in the synthesis of this amine. The metabolism of 5-hydroxytryptamine is prevented or reduced by monoamine oxidase inhibitors such as phenelzine and tranylcypromine.

5-Hydroxytryptamine Receptors

5-Hydroxytryptamine produces its effect in the body by binding to 5-HT receptors. These receptors are present in the central and peripheral nervous systems. There are four 5-HT receptor subtypes: type 1 (5-HT_1), type 2 (5-HT_2), type 3 (5-HT_3), and type 4 (5-HT_4). In addition, the type 1 (5-HT_1) receptors have been divided into five more classifications: 5-HT_{1A}, 5-HT_{1B}, 5-HT_{1C}, 5-HT_{1D}, and 5-HT_{1E}. Of this latter group, much interest has centered around the 5-HT_{1D} receptor because of its association with the therapy of migraine headaches. The 5-HT_{1B} receptor is found in rodents and may not be present in humans.

Effects of Tissues

Tryptaminergic (serotonergic) neurons are present in the CNS. The various receptors for 5-hydroxytryptamine are distributed throughout the brain and spinal cord where they are located on presynaptic terminals and postsynaptic membranes. It appears that 5-HT_1 receptors are primarily inhibitory while 5-HT_2 receptors are mostly excitatory in their function. The central arteries possess predominantly 5-HT_1 receptors, whereas the temporal arteries contain mainly 5-HT_2 receptors. The meningeal arteries contain all the subgroups of 5-HT receptors.

In the heart, 5-HT_1 receptor activation produces an increase in the force of contraction and enhances heart rate. Stimulation, however, of 5-HT_3 receptors may lead to bradycardia and hypo tension via chemoreflex (Bezold-Jarisch effect). Most blood vessels undergo vasoconstriction by agonistic activity at 5-HT_1 and 5-HT_2 receptors. The 5-HT_1 receptors cause contraction of such blood vessels as cerebral, basilar, renal, and pulmonary. Most other vascular smooth muscles are constricted by stimulation of 5-HT_2 receptors. In addition, vasodilatation is produced in arterioles and small vessels by the activation of 5-HT_1 receptors.

It should be mentioned that 5-HT_1 receptors are present on the nerve terminals of the sympathetic nervous system. These receptors, when stimulated by agonists, cause an inhibition of the release of norepinephrine. 5-HT receptors are also present on other neuronal terminals and produce a negative-feedback to prevent neurotransmitter release. The effect of 5-hydroxytryptamine on bronchiolar, uterine, and small intestinal muscles is contraction, whereas it may produce inhibition of gastric and large intestinal motility.

5-HYDROXYTRYPTAMINE AGONISTS

Sumatriptan

This drug is an indole derivative that is closely related to 5-hydroxytryptamine in structure. Sumatriptan is recommended in the acute treatment of migraine headaches. Pharmacologically, it acts as a selective agonist on the 5-HT_1 subgroup of receptors and more specifically at 5-HT_{1D} receptors. This compound does not appear to bind to other 5-HT receptor types, nor to adrenergic, dopaminergic, or muscarinic receptor sites.

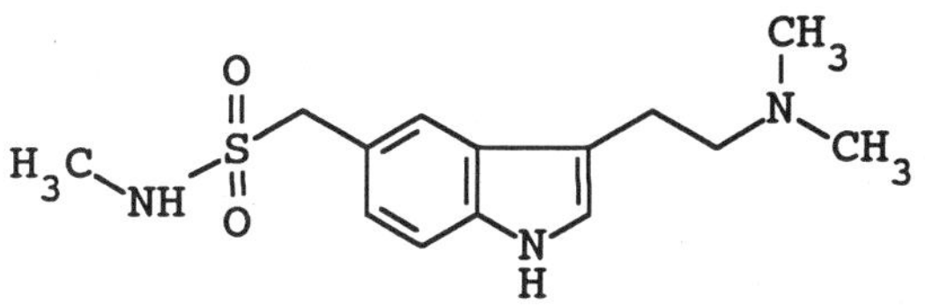

Mechanism of Action The efficacy of this drug is related to its effect at 5-HT_{1D} receptors. In addition, receptor binding studies have shown that not only does sumatriptan have high affinity for the 5HT_{1D} receptor but the antimigraine drugs, ergotamine and dihydroergotamine, also exhibit similar affinities to this receptor. It appears that the efficacy of ergotamine and dihydroergotamine in migraine attacks is partly or completely related to an effect at 5HT_{1D} receptors.

The pain of migraine headaches has been suggested to be due to vasodilation of intracranial blood vessels and stimulation of trigeminovascular axons which cause pain and release vasoactive neuropeptides to produce neurogenic inflammation and edema. Nociceptive impulses are transmitted from the dilated, edematous vessels to the CNS. 5-HT_{1D} receptors are present on cerebral and meningeal arteries. In addition, 5-HT_{1D} receptors are on presynaptic nerve terminals and function to inhibit the release of neuropeptides and other neurotransmitters.

Although the exact mechanism of sumatriptan is not fully understood, research evidence suggests that sumatriptan is an agonist at 5-HT_{1D} receptors. This results in vasoconstriction of dural blood vessels and inhibits the release of neuropeptides, thereby reducing the pain associated with the migraine attack. Further research is needed to delineate more fully the factors and events associated with the pathophysiology of the migraine headache and to determine more specifically the effects of antimigraine drugs when they bind to 5-HT_{1D} receptors.

Pharmacokinetics Sumatriptan is administered by subcutaneous injection; the bioavailability from the injection site is 97 percent. In the blood, the degree of protein binding is between 14 and 21 percent. The elimination half-life of sumatriptan is about 2 hours. The biotransformation of this compound occurs in the liver with the production of an indoleacetic acid metabolite. Both the parent compound and the inactive metabolite are excreted in the urine.

Adverse Reactions This antimigraine drug has been reported to cause a number of untoward effects such as pain at the injection site, dizziness, chest discomfort, and transient elevation of blood pressure. Coronary spasms have occurred, particularly in individuals with coronary artery disease. Although rare, cardiac arrhythmias can occur. Sumatriptan should be administered with caution to patients with liver and renal dysfunction. The drug is contraindicated in patients with ischemic heart disease, Prinzmetal's angina, or uncontrolled hypertension. Furthermore, sumatriptan should not be administered intravenously due to the fact that it may cause coronary vasospasms when given by this route.

Therapeutic Use Sumatriptan is indicated in the abortive treatment of migraine headaches. This drug is an effective agent in the treatment of acute migraine attacks and is effective even up to two hours after their onset. However, in a number of individuals (approximately 40 percent) the migraine pain can return within 24 to 48 hours after the successful termination of the migraine attack by sumatriptan. The drug is not recommended for hemiplegic or basilar migraine. In addition, this antimigraine drug should not be used in combination with ergotamine or products that contain ergotamine.

Ergot Alkaloids

Ergotamine, ergonovine, and a variety of other alkaloids were isolated from ergot, which is a product of a fungal infestation of grains, particularly rye. In the early history of civilization and during the Middle Ages, the consumption of grain contaminated with ergot resulted in gangrene of the extremities, abortions, and convulsions. In the Middle Ages ergot poisoning was known as *St. Anthony's fire*. In the early 1900s the ergot alkaloids were the first adrenergic blocking drugs to be investigated. Although most of the ergot alkaloids possess α-adrenergic blocking activity, their pharmacology is somewhat diversified and it appears that agonistic activity of ergotamine, dihydroergotamine, and ergonovine at 5-HT receptors plays a significant role in the therapeutic efficacy of these drugs. Chemically, these drugs are related to D-lysergic acid (see Chapter 19).

Ergotamine

Ergotamine is used in therapy because of its ability to produce vasoconstriction. Ergotamine is used to terminate the acute attacks of a migraine headache. Although ergotamine has several pharmacologic properties such as α-adrenergic blocking activity, its mechanism of action in treating migraine headaches is primarily related to its agonistic interaction with 5-HT_{1D} receptors resulting in vasoconstriction. Research investigations have shown that ergotamine has high binding affinity to 5-HT_{1D} receptors similar to that of sumatriptan and the mechanism of action may be the same as for that described above for sumatriptan. In addition, it is suggested that ergotamine depresses second-order neurons in the CNS that carry the nociceptive impulse from the distended and edematous cerebral vessels; thus, the drug may have a secondary mechanism of action.

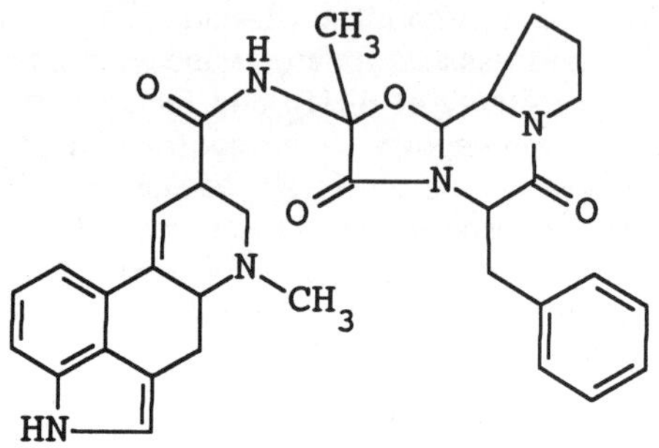

The absorption of ergotamine from the gastrointestinal tract is poor. To achieve a therapeutic effect by oral administration, ergotamine is often combined with caffeine, which appears to enhance its absorption. In addition, the vasoconstrictor effect of caffeine on cranial blood vessels may contribute to the desired therapeutic effect. Other routes of administration of ergotamine in the treatment of migraine headaches are inhalation and sublingual. Suppositories which contain ergotamine and caffeine may also be used. In addition, ergotamine may have value in the treatment of acute attacks of cluster headache.

Adverse reactions of ergotamine may include nausea, vomiting, diarrhea, paresthesia of limbs, and cramps. In the absence of peripheral vascular disease, gangrene is rare. The drug is contraindicated in severe hypertension, peripheral vascular disease, ischemic heart disease, and pregnancy.

Ergotamine cannot be used for the chronic or prophylactic treatment of migraines because of its potential adverse reactions such as the induction of gangrene. Drugs such as propranolol, methysergide, and amitriptyline may be used on a prophylactic basis to prevent or reduce the incidence of migraine headaches in patients. Calcium channel blockers may also be of some value.

Dihydroergotamine

This compound is a hydrogenated form of ergotamine. It is indicated in the treatment of acute migraine headaches as is ergotamine. Its mechanism of action is similar to that of ergotamine. Dihydroergotamine is generally given by intramuscular injection at the first warning signs of headache. The adverse reactions and contraindications for this drug are similar to those of ergotamine.

Ergonovine and Methylergonovine

These ergot alkaloids are used in the treatment of postpartum bleeding. The mechanism of action for the uterine-stimulating activity of ergonovine and its methylated derivative seems to be related to a direct musculotropic spasmogenic effect on the uterus (oxytocic effect) possibly by agonistic (or partial agonistic) activity at 5-HT_2 receptors and at α-adrenergic receptor sites. Although these drugs are ergot alkaloids, they do not have significant α-adrenergic blocking activity.

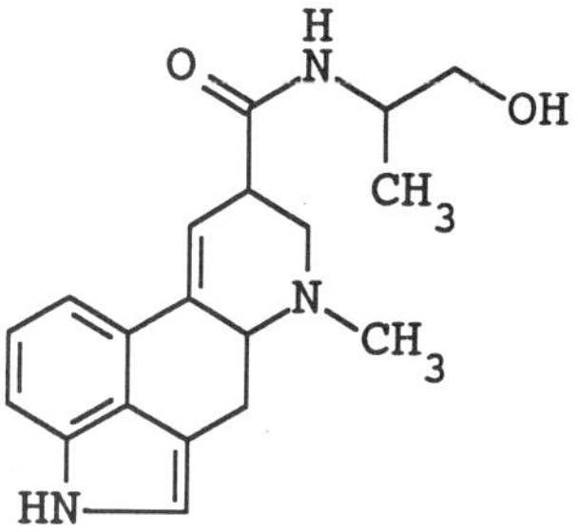

Ergonovine

Upon oral administration, ergonovine and methylergonovine have adequate bioavailability in contrast to ergotamine. In addition, these drugs may be injected by the intramuscular and intravenous routes. The intravenous route is used for emergency situations of excessive postpartum bleeding.

Adverse reactions of these compounds that may occur are nausea, vomiting, blurred vision, headache, hypertension, and convulsions. The use of both ergonovine and methylergonovine is contraindicated in pregnant women.

5-HYDROXYTRYPTAMINE ANTAGONISTS

Cyproheptadine

This drug is a tricyclic compound in which the middle ring contain seven carbons and has an ethylene bond. The structure is:

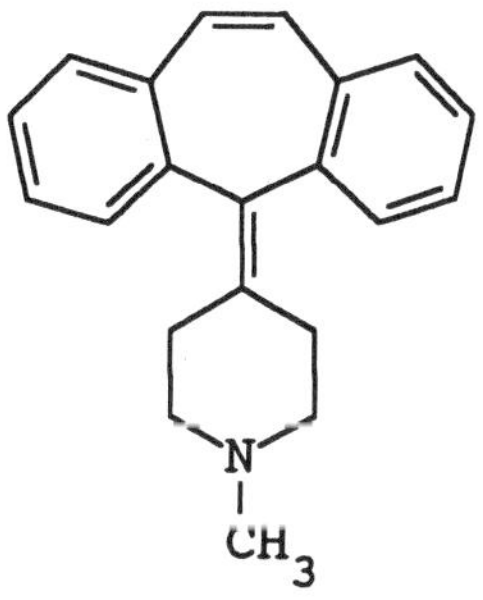

Cyproheptadine is an antagonist at 5-HT and H_1 receptors. In addition, it has antimuscarinic and mild sedative effects. The biotransformation of cyproheptadine results in the production of a quaternary ammonium glucuronide which is excreted in the urine. Drug excretion is reduced in the presence of kidney impairment.

Cyproheptadine is recommended for allergic conditions such as allergic and vasomotor rhinitis, conjunctivitis, urticaria, and pruritus. The drug also has been used in treating increased hypermotility of the gastrointestinal tract associated with carcinoid tumors, in postgastrectomy dumping syndrome, and in the prophylactic treatment of severe headaches in children.

Some adverse reactions of cyproheptadine include sedation, ataxia, confusion, hypotension, tachycardia, blood dyscrasias, xerostomia, and excessive perspiration. The drug is contraindicated in newborn and premature infants, in nursing mothers, in patients with prostatic hypertrophy or angle-closure glaucoma, and in elderly, debilitated patients.

Methysergide

This drug has been shown to block the effects of 5-hydroxytryptamine on both vascular and nonvascular smooth muscle. Although methysergide is a semisynthetic ergot derivative and structurally related to methylergonovine, it has only a weak oxytocic effect. The mechanism of action of methysergide is believed to be related to blockade of peripheral 5-HT receptors; however, some data indicate that it acts as an agonist at certain 5-HT receptors in the brain. Therefore, the mechanism of action has not be completely established.

Methysergide is indicated for the prevention of vascular headaches, including migraine headaches. Since the onset of action takes 1 to 2 days to develop, the drug is not useful for acute attacks, but for prophylactic treatment.

Ondansetron

This drug, which is an indole derivative, is classified as a selective blocker of 5-HT_3 receptors. Ondansetron is used to prevent nausea and vomiting that can accompany chemotherapy. The mechanism of action of ondansetron may involve blockade 5-HT_3 receptors in the chemoreceptor trigger zone and on the vagal nerve terminals. It is known that 5-hydroxytryptamine can activate vagal afferent fibers and induce the vomiting reflex.

Ondansetron is administered orally or by intravenous injection. The oral preparation has a bioavailability of about 55 percent and the elimination half-life is 3 hours. For the intravenous preparation, the mean elimination half-life is 4 hours in adult cancer patients. The major biotransformation pathway for the ondansetron involves hydroxylation followed by glucuronide or sulfate conjugation.

Some of the adverse reactions reported for ondansetron include constipation; headache; xerostomia; rash; and although rare, tachycardia, bronchospasms, hypokalemia, and tonic-clonic seizures have occurred. The drug is to be used with caution in pregnancy and in nursing mothers. There appears to be no increase in adverse reactions when younger patients were compared to patients who were 65 years or older.

Ketanserin

This antagonist of 5 hydroxytryptamine is classified as a selective blocker of 5-HT_2 receptors. In addition to this action, ketanserin also has α-adrenergic blocking properties. Although ketanserin is not approved for use in this country, it is used in other countries for the treatment of hypertension and in the therapy of Raynaud's syndrome.

BIBLIOGRAPHY

Histamine and Antihistamines

Black, J.W., W.A.M. Duncan, C.J. Durant, C.R. Ganellin, and E.M. Parsons: "Definition and Antagonism of Histamine H_2-Receptors," *Nature* **236**: 385-390 (1972).

Callaghan, J.T., R.F. Bergstrom, A. Rubin, et al.: "A Pharmacokinetic Profile of Nizatidine in Man," *Scand. J. Gastrol.* **22 (Suppl. 136)**: 9-17 (1987).

Ganellin, C.R., and M.E. Parsons: *Pharmacology of Histamine Reception*, Wright-PSG, Bristol, England, 1982.

Dammann, H.G., W.R. Gottlieb, T.A. Walter, P. Muller, D. Simon, and P. Keohane: "The 24-Hour Acid Suppression Profile of Nizatidine," *Scand. J. Gastenterol.* **22 (Suppl. 136)**: 56-60 (1987).

Hill, S.J.: "Distribution, Properties, and Functional Characteristics of Three Classes of Histamine Receptors," *Pharmacol. Rev.* **42**: 45-83 (1990).

Jensen, R.T., M.J. Collen, S.J. Pandel, et al.: "Cimetidine-Induced Impotence and Breast Changes in Patients with Gastric Hypersecretory States," *N. Engl. J. Med.* **308**: 883-887 (1983).

Klotz, U., P. Arvela, M. Pasanen, H. Kroemer, and O. Pelkonen: "Comparative Effects of H_2 Receptor Antagonists on Drug Metabolism in Vitro and in Vivo," *Pharmacol. Ther.* **33**: 157-162 (1987).

Powell, J.R., and K.H. Donn: "The Pharmacokinetic Basis for H_2-Antagonist Drug Interactions: Concepts and Implications," *J. Clin. Gastroenterol.* **5 (Suppl. 1)**: 95-113 (1983).

van Hecken, A.M., T.B. Tjandramaga, A. Muller, R. Verbesselt, and P.J. de Schepper: "Ranitidine: Single Dose Pharmacokinetics and Absolute Bioavailability in Man," *Br. J. Clin. Pharmacol.* **14**: 195-200 (1982).

5-Hydroxytryptamine and Its Congeners

Deliganis, A.V., and S.J. Peroutka: "5-Hydroxytryptamine$_{1D}$ Receptor Agonism Predicts Antimigraine Efficacy," *Headache* **31**: 228-231 (1991).

Hsu, V.D.: "Sumatriptan: A New Drug for Vascular Headache," *Clin. Pharm.* **11**: 919-929 (1992).

Humphrey, P.P.A., and W. Feniuk: "Mode of Action of the Anti-migraine Drug Sumatriptan," *Trends Pharmacol. Sci.* **12**: 444-446 (1991).

Lance, J.W.: "5-Hydroxytryptamine and Its Role in Migraine," *Eur. Neurol.* **31**: 279-281 (1991).

Moskowitz, M.A., and R. MacFarlane: "Neurovascular and Molecular Mechanisms in Migraine Headache," *Cerebrovas. Brain Metab. Rev.* **5**: 159-177 (1993).

CHAPTER 14

Prostaglandins and Related Eicosanoids

J. Bryan Smith

The prostaglandins and related eicosanoids are a family of oxygenated, unsaturated 20-carbon fatty acids that are implicated in a great many biologic systems. The discovery of prostaglandins followed early studies of biologically active substances present in prostate glands and semen of various species. In 1934, smooth muscle-stimulating material that was both acidic and lipid in nature was isolated from human semen and was given the name *prostaglandin*, owing to the mistaken belief that it came from the prostate gland. The isolation and identification of a family of prostaglandins from sheep seminal vesicles and from human semen was accomplished by the mid-1960s. Subsequently, other prostaglandins, such as *prostacyclin*, and related eicosanoids, such as *thromboxanes* and *leukotrienes*, were discovered.

It is now known that many cells in the body are capable of producing eicosanoids. The cells can do this because they contain both the appropriate fatty acid precursors (e.g., arachidonic acid), as esters in their membrane phospholipids, as well as the enzymes that are involved in the oxygenizing transformation of these fatty acids once they are released from ester linkage. In part because of this almost ubiquitous biosynthetic potential of cells and in part because of their diversity of effects, the eicosanoids are involved in a great number of physiologic and pathologic processes including reproduction, blood pressure regulation, bronchoconstriction, inflammation, nerve transmission, gastric secretion, urine formation, and platelet aggregation. The participation of the eicosanoids in each of these areas is briefly discussed in this chapter.

The prostaglandins and related compounds can be used as drugs themselves to mimic the effects of endogenously produced eicosanoids. However, the use of prostaglandins as drugs has not become widespread because of the multiplicity of side effects due to the fact that prostaglandins act on so many systems. Alternatively, other drugs (most notably nonsteroidal anti-inflammatory drugs) can act by inhibiting the biosynthesis of the endogenous eicosanoids. An increasing number of experimental agents which inhibit the effects of endogenous eicosanoids at the receptor level are being synthesized.

CHEMISTRY

Biosynthesis of Eicosanoids

The fatty acid precursors of the eicosanoids are not freely available in cells, but they are abundant in ester linkage in phospholipids in the membranes of many cell types. The initiation of the biosynthesis of prostaglandins and related eicosanoids therefore depends on the release of the fatty acid precursors by enzymatic hydrolysis of the phospholipids. In general, it appears that this hydrolysis is catalyzed by phospholipase A_2, an enzyme that acts on most phospholipids and whose activity is enhanced by an increase in intracellular free calcium ions as occurs during cellular stimulation. In addition, there is some evidence that small amounts of the precursor fatty acids also may be released from one particular phospholipid, phosphatidylinositol, by the combined actions of phospholipase C (which produces diacylglycerol) and diacylglycerol lipase. Examples of stimuli which cause eicosanoid synthesis in cells include mechanical distortion of cell membranes, changes in ion fluxes, ischemia, hormones, enzymes such as thrombin, and antigens. It is important to remember that the prostaglandins and related eicosanoids (1) are not stored for later release like the catecholamines but are biosynthesized within seconds

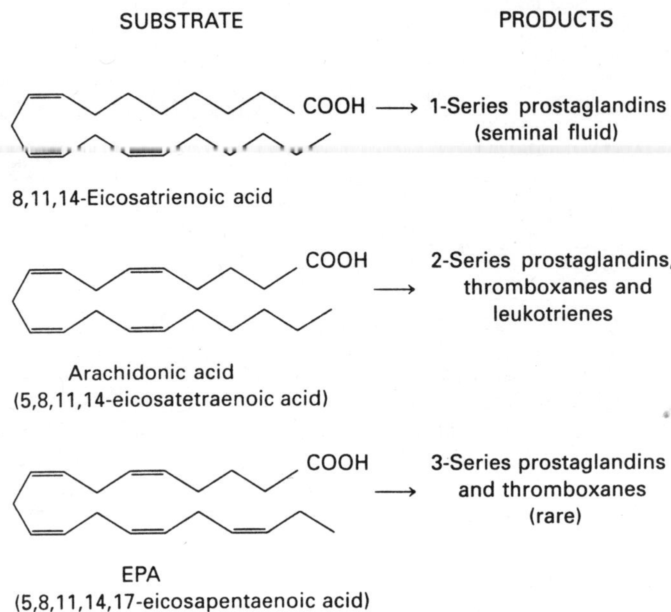

FIGURE 14-1 *Precursor substrates of the eicosanoids.*

of the activation of phospholipase A_2 and (2) usually act as autocoids because they are rapidly metabolized.

The fatty acid precursors of the prostaglandins and related eicosanoids all contain 20 carbon atoms, which is signified by *eicosa*. In addition, these precursors contain three, four, or five double bonds; hence the names 8,11,14-eicosatrienoic acid, 5,8,11,14-eicosatetraenoic acid (arachidonic acid) and 5,8,11,14,17-eicosapentaenoic acid (EPA), where the numbers 5, 8, 11, 14, and 17 refer to the position of the double bonds with the carbon atom of the carboxyl group being numbered as 1 (Fig. 14-1). Of these three eicosanoid precursors, human cells and tissues contain almost exclusively arachidonic acid esterified to phospholipids with the major exception of human seminal vesicles, which contain equal amounts of 8,11,14-eicosatrienoic acid and arachidonic acid and lesser amounts of EPA in their phospholipid membranes. The first two eicosanoid precursor fatty acids either are derived from dietary linoleic acid, an essential fatty acid which cannot be biosynthesized by humans, or are ingested as constituents of meat. The third, EPA, is almost entirely assimilated by the ingestion of cold-water fish.

Once released, eicosanoid precursors (usually arachidonic acid) are rapidly transformed into oxygenated products by one or both of two distinct pathways involving either prostaglandin endoperoxide synthase or lipoxygenases (Fig. 14-2). A third pathway of transformation of arachidonic acid involves cytochrome P-450-dependent monooxygenases with the formation of *epoxyeicosatrienoic acids*.

Prostaglandins and Thromboxanes All prostaglandins (PGs) are analogs of the hypothetical compound *prostanoic acid*, a 20-carbon fatty acid which contains a five-membered ring consisting of carbons 8, 9, 10, 11, and 12 (Fig. 14-3). The different prostaglandins are divided into several types or classes (A through I) according to the substituents present in the cyclopentane ring. They are further divided by a subscript (1, 2, or 3) which indicates the number of double bonds in the side chains. Prostaglandins D, E, F, and I are considered to be the compounds of primary interest since they are released from the activated cells. Prostaglandins A, B, and C can be derived chemically from prostaglandin E (PGE), but probably none of them occurs biologically. Prostaglandins G and H are intermediate cyclic endoperoxide derivatives that occur during prostaglandin biosynthesis as discussed below.

Prostaglandin endoperoxide synthase is a membrane-associated enzyme present in almost all cells. It consists of two subunits and possesses

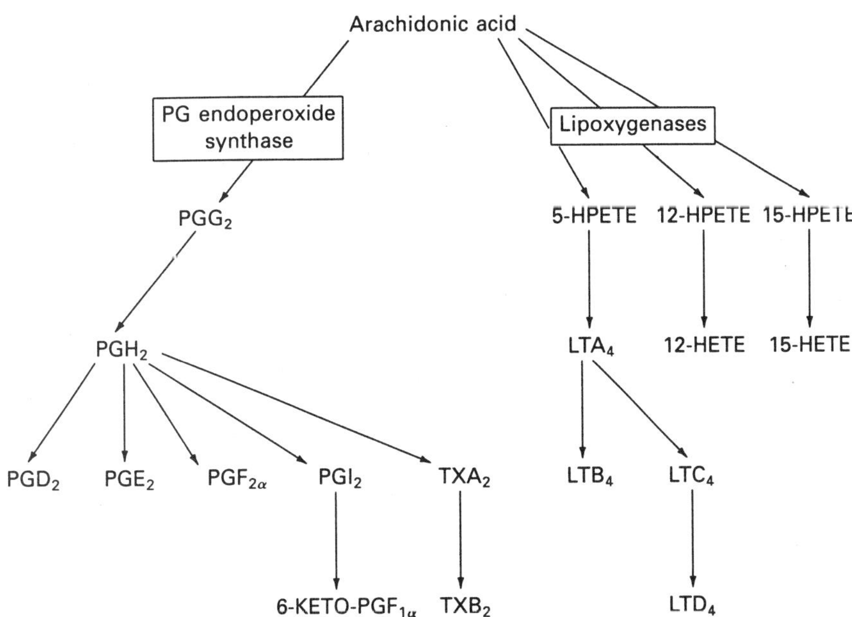

FIGURE 14-2 *Overall schematic for the biosynthesis of prostaglandins and related eicosanoids. PG = prostaglandins; TX = thromboxane; HPETE = hydroperoxyeicosatetraenoic acid; HETE = hydroxyeicosatetraenoic acid; and LT = leukotriene.*

both cyclooxygenase and peroxidase activities. Cyclooxygenase inserts two molecules of oxygen into arachidonic acid and causes an intramolecular rearrangement to yield an intermediate, PGG_2. The peroxidase then reduces PGG_2 to another chemically unstable ($t_{1/2}$ = 5 min at 37 °C and pH 7.5) intermediate, PGH_2. PGH_2 is the precursor of all other known prostaglandins and thromboxanes containing two side-chain double bonds (see below). Prostaglandin endoperoxide synthase also will convert 8,11,14-eicosatrienoic acid into PGH_1 and 5,8,11,14,17-eicosapentaenoic acid into PGH_3, and these endoperoxides can likewise be converted into other prostaglandins containing either one or three double bonds in their side chains, respectively.

Recently it has been shown that there are two distinct prostaglandin endoperoxide synthases (or cyclooxygenases), one of which is a constitutive form (*cyclooxygenase-1*) and one of which is induced in certain cells during inflammation (*cyclooxygenase-2*). Corticosteroids suppress induction of this latter form, suggesting a mechanism for their anti-inflammatory action.

The prostaglandin endoperoxides are isomerized enzymatically to a number of different products (Fig. 14-3). These products include PGD, PGE, PGF, PGI, and thromboxanes, and their formation depends on the presence of the appropriate isomerase or synthase within the cell. Brain tissue and mast cells contain a *PGH-PGD isomerase*, which can convert PGH_2 into PGD_2. Seminal vesicles contain *PGH-PGE isomerase* explaining the occurrence of large amounts of PGE_1 and PGE_2 in human semen. The precise mechanism of formation of $PGF_{2\alpha}$, by the uterus, for example, is still unclear. $PGF_{2\alpha}$ can be formed by the action of a reductase on PGH_2, PGD_2, or PGE_2. Endothelial cells contain *prostacyclin synthase* and convert PGH_2 primarily to prostacyclin (PGI_2). PGI_2 is unstable ($t_{1/2}$ = 3 min) and breaks down nonenzymatically to 6-keto-$PGF_{1\alpha}$. Blood platelets (thrombocytes) contain primarily *thromboxane synthase* and convert PGH_2 almost exclusively into thromboxane A_2 (TXA_2). TXA_2 has a very short half-life ($t_{1/2}$ = 30 sec) and converts nonenzymatically to thromboxane B_2 (TXB_2). Both prostacyclin and thromboxane synthases are cytochrome P-450 enzymes. Although thromboxanes are derived from prostaglandin endoperoxides, they are not prostaglandins because they contain a six-membered oxane ring rather than the cyclopentane ring of prostanoic acid.

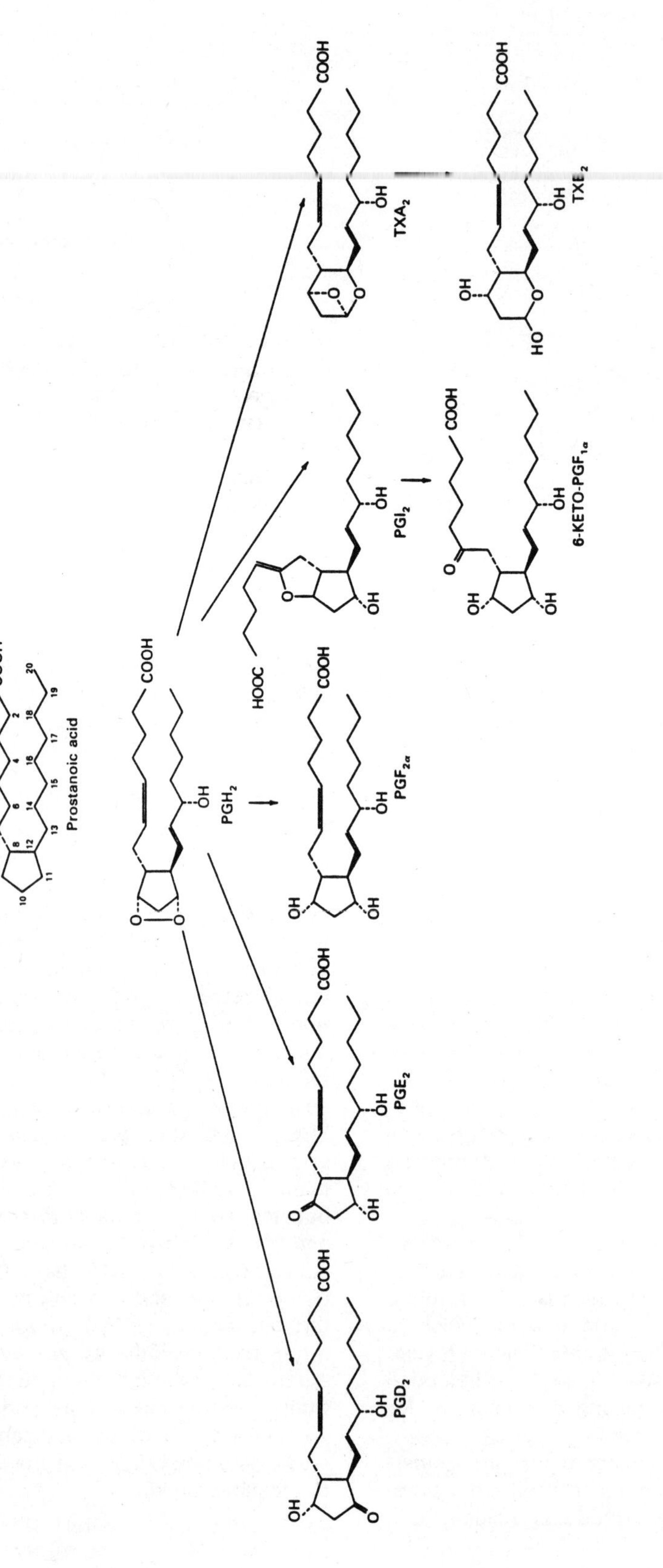

FIGURE 14-3 *Structures of the hypothetical compound prostanoic acid and of prostaglandins and thromboxanes derived from arachidonic acid.*

Leukotrienes In contrast to prostaglandin endoperoxide synthase, which is present in the membranes of almost all cells, the *lipoxygenases* appear to be cytoplasmic and are almost entirely restricted to circulating or resident white blood cells. Three major mammalian lipoxygenases have been discovered, namely, those that catalyze the incorporation of a molecule of oxygen into the 5-, 12-, or 15-positions of arachidonic acid with the formation of the corresponding 5-, 12-, and 15-hydroperoxyeicosatetraenoic acids (HPETEs). Platelets contain *12-lipoxygenase* and produce 12-HPETE and its reduction product 12-hydroxyeicosatetraenoic acid (12-HETE). The function of this enzyme is unknown. However, recent evidence suggests that it is involved in the formation of *lipoxins*, tetraene-containing eicosanoids with selective biological actions. Polymorphonuclear leukocytes, macrophages, basophils, and mast cells contain *5-* and *15-lipoxygenases* and produce potent biologically active substances as a result of this activity. These substances include the *leukotrienes*.

The term *slow-reacting substance (SRS)* was first introduced in 1938 to describe a factor appearing in the perfusate of guinea pig lung following treatment with cobra venom. The factor produced a slow, prolonged contraction of a smooth muscle preparation, in contrast to the rapid and transient action of histamine. A chemically and biologically similar material was subsequently found in the perfusate of sensitized guinea pig lungs following challenge with antigen. This immunologically released SRS was designated as *slow-reacting substance of anaphylaxis* (SRS-A) and was considered to be released together with other mediators (e.g., histamine and chemotactic factors) from mast cells after interaction between antigens, such as pollens, with immunoglobulin E (IgE) molecules bound to membrane receptors.

Studies of the transformation of arachidonic acid by polymorphonuclear leukocytes obtained from the peritoneal cavity of rabbits led initially to the identification of the major product as 5-hydroxyeicosatetraenoic acid (5-HETE). Further studies showed, however, that additional products also were formed; the major one was identified as 5,12-dihydroxyeicosatetraenoic acid and it was given the name leukotriene B_4 (LTB_4). It appears that, for the formation of LTB_4, arachidonic acid is first transformed by a 5-lipoxygenase into 5-HPETE. This requires the involvement of *5-lipoxygenase activating protein* (FLAP), an 18 kDa protein with three putative transmembrane domains, that is responsible for translocation of the enzyme from the cytoplasm to the membrane. The 5-HPETE then is converted into an intermediate, leukotriene A_4 (LTA_4). This compound is converted into LTB_4 by enzymatic hydrolysis (see Fig. 14-2). The name *leukotriene* was chosen to denote the cellular origin of these products (leukocytes) as well as the fact that they contained a conjugated double bond (triene) structure.

Physicochemical data on LTB_4 and SRS-A were similar and led to the hypothesis that there was some link between the two. After intensive study it was determined that the initial step in the biosynthesis of SRS-A is the formation of LTA_4. However, this LTA_4, instead of being converted into LTB_4 by hydrolysis, as in polymorphonuclear leukocytes, is transformed in mast cells by the addition of glutathione to produce the peptide-leukotriene LTC_4. Removal of glutamate from LTC_4 by a peptidase generates LTD_4, a peptide-leukotriene containing cysteinyl-glycine. It now appears that SRS-A is a mixture of LTC_4 and LTD_4 (Fig. 14-4). LTD_4 can be further metabolized to LTE_4 by a peptidase. LTE_4 has about one-tenth the myogenic activity of LTC_4 or LTD_4.

Inhibition of Eicosanoid Biosynthesis

Corticosteroids can inhibit prostaglandin biosynthesis in fibroblasts, endothelial cells, monocytes, macrophages, and certain other cell types by preventing the induction of cyclooxygenase-2 (and possibly phospholipase A_2) in response to cytokines such as interleukin-1 during inflammation. Alternatively, there are data that suggest that the corticosteroids prevent the release of precursor arachidonic acid from membrane phospholipids by inducing the synthesis of a protein inhibitor of phospholipase A_2 called *lipocortin*. As described in greater detail in Chapter 42, corticosteroids induce the synthesis of many proteins, and it seems likely that the synthesis of lipocortin is at best only partly responsible for their anti-inflammatory action.

On the other hand, the action of the nonsteroidal anti-inflammatory drugs (NSAIDs) such as aspirin, indomethacin, naproxen, and ibuprofen, depends to a great extent on their ability to selectively inhibit the activities of both cyclooxygenase-1 and cyclooxygenase-2, and therefore block the synthesis of both prostaglandins and thromboxanes (see Fig. 14-2). It is known that aspirin acts by acetylating a hydroxyl group of a serine located in the active center of cyclooxygenase. The other agents act by complex mechanisms which seem to

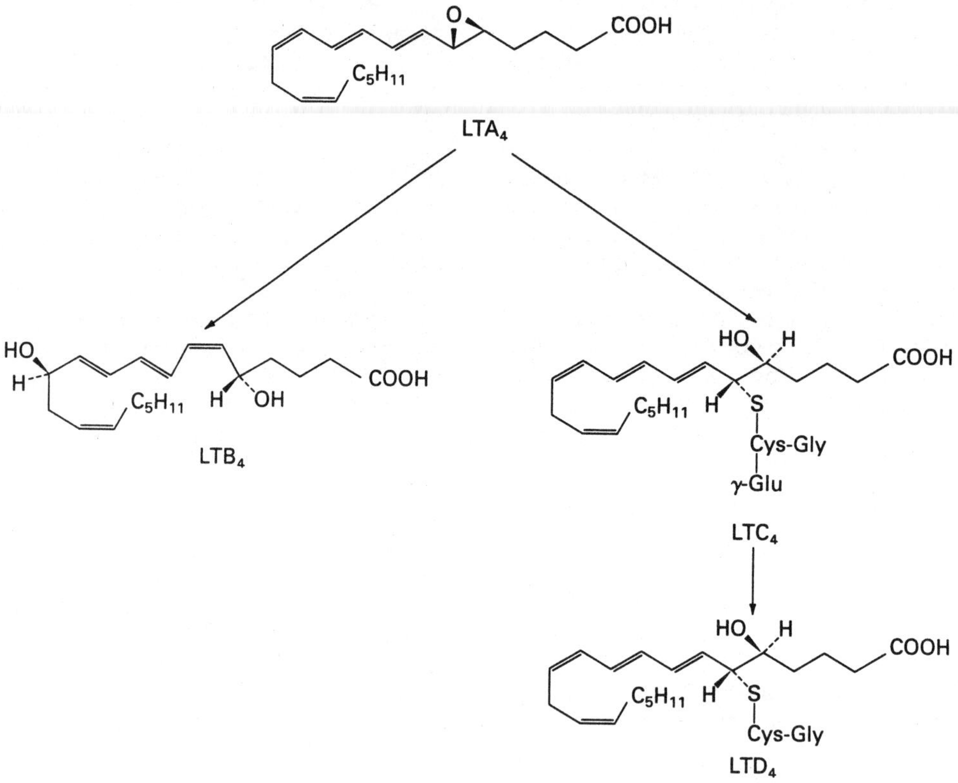

FIGURE 14-4 *Structures of the leukotrienes.*

involve, in part, competition with arachidonic acid for access to the active site of the enzyme. Interestingly, salicylate, although closely related in structure to aspirin, has no acetylating capacity and is almost inactive as an inhibitor of cyclooxygenase. It is important to note that NSAIDs inhibit prostaglandin endoperoxide synthase but not lipoxygenases. Therefore, it is possible that under certain conditions (for example, in mast cells which contain both prostaglandin endoperoxide synthase and 5-lipoxygenase activities) NSAIDs can actually increase the production of leukotrienes by diverting arachidonic acid to the 5-lipoxygenase pathway.

MECHANISM OF ACTION OF EICOSANOIDS

Prostaglandins, thromboxanes, and leukotrienes produce their effects on smooth muscle and other cells via interaction with membrane-bound G-protein linked receptors, which not only are specific for eicosanoids, as opposed to other hormones, but they also differentiate between the individual eicosanoids. Different cells contain specific receptors for many eicosanoids including PGE_1, PGE_2, $PGF_{2\alpha}$, LTB_4, and LTD_4, for example. The overall effect elicited by the eicosanoid-receptor interaction frequently appears to be mediated intracellularly by (1) changes in the activity of adenylate cyclase, or (2) stimulation of phospholipase C leading to the formation of diacylglycerol and inositol triphosphate (which causes an increase in the level of free intracellular calcium ions). For example, PGE_1, PGD_2, and PGI_2 inhibit platelet aggregation by increasing the intracellular concentration of cyclic AMP, whereas PGG_2, PGH_2, and TXA_2 induce platelet aggregation by increasing the level of intracellular ionized calcium. Other eicosanoids such as PGE_2, $PGF_{2\alpha}$, 6-keto-$PGF_{1\alpha}$, TXB_2, LTB_4, and LTD_4 have little or no effect on platelets, although some of these eicosanoids have important effects on other cells.

PHARMACOKINETICS

As was previously mentioned, prostaglandins and other eicosanoids are not stored; rather they are formed quickly after the activation of phospholipase A_2 and are rapidly metabolized to inactive products after they enter the circulation. The lungs remove PGE_2 and $PGF_{2\alpha}$, from the circulation by an active uptake mechanism and subject them to enzymatic deactivation by *15-hydroxyprostaglandin dehydrogenase* and *prostaglandin reductase*. The first enzymatic product, i.e., 15-keto-PGE_2, is less biologically active than its precursor, and the second metabolite, i.e., 15-keto-13,14-dihydro-PGE_2, is almost totally inactive. It has been estimated that 95 percent of E-type prostaglandins and 80 percent of F-type prostaglandins are inactivated in one single passage through the lungs. The prostaglandins are also biotransformed in the liver and elsewhere by beta and omega oxidation, and many of the metabolites of prostaglandins that appear in urine are dicarboxylic acids. Under certain unusual circumstances, prostaglandins may reach relatively high concentrations in circulating blood, e.g., PGD_2 in mastocytosis, PGE_2 in association with some solid tumors with metastases to bone, and PGI_2 in pregnancy.

PHYSIOLOGIC AND PHARMACOLOGIC EFFECTS

The physiologic and pharmacologic effects of prostaglandins and other eicosanoids are summarized briefly in Table 14-1 and are discussed in greater detail below.

The Reproductive System

The fact that there are large (microgram) amounts of PGE_1, PGE_2, $PGF_{1\alpha}$, and $PGF_{2\alpha}$ present in human semen has led to the "joint effort" hypothesis. This theory states that in males the prostaglandins stimulate the smooth muscle contraction necessary for ejaculation, whereas in females the prostaglandins are absorbed by the vagina and contract the myometrium and oviducts. It should be pointed out, however, that, while there does seem to be some correlation between the levels of prostaglandins in semen and male fertility, the requirement for the prostaglandins does not seem to be absolute and their precise role remains to be determined.

In many subprimate species, luteolysis (destruction of the corpus luteum in the ovary) is undoubtedly caused by $PGF_{2\alpha}$. This prostaglandin is released in a pulsatile manner from the uterus at term and passes by local vascular transfer from the utero-ovarian vein into the closely positioned ovarian artery whereby it reenters the ovary. The parenteral injection of $PGF_{2\alpha}$ is associated with decreased output of progesterone by the corpus luteum and interrupts early pregnancy, which is dependent on luteal rather than placental progesterone. The luteolytic activity of prostaglandins of the F-type has been put to veterinary use in synchronizing estrus in farm animals such as sheep, cattle, and pigs, which has simplified the breeding of the animals. The prostaglandins also can be used to provide safe, early abortions before the animals are put to market.

PGE_2 and $PGF_{2\alpha}$ can cause contraction of uterine smooth muscle of primates including that of the human uterus. It is thought that the increased synthesis of one or both of these prostaglandins may modulate menstruation in the human female. In keeping with this concept, NSAIDs (e.g., ibuprofen) are now prescribed for relieving menstrual cramps (dysmenorrhea).

Increased concentrations of prostaglandins have been found in the circulating blood of females during labor or spontaneous abortion. Thus, it is thought that increased intrauterine synthesis of prostaglandins initiates and maintains uterine contractions during labor. Labor may actually be induced by PGE_2 given orally (0.5 mg/h); if labor is not established by 12 h, an intravenous infusion of oxytocin is substituted. However, since this practice is accompanied by increased risk of uterine hypertonus and fetal bradycardia, the primary use of prostaglandins in gynecologic practice has been as abortifacients (see "Therapeutic Uses").

Inflammatory and Immune Responses

Prostaglandins of the E-type are inflammatory, i.e., they can cause erythema, pain, and hyperalgesia (increased tenderness). They are produced locally in response to many different types of stimuli such as heat, foreign particles, and bacteria, and, by sensitizing nerve endings and increasing local blood flow, enhance the pain and increased vascular permeability induced by other agents such as complement, bradykinin, serotonin, and histamine. PGE_1 and PGE_2 have been shown to elicit pain and induce a wheal and flare responses when injected

TABLE 14-1 Physiologic and pharmacologic effects of prostaglandins and related eicosanoids

Biologic Process	Eicosanoid	Effect
Reproduction	PGE_2	Contract pregnant uterus
	$PGF_{2\alpha}$	Destruct corpus luteum
		Contract pregnant uterus
Blood pressure regulation	PGE_1, PGE_2, PGI_2	Dilate blood vessels
	$PGF_{2\alpha}$	Constrict veins
	TXA_2	Constrict arteries
Gastric secretion	PGE_1, PGE_2	Contract longitudinal smooth muscle, stimulate bicarbonate secretion
	$PGF_{2\alpha}$, LTC_4, LTD_4	Contract smooth muscle
Inflammation	PGE_1, PGE_2, PGI_2	Increase local blood flow, increase vascular permeability
	LTB_4	Chemotactic for leukocytes
	LTC_4, LTD_4	Increase vascular permeability
Bronchoconstriction	PGD_2, $PGF_{2\alpha}$, TXA_2, LTC_4, LTD_4	Cause bronchoconstriction
	PGE_1, PGE_2, PGI_2	Cause bronchodilation
Platelet aggregation	PGE_1, PGD_2, PGI_2	Inhibit platelet aggregation
	PGG_2, PGH_2, TXA_2	Induce platelet aggregation

into human skin in nanogram amounts and to directly increase vascular permeability when injected subcutaneously in animals. PGI_2 also is likely to be generated during inflammation and it, too, can cause erythema and increase local blood flow, but other prostaglandins such as PGD_2 (the major prostaglandin from mast cells) and $PGF_{2\alpha}$, have not been implicated to any great extent in the inflammatory response. In contrast to the short-lived effects of other inflammatory mediators, E-type prostaglandins produce long-lasting effects (up to 10 h) upon subcutaneous blood vessels after intradermal injection. The release of prostaglandins during the inflammatory process thus produces both a direct response as well as a mechanism for the amplification of the effects of other inflammatory mediators.

The leukotrienes may also be involved in inflammation; LTB_4 is an extremely potent chemotactic agent for polymorphonuclear leukocytes, and LTC_4 and LTD_4 have the capacity to increase vascular permeability. It is known that, early in the inflammatory process, leukocytes migrate into the injured area and phagocytize the bacteria, antigen-antibody particles, or other noxious agents that may be present. During this process, the leukocytes release lytic enzymes from their lysosomes and synthesize and release LTB_4. The lysosomal enzymes then cause damage to surrounding tissue, while the LTB_4 recruits more leukocytes to the scene. Furthermore, there is evidence that the peptide-leukotrienes, LTC_4 and LTD_4 not only are formed in response to the combination of antigen with the IgE bound to the membranes of mast cells but also can be produced in increased amounts following mechanical trauma such as in surgery.

The fact that NSAIDs inhibit the formation of prostaglandins, but not the formation of leukotrienes, specifically implicates the prostaglandins as contributing to the symptoms of inflammation. Furthermore, NSAIDs have little or no effect on the release or activity of histamine, serotonin, or lysosomal enzymes and, similarly, potent antagonists of serotonin or histamine have little or no therapeutic effect in inflammation. Consequently, the contribution of these latter mediators in inflammation is of doubtful importance. However, this does not exclude the leukotrienes as making a contribution to the inflammatory response. It is possible that the steroidal anti-inflammatory drugs may act by inhibiting the production of both prostaglandins and leukotrienes by inducing the synthesis of the inhibitor of phospholipase A_2, lipocortin.

Human blood monocytes have the capacity to produce PGE_2. This prostaglandin has been implicated in the control of the immunologic response as it elevates cyclic AMP in T lymphocytes and thereby inhibits mitogenesis. The production of interleukin 2 (T-cell growth factor) is inhibited indirectly via PGE_2-induced activation of an $OKT8^+$ (T-suppressor) population of lymphocytes.

Platelet Aggregation

Platelets respond to vessel injury by adhering to exposed connective tissue and clumping together to form a hemostatic plug to stem blood loss. A very similar series of events seems to occur in arterial thrombosis, with the formation of a thrombus that can lead to stroke or myocardial infarction. During the adhesion of platelets to collagen, they synthesize and release TXA_2, which can induce platelet aggregation and constrict brain and coronary arteries. The coagulation protein thrombin also is a powerful stimulus for platelet TXA_2 formation. TXA_2 acts together with adenosine diphosphate, another aggregating agent released from the platelets, to recruit passing platelets to build up the thrombus.

A single tablet of aspirin (325 mg) totally inhibits platelet thromboxane production and hence considerably reduces the aggregation induced by collagen. The effect of aspirin on platelet aggregation lasts for 3 to 4 days because platelets (unlike most other cells) have little or no capacity for the synthesis of new protein. The return of cyclooxygenase activity, and the associated thromboxane formation, must await the entry of fresh platelets (with cyclooxygenase that has not been acetylated) from the bone marrow. It has been shown in clinical trials that aspirin reduces the incidence of transient ischemic attacks in the brain, as well as myocardial infarctions in men with unstable angina. These benefits presumably result from the ability of aspirin to inhibit collagen-induced platelet aggregation.

Prostacyclin (PGI_2) is much more potent than aspirin as an inhibitor of platelet aggregation and also dilates coronary arteries. PGD_2 and PGE_1 also inhibit platelet aggregation but are less potent and seem to be less important. Endothelial cells and smooth muscle cells can synthesize PGI_2 in response to certain stimuli such as bradykinin, but the circulating levels are too low to produce systemic effects. Prostacyclin has been used clinically to prevent platelet loss during extracorporeal circulation of blood during dialysis, cardiopulmonary bypass, and hemoperfusion through charcoal. However, prostcyclin has to be infused continuously because of its rapid metabolism, and its use is complicated by a profound hypotensive effect.

Substitution of the eicosapentaenoic acid (EPA; in fish oil) for arachidonic acid in the diet seems to reduce plasma triglycerides and cholesterol and inhibits platelet aggregation. This, coupled with the knowledge that Eskimos who eat a lot of fish have a reduced incidence of atherosclerosis, has led to the hypothesis that the formation of more derivatives of PGH_3 and fewer derivatives of PGH_2 is beneficial. However, the evidence obtained to support this hypothesis is presently inconclusive.

The Gastrointestinal Tract

Longitudinal smooth muscle from stomach to colon contracts in response to prostaglandins of the E- and F-type. Circular smooth muscle contracts in response to $PGF_{2\alpha}$ but is relaxed by PGE_2. Leukotrienes C_4 and D_4 are very potent in contracting gastrointestinal smooth muscle. Prostaglandins are also involved in normal and abnormal gastrointestinal motility. Administration of PGE_2 or $PGF_{2\alpha}$ orally or intravenously often causes diarrhea, and endogenously produced prostaglandins are implicated in diarrhea associated with medullary carcinoma of the thyroid and with cholera. In contrast to PGE_2 and $PGF_{2\alpha}$, PGI_2 does not cause diarrhea.

Prostaglandins E_1 and E_2 inhibit basal as well as stimulated gastric acid production and pepsin secretion in response to feeding or administration of histamine or pentagastrin. These compounds also stimulate bicarbonate secretion in the stomach and duodenum and increase the production of the protective mucin in the stomach. Prostaglandin analogs are being developed to take advantage of these protective properties; one such analog, misoprostol (15-deoxy-16-hydroxy-16-methyl-PGE_1 methyl ester) is approved and marketed in over 20 countries for the treatment of ulcers.

The use of NSAIDs increases fecal blood loss and is sometimes associated with gastrointestinal disturbances. This may be due in part to their ability to inhibit the formation of prostaglandins by the stomach.

Blood-Flow Regulation

Prostaglandins E_1, E_2, and I_2 are potent dilators of almost all blood vessels. Intravenous infusion of PGE_2 and PGI_2 in humans induces facial flushing, vasodilatation in the systemic and pulmonary vascular beds, and hypotension. Endogenously produced PGE_2 and PGI_2 may be local regulators of blood flow in many vascular beds. For example, PGE_2 is synthesized by the kidney medulla and can regulate blood flow to the inner and outer cortex. Renal synthesis of PGE_2, a vasodilator, increases in response to angiotensin II, a vasoconstrictor, thereby causing negative feedback. Inhibition of prostaglandin synthesis by NSAIDs reduces blood flow to the inner cortex and increases flow to the outer cortex.

It is thought that renal prostaglandins are involved in Bartter's syndrome. In this rare condition there are increased levels of renin and aldosterone in blood and increased amounts of potassium and prostaglandins (PGE_2 and PGI_2) in urine. However, the patients are normotensive. If the patients are given indomethacin chronically, the urinary excretion of prostaglandins is inhibited and aldosterone returns to normal.

$PGF_{2\alpha}$ constricts superficial veins of the hand, and TXA_2 constricts cerebral and coronary arteries; their metabolites, 6-keto-$PGF_{1\alpha}$, and TXB_2, respectively, are inactive on the cardiovascular system. It is possible that Prinzmetal's angina, a vasoconstrictive problem in coronary arteries, may in part be due to TXA_2 release from platelets. The peptide-leukotrienes C_4 and D_4 also have been shown to have the ability to constrict coronary arteries.

Bronchoconstriction

Not only can lungs remove prostaglandins from the circulation and inactivate them as noted above, but they can also produce $PGF_{2\alpha}$, PGE_2, PGI_2, TXA_2, LTC_4, and LTD_4. The source of PGD_2 and the leukotrienes is most likely the mast cells which line the respiratory passages. Overproduction of PGD_2 or the leukotrienes will result in bronchoconstriction, and both are thought to be potential mediators of asthma. $PGF_{2\alpha}$, and TXA_2 also are potent constrictors of bronchial and tracheal muscle. On the other hand, PGE_1, PGE_2, and PGI_2 are potent bronchodilators, with PGE_2 being much more active than PGI_2. Unfortunately prostaglandins are irritant to the airways and cause coughing when inhaled, which has precluded their use as antiasthmatic drugs.

Nerve Transmission

Prostaglandins E_1 and E_2, but not prostacyclin, have been found to be potent inhibitors of norepinephrine output from nerve endings and to depress the responses of the innervated tissues. However, these effects vary greatly depending on the species, tissue, and experimental conditions used for the studies. Many stimulant and depressant effects of prostaglandins on the central nervous system also have been reported. In general, these effects have been elicited with rather high concentrations of prostaglandins, and they require further study to shed light on their relevance to physiologic or pathologic conditions.

THERAPEUTIC USES

Abortifacients

In contrast to oxytocin, prostaglandins will induce contractions of human uterus at all stages of pregnancy. However, the state of contractile responsiveness of the uterus to the prostaglandins is at its greatest at term and at its lowest early in pregnancy. Thus, larger doses of PGE_2 or $PGF_{2\alpha}$ are needed to induce early, second trimester abortion, as compared with producing labor.

Since they stimulate the uterus to contract, certain prostaglandins, specifically PGE_2 (generic name dinoprostone) and 15-methyl $PGF_{2\alpha}$ (carboprost), are available for use as abortifacients.

Dinoprostone is indicated for use between the 12th and 20th gestational weeks. It is also used to evacuate the uterus in intrauterine fetal death up to 28 gestational weeks. This drug is administered by vaginal suppository (20 mg) given every 3 to 5 h until abortion occurs. Continuous administration for more than 48 h is not recommended.

Carboprost is available only for intramuscular administration and is recommended for use during the 13th to 20th gestational weeks. The drug is also indicated for second trimester abortions following the failure of other methods to expel the fetus. Typically 250 µg of the drug is given every 1.5 to 3.5 h based on the uterine response. Carboprost is also used for refractory postpartum bleeding of uterine atony; usually a satisfactory response occur after a single injection.

Regardless of which drug is used, the response that occurs takes the form of a sharp rise in tonus with superimposed rhythmic contractions. This abortifacient action of prostaglandins in early human pregnancy is not associated with a decreased output of progesterone, and luteolysis does not seem to be a significant factor.

Neither of these drugs are specific for the gravid uterus and they will elicit all the effects associated with the prostaglandins throughout the body. A high incidence of gastrointestinal upset (nausea, vomiting, and diarrhea) has been observed with both drugs.

Cervical Ripening

Dinoprostone is also indicated for cervical ripening (softening, effacement and dilation) in pregnant women at or near term who have a medical or obstetrical need for induction of labor. The effect is thought to be due in part to collagen degradation resulting from collagenase secretion as a response to PGE_2. The drug (0.5 mg in a gel) is introduced into the cervical canal just below the internal os. If the required response is obtained, labor is induced after 6 to 12 hours with IV oxytocin.

Ductus Arteriosus

Especially in premature deliveries, sometimes the ductus arteriosus of the newborn will remain patent (open) such that 90 percent of the cardiac output is shunted away from the lungs. The delayed spontaneous closure of the ductus is almost certainly due to the continued high production of prostaglandins (probably PGI_2) after delivery. Indomethacin inhibits prostaglandin formation and closes the patent ductus arteriosus, and the IV use of this drug is approved by the FDA for this purpose.

Conversely, certain neonates with congenital heart defects including pulmonary atresia or stenosis, tricuspid atresia, tetralogy of Fallot, interruption of the aortic arch, coarctation of the aorta, or transposition of the great vessels, depend on an open ductus for survival. The smooth muscles of the ductus are especially sensitive to PGE_1, and the compound causes dilatation to occur.

Prostaglandin E_1 (generic name alprostadil) is useful therapeutically to temporarily maintain the patency of the ductus arteriosus until corrective surgery is performed. Alprostadil is administered by continuous IV infusion or by catheter through the umbilical artery and should only be used in pediatric intensive care facilities. Commonly 0.05 to 0.1 μg/kg/min is used; this dose may be reduced as the therapeutic response is achieved. The more common adverse reactions to this drug include fever, flushing, bradycardia or tachycardia, hypotension, and apnea.

Prevention of Gastric Ulcers

Endogenous prostaglandins secreted by the gastric mucosa, i.e., PGE_2 and PGI_2, inhibit gastric acid output and the volume of gastric acid secretions. In addition, they stimulate the secretion of bicarbonate and mucin from the stomach and, therefore, protect the mucosa from the ulcerogenic effects of acid. The most common adverse effect of NSAIDs is gastric irritation, which may lead to gastric ulceration and bleeding. These effects result from the ability of NSAIDs to inhibit prostaglandin formation in the gastrointestinal tract.

Misoprostol is a synthetic analog of PGE_1 (15-deoxy-16-hydroxy-16-methyl-PGE_1 methyl ester). In the United States it is indicated for the prevention of gastric ulcers in patients taking NSAIDs (see Chapter 37); in other countries the drug is approved and marketed for the treatment of idiopathic septic ulcers unrelated to NSAIDs.

Misoprostol is available as tablets (100 and 200 μg) and is administered orally in a dosage of 100 to 200 μg 4 times daily. It is rapidly absorbed in the intestine and is biotransformed to its free acid, which is the product responsible for the drug's activity. The half-life of the compound is only 20 to 40 min; excretion is mainly via the urinary tract and partly through the feces.

The most common adverse effects of this drug are diarrhea and abdominal pain, which are usually transient. Gynecological disturbances, e.g., spotting, cramps, and dysmenorrhea, have also been reported. Rarely do the adverse effects of misoprostol require cessation of therapy.

BIBLIOGRAPHY

Bergstrom, S.: "Prostaglandins: Members of a New Hormonal System," *Science* **157**: 382-391 (1967).

DiPalma, J.R.: "Misoprostol: Prostaglandin for Peptic Ulcer," *Am. Fam. Physician* **40**: 217-219 (1989).

Dunn, M.J., and V.L. Hood: "Prostaglandins in the Kidney," *Am. J. Physiol.* **233**: F169-F184 (1977).

Fischer, S.: "Dietary Polyunsaturated Fatty Acids and Eicosanoid Formation in Humans," *Advances Lipid Res.* **23**: 169-198 (1989).

Flower, R.J.: "Drugs Which Inhibit Prostaglandin Biosynthesis," *Pharmacol. Rev.* **26**: 33-67 (1974).

Kujubu, D.A., and H.R. Herschman: "Dexamethasone Inhibits Mitogen Induction of the T1S10 Prostaglandin Synthase/Cyclooxygenase Gene," *J. Biol. Chem.* **267**: 7991-7994 (1992).

Piper, P.J.: "Formation and Actions of Leukotrienes," *Physiol. Rev.* **64**: 744-761 (1984).

Smith, J.B.: "The Prostanoids in Hemostasis and Thrombosis," *Am. J. Pathol.* **99**: 742-804 (1980).

Smith, W.L.: "The Eicosanoids and their Biochemical Mechanisms of Action," *Biochem. J.* **259**: 315-324 (1989).

PART IV

Central Nervous System Drugs

SECTION EDITOR

G. John DiGregorio

CHAPTER 15

General Anesthetics

Jan C. Horrow and Ruby M. Padolina

Anesthesia, literally, denotes a loss of sensibility. In current practice, general anesthesia is a controlled degree of central nervous system (CNS) depression with the following components: analgesia (lack of pain), amnesia (lack of memory), inhibition from reflexes such as bradycardia and laryngospasm, and skeletal muscle relaxation. Although frequently called sleep, anesthesia is an altered state of consciousness quite different from sleep. The general anesthetics depress or block neurologic impulses throughout the CNS. An ideal anesthetic would possess all the above properties, including a wide margin of safety without serious adverse effects. Presently, there are two types of general anesthetics. They are the inhaled or gaseous agents and the intravenous anesthetics.

This chapter includes a discussion of the inhaled anesthetic agents (nitrous oxide, halothane, enflurane, isoflurane, methoxyflurane, desflurane, and sevoflurane) and the intravenous anesthetic agents (ultrashort-acting barbiturates, ketamine, etomidate, and propofol). Included also are the adjuncts to anesthesia such as fentanyl, sufentanil, alfentanil, diazepam, lorazepam, and midazolam. This chapter also contains discussion of the following three major principles underlying the use of general anesthetics:

1. *Minimum alveolar concentration (MAC)* This concept explains and quantitates the pharmacodynamic properties of inhaled anesthetics.
2. *Uptake and distribution* These topics describe the pharmacokinetics of the inhaled agents.
3. *Mechanism of action* A theory of action is presented explaining how anesthetics produce graded depression of the CNS.

Minimum Alveolar Concentration

The effects of any oral or parenteral drug are characterized by a dose-response curve relating serum concentration to a measured organ response. With inhalation anesthetics, the end organ of interest is the brain, and its desired response is unconsciousness to a noxious stimulus such as surgical incision.

Drugs administered as gases are unusual in that most of the drug inspired is immediately exhaled with only a fraction being absorbed and retained. The dose administered is measured not by weight but by that percent of an atmosphere containing the drug. Since gases in the alveoli are equilibrated with blood, the dose of anesthetic is measured by its alveolar concentration. End-tidal gas concentrations reflect alveolar gas concentrations. Thus anesthetic dose (alveolar concentration) is conveniently measured by analyzing exhaled gas.

The anesthetic potency is characterized by the minimal alveolar concentration (MAC) of a drug that abolishes motion in response to a noxious stimulus in 50 percent of people. The more potent an anesthetic, the lower its value for MAC. The dose-response curve is steep: 99 percent of people remain immobile when given 1.3 times the MAC of an anesthetic.

Why is MAC important? Just as uptake and distribution (see the next section) describe the pharmacokinetics of inhaled anesthetics, MAC describes their pharmacodynamics. The analog of MAC for non-inhalation drugs is the steady-state plasma concentration at 50 percent effect, or $Cpss_{(50)}$. Inhaled anesthetics have very low therapeutic indices, ranging around 2 to 4. Safe use thus requires accuracy in choosing and administering a dose. MAC allows safe selection of an initial dose (concentration) of drug. The MACs for

TABLE 15-1 Properties of some modern inhalation anesthetics

Drug	MAC, % atm	Vapor pressure at 20 °C, mmHg	Partition coefficients at 37 °C			
			Blood-gas	Brain-blood	Fat-blood	Oil-gas
Nitrous oxide	110.00	—	0.47	1.06	2.3	1.4
Halothane	0.77	243	2.40	2.30	60.0	224.0
Enflurane	1.68	175	1.90	1.45	36.2	98.5
Isoflurane	1.15	238	1.40	2.60	45.0	90.8
Desflurane	6.00	664	0.42	1.29	27.2	18.7
Sevoflurane	1.71	160	0.60	1.70	47.5	53.4
Methoxyflurane	0.16	23	12.00	2.00	49.0	970.0

currently used agents are listed in Table 15-1. Note that the MAC of nitrous oxide is very different from the MACs of volatile anesthetics.

MAC is highest in infants and steadily decreases with age to a value in the elderly of about one-half that of the infant. MAC decreases during pregnancy. It also declines as body temperature drops. There is no synergism or antagonism among inhalation anesthetics when they are administered concurrently: MAC is additive. Thus 1.3 MAC may be provided by adding 0.7 MAC of nitrous oxide to 0.6 MAC of halothane. MAC is increased in the presence of increased sympathetic neurotransmitter activity in the CNS. Thus agents that increase the concentration and release of catecholamines centrally, such as cocaine and amphetamines used acutely, will elevate MAC. MAC is decreased by agents depleting CNS catecholamines, such as methyldopa, clonidine, and chronic amphetamine use. Concurrent administration of intravenous anesthetics, sedatives, or opioids will lower the MAC of inhaled agents. Acute ethanol intoxication decreases MAC (with ethanol providing the balance of CNS depression in additive fashion), while tolerance to alcohol elevates MAC.

Uptake and Distribution of Inhaled Agents

The effect of a given concentration of an anesthetic agent on humans is dependent on its anesthetic potency (MAC) and the manner in which it is handled by the transport mechanisms and storage depots of the body. The process governing uptake of inhalation anesthesia can be divided into several sections (Fig. 15-1).

Since uptake and distribution depend on the tension or pressure of the dissolved gas in blood and tissues, these aspects of inhalation anesthesia are presented in terms of the partial pressure of

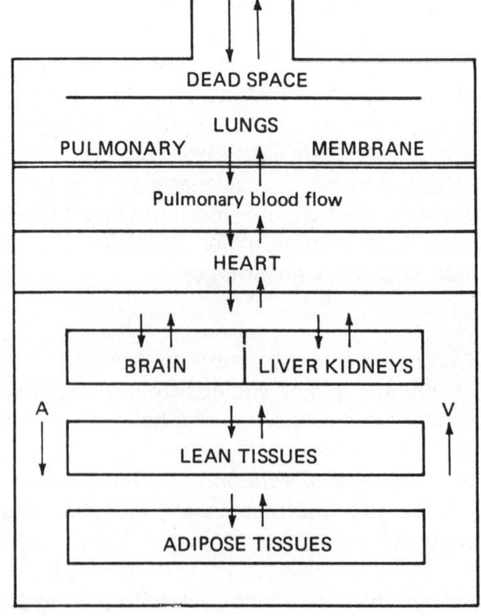

FIGURE 15-1 *Diagram illustrating some of the physiologic and physical factors underlying the uptake of inhalation anesthetics by the body.*

anesthetics rather than their concentrations. The partial pressure of the inhaled anesthetic depends on the vapor pressure and the volume of gas in which the anesthetic is mixed.

After volatilization and mixing in the anesthesia machine, gases are delivered via a breathing circuit. The patient inhales the anesthetic agent, producing an alveolar partial pressure with which each tissue equilibrates. The target tissue in which an anesthetizing partial pressure must develop is the brain. In order to increase the fraction of anesthetic in the alveolus (F_A), the anesthesiologist must deliver a suitable inspired fraction of anesthetic agent (F_I) and the patient must breathe. Ventilation delivers anesthetic to the alveoli, while uptake removes anesthetic from the alveoli. The alveolar concentration results as a balance between these two forces.

Uptake into blood is a product of three factors: anesthetic solubility, cardiac output, and the difference of anesthetic partial pressure between alveolar gas and venous blood. An increase in any of these causes a proportional increase in uptake, presuming the other two factors remain constant. If any of these approaches zero, uptake approaches zero and F_A rapidly approaches F_I.

Anesthetic solubility is a specific type of partition coefficient. If the affinity of gas anesthetic for phase A is twice the affinity for phase B, then we say that gas anesthetic has an A/B partition coefficient of 2. Partition coefficients are measured by determining the relative concentration of gas anesthetic in phases A and B when the partial pressure of gas anesthetic is the same in both phases. Table 15-1 gives representative values for the blood-gas partition coefficient, for the tissue-blood partition coefficients for two tissues (brain and fat), and for the oil-gas partition coefficient.

On the first inspiration of an anesthetic, the blood coming to the alveolus via the pulmonary capillaries is suddenly exposed to the tension of the anesthetic present in the alveolus. If the anesthetic is totally insoluble in blood (i.e., blood-gas partition coefficient = 0), then none of it will be taken up by the circulation and alveolar concentration rises rapidly as permitted by ventilation.

Anesthetics with high blood solubility produce high uptake but slow induction, since alveolar partial pressure rises slowly. With anesthetics of low blood solubility only a small quantity is dissolved in blood, so the alveolar concentration rises rapidly. This process is somewhat analogous to a drug administered intravenously that is highly bound to plasma proteins: more drug must be given to saturate binding sites so that enough unbound, free drug remains to exert its effect.

An increase in cardiac output presents more blood to the anesthetic within the alveolus, leading to an increase in uptake, a slower rise of alveolar partial pressure, and prolonged induction.

The uptake of an anesthetic agent by the tissue depends on the same factors as described for the blood — the tension gradient between the blood and the tissue, the solubility of the agent in a particular organ, and finally the blood flow. A high tissue solubility (a high tissue-blood partition coefficient), a high tissue volume relative to blood flow, and a high arterial to tissue anesthetic partial pressure difference all increase uptake by tissue.

Subsequent distribution throughout the body is shown by the directional arrows of Fig. 15-1. On the arterial side (A), the tension of anesthetic reaching tissues is the same. The volume of blood flow to the brain, heart, and kidneys is high compared with their mass. Diffusion of anesthetic gas into and out of tissues occurs according to the prevailing partial pressure gradient on the venous side (V) of the circulation. The tension of anesthetic returning to the right heart and lungs represents the flow-weighted average of tensions of anesthetic returned from the various tissues.

In Fig. 15-2, curves demonstrate the rate of the increase in arterial partial pressure of several anesthetics expected to occur during administration of anesthetics. The curves show how arterial anesthetic gas tensions approach a constant inhaled tension of the gas or vapor which would be expected to produce anesthesia. Because of the excellent blood supply of the brain and the rapid exchange of dissolved gas between brain and blood, the curves also indicate the partial pressures reached in the brain, leading to the induction of the anesthetic state. It is assumed that the minute volume of respiration, the size of the lung compartments, and the cardiac output are average normal values for adults. The general shape and direction of the curves in Fig. 15-2 are similar for each anesthetic, indicating the constancy of the physiologic conditions. The variations are explained by differences in the physical properties of the anesthetics. Initially, within 2 to 3 min, there is a sharp rise in the arterial curve and a leveling off at the knee of the curve, with a different height for each anesthetic. The heights reached indicate that nitrous oxide approaches the inhaled tension most rapidly. This reflects the relative solubilities in blood, those anesthetics with the lesser solubilities maintaining an alveolar pressure close to the inhaled tension. Thus the *height of*

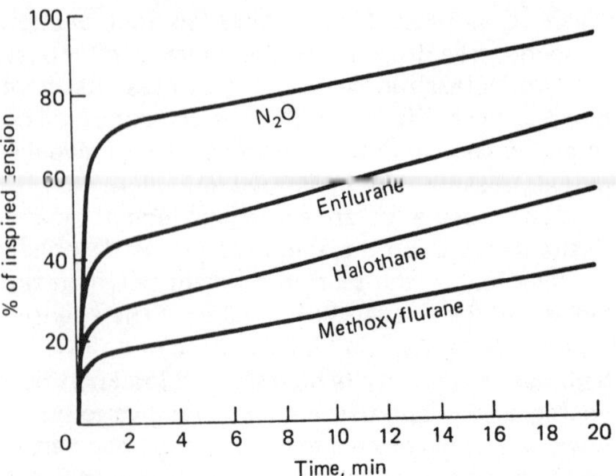

FIGURE 15-2 *Exchange of gas at lungs and tissues. Graphic representation of how the tension of anesthetic gas in arterial blood approaches inspired tension during the course of inhalation anesthesia (values calculated from a formula derived by Kety). With the inspired tension of anesthesia gas shown as 100 percent, the tension of anesthetic in arterial blood is read from the ordinate as a percentage of the inspired tension. Time in minutes is shown on the abscissa.*

the knee for each anesthetic inversely corresponds to its solubility in the blood, so that nitrous oxide may be expected to induce anesthesia quickly, methoxyflurane more slowly.

It appears from Fig. 15-2 that anesthesia is never reached with the anesthetics that are most soluble. Practically, however, the anesthesiologist does not maintain a constant inhaled partial pressure of anesthetic, as the diagram suggests, but increases the partial pressure for rapid induction and subsequently varies the level according to the patient's reactions and the surgical needs. When saturation of tissues is approached, the arterial anesthetic tension approximates that of the inhaled tension. The process of desaturation and emergence from anesthesia can be followed graphically by inverting the curves shown in Fig. 15-2, but this is true only if equilibration had been reached; otherwise, redistribution among tissues could still be most rapid with the agents that are least soluble in blood, e.g., nitrous oxide. At the same time, rapid diffusion into the alveoli lowers the blood level quickly, and within the period of lung washout there should be an approach to recovery of consciousness. Even in this case, however, a residual concentration is present in blood as long as the tissues retain the anesthetic, this again being a function of circulation and distribution between blood and tissues.

The actual sequence of anesthesia induction provides insight into the choice of modern anesthetic agents. The anesthesiologist employs a precision calibrated vaporizer to increase gradually the inspired concentration of volatile anesthetic in oxygen. Corrugated tubing delivers this gas mixture to a mask placed snugly over the patient's mouth and nose. Anesthetic concentration is increased by about 0.5 percent with every other breath. The patient passes through several "stages" of anesthesia. In the first stage, the stage of analgesia, sensation to pain is blunted while consciousness remains intact. During stage 2, the stage of excitability, inhibitory reflexes are depressed, and the patient is unable to follow commands. Respirations become irregular, heart rate increases, and cardiac dysrhythmias may appear. The patient may attempt to sit up and leave the room, or may pull out intravenous catheters and disengage monitoring devices. Vomiting and regurgitation may occur; inhibition of the appropriate reflex laryngeal closure to entry of this foreign material may result in pulmonary aspiration of gastric secretions, an event associated with high mortality. For these reasons, clinicians strive to minimize the intensity and duration of stage 2.

As delivery of anesthetic to the brain progresses, stage 3, the stage of surgical anesthesia, begins. Anesthesiologists refer to the planes, or levels, of this stage as being light or deep, with deep indicating greater depression. Finally, if administration of large doses of anesthetic continues, stage 4 results. At this stage, depressant effects produce cardiovascular collapse and death.

Mechanism of Action

From 1899 to 1901, Meyer and Overton proposed a theory regarding "the action of the anesthetic agents." They correlated the potency of anesthetics with their degree of solubility in olive oil, the more fat-soluble anesthetic agents being more potent. Others related anesthetic potency to surface tension reducing properties or to the ease of formation of "icebergs" within the cell. Anesthetics most likely act by changing the physical properties of the phospholipid matrix of the biologic membrane, resulting in altered function of receptors and ion channels.

General anesthetics have physiologic effects on the neurons of the CNS. These compounds decrease the firing rate of nerve cells by decreasing the rise of the action potential. The proposed molecular mechanism is based on the effects of these agents on sodium movement across the membrane. The general anesthetics apparently attach to the sodium channels by interacting with the lipid and hydrophilic areas of the channel causing a distortion of this structure. The resulting distortion of the channel causes an interference in sodium conductance across the membrane.

INHALED ANESTHETIC AGENTS

Nitrous Oxide

Chemistry Nitrous oxide, N_2O, the only inorganic gas used to produce anesthesia in humans, has a molecular weight of 44 and specific gravity of 1.527 (air = 1). It is neither flammable nor explosive but will support combustion of other agents, even in the absence of oxygen, owing to its decomposition to N_2 and O_2 at temperatures about 450 °C. The oil-water solubility ratio is 3.2. The blood-gas solubility coefficient is 0.47.

Pharmacokinetics Despite the relative insolubility of nitrous oxide in blood, a large amount is rapidly taken up because high concentrations are given. Within 20 min of administration, as much as 30 L may be absorbed via the lungs and distributed to body tissue. At the termination of anesthesia, if the patient is abruptly permitted to breathe room air, a correspondingly large volume of nitrous oxide diffuses outward, thus lowering alveolar P_{O2}, and temporarily causing hypoxemia (diffusion hypoxia). The large volume of nitrous oxide also decreases alveolar P_{CO2}, causing respiratory depression. This undesirable sequence is avoided by administration of pure oxygen for a few minutes before permitting inhalation of room air. The drug is not metabolized; it is eliminated from the body unchanged through the lungs.

Pharmacodynamics Nitrous oxide is a weak anesthetic agent. Clinical doses are limited to 80 percent, an amount not sufficient to progress beyond stage 2 in most patients. With a MAC of over 100 percent, it cannot be used as the sole anesthetic agent. Nitrous oxide is considered an *incomplete general anesthetic*. However, when combined with another agent, nitrous oxide provides additive anesthetic action: 30 percent nitrous oxide (0.3 MAC) reduces the amount of enflurane needed by 0.3 MAC, from 1.68 to 1.17 percent. Likewise, 70 percent nitrous oxide reduces enflurane requirement to 0.5 percent, which is 0.7 of its MAC.

Adverse Reactions *Hematologic Effects* There is evidence of interference with production of both leukocytes and red blood cells by the bone marrow, following very prolonged administration of nitrous oxide. Nitrous oxide can oxidize the cobalt atom in vitamin B_{12} and, thereby, cause megaloblastic changes in the bone marrow and a neuropathy in experimental animals.

Teratogenic Effects Many epidemiologic surveys have investigated the possible adverse reproductive effects of working in operating or dental suites. The most consistent finding is a higher than expected incidence of spontaneous abortion among female personnel directly exposed to waste anesthetic gases. Spontaneous abortion may be 25 percent more frequent among exposed pregnant women. Spontaneous abortion rates for chairside assistants of dentists increase with increasing duration of exposure to nitrous oxide, reaching a maximum of 2 times the control rate. The data from studies on congenital abnormalities are less consistent. Malformations may be slightly more frequent in the offspring of exposed women.

Diffusion into Air Containing Spaces The blood-gas partition coefficient of nitrous oxide (0.47) is 34 times greater than that of nitrogen (0.014). This differential solubility means nitrous oxide can leave the blood to enter an air (79% nitrogen) filled cavity 34 times more rapidly than nitrogen can leave the cavity to enter the blood. Hence, either the volume or pressure within the cavity increases. Air filled cavities surrounded by a complaint wall (intestinal gas, pneumothorax, lung distal to a pulmonary embolus, and pulmonary vascular air embolism) will expand; for those cavities surrounded by a noncompliant wall (middle ear, cerebral ventricles, and supratentorial subdural space), intra-cavity pressure will increase.

Therapeutic Uses *Analgesia* At a concentration of 6 to 25 percent, nitrous oxide achieves analgesia (stage 1), but patients remain in full contact with their surroundings. As a sole agent, nitrous oxide may thus be used intermittently to provide analgesia for dental procedures and during the first stage of parturition. The drug is used in some countries in this manner to produce postoperative analgesia.

Surgical Anesthesia Since nitrous oxide is an incomplete anesthetic, it must be administered with adjuvant drugs, including neuromuscular blocking agents. Commonly, volatile anesthetics are used, but not infrequently large doses of a short-acting opioid such as fentanyl are given in order to produce an anesthetic state.

Abuse Potential Recreational inhalation of nitrous oxide, which began with the early experiments of Humphrey Davy, gained popularity in recent years owing to the extensive use of nitrous oxide analgesia in dentistry. Nitrous oxide possesses a (false) reputation as a harmless, chemically inert substance.

A survey of medical and dental students at a university via anonymous questionnaire disclosed that up to 20 percent of medical and dental students abused nitrous oxide to produce euphoria. Nitrous oxide had been obtained from a variety of sources, most often the cylinders used for producing whipped cream. Health professionals with easy access to the agent are especially vulnerable to this practice. Some of the 524 students responding to the questionnaire reported nausea, diarrhea, cyanosis, and syncope. Hypoxia and asphyxia leading to malignant dysrhythmias and death may occur when adequate concentrations of inspired oxygen do not accompany inhalation of nitrous oxide.

Halothane

The ongoing research for a potent inhalation agent that was neither explosive nor highly toxic led to the development 40 years ago of halothane, a halogenated hydrocarbon. Halothane was one of the most significant advances in general anesthesia since the introduction of diethyl ether over 100 years earlier.

Chemistry Halothane resembles the pioneering anesthetic chloroform, a substituted alkane. In contrast to halothane are the substituted methyl-ether ethers, including enflurane and isoflurane.

```
 F     Br
  \   /
   C—CH
F/ |   \
   F    Cl
```

At room temperature, halothane exists as a volatile liquid with a vapor pressure of 243 mm Hg, about one-third of an atmosphere at sea level. Since low concentrations of inspired halothane provide surgical anesthesia, the mixture of inspired gases containing halothane must be controlled accurately. A precision, calibrated vaporizer provides this control with correction for changes of vapor pressure with temperature. Halothane is administered only by inhalation of vaporized liquid, never intravenously.

Halothane corrodes many metals and some plastics. Addition of thymol to liquid halothane prevents degradation during storage. Halothane has a sweet, pleasant odor and is not irritating to respiratory mucosa.

Pharmacokinetics Halothane undergoes significant metabolism in humans, with about 20 percent of the absorbed dose recovered as metabolites. Both oxidative and reductive metabolism occur, but oxidative metabolism predominates.

The major metabolite of oxidative metabolism is trifluoroacetic acid, which is excreted in the urine. Other oxidative metabolites that appear in the urine are chloride and bromide. Trifluoroacetic acid has no known adverse effects. However, serum bromide concentration will increase approximately 0.5 mEq/L per MAC per hour of halothane administration. Signs of bromide toxicity (such as somnolence, mental confusion) occur when the serum bromide concentration exceeds 6 mEq/L.

Reductive metabolism of halothane is more likely to occur in the presence of inadequate oxygen delivery to hepatocytes and stimulation of hepatic microsomal enzyme activity by drugs (e.g., phenobarbital) or chemicals (e.g., polychlorobiphenyls). This results in the formation of reactive intermediary metabolites and fluoride. The reactive intermediaries may produce liver damage either directly or via an immune-mediated hypersensitivity reaction.

Pharmacodynamics *Central Nervous System* Inhalation of increasing concentrations of halothane results in progressive obtundation leading to the state of surgical anesthesia and, if continued, on to cardiovascular collapse and death. Halothane produces analgesia and amnesia in sub-MAC concentrations. The EEG reflects these CNS events. The baseline EEG consisting of a fast, low voltage signal becomes a slow, higher voltage signal with clinical doses of halothane. Cerebral blood flow increases even though the cerebral metabolic rate of oxygen use declines: this disparity defines a state of impaired cerebral autoregulation. Halothane increases intracranial (cerebrospinal fluid) pressure.

Cardiovascular System Halothane induces a dose-dependent decrease in systemic blood pressure: mean arterial pressure is halved at 2 MAC. Cardiac output is decreased while systemic vascular resistance changes little. Myocardial blood flow and extraction of oxygen and lactate decrease proportionally, indicating preservation of coronary vascular autoregulation. Heart rate decreases during halothane inhalation secondary to diminished sympathetic tone. Obtunding of the baroreceptor reflex permits heart rate to remain constant or decrease despite a fall in systemic blood pressure. Adrenergic stimulation during halothane inhalation induces ventricular dysrhythmias. The source of this stimulation may be extrinsic, as from a surgical incision or administration of epinephrine, or intrinsic, as occurs with hypercarbia and light planes of anesthesia. Although overall systemic vascular resistance remains unchanged, splanchnic beds constrict while skin and muscle beds dilate.

Respiratory System Halothane decreases tidal volume and increases respiratory rate in humans, yielding a net decrease in minute ventilation. As a consequence, the arterial P_{CO2} rises to almost 50 mmHg at 1 MAC. The normal ventilatory response to carbon dioxide is attenuated: the curve is shifted to the right (decreased minute ventilation for a given P_{CO2}), and its slope is less steep (smaller increase in ventilation per mmHg increase in P_{CO2}). These alterations are centrally mediated and not secondary to an effect on peripheral chemoreceptors. The ventilatory response to hypoxia is also obtunded by halothane. Only 1.1 MAC obliterates the normal hyperventilatory response to hypoxia. Unlike halothane's attenuation of the effects of hypercarbia, halothane depresses the hypoxic respiratory drive by directly affecting peripheral chemoreceptors.

Halothane dilates a constricted airway via direct action on bronchial smooth muscle as well as via depression of local reflex arcs: its effect is not dependent on obtaining blood concentrations of drug. A resting, unstimulated airway with normal bronchial tone is not further dilated by halothane. Mucociliary function is depressed during halothane inhalation.

Neuromuscular Junction By itself, halothane provides inadequate muscle relaxation for surgery, although it does potentiate the action of nondepolarizing muscle relaxants. At 1 MAC of halothane, the dose of neuromuscular blocking drug may be reduced by about one-third to one-half. The site of action appears to be the muscle membrane.

Other Effects Renal blood flow and glomerular filtration rate both decrease during halothane inhalation. Renovascular autoregulation is not disturbed. The rate of urine production decreases by more than half. Hepatic blood flow and hepatic enzymatic activity decrease. Halothane relaxes the uterus: it is used clinically to treat uterine tetany during labor.

Adverse Reactions *Halothane Hepatotoxicity* Soon after the discovery of halothane, reports of postoperative jaundice and hepatic necrosis appeared with findings similar to those caused by chloroform. Repeated administration of halothane has been associated with liver damage in rare instances. Prolonged exposure to halothane, even following enzyme induction with phenobarbital, has failed to produce liver damage. However, both pretreatment and hypoxia produce centrilobular necrosis following exposure to halothane.

Sustained exposure to halothane permits significant acetylation of the compound which may increase the risk of liver damage. The acetylated molecule participates in an immune mechanism resulting in damage to hepatic proteins and cells. The U.S. National Halothane Study reviewed 85,000 anesthesias. It concluded that the incidence of massive hepatic necrosis associated with halothane is 1 in 10,000 and recommended that unexplained fever and jaundice following halothane might reasonably be considered a contraindication to subsequent use.

Dysrhythmias Theophylline, like epinephrine and other sympathomimetic agents, may cause ventricular tachycardia or fibrillation during halothane anesthesia. The use of alternative inhalation agents with a bronchodilator effect, such as enflurane or isoflurane, is recommended for asthmatic patients who must receive theophylline (or aminophylline) before or during surgery. Patients who are being treated for depression with the tricyclic compound amitriptyline may suffer life-threatening ventricular dysrhythmias when given halothane and pancuronium, probably related to the blocking effect of tricyclic compound on reuptake of the neurotransmitter norepinephrine.

Malignant Hyperthermia A rare patient (one in 10,000 to 20,000) experiences rapid temperature elevation upon exposure to volatile anesthetics or the depolarizing muscle relaxant succinylcholine.

This syndrome, which occurs only in genetically susceptible individuals, arises from a primary disorder of muscle involving poor control of intracellular calcium sequestration during muscle contraction. Although malignant hyperthermia is of little consequence when a susceptible individual is not anesthetized, when it occurs untreated under anesthesia, death is likely. Metabolic acidemia, cardiac dysrhythmias, and hyperkalemia accompany episodes of malignant hyperthermia. Prophylaxis for susceptible patients and treatment of ongoing episodes utilize dantrolene, a drug which interferes with the release of calcium from the sarcoplasmic reticulum (see Chapter 12).

Therapeutic Use Halothane induces analgesia, amnesia, loss of consciousness, and obtunds noxious reflexes such as bradycardia and laryngospasm. These properties define a complete anesthetic. Halothane may serve as the sole agent in providing anesthesia in suitable patients for procedures not requiring muscular relaxation although, for reasons already discussed, a single drug is rarely used to provide anesthesia. Despite the attraction of a certain simplicity in providing anesthesia with a single drug, one agent, such as halothane, is rarely administered by itself. More commonly, other anesthetic agents and adjuvants combine with halothane to provide a smoother and safer passage from consciousness to stage 3. A rapid acting intravenous agent such as thiopental will bypass stages 1 and 2 altogether; the term *induction agent* is suitably applied. Addition of nitrous oxide to a halothane oxygen gas mixture utilizes the additive properties of MAC and the more favorable blood-gas partition coefficient of nitrous oxide to accelerate anesthetic delivery to brain and shorten stage 2. Following induction of anesthesia, controlled ventilation, as opposed to spontaneous breathing, prevents the adverse consequences of hypercarbia attendant with inhalation of volatile anesthetic (see below).

The factors determining choice of volatile anesthetic agent are varied and complex. The patient's pathophysiologic derangements related to concurrent disease states provide the primary motivations to select or avoid particular drugs. For example, severe asthmatics who require general anesthetics often do best with a volatile agent, which dilates constricted bronchi. Patients with congestive heart failure, on the other hand, may develop worsening failure with the volatile anesthetics owing to myocardial contractile depression. Some clinicians avoid halothane in patients with a history of abnormal liver function, so that in the event of postoperative worsening of hepatic function, the differential diagnosis is not complicated by the specter of halothane hepatitis.

During a mask induction of anesthesia using halothane and oxygen, with or without nitrous oxide, large concentrations of halothane, up to 5 percent or even higher, will be administered transiently. The purpose of this "over-pressuring" is to establish as quickly as possible a brain partial pressure of anesthetic that is consistent with stage 3 anesthesia. Following induction, inspired concentrations are decreased to match the level of surgical stimulation. For example, during placement of surgical drapes, stimulation is minimal; the anesthetic requirement may be less than 1 MAC, say 0.5 percent. In contrast, the deeper plane of anesthesia needed for manipulation of the peritoneum often demands concentrations around 1.5 percent, or about 2 MAC.

Enflurane

Following synthesis of halothane, a substituted ethane, the search continued for a halogenated anesthetic similar in structure to diethyl ether. A series of substituted ethers emerged, including fluroxene, methoxyflurane, enflurane, and isoflurane. Of these, enflurane and isoflurane remain in common use today.

Chemistry Enflurane is a substituted methyl ethyl ether. The oxygen linkage combined with increased fluorine substitution yields greater molecular stability compared with halothane. Enflurane is less volatile and less potent than halothane. Its room temperature vapor pressure of 175 mmHg is about one-quarter of an atmosphere at sea level. MAC for enflurane is 1.68 percent, more than twice that of halothane. Like halothane, enflurane has a sweet odor, although enflurane inhalation is slightly less pleasant and more irritating to respiratory mucosa.

```
F         F  F
 \   O    /  /
 HC     C--CH
 |     /     \
 F    F       Cl
```

Pharmacokinetics The lower blood-gas partition coefficient for enflurane allows for more rapid onset and offset of anesthesia compared with halothane. A lower solubility in fat results in more rapid excretion and less time for metabolism to occur. Small amounts of enflurane are defluorinated in the liver yielding several metabolic products including fluoride ion. While excessive fluoride is nephrotoxic, peak fluoride levels rarely exceed even half the threshold for toxicity.

Pharmacodynamics The increase in cerebral blood flow during enflurane inhalation is less than that during halothane administration. Enflurane profoundly depresses the oxygen and glucose needs of the brain. Like halothane, enflurane increases intracranial pressure. Large doses of enflurane result in seizure-like activity, especially in the presence of hypercarbia. Both abnormal muscular contraction and spike-and-dome complexes on the EEG can occur. Enflurane-induced seizure activity markedly elevates the cerebral metabolic rate.

Blood pressure decreases during enflurane administration secondary to decreases in both cardiac output and systemic vascular resistance. Heart rate remains unchanged. Junctional rhythm occurs on occasion, while ventricular ectopy is rare even during sympathetic stimulation.

Tidal volume and respiratory rate both decrease, producing profound ventilatory depression and arterial P_{CO2} values greater than 60 mmHg at 1 MAC. Like halothane, enflurane dilates a constricted airway and obtunds the ventilatory responses to hypercarbia and hypoxia. Potentiation of nondepolarizing muscle relaxants is greater with enflurane than with halothane, thus reducing the dose of relaxant by two-thirds. Enflurane and halothane have similar effects on the kidney, liver, and uterus.

Isoflurane

Chemistry Isoflurane is an isomer of enflurane. The MAC of isoflurane is about 1.15 percent, which is lower than the MAC of its isomer enflurane (1.68 percent). The blood-gas and oil-gas partition coefficients are 1.4 and 98, respectively. Isoflurane is more pungent than both halothane and enflurane.

```
F        H   F
 \      /   /
 HC--O-C---C--F
 |     \    \
 F      Cl   F
```

Pharmacokinetics Isoflurane causes direct coronary vascular dilatation leading to redistribution of coronary blood flow away from diseased vessels that had already been maximally dilated, thereby worsening ischemia. However, the existence of this syndrome has not been proven in humans, and its effect on the outcome in humans undergoing anesthesia with isoflurane appears small.

Insignificant metabolism of isoflurane occurs in the body, yielding negligible amounts of fluoride ion and trifluoroacetic acid. Although enzyme induction by phenobarbital, ethanol, and isoniazid increases the metabolism of isoflurane, the amount of fluoride ion released is of no clinical significance.

Pharmacodynamics Isoflurane increases cerebral blood flow and decreases cerebral metabolic rate for oxygen (CMR_{O2}). At 1.5 to 2 MAC, isoflurane decreases CMR_{O2} by 50 percent and produces an isoelectric EEG. Further increases do not produce deeper metabolic depression. The effect of isoflurane on the EEG is dose dependent: fast activity with low amplitude occurs at 0.5 MAC, progressing with increasing dose through slow waves and burst suppression to an isoelectric tracing at 2 MAC. Isoflurane promotes muscle relaxation and enhances the effects of muscle relaxants on the neuromuscular junction to the same extent as enflurane. This characteristic is attributed to the increase in the effects on the CNS and the neuromuscular junction. Mean arterial pressure decreases with the administration of isoflurane in a dose-dependent fashion, due mostly to a decrease in systemic vascular resistance.

Desflurane

This inhalation anesthetic features low blood solubility, permitting rapid recovery from anesthesia. It has a low molecular weight (168 Da). At one atmosphere, desflurane boils at room temperature; this results from the substitution of a fluorine atom for the chlorine in isoflurane. The drug is considerably less potent than isoflurane, with a highly variable MAC (3 to 10 percent; average of approximately 6).

```
F        H   F
 \      /   /
 HC--O-C---C--F
 |     \    \
 F      F    F
```

The low blood-gas partition coefficient of desflurane (0.42), close to that of nitrous oxide, produces an exceptionally rapid induction of and recovery from anesthesia. However, airway irritation limits the usefulness of the drug as an induction agent, since coughing and breath holding ensue. Extreme volatility of the liquid requires specially constructed precision vaporizers for delivery. The rapid elimination of desflurane via the lungs decreases the risk of toxicity from biodegradation.

Like its congeners, desflurane depresses the ventilatory response to both carbon dioxide and to hypoxia. It produces a dose-dependent decrease in blood pressure and systemic vascular resistance. The cardiovascular depressant effects of desflurane manifest during controlled ventilation as increased cardiac filling pressure and decreased stroke volume, but not until concentrations exceed 1.66 times MAC.

Desflurane potentiates the action of neuromuscular relaxants as extensively as do enflurane and isoflurane. Cerebrovascular resistance and the CMR_{O2} decrease in dose-dependent fashion. The resulting cerebral vasodilation increases intracranial pressure. Like isoflurane, desflurane depresses the electroencephalogram. Toxicity to liver or kidney has not been elicited with desflurane.

Sevoflurane

Like desflurane, the volatile anesthetic sevoflurane features very low solubility in blood. The blood-gas partition coefficient of 0.60 produces rapid induction and emergence from anesthesia and the ability to change anesthetic depth rapidly. The MAC of sevoflurane, 1.7 percent, resembles those of enflurane and isoflurane. Unlike desflurane, inhaled induction appears to be pleasant.

Metabolism of sevoflurane produces fluoride ion. However, rapid removal of sevoflurane from the body via pulmonary excretion yields only transient increases in serum fluoride concentration. About 2 or 3 percent of sevoflurane undergoes metabolism during a one hour anesthetic procedure. Isoniazid and ethanol induce the metabolism of sevoflurane.

Like halothane, sevoflurane increases respiratory rate, yet decreases minute ventilation, thus increasing P_{CO2}. Sevoflurane decreases cardiac output and blood pressure with little effect on heart rate. Similar to other newer inhaled agents (enflurane, isoflurane, and desflurane), it does not sensitize the myocardium to dysrhythmic effects of epinephrine. Cerebral blood flow increases less so than with other volatile anesthetics. Liver, kidney, or bone marrow toxicity is rare.

Methoxyflurane

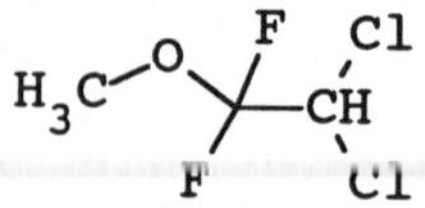

H_3C—O F Cl CH F Cl

Another substituted methyl ethyl ether, methoxyflurane, has a characteristic fruity odor. With a MAC of 0.16 percent, it is the most potent anesthetic available. Its high blood-gas solubility coefficient of about 12 yields prolonged induction and emergence from anesthesia. Clinicians employ methoxyflurane rarely owing to the drug's potential for nephrotoxicity. Biotransformation liberates a significant amount of fluoride ion, which can produce high output renal failure.

INTRAVENOUS ANESTHETICS

The first attempt at producing insensibility by means of intravenous injection occurred in 1656, when Percival Christopher Wren, with the encouragement of Dr. Robert Boyle, injected tincture of opium into the vein of a dog. Since then, many drugs have been tried with varying degrees of success. But it was not until the introduction of thiopental, a sulfur derivative of pentobarbital, independently by Lundy and Waters in 1934, that the intravenous method began to achieve popularity. The simplicity of the intravenous induction technique, combined with its ready acceptance by patients, has created widespread popularity among clinicians. However, its utility is limited by side effects and a lack of rapid reversibility.

These agents are discussed here briefly, highlighting their uses in the practice of anesthesia. Full presentations for several drugs appear in other chapters (see Chapters 16, 17, and 23).

Ultrashort-Acting Barbiturates

The ultrashort-acting barbiturates are highly lipid soluble. Therefore, they are suitable for induction of anesthesia. The two most commonly used are thiopental and methohexital. The uptake by brain is very rapid and reaches a maximum within 30 sec. Anesthesia lasts for 5 min. This short duration of action is due to rapid redistribution of the drug from brain to muscle and skin. Redistribution to fatty tissue is much slower owing to minimal perfusion of this tissue group.

Thiopental has a profound, direct, and dose-dependent depressant effect on the myocardium. An induction dose decreases stroke volume and cardiac output, resulting in hypotension. Thiopental decreases venous tone, thus decreasing venous return to the heart. This effect is mediated through depression of the CNS and, to a lesser degree, through direct relaxation of venous smooth muscle.

Barbiturates decrease cerebral blood flow (CBF) and CMR_{O2} in a dose-dependent fashion. Both components are reduced by 30 percent with an induction dose of thiopental. Larger doses of thiopental decrease these parameters by 50 percent and produce an isoelectric EEG. Doses greater than those which provide an isoelectric EEG do not further decrease CBF and CMR_{O2}. Cerebral blood flow autoregulation and its response to carbon dioxide remain intact at a mean arterial pressure above 60 mmHg. The depressant effect of barbiturates on CBF makes these drugs ideal for induction of anesthesia and management of patients within increased intracranial pressure. The salutary effects of barbiturates on CBF, CMR_{O2}, and intracranial pressure suggest that patients predisposed to cerebral ischemia, such as those with carotid occlusive disease, may benefit from their use. This approach remains controversial. Limited protection can be achieved with barbiturates in incomplete ischemia, while in complete ischemia the brain does not benefit from the effect of barbiturates.

The termination of action of thiobarbiturates depends on redistribution of the drug away from the brain (see Fig. 15-3). Accumulation of the drug in other tissue depots accrues, however, which may lead to continued low levels of drug entering the bloodstream. Thus, if given in sufficiently high doses, ultrashort-acting hypnotics may have a long duration of action.

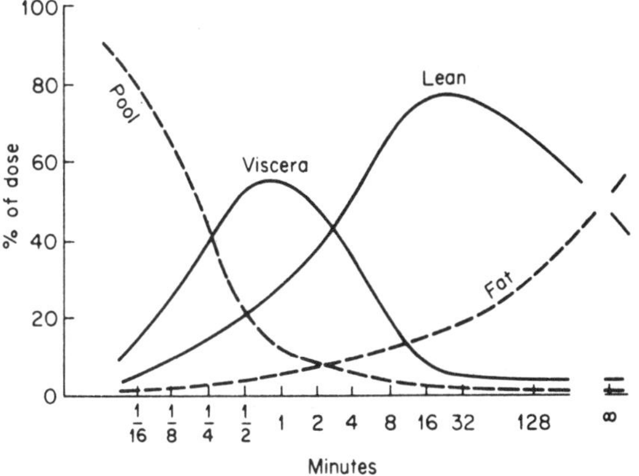

FIGURE 15-3 *Distribution of thiopental in different body tissues at various times after intravenous injection. Time scale (in minutes) progresses geometrically. Final values are at infinity.*

Ketamine

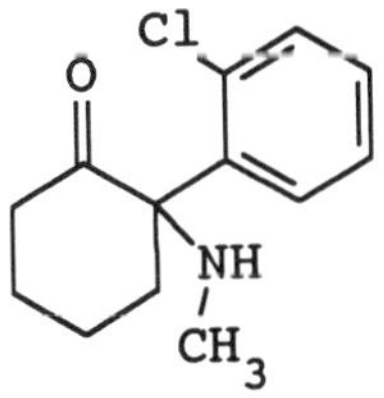

Phencyclidine (PCP) and ketamine produce a state called *dissociative anesthesia*, which provides amnesia and analgesia while preserving respiratory drive and muscle tone and augmenting sympathetic nervous system tone. Phencyclidine has been abandoned owing to the high frequency of its side effects: hallucinations, unpleasant dreams, and excitement. Phencyclidine is abused by individuals for its hallucinogenic property. These dysphoric sequelae occur less frequently with ketamine, which is still used for anesthesia. Induction is complete within 30 sec and lasts for 15 min. Analgesia is profound and lasts about 40 min. The amnestic effect may linger for 1 to 2 h.

Premedication with morphine and scopolamine, benzodiazepines, or butyrophenones reduces the dysphoric effects of ketamine. Young adults and children have a lower incidence of these side effects than adult patients. Ketamine is a valuable induction agent for critically ill and pediatric patients and as an analgesic during parturition. It enjoys an expanding role in outpatient procedures.

Etomidate

Etomidate is an imidazole-containing molecule not structurally similar to other anesthetics.

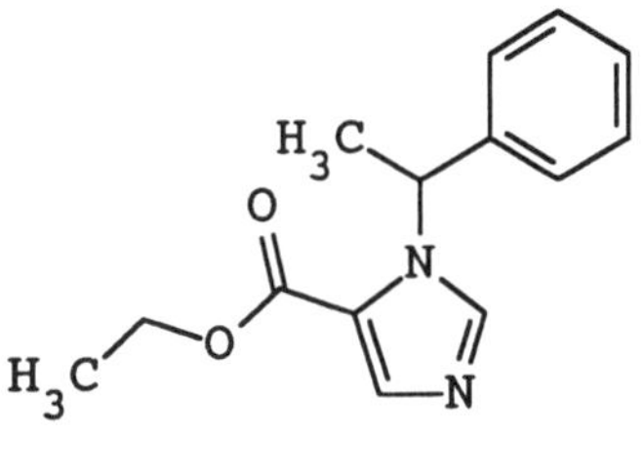

Since intravenous bolus doses provide rapid loss of consciousness, etomidate is classified as a sedative-hypnotic agent. Owing to poor solubility in water above pH 3, clinical preparations employ a propylene glycol solvent, which often engenders pain on injection.

The speed of onset and offset of unconsciousness is slightly less rapid than that of the thiobarbiturates. Rapid redistribution from brain to other tissues provides the rapid offset, as with the thiobarbiturates. Both hepatic microsomal enzymes and plasma esterases participate in metabolism of etomidate. The cerebral effects of etomidate and thiopental are similar: cerebral blood flow, CMR_{O2}, and intracranial pressure all decrease; both drugs are anticonvulsant; neither drug is analgesic. Unlike thiopental, etomidate occasionally causes transient myoclonic activity, which is not accompanied by seizure activity on the EEG.

Heart rate remains unchanged while systemic vascular resistance and blood pressure decrease slightly. There is a high incidence of nausea and vomiting postoperatively. Steroid production in the adrenal gland is inhibited for several hours following induction doses of etomidate. Inhibition of steroid synthesis can lead to an Addisonian crisis in patients maintained on continuous infusion of etomidate for long-term sedation in intensive-care units.

Etomidate is useful for rapid induction of anesthesia in patients with cardiovascular instability, particularly in patients with elevated intracranial pressure. Pain on injection and postoperative nausea and vomiting limit its widespread use.

Propofol

This newer hypnotic agent requires a vehicle of soybean oil, glycerol, and egg lecithin for intravenous administration. It is stable at room temperature.

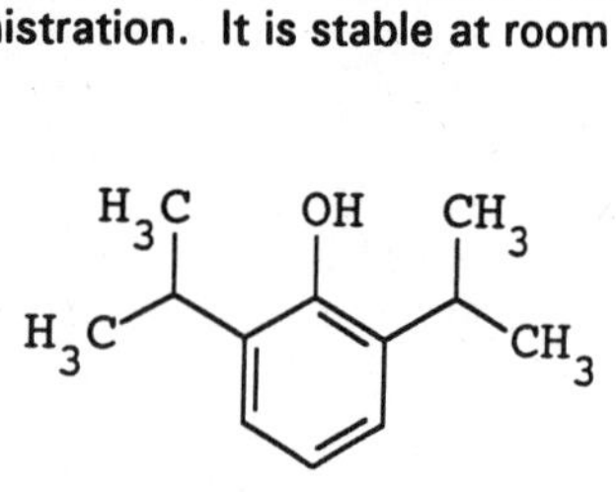

H_3C OH CH_3
H_3C CH_3

A dose of 1.5 to 3 mg/kg causes unconsciousness within seconds. High lipid solubility permits ready penetration of the blood-brain barrier, resulting in rapid induction. Recovery occurs in about 5 min at a plasma concentration of about 1 mg/mL. Propofol is 96 percent bound to plasma proteins, with a distribution half-life of 2.2 min and elimination half-life of 70 min. Its brief action after a single injection results from redistribution and hepatic metabolism. Active metabolites are not known. Clinical applications include induction of general anesthesia and continuous infusion for maintenance of general anesthesia. Patients awaken from propofol anesthesia devoid of nausea and with exceptional clear-headedness.

Propofol is a respiratory depressant. Like other induction agents, it may produce brief periods of apnea. Systemic blood pressure, stroke volume, and systemic vascular resistance decrease minimally. Cardiac output remains unchanged. Propofol reduces cerebral blood flow, CMR_{O2}, and intracranial pressure in dose-dependent fashion. Intraocular pressure decreases after propofol administration. The drug has few adverse effects in the liver or kidneys.

Potent Opioids

Use as Adjuvants Opioids are used widely in the practice of anesthesia as adjuvant drugs. Since opioid analgesics are essential for relief of pain after an operation, patients often receive an opioid prior to the termination of anesthesia. Clinical doses of opioids permit the use of smaller doses of anesthetic agents. Patients frequently receive an opioid prior to surgery as part of their premedication. The usual choice in this regard is intramuscular morphine. Clinical trials have shown sufentanil-impregnated lollipops to be equally successful in small children.

Use in Balanced Anesthesia Opioid analgesics form an essential part of the "balanced" anesthetic technique, in which about 0.7 MAC of nitrous oxide, a skeletal muscle relaxant, and an opioid are administered together. Other components of balanced anesthesia are a thiobarbiturate for induction, hyperventilation, and a potent sedative-amnestic such as scopolamine. Balanced anesthesia provides selected patients with rapid awakening to a lucid, intensely analgesic state. The analgesics that are currently used for anesthesia are morphine, fentanyl, sufentanil, and alfentanil. Morphine 0.1 to 0.3 mg/kg is usually employed in long procedures. However, fentanyl 8 to 20 μg/kg is the drug of choice for shorter surgical procedures.

Fentanyl is a synthetic opioid that is approximately 80 percent bound to plasma proteins, has a volume of distribution of 40 L/kg, and an elimination half-life of 3 to 4 h. Redistribution of fentanyl from brain to other tissues accounts for its shorter duration of action. Unlike morphine, fentanyl does not release histamine upon rapid injection. Its structure is:

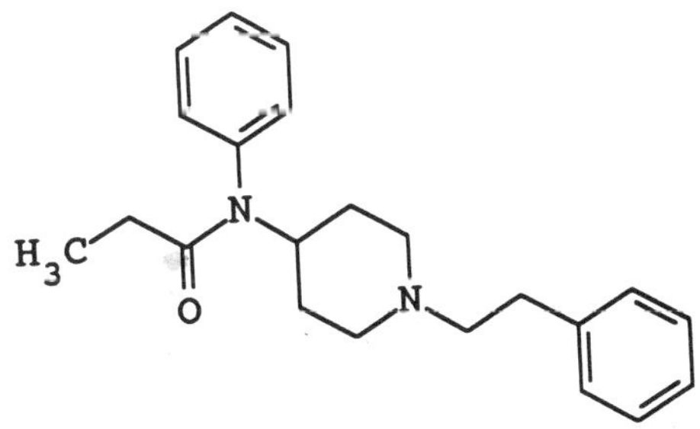

$$H_3C-CH_2-C(=O)-N(C_6H_5)-C_5H_9N-CH_2CH_2-C_6H_5$$

Compared with fentanyl, sufentanil is more lipophilic and 10 times more potent. Induction is more rapid, and histamine release is likewise absent. Alfentanil is less potent than fentanyl (1:4 ratio) but much more lipophilic; its short duration of action makes it inappropriate for procedures lasting many hours.

Use as Sole Anesthetic Agents High doses of potent opioids produce profound analgesia and anesthesia in most patients. The opioid is given intravenously while the patient inhales pure oxygen. As with balanced anesthesia, an amnestic agent is frequently employed. Morphine, 1 to 2 mg/kg, was the first opioid to gain widespread use as the sole anesthetic for patients with cardiovascular compromise. The rapidity of injection is limited severely by histamine release and need for fluid administration. Compared with morphine, fentanyl is more lipophilic and 80 times more potent; furthermore, it does not release histamine. Intravenous induction doses of fentanyl vary from 20 to 100 μg/kg. With these large doses, duration of action is no longer determined by redistribution but rather by elimination half-life. Both alfentanil and sufentanil are also used both intravenous injection as primary anesthetics for the induction of anesthesia.

Opioids given rapidly act in the CNS to cause bradycardia and muscular rigidity, the latter most notably affecting the chest wall, thus impairing ventilation. Cardiovascular stability is prominent with all opioids except meperidine. Partial agonist-antagonist agents do not provide satisfactory oxygen-opioid anesthesia owing to their limited efficacy. Respiratory depression is profound and long lasting, necessitating controlled ventilation for as long as 24 h. An occasional patient is not completely anesthetized with this technique and exhibits a hyperdynamic circulatory state characterized by tachycardia, hypertension, and high cardiac output. Sub-MAC doses of volatile anesthetics usually control these undesirable hemodynamics.

Benzodiazepines

The primary use of these drugs is the treatment of anxiety. CNS effects of benzodiazepines include anxiolysis, sedation, anticonvulsant activity, amnesia, and skeletal muscle relaxation. Three compounds in the group are of particular interest to anesthesiologists: diazepam, lorazepam, and midazolam. These drugs are utilized in various surgical procedures as preanesthetic medications for their calming effect. All three potentiate the action of γ-aminobutyric acid (GABA), an inhibitory neurotransmitter in the cerebrum, substantia nigra, hippocampus, cerebellum, and spinal cord.

Diazepam Diazepam is used widely as a preanesthetic medication, an adjunct to regional anesthesia, and an induction agent for minor procedures including endoscopy. Owing to poor solubility in water, the parenteral form is a glycol-alcohol solution that causes pain and venous irritation upon intravenous administration as well as unpredictable absorption when given by intramuscular injection. Diazepam has a high volume of distribution and a low clearance rate, resulting in an elimination half-life of 20 to 40 h. Oxidative metabolism in the liver yields active metabolites. Elderly patients exhibit prolonged excretion owing to changes in tissue distribution and protein binding.

Diazepam has minimal circulatory effects. It produces less depression of ventilation than barbiturates. However, in combination with opioids and anesthetics, significant respiratory depression will occur. It is highly effective as an anticonvulsant and useful to control the skeletal muscle rigidity and spasm in patients with tetanus or cerebral palsy.

Lorazepam Lorazepam is slow in onset of action (10 to 20 min). Its chief use has been as a preanesthetic medication and as an adjuvant to regional anesthesia due to its profound anxiolytic, amnesic, and tranquilizing effects. Pharmacologic actions are similar to those of diazepam. Although its elimination half-life (16 h) is shorter than that of diazepam, its clinical duration of action is longer than the action of diazepam, since the less lipid soluble lorazepam terminates more by elimination than redistribution.

Midazolam This drug is used by intramuscular injection as a pre-operative sedative, and by the intravenous route for induction of anesthesia and to produce conscious sedation prior to short diagnostic or endoscopic procedures. Midazolam is a water-soluble benzodiazepine. Pain on intramuscular injection and post-injection phlebitis are rare. Despite a large volume of distribution, the elimination half-life is 2 to 4 h owing to rapid hepatic clearance. Midazolam has little effect on the cardiovascular system. Ventilation is usually preserved, although intravenous administration demands the presence of equipment to control ventilation in case apnea ensues. Midazolam is approximately 1.5 to 2 times more potent than diazepam.

Flumazenil Flumazenil is a competitive benzodiazepine receptor antagonist (see Chapter 17 for a more complete discussion). The drug reverses the CNS sedative effects of benzodiazepines and is indicated where general anesthesia has been induced by or maintained with benzodiazepines such as diazepam, lorazepam, or midazolam.

BIBLIOGRAPHY

Buffington, C.W., J.L. Romson, A. Levine, N.C. Duttlinger, and A.H. Huang: "Isoflurane Induces Coronary Steal in a Canine Model of Chronic Coronary Occlusion," *Anesthesiology* **66**: 280-292 (1987).

Edwards, R.P., R.D. Miller, M.F. Roizen, J. Ham, W.L. Way, C.R. Lake, and L. Roderick: "Cardiac Responses to Imipramine and Pancuronium During Anesthesia with Halothane or Enflurane," *Anesthesiology* **50**: 421-425 (1979).

Holaday, D.A., and F.R. Smith: "Clinical Characteristics and Biotransformation of Sevoflurane in Healthy Human Volunteers," *Anesthesiology* **54**: 100-106 (1981).

Morison, D.H.: "New IV Induction Anaesthetics," *Can. J. Anaesth.* **40**: R9-R18 (1993).

Nakajima, R., Y. Nakajima, and K. Ikeda: "Minimum Alveolar Concentration of Sevoflurane in Elderly Patients," *Br. J. Anaeth.* **70**: 273-275 (1993).

Newburg, L.A., J.H. Milde, and J.D. Michenfelder: "The Cerebral Metabolic Effects of Isoflurane at and Above Concentrations That Suppress Cortical Electrical Activity," *Anesthesiology* **59**: 23-28 (1983).

Nussmeier, N.A., C. Arlund, and S. Slogoff: "Neuropsychiatric Complication after Cardiopulmonary Bypass: Cerebral Protection by a Barbiturate," *Anesthesiology* **64**: 165-170 (1986).

Rampil, I.J., S.H. Lockhart, M.S. Zwass, N. Peterson, N. Yasuda, E.I. Eger II, R.B. Weiskopf, and M.C. Damask: "Clinical Characteristics of Desflurane in Surgical Patients: Minimum Alveolar Concentration," *Anesthesiology* **74**: 429-433 (1991).

Roizen, M.F., and V.C. Stevens: "Multiform Ventricular Tachycardia due to Interaction of Aminophylline and Halothane," *Anesth. Analg.* **57**: 738-741 (1978).

Rosenberg, H., F.K. Orkin, and J. Springstead: "Abuse of Nitrous Oxide," *Anesth. Analg.* **58**: 104-106 (1979).

Szenohradszky, J., D.M. Fisher, V. Segredo, J.E. Caldwell, P. Bragg, M.L. Sharma, L.D. Gruenke, and R.D. Miller: "Pharmacokinetics of Rocuronium Bromide (ORG 9426) in Patients with Normal Renal Function or Patients Undergoing Cadaver Renal Transplantation," *Anesthesiology* **77**: 899-904 (1992).

White, P.F., W.L. Wary, and A.J. Trevor: "Ketamine — Its Pharmacology and Therapeutic Uses," *Anesthesiology* **56**: 119-136 (1982).

Wood, M., M.L. Berman, R.D. Harbison, P. Hoyle, J.M. Pythyon, and A.J. Wood: "Halothane-Induced Hepatic Necrosis in Triiodothyronine-Pretreated Rats," *Anesthesiology* **52**: 470-476 (1980).

CHAPTER 16

Sedatives and Hypnotics

Laurence A. Carr

The sedative-hypnotic agents are classified into the barbiturates, the benzodiazepine hypnotics, and a miscellaneous group. These drugs, which possess sedative and hypnotic properties, are frequently used as adjuncts in the treatment of organic and emotional disorders to provide a calming effect and induce sleep. The majority of drugs in this chapter are indicated in the treatment of insomnia. With some exceptions the same drugs can be utilized for sedation and hypnosis. The differences in effects are dependent on the dose. Sedation is characterized by mild depression of the central nervous system (CNS), while hypnosis is a greater depth of CNS depression that resembles natural sleep.

BARBITURATES

The barbiturates are derivatives of barbituric acid, which is formed by the condensation of malonic acid (HOOC-CH_2-COOH) with urea (NH_2-CO-NH_2). Barbiturates are weak acids, and salts of the compounds are formed at position 2. The structures of some barbiturates, as well as their relative durations of action, are shown in Table 16-1.

In order for derivatives of barbituric acid to have central depressant activity, they must have two substitutions at position 5. Barbital, which is a 5,5-diethyl derivative, is a weak hypnotic, while barbiturates with an ethyl group and a longer chain are more potent than barbital. Compounds with a branched chain at position 5 usually have greater hypnotic activity than the corresponding drug with a straight chain. Barbiturates containing a phenyl group at position 5 are less potent hypnotics than their aliphatic or alicyclic analogs, but they have enhanced anticonvulsant and antiepileptic activity. N-Methylation of the barbituric acid nucleus increases lipid solubility and decreases duration of action. It also may confer antiepileptic activity, while alkylation of both nitrogens yields derivatives that show convulsant activity. Replacement of the oxygen at position 2 by sulfur (creating thiobarbiturates) causes a marked increase in the lipid-to-water partition coefficients of 5,5-disubstituted barbiturates (Table 16-2). The resulting drugs have greater hypnotic potency than their oxygen analogs when given intravenously, but their low water solubility and their localization in depot fat make them unsuitable for oral administration as hypnotics. Their greatest usefulness is as intravenous anesthetics (ultrashort-acting barbiturates).

Mechanism of Action

Actions of barbiturates on the CNS are expressed in many ways, ranging from subtle changes in mood to more profound effects such as sedation, sleep, or anesthesia, depending on the dose administered. The pharmacologic basis of such CNS depression appears to be complex in its nature.

Although a detailed mechanism of action for the barbiturates is not fully delineated at the present time, it appears that γ aminobutyric acid (GABA) receptor-mediated chloride ion fluxes have a role in the central depressant properties of these drugs.

GABA is an inhibitory neurotransmitter in the CNS. It binds to both $GABA_A$ and $GABA_B$ receptors. $GABA_A$ receptors are associated with the chloride ionophore, which is a macromolecular complex that also contains receptor sites for GABA, barbiturates, and benzodiazepines. $GABA_A$ receptors are believed to be a complex of 5 subunits containing proteins designated α, β, and γ in various combinations (see Chapter 3). The binding of benzodiazepines appears to occur on the α

TABLE 16-1 Classification and structures of some clinically useful barbiturates

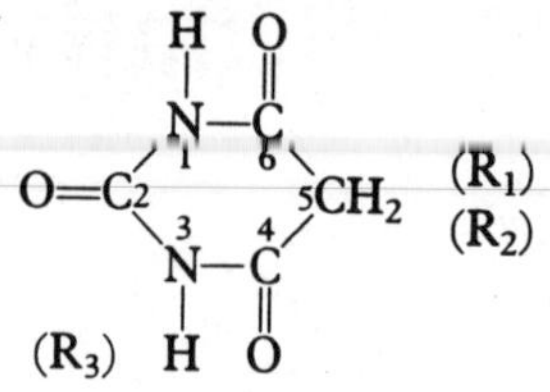

$$
\begin{array}{c}
\text{H} \quad \text{O} \\
| \quad \| \\
\text{N}_1\text{—C}_6 \\
\text{O=C}_2 \qquad {}_5\text{CH}_2 \ (R_1)(R_2) \\
\text{N}_3\text{—C}_4 \\
| \quad \| \\
(R_3)\ \text{H} \quad \text{O}
\end{array}
$$

Barbituric acid

Barbiturate	R_1	R_2	R_3
Ultrashort-acting			
Methohexital	Allyl	1-Methyl-2-pentynyl	CH_3
Thiopental[a]	Ethyl	1-Methylbutyl	H
Short to intermediate-acting			
Amobarbital	Ethyl	Isopentyl	H
Butabarbital	Ethyl	*sec*-Butyl	H
Pentobarbital	Ethyl	1-Methylbutyl	H
Secobarbital	Allyl	1-Methylbutyl	H
Long-acting			
Mephobarbital	Ethyl	Phenyl	CH_3
Phenobarbital	Ethyl	Phenyl	H

[a] Sulfur is present at position 2 instead of oxygen.

subunit(s), while the γ subunit appears to be an absolute requirement for benzodiazepine binding. The GABA recognition sites, the barbiturate receptor, and the binding sites for picrotoxin appear to be carried on the β subunit(s).

When GABA binds to the $GABA_A$ receptor site in the postsynaptic chloride ionophore, an influx of chloride ions into neuronal tissue occurs, which results in hyperpolarization of the membrane. Barbiturates and benzodiazepine derivatives, such as the benzodiazepine hypnotics discussed in this chapter, potentiate $GABA_A$ receptor-mediated chloride influx by binding to their specific receptor sites on the chloride ionophore. In the presence of GABA, barbiturates prolong the duration of the $GABA_A$-activated chloride ion influx. In addition, barbiturates can enhance the affinity of GABA for its receptor site on the chloride ionophore. The benzodiazepines potentiate the activity of GABA on chloride influx by increasing the frequency of the openings of the $GABA_A$ receptor-mediated chloride channels.

Another effect of barbiturates in the CNS that is also possibly related to their mechanism of action is the ability of barbiturates to increase membrane fluidity when they are administered acutely. The drug molecules appear to position themselves into the lipid components of the membrane and reduce the rigidity of the structural arrangement. By increasing neuronal membrane fluidity, the barbiturates may alter (1) the conformation of enzymes, (2) ion fluxes, and (3) neurotransmitter release. Other drugs such as ethanol and the general anesthetics are also reported to produce their pharmacologic effects by increasing neuronal membrane fluidity. These drugs alter membrane fluidity not by a receptor mechanism but by their physical presence in the membrane.

Although some barbiturates have been demonstrated to alter membrane fluidity, it is not known whether this action is related to their sedative or hypnotic effects.

TABLE 16-2 Barbiturates: some pharmacokinetic data

Barbiturate	Elimination half-life[a]	Partition coefficient[b]	Plasma protein binding[c]
Amobarbital	16 - 24	——	——
Butabarbital	62 - 138	——	——
Pentobarbital	21 - 48	39	35
Phenobarbital	72 - 96	3	20
Secobarbital	20 - 28	52	44
Thiopental	——	580	65

[a] Plasma half-life in adults.
[b] Concentration in methylene chloride / concentration in water.
[c] Percent binding to bovine serum albumin.

Pharmacodynamics

Central Nervous System The central depressant actions of the barbiturates resemble those of the general anesthetics, ethanol, and most of the hypnotic drugs discussed in subsequent sections of this chapter. Although barbiturates are uniformly distributed within the CNS, the reticular activating system appears to be the most sensitive area to the depressant effects. Depending on the dose administered, all of the clinically useful drugs produce a broad range of effects extending from mild sedation to deep coma or anesthesia. The degree of CNS depression is also dependent on the level of excitability or arousal in the individual.

Sedation and Hypnosis Although the doses employed for hypnosis are larger than those for sedation, the therapeutic goal is the same: to reduce awareness of external stimuli and, in appropriate circumstances, to promote sleep. The barbiturates most favored for daytime sedation are those which have a long or intermediate duration of action, for example, phenobarbital or butabarbital, respectively.

In general, barbiturates with a short to intermediate duration of action, such as secobarbital or amobarbital, are employed as hypnotic agents. The hypnotic action is sometimes apparent as early as 15 min after ingestion of the drug, but usually 30 to 60 min is needed. Sleep is usually maintained uninterrupted for 5 to 6 h. The incidence of rapid eye movement (REM) sleep and dreams is reduced. In REM sleep, also called *paradoxical* sleep, periods of rapid eye movements under closed eyelids alternate with periods of quiescence during physiologic sleep. Episodes of rapid eye movement have been correlated and associated with dreaming. Prolonged deprivation of REM sleep may result in reversible gross behavioral effects.

Anesthesia In sufficiently large doses, all of the barbiturate hypnotics are capable of producing surgical anesthesia. However, only ultrashort-acting barbiturates are useful anesthetics (see Chapter 15).

Anticonvulsant Effects All of the sedative-hypnotic barbiturates are effective antidotes to convulsant drugs, and in anesthetic doses they suppress the convulsions of tetanus and status epilepticus. Phenobarbital, in particular, is utilized in the prevention of epileptic seizures, particularly of the generalized tonic-clonic seizure type. The pharmacology of antiepileptic drugs is discussed in Chapter 22.

Analgesia The barbiturates differ from opioids and non-opioid analgesics in that they lack significant ability to obtund pain in doses not impairing consciousness. In fact, they may induce excitability and restlessness when pain is present. However, increased pain relief is occasionally achieved by combining barbiturates with aspirin or small doses of opioid analgesics.

Respiratory System Sleep induced by hypnotic doses of barbiturates is usually not associated with more depression of the respiratory system than occurs in normal sleep. Larger doses cause progressive reduction of the minute volume; the rate may be increased or decreased. The respiratory-stimulating action of 5 to 10 percent carbon dioxide becomes progressively weaker and finally disappears. Death from acute barbiturate poisoning is usually attributed to respiratory failure. With toxic doses the mechanism appears to be a direct paralysis of the medullary respiratory center as a result of the loss of the response to the carbon dioxide drive. However, in abusers who chronically overdose with barbiturates, pulmonary edema or hypostatic pneumonia often plays a role in decreasing the respiration. Laryngospasm appears to be a rare complication of ordinary barbiturate poisoning but is of considerable importance in connection with the intravenous administration of the ultrashort-acting thiobarbiturates.

Circulatory System The circulation is not significantly affected by sedative or hypnotic doses of barbiturates. Doses large enough to cause coma or anesthesia may produce a sustained decrease in the mean arterial pressure and pulse pressure.

Liver Hypnotic doses do not alter the results of any of the usual clinical tests of hepatic function. Even in patients with severe liver disease, the tests reveal no changes suggestive of deleterious effects of the drugs.

Barbiturates may cause a striking enhancement of the activity of hepatic microsomal enzymes involved in the biotransformation of a variety of drugs and certain normal body constituents. The mechanism of this effect is not fully understood but appears to involve increased synthesis of enzymes in the endoplasmic reticulum. This action of barbiturates may be of clinical significance (see Chapter 5).

Enzyme induction may extend beyond microsomal enzymes to include aldehyde dehydrogenase and δ-aminolevulinic acid synthetase. The barbiturates may also competitively interfere with the biotransformation of a number of substrates of cytochrome P-450.

Pharmacokinetics

The barbiturates are readily absorbed from the stomach, small intestine, rectum, and intramuscular sites. The mechanism of absorption from the gastrointestinal tract is simple passive diffusion. Following absorption, the drugs are distributed to all tissues and fluids of the body. Barbiturates readily cross the placental barrier and become widely distributed in the fetal tissues. The drugs differ considerably in their binding to plasma protein (Table 16-2). Binding to tissue proteins parallels the binding to plasma proteins. Therefore, the drugs are rather uniformly distributed throughout the body. Ultrashort-acting barbiturates such as thiopental attain much higher concentrations in depot fat than in other tissues of the body due to their high lipid solubility.

Barbiturate hypnotics are biotransformed primarily in the liver by oxidation of the substituents at position 5. Ethyl groups are quite resistant to oxidation. Therefore, barbital, which contains two ethyl groups, is excreted almost completely unchanged. Longer alkyl chains are oxidized to form secondary alcohols, ketones, or carboxylic acid derivatives; the latter are sometimes subjected to β-oxidation to form carboxylic acids with two fewer carbon atoms. The phenyl group in phenobarbital is hydroxylated in the para position. N-dealkylation and desulfuration may occur when the appropriate substituents are present. Phenolic as well as alcoholic biotransformation products are conjugated with glucuronic acid to varying extent. The allyl ($CH_2{=}CH\text{-}CH_2$) group present in a few of the barbiturates usually escapes biotransformation, but in secobarbital it is converted in part to a 2,3-dihydroxypropyl ($CH_2OH\text{-}CHOH\text{-}CH_2$) group. Hydrolysis of the barbituric acid ring is generally only a minor reaction.

The barbiturates and their biotransformation products are eliminated primarily by renal excretion. Alkalinization of the urine does little to expedite the elimination of most barbiturates, but does have an effect on the excretion of phenobarbital. The basis for this difference is that phenobarbital has a lower pK_a (7.2) than do the other barbiturates. Therefore, increasing the pH in the physiologic range converts a greater fraction of phenobarbital to the anionic form, to which renal tubules are impermeable.

Barbiturates are administered orally, rectally, intramuscularly, or intravenously. The oral route should be employed whenever possible. In infants or in patients who are vomiting, the drugs may be given rectally in the form of a suppository or retention enema. When rapid onset of action is needed, as in patients with convulsions, the drugs may be injected intramuscularly or intravenously.

Adverse Reactions

Acute Poisoning The wide availability of barbiturate hypnotics provides ample opportunities for accidental intoxication and suicide attempts. Most cases of barbiturate poisoning stem from attempted suicide, but some are accidental, and a few may result from what has been called *automatism*. This is a state of drug-induced confusion in which the patient forgets having taken the medication and ingests more of it.

The diagnosis of barbiturate intoxication is based on the history, physical examination, and detection of drugs in the blood, urine, or gastric contents. Poisoning by barbiturates seldom can be distinguished on purely clinical grounds from that caused by other hypnotic drugs. The cardinal signs are stupor or coma and respiratory depression. The respiration is affected early in the course of intoxication. The minute respiratory volume is decreased, sometimes sufficiently to cause cyanosis. The rhythm may be slow or rapid or may, have a Cheyne-Stokes pattern. Ordinarily the blood pressure falls appreciably only in the presence of marked respiratory depression. Undoubtedly, hypoxia plays an important role in causing the hypotension, since merely providing adequate ventilation often restores blood pressure to normal. However, severely poisoned patients may develop circulatory shock.

The treatment of barbiturate poisoning includes removing any unabsorbed drug from the stomach, supporting the respiration and circulation, performing hemodialysis, and preventing complications. It should always be kept in mind that acute intoxication may be superimposed upon chronic intoxication. After emerging from coma, every patient poisoned by barbiturates should be questioned about chronic use of the drugs and treated accordingly.

Chronic Toxicity The clinical picture of chronic barbiturate intoxication resembles that of mild acute barbiturate or alcohol intoxication. Barbiturate abusers differ from alcoholics in that they usually maintain a good state of nutrition. The signs and symptoms vary considerably in different individuals and in the same subject at different times. The effects are greatest when the drug is taken on an empty stomach. They are least marked upon arising and increase during the day as successive doses are consumed. The mental changes include impairment of intellectual ability, defective judgment, loss of emotional control, and accentuation of pathologic features of the personality. Most abusers prefer shorter acting barbiturates such as pentobarbital, secobarbital, or amobarbital to phenobarbital. The drugs are usually taken by mouth, although some abusers inject them intravenously.

The severity of the abstinence syndrome depends on the individual patient as well as on the daily dosage and the duration of the intoxication. Abrupt withdrawal of barbiturates from chronically intoxicated individuals is absolutely contraindicated. The patient should be hospitalized and stabilized on the smallest amount of the drug which maintains a continuous state of mild intoxication. A period of two to three weeks is usually required to withdraw barbiturates safely. Rehabilitation and psychotherapeutic treatment of recovered barbiturate abusers is the same as that for alcoholics or opioid abusers.

Idiosyncratic Reactions Abnormal reactions to the barbiturates may be encountered in certain patients who have not had prior experience with the drugs. In some individuals, particularly children or elderly patients, hypnotic doses of the barbiturates consistently produce excitement and inebriation. Others respond with headache, nausea and vomiting, or diarrhea. Occasionally the drugs appear to be responsible for myalgia, neuralgia, or arthralgia, which may persist for several days after discontinuation of medication.

Hypersensitivity Hypersensitivity reactions to the barbiturates most commonly involve the skin, although the blood and blood-forming organs may also be affected. In rare instances, phenobarbital may cause exfoliative dermatitis, accompanied by parenchymatous hepatitis. A few cases of agranulocytosis and thrombocytopenic purpura have also been attributed to the drug.

Drug Interactions When a barbiturate is administered to an individual who has received opioids, other sedatives or hypnotics, general anesthetics, neuromuscular blocking agents, alcohol, or antianxiety agents, an additive respiratory depressant effect may occur. When a barbiturate is used by a chronic alcohol abuser, in the absence of ethanol, there is a decreased sedative effect from the barbiturate due to its increased biotransformation by the drug-metabolizing microsomal system (DMMS), which is induced by the chronic use of ethanol. Acute ethanol administration can also inhibit the metabolism of barbiturates, further enhancing CNS depression. Rifampin will decrease the effect of barbiturates because of induction of the DMMS. Barbiturates may also diminish the response to coumarin anticoagulants, resulting in less suppression of prothrombin. This effect is due primarily to the increased activity of the drug-metabolizing microsomal enzymes and increased biotransformation of the coumarin anticoagulant. Withdrawal of the barbiturate without a dose alteration of the anticoagulant may result in hemorrhage. Other drugs biotransformed by the DMMS may similarly have their therapeutic activity adversely affected by barbiturates; these include tricyclic antidepressants, corticosteroids, digitoxin, phenothiazines, quinidine, and tetracyclines.

Contraindications The barbiturates are definitely contraindicated in patients who have become sensitized to them. Severe pulmonary insufficiency constitutes a contraindication, since patients with disorders such as chronic emphysema are often extremely sensitive to the respiratory-depressant effect of ordinary hypnotic doses. Barbiturates are contraindicated in patients with intermittent porphyria. This metabolic disorder involves a defect in the regulation of δ-aminolevulinic acid synthetase, and the administration of a barbiturate which increases this enzyme may cause a dangerous and precipitous increase in the level of porphyrins, which may result in paralysis and death.

Barbiturates should be used with caution in patients with decreased liver function or renal insufficiency because these conditions will impair the biotransformation and excretion, respectively, of the barbiturate. Great caution must be exercised in prescribing barbiturates for the individual with a suicidal tendency or a predisposition to abuse them.

Clinical Uses

Sedation and Hypnosis Although barbiturates are effective sedatives and hypnotics, there is little rationale to justify their use in most patients. The barbiturates generally have a greater potential to cause dangerous adverse reactions, dependence, and abuse than the benzodiazepines, which are generally considered to be the drugs of choice.

When the barbiturates are used to treat ordinary insomnia, they should not be regarded as a substitute for a concerted effort to discover and treat the basic causes of the disorder. Patients should be urged to provide an environment maximally conducive to sleep and to seek methods of relaxing at bedtime. In recommending drugs to be administered during the night, it is advisable that the dose to be taken be isolated from the main supply to guard against accidental ingestion of an excessive amount. Continuous use of barbiturates in recommended doses may result in tolerance and dependence. The patient should be told that the first night after discontinuing the drug may be less restful than usual. Sleep laboratory research on most hypnotics has found them to lose their sleep-promoting properties within 3 to 14 days of continuous use. Physicians should look for and treat underlying disorders causing insomnia and follow a conservative approach in the prescribing of hypnotics.

Anticonvulsant and Antiepileptic Uses The barbiturates may be used in the treatment of acute convulsions arising from various disease processes or from the ingestion of poisons. Thus they have been employed in the therapy of status epilepticus, eclampsia, and cerebral hemorrhage. The therapeutic use of phenobarbital and mephobarbital in the treatment of epilepsy is discussed in Chapter 22.

Preanesthetic Medication Pentobarbital, amobarbital, and secobarbital are employed as preanesthetic medication. In the absence of pain, they provide the serenity desired before anesthesia.

BENZODIAZEPINES

Estazolam, flurazepam, quazepam, temazepam, and triazolam are all benzodiazepine derivatives that are used exclusively for their hypnotic effect in the treatment of sleep disorders. Other benzodiazepines that are used primarily for their antianxiety effect are discussed in Chapter 17. All of the benzodiazepine compounds have the same basic structural nucleus as is illustrated by flurazepam.

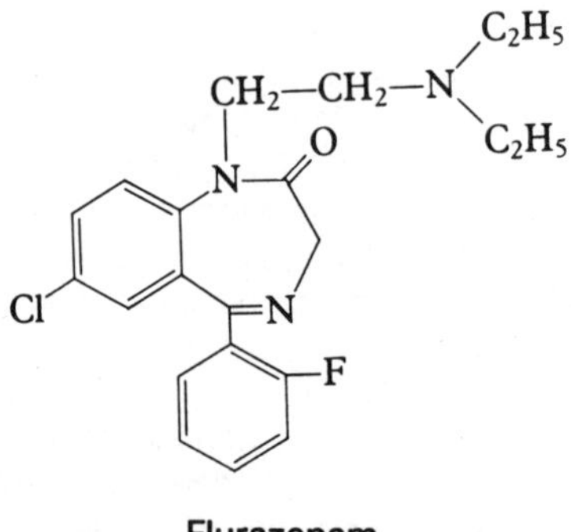

Flurazepam

Mechanism of Action

Most of the evidence in the literature suggests that the central effects of these hypnotic agents result from a neurochemical action similar to that described above for barbiturates. Estazolam, flurazepam, quazepam, temazepam, and triazolam are believed to increase the inhibitory effect of

GABA on neurons in the CNS. Specifically, they appear to potentiate the activity of GABA on chloride ion influx by increasing the frequency of the openings of the $GABA_A$ receptor-mediated chloride channels by binding to specific benzodiazepine (BZ) receptors on the chloride ionophore.

Two BZ receptor subtypes have been identified in brain, i.e., BZ_1 (believed to be associated with sleep) and BZ_2 (thought to be involved with motor, sensory, and cognitive functions). Estazolam, flurazepam, temazepam, and triazolam are nonselective agonists at both receptor subtypes; quazepam and its active metabolite 2-oxoquazepam have a greater affinity for BZ_1 receptors.

Pharmacokinetics

These benzodiazepine hypnotics are well absorbed from the gastrointestinal tract after oral administration and exhibit very good bioavailability. Plasma protein binding of triazolam is approximately 85 percent; the other four compounds have a plasma protein binding of at least 93 percent. All are biotransformed in the liver by the DMMS. Flurazepam undergoes an N-dealkylation reaction to yield N-desalkylflurazepam, a major active metabolite which has an elimination half-life of 76 to 160 h. Quazepam is biotransformed to 2-oxoquazepam (an active product) which is then converted to N-desalkyl-2-oxoquazepam (which is identical to N-desalkylflurazepam and, therefore, active). The half-life of quazepam is 25 to 41 h. The other compounds do not form active metabolites. For estazolam, temazepam, and triazolam the elimination half-lives are 10 to 24 h, 8 to 38 h, and 1.6 to 5.4 h, respectively. All of these drugs and their metabolites are eliminated from the body primarily by renal excretion.

Adverse Reactions

Drowsiness, dizziness, lethargy, and ataxia may occur particularly in elderly and debilitated patients. Confusion, dry mouth, headache, and gastrointestinal disturbances have been observed. Idiosyncratic excitement, stimulation, hyperactivity, and hallucinations have been reported, especially in elderly patients.

Tolerance to the hypnotic effect has not been observed following one or two months of continuous nightly usage. Dependence does not appear to develop in individuals taking therapeutic doses of these drugs. However, as with any CNS depressant, there is always the possibility that dependence may occur. In cases of overdosage, ataxia, hypotension, respiratory depression, and coma have been reported. The benzodiazepine hypnotics have an additive depressant effect with other CNS depressants, including alcohol. Benzodiazepines should be avoided during pregnancy.

Clinical Uses

Estazolam, flurazepam, quazepam, temazepam, and triazolam are used for the treatment of insomnia. They are of value in treating persons who have difficulty in falling asleep, frequent nocturnal awakenings, or early morning awakening. When the drugs are taken at bedtime, the least preferred hypnotic to use in patients who have difficulty in falling asleep is temazepam. In order for temazepam to influence a patient's sleep latency the compound should be taken 1 to 2 h before bedtime.

These benzodiazepines decrease time to onset of sleep and number of awakenings and increase total sleep time. At ordinary therapeutic doses flurazepam and the other benzodiazepine drugs neither suppress REM sleep nor cause a rebound after withdrawal; however, the percentage of REM sleep is decreased because there is an increase in total sleep time. Stages 3 and 4 of sleep are reduced but stage 2 is lengthened. In general, little or no rebound insomnia occurs when the drug is discontinued. In some patients as little as one-half of the recommended dose may be effective.

MISCELLANEOUS GROUP

Chloral Hydrate

Chloral hydrate (CCl_3-$CH(OH)_2$) is an aldehyde hydrate which has a pungent odor and somewhat caustic taste. Chloral hydrate is usually taken by mouth but is sometimes given rectally. Its irritant action precludes subcutaneous or intramuscular injection.

The sedative-hypnotic action of chloral hydrate can be attributed almost entirely to trichloroethanol formed by the enzymatic reduction of the drug in the liver. Although the exact mechanism of action of chloral hydrate is unknown, the drug probably acts in a manner similar to ethanol in the CNS which results in sedation or sleep (see Chapter 18).

Pharmacokinetics Very little chloral hydrate is available to the central and systemic circulations because of a high first-pass effect in the liver that transforms it to trichloroethanol by the enzyme alcohol dehydrogenase. The drug and its products of biotransformation appear to be widely distributed throughout the body. A small fraction of chloral hydrate is partly oxidized to trichloroacetic acid. This active metabolite has a half-life of 4 to 12 h. Chloral hydrate and trichloroethanol are biotransformed by the liver to trichloroacetic acid and urochloralic acid, both of which are excreted by the kidney.

Pharmacodynamics The central depressant actions of chloral hydrate resemble those of alcohol, the barbiturates, and the general anesthetics. In small doses, the principal effect is sedation. Somewhat larger doses taken under appropriate circumstances induce sleep. In ambulatory individuals, the drug may produce the signs and symptoms of drunkenness. Larger doses lead to coma or anesthesia. However, the drug is not used for anesthesia because the margin of safety is too narrow.

Controlled clinical studies have proved the effectiveness of choral hydrate in inducing and maintaining sleep. In most individuals sleep occurs within 1 h after swallowing the drug and continues for 5 h or longer. At any time during the hypnotic response, the patient can be readily aroused. The duration of action of chloral hydrate is short enough so that the incidence of after effects (hangover) is insignificant.

Chloral hydrate has minimal effects on the various stages of normal sleep, including REM sleep, when given in therapeutic doses. At high doses REM sleep may be suppressed.

Doses of chloral hydrate larger than the therapeutic dose cause deeper and longer sleep and increase the incidence of hangover. Pain is obtunded, and the body temperature may fall. Loss of all reflexes and depression of the medullary respiratory and vasomotor centers occur after doses in the lethal range.

Therapeutic doses of chloral hydrate ordinarily cause no changes in the respiration, blood pressure, or heart rate beyond those occurring in normal sleep. However, extremely large doses may cause myocardial depression or arrhythmias, in which central vagal stimulation appears to be involved. Chloral hydrate has an irritant action on the gastric mucosa and therefore should be taken well diluted; otherwise it may cause nausea and vomiting.

Adverse Reactions Undesirable reactions occurring in individuals taking chloral hydrate include hangover, drowsiness, headache, nausea, vomiting, flatulence, staggering gait, and ataxia. Idiosyncratic excitement and delirium may also occur.

Chloral hydrate has additive CNS depressant effects with other drugs such as alcohol, barbiturates, and antianxiety agents. It may also alter the therapeutic response of any drug which is biotransformed by the DMMS.

Acute Poisoning The signs of poisoning by choral hydrate resemble those from alcohol or the barbiturates. The usual features are coma, depressed respiration, hypotension, and hypothermia. The ingestion of large doses may cause death almost immediately. If the patient survives for several hours, the prognosis is generally good, although transient jaundice or albuminuria may be present during recovery. The average *lethal* dose has been estimated to be about 10 g. In the past, many cases of poisoning occurred from choral hydrate added illicitly to alcohol beverages ("Mickey Finn," "knockout drops"); however, the belief that the activity of chloral hydrate is enhanced by a chemical reaction with alcohol is erroneous. The metabolism of ethanol is not appreciably altered by choral hydrate. However, blood trichloroethanol reaches earlier and higher peak levels when chloral hydrate is administered with ethanol, an effect attributed to decreased oxidation of the halogenated drug to trichloroacetic acid.

Treatment of acute poisoning consists of gastric lavage, support of respiration and circulation, and maintenance of normal body temperature.

Chronic Poisoning Chloral hydrate is very similar to alcohol, the barbiturates, and other hypnotics with respect to tolerance and psychological and physical dependence. Dependence on chloral hydrate is uncommon, and protocols for treatment have not been formulated in detail, although experience with barbiturate dependence suggests that gradual reduction of the daily dose would be preferable to abrupt withdrawal of the drug. Delirium, mania, or convulsions occurring during withdrawal should receive the same treatment as that given for alcohol or barbiturate abstinence.

Precautions The drug should be used cautiously in the presence of severe hepatic, renal, or cardiac disease. Oral administration is wisely avoided in patients with esophagitis, gastritis, or gastric or duodenal ulcers. Continued administration of chloral hydrate may increase the activity of the DMMS. This effect is of particular importance in patients receiving coumarin anticoagulants because withdrawal of the hypnotic may decrease the rate of biotransformation of the anticoagulant and thereby increase bleeding tendency.

Trichloroacetic acid binds strongly to plasma proteins. Therefore it may interact with other drugs or natural substances which bind to plasma proteins by displacing them, resulting in a sharp rise in blood level of the free drug or natural substance.

Clinical Use Chloral hydrate is used in adults and children for the short-term treatment of insomnia. Its rapid onset of action and short duration of effect make it suitable for individuals whose main difficulty is failing asleep. In certain patients chloral hydrate may be considered as an alternative to the benzodiazepine hypnotics. The drug is also indicated as a sedative in children and adults.

Paraldehyde

Paraldehyde, a trimer of acetaldehyde, has the following structure:

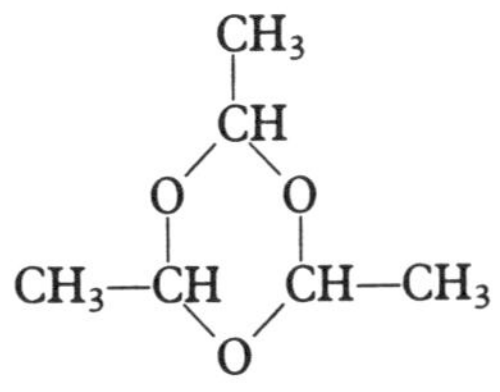

```
          CH3
          |
          CH
         /  \
        O    O
        |    |
CH3—CH    CH—CH3
        \  /
          O
```

Paraldehyde

It is a colorless liquid with a characteristic penetrating odor and a disagreeable burning taste.

The exact mechanism for the hypnotic action of paraldehyde is unknown. It appears likely that the central depressant actions of paraldehyde can be attributed to the drug rather than one of its biotransformation products.

Paraldehyde is absorbed rapidly from the gastrointestinal tract including the rectum. The drug is extensively metabolized in the body; 11 to 28 percent is excreted unchanged through the lungs and 0.1 to 2.5 percent through the kidneys. The fate of the remaining drug appears to involve conversion to acetaldehyde and subsequent oxidation via the tricarboxylic acid cycle to carbon dioxide and water.

The liver seems to be the principal organ involved in the metabolism of paraldehyde. In some patients with severe hepatic disease, the drug is detoxified at an abnormally slow rate, and the hypnotic effects are prolonged. The abstinence syndrome resembles delirium tremens.

Paraldehyde is quite similar to chloral hydrate, alcohol, and the barbiturates in regard to tolerance and dependence. The usual features of acute poisoning are coma, depressed respiration, and hypotension.

The treatment of acute poisoning by paraldehyde consists of gastric or rectal lavage to remove unabsorbed drug, maintenance of body temperature, and support of respiration and circulation. The patient may remain in coma for many hours, since the rate of biotransformation of paraldehyde is low.

Because of its irritant action, oral administration of paraldehyde is contraindicated in esophagitis, gastritis, or gastric or duodenal ulcers, and rectal administration should be avoided in the presence of inflammatory conditions of the anus or lower bowel. Some physicians consider the drug contraindicated in patients with asthma or other bronchopulmonary diseases. Paraldehyde is also contraindicated in patients taking disulfiram, a drug that inhibits acetaldehyde biotransformation. The use of decomposed paraldehyde, which contains acetic acid, has been responsible for several cases of serious corrosion of the stomach and rectum.

The odor it imparts to the breath restricts the use of paraldehyde for most ambulatory patients; thus the drug has found limited use as a sedative and hypnotic.

Ethchlorvynol

The sedative-hypnotic ethchlorvynol has approximately the same potency and toxicities as phenobarbital, but its hypnotic effects are achieved more rapidly (within 30 min) and disappear more quickly (5 h).

After oral administration, ethchlorvynol is rapidly absorbed from the gastrointestinal tract. It is highly localized in body lipids, biotransformed primarily by the liver, and slowly excreted by the kidney. The compound can induce the liver DMMS.

Acute toxicity of ethchlorvynol produces an array of signs and symptoms indistinguishable from those caused by other hypnotics, and chronic intoxication resembles chronic poisoning by alcohol or the barbiturates. Patients may exhibit ataxia, confusion, disorientation, and occasionally visual or auditory hallucinations. A daily dose of 2 g appears sufficient to cause physical dependence. Withdrawal of the drug may result in generalized tonic-clonic seizures or psychotic behavior.

Due to the availability of other hypnotics such as the benzodiazepine derivatives, ethchlorvynol is seldom used in the treatment of insomnia.

Glutethimide

Glutethimide has hypnotic and sedative properties. The hypnotic effect is about the same as that of pentobarbital. Its abuse can lead to psychological and physical dependence and acute poisoning.

After oral absorption, the drug is widely distributed and reaches somewhat higher concentrations in fat than in other tissues because of its lipid solubility. Glutethimide is almost completely biotransformed by hydroxylation. It has a half-life of 45 h.

Glutethimide was originally indicated for the treatment of insomnia in individuals who could not tolerate barbiturates. However, the drug offers no therapeutic advantages over the benzodiazepine hypnotic and is rarely used.

Methyprylon

Methyprylon is a hypnotic agent whose pharmacologic effects closely resemble those of pentobarbital and secobarbital. Large doses of the drug cause coma, which may be accompanied by respiratory depression or hypotension or both. Chronic abuse of methyprylon results in the development of tolerance and physical dependence. As with glutethimide this drug is now rarely used in the treatment of insomnia.

Zolpidem

Zolpidem is a non-benzodiazepine hypnotic. Chemically it belongs in the imidazopyridine class and is unrelated to the barbiturate or benzodiazepine structure. Zolpidem selectively binds to the benzodiazepine receptor site, and produces its hypnotic activity similar to the benzodiazepines, but differs from them by not possessing muscle relaxant and anticonvulsant effects.

Zolpidem is readily absorbed from the gastrointestinal tract. Plasma protein binding is approximately 93 percent. The drug is metabolized to inactive products which are eliminated in the urine. The mean half-life is 2.5 h.

The drug is indicated for short-term treatment of insomnia. There is no evidence to suggest that zolpidem causes memory impairment, effects on REM sleep, rebound insomnia or next day residual effects. The major adverse effects include: headaches, confusion, drowsiness, ataxia and vertigo. Overdose symptoms include both respiratory and cardiovascular collapse.

Nonprescription Sleep Medication

There are several over-the-counter (OTC) products which may promote the induction of sleep at bedtime. The active ingredient in these preparations is an antihistamine (diphenhydramine or doxylamine) which has prominent sedative properties.

The sedative effect of antihistamines is enhanced by the concurrent administration of other CNS depressants and ethanol. If satisfactory results are not obtained by the use of an OTC sleep medication, the individual should seek medical treatment for the insomnia. For more information about these antihistamines see Chapter 13.

BIBLIOGRAPHY

Bliwise, D., W. Seidel, I. Karacan, M. Mitler, T. Roth, F. Zovick, and W. Dement: "Daytime Sleepiness as a Criterion in Hypnotic Medication Trials: Comparison of Triazolam and Flurazepam," *Sleep* **6**: 156-163 (1983).

Eldefrawi, A.T., and M.E. Eldefrawi: "Receptors for γ-Aminobutyric Acid and Voltage-Dependent Chloride Channels as Targets for Drugs and Toxicants," *FASEB J.* **1**: 262-271 (1987).

Lader, M., and H. Petursson: "Long-Term Effects of Benzodiazepines," *Neuropharmacol.* **22**: 527-533 (1983).

Owen, R.T., and P. Tyrer: "Benzodiazepine Dependence: Review of the Evidence," *Drugs* **25**: 385-398 (1983).

Richter, J.A., and J.R. Holman: "Barbiturates: Their *in vivo* Effects and Potential Biochemical Mechanisms," *Prog. Neurobiol.* **18**: 275-319 (1982).

Rickels, K.: "Clinical Trials of Hypnotics," *J. Clin. Psychopharmacol.* **3**: 133-139 (1983).

Sellers, E.M., and U. Basto: "Benzodiazepines and Ethanol: Assessment of Effects and Consequences of Psychotropic Drug Interaction," *J. Clin. Psychopharmacol.* **2**: 249-262 (1982).

Shiromani, P.J., J.C. Gillin, and S.J. Henriksen: "Acetylcholine and the Regulation of REM Sleep: Basic Mechanisms and Clinical Implications for Affective Illness and Narcolepsy," *Annu. Rev. Pharmacol. Toxicol.* **27**: 137-156 (1987).

Smith, A.G., and F. DeMatteis: "Drugs and Hepatic Porphyria," *Clin. Haematol.* **9**: 399-424 (1980).

Snyder, S.H.: "Drug and Neurotransmitter Receptors in the Brain," *Science* **224**: 22-31 (1984).

Stephenson, F.A.: "Understanding the $GABA_A$ Receptor: A Chemically Gated Ion Channel," *Biochem. J.* **249**: 21-32 (1988).

Trifiletti, R.R., A.M. Snownan, and S.H. Snyder: "Barbiturate Recognition Site on the GABA/Benzodiazepine Receptor Complex Is Distinct from the Picrotoxin/TBPS Recognition Site," *Eur. J. Pharmacol.* **106**: 441-447 (1985).

CHAPTER 17

Antianxiety Drugs

Lynn Wecker

The term *anxiety* refers to a pervasive feeling of apprehension that is associated with specific anxiety disorders, and may be manifest with other medical conditions such as coronary heart disease, cancer or impending surgery. In the realm of psychiatry, anxiety disorders include generalized anxiety disorder, panic attacks, phobic disorders and obsessive-compulsive disorders. All anxiety disorders share two cardinal features, i.e., anxiety symptoms and avoidance behavior. Anxiety is characterized by diffuse symptoms such as feelings of helplessness, difficulties concentrating, irritability and insomnia, as well as somatic symptoms including gastrointestinal disturbances, muscle tension, excessive perspiration, tachypnea, tachycardia, nausea, palpitations, and dry mouth. While these symptoms are associated with both generalized anxiety disorder and panic attacks, the latter are characterized by the spontaneous occurrence of symptoms including an intense fear that cannot be associated with an identifiable situation.

Many times anxiety symptoms may be mild and require little or no treatment. However, at other times, symptoms may be severe enough to cause patients considerable distress. When patients exhibit anxiety so debilitating that lifestyles, work, and interpersonal relationships are severely impaired, they may be treated with antianxiety or anxiolytic agents. Although the anxiolytics have been of great benefit, concurrent psychological support and counseling are absolute necessities for the treatment of anxiety and cannot be overemphasized.

BENZODIAZEPINES

The benzodiazepines represent the most commonly prescribed anxiolytics in the U.S. Prior to the introduction of the benzodiazepines for anxiety in the 1960's, the major drugs used for the treatment of anxiety were primarily sedatives and hypnotics and included meprobamate, glutethimide, barbiturates, and alcohols. Unfortunately, these compounds have a strong abuse potential and potent respiratory depressant effects and led to a high incidence of drug dependency, drug overdose, and death. Although the benzodiazepines are not devoid of adverse effects or abuse potential, they have a wide margin of safety with anxiolytic activity achieved at dosages that do not induce respiratory depression. Thus, the benzodiazepines are considered much safer than the previously used compounds.

During the last 40 years, over a dozen benzodiazepines have been introduced successfully into clinical medicine for the treatment of anxiety, insomnia, seizure disorders, and for the induction and facilitation of anesthesia. The term *benzodiazepine* reflects the structure of these compounds which contains a benzene ring fused to a 7-membered diazepine ring (Fig. 17-1). In addition, the benzodiazepines contain a 6-membered ring at the C-5 position of the diazepine ring, and an electronegative group (such as a halogen or nitro group) at the C-7 position on the benzene ring, the latter necessary for sedative-hypnotic activity and conferring optimal anxiolytic activity. Some benzodiazepines such as alprazolam, estazolam, and triazolam, contain a triazolo ring fused at positions 1 and 2 on the diazepine ring. These compounds are referred to as the triazolobenzodiazepines, and cause more serious withdrawal reactions than the other benzodiazepines.

Mechanism of Action

The benzodiazepines are believed to exert their effects through an interaction with a specific site

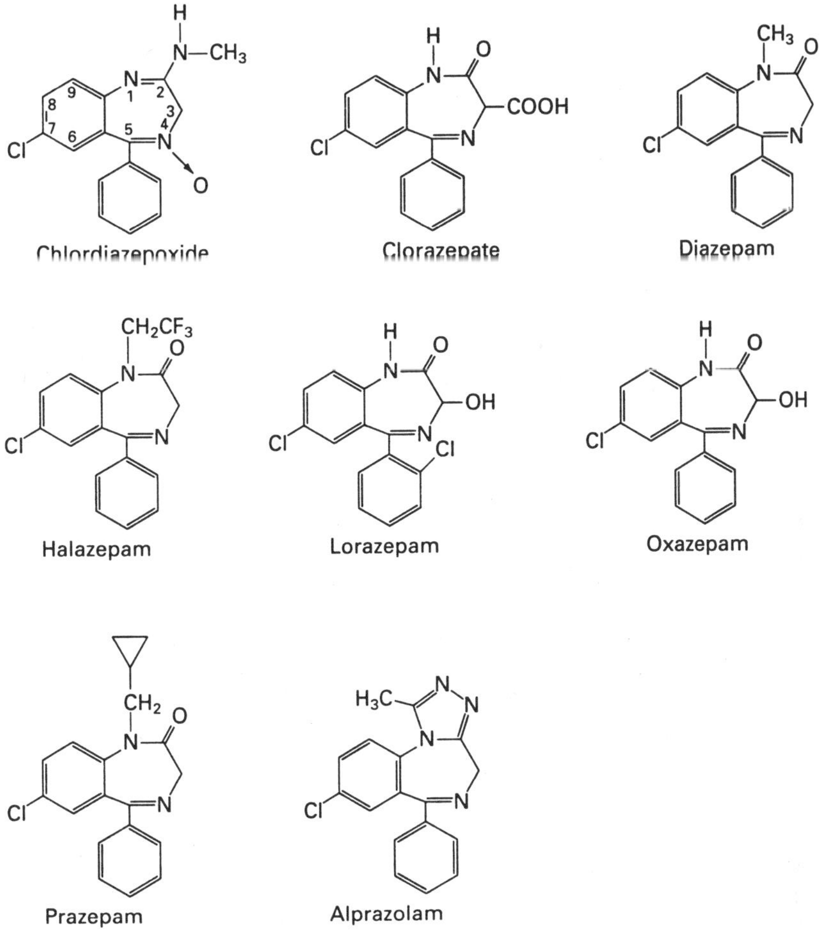

Chlordiazepoxide

Clorazepate

Diazepam

Halazepam

Lorazepam

Oxazepam

Prazepam

Alprazolam

FIGURE 17-1 *Chemical structures of some benzodiazepines.*

on chloride channels. Chloride channels are oligomeric, integral membrane glycoprotein complexes that belong to the family of ligand-gated ion ion channels. Stimulation by GABA (γ-aminobutyric acid) of $GABA_A$ receptors on the protein complex leads to an increased chloride ion influx, resulting in hyperpolarization of the neuronal membrane (see Chapters 3 and 16). In addition to the GABA receptor, the chloride ionophore complex contains numerous allosteric modulatory sites. The benzodiazepines are thought to bind to one type of these modulatory sites referred to as the benzodiazepine receptor. When the drugs bind to this site, they induce an allosteric change in the protein complex, resulting in an increased frequency of chloride ion channel openings. The benzodiazepines do not alter channel open time like the barbiturates (see Chapter 16).

Three types of compounds are known to interact with benzodiazepine binding sites on the chloride channel. Full agonists such as the benzodiazepines, enhance the effects of GABA. In contrast, full antagonists such as flumazenil have no intrinsic activity and do not affect GABA-mediated chloride ion influx, but rather, competitively antagonize the actions of the benzodiazepines. A third group of compounds that interact with the benzodiazepine receptors are the inverse agonists such as the β-carbolines. These compounds are termed agonists because they have intrinsic activity. However, they produce anxiety and seizures and decrease GABA-induced chloride ion influx, actions opposite those of the benzodiazepines. The inverse agonists also block the effects of the benzodiazepines, and the effects of the inverse agonists are competitively antagonized by flumazenil.

Although all benzodiazepines are believed to act at benzodiazepine receptor sites on the chloride channel, these compounds differ in their pharmacological profiles. For example, some anxiolytic benzodiazepines are non-sedating, while other benzodiazepines are used selectively for their sedative properties. Similarly, the incidence of muscle relaxation differs among compounds, and not all benzodiazepines have anticonvulsant activity. During the past several years attempts have been made to explain the differences in the behavioral and pharmacological profiles of these drugs. Recent studies suggest that these differences may be attributed to two primary factors. The first is the subtype of benzodiazepine receptor involved, and the second is the nature of the interaction of the benzodiazepine with the binding site.

Current evidence indicates that at least two subpopulations of benzodiazepine binding sites exist in the brain, defined on the basis of different affinities for certain compounds. Type I (or BZ_1) receptors appear to be enriched in the cerebellum, cerebral cortical layer IV, and the substantia nigra; type II (BZ_2) receptors are concentrated in the hippocampus, superior colliculus, and cerebral cortical layers I to III. Evidence suggests that full agonists at the BZ_1 receptor have a lower propensity to induce muscle relaxation, suggesting that pharmacological selectivity may be related to the subtype of receptor and location involved.

In addition to receptor subtype selectivity, the divergent pharmacological and behavioral profiles of the benzodiazepines may be explained on the basis of differences in intrinsic efficacy. The benzodiazepines exhibit a broad range of intrinsic efficacies, and studies have shown that partial agonists with anxiolytic and anticonvulsant activities are non-sedating and do not cause muscle relaxation. Thus, as more is learned about benzodiazepine receptor subtypes, and the nature of the interactions between these receptors and the benzodiazepines, therapeutic compounds with selective and specific pharmacological and behavioral profiles will be developed.

Pharmacokinetics

Currently available benzodiazepines, their onset and duration of action, and their therapeutic indications are presented in Table 17-1. The drugs differ with respect to absorption, plasma protein binding, lipid solubility and biotransformation to active as well as inactive metabolites. All anxiolytic benzodiazepines are administered orally, but within this group, diazepam, chlordiazepoxide and lorazepam are also available for injection. Lorazepam is well absorbed by both the oral and intramuscular routes, but the absorption of diazepam and chlordiazepoxide is poor and erratic following intramuscular injection, and should be avoided. When administered intravenously as an anticonvulsant or for induction of anesthesia, diazepam may induce pain and phlebitis. Generally, all the benzodiazepines are completely absorbed with the exception of clorazepate, which is the only benzodiazepine that is rapidly converted by gastric acid in the stomach to the active product N-desmethyldiazepam. The rate of conversion of clorazepate is inversely proportional to gastric pH.

In general, the benzodiazepines and their active metabolites are highly bound to plasma proteins. Plasma protein binding correlates with lipid solubility and is greatest for diazepam (99 percent) and lowest for alprazolam (70 percent). Binding for the remaining agents varies from 88 to 97 percent. The distribution of diazepam and other benzodiazepines is complicated somewhat by a considerable degree of biliary excretion, which occurs early in the distribution of these agents. This enterohepatic recirculation occurs with metabolites as well as parent compounds and may be important clinically for compounds with a long elimination half-life. The presence of food in the upper intestine delays reabsorption and contributes to the late resurgence of plasma drug levels and activity.

The benzodiazepines are metabolized extensively by the hepatic microsomal cytochrome P-450 monooxygenase system (P-450) as depicted in Figure 17-2. The major biotransformation reactions are N-dealkylation and aliphatic hydroxylation, followed by conjugation to inactive glucuronides which are excreted in the urine. The long-acting benzodiazepines clorazepate, diazepam, chlordiazepoxide, prazepam and halazepam are dealkylated to the active compound N-desmethyldiazepam (nordazepam) which has an elimination half-life of 30 to 200 hours and is responsible for the long duration of action of these compounds. N-Desmethyldiazepam undergoes hydroxylation to oxazepam which forms a glucuronide conjugate. Alprazolam undergoes hydroxylation followed by glucurondation, and lorazepam is directly glucuronidated.

Because the benzodiazepines are metabolized extensively by P-450 in the liver, alterations in hepatic function can alter the clearance of these compounds. An increased elimination half-life of

TABLE 17-1 Pharmacokinetic characteristics and therapeutic indications of benzodiazepines

Drug	Onset of action[a]	Duration of action[b]	Therapeutic Indications
Alprazolam	Intermediate	Intermediate	Anxiety
Chlordiazepoxide	Intermediate	Long	Anxiety
Clonazepam	Intermediate	Intermediate	Seizures
Clorazepate	Rapid	Long	Anxiety Seizures
Diazepam	Rapid	Long	Anxiety Seizures Skeletal muscle spasms
Estazolam	Slow	Intermediate	Insomnia
Flurazepam	Rapid	Long	Insomnia
Halazepam	Intermediate	Long	Anxiety
Lorazepam	Intermediate	Intermediate	Anxiety
Midazolam	Rapid	Ultrashort	Preoperative sedation Induction of anesthesia
Oxazepam	Slow	Short	Anxiety
Prazepam	Slow	Long	Anxiety
Quazepam	Rapid	Long	Insomnia
Temazepam	Slow	Intermediate	Insomnia
Triazolam	Intermediate	Short	Insomnia

[a] Rapid: 15 to 30 minutes; Intermediate: 30 to 45 minutes; Slow: 45 to 90 minutes.
[b] Ultrashort: $<$ 5 hours; Short: 5 to 24 hours; Intermediate: 24 to 48 hours; Long: $>$ 48 hours.

the benzodiazepines that are biotransformed by the liver occurs in patients with hepatic dysfunction, in the elderly, and in patients concurrently on other therapeutic agents that alter hepatic metabolism. Of particular significance is the interaction between these benzodiazepines and therapeutic agents that inhibit P-450. The histamine (H_2) receptor antagonist cimetidine, as well as oral contraceptives, prolong the elimination half-life of the benzodiazepines by inhibiting their metabolism. Conversely, compounds that induce P-450 such as the barbiturates, will increase the rate of metabolism of these benzodiazepines. Of course, the biotransformation of benzodiazepines that proceed by a route other than hepatic oxidation is unaltered. Although the benzodiazepines are biotransformed via P-450, they do not significantly induce P-450 activity, and consequently do not accelerate the metabolism of other agents that are biotransformed via this system.

Pharmacodynamics

All the effects of the benzodiazepines are a consequence of their actions in the CNS to enhance GABAergic neurotransmission and thereby cause CNS depression. The generalized CNS depressant effects of the benzodiazepines are manifest by constant tiredness, difficulty concentrating and staying awake, decreased visual accommodation, decreased psychomotor performance, delayed reaction time, and ataxia.

Sedation is the most common effect of the benzodiazepines, and the intensity and duration of sedation depends on the dose and the concentra-

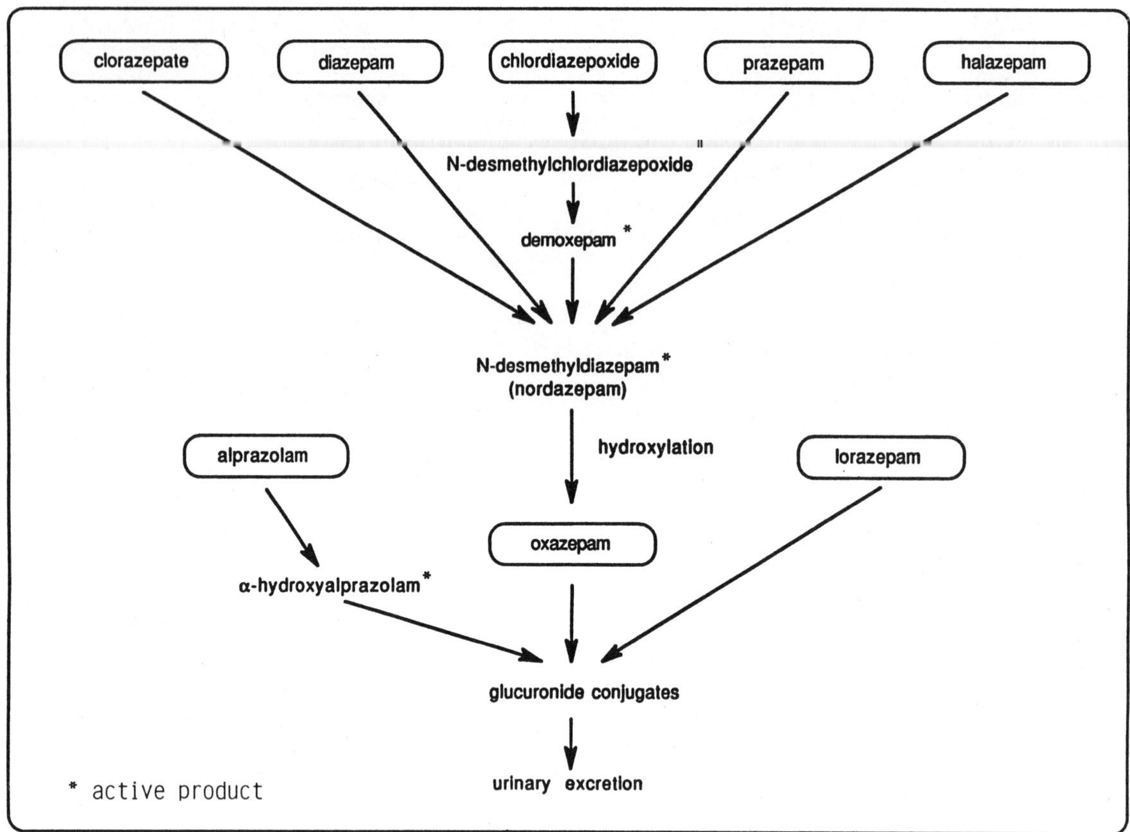

FIGURE 17-2 *Major metabolic interrelationships of benzodiazepines used as antianxiety drugs. Names circled represent those compounds that are available for therapeutic use; active biotransformation products are indicated by an asterisk.*

tion of drug in plasma and brain. Sedation is present at therapeutic doses of the drugs, and this effect is more severe and disabling in the elderly. With increasing doses, sedation proceeds to a hypnotic state and stupor. However, awareness persists, and thus, a general anesthetic state cannot be achieved. Benzodiazepines with a shorter duration of action (e.g., oxazepam) are less likely to cause daytime sedation than compounds with a long duration of action, such as diazepam. It is important to note that tolerance occurs to the sedative, but not the anxiolytic effect of the benzodiazepines.

The depressant actions of these drugs are manifest by alterations in sleep patterns. The latency of sleep onset (time to go to sleep) decreases, the amount of time spent in stage 2 sleep increases, and there is an overall increase in total sleep time. However, REM sleep, as well as stage 4 (slow wave sleep), are depressed, and if the benzodiazepines are discontinued, a rebound increased REM sleep occurs, characterized by "bizarre" dreams.

The benzodiazepines, particularly lorazepam, have been shown to impair memory and cause anterograde amnesia. Thus, patients cannot recall information acquired after drug administration. This effect has been attributed to interference with the memory consolidation process, and may be of benefit when the benzodiazepines (e.g., diazepam) are administered parenterally for various presurgical or diagnostic procedures such as endoscopy. In this situation, patients should be warned of this effect, especially if they are being treated as an outpatient. When administered orally, most benzodiazepines do not cause this effect.

The benzodiazepines produce skeletal muscle

relaxation by inhibiting polysynaptic reflexes. However, most evidence suggests that, with the exception of diazepam, skeletal muscle relaxation occurs only with doses of the benzodiazepines that have significant CNS depressant effects. Diazepam has a direct depressant effect on monosynaptic reflex pathways in the spinal cord, and thus, produces skeletal muscle relaxation at doses that do not induce sedation. This effect renders diazepam of benefit for treating the spasticity associated with cerebral palsy.

The ability of the benzodiazepines to increase the convulsive seizure threshold is well documented and is discussed in Chapter 22.

Adverse Effects

The adverse reactions most frequently encountered with benzodiazepine therapy are an extension of their CNS depressant effects and include sedation, lightheadedness, ataxia, and lethargy. The mild sedative actions of these drugs vary quantitatively. For example, lorazepam has a prolonged sedative action compared with the other benzodiazepines even though it clears the body rapidly. Occasional reactions observed with hypnotic doses of the benzodiazepines include impaired mental and psychomotor function, confusion, euphoria, delayed reaction time, uncoordinated motor function, dysarthria, headache, and xerostomia. Rare reactions may include syncope, hypotension, blurred vision, altered libido, skin rashes, nausea, menstrual irregularities, agranulocytosis, lupus-like syndrome, edema, and constipation.

Adverse reactions associated with the intravenous use of the injectable benzodiazepines include pain during injection, thrombophlebitis, hypothermia, restlessness, cardiac arrhythmias, coughing, apnea, vomiting, and a mild anticholinergic effect. Deaths from overdose of benzodiazepines alone rarely occur. Patients have taken as much as 50 times the therapeutic doses of these drugs without causing mortality. This particular property of these drugs is another example of how they differ from the potent respiratory depressant sedative-hypnotics. Unlike the barbiturates, the benzodiazepines have only a mild effect on respiration when given by the oral route, even with toxic doses. However, when the benzodiazepines are administered parenterally or when they are taken in conjunction with other depressants like alcohol, all the compounds have the potential of causing significant respiratory depression and death.

Drug Withdrawal and Dependence

The benzodiazepines are well known to produce physical dependence, and withdrawal reactions ensue upon abrupt discontinuation. However, the dependence associated with the benzodiazepines is not identical to that observed with alcohol, opioids or the barbiturates. Although physical dependence is more likely to occur with high drug doses and long term treatment, it has been reported to occur after usual therapeutic regimens. The onset of withdrawal symptoms is related to the elimination half-life of the benzodiazepines and is more rapid in onset and more severe after discontinuation of the shorter-acting benzodiazepines such as oxazepam, lorazepam, and alprazolam. With the longer-acting benzodiazepines, the onset is much slower due to their longer half-lives and slower disappearance from the plasma. Therefore, doses of the benzodiazepines with short half-lives should be decreased gradually and not abruptly.

The withdrawal symptoms accompanying abrupt discontinuation from the benzodiazepines are generally autonomic in nature and include tremulousness, sweating, insomnia, abdominal discomfort, tachycardia, systolic hypertension, muscle twitching, and sensitivity to light and sound. In rare instances, severe withdrawal reactions may develop characterized by convulsions. These reactions are usually manifest in individuals maintained on high doses of the benzodiazepines for prolonged (more than 4 months) periods of time. In addition to these autonomic manifestations, abrupt withdrawal of the benzodiazepines can often cause patients to "rebound" exhibiting symptoms of anxiety and insomnia sometimes worse than before drug treatment was initiated.

The benzodiazepines have been reported to have a high abuse potential. However, evidence suggests that psychological dependence occurs mainly with individuals with a history of drug abuse; appropriate therapeutic use by persons not predisposed to drug abuse should not lead to abuse of the benzodiazepines.

Drug Interactions

The benzodiazepines are powerful CNS depressants and additive effects can occur when they are administered with other CNS depressant agents including ethanol, antihistamines, other sedative-hypnotic agents, antipsychotics, antidepressants, and opioid analgesics. Because ethanol is readily available and has a widespread use, the CNS depressant interaction between the benzodiazepines and ethanol is common. Individuals may experience episodes of mild to severe ataxia and "drunkenness" which severely retards performance levels. No single benzodiazepine is considered safer than another in combination with ethanol. Therefore, it is imperative that physicians inform their patients of this potential interaction and caution them not to drink alcoholic beverages while taking benzodiazepines. This is especially important for patients not previously exposed to the benzodiazepines. Individuals who have been drinking alcohol and taking benzodiazepines for long periods of time experience this interaction, but to a milder degree.

As mentioned previously, another drug interaction is a consequence of the biotransformation of the benzodiazepines. Because many of the benzodiazepines are metabolized by the hepatic P-450 monooxygenase system, compounds that inhibit P-450, such as cimetidine or the oral contraceptives, decrease the biotransformation of the long-acting benzodiazepines.

Contraindications and Precautions

As with any drug or class of drugs, the benzodiazepines should be avoided in patients with a known hypersensitivity to these agents. Alprazolam, clorazepate, diazepam, halazepam, lorazepam, and prazepam are contraindicated in individuals with acute narrow-angle glaucoma because of their anticholinergic side effects. In addition, due to the considerable lipid solubility of most benzodiazepines, these agents cross the placenta and are secreted in maternal milk. Consequently, they should be avoided in pregnant and nursing women.

Again, due to the hepatic biotransformation on these compounds, caution should be used in individuals with hepatic dysfunction and the elderly and debilitated population. Dose adjustments must be made, and initial doses should be limited to the smallest effective amount.

As with other psychoactive medications, precautions should be given with respect to administration of the drug and the amount of the prescription for severely depressed patients or for those in whom there is reason to expect concealed suicidal ideation or plans.

Therapeutic Uses

The primary indications for the benzodiazepines are anxiety, insomnia, seizure disorders, for preoperative sedation, and induction of anesthesia (see Table 17-1). The benzodiazepines useful for the treatment of insomnia include estazolam, flurazepam, quazepam, temazepam, and triazolam, and are discussed separately in Chapter 18.

Generalized anxiety disorder is managed effectively with all the benzodiazepines, while panic attacks respond favorably to alprazolam and the anticonvulsant benzodiazepine clonazepam. In addition, alprazolam has been shown to posses antidepressant activity similar to the tricyclics, which are also used for the treatment of panic attacks.

The intravenous administration of benzodiazepines provides immediate relief for uncontrolled seizures such as status epilepticus with less respiratory depression than other sedatives. However, because the duration of action is brief following this route of administration, loading doses of the anticonvulsant phenytoin should be used following the administration of the benzodiazepine. Although diazepam was the preferred drug of choice for status epilepticus, lorazepam and midazolam (not approved for the treatment of seizures by the FDA) are better tolerated following intravenous administration and are often used. The use of clonazepam for the treatment of convulsive disorders is discussed in Chapter 22.

Owing to their ability to produce sedation and anterograde amnesia, and reduce the anxiety, stress and tension associated with surgical or diagnostic procedures, the benzodiazepines are also used both as preanesthetic medication and for the induction and maintenance of general anesthesia. For procedures that do not require anesthesia such as endoscopy, cardioversion, cardiac catheterization, specific radiodiagnostic procedures, and reduction of minor fractures, the benzodiazepines may be administered orally, intramuscularly or intravenously. For anesthesia induction, the benzodiazepines are administered intravenously. Again, although diazepam used to be the agent of choice, lorazepam and midazolam are now the preferred compounds for the induction and maintenance of general anesthesia.

In addition to these major indications, the benzodiazepines have also been found to be of use for the treatment of alcohol withdrawal. Because the benzodiazepines exhibit cross-tolerance with alcohol, have anticonvulsant activity, and do not have major respiratory depressant effects, these compounds have become the drugs of choice for the treatment of acute alcohol withdrawal symptoms. In particular, chlordiazepoxide, clorazepate, diazepam and oxazepam have now replaced other sedatives for this purpose.

Diazepam is of use for relief of skeletal muscle spasms, spasticity, and athetosis, while lorazepam, administered intramuscularly with an antipsychotic, is useful for controlling agitation in psychotic individuals.

BENZODIAZEPINE ANTAGONIST

As mentioned in the beginning of this chapter, flumazenil is a competitive antagonist at benzodiazepine receptors on the chloride ionophore complex. The drug reverses the sedative effects of the benzodiazepines following overdose, anesthesia or sedation for brief surgical or diagnostic procedures. Flumazenil does not have any activity on its own, and does not antagonize the effects of the opioids, non-benzodiazepine sedatives or anesthetic agents. In addition, although flumazenil can antagonize the sedative effects of the benzodiazepines, it may not be effective in reversing the respiratory depression.

Flumazenil has a very short duration of action and is metabolized by the liver to inactive products and excreted in the urine with a half-life of approximately 1 hour. Its antagonist activity is manifest within 1 to 2 minutes after intravenous administration, a peak effect is seen in 6 to 10 minutes, and the duration of action is about an hour. Flumazenil has been found to be of great benefit in cases of overdose, and it has been reported that in unconscious adults, flumazenil causes regain of consciousness sufficient such that gastric lavage, bladder catheterization, electroencephalography and other procedures could be avoided.

Adverse reactions which can occur include nausea, dizziness, headache, blurred vision, increased sweating, and anxiety. In addition, a panic attack has been reported to occur in some patients. Flumazenil can precipitate convulsions in individuals physically dependent on benzodiazepines as well as in patients maintained on benzodiazepines for seizure disorders. Cardiac arrhythmias have been reported in some instances.

Flumazenil must be used with caution in patients taking benzodiazepines and tricyclic antidepressants because flumazenil will antagonize the anticonvulsant effect of the benzodiazepines and unmask the epileptogenic effect of the tricyclic antidepressant.

In patients with mild to moderate liver dysfunction, the clearance of flumazenil is reduced and caution is indicated on repeated administration of the drug. In this circumstance, the dose of flumazenil should be decreased as well as the frequency of administration.

BUSPIRONE

Buspirone is a member of a new series of antianxiety drugs that is unrelated chemically to the benzodiazepines or the barbiturates. Buspirone is not a general CNS depressant, does not potentiate alcohol-induced depression, and has little addiction liability. In addition, buspirone is as effective as the benzodiazepines as an anxiolytic, but lacks the anticonvulsant and muscle relaxant effects. It also has minimal sedative effects as compared with other antianxiety drugs.

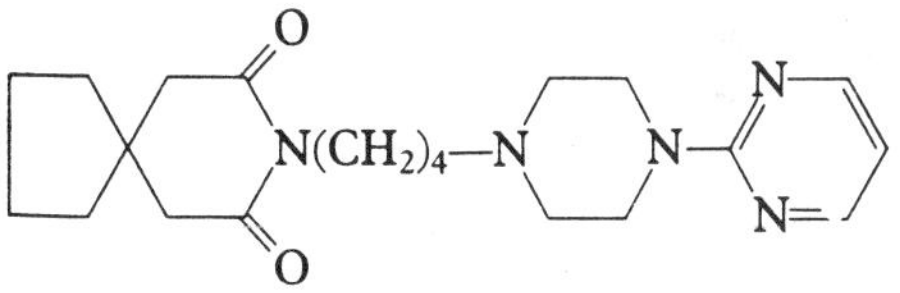

The mechanism of action of buspirone does not involve an interaction at the $GABA_A$ receptor complex like the benzodiazepines and barbiturates. Rather, evidence suggests that the actions of buspirone may be attributed to its partial agonist activity at the $5\text{-}HT_{1A}$ subtype of serotonin (5-HT) receptors.

Buspirone is rapidly absorbed and undergoes a first-pass effect. Approximately 95 percent of the drug is bound to plasma proteins, and it is metabolized by oxidation to an active metabolite, 1-pyrimidinyl piperazine. The elimination half-life of buspirone is about 2 to 3 hours, and less than 50 percent of the drug is excreted in the urine unchanged.

Adverse reactions of buspirone include dizziness, drowsiness, dry mouth, headaches, nervousness, fatigue, insomnia, weakness, lightheadedness, and muscle spasms. When administered chronically, buspirone causes less tolerance and potential for abuse than other anxiolytic drugs, and unlike the benzodiazepines, buspirone does not produce a rebound effect after discontinuation.

Buspirone is indicated for the management of generalized anxiety disorder and appears to be more effective than the benzodiazepines for chronic states of anxiety in which irritability and hostility are manifest. However, patient compliance with buspirone has been poor, especially in individuals who have previously been treated with benzodiazepines.

MEPROBAMATE

Meprobamate is the prototype drug for a group of antianxiety agents (the propanediol carbamates) which were used extensively for the treatment of anxiety and for daytime sedation prior to the advent of the benzodiazepines. The effects of meprobamate are somewhat similar to those of the barbiturate, phenobarbital, although shorter in duration. The precise mechanism by which meprobamate produces these effects is unknown. Meprobamate produces a widespread but uneven depression of the CNS; polysynaptic reflexes are depressed, while monosynaptic reflexes are undisturbed. Little skeletal muscle relaxation is produced at therapeutic doses. Meprobamate has no analgesic effect of its own, but has been reported to enhance the analgesia produced by other agents when used in combination for musculoskeletal pain. Meprobamate promotes sleep in patients with insomnia; however, in a fashion similar to the barbiturates, it depresses REM sleep.

The untoward effects most commonly associated with meprobamate are drowsiness and ataxia. Anaphylaxis, allergic reactions, hypotension, and syncope have also been reported. Long-term high-dose use of meprobamate has been shown to cause psychological and physical dependence and abrupt discontinuation may produce withdrawal symptoms. Meprobamate may precipitate seizures in epileptic patients.

Patients should be warned that meprobamate may impair the mental and physical abilities required for the performance of potentially hazardous tasks such as driving a motor vehicle or operating machinery.

OTHER ANXIOLYTICS

Beta-adrenergic blockers such as propranolol (see Chapter 9) have been found to be of use for the treatment of performance anxiety or "stage fright." These compounds are effective in suppressing the somatic and autonomic symptoms of anxiety, but do not alter emotional symptoms. The α_2-adrenergic agonist, clonidine, has also been reported to have anxiolytic properties.

The antihistamine hydroxyzine has been used for its anxiolytic activity, sedative properties, for motion sickness, as a preanesthetic medication, for alcohol addiction, and in allergic reactions. The most common side effects are drowsiness (25 percent of patients), headaches, nausea, and xerostomia. Hydroxyzine enhances the depressant effects of the opioids and barbiturates. This compound does not exhibit cross-tolerance with the benzodiazepines, barbiturates, meprobamate, or alcohol, and does not produce physical or psychological dependence.

BIBLIOGRAPHY

Doble, A., and I.L. Martin: "Multiple Benzodiazepine Receptors: No Reason for Anxiety," *Trends Pharm. Sci.* **13**: 76-81 (1992).

Heafely, W.: "The GABA-Benzodiazepine Interaction Fifteen Years Later," *Neurochem. Res.* **15**: 169-174 (1990).

Olsen, R.W., and A.J. Tobin: "Molecular Biology of $GABA_a$ Receptors," *FASEB J.* **4**: 1469-1480 (1990).

Shader, R.I., and D.J. Greenblatt: "Use of Benzodiazepines in Anxiety Disorders," *New Eng. J. Med.* **328**: 1398-1405 (1993).

Sieghart, W.: "$GABA_A$ Receptors: Ligand-gated Cl^- Ion Channels Modulated by Multiple Drug-Binding Sites. *Trends Pharm. Sci.* **13**: 446-450 (1992).

CHAPTER 18

Ethanol and Related Alcohols

Andrew P. Ferko

Ethanol is classified as a central nervous system depressant. Although ethanol is chemically a simple compound, it produces numerous pharmacologic and toxicological effects which can be complex and diverse. It has become one of the most widely abused drugs in our society. Acute usage of ethanol leads to intoxication while chronic usage of ethanol results in alcohol dependence and serious damage to various organ systems in the body. In this chapter the basic concepts of the effects of ethanol are discussed. In addition, other alcohols, methanol, ethylene glycol, and isopropyl alcohol, are presented from the standpoint of their toxicology when they are accidentally or intentionally ingested.

ETHANOL

Ethanol is one of the oldest drugs used by humans in the course of civilization. The drug is employed for both medicinal and social uses. Although ethanol has several therapeutic indications, its primary medical interest today is related to the fact that ethanol is commonly used as a drug of abuse. Ethanol produces central nervous system euphoria and depression. On repeated administration over a period of time, tolerance and physical dependence can develop. Prolonged ingestion of ethanol can lead to pathologic changes in body organs, e.g., cirrhosis of the liver, pancreatitis, cardiac dysfunction, and brain damage. Approximately 10 percent of the population exhibits alcohol abuse and alcoholism. Ethanol consumption can seriously affect the lives of alcoholics and their families. Alcoholics have 15 times the suicide rate of the general population. Ethanol is significantly involved in many cases of wife and child abuse. In addition, the drinking of ethanol is associated with about 50 percent of all deaths that occur in automobile accidents. Although ethanol has many social implications in its use, the intent of this chapter is to be an introduction to the basic pharmacology of ethanol that is associated with its acute and chronic effects.

Chemistry and Source

Ethanol (CH_3-CH_2-OH) is a water-soluble aliphatic alcohol; it is also referred to as *ethyl alcohol*, or *alcohol*. Ethanol is manufactured by the process of fermentation. In the presence of yeast, sugar is converted to ethanol. If the starting product is a cereal which contains starch, the starch is first malted so that the starch is converted to the sugar maltose.

The ethanol content of alcoholic beverages such as wines and distilled liquors are listed as the percentage of alcohol expressed by volume or as a number followed by the word *proof*. In the United States the proof number is twice the percentage of alcohol by volume.

The term proof originated in an old English custom of testing the alcohol content of whiskey. The whiskey was poured over gunpowder and a flame applied to it. If the gunpowder exploded, the whiskey was said to be of "proof strength." For whiskey to ignite, it must contain at least 50 percent ethanol by volume.

Mechanism of Action

Ethanol is a central nervous system depressant. Depending on the dose, there may occur sedation, ataxia, analgesia, hypnosis, anesthesia, or even death due to respiratory paralysis. At the present time, the exact mechanism of action for ethanol in the central nervous system is not fully delineated, however, it is proposed that the site of action for ethanol is the cellular membrane. It is suggested that acute ethanol administration acts in a physical manner to cause the disordering of membranes and thereby increase membrane fluidity in areas of the membrane associated with receptors and ion channels. The ethanol molecules dissolve into cell membranes and cause the lipid bilayer of the membrane to become less rigid in its structural arrangement. The enhanced fluidity of neuronal membranes produced by ethanol may alter such events as (1) ion fluxes across the membrane, (2) conformational changes in enzymes, or (3) neurotransmitter mechanisms.

It is reported that some behavioral effects of ethanol are attributed to an enhancement of chloride ion influx, resulting in hyperpolarization of membranes. In neuronal membranes this stimulated influx of chloride ions occurs through the chloride ionophore, a macromolecular complex that contains receptors for gamma-aminobutyric acid (GABA), benzodiazepines, and barbiturates. It appears that ethanol modifies the microenvironment of the postsynaptic $GABA_A$ receptor-mediated chloride ion channel to augment the influx of chloride ions which results in inhibition of neuronal function. Although chloride ions have been implicated in some of the behavioral actions of ethanol such as antianxiety, intoxication and loss of motor coordination, this chloride ion proposal does not explain fully the pharmacologic effects of ethanol. Ethanol also alters the fluxes of other ions such as sodium and calcium. In addition, a variety of neurotransmitters such as glutamate, serotonin, glycine, and dopamine, are affected by the administration of ethanol.

The glutamate receptors, particularly the NMDA (N-methyl-D-aspartate) receptor, appears to be involved with learning, memory, neuronal development and physical dependence on ethanol. In addition, some evidence suggest that a interaction between the GABAergic and glutamatergic systems may be associated with the central depressant action of ethanol. The neurotransmitter serotonin may play a part in the desire to consume ethanol. In the CNS ethanol can affect signal transduction and second messengers such as dopamine-stimulated cyclic-AMP production. In addition, glycine, an inhibitory amino acid neurotransmitter, appears to enhance the central depressant properties of ethanol.

When ethanol is administered in repeated doses over a period of time, it has been shown that the drug induces less alteration of membrane fluidity as compared with single-dose administration of it. This adaptation of the components of membranes to repeated exposure of ethanol may play a role in the phenomena of tolerance and physical dependence that are associated with ethanol along with changes in ion fluxes and alteration of certain cellular functions.

The various actions of ethanol occur in a complex manner and probably involve interaction between neurotransmitter, neuromodulator and diverse integrations of various neural systems in the brain. Further research is required before a more definitive statement can be made about a detailed mechanism for the action of ethanol.

Pharmacokinetics

Upon oral administration, ethanol is initially absorbed in the stomach, but the major portion of the drug is absorbed in the small intestine. This neutral, low molecular weight compound is transported across membranes by simple diffusion. The absence of food in the stomach and increasing the concentration of ethanol up to 40 percent enhance the rate of ethanol absorption. High concentration of ethanol (40 percent or greater) can produce gastric irritation, pylorospasm, and gastric mucous secretion, which tend to impede the absorption of ethanol from the gastrointestinal tract.

Ethanol is widely distributed in the body according to the water content of tissues. The rate of ethanol accumulation in the various tissues depends on the blood supply to them. As blood level of ethanol increases, ethanol tissue concentrations build up quite readily in the brain but more slowly in skeletal muscle and adipose tissue. At equilibrium the exhaled air from the lungs contains 0.05 percent of the ethanol concentration that is present in the blood. Therefore, the analysis of expired air serves as a method for the determination of the concentration of ethanol in the blood.

Over 90 percent of ethanol is biotransformed, primarily in the liver. The remainder is eliminated unchanged in the urine, exhaled air, sweat, and saliva. For humans the average rate at which this occurs is 100 mg/kg/h and is reflected as a corresponding fall in blood ethanol in the body. In other words, a 150 lb person can eliminate 7 g (9 mL) of absolute ethanol or about 2/3 oz. of 100 proof whiskey every hour. For each gram of ethanol biotransformed, 7 kcal is made available to the body.

The biotransformation of ethanol may be divided into three stages, which take place concurrently (Fig. 18-1).

Stage I $$CH_3\text{-}CH_2OH + NAD^+ \xrightarrow[\text{dehydrogenase}]{\text{alcohol}} CH_3\text{-}CHO + NADH + H^+$$

Stage II $$CH_3\text{-}CHO + H_2O \xrightarrow[\text{dehydrogenase}]{\text{aldehyde}} CH_3\text{-}COOH + (2H)$$

Stage III $$CH_3\text{-}COOH + 4(O) \longrightarrow 2CO_2 + 2H_2O$$

FIGURE 18-1 *Biotransformation of ethanol by the alcohol dehydrogenase pathway.*

Stage I During this stage, ethanol is oxidized to acetaldehyde by alcohol dehydrogenase, with nicotinamide adenine dinucleotide (NAD^+) acting as the immediate hydrogen acceptor. Alcohol dehydrogenase, a zinc-containing enzyme, is present in the liver to a large extent, and smaller concentrations are found in the gastrointestinal tract and kidney. Stage I occurs almost exclusively in the liver. The rate at which alcohol is converted to acetaldehyde is constant, and it essentially follows zero-order kinetics. It appears that the velocity of the reaction, and therefore the ethanol elimination rate, are primarily dependent on the concentration of NAD^+, that is the rate at which NADH is converted to NAD^+ and the total enzyme activity of alcohol dehydrogenase. In addition, atypical alcohol dehydrogenase has been identified in several populations and is responsible for the enhanced biotransformation of ethanol and the subsequence accumulation of acetaldehyde.

Stage II In this step the acetaldehyde is oxidized to acetic acid and the latter buffered to form acetate. The enzyme responsible for the oxidation of acetaldehyde to acetate is a mitochondrial aldehyde dehydrogenase, and the hydrogen acceptor is NAD^+. Stage II is a very rapid reaction, so that only small traces of acetaldehyde appear in the blood, even after excessive consumption of alcohol. Studies have shown that aldehyde dehydrogenase can also exit in a high-affinity form and low-affinity form. Individuals, e.g., some Orientals, with the low-affinity aldehyde dehydrogenase tend to accumulate blood acetaldehyde and can experience untoward effects such as facial flushing.

Stage III The acetate formed in stage II increases the body's pool of acetate, which is finally oxidized to CO_2 and H_2O. The actual reaction is much more complicated, and most of the acetate probably goes through the Krebs cycle. The CO_2 formed then enters the body's pool of bicarbonate, almost all of which finally exists as pulmonary CO_2.

Two other biotransformation systems have been implicated in the oxidation of ethanol to acetaldehyde (Fig. 18-2). They are the hepatic microsomal ethanol oxidizing system (MEOS) and the catalase system. The MEOS requires NADPH-cytochrome P-450 reductase, cytochrome P-450, molecular oxygen, and phospholipids. The catalase system, which is also present in the liver,

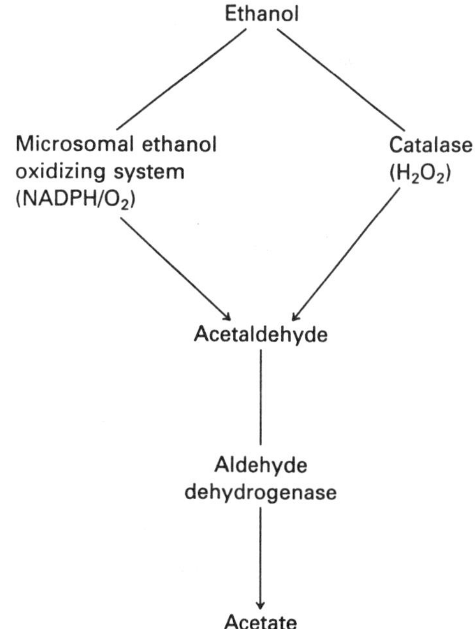

FIGURE 18-2 *Alternate pathways for the oxidation of ethanol to acetaldehyde.*

requires the availability of hydrogen peroxide. Although the major pathway for oxidation of ethanol to acetaldehyde is by alcohol dehydrogenase, under normal conditions the MEOS seems to participate in the oxidation of ethanol when high blood levels are present in the body and during chronic consumption of ethanol. The increased rate of ethanol biotransformation that is observed during chronic use of ethanol is believed to be due to enhanced activity of the MEOS. Catalase may have some role in the biotransformation of ethanol; however, its contribution has not been fully delineated.

Pharmacodynamics

The main effect of ethanol is depression of the central nervous system. This depressant effect begins with the higher functions and later extends to the lower centers of the brain as the concentration of ethanol in the central nervous system increases. The reticular activating system is most sensitive to the depressant action of ethanol. The common misconception that ethanol is a stimulant is due to its effect to lessen inhibitory influences in other areas of the brain, particularly the cortex, by suppression of the integration function of the reticular activating system. Some important effects of ethanol on the central nervous system are as follows:

1. *Euphoria* Drinkers see the world and themselves through rose-colored glasses. The desire to secure this effect is the chief reason for the popularity of alcoholic beverages, except for those who use these beverages sparingly as a condiment. Euphoria usually begins at levels of blood ethanol below those causing definite muscular incoordination.

2. *Removal of inhibitions* Ethanol, even in rather small amounts, causes loss of inhibitions, and the individual responds to many impulses which are ordinarily repressed. The resultant behavior may consist of silly speech and harmless antics, but sometimes becomes vicious and antisocial.

3. *Impairment of vision* Ethanol reduces visual acuity. The ethanol in two or three cocktails may cause a reduction in visual acuity of more than 50 percent. Diplopia may occur if the blood ethanol concentration reaches 200 to 300 mg per 100 mL.

4. *Muscular incoordination* Small doses of ethanol impair the ability of the brain to coordinate muscular activity. With high concentrations of ethanol in the body, the manifestations of muscular incoordination are slurred speech and staggering gait, the complete loss of the power of speech and locomotion, and finally coma and general anesthesia.

5. *Lengthened reaction time* The mean normal reaction time is around 0.29 sec to light and 0.19 sec to sound. Blood ethanol concentrations below 100 mg per 100 mL have very little effect on reaction time. Levels between 100 and 200 mg per 100 mL usually lengthen the reaction time from 10 to 50 percent.

In the posterior pituitary, ethanol produces depression, and this results in a reduction in the release of antidiuretic hormone. As a consequence of the suppression of antidiuretic hormone, less water is reabsorbed from the collecting duct of the nephron of the kidney and diuresis ensues. This diuretic effect occurs primarily as blood ethanol concentrations are increasing. Another area of the brain that is affected by ethanol is the hypothalamus. Higher concentration of ethanol (greater than 1 g/kg) can induce hypothermia, and this effect is enhanced when the environmental temperature is low. In addition, when blood ethanol concentrations are increasing, depression of the vasomotor center and the respiratory center leads to a decrease in blood pressure and a suppression of respiration. The lethal effect of ethanol is attributed to respiratory depression.

Ethanol exerts effects on the gastrointestinal tract and liver. In the gastrointestinal tract ethanol increases in gastric acid secretion; however, when concentrations of ethanol are greater than 20 percent, there is a reduction in gastric acid and pepsin secretion. Gastritis can be produced by ethanol and can lead to acute gastric hemorrhage. Ethanol also enhances salivary secretion. In the liver, following ethanol ingestion, high concentrations of ethanol reach the liver via the portal vein, and since the liver bears the brunt of oxidizing ethanol to acetaldehyde, it is apparent that ethanol may eventually produce hepatic dysfunction. It appears that females are more susceptible to hepatic dysfunction than males. In the chronic abuse of ethanol, the hepatic cirrhosis that can develop is due to prolonged high intake of ethanol rather than to the associated dietary deficiencies, and therefore ethanol has a direct hepatotoxic action.

Adverse Reactions

Acute There is a direct correlation between the concentration of ethanol in the blood and pharmacologic effects leading to impairment. One type of impairment, frank intoxication, exhibits the common signs of drunkenness, including slurred speech, difficulty of locomotion, and obvious loss of inhibitions. The results of several studies have been summarized as follows: For six zones of blood ethanol concentration (expressed in mg per 100 mL), the average percentage of subjects judged to be intoxicated were 0 to 50, 10 percent; 51 to 100, 34 percent; 101 to 150, 64 percent; 151 to 200, 86 percent; 201 to 250, 96 percent and 251 to 300, 99 percent. These studies agree that almost all subjects with blood alcohol levels above 200 mg per 100 mL were definitely drunk. The blood ethanol level to be considered intoxicated for operating a motor vehicle from a legal standpoint is 100 mg per 100 mL.

The symptoms of severe, acute toxicity are much like those of an overdose of any general CNS depressant drug, with shallow respiration and some impairment of circulation. The face and body surface are pale, and the extremities are cold. Depression of the respiratory and vasomotor centers is observed at 350 mg per 100 mL of ethanol. Although deaths have been reported at this blood ethanol concentration, it is uncommon. Greater suppression of the respiratory, cardiac, and vasomotor centers occurs when the blood ethanol concentration increases to 550 mg per 100 mL. Acidosis, hypoglycemia, and elevated intracranial pressure are noted. The patient may be in a stupor or coma at this point, and if not treated, death can occur. Death is due to respiratory failure. Chief postmortem findings are hyperemia of the stomach mucosa and edema at the base of the brain.

No specific treatment for severe acute intoxication has been found. Treatment is symptomatic, such as the administration of pressor amines, glucose, or mannitol, and the correction of metabolic acidosis by sodium bicarbonate. If the patient can be kept alive and hypoxia avoided, he or she will usually recover as the absorbed ethanol is biotransformed.

The consumption of ethanol in a very cold environment, which can induce hypothermia, is dangerous under certain circumstances. Ingestion of moderate quantities causes dilation of skin blood vessels, with flushing of the face, neck, and upper trunk area. This effect prevents normal cutaneous vasoconstriction on exposure to cold, so that intoxication hastens the fatal outcome in "freezing to death." Central vasomotor depression probably plays a role in the production of this vasodilatation as well as a direct effect of ethanol to relax cutaneous blood vessels.

Chronic Alcoholism presents a serious medical, social, and economic problem. At present there is no scientific explanation for the fact that some persons continue excessive drinking to the point where their lives become "utterly unmanageable," to quote a phrase from Alcoholics Anonymous.

The alcoholic cannot refrain from excessive drinking and is distressed and upset without the euphoria produced by alcohol in his or her system. Some chronic alcoholics often do not drink to the point of marked intoxication; others are quite drunk most of the time. The outstanding symptom is an intense craving for ethanol, the desire to drink being about the only interest in life. There are, of course, varying gradations of the affliction. Alcohol abuse and alcoholism affect approximately 10 percent of the adult population in the United States. Although genetic factors may play some role in the development of alcoholism, many other factors are involved in this complex issue such as peer pressure, stress, cultural values, family situation, adolescent drinking, depression, and anxiety.

Chronic consumption of ethanol produces tolerance and physical dependence. The degree and severity of the withdrawal syndrome that occurs upon abrupt discontinuation of ethanol drinking depends on the amount of ethanol ingested and the duration of time that the ethanol was used. On termination of ethanol consumption, the individual can have *acute alcoholic hallucinosis*. These hallucinations can be auditory, visual, tactile, or olfactory in their manifestation. In most severe cases of physical dependence, *delirium tremens* occurs. Delirium tremens usually occurs as a sequel to heavy, excessive drinking over a period of 2 to 6 weeks. The initial symptoms are restlessness, insomnia, tremor, fear, perspiration, and headache. This is followed by the second stage, which is characterized by hallucinations and delirium. The hallucinations are predominantly visual but may be tactile and auditory; they generally involve great fear. Alcoholics call the first stage the "shakes" and the second stage the "horrors." Convulsions may occur. The delirium usually lasts 3 or 4 days. Delirium tremens can be a life-threatening situation. Management of delirium tremens may involve the use of benzodiazepines such as diazepam and chlordiazepoxide.

Other chronic effects from ethanol abuse include morning nausea and vomiting, gastritis, ulceration of the gastrointestinal tract, pancreatitis, cardiomegaly, hypertension, fatty liver, alcoholic hepatitis, and cirrhosis of the liver. Ethanol may alter male fertility by reducing serum testosterone levels and decreasing sperm motility. *Alcoholic polyneuropathy*, which is associated with numbness, pain, and muscle wasting in the legs, may be produced. *Wernicke's Disease* is the result of excessive ethanol use and a deficiency of thiamine. This disorder is characterized by ocular abnormalities, e.g., nystagmus, ataxia, and mental confusion.

Wernicke-Korsakoff's syndrome appears in a few alcoholics, the incidence of this disorder being about one-tenth that of delirium tremens. The chief signs of Wernicke-Korsakoff's syndrome are impairment of memory of recent events, lessened learning ability, disorientation in space and time, and polyneuritis involving pain in the extremities and partial or total paralysis of the arms and legs. The polyneuritis appears to be due to a marked deficiency of vitamin B_1 (thiamine).

In pregnancy, the daily consumption of ethanol increases the risk of birth defects. As little as 1 oz. of ethanol (two drinks), but definitely 3 oz. (six drinks) or more, daily is associated with a significant incidence of congenital anomalies which are referred to as the *fetal alcohol syndrome* (FAS). The neonate may exhibit such signs as growth deficiency, developmental delay or mental retardation, craniofacial abnormalities, and structural anomalies of the heart and genitals. A second condition that may result from prenatal exposure to ethanol is called *fetal alcohol effects* (FAE). The children exhibit behavioral problems and learning disabilities. Children diagnosed with FAE have less physical and mental impairment than children with FAS. Complete safety from the threat of FAS or FAE can be assured only by abstinence from ethanol during the entire pregnancy.

Some cases of chronic alcoholism, both psychotic and nonpsychotic, terminate fatally in a few months or years. However, many chronic alcoholics have a fairly normal life expectancy, aside from being bad safety risks. Chronic alcoholics have a serious illness and should be treated as such.

Attempts have been made to identify some biochemical marker in the body that would be reliable than self-reporting of ethanol usage by individuals with alcoholism. During high ethanol consumption isomeric forms of serum transferrin which are deficient in their carbohydrate constituents are produced. Elevation in the levels of carbohydrate-deficient transferrin (CDT) is indicative of continuous ethanol ingestion. Another marker is urinary 5-hydroxytryptophol (5-HTOL) which appears to be useful to reveal recent ethanol drinking. The use of these biochemical markers and possibly others may aid in the early detection of relapse and be useful in alcohol treatment monitoring.

Drug Interactions

Since ethanol causes central nervous system depression and can influence the drug-metabolizing microsomal system (DMMS), various drugs, when taken in combination with ethanol, may produce altered therapeutic responses or adverse reactions in the patient. Acute ethanol administration increases the central depressant properties of barbiturates, benzodiazepines, H_1-antihistamines with sedative effects, and opioid analgesics. This effect is due to the fact that these drugs and ethanol depress the central nervous system and their combined effect is additive. Ethanol can have an additive effect on the adverse reaction of sedation that is associated with phenothiazines and tricyclic antidepressants, particularly those antidepressants with significant sedative properties, e.g., amitriptyline and doxepin. Also acute ethanol consumption may inhibit the microsomal biotransformation of these drugs listed above and thus enhance their effects, particularly on the central nervous system. Chronic ethanol administration, however, induces the microsomal system and may accelerate drug metabolism, thereby possibly attenuating their pharmacologic action.

Chronic ingestion of ethanol can enhance the hepatotoxic effect of acetaminophen, particularly when acetaminophen is taken in large doses or in an overdose situation. It appears that ethanol increases the formation of metabolites that are toxic to the liver, e.g., N-acetyl-p-benzoquinone. Aspirin and related nonsteroidal anti-inflammatory drugs (NSAIDs) may exhibit a greater tendency to cause gastrointestinal bleeding in the presence by ethanol. These analgesics and ethanol can adversely affect the gastric mucosal barrier. Ethanol can also enhance bleeding time. Cimetidine may increase the intoxication of ethanol by inhibiting ethanol's biotransformation and possibly enhancing its absorption from the gastrointestinal tract. The greater degree of central nervous system depression that is noted with chloral hydrate and

TABLE 18-1 Some drug interactions with ethanol

Drug	Reaction
Chlorpropamide	Facial flushing
Cyclobenzaprine	Enhanced CNS depression
Nitrates	Enhanced hypotensive effect
Nitrates (IV preparations)	Ethanol content may cause CNS and cardiac depression
Phenytoin	Decreased phenytoin serum levels
Oral hypoglycemics (sulfonylureas)	Risk of hypoglycemia

ethanol appears to be related to a reduction in the biotransformation of ethanol and an increased rate of metabolism of chloral hydrate to trichloroethanol, which is the active component of chloral hydrate. Ethanol can increase or decrease the prothrombin time of a patient who is receiving anticoagulants. Other drug interactions with ethanol are listed in Table 18-1.

Several drugs appear to interfere with the oxidation of ethanol and increase the blood levels of acetaldehyde which produces a disulfiram-like reaction in the patient (see "Disulfiram" below). This reaction is associated with such symptoms as sweating, vomiting, weakness, and tachycardia. Some drugs that may produce a disulfiram-like reaction, are listed in Table 18-2. Since the drugs that are capable of interaction with ethanol are so numerous, it is reasonable to suggest that when patients are on any medication they should refrain from the consumption of ethanol.

TABLE 18-2 Drugs which cause a disulfiram-like reaction in the presence of ethanol

Acetohexamide	Metronidazole
Cefoperazone	Phentolamine
Ceftriaxone	Procarbazine
Chloramphenicol	Tolazamide
Griseofulvin	Tolbutamide

Clinical Uses

Ethanol is used as an antiseptic in solutions of 50 to 95 percent. A 70 percent solution is generally considered the optimum concentration for penetration and denaturation of bacterial protein. Ethanol evaporates readily from the skin, producing a cooling effect. It lowers surface tension and is also a good solvent for many substances on the skin. Sponge baths with ethanol or isopropyl alcohol are sometimes useful for cleansing and as an aid in reducing fevers.

The use of alcohol to dilate coronary vessels and for treating peripheral vascular diseases is unreliable. However, alcoholic drinks may be of benefit to patients with cardiac disease in that the mild sedation permits rest and relaxation.

Ethanol is used as an antidote in methanol and ethylene glycol poisoning. These uses of ethanol are discussed later in the chapter.

Ethanol and hydroalcoholic solutions are excellent solvents and preservatives for many drugs.

DISULFIRAM

Many physicians refer their alcoholic patients to Alcoholics Anonymous. However, sometimes disulfiram is employed to bolster sobriety by the production of unpleasant symptoms.

$$(C_2H_5)_2N-\underset{\underset{S}{\|}}{C}-S-S-\underset{\underset{S}{\|}}{C}-N(C_2H_5)_2$$

When taken by itself in small doses, disulfiram produces no apparent pharmacologic effects. If, however, after several days of such medication, small amounts of alcohol are imbibed, a toxic reaction follows, which persists as long as the alcohol is being metabolized. Roughly in order of their appearance, the symptoms and signs are a cutaneous sensation of heat, flushing, vasodilatation, hypotension, palpitation, increased heart rate, dizziness, vomiting, unconsciousness, and collapse. The magnitude of these symptoms is subject to individual variation and is proportional to the dosage of both disulfiram and alcohol. In some patients only discomfort has been observed; in a few instances death has occurred.

The mechanism by which disulfiram produces this unpleasant reaction or the "acetaldehyde syndrome," as it is sometimes called, is due to interference with the oxidation of ethanol. Disulfiram irreversibly inhibits the enzyme aldehyde dehydrogenase by binding to sulfhydryl groups of the enzyme and also chelating zinc, which is present in the enzyme. In addition, disulfiram is biotransformed to active metabolites, which also inhibits aldehyde dehydrogenase. As a result of the inhibition of aldehyde dehydrogenase, the blood acetaldehyde level can be 5 to 10 times higher than with the consumption of ethanol in the absence of disulfiram.

The drug is adequately absorbed (80 percent) from the gastrointestinal tract and achieves a peak plasma concentration within 1 to 2 h. The drug is widely distributed in the body because of its lipid solubility; however, only small concentrations of the drug are present in the brain. Disulfiram is reduced in the body to diethyldithiocarbamic acid. In addition, this metabolite undergoes several other reactions such as methylation, oxidation, and conjugation with glucuronic acid.

Disulfiram is contraindicated in patients with a history of severe myocardial disease or coronary occlusion, psychosis, or hypersensitivity reaction to disulfiram. This drug should be used only in selected patients to bolster their determination not to drink and should be accompanied by good psychiatric and medical treatment.

METHANOL

Methanol is a simple compound with the following chemical structure: CH_3-OH. This aliphatic alcohol is also known as methyl alcohol, wood spirit, and wood alcohol. It is used mainly as an industrial solvent and is found also in such products as paint thinner, solid canned heat, gasoline (as an additive), and paint remover. Methanol poisoning can result from industrial exposure and accidental or intentional ingestion of products containing it.

After oral ingestion of methanol, the compound is readily absorbed from the gastrointestinal tract and distributed in the body. Methanol is oxidized by the alcohol dehydrogenase system, the same pathway that biotransforms ethanol. The oxidation of methanol follows zero-order kinetics, but the rate of disappearance of methanol from the blood occurs at a much slower rate than that of ethanol elimination (about one-seventh). Methanol is biotransformed to formaldehyde and formic acid. The metabolite, formic acid, appears to be responsible for the blindness that is associated with methanol ingestion. The possibility of blindness is enhanced in the presence of acidosis. It has been suggested that some of the methanol may be metabolized by the catalase system. If the catalase system does play a role in the oxidation of methanol, it is probably a minor component when compared with the alcohol dehydrogenase system.

The symptoms of methanol poisoning include initial visual disturbances, which may lead to partial or complete blindness due to damage of retinal cells and degeneration of the optic nerve by the metabolite of methanol, formic acid. Central nervous system depression occurs along with nausea, vomiting, slowed respiration, bradycardia, and coma.

Therapeutic measures that are taken to treat methanol toxicities can include (1) correction of acidosis, (2) maintenance of respiration, (3) monitoring of electrolytes and providing nutrition, and (4) administration of ethanol. Ethanol is given to the patient to reduce the rate of methanol metabolism. Ethanol competes with methanol for alcohol dehydrogenase and, therefore, decreases the formation of formaldehyde and formic acid. In serious methanol poisoning, hemodialysis is also employed. Another antidote that has been proposed for the treatment of methanol poisoning is 4-methylpyrazole. This compound is an inhibitor of alcohol dehydrogenase and prevents the formation of the toxic metabolite of methanol.

ETHYLENE GLYCOL

Ethylene glycol (CH_2OH-CH_2OH) is a dihydroxy-alcohol. This agent is found in antifreeze solutions and as an industrial solvent for plastics and paints. Ethylene glycol is discussed in this chapter because of the toxicities that can occur upon accidental or intentional ingestion.

In the body, ethylene glycol is first oxidized by alcohol dehydrogenase and then further metabolized to oxalic acid and other products (glycolic and formic acids). Calcium oxalate crystals that are formed, deposit in a variety of tissues, particularly the kidney, where they are nephrotoxic. Oxalate crystals also appear in the urine.

The symptoms of ethylene glycol poisoning may be central nervous system depression, convulsions, acidosis, renal damage, and respiratory failure. Management of ethylene glycol intoxication can include (1) gastric lavage, (2) maintenance of airway, (3) maintenance of body temperature (4) vigorous diuresis, (5) correction of acidosis, (6) hemodialysis, and (7) administration of ethanol. Ethanol will slow the biotransformation of ethylene glycol and reduce the formation of toxic metabolites. Another compound that has been suggested for the treatment of ethylene glycol intoxication is 4-methylpyrazole. This antidote reduces the biotransformation of ethylene glycol into oxalate by inhibition of the enzyme alcohol dehydrogenase, which is the first step in its biotransformation.

ISOPROPYL ALCOHOL

Isopropyl alcohol (isopropanol, 2-propanol) is available as a rubbing alcohol (a 70 percent solution), an antiseptic, and a topical agent to reduce fever. It readily evaporates from the skin and lowers elevated body temperature. This alcohol, however, is probably a better antibacterial agent than ethanol.

Isopropyl alcohol is about twice as potent as a CNS depressant when compared with ethanol. It is slowly biotransformed in body, possibly by alcohol dehydrogenase to acetone, which also possesses depressant properties. The half-life of isopropyl alcohol is 2.5 to 3 h.

Isopropyl alcohol produces toxicities when it is intentionally or accidentally ingested or inhaled. Toxicities of isopropyl alcohol can include nausea, vomiting, dizziness, CNS depression, coma, and respiratory depression. Treatment of isopropyl alcohol poisoning consists of supportive measures to maintain vital functions and hemodialysis.

BIBLIOGRAPHY

Berglund, M.: "Alcoholics Committed to Treatment: A Prospective Long-Term Study of Behavioral Characteristics, Mortality, and Social Adjustment," *Alcoholism: Clin. Exp. Res.* **12**: 19-24 (1988).

Bloom, F.E., and G.R. Siggins: "Electrophysiological Action of Ethanol at the Cellular Level," *Alcohol* **4**: 331-337 (1987).

Bosron, W.F., L. Lumeng, and T.K. Li: "Genetic Polymorphism of Enzymes of Alcohol Metabolism and Susceptibility to Alcohol Liver Disease," *Mol. Aspects Med,* **10**: 147-158 (1988).

Carlsson, A., A.J. Hiltunen, O. Beck, H. Stibler, and S. Borg: "Detection of Relapses in Alcohol-dependent Patients: Comparison of Carbohydrate-deficient Transferrin in Serum, 5-Hydroxytryptophol in Urine, and Self-reports," *Alcoholism: Clin and Exp. Res.* **17**: 703-708 (1993).

Chin, J.H., and D.B. Goldstein: "Membrane-Disordering Action of Ethanol," *Mol. Pharmacol.* **19**: 425-431 (1981).

Crabb, D.W., W.F., Bosron, and T.K. Li: "Ethanol Metabolism," *Pharmacol. Ther.* **34**: 59-73 (1987).

deWit, H., E.H. Whlenhuth, J. Pierri, and C.E. Johanson: "Individual Differences in Behavioral and Subjective Responses to Alcohol," *Alcoholism: Clin. Exp. Res.* **11**: 52-59 (1987).

Ferko, A.P.: "NMDA Enhances the Central Depressant Properties of Ethanol in Mice," *Pharmacol. Biochem. Behav.* **43**: 297-301 (1992).

Freund, R.K., C.G. van Horne, T. Harlam, and M. R. Palmer: "Electrophysiological Interaction of Ethanol with GABAergic Mechanisms in Rat Cerebellum In Vivo," *Alcoholism: Clin. Exp. Res.* **17**: 321-328 (1993).

Lieber, C.S.: "Biochemical and Molecular Basis of Alcohol-induced Injury to Liver and Other Tissues," *N. Engl. J. Med.* **31**: 1639-1650 (1988).

Mattucci-Schiavone, L., and A.P. Ferko: "Effect of Muscimol on Ethanol-Induced Central Nervous System Depression," *Pharmacol. Biochem. Behav.* **27**: 745-748 (1987).

Suzdak, P.D., and S.M. Paul: "Ethanol Stimulated GABA Receptor-Mediated Cl^- Ion Flux In Vitro: Possible Relationship to Anxiolytic and Intoxicating Actions of Alcohol," *Psychopharmacol. Bull.* **23**: 445-451 (1987).

Wood, W.G., and F. Schroeder: "Membrane Effects of Ethanol: Bulk Lipid Versus Lipid Domain," *Life Sci.* **43**: 467-475 (1988).

Wright, C., and R.D. Moore: "Disulfiram Treatment of Alcoholism," *Amer. J. Med.* **88**: 647-655 (1990).

CHAPTER 19

Psychotomimetic Drugs

Alan S. Bloom

The nonmedical use and abuse of psychoactive substances continues to be a significant medical and social problem. Among those psychoactive drugs that are commonly abused are a diverse group of compounds often referred to as *psychotomimetics*. As a group, they possess the ability to induce psychic and behavioral patterns that are in some ways characteristic of psychosis. From time to time, these drugs have been proposed and/or investigated for the treatment of alcoholism, drug addiction, and a variety of mental disorders. Currently many of these drugs have no generally accepted medical use and are classified as Schedule I drugs under the Controlled Substances Act. Other drugs discussed in this chapter such as cocaine and Δ^9-tetrahydrocannabinol have very limited medical indications and are classified as Schedule II drugs. Many of these compounds are also classified as *hallucinogens*. They are often abused "recreationally"; possibly for their novel sensory and hallucinogenic effects. The recreational and experimental use of lysergic acid diethylamide (LSD) type hallucinogens spans the last half of this century and is still prominent in many areas of the United States. Similarly, the use and abuse of other psychoactive drugs such as phencyclidine, marijuana, amphetamine, and cocaine are causing significant health and social problems.

CLASSIFICATION OF PSYCHOTOMIMETIC AND HALLUCINOGENIC SUBSTANCES

As a group, the drugs discussed in this chapter have been referred to by a variety of names in addition to hallucinogens or psychotomimetics. For example, the term *psychedelic* has also been used to describe the effects of some of these (LSD-type) drugs. It means the heightening or expansion of consciousness. Most have effects on mood and perception. Psychotomimetic drugs do not form a distinct drug class based on either chemistry or action. Rather, they are commonly grouped based on psychopharmacologic drug profiles and the ability of some drugs to display cross-tolerance.

Psychotomimetic drugs can be divided into three general groups. The first group consists of the hallucinogens which includes LSD, psilocybin, N,N-dimethyltryptamine (DMT), mescaline, 2,5-dimethoxy-4-methylamphetamine (DOM), and 3,4-methylenedioxymethamphetamine (MDMA). Cross-tolerance exists between drugs. Neurochemical studies indicate that these drugs act on a specific serotonin receptor subtype. Consequently, they appear to share a common mechanism of action and constitute one group, the LSD-type hallucinogens. A second group is composed of centrally-acting anticholinergic drugs such as atropine and scopolamine. A third, miscellaneous group of abused drugs, includes phencyclidine, the psychomotor stimulants (amphetamine, cocaine), and marijuana. These drugs do not share cross-tolerance with the LSD-type drugs and each has their own pharmacology which differs qualitatively from each other and the other two groups.

LSD-TYPE HALLUCINOGENS

This group of drugs share many pharmacological properties, including mechanism of action, psychotomimetic effects, and development of tolerance and cross-tolerance. Chemically, they are either indoleamine or substituted phenylethylamine derivatives. The prototype of this group is LSD. Structurally, LSD, psilocybin, and DMT are all indoleamines and possess a tryptamine nucleus, as does the centrally-acting neurotransmitter serotonin (5-hydroxytryptamine or 5-HT). The structure of LSD is shown below, the broken line indicating the tryptamine structure within the LSD molecule.

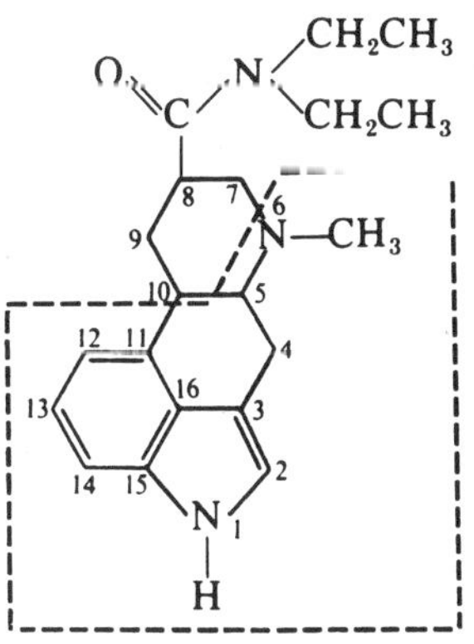

LSD

Mescaline and DOM are phenylethylamine or phenylisopropylamine rather than indole derivatives. However this does not appear to produce significant qualitative differences in the hallucinogenic properties of these drugs. This section will concentrate on the pharmacology of LSD and point out significant differences in the other compounds in this group.

Mechanism of Action

The exact mechanism by which this group of drugs produce its hallucinogenic actions is still not completely understood at a cellular level. Early theories emphasized the central nervous system (CNS) interactions of LSD with catecholamine and 5-HT neurotransmitters. Structural similarities of LSD to 5-HT (both contain an indole nucleus) and the finding that LSD was a potent antagonist of the peripheral actions of 5-HT, led investigators to propose that the hallucinogenic effects were due to antagonism of 5-HT within the CNS. Subsequent investigations revealed that the peripheral and central interactions of LSD with 5-HT differed. In the CNS, LSD suppressed the activity of serotonergic neurons — a presynaptic effect. Additional experiments, however, show that the effects of LSD persisted and were even enhanced after destruction of serotonergic neurons. This suggested that the site of action of LSD's hallucinogenic effects was postsynaptic.

Based on the results of receptor binding studies it is now known that LSD displays high-affinity binding to one of the several subtypes of serotonin receptors, the 5-HT_2 receptor, which is found in the cerebral cortex and other brain areas. LSD acts as an *agonist* at this receptor. LSD also acts on 5-HT autoreceptors to decrease the release of serotonin from neurons.

Numerous serotonergic pathways originate in the brain stem and project to all major areas of the brain. The agonist actions of LSD on 5-HT_2 receptors are thought to trigger a series of neuronal actions involving other neurotransmitter systems (especially noradrenergic and dopaminergic), which then, by some yet unexplained mechanism, contribute to the hallucinogenic actions of this group of drugs. For example, LSD has been shown to increase the concentration of dopamine in terminal fields of the mesocortical and mesolimbic pathways. The other drugs of this group including psilocybin and mescaline have also been shown to bind to 5-HT_2 receptors.

LSD Syndrome

Following administration of LSD and similar hallucinogens, a common sequence of dose-related effects occur. They have been divided into three phases: (1) the *somatic phase* occurs initially after absorption and consists of CNS stimulation and autonomic changes which are predominantly sympathomimetic in nature; (2) the *sensory phase* is characterized by sensory distortions and pseudohallucinations, which are the effects desired by the drug user; and (3) the *psychic phase* signals a maximum drug effect where disruption of thought processes, depersonalization, true hallucinations, and psychotic episodes may occur. For some users, experiencing the latter phase may be considered a "bad trip".

Pharmacokinetics of LSD

After oral administration, LSD is readily absorbed from the gastrointestinal tract and widely distributed throughout the body. The typical hallucinogenic dose ranges from 50 to 100 µg with less than 1 percent reaching the brain. Since it is assumed the psychoactive effects of LSD are due to actions in the brain, this makes its potency all the more impressive. The duration of action is about 12 h, with peak effects occurring 1 to 2 h after oral administration. The plasma half-life of LSD is approximately 3 h.

LSD is biotransformed in the liver by hydroxylation, with subsequent conjugation to glucuronide. Excretion is primarily through the biliary tract into the intestinal tract (80 to 90 percent), with the remainder eliminated by urinary excretion.

Pharmacological Effects of LSD

LSD is a very potent stimulant of the CNS; individuals may remain sleepless for many hours after ingesting it. The predominant somatic effect of LSD is sympathetic stimulation. This effect may be even more prominent with the phenylethylamine-derived hallucinogens. They include pupillary dilation, increases in heart rate and blood pressure, increased body temperature, piloerection, tremor, and hyperreflexia. Pupillary inequality (anisocoria) is common, as is hippus, a rhythmic dilation and contraction of the pupils, often synchronous with respiration. The pupillary effects and the hyperreflexia are inversely correlated with age, being greater in young adults and lesser in older subjects. Euphoria and/or excitement can be seen. There may also be nausea, weakness, and paresthesia.

Street LSD was believed to have the potential to cause both mutagenic and teratogenic effects. In the laboratory, the genetic toxicity of LSD is not a robust phenomenon. Reports of chromosomal damage and birth defects involving limb deformities and spina bifida have yet to be adequately investigated. Lethalities due directly to LSD overdose are believed to be rare.

Sensory and Subjective Effects of LSD

Along with the autonomic and other somatic effects described above, sensory distortions occur regularly. A sense of variation in lighting progresses to vivid visual illusions, pseudohallucinations, and, after sufficiently large doses, true hallucinations. Typically, the hallucinations are visual, in contrast to schizophrenia where the hallucinations are often auditory. Colors are reported to be heard and sounds seen. Often, moving objects seem to be followed by a stream of color. Bizarre paresthesia and distorted proprioception are frequent, ranging from formication to sensations of walking on a pebbly or hot surface.

Distortions in perceptions of size and distance and other spatial distortions are very common and are often associated with distortions of body image. Feelings of separation of part of the body, or loss of a part, or failure to recognize a part as one's own are also common. Depersonalization can also be seen.

LSD possesses a unique pharmacological property known as *flashback* which is seen in more than 15 percent of users. This phenomenon, which can occur at any time (months to years) after single or multiple exposures to LSD, is characterized by many of the sensory and subjective effects of LSD without readministration of the drug. Flashbacks often occur after the use of other psychoactive drugs, which may somehow trigger the flashback episode.

Tolerance and Physical Dependence

Tolerance develops rapidly to the behavioral effects of LSD, usually after 3 or 4 daily doses. It may be due to a down regulation of 5-HT receptors. Cross-tolerance exists between LSD and the other drugs of this group so that subsequent doses of one drug taken shortly after another drug will produce decreased effects. There is no cross-tolerance between LSD and anticholinergic drugs or marijuana. The tolerance is not accompanied by physical dependence, and abrupt discontinuance after chronic use does not precipitate withdrawal symptoms.

Treatment of Adverse Reactions

The most common adverse reaction to LSD is known as the "bad trip". It is characterized by a period of anxiety, hallucinations, and possibly psychotic behavior. Other signs and symptoms of LSD intoxication including elevated body temperature and blood pressure, tachycardia and hyperreflexia, may be present. The duration of a "bad trip" is usually less than 24 hours. LSD has a high therapeutic index, virtually no known cases of death have been directly caused by an overdose of LSD alone. Consequently, treatment is aimed at protecting the patient from accidental injury until drug effects subside. The individual should be placed in a quiet, non-threatening environment and given reassurance that everything will be all right. Benzodiazepine antianxiety agents can be used for their sedative effects. Antipsychotic drugs are pharmacologic antagonists of LSD, but may cause additional undesirable effects and are generally avoided. These drugs are indicated when individuals are uncontrollable. This approach to treatment is considered standard therapy for most hallucinogenic drug intoxication.

Other LSD-Type Hallucinogens

As discussed earlier in this chapter, there are several other drugs that are pharmacological similar to LSD and demonstrate cross-tolerance with it. Chemically they can be classified as indoleamines or phenylethylamines.

Indoleamine Derivatives Psilocybin and N,N-dimethyltryptamine (DMT) are obtained from natural sources. Psilocybin is found in a variety of *Psilocybe* mushroom species, which have been eaten ceremonially by primitive cultures for centuries. Psilocybin is converted to an active metabolite, psilocin, which is believed to be responsible for the majority of psychotomimetic effects. The hallucinogenic dose of psilocybin is approximately 25 mg, which produces effects lasting 3 to 6 h.

DMT occurs in many plants and has been used as a snuff by various Indian cultures. It is ineffective when taken orally and must be inhaled or administered parenterally. The usual hallucinogenic dose given by injection is 1 mg/kg of body weight, which produces psychotomimetic effects lasting approximately 1 h.

Phenylethylamine Derivatives Mescaline, 2,5-dimethoxy-4-methylamphetamine (DOM) and 3,4-methylenedioxymethamphetamine (MDMA) are phenylethylamine derivatives similar in structure to norepinephrine and amphetamine. CNS stimulation and sympathomimetic effects are prominent features of these drugs.

Mescaline, found in the peyote cactus, is among the least potent (4000 times less potent than LSD) of the hallucinogenic drugs. It is readily absorbed from the gastrointestinal tract and produces effects which last about 6 h.

DOM or STP (serenity, tranquility, peace) is a synthetic compound. The usual hallucinogenic dose is 3 to 5 mg, which produces effects lasting 6 to 8 h. A more recent addition to this group of drugs is MDMA or "ecstasy". It is referred to as a "designer drug" since it was initially synthesized to avoid regulation by the Controlled Substances Act. (Other designer drugs have appeared as phencyclidine and heroin substitutes.) It demonstrates both hallucinogenic and amphetamine like properties. There is experimental evidence demonstrating that both of these drugs are neurotoxic and damage serotonergic neurons. The chemical structures of mescaline, and DOM are compared to norepinephrine and amphetamine in Fig. 19-1.

ANTICHOLINERGIC PSYCHOTOMIMETIC DRUGS

The prototypes of this group are atropine and scopolamine. Their basic pharmacology is given in Chapter 11. At present, the most plausible explanation for the actions of these compounds is that, by blocking cholinergic muscarinic mechanisms in the brain, they allow predominance of other neurotransmitter systems, most likely adrenergic, dopaminergic, and serotonergic. They have been used ritually and situationally by certain tribes in the Americas and Australia. The anticholinergic drugs are not widely abused, and psychic effects can occur when these drugs are used therapeutically.

The peripheral effects of anticholinergic psychotomimetics resemble those of the parent compound atropine and include dilated pupils; dry, hot, flushed skin; dry mouth; and tachycardia. Blood pressure changes are those of postural

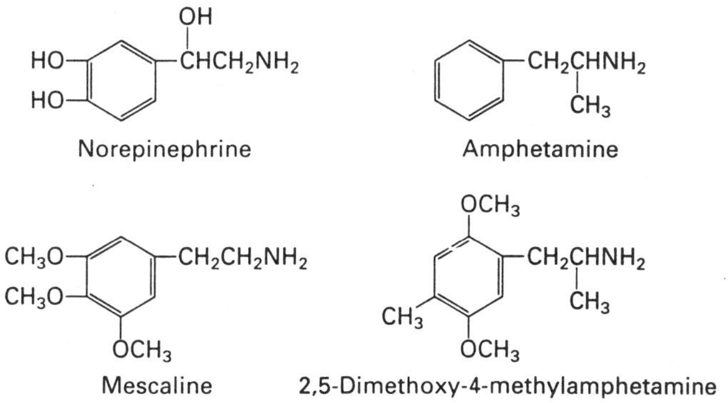

Norepinephrine Amphetamine

Mescaline 2,5-Dimethoxy-4-methylamphetamine

FIGURE 19-1 *Comparison of the chemical structures of norepinephrine, amphetamine, mescaline, and 2,5-dimethoxy-4-methylamphetamine (DOM).*

hypotension and are usually unimpressive except in severe toxicity when hypotension occurs because of ganglionic blockage.

The psychotomimetic effects are similar to those of a toxic psychosis. The most marked effects are delirium, mental confusion, and disorientation. Attention span is reduced along with loss of memory for recent events. Auditory and visual hallucinations can occur. Restlessness and hyperactivity may continue for many hours. In advanced toxicity, CNS depression, respiratory failure, cardiovascular collapse, and hyperpyrexia are contributing factors in fatalities due to these compounds. Treatment of anticholinergic poisoning includes: gastrointestinal tract decontamination via emesis, lavage, and saline cathartics; cardiopulmonary support; and administration of physostigmine, a reversible cholinesterase inhibitor with CNS activity.

MISCELLANEOUS DRUGS

Phencyclidine

Phencyclidine (PCP) was initially used as a general anesthetic in humans. However, because of the high incidence of emergence delirium, it was dropped from further consideration for this purpose. Ketamine, a PCP analog, is still used occasionally as a human anesthetic (see Chapter 15) and in veterinary practice to immobilize nonhuman primates. Because of its psychoactive properties, phencyclidine gained wide popularity as a drug of abuse. Initially it was used as a substitute for other hallucinogens or to "improve" low potency marijuana, but later was sold as a street drug in its own right. Street names for phencyclidine include Angel Dust, Elephant or Horse Tranquilizer, Hog, and Peace Pill.

Phencyclidine [N-(1-phenylcyclohexyl) piperidine] is a white, stable solid. It is a weak base and is readily soluble in water, alcohol, and lipids.

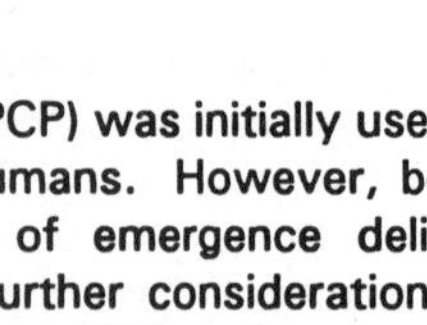

Mechanism of Action The pharmacology of phencyclidine is very complex. PCP produces multiple pharmacologic actions including CNS stimulation, CNS depression, peripheral autonomic effects, analgesia, and anticonvulsant activity. The psychoactive actions which occur at nonanesthetic doses is varied and the result of mixed CNS stimulant and depressant actions exerted at multiple brain sites. PCP interacts with several neurotransmitters including dopamine, norepinephrine, acetylcholine, 5-hydroxytryptamine, and the excitatory amino acids glutamate and aspartate. These interactions have been used to account for many of the actions of PCP. In addition, a specific receptor site has been identified which is believed to mediate many of the behavioral effects caused by PCP and PCP-like drugs.

PCP, more than any other drug, appears to produce psychic disturbances that closely mimic those of schizophrenia. Since antipsychotic drugs affect dopamine activity, an interaction between PCP and dopamine was suggested to explain the psychotomimetic effects of PCP. Some of the effects of PCP such as increased motor activity, suppression of appetite, stereotyped behavior, and suppression of prolactin secretion are common to dopamine agonists, like the amphetamines. Antipsychotic drugs, which block dopamine receptors, have been shown to antagonize the dopamine-related actions which both PCP and amphetamine produce. This indicates that some of the effects of PCP are mediated by a dopaminergic action. Additionally, PCP has been demonstrated to block the reuptake of dopamine and possibly enhance its release.

Structure-activity relationships among PCP and several PCP-like drugs (e.g., ketamine) and the ability of various animal species to discriminate between these drugs has contributed to the hypothesis that a specific receptor may mediate some aspects of the behavioral actions of PCP. These drugs block a cation channel that is regulated by one type of excitatory amino acid receptor known as the N-methyl-D-aspartate (NMDA) receptor (see Chapter 3). Further research will be needed to elucidate the role of this receptor in the actions of PCP. PCP also binds to the sigma (σ) opioid site, the function of which is unclear (see Chapter 23).

Pharmacokinetics PCP is active when administered by most routes including inhalation (smoking), oral, insufflation (snorting), and injection. It is lipid-soluble and widely distributed to peripheral tissues where it accumulates and persists in fat. PCP is also secreted into gastric acid and then reabsorbed in the intestine. This recycling, combined with the persistence of PCP in fat tissue, contributes to a prolonged half-life (48 to 72 h) and protracted systemic effects, particularly after an overdose. PCP is readily metabolized by the liver to various hydroxylated derivatives, which are then conjugated with glucuronic acid and excreted in the urine.

Pharmacologic Effects The effects of PCP are dose related. At low doses there is CNS stimulation, euphoria, and sympathetic stimulation similar to the effects produced by amphetamines. PCP is one of the few hallucinogenic drugs to be self-administered by nonhuman primates, which may be due to its stimulant effect. With increasing dosage, thought processes become disoriented and speech is slurred. This is followed by paresthesia, slowed reflexes, and ataxia. This state may last 4 to 6 hours; longer with an overdose where it may take days before the affected individual returns to normal. Violent and suicidal behavior has been associated with PCP use. In acute toxicity, the individual will exhibit marked anxiety, agitation, hallucinations, and increased body temperature. This may progress to dysphoria, catatonia, muscle rigidity, convulsions, nystagmus, hypertensive crisis, coma, and death.

Treatment of Intoxication Initial treatment of adverse reactions should include placing the patient in a quiet environment and minimizing sensory stimulation. At present, there is no specific antagonist for this class of drugs; therefore, overdoses must be treated symptomatically when necessary. α-Adrenergic receptor blockers may be used to treat hypertension and sedative agents may be appropriate. If an antipsychotic agent is deemed necessary, a drug with low anticholinergic activity such as haloperidol should be used. Acidification of the urine to pH 5.5 with ammonium chloride will increase elimination of PCP from the body. Continuous gastric suction also will increase elimination of PCP by interfering with intestinal reabsorption after gastric secretion since PCP has anticholinergic activity and can delay gastric emptying. Seizures can be treated with phenytoin or diazepam.

Chronic use of PCP can give also give rise to a psychotic syndrome that is different from that seen with other hallucinogens. It can occur long after withdrawal from the drug and may last for several weeks. This psychosis can be mistaken for schizophrenia, particularly if a drug history is not available.

Tolerance and Dependence Tolerance develops fairly rapidly to the behavioral and toxic effects of PCP during chronic use. PCP has been demonstrated to be a positive reinforcer of behavior in some animal species. This suggests the development of some degree of dependency. The drug dependence appears to be predominantly psychological rather than physical. Withdrawal symptoms, when present, include a craving for the drug, increased anxiety and mental depression.

Psychomotor Stimulants

Amphetamine and cocaine are potent CNS stimulants which are widely abused. At higher doses these drugs produce psychotic symptoms. The basic pharmacology of amphetamines and cocaine related to their therapeutic uses is given in Chapters 8 and 25, respectively, and only the stimulant and psychotomimetic properties will be presented here. The central actions of these drugs are very similar, and many experienced drug users have difficulty discriminating between them following intravenous administration.

Mechanism of Action The psychoactive properties of amphetamine and cocaine are due to an action within the brain. Both drugs increase the amounts of norepinephrine (NE) and dopamine (DA) that are available for stimulation of adrenergic and dopaminergic receptors. Amphetamine enhances the release of NE and DA from presynaptic nerve terminals and, in addition, blocks the neuronal reuptake of both neurotransmitters. It also can act as a direct adrenergic receptor agonist. The stimulant actions of cocaine are related to its ability to block the neuronal reuptake of NE and DA. There is also evidence that both drugs affect the levels of 5-hydroxytryptamine. The increased levels of NE produce prominent peripheral and central sympathomimetic effects and mediate some behavioral actions. The higher levels of DA influence behavioral activity, particularly that involving the limbic system. This enhancement of dopaminergic neurotransmission accounts for the ability of these drugs to act as potent reinforcers of behavior. In animal studies, this is defined by the rapidity of acquisition of self-administration. Cocaine has been shown to be one of the most potent drug reinforcers of behavior yet studied. Supporting this action on DA is the finding that dopamine receptor antagonists will eliminate the reinforcing properties of both amphetamine and cocaine. The dopamine pathway involved has its cell bodies in the ventral tegmental area and nerve terminals in the limbic forebrain.

Amphetamines

A number of drugs are referred to as the "amphetamines." This includes amphetamine itself (racemic form), dextroamphetamine (dextrorotatory isomer of amphetamine), methamphetamine, and a few related drugs. Other agents such as methylphenidate, phenmetrazine, and most recently methcathinone ("cat") have a similar behavioral pharmacology, varying only in potency. There may be slight differences in their actions at a cellular level. The amphetamines are basically sympathomimetic amines with chemical structures very similar to NE and DA. They are lipophilic compounds that are weak bases.

Pharmacokinetics The amphetamines are well absorbed orally, readily pass into the brain, and produce effects lasting several hours. Intravenous injection of amphetamines, especially methamphetamine ("speed"), was a significant problem in the past. Large amounts were often injected repeatedly over several days. It is during these sustained high-dosage bouts that the psychotomimetic effects of the drug frequently occur.

Biotransformation of the amphetamines occurs in the liver with formation of several metabolites; some of which are active and produce pharmacologic actions similar to the parent compounds. One of these is parahydroxyamphetamine, which is subsequently converted to another active metabolite, parahydroxynorephedrine. Following deamination and conjugation, the metabolites are excreted primarily in the urine along with 20 to 40 percent of the unmetabolized parent compound.

Pharmacologic Effects The amphetamines have central stimulant and peripheral sympathomimetic activity. After oral administration, people feel more confident, alert, talkative, and generally show an increased activity level. Amphetamines increase endurance and reduce feelings of fatigue. They also have an anorexic (decreased appetite) effect. Following intravenous administration, the user often experiences an initial "rush" which has been described as orgasm-like. The euphoria and excitement produced by amphetamines are important for their reinforcing properties. This causes the user to repeat the drug again and again in order to maintain the good feelings, "the reward."

Initially, amphetamine may produce an increase in performance, particularly on less complex tasks, but eventually performance deteriorates. Activity may continue for hours but may also become compulsive and highly stereotyped. The user gets "hung up" doing one thing over and over again. As amphetamine usage increases and the dosages become larger, the psychotomimetic effects become apparent and can lead to psychotic behavior.

The amphetamine psychosis is paranoid in character and similar to paranoid schizophrenia. Although the users may feel elated, they appear glum, depressed, and withdrawn. Suspicion, hostility, and aggressive behavior may lead to violent acts. Sensory illusions and tactile, auditory and visual hallucinations may occur. The psychosis can occur after only a few very high doses but usually occurs after chronic use of high doses.

After discontinuance of the drug, profound sleep usually occurs. Upon awakening, the user experiences disagreeable depressed feelings ("crash") and wants to resume drug taking.

Tolerance and Dependence Tolerance to the amphetamines, especially after prolonged intravenous use, develops rapidly, and larger amounts are usually administered with continuous use. The peripheral sympathomimetic effects show greater tolerance than the central effects. Tolerance does develop to some of the central effects such as the euphoria and appetite suppression. Other CNS effects, however, do not appear to develop tolerance and may demonstrate sensitization (reverse tolerance). The development of tolerance to amphetamines is not completely understood.

Abrupt discontinuance of amphetamines after chronic use results in only mild physical withdrawal symptoms. Withdrawal effects appear to be predominantly psychological in nature and include extreme fatigue, mental depression, and a strong desire for the drug.

Intoxication and Treatment There are a number of adverse effects and potential complications caused by overstimulation of the sympathetic and central nervous systems. The psychotomimetic effects and the paranoid behavior have already been described. Sympathetic stimulation produces hyperthermia and profuse sweating, respiratory difficulties, tremors, and various cardiovascular effects. Intense cardiovascular stimulation results in tachycardia, arrhythmias, and hypertension. After prolonged intravenous use, severe fatigue and exhaustion may be followed by convulsions, coma, and death. Chronic intoxication can produce all of these effects, and, in addition, there may be extreme weight loss due to the anorexic effect of these drugs.

Treatment of amphetamine intoxication is aimed at supporting vital functions and providing symptomatic therapy. Acidification of the urine increases excretion since amphetamine is a weak base. Adrenergic blockers and vasodilators can be administered to control excessive sympathetic and cardiovascular stimulation. Highly agitated individuals can be given antipsychotic drugs, which reduce psychotic symptoms by antagonizing the actions of DA and NE.

Cocaine

Cocaine is extracted from the leaves of *Erythroxylon coca* which is found primarily in South America. Native Indians of South America have chewed coca leaves for centuries to ward off fatigue and hunger. In the late nineteenth century, cocaine was considered a "wonder drug" and advocated for numerous medical conditions, including the treatment of morphine and alcohol addiction. After recognizing the potential dangers of cocaine abuse, the government enacted legislation in 1914, which restricted and controlled the use of cocaine. Cocaine was "rediscovered" in the 1970s as the phenomenon of recreational drug use dramatically increased. Presently, cocaine is considered the "illicit drug of choice," and widespread abuse has generated major social and medical problems.

The pharmacologic effects of cocaine are similar to those of the amphetamines. However, cocaine possesses a number of features which make it more popular with drug users. Cocaine is prepared in different forms, which can be administered by a variety of methods. The intensity and duration of drug effects are highly dependent on the preparation used and the route of administration. The structure of cocaine is shown below.

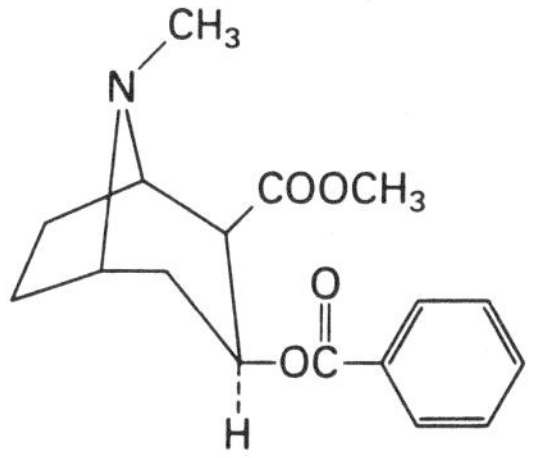

Preparations Cocaine base (benzoylmethylecgonine) is extracted from coca leaves and converted to the water-soluble hydrochloride salt. It is in this form that cocaine is exported and adulterated with other substances such as sugars and local anesthetics. Cocaine hydrochloride can be administered orally, intranasally, and intravenously. It is, however, destroyed by the high temperatures generated during smoking. Several methods exist for conversion of cocaine hydrochloride back into the free-base form. Free-base cocaine possesses greater lipid solubility and can be volatilized at a lower temperature than the hydrochloride salt. Consequently, it can be smoked, which allows for very rapid delivery of cocaine to the brain. The intensity of effect is greatly increased. One form of free-base cocaine, "crack", is prepared by an alkalinization-water process, which forms a crystalline rocklike substance that makes a cracking sound when it is smoked.

Pharmacokinetics Cocaine is absorbed from all mucous membranes including the intestinal tract. Pharmacologic effects are delayed (30 to 60 min) and less intense after oral administration compared to other routes. Drug effects are detectable 3 to 5 min after intranasal administration, peak in 20 to 30 min, and last 60 to 90 min. Intravenous injection and smoking both provide immediate effects of high intensity, but of shorter duration. Peak effects by these routes occur in minutes and last about 20 min. Smoking cocaine is the most popular route of administration. It is more convenient than making injections, and there is less nasal irritation and septal perforation than when cocaine is used intranasally.

The plasma half-life of cocaine is approximately 40 to 60 min; however, there is considerable variability. Cocaine is metabolized primarily by serum and liver cholinesterases. Serum cholinesterase or pseudocholinesterase is genetically influenced, and variations in enzyme activity may account for individual sensitivities to cocaine. The major metabolites which are excreted in the urine are benzoylecgonine and ecgonine methyl ester, which can be further metabolized to ecgonine, benzoic acid, and methanol. Demethylation also occurs in the liver, and one metabolite, norcocaine, possesses some ability to inhibit reuptake mechanisms. The persistence of these metabolites in the plasma and urine is much greater than that of the parent compound.

Cocaine has also been detected in parotid saliva and hair along with its major metabolite, benzoylecgonine. If taken with ethanol, cocaine is converted to cocaethylene by the liver. This compound has been detected and quantified in plasma, parotid saliva, and hair, and represents the presence of ethanol and cocaine in an individual.

Most urine tests screening for cocaine use look for the presence of benzoylecgonine, which can be detected for a day or more after drug use.

Pharmacological Effects The mechanism of action of cocaine for its central pharmacological effects is related to its ability to block the reuptake of norepinephrine and dopamine into nerve terminals. In the CNS, cocaine is a powerful stimulant, producing marked euphoria, self-confidence, and heightened feelings of physical and mental ability. These effects can lead to delusions of grandeur, which have been referred to as "cocainomania". These positive psychological effects can be followed by dysphoria, anxiety, and feelings of depression as the drug effect wears off, which are sometimes called "cocaine blues". This creates a desire in the user to repeat the drug again, which often leads to prolonged binges where cocaine use becomes compulsive. This is similar to the situation which develops with amphetamines. However, the duration of action after smoking or injecting cocaine is only 20 to 30 min, compared to several hours for amphetamines. Consequently, cocaine must be administered much more frequently in order to maintain the "good feelings".

As doses of cocaine are increased, CNS stimulation becomes excessive. Tremors and myoclonic jerks develop and may progress to tonic-clonic convulsions. Peripheral sympathomimetic effects increase, and cardiovascular stimulation resulting in hypertension, tachycardia, and arrhythmias may occasionally result in sudden death. A toxic psychosis, similar to that caused by amphetamines, can develop after high doses or prolonged use. Symptoms include hostility, social withdrawal, paranoid ideation, hallucinations, delusions, and violent behavior.

Tolerance and Dependence The question of tolerance to cocaine is not entirely clear. Acute tolerance does develop to sympathomimetic and psychological effects when cocaine is used frequently within short periods of time. The tolerance does not appear to involve any changes in metabolism or distributional disposition. Users often purposefully increase dosage in an attempt to supersede the "high" of the previous dose. There is also evidence that reverse tolerance or "kindling" may develop to some of the effects of cocaine after chronic use.

Before widespread abuse in the 1970s, cocaine was considered a relatively safe drug which did not cause physical dependency. However, with the technique of free-basing where higher doses are administered frequently on a daily basis, the evidence suggests that cocaine does produce some degree of physical dependence. The symptoms of withdrawal from cocaine include a craving for the drug, dysphoria, irritability, anxiety, depression, tremors, and eating and sleeping disturbances.

Intoxication and Treatment Depending on the dosage and time since administration, the user may be euphoric and excited or dysphoric, anxious, and depressed. After prolonged binges of cocaine use, extreme fatigue, exhaustion, hyperthermia, seizures, and coma may occur. The most serious effects of acute cocaine poisoning are on the CNS and cardiovascular system, leading to convulsions and cardiac complications. Tachycardia and arrhythmias may precipitate ventricular fibrillation and sudden death. CNS stimulation is followed by severe depression resulting in respiratory failure and cardiovascular collapse. Individuals with underlying cardiovascular disease are at greater risk of complication and sudden death. The psychotic reactions which usually occur after prolonged use are similar to those observed with amphetamines.

Treatment of cocaine intoxication is similar to that of amphetamine poisoning, supportive and symptomatic. Diazepam is useful to control seizures and for sedation. Since the half-life of cocaine is short, the greatest danger in acute intoxication occurs within the first few hours. Antipsychotic drugs, such as chlorpromazine and haloperidol, are useful because of their multiple effects to antagonize DA and NE.

Treatment of cocaine dependence usually involves education of the individual to the dangers of continued use and behavioral modification to control impulsive desires for the drug. A newer approach to the treatment of cocaine dependence is the use of drugs to control the craving for it and to replenish dopamine that it may deplete. Drugs used include tricyclic antidepressants such as desipramine. Treatment with desipramine has been reported to lessen the euphoric effects of cocaine and reduce cravings for continued use of the drug. Other drugs including the agonist-antagonist opioids and anticonvulsant agents are also being tested.

Marijuana

Marijuana comes from the hemp plant, *Cannabis saliva*. The marijuana plant is dioecious; the flowering tops of the female plant are particularly rich in a sticky resin in which the active psychotropic principle, Δ^9-tetrahydrocannabinol (THC) is found in highest concentrations. The resin can be extracted from the plant and is known as *hashish*. Marijuana generally refers to the dried, chopped plant (seeds, flowers, twigs, leaves) which is usually smoked. The psychoactive and medicinal effects of the marijuana plant have been known for many centuries and in many cultures. This is reflected in the many names given to different preparations by different countries: Bhang (India), Ganja (Jamaica), Kif (North Africa), Kabak (Turkey), and Grass or Pot (United States).

Various preparations from the marijuana plant have been tried medicinally over the centuries for anesthesia, analgesia, hypnosis, bronchodilation, and antiemetic effects. Tinctures and extracts of cannabis were used officially in the United States until 1937, when the Marijuana Tax Act eliminated further widespread use. Marijuana has the distinction of being the most frequently used illicit drug, having been used at least once by well over 60 million Americans.

Chemistry The pharmacologically active substances in marijuana are nitrogen-free tricyclic compounds referred to as *cannabinoids*. Two systems of nomenclature are used to describe these compounds: the formal or dibenzopyran system and the monoterpene system. The dibenzopyran system is used in this chapter. Cannabinoids of major interest that are found naturally in the marijuana plant are shown in Fig. 19-2. The major active cannabinoid present in the plant is (-)-Δ^9-*trans*-tetrahydrocannabinol (Δ^9THC), hereafter referred to as THC. Another isomer, Δ^8THC, is similar in potency to THC but is found in very small quantities in fresh plant material. Cannabinol possesses less than one tenth the potency of THC, while cannabidiol, a THC precursor in the plant, is devoid of marijuana-like behavioral activity. It may have other pharmacological properties of potential clinical interest.

Marijuana typically contains between 1 and 4 percent THC. The resin, hashish, usually contains about 10 percent of THC. It should be noted that there are hundreds of chemical compounds in the marijuana plant, with more than 60 that are unique to the plant and referred to as cannabinoids. During the pyrolysis of smoking, many chemical conversions occur, including conversion of the inactive monocarboxylic acid of THC to the active THC. Also, about 30 percent of THC is estimated to be destroyed during the smoking process. Thus the pharmacology of THC may not be identical to that of smoking marijuana.

Pharmacokinetics The cannabinoids are highly lipid-soluble compounds. The most common route of administration of marijuana is smoking, which provides bioavailability of 10 to 25 percent, depending on the efficiency of smoking technique. Effects after smoking begin within 5 to 15 min, peak in 30 to 90 min, and generally last 3 to 4 h. Bioavailability after oral administration averages only 6 percent. Effects begin within 30 to 60 min, peak in 1 to 2 h, and last about 4 to 6 h.

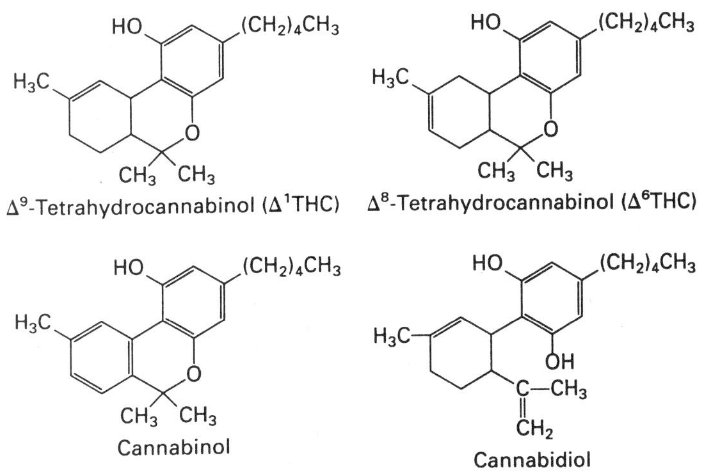

Δ^9-Tetrahydrocannabinol (Δ^1THC)

Δ^8-Tetrahydrocannabinol (Δ^6THC)

Cannabinol

Cannabidiol

FIGURE 19-2 *Natural cannabinoids of Cannabis sativa. The monoterpene numbering system is shown in parentheses for Δ^9THC and Δ^8THC.*

THC is widely distributed throughout the body; however, the initial volume of distribution is small because of high plasma protein binding (97 to 99 percent). With continued use, the volume of distribution increases as the highly lipid-soluble THC is taken up by peripheral body compartments and sequestered in adipose tissue. The initial plasma level of THC decreases rapidly after absorption as distribution to peripheral tissues occurs.

Biotransformation of THC occurs predominantly in the liver by the microsomal enzyme system. Metabolic degradation is complex, with approximately 80 different metabolites already identified. The primary metabolite of THC is 11-hydroxy-Δ^9THC (11-OH-Δ^9THC), which is active and at least as potent as THC. This compound is subsequently biotransformed to a number of inactive metabolites, which are then excreted. Figure 19-3 shows the principal THC metabolites.

Approximately 60 to 70 percent of THC metabolites are slowly eliminated, via the bile, into the feces with the remainder excreted in the urine. THC is readily metabolized when it is in the plasma. However, rapid redistribution from the plasma to peripheral tissue compartments removes approximately 70 percent of the THC administered. Because of its high lipid solubility, THC is released slowly back to the plasma, biotransformed by the liver, and excreted in the feces and urine. After 72 h, approximately 50 percent of an original dose is still present in the tissues and organs. The elimination half-life of THC ranges from 20 to 36 h, and THC can persist to some extent in adipose tissue for 2 weeks or more, particularly after heavy use.

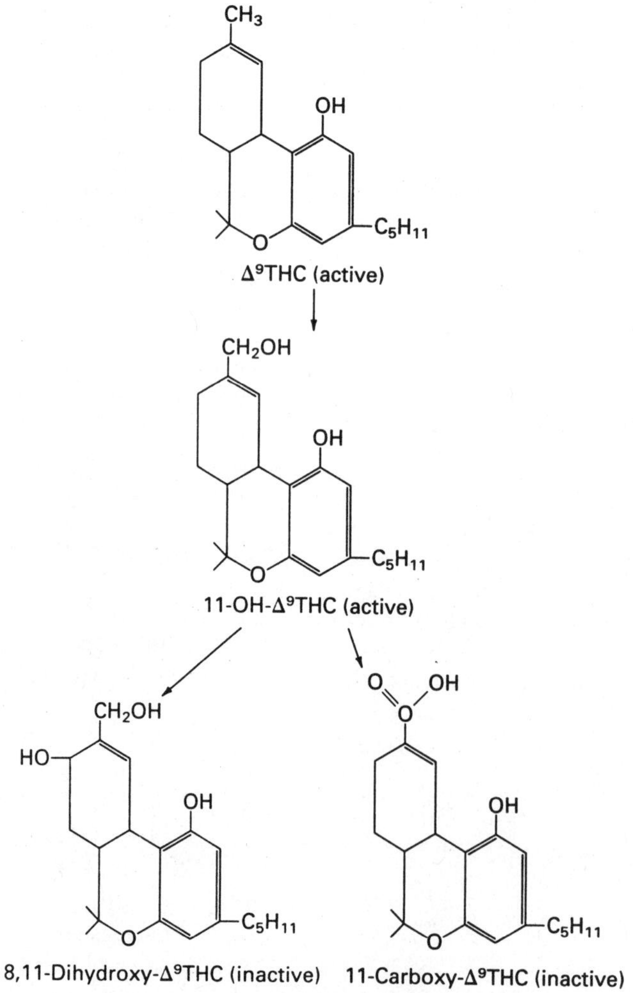

CH_3 OH C_5H_{11} O

Δ^9THC (active)

CH_2OH OH C_5H_{11} O

11-OH-Δ^9THC (active)

CH_2OH HO OH C_5H_{11} O

8,11-Dihydroxy-Δ^9THC (inactive)

O OH O OH C_5H_{11} O

11-Carboxy-Δ^9THC (inactive)

FIGURE 19-3 *Principal metabolites of Δ^9THC.*

There is significant medical and legal interest in the detection of marijuana use through the measurement of Δ^9THC or its metabolites in blood and urine. The most common method is identification of the urinary metabolites of THC. One of the metabolites frequently measured is 11-nor-Δ9THC carboxylic acid. THC metabolites can be identified in the urine and feces for more than a week.

Mechanism of Action Tremendous gains have been made in our understandings of the mechanism of action of the cannabinoids in recent years. A cannabinoid receptor has been identified. A cDNA that codes for a cannabinoid receptor has also been isolated and its expression studied. The receptor has a unique distribution in the brain and is negatively coupled to adenylate cyclase. Recently, an endogenous ligand for the receptor, anadamide, which is related to arachidonic acid, has been discovered.

Pharmacologic Effects *Acute Effects* Conjunctival reddening and increases in heart rate have been the most consistently reported effects of marijuana in humans. Heart rate increases of 20 to 50 beats per minute may occur and are dose-related. After smoking marijuana, there is usually physical and mental relaxation, feelings of euphoria, and increased sociability. There is often a sense that time is passing slowly. With moderate intoxication, there is drowsiness and lapses of attention. Impairment of short-term memory is very common. Perceptual motor skills such as those involved in driving are also impaired. At high levels of intoxication, reflexes are slowed, muscle coordination decreases, ataxia is evident, and speech and the ability to concentrate become more difficult. Performance of a variety of tasks deteriorates. The more complex the task, the greater the degree of disruption produced. Dream-like states with alterations of auditory and visual perceptions can also be produced. Acutely, the primary psychiatric symptom seen is panic and anxiety attacks. There is occasionally a transient paranoia. Anecdotal evidence suggests that marijuana use may exacerbate or unmask schizophrenia that is in remission or latent.

Chronic Effects Chronic use of marijuana in the young has frequently been related to the development of an "amotivational syndrome". This is a highly controversial issue. Many studies have concluded that the lack of interest and motivation demonstrated by many heavy users of marijuana was present before drug use and the effect on motivation is not a specific effect of marijuana. At low doses, marijuana produces a slight bronchodilatation. However, marijuana smoke contains higher concentrations of tar and some carcinogens than tobacco smoke. Chronic use can produce hoarseness, cough, and bronchitis.

Marijuana alters the plasma levels of some reproductive hormones. In males, lower testosterone levels decrease the sperm count and motility. In females, levels of luteinizing hormone and prolactin are suppressed resulting in sporadic ovulation and irregular menstrual cycles. THC readily crosses the placenta, and teratogenic effects have been demonstrated in animal studies. Specific birth defects have not been observed in humans. Marijuana appears to have some teratogenic potential, and use during pregnancy should be strongly discouraged. Experimental studies have shown marijuana to cause a mild, transitory immunosuppressant effect. The clinical significance of this effect has not been determined.

Tolerance and Dependence Tolerance to marijuana, i.e., diminished response to a given dose when repeated, has been demonstrated. However, the development of tolerance usually occurs only in the laboratory after use of high doses of marijuana or THC. The tolerance is variable and develops to a greater degree for some effects such as tachycardia, CNS depression, and euphoria. Tolerance is rapidly reversed after cessation of marijuana use. Cross-tolerance with other psychoactive drugs has not been demonstrated.

Abrupt cessation of marijuana after prolonged use has been associated with the development of some dependency. The dependence appears to be more psychological than physical and of considerably less intensity than observed with cocaine and amphetamines.

Intoxication and Treatment The most common intoxication reaction requiring treatment is the acute panic-anxiety reaction where the users appear to lose control and feel great anxiety. This reaction occurs most frequently with inexperienced users who are unfamiliar with the effects of marijuana. The effects rarely last more than a few hours. Very high doses have been reported to occasionally produce a diffuse acute brain syndrome which includes such symptoms as clouding of consciousness and disorders of memory, perception and sleep.

Therapeutic Uses THC is currently used as an antiemetic for cancer patients who are receiving chemotherapy. Dronabinol is the generic name for THC for use in cancer patients. The compound is used by the oral route. Other properties of THC including analgesia, bronchodilation, and anticonvulsant effects have also been investigated.

BIBLIOGRAPHY

Agurell, S., M. Halldin, J.E. Lindgren, A. Ohlsson, M. Widman, H. Gillespie, and L. Hollister: "Pharmacokinetics and Metabolism of Δ^9-Tetrahydrocannabinol and Other Cannabinoids with Emphasis on Man," *Pharm. Rev.* **38**: 21-43 (1986).

Anderson, P.O., and G.G. McGuire: "Delta-9-Tetrahydrocannabinol as an Antiemetic," *Am. J. Hosp. Pharm.* **38**: 639-646 (1981).

Barbieri, E.J., G.J. DiGregorio, A.P. Ferko, and E. K. Ruch: Rat Cocaethylene and Benzoylecgonine Concentrations in Plasma and Parotid Saliva after the Administration of Cocaethylene," *J. Anal. Toxicol.* **18**: 60-61 (1994).

Brawley, P., and J.C. Duffield: "The Pharmacology of Hallucinogens," *Pharm. Rev.* **24**: 31-66 (1972).

Clonet, D.H. (ed.): "Phencyclidine: An Update," *Research Monograph 64, NIDA*, Washington, D.C., 1986, pp. 1-260.

Cohle, S.D., and J.T. Lie: "Dissection of the Aorta and Coronary Arteries Associated with Acute Cocaine Intoxication," *Arch. Pathol. Lab. Med.* **116**: 1239-1242 (1992).

Cone, E.J., D. Yousefnejad, W.D. Darwin, and T. Maguire: "Testing Human Hair for Drugs of Abuse. II. Identification of Unique Cocaine Metabolites in Hair of Drug Abusers and Evaluation of Decontamination Procedures," *J. Anal. Toxicol.* **15**: 250-255 (1991).

DiGregorio, G.J., E.J. Barbieri, A.P. Ferko, and E.K. Ruch: "Prevalence of Cocaethylene in the Hair of Pregnant Women," *J. Anal. Toxicol.* **17**: 445 (1993).

Ferko, A.P., E.J. Barbieri, G.J. DiGregorio, and E.K. Ruch: "The Presence of Cocaine and Benzoylecgonine in Rat Parotid Saliva, Plasma, and Urine after Intravenous Administration of Cocaine," *Res. Commun. Substance Abuse* **11**: 11-25 (1990).

Grabowski, J. (ed.): "Cocaine: Pharmacology, Effects and Treatment of Abuse," *Research Monograph 50, NIDA*, Washington, D.C., 1984, pp. 1-9.

Hollister, L.E.: "Health Aspects of Cannabis," *Pharm. Rev.* **38**: 1-20 (1986).

Jacobs, B.L.: "How Hallucinogenic Drugs Work," *Am. Sci.* **75**: 386 (1987).

Meltzer, H.Y. (ed.): *Psychopharmacology: The Third Generation of Progress*, Raven Press, New York, 1987.

Pertwee, R.G.: "The Central Neuropharmacology of Psychotropic Cannabinoids," *Pharmac. Ther.* **36**: 189-261 (1988).

Ray, O. (ed.): *Drugs, Society and Human Behavior*, Mosby, St. Louis, 1978.

Schultes, R.E., and A. Hofmann: *The Botany and Chemistry of Hallucinogens*, Charles C. Thomas, Springfield, 1980.

CHAPTER 20

Antipsychotic Drugs and Lithium

Martin D. Schechter

Antipsychotic drugs are used to treat psychosis, i.e., abnormalities of mental function. The pharmacological terms used to describe this class of drugs include: ataractics, neuroleptics, neuroplegics and major tranquilizers. This latter term is perhaps the poorest choice as it may connote a continuum of effect from minor tranquilizers which, in fact, does not exist. Thus, minor tranquilizers are specifically used as anxiolytics and are ineffective in the treatment of psychosis, whereas antipsychotics are not generally used for the treatment of anxiety. As a class, antipsychotic drugs produce emotional calmness and mental relaxation and are, therefore, highly effective in controlling the symptoms of acutely and chronically disturbed patients. Many of these drugs are also used in the treatment of conditions other than psychoses, including the control of nausea, emesis, hiccoughs, itching, and potentiation of the action of other drugs. In Europe, these drugs are called *neuroleptics* because they have diffuse activities throughout the central nervous system (CNS), including suppression of spontaneous movement and complex behavior.

CLASSIFICATION

The antipsychotic drugs are subdivided into groups based on their chemical structure: phenothiazines, butyrophenones, thioxanthenes, dihydroindolones, dibenzoxazepines, dibenzodiazepines, diphenylbutylpiperidines, and benzisoxazoles.

PHENOTHIAZINE DERIVATIVES

The phenothiazines are historically and currently of the greatest importance and, as a group, have a complex pharmacology with effects on both central and peripheral nervous systems, in addition to important metabolic and endocrine effects. Each compound differs quantitatively and qualitatively in the extent to which it produces each of these pharmacologic effects. With few exceptions, all of them act on the CNS to produce (1) mild sedation; (2) antiemetic effects, (3) alteration of temperature regulation, which may result in either hypothermia or hyperthermia, depending on environmental temperature; (4) alteration of skeletal muscle tone; (5) endocrine alterations; and (6) potentiation of analgesics. They can also act on the autonomic nervous system to produce (1) α-adrenergic receptor blockade, (2) inhibition of biogenic amine uptake and adrenergic potentiation, and (3) cholinergic blocking effects at both nicotinic and muscarinic receptor sites. They also block serotonin and histamine receptors.

Chemistry

The basic chemical structure of the phenothiazines consists of three rings in which two benzene rings are linked by a sulfur and a nitrogen as illustrated in Table 20-1. It is the substitutions on the nitrogen at position 10 (R_1) that yields the subclasses of phenothiazines that may be divided into aliphatic (straight-chain), piperazine, and piperidine derivatives, with members of each subclass having distinct pharmacological properties. Substitutions at the carbon in position 2 (R_2) tend to render the rings more asymmetrical enhancing lipid solubility and, thus, increasing potency.

Sites and Mechanism of Action

The specific etiology of psychotic disorders is presently unknown. However, an imbalance of

TABLE 20-1 Some therapeutically useful phenothiazine derivatives

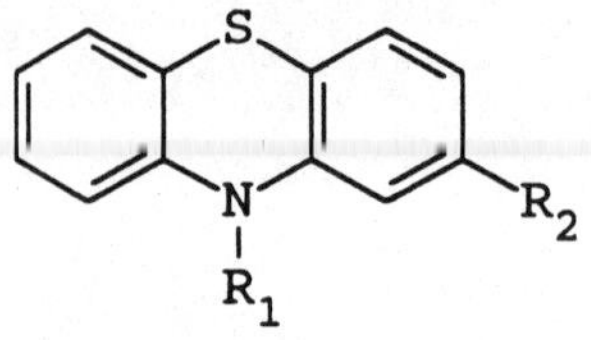

(Phenothiazine nucleus: ring N bears R_1; position 2 bears R_2)

Subgroups and drugs	R_1	R_2
Aliphatics		
Promazine	$CH_2CH_2CH_2N(CH_3)_2$	H
Chlorpromazine	$CH_2CH_2CH_2N(CH_3)_2$	Cl
Triflupromazine	$CH_2CH_2CH_2N(CH_3)_2$	CF_3
Promethazine	$CH_2CH(CH_3)N(CH_3)_2$	H
Piperazines		
Prochlorperazine	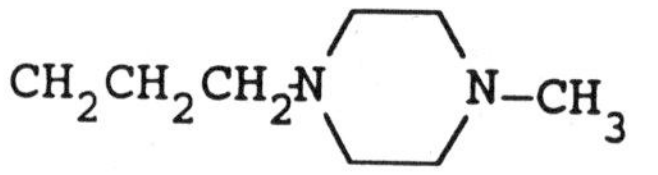 $CH_2CH_2CH_2N$(piperazine)$N-CH_3$	Cl
Trifluoperazine	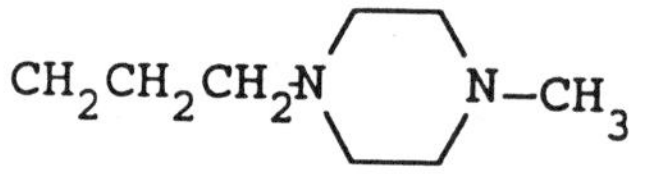 $CH_2CH_2CH_2N$(piperazine)$N-CH_3$	CF_3
Fluphenazine	$CH_2CH_2CH_2N$(piperazine)$N-CH_2CH_2OH$	CF_3
Piperidines		
Thioridazine	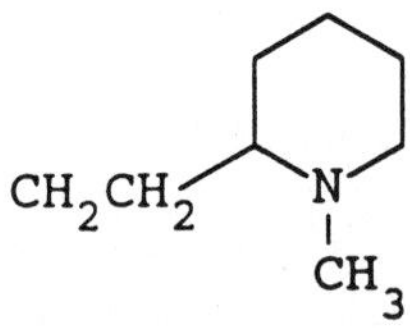 CH_2CH_2-(2-piperidyl, $N-CH_3$)	SCH_3

dopaminergic function in the central nervous system has been suspected as one of the primary causes of psychotic behavior. Most investigators believe that increased dopaminergic activity in specific areas of the CNS, e.g., the limbic system, is responsible for this abnormal behavior pattern. The site of antipsychotic activity for phenothiazines is the mesolimbic and hippocampal areas of the CNS. These compounds appear to block the activity of dopamine on dopaminergic receptor sites, thus decreasing psychotic activity.

The central dopamine receptors may be divided into D_1 and D_2 receptors. Both receptors have a high affinity for dopamine but differ in their sensitivity to antipsychotic drugs. The D_1 receptor site is excitatory and activates the adenylate cyclase system. The D_2 receptor is also related to the adenylate cyclase system and may be inhibitory in some brain tissues. Phenothiazines are nonselective, competitive D_1, and D_2 antagonists. Butyrophenone antipsychotics, such as haloperidol, are known to selectively antagonize D_2 receptors. This suggests that the antipsychotic activity of these drugs is primarily related to the blockade of the D_2 receptors.

The blockade of dopamine receptors is also responsible for at least some of the adverse effects of these drugs. For example, by blocking the action of dopamine in the nigrostriatal pathway, these compounds cause a parkinsonism-like syndrome. Blockade of other dopamine receptors in the tuberoinfundibular dopamine pathway by these drugs releases prolactin, resulting in hyperprolactinemia.

The antipsychotic drugs also possess antiserotonergic, antihistaminic, and α-adrenergic blocking activities. Some researchers believe that these activities also contribute to the therapeutic effectiveness of these drugs. For example, the antihistaminic effect may be related to the sedative activity of these drugs. The α-adrenergic blocking activity may be related to the decrease in CNS stimulation as well as the cause for the orthostatic hypotension. Still it remains to be established whether any of the non-dopaminergic mechanisms play a major role in the antipsychotic activity of the phenothiazines.

Effects on Organ Systems

Central Nervous System The administration of chlorpromazine and related phenothiazines produces depression of CNS activity. The aliphatic phenothiazines and the piperidines tend to be more sedative than the piperazine derivatives (Table 20-2). Depression resulting in anesthesia, however, is seldom produced even with large doses. After receiving large doses of phenothiazines, psychotic patients appear less severely disturbed and have fewer hallucinations and delusions. However, the antipsychotic effects are not generally seen for several weeks or months after initiation of chronic therapy. Administration of these agents for acute conditions produces a quieting effect in grossly agitated and disturbed patients. After long-term administration of phenothiazines, tolerance develops to their sedative effect with no reduction in antipsychotic activity.

The piperazine phenothiazines (for example, trifluoperazine) has the greatest antipsychotic potency when compared, on a weight basis, with the aliphatic or piperidine derivatives; however, none of the subgroups of phenothiazines differ in efficacy in the management of psychosis. Thus, the delusions, hallucinations, distorted thought processes and bizarre behavior associated with psychosis are generally diminished with any of the antipsychotic agents administered in an adequate dose for an appropriate duration of time.

Antiemetic Actions There is a bilateral area on the floor of the fourth ventricle known as the area postrema which, when stimulated by chemical agents will cause emesis. This area is thought to be dopamine rich and is referred to as the *chemoreceptor trigger zone*. The phenothiazines, with the exception of thioridazine, act as antiemetics by suppression of the chemoreceptor trigger zone. They cannot prevent vomiting induced by vestibular dysfunction (motion sickness) but are effective when emesis is produced by gastrointestinal conditions, e.g., gastroenteritis.

Alteration of Temperature Regulation The phenothiazines depress hypothalamic temperature-regulating mechanisms. They may produce hypothermia or hyperthermia, depending on the environmental temperature. In climates where the temperature is high, patients on phenothiazine medication may suffer a hyperthermic episode because of failure to lose body heat and this poikilothermic phenomenon resulted in deaths early in the use of phenothiazines during the summer in non-air-conditioned hospitals. In cold environmental temperatures, phenothiazines can produce hypothermia.

Endocrine Effects The endocrine effects of the phenothiazines are due primarily to their action on the hypothalamus and pituitary. Dopamine normally inhibits prolactin release. Phenothiazines, which are dopamine receptor antagonists, block this action of dopamine. They may, as a result of this activity, increase prolactin levels and lactation. The chronic use of phenothiazines may, thus, increase lactation in female patients and produce gynecomastia in male patients.

The effects of the phenothiazines on ovulation and menstruation depend on the dose and duration of treatment. Therapeutic doses delay ovulation, basal body temperature, and menstruation. It has been shown that some phenothiazines, especially in high doses, produce amenorrhea by decreasing gonadotropin liberation.

False-positive human chorionic gonadotropin

TABLE 20-2 Comparison of some pharmacodynamic properties of antipsychotics

	Equivalent doses, mg, for antipsychotic activity	Sedation	EPR[a]	Anti-cholinergic effects	α-Adrenergic blocking activity (orthostatic hypotension)
Phenothiazines					
Aliphatics					
Chlorpromazine	50	High	Moderate	Moderate	High
Promazine	100	Moderate	Moderate	High	Moderate
Piperazines					
Prochlorperazine	8	Moderate	High	Low	Low
Trifluoperazine	2.5	Low	High	Low	Low
Fluphenazine	1	Low	High	Low	Low
Piperidines					
Thioridazine	50	High	Low	High	High
Mesoridazine	25	High	Low	Moderate	Moderate
Butyrophenones					
Haloperidol	1	Low	High	Low	Low
Thioxanthenes					
Thiothixene	2	Low	High	Low	Low
Dihydroindolones					
Molindone	5	Low	High	Low	Low
Dibenzoxazepines					
Loxapine	8	Moderate	High	Low	Moderate
Dibenzodiazepines					
Clozapine	25	High	Low	High	High
Diphenylbutylpiperidines					
Pimozide	0.2	Moderate	High	Moderate	Low

[a] EPR = extrapyramidal reactions (excluding tardive dyskinesia).

pregnancy tests may also result with phenothiazine use. This may be due to the stimulation of hypothalamic release of pituitary hormones. Phenothiazines also interfere with the release of corticotropin from the pituitary.

Dopamine also inhibits the release of melanocyte-stimulating hormone (MSH). The phenothiazines, therefore, stimulate the release of MSH from the pituitary, which results in abnormal pigmentation. This production of a grey metal discoloration of the skin may be more pronounced after exposure to the sun.

Peripheral Nervous System The phenothiazines have multiple actions on the peripheral nervous system. These compounds produce differing degrees of α-adrenergic receptor blockade, depending on the dose and duration of therapy. With a single small dose, especially with chlorpromazine, the α-adrenergic blockade is more consistent. Owing to the blockade of these receptor sites, orthostatic hypotension will occur in a significant number of patients (Table 20-2). Although most of the phenothiazines produce α-adrenergic receptor blockade, their actions are considered to be much less specific compared with a classic α-adrenergic blocking agent. The phenothiazines also block cholinergic receptors, primarily muscarinic (Table 20-2). These actions are weak and are seen primarily as annoying side effects. However, some phenothiazines such as thioridazine are effective anticholinergics. The phenothiazines also vary widely in antihistaminic actions. Those phenothiazines having an ethyldiethylamino group on the nitrogen, e.g., promethazine, generally have higher antihistaminic activity and are used mainly for that purpose.

Skeletal Muscle It is believed that phenothiazines have skeletal muscle relaxant properties. This activity is probably mediated centrally through the basal ganglia, but the drugs may also block nicotinic skeletal muscle receptors. Shivering, which is a protective action against cold weather, may be diminished. This may contribute to the hypothermia of patients taking phenothiazines in cold weather.

Pharmacokinetics

Many of the phenothiazines can be given intravenously, subcutaneously, intramuscularly, rectally, and orally. They must be given very slowly intravenously because of local irritation and possible severe hypotension due to central vasomotor depression and α-adrenergic receptor blockade.

Ordinarily, the oral absorption of phenothiazines is slow and incomplete; peak plasma levels are reached within 2 to 4 h. The effect of intramuscular and/or intravenous injection is immediate and may persist for 4 h. Fluphenazine, as the decanoate or enanthate salt is available in a depot form, with a duration of action of 3 to 4 weeks after intramuscular administration.

The biotransformation of chlorpromazine and similar phenothiazines is accomplished by the drug-metabolizing microsomal system in the liver. The most common pathway is hydroxylation of the ring and subsequent conjugation with glucuronic acid. The second most common pathway is the formation of sulfoxides. In addition, demethylation and side-chain oxidation can occur. The half-life of chlorpromazine is between 16 and 30 h, and its plasma protein binding is more than 90 percent. About 1 percent of chlorpromazine appears in the urine unchanged. However, at least five biotransformation products of chlorpromazine are found: chlorpromazine sulfoxide, desdimethylchlorpromazine sulfoxide, glucuronide conjugates, hydroxyl derivatives, and promazine (via dechlorination). There are more than 150 proposed metabolites of chlorpromazine and some can be found in the body months after cessation of administration.

Thioridazine undergoes sulfoxidation to sulfoxide and sulfone metabolites. Mesoridazine and sulforidazine are active metabolites. The metabolism of the piperazine phenothiazines is similar to that of chlorpromazine. There are apparently no active metabolites from this group.

Although the elimination of chlorpromazine and related phenothiazines may take many weeks, the duration of action of these drugs is relatively short, especially on single-dose administration. Compounds such as chlorpromazine have a duration of action after oral administration of 6 h; it is necessary to medicate 3 to 4 times a day to maintain an adequate blood level. In the case of some phenothiazines, such as trifluoperazine, drug administration twice a day is sufficient. The use of depot forms of antipsychotics preclude these multiple dosing regimens and can increase patient compliance.

Correlations of plasma concentrations of phenothiazines and efficacy are difficult to establish. Chlorpromazine causes an improvement in clinical situations with plasma levels in wide range of 50 to 300 ng/mL. Higher concentrations may not increase efficacy.

Therapeutic Uses

The phenothiazines are used widely as antipsychotics and, although these agents are not curative, they do reduce psychiatric symptoms sufficiently to allow mentally disturbed patients to have better contact with reality and to be discharged to a home and family environment. Therapeutic use of these drugs has made community psychiatric treatment a reasonable possibility and the sight of unkempt, violent, catatonic, incontinent and actively hallucinating patients in mental hospitals is almost non-existent today. The course of therapy using antipsychotic drugs to treat schizophrenia may be divided into three phases: (1) the initial phase which has been termed the "pharmacolysis of psychosis" is a period of a few weeks when there is a need to rapidly reverse the behavior of an agitated, manic patient so as to control the hostility, hallucinations, delusions and disordered thinking. At this time, the high doses of antipsychotics can best be given at night to allow for sleep onset; (2) the second phase involves stabilization of dose with resolving the abnormal behavior. This phase follows the 1 to 3 week period of higher dosing with a gradually reducing regimen over the next 2 to 4 weeks. This dosing schedule is in place to maintain control at the same time as minimizing side effects. Generally dosages are reduced to 1/4 to 1/2 of the maximal dose used during the initial phase; (3) the maintenance phase involves further reduction to the lowest dose necessary to continue management. Reappearance of psychotic symptoms may be countered with temporary increases in dosage.

Occasionally phenothiazines are used for purposes other than the treatment of psychosis. For example, they have been employed to relieve very severe anxiety and especially panic reactions induced by abuse of amphetamines and lysergic acid diethylamide (LSD). Children having serious behavioral problems which cannot be controlled by psychotherapy or other non-neuroleptic drugs may be given small doses of antipsychotics. The drugs are also useful as preanesthetic medications because of the following reasons: (1) they reduce anxiety and apprehension; (2) they control nausea and vomiting, which are very common in surgical patients; (3) they cause muscle relaxation during surgery. Phenothiazines administered intramuscularly, rectally as a suppository, or orally (if the patient can retain the drug) are useful antiemetics. The antiemetic effect of the drug may suppress vomiting from illnesses such as intestinal obstruction and brain tumors and thus obscure their signs and symptoms. This fact must be borne in mind when they are prescribed. Other uses include the treatment of intractable hiccough, tetanus, and in Tourette's Disorder.

Adverse Reactions

The phenothiazines affect many organ systems and, thus, produce numerous undesirable side effects. These include CNS disturbances (extrapyramidal symptoms), endocrine disorders, autonomic nervous system disturbances, hematologic abnormalities, jaundice, and skin pigmentation. The potency of the substituted phenothiazines as antipsychotics correlates inversely with sedation, undesirable autonomic effects, seizures, dermatitis, jaundice, and agranulocytosis. It follows that the autonomic nervous system effects are most prevalent with less potent antipsychotic drugs such as chlorpromazine and that autonomic side effects are less frequent with the potent agents such as trifluoperazine and fluphenazine.

Allergic reactions to the phenothiazines generally occur in the first few weeks of treatment. These include various forms of dermatitis, urticaria, photosensitivity, asthma, laryngeal edema, angioneurotic edema, and anaphylaxis.

Most blood dyscrasias also occur within the first few weeks of therapy. Agranulocytosis, although very rare, is more prevalent with chlorpromazine than with the other more potent phenothiazines. If this is recognized and the drug is stopped, the patient will recover completely. Eosinophilia, leukopenia, aplastic anemia, and thrombocytopenia have also been reported.

Phenothiazines can produce a wide range of metabolic and endocrine effects. Weight gain, one major adverse effect, may be due to increased appetite. Galactorrhea is observed in chronically treated women and is due to increased levels of prolactin. Amenorrhea is also produced owing to variable concentrations of luteinizing hormone (LH). In males, there is gynecomastia and a decrease in libido. Impotence and sterility may occur. These effects are probably associated with hyperprolactinemia.

Usually following chronic, but occasionally after acute, administration of some phenothiazines, extrapyramidal side effects may develop. The phenothiazines produce extrapyramidal symptoms presumably by blocking dopamine receptors in the basal ganglia. The extrapyramidal reactions may be divided into three areas: (1) parkinsonism, (2) akathisia, and (3) dystonic reactions. The phenothiazines with the greatest antipsychotic potency, i.e., the piperazine derivatives, produce the highest incidence of extrapyramidal reactions. The reduction in dopaminergic activity produced by the phenothiazines results in a relative increase in cholinergic activity in the basal ganglia. Therefore, anticholinergic therapy, e.g., benztropine, can control these symptoms. Those substituted phenothiazines with the highest anticholinergic activity (e.g., thioridazine) produce the lowest incidence of parkinsonian-like symptoms (Table 20-2). Extrapyramidal symptoms induced by the phenothiazines are frequently dramatic. In one study, akathisia (motor restlessness) occurred in approximately 21 percent, tremors in 15 percent, and dystonic reactions in 2 percent of cases. A correlation has been found between the percentage of occurrence of such reactions and the milligram potency of the drugs. Some interesting sex differences have also been observed. Akathisia and tremors occur twice as often in women as in men. In men, dyskinesia occurred earliest (90 percent within 4.5 days), akathisia next, and tremors last. Dystonic reactions include bizarre neuromuscular manifestations which could be mistaken for seizures, tetanus, meningitis, encephalitis, and poliomyelitis. These extrapyramidal symptoms are completely reversible upon discontinuation of the drug or by reduction of dose.

A life-threatening syndrome known as *neuroleptic malignant syndrome* has also been reported. This syndrome is characterized by muscular rigidity, hyperthermia (as high as 42 °C), altered consciousness, and autonomic dysfunction. It develops suddenly over 24 to 72 hours and can occur within hours to weeks after initial drug therapy. Mortality has been 20 percent in reported cases due to respiratory or cardiovascular complications. Management consists of immediate discontinuance of the antipsychotic agent and supportive medical care. Usually, the symptoms improve within 5 to 10 days of stopping the drug. Some reports indicate that bromocriptine and/or dantrolene sodium may improve the outcome.

Tardive dyskinesia is a syndrome associated with administration of large chronic doses of phenothiazines. It appears to be caused by an imbalance of acetylcholine and dopamine in which there is an increase in dopaminergic activity and a relative decrease in cholinergic activity. However, there is no direct relationship between the potency of the phenothiazines and their ability to produce this syndrome. This phenomenon appears to be a consequence of a decrease in dosage or increase in tolerance to the phenothiazine effects possibly due to supersensitivity of dopamine receptors. Anticholinergics have been found to intensify the symptoms of tardive dyskinesia while the administration of higher doses of the phenothiazines or a cholinergic drug has been found to be useful in decreasing the symptoms of this syndrome. This syndrome usually occurs in older patients and more commonly in women after administration of large doses of phenothiazines for long periods, yet it can be seen in any patient or after any dosage or regimen. The onset is insidious, and the movements are rhythmic and coordinated rather than spasmodic. The tongue, lips, face, and jaw are most commonly involved. The late (i.e., "tardive") dyskinesia is not only irreversible, but it is usually intensified when the phenothiazine is withdrawn. This reaction is difficult to reverse and there is no current effective therapy to treat tardive dyskinesia. Present treatment consists of slowly reducing the dose of the phenothiazine and removing or stopping all anticholinergic agents.

Large doses of most antipsychotic drugs are capable of causing convulsions. Epileptics are more susceptible because of the ability of the phenothiazines to decrease the seizure threshold. Although this is rarely seen, the seizure history of the patient should be carefully noted prior to onset of therapy.

Thioridazine appears to produce significantly fewer untoward side effects such as extrapyramidal symptoms, lethargy, drowsiness, orthostatic hypotension, convulsions, and photosensitivity, compared with other phenothiazines. However, this compound has its own side effects including atropine-like effects and when given in doses over 800 mg in 1 day, pigmentary retinopathy and lens opacities may occur. Temporary failure of ejaculation without affecting erection has also been described following this medication.

Three types of pathologic liver conditions are associated with phenothiazine medication. The most frequent type is a diffuse inflammatory change associated with biliary stasis. The clinical picture is that of obstructive jaundice with a moderate elevation of alkaline phosphatase level. The next type of liver-induced ailment resembles acute hepatitis with evidence of parenchymal liver damage. In the third and least common type of reaction, early cirrhosis is observed.

Autonomic nervous system disturbances can be either anticholinergic, antiadrenergic (α-adrenergic receptor blocking), or both depending on the drug administered. Antiadrenergic symptoms include nasal stuffiness, dry mouth, hypotension, ejaculatory disorders, and miosis. Anticholinergic side effects can be obstipation, constipation, impotence, urinary retention, and mydriasis.

Exposed portions of the skin may develop pigmentation. Eye complications consisting of corneal and lenticular deposits, epithelial keratopathy, and pigmentary retinopathy may also occur.

The most common adverse effects in children are extrapyramidal reactions, which may be confused with encephalitis or other neurologic syndromes. The less common complications of phenothiazine therapy in children include jaundice, granulocytopenia, cutaneous eruptions, and hyperpyrexia.

Patients who take an excessive amount of phenothiazines present with two different clinical pictures. The first is related to extreme somnolence: with prodding, the patient can be aroused but promptly falls back into a deep sleep. The second is hypotension. There may be a mild to moderate drop in blood pressure; the patient may or may not be conscious. The skin may be markedly gray but warm and dry. The nail beds are usually still pink, and the pulse is strong but more rapid than normal. Respiration usually is slow and regular. Hypotension may be severe, in which case the patient may present symptoms of shock, including weakness, cyanosis, perspiration, and a rapid, thready pulse.

Drug Interactions

By induction of liver microsomal enzymes, chlorpromazine can accelerate its own biotransformation. Similarly, potent enzyme inducers such as phenobarbital and other barbiturates will increase the biotransformation of chlorpromazine and possibly lead to a reduced antipsychotic effect. There is also evidence that phenothiazines and haloperidol can inhibit the biotransformation of tricyclic antidepressants and vice versa. CNS depressants such as barbiturates, opioids, general anesthetics, and anticholinergics (e.g., atropine) should not be used or be used very cautiously in patients taking neuroleptics because of additive sedative effects. Chlorpromazine has been shown to depress the level of alcohol dehydrogenase causing increasing blood levels of ethanol.

The concurrent administration of antidiarrheal mixtures or a colloidal antacid, such as aluminum hydroxide gel, with chlorpromazine could decrease the absorption of chlorpromazine and lead to reduced plasma levels. Similarly, the combination of a potent anticholinergic agent and chlorpromazine could decrease chlorpromazine plasma levels by decreasing gastric motility and allowing more chlorpromazine to be biotransformed in the gastrointestinal tract before it is absorbed. By an unknown mechanism, caffeine can diminish the antipsychotic effect of the drugs, so drinks containing caffeine should not be taken. Phenothiazines can block the therapeutic response to levodopa in patients with parkinsonism by blocking dopamine receptors at the target sites. These drugs can also interact with guanethidine and negate its antihypertensive action. The combination of methyldopa with phenothiazines can lead to a decreased antihypertensive effect. When epinephrine is used with phenothiazines there is predominant activity of β-adrenergic receptors because α-adrenergic receptors are blocked by the later drug. This can be dangerous, and so epinephrine should be avoided. Propranolol and phenothiazine together increase plasma levels of both drugs by an unknown mechanism. Cardiac depression caused by quinidine can be enhanced by phenothiazines. Encephalopathy has been reported in a few patients receiving both haloperidol and lithium carbonate. When the phenothiazines are administered along with lithium, the phenothiazine blood level decreases. Phenytoin toxicity may be increased by phenothiazines via altered hepatic metabolism. The use of benzodiazepines with antipsychotics, in the treatment of psychosis with a large anxiety component, increases sedation and requires lower doses of antipsychotics to be prescribed which may, in turn, prevent improvement of the patient's condition.

Contraindications

Phenothiazine antipsychotics are contraindicated in individuals with previous hypersensitivity reactions to these agents. The possibility of cross-sensitivity among various phenothiazines exists. All antipsychotic compounds are contraindicated in comatose patients or in those with CNS depression due to alcohol or other centrally acting depressants. The presence of liver disease or bone marrow depression is a relative contraindication to the use of these agents. The more potent agents should not be used in patients with Parkinson's disease of an extreme degree. Thioridazine should be avoided in patients with severe heart disease. The drugs should be avoided in children suspected to have Reye's syndrome since confusion may arise between the disease and the extrapyramidal symptoms produced by the drug.

The safety of all antipsychotic compounds for use during pregnancy has not been established. Therefore, these drugs should be given to pregnant patients only when, in the judgment of the physician, the expected benefits from treatment exceed the possible risks to mother and fetus.

THIOXANTHENE DERIVATIVES

Structurally, the thioxanthenes differ from the phenothiazines only in that they have a carbon in place of a nitrogen at position 10 in the center ring. Thiothixene is very similar pharmacologically to its corresponding phenothiazine analogs. It has the same mechanism of action and similar effects on the central and peripheral nervous systems. The difference is quantitative. Thiothixene is a more potent antipsychotic agent than most phenothiazine derivatives. Compared to chlorpromazine, thiothixene produces a higher incidence of extrapyramidal symptoms, but less sedation, anticholinergic effects, and orthostatic hypotension.

TABLE 20-3 Therapeutically useful thioxanthene derivative

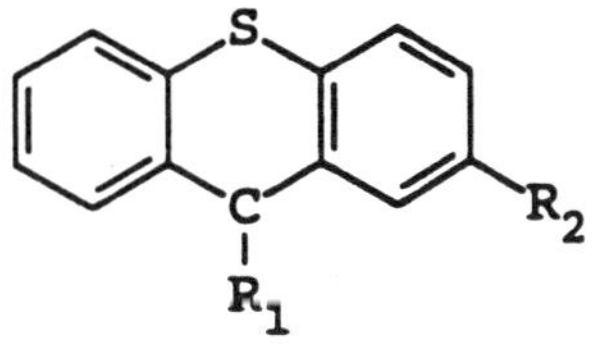

Generic name	R_1	R_2
Thiothixene	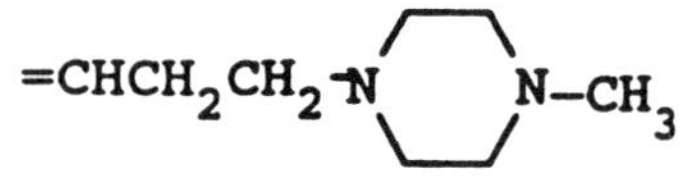 $=CHCH_2CH_2-N$ (piperazine) $N-CH_3$	$O_2S-N(CH_3)_2$

Thiothixene is rapidly absorbed, and peak plasma levels are obtained in 1 to 2 h. The drug has a half-life of 34 h.

BUTYROPHENONE DERIVATIVES

Although the butyrophenone derivatives have pharmacologic properties which are very similar to those of the phenothiazines and thioxanthenes, they are chemically quite different. Haloperidol, a potent butyrophenone antipsychotic agent, has the following structure:

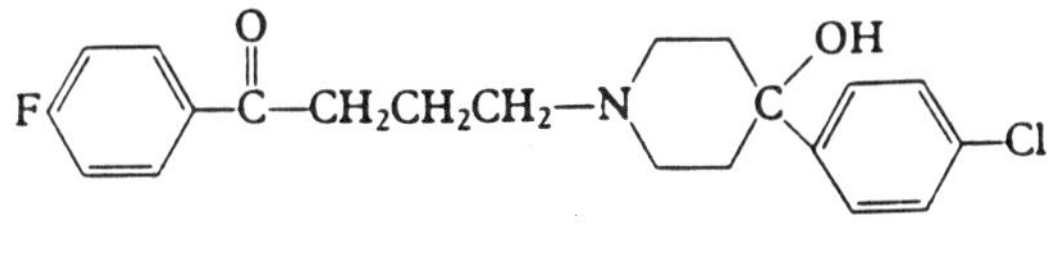

Haloperidol has a mechanism of action that is identical with that of the phenothiazines, that is, blockade of dopaminergic receptors. However, it is more selective for D_2 receptors.

Haloperidol has good oral absorption with peak plasma levels in 3 to 6 h. It has an elimination half-life of 12 to 20 h. The major metabolites are inactive. Unlike the many metabolites of chlorpromazine found, haloperidol has no active metabolites. Approximately 40 percent of the drug is eliminated in the urine unchanged. Correlation of haloperidol blood levels and therapeutic effect is poor. The drug is used orally, and by intramuscular and intravenous injection. Intramuscular injection of the decanoate salt provides a long duration of action.

Haloperidol has similar pharmacodynamic properties to chlorpromazine (see Table 20-2), yet it is more potent as an antipsychotic drug than chlorpromazine. It produces less sedation, anticholinergic effects, and orthostatic hypotension than chlorpromazine. Haloperidol, however, produces a greater incidence of extrapyramidal reactions. Haloperidol is indicated for the treatment of psychosis associated with acute schizophrenia or delirium. It is also used in suppressing the symptoms (tics and vocal utterances) of Tourette's Disorder and in hyperactive children showing excessive motor activity with conduct disorder. Neuroleptics should be used in children only after failure of psychotherapy and other medications.

Haloperidol is the only butyrophenone derivative used as an antipsychotic in the USA. A derivative, droperidol, is indicated (1) to produce tranquilization and reduce nausea and vomiting in surgical and diagnostic procedures, (2) as an adjunct in the maintenance of anaesthesia, and (3) to produce tranquilization and reduce anxiety as an adjunct to opioids in the therapy of chronic pain, a procedure known as *neuroleptanalgesia*.

DIHYROINDOLONE DERIVATIVE

Molindone is a dihydroindolone drug whose structure is unrelated to the phenothiazines, the butyrophenones, or the thioxanthenes.

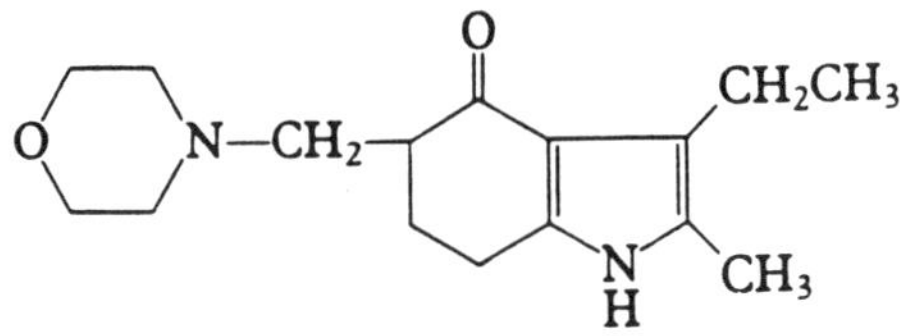

The mechanism of action of this drug is similar to that of the phenothiazines. Molindone is more potent as an antipsychotic drug when compared with chlorpromazine (see Table 20-2). It produces less sedation, anticholinergic effects, and orthostatic hypotension, but causes a greater incidence of extrapyramidal reactions than chlorpromazine. It is well absorbed orally, with peak levels reached in 60 to 90 min. It is believed to be metabolized in the liver and has 36 recognizable metabolites. The metabolites are excreted in the urine. Less than 3 percent of the parent drug is excreted in the urine. Elimination by hemodialysis or peripheral dialysis is insignificant.

The adverse reactions are similar to the phenothiazines, but molindone has no effect upon the seizure threshold and may actually decrease appetite and facilitate weight loss. It is indicated only for the management of psychotic disorders.

DIBENZOXAZEPINE DERIVATIVE

Loxapine is a dibenzoxazepine compound which represents a tricyclic antipsychotic agent similar to the phenothiazines.

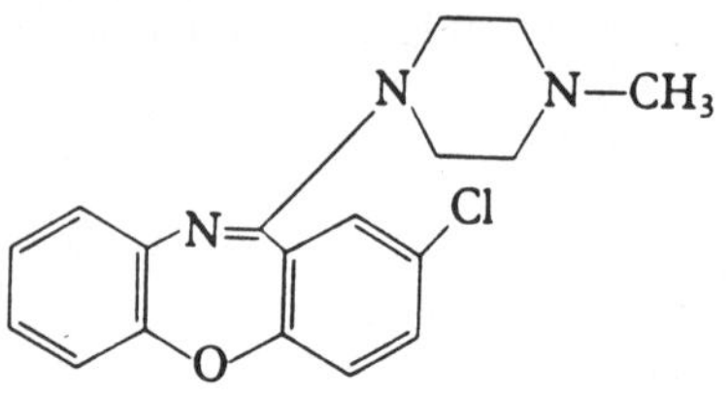

N N—CH_3 N= Cl O

The mechanism of action is identical with that of the phenothiazines. Loxapine is more potent as an antipsychotic drug than chlorpromazine. It is somewhat less sedative and induces less anticholinergic effects and orthostatic hypotension than chlorpromazine; however, molindone tends to cause a higher incidence of extrapyramidal reactions. The drug is completely absorbed orally, and after absorption it is rapidly distributed to tissues. The drug has a half-life of 6 to 8 h. It is metabolized in the liver and has both conjugated and unconjugated metabolites. The conjugated metabolites are excreted in the urine, while unconjugated metabolites are excreted in the feces.

The adverse reactions of loxapine are similar to those of the phenothiazines. Like molindone, loxapine has a lower incidence of anticholinergic effects than chlorpromazine, but extrapyramidal effects are more common (see Table 20-2). It is used either orally or by intramuscular injection to treat a variety of psychoses.

DIBENZODIAZEPINE DERIVATIVE

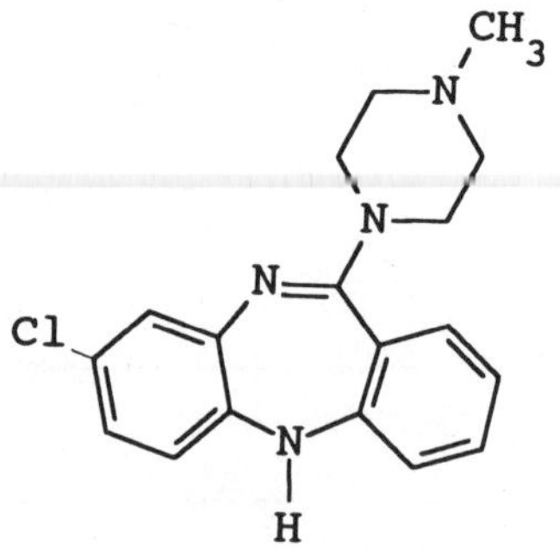

CH_3 N N N= Cl N H

Clozapine may be unique among antipsychotics in that it appears to be only minimally active at dopamine receptors. Therefore, it has received a designation as an "atypical" antipsychotic agent. Experimental evidence suggests that the drug is more active at limbic dopamine receptors than at striatal dopamine receptors. This may reflect the fact that it produces little, if any, extrapyramidal effects in the recommended dosage range and, therefore, may not allow for the development of tardive dyskinesia. The relative lack of extrapyramidal effects may be a distinct advantage in the use of clozapine. Unfortunately, clozapine has been shown to produce, on rare occasions, granulocytopenia or agranulocytosis whereby several fatalities occurred in a Finnish study prior to its approval in the USA. Because of this, the use clozapine is regulated by the need for weekly blood counts for patients on this medication and for 4 weeks following discontinuation of therapy with the drug. The cost of the hematology tests added to that of the antipsychotic itself makes clozapine a very expensive drug. Clozapine is useful (at this writing) only for treatment of refractory, severely ill schizophrenics or in those patients very susceptible to extrapyramidal reactions.

Clozapine is adequately absorbed following oral administration, with peak plasma concentrations occurring at 2.5 h. The drug is approximately 95 percent bound to plasma proteins. Clozapine is almost completely biotransformed to several weakly active and inactive products. Drug elimination is via the urine and feces. The mean elimination half-life of the drug is 8 h after single doses and 12 h after steady-state has been attained.

In addition to the blood dyscrasias discussed above, clozapine produces a high incidence of CNS (sedation, dizziness, headache), cardiovascular (tachycardia, orthostatic hypotension), and gastrointestinal (constipation) adverse effects. In addition, the drug appear to induce a high incidence of seizures, probably by reducing the seizure threshold similar to the phenothiazines.

DIPHENYLBUTYLPIPERIDINE DERIVATIVE

Pimozide is a diphenylbutylpiperidine, which is approved in the USA solely for use in patients having uncontrolled Tourette's Disorder.

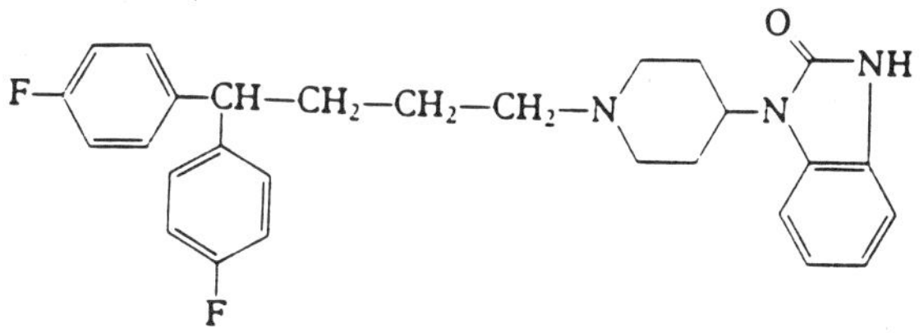

The drug has a number of adverse effects, many of which are similar to the phenothiazines. In addition to the extrapyramidal symptoms, neuroleptic malignant syndrome, tardive dyskinesia, and allergies, it can cause prolongation of the ST segment, flattening or inversion of T wave, nausea, vomiting, dizziness, blurred vision, chest pain, periorbital edema, and urinary frequency. The mechanism of action is believed to be blockade of dopaminergic receptors. The use of the drug is contraindicated in patients having hypersensitivity to it, CNS depression, prolonged QT interval or cardiac arrhythmias, in patients taking drugs known to cause motor tics, and in patients having tics from disorders other than Tourette's Disorder.

BENZISOXAZOLE DERIVATIVE

Risperidone is the only antipsychotic drug under this chemical class that is available in the United States. Its mechanism of action is apparently related to its antagonism of D_2 and serotonergic type 2 ($5\text{-}HT_2$) receptors. The compound also has high affinity for and antagonism of α-adrenergic and histaminic (H_1) receptors, which helps to explain some of the major adverse effects of the drug. Other receptors, including D_1 and subtypes of serotonergic receptors (e.g., $5\text{-}HT_{1A}$, $5\text{-}HT_{1C}$, and $5\text{-}HT_{1D}$), are blocked to a lesser extent. The drug does not block muscarinic receptors; therefore, anticholinergic effects are insignificant.

Risperidone is well absorbed orally, with an oral bioavailability of 70 percent. It is biotransformed in the liver by hydroxylation to an equally-active product, 9-hydroxyrisperidone. The elimination half-lives of risperidone and 9-hydroxyrisperidone are 3 and 21 h, respectively. Plasma protein binding of risperidone and 9-hydroxyrisperidone are 90 percent and 77 percent, respectively.

The most common adverse effects of this drug include extrapyramidal symptoms, dizziness, somnolence, and nausea. Other adverse reaction that have been reported include the neuroleptic malignant syndrome, tardive dyskinesia, electrocardiographic changes, orthostatic hypotension, thrombocytopenic purpura, body temperature abnormalities, and photosensitivity.

The major indication for the use of risperidone is in the management of psychotic disorders. At present, risperidone shows no major advantages over previously discussed antipsychotic drugs.

SELECTION OF AN ANTIPSYCHOTIC

The so-called "positive" psychotic symptoms, including delusional and hallucinatory behavior, distorted thought processes, and bizarre behaviors including mutism, are all diminished with any of the antipsychotic agents listed above and no antipsychotic agent is superior to another in this regard. The question is: how to choose one or the other antipsychotic medication? In truth, a specific antipsychotic agent may be selected to treat a given patient if that patient has received palliative effects with the drug during a previous acute psychotic episode. In addition, a specific antipsychotic drug may be selected because the adverse effects of that drug, as they are known, may be "tailored away" from the symptoms present or expected in the individual patient. To illustrate this, the piperazine phenothiazine derivatives, which carry a greater risk of extrapyramidal effects, should be avoided in the elderly who are more prone to idiopathic Parkinson's disease. In manic, agitated psychotic patients, an antipsychotic with potent histamine antagonistic effects may be better used as the side effect of sedation may, in fact, help the behavioral adaptation of the patient. Thioridazine, a drug that produces less extrapyramidal effects than other phenothiazines, should be avoided in patients with a tendency to attempt suicide, since this particular phenothiazine derivative has been shown to produce a greater occurrence of cardiac conduction difficulties when taken in overdose. Lastly, the two compounds presently available for depot administration, i.e., fluphenazine and haloperidol, should be considered for those patients who may be non-compliant. Thus, a thorough understanding of the advantages (pharmacological effects) and disadvantages (adverse effects) of each of the antipsychotic drugs will allow the prescribing physician to best choose the most appropriate drug for the individual patient.

LITHIUM CARBONATE

Bipolar affective disorder is a mental disorder which combines episodes of alternating mania and depression and, thus, its other name "manic depression". The mania is characterized by elation of mood, grandiosity, irritability, distractibility and hyperactivity. It may either precede or follow a period of normal mood or a depressed phase. Lithium (as the carbonate or citrate) is effective prophylactically in decreasing the cycling of manic depression and this is the only FDA approved use of this agent. Lithium is a monovalent cation that belongs chemically to the same family as sodium and potassium.

Mechanism of Action

In normal patients, therapeutic levels of lithium have no sedative, depressant, or euphoric effects on the CNS. However, in those correctly diagnosed with bipolar affective disorder lithium is mood-stabilizing.

Lithium is absorbed and apparently exerts its effects as the lithium ion. Lithium ion increases neuronal reuptake of norepinephrine and serotonin. Electrolytes may play a key role in maintaining the synthesis, storage release and inactivation of neurotransmitters. Lithium could induce changes in these electrolytes, which may induce changes of neurotransmitters such as mentioned previously with norepinephrine and serotonin. Other possibilities exist that indicate that lithium's antimanic effects may be due to increased cholinergic activity or by inhibiting cyclic AMP.

Pharmacokinetics

Absorption of lithium ion is virtually 100 percent. Food does not impair this absorptive process. Peak serum levels are reached in 2 to 4 h with complete absorption in 8 h. The mean serum half-life is approximately 24 h; steady-state is reached within 5 to 7 days.

Lithium is not bound to plasma proteins or metabolized, but is freely filtered through the glomerular membrane. The volume of distribution is equal to that of total body water. When steady-state is reached, the concentration in the cerebrospinal fluid is about 40 to 50 percent of the concentration in plasma. Lithium concentrations in blood are easily measured with flame photometry. The therapeutic serum level ranges from 0.4 to 1.0 mEq/L. Adverse and toxic reactions usually occur when serum lithium levels exceed 2 mEq/L. Approximately 95 percent of a single dose of lithium is eliminated in the urine. About 80 percent of filtered lithium is reabsorbed by the renal tubules; lithium clearance by the kidney is about 20 percent of that for creatinine, ranging between 15 and 30 mL per minute. This is lower in elderly persons and in patients with renal impairment.

Therapeutic Use

Lithium levels are measured as mEq/L and a useful guide is that each 300 mg oral dosage of lithium raises its plasma level by 0.3 mEq/L. During the generally extended lag-time of approximately two weeks between the start of lithium treatment and the beginning of adequate therapeutic levels, an antipsychotic agent can be prescribed along with lithium in an effort to control manic episodes and later withdrawn as lithium blood levels rise.

Adverse Effects

Adverse reactions are seldom seen when lithium levels are below 2 mEq/L but can be observed in patients sensitive to the drug. Blood samples for serum lithium levels should be drawn prior to the next dose. Levels should be determined daily until serum levels are stabilized. The following adverse reactions have been reported to be related to serum lithium levels, including therapeutic levels:

Neuromuscular/central nervous system Tremor, muscle hyperirritability (fasciculation, twitching, clonic movements of whole limbs), ataxia, choreoathetotic movements, hyperactive deep tendon reflexes, extrapyramidal symptoms, blackout spells, epileptiform seizures, slurred speech, dizziness, vertigo, incontinence of urine or feces, somnolence, psychomotor retardation, restlessness, confusion, stupor, coma, tongue movements, tics, tinnitus, hallucinations, poor memory, slowed intellectual functioning, startled response.

Cardiovascular Cardiac arrhythmias, hypotension, peripheral circulatory collapse, bradycardia, sinus node dysfunction.

Gastrointestinal Anorexia, nausea, vomiting, diarrhea, gastritis, salivary gland swelling, abdominal pain, excessive salivation, flatulence, indigestion.

Genitourinary Albuminuria, oliguria, polyuria, glycosuria, decreased creatinine clearance.

Dematologic Drying and thinning of hair, alopecia, anesthesia of skin, chronic folliculitis, xerosis cutis, psoriasis or its exacerbation, itching, angioedema.

Autonomic Blurred vision, dry mouth.

Thyroid abnormalities Euthyroid goiter and/or hypothyroidism (including myxedema) accompanied by lower T_3 and T_4. ^{131}I uptake may be elevated. Paradoxically, rare cases of hyperthyroidism have been reported as diffuse nontoxic goiter with or without hypothyroidism.

EEG changes Diffuse slowing, widening of the frequency spectrum, potentiation and disorganization of background rhythm.

EKG changes Reversible flattening, isoelectricity, or inversion of T waves.

Miscellaneous Fatigue, lethargy, dehydration, weight gain, tendency to sleep, leukocytosis, headache, transient hyperglycemia, generalized pruritus with or without rash, cutaneous ulcers, albuminuria, worsening of organic brain syndrome, edematous swelling of ankles or wrists, thirst or polyuria (sometimes resembling diabetes insipidus), metallic taste, impaired or distorted taste, salty taste, swollen lips, tightness in chest, impotence and sexual dysfunction, swollen and/or painful joints, fever, polyarthralgia, dental caries.

A few reports have been received of the development of painful discoloration of fingers and toes and coldness of the extremities within one day of the starting of treatment with lithium. The mechanism through which these symptoms (resembling Raynaud's syndrome) developed is not known. Recovery followed discontinuance of the drug.

Lithium should generally not be given to patients with significant renal or cardiovascular disease, severe debilitation or dehydration, or sodium depletion, and to patients receiving diuretics, since the risk of lithium toxicity is very high in such patients. If the psychiatric indication is life-threatening, and if such a patient fails to respond to other measures, lithium treatment may be undertaken with extreme caution, including daily serum lithium determinations and adjustment to the usually low dose ordinarily tolerated by these individuals. In such instances, hospitalization is a necessity.

Chronic lithium therapy may be associated with diminution of renal concentration ability, occasionally presenting as nephrogenic diabetes insipidus, with polyuria and polydipsia. Such patients should be carefully managed to avoid dehydration with resulting lithium retention and toxicity. This condition is usually reversible when lithium is discontinued.

Morphologic changes with glomerular and interstitial fibrosis and nephron atrophy have been reported in patients on chronic lithium therapy. Morphologic changes have also been seen in patients never exposed to lithium. The relationship between renal function and morphologic changes and their association with lithium therapy have not seen established.

Lithium may cause fetal harm when administered to a pregnant woman. Data from lithium birth registries suggest an increase in cardiac and other anomalies, especially Ebstein's anomaly. If this drug is used during pregnancy, or if a patient becomes pregnant while taking this drug, the patient should be apprised of the potential hazard to the fetus.

Drug Interactions

Acetazolamide, aminophylline, mannitol, sodium bicarbonate, and urea can substantially increase renal clearance of lithium.

Lithium excretion decreases with sodium depletion and increases when large doses of sodium chloride are given. Thus, because lithium is treated by the kidneys as if it were sodium, any type of sodium depletion can drop sodium levels below normal and cause a selective retention of lithium with potential for toxicity.

Long-term therapy with ethacrynic acid, furosemide, or thiazide diuretics has been shown to decrease renal clearance of lithium. Reduced urine output, paradoxical fluid retention, and a rise in serum lithium levels to toxic concentrations may occur during concomitant therapy. Dosage modification may be necessary. Spironolactone and triamterene appear to have little or no effect on lithium clearance.

Lithium may prolong the effects of neuromuscular blocking agents. Therefore neuromuscular blocking agents should be given with caution to patients receiving lithium.

Management of Intoxication

The best therapy is prophylactic avoidance of toxicity. Periodic serum lithium measurements are mandatory along with dosage adjustments. Ordinarily 6 days are required to stabilize the serum level after a change in dose.

Water and sodium intake must not be restricted at any time. Excessive sweating such as during exercise in hot weather may lead to lithium intoxication because of sodium and water loss.

Severe lithium intoxication is a medical emergency and requires hospitalization. Lithium and diuretics are to be discontinued immediately. The condition is treacherous and despite corrective measures may worsen. The primary aim of therapy is to restore water and sodium balance. This can be cautiously accomplished by mild diuresis and sodium infusion. Experience has shown that caution is to be exercised, and sometimes half-normal saline is a wiser choice.

In extreme cases, hemodialysis is the preferred therapy. If this is not available, peritoneal dialysis is a good substitute. Complete recovery may be prolonged, and some instability of water balance and renal and neurologic function may persist for weeks or months.

BIBLIOGRAPHY

Black, J.L.: "Antipsychotic Agents: A Clinical Update," *Mayo Clin. Proc.* **60**: 777-789 (1985).

Carlton, P.L., and P. Manowitz: "Dopamine and Schizophrenia: An Analysis of the Theory," *Neurosci. Biobehav. Rev.* **8**: 137-151 (1984).

Delini-Stula, A.: "Neuroanatomical, Neuropharmacological and Neurobiochemical Target Systems for Antipsychotic Activity of Neuroleptics," *Pharmacopsychiat.* **19**: 134-139 (1986).

Ellenbroek, B.A.: "Treatment of Schizophrenia: A Clinical and Preclinical Evaluation of Neuroleptic Drugs," *Pharmacol. Ther.* **57**: 1-79 (1993).

Hashimoto, F., C.B. Sherman, and W.H. Jeffrey: "Neuroleptic Malignant Syndrome and Dopaminergic Blockade," *Arch. Intern. Med.* **144**: 629-630 (1984).

Hollister, L.E.: "Drug Treatment of Schizophrenia," *Psychiatric Clin. North Am.* **7**: 435-452 (1984).

The Medical Letter on Drugs and Therapeutics. "Drugs for Psychiatric Disorders," **33**: 43-50 (1991).

Pirodsky, D.M., and J.S. Cohn: *Clinical Primer of Psychopharmacology: A Practical Guide, 2nd Ed.*, McGraw-Hill, New York, 1991, pp. 1-32.

CHAPTER 21

Antidepressant Drugs

Beth Hoskins

Affective disorders, or disorders of mood, are a very common occurrence. At some time, almost everyone has felt "blue" or "down in the dumps." In most people, this mood state is quite transient (hours to several days) and can clearly be identified with some precipitating event. Therefore, it deserves emphasis that major affective disorder, which is the state of clinical depression for which antidepressant drugs should be prescribed, is a distinct psychiatric diagnosis which is not made on the basis of a transient dysphoric mood. Rather, the mood disturbance should be prominent and persistent and be accompanied by other symptoms like sleep disturbance, change in appetite, psychomotor disturbances, pervasive loss of interest and of pleasure, feelings of worthlessness or guilt, and even thoughts of death or suicide. The use of an antidepressant drug should be limited to patients with major affective disorder and not to those experiencing relatively transient feelings of sadness. The magnitude of importance can be realized by the fact that about 15 percent of adults in the United States may suffer from significant depressive symptomatology in any given year, and about 40 to 80 percent of suicides are by individuals who have a major affective disorder.

There are four classes of antidepressant drugs. They are the tricyclic antidepressants (TCAs), selective serotonin uptake blockers, other cyclic drugs, and monoamine oxidase inhibitors (MAOIs).

TRICYCLIC ANTIDEPRESSANTS

Chemistry

These drugs have been, until recently, the most commonly prescribed antidepressants and are called "tricyclic" because of their similar three joined-ring structures as shown in Fig. 21-1. Their structures consist of two benzene rings attached to a central seven-membered ring. An amine-containing side chain is attached to the central ring. Based on the substituents on the terminal nitrogen, there are two groups of tricyclic antidepressants: the tertiary amines and the secondary amines. Examples of tertiary amines are imipramine, amitriptyline, trimipramine, and doxepin. Desipramine, nortriptyline, and protryptyline are examples of secondary amines. The tricyclic antidepressants are closely related chemically to the phenothiazines, which are used widely as antipsychotic agents. Indeed, the side effects caused by blockade of α-adrenoceptors, histamine receptors (H_1), and muscarinic receptors are typical of those caused by the phenothiazines.

Mechanism of Action

The tricyclic compounds that are presented in this chapter are effective agents in the treatment of endogenous depression. Studies showed that tricyclic antidepressants blocked reuptake of norepinephrine and/or serotonin (Table 21-1) into the presynaptic nerve terminal. In order for the tricyclic antidepressants to start to alleviate depression in a patient, these drugs must be administered for 2 to 4 weeks; however, their ability to block the reuptake of biogenic amines occurs immediately. It appears that some other biochemical events, although related to the increased presence of amines in the synapse, may be responsible for the antidepressant activity of these agents. Recent evidence indicates that upon chronic administration of tricyclic antidepressants, the blockade of the reuptake of biogenic amines leads to prolonged increased levels of amines in

I. TRICYCLIC ANTIDEPRESSANTS

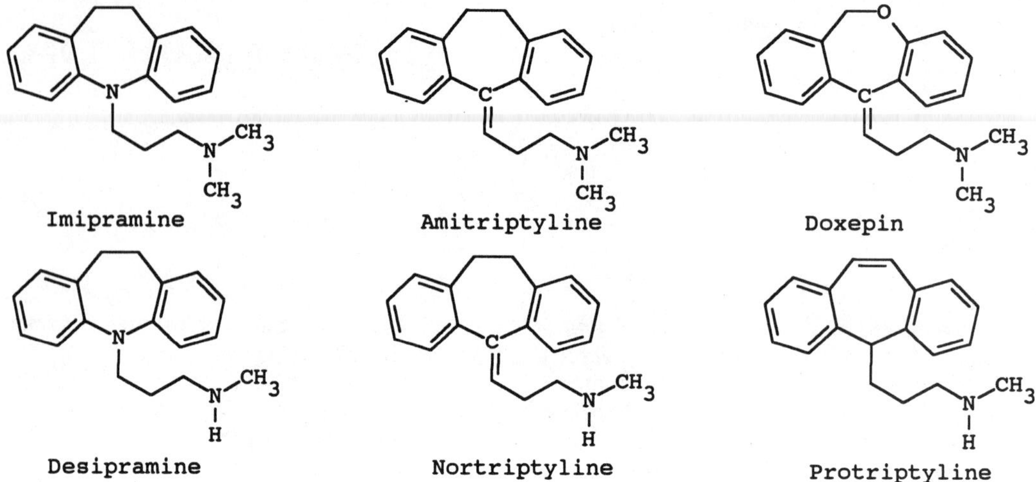

II. SEROTONIN UPTAKE BLOCKERS

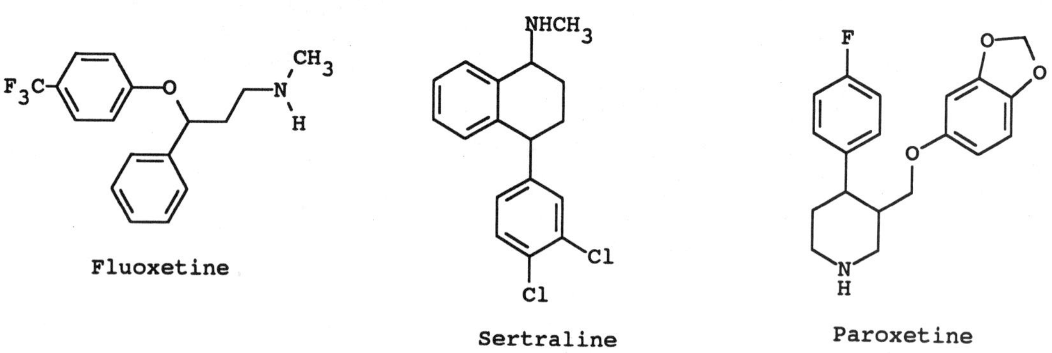

III. OTHER CYCLIC ANTIDEPRESSANTS

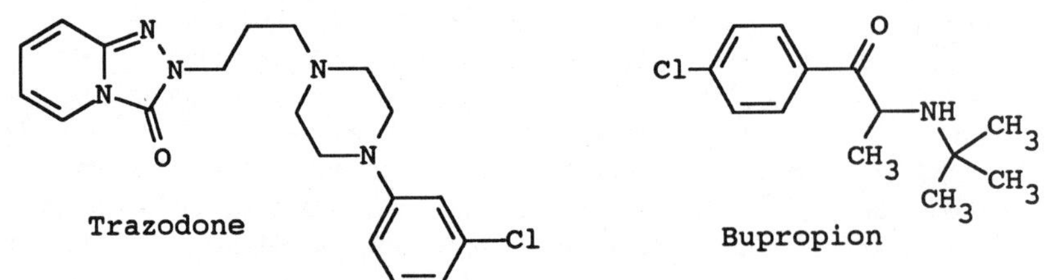

IV. MONOAMINE OXIDASE INHIBITORS

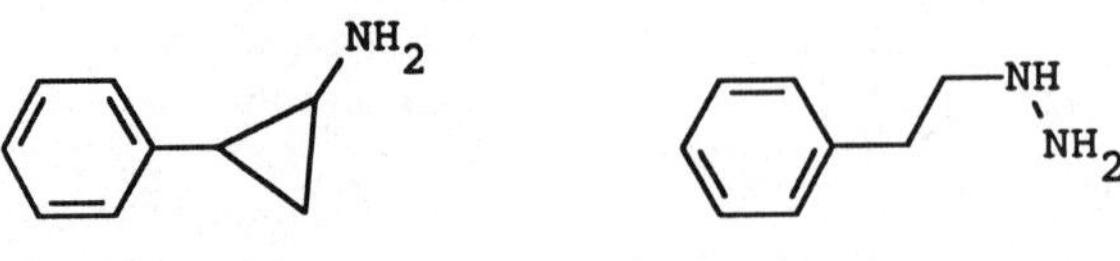

FIGURE 21-1 *Chemical structures of representative antidepressant drugs.*

TABLE 21-1 Potency of antidepressants to block either monoamine uptake or receptors

Drug	Blockade of Monoamine uptake		Blockade of receptors			
	NE[a]	5-HT[b]	$Histamine_1$	Muscarinic	$Alpha_1$	$Serotonin_2$
TRICYCLIC ANTIDEPRESSANTS (TCAs)						
Amitriptyline	Low	Moderate	High	Moderate	Moderate	Moderate
Desipramine	High	Low	Moderate	Low	Low	Low
Doxepin	Low	Very low	Very high	Moderate	Moderate	Moderate
Imipramine	Moderate	Moderate	High	Moderate	Moderate	Moderate
Nortriptyline	High	Low	High	Low	Moderate	Moderate
Protriptyline	High	Low	Moderate	Moderate	Low	Moderate
Trimipramine	Very low	Very low	Very high	Moderate	Moderate	Moderate
Amoxapine	Moderate	Low	Moderate	Very low	Moderate	High
Maprotiline	Moderate	Very low	High	Low	Moderate	Low
SEROTONIN UPTAKE BLOCKERS						
Fluoxetine	Very low	High	Very low	Very low	Very low	Low
Sertraline	Very low	High	Very low	Very low	Very low	Very low
Paroxetine	Very low	High	Very low	Very low	Very low	Very low
OTHER CYCLIC ANTIDEPRESSANTS						
Bupropion	Low	Low	Very low	Very low	Very low	Low
Trazodone	Very low	Low	Low	Very low	Moderate	High

[a] NE: norepinephrine
[b] 5-HT: 5-hydroxytryptamine (serotonin)

the synapse which, in turn, produce a down-regulation of β-adrenergic and serotonin receptors that are present in the postsynaptic membrane. This down-regulation of biogenic amine receptors, which can cause a modification of cellular responses, is suggested as a mechanism of action of these antidepressants.

Another effect of the tricyclic antidepressants that may be involved in their therapeutic effect is their action on α_2-adrenergic receptor sites. These drugs may antagonize the effect of norepinephrine at the presynaptic α_2-adrenergic receptor and cause an enhanced release of norepinephrine from the adrenergic nerve terminal. This increased release of norepinephrine possibly enhances the eventual down-regulation of β-adrenergic receptors.

It also should be mentioned that the antimuscarinic effect of some tricyclic antidepressants may contribute to their mechanism of action. By blocking cholinergic activity there can be an increase in the activity of the sympathetic neurons in the central nervous system (CNS). Some investigators have suggested that this antimuscarinic effect, if it occurs, plays a minor role in the overall antidepressant effect and is more likely related to the adverse reactions produced by these drugs.

The mechanism of action of the tricyclic antidepressants is not completely known; it appears that the antidepressant effect of these drugs is complex in nature. However, down-regulation of biogenic amine receptors appears to be associated with the elevation of mood in the patient.

Pharmacologic Effects

Antidepressant Effects The antidepressant effects of the tricyclic drugs are not akin to the acute stimulant or mood elevating effects produced in normal subjects by drugs such as amphetamine or methylphenidate. Tricyclic antidepressants do not cause mood-elevating effects in nondepressed persons. The acute effect of the tricyclic antidepressants in normal subjects is sedation, often accompanied by unpleasant anticholinergic effects. Repeated administration of these drugs to nondepressed subjects usually accentuates these symptoms and can lead to difficulty in concentrating. By contrast, repeated administration of the same drugs to depressed patients results in an elevation of mood. Thus, in contrast to stimulant drugs, the mood-elevating properties of antidepressants are dependent on the initial behavioral state. In general, this seems to be true for monoamine oxidase inhibitors as well, although tranylcypromine may have some stimulant properties, probably owing to its structural similarity to amphetamine. Further distinguishing antidepressants from stimulants is the fact that drugs such as amphetamine, cocaine, and methylphenidate are not effective antidepressants and that the antidepressants do not have abuse potential as do the stimulants.

It is widely believed that the beneficial therapeutic effect of all types of chemical antidepressants may take 2 to 4 weeks before becoming evident. This lag period has been interpreted as indicating that there is a time delay in the onset of action of antidepressants. Although claims have been made that some of the newer compounds have a faster onset of action, there is no conclusive evidence that this is so. However, what most clinical trials also show is that there is clinical improvement in patients on an antidepressant drug within the first couple of weeks of treatment, but that the response to the antidepressant is no better than the response to placebo. From such data, it is difficult to determine when the *onset* of drug-induced antidepressant effects occurs. In reality, the lag period really seems to pertain to maximal therapeutic benefit derived from antidepressants and all studies show that this takes 4 weeks or longer to occur. Still there is no drug that rapidly produces maximal amelioration of depressive symptomatology.

Not all depressed patients respond equally well to the tricyclic antidepressants. Melancholic patients with symptoms such as loss of appetite and weight loss, early morning awakening, psychomotor retardation or agitation, and lack of reactivity tend to respond well to these drugs. By contrast, depressions that are accompanied by delusions or hallucinations (i.e., psychotic depressions) tend to respond poorly to the tricyclics.

One final point about the clinical use of antidepressants is noteworthy. At least one-half of the individuals with an initial episode of major depression have at least one recurrence during their lifetime. There is an accumulating body of data that tricyclic antidepressants are effective in preventing or attenuating new episodes and are beginning to be used as preventative treatments. Also, patients are being continued on these drugs longer than they were previously in order to maintain control of an acute episode after the initial symptomatology has subsided. Such continuous treatment may often take place for up to 16 to 20 weeks. Because of this longer duration of treatment with tricyclic antidepressants, it is likely that all types of physicians will encounter patients being treated with these drugs in their clinical practices.

Anticholinergic Effects Apart from antidepressant effects, the tricyclics have anticholinergic effects such as dry mouth, constipation, mydriasis, blurred vision, and retention of urine. The degree of anticholinergic effect varies with the choice of drug (see Table 21-2).

Cardiovascular Effects The most important and troublesome action is the production of orthostatic hypotension by blockade of α_1-adrenergic receptors (Table 21-2). Although tricyclic antidepressants can cause severe arrhythmias in overdosage, they actually have strong antiarrhythmic activity at usual plasma concentrations. These effects are best documented for imipramine and nortriptyline but may pertain to the other tricyclic compounds as well. The antiarrhythmic activity seems mainly

TABLE 21-2 Some pharmacologic effects of antidepressant drugs

Drug	Sedative or stimulant	Anticholinergic effect	Cardiovascular effects	
			Potential for causing orthostatic hypotension	Potential for causing conduction disturbances[a]
TRICYCLIC ANTIDEPRESSANTS				
Amitriptyline	Sedative[b]	Marked	High	High
Desipramine	Sedative[c]	Moderate	Low	High
Doxepin	Sedative[b]	Marked	High	Moderate
Imipramine	Sedative	Moderate	Moderate	High
Nortriptyline	Sedative[c]	Moderate	Low	Moderate
Protriptyline	Sedative[c]	Moderate	Low	High
Trimipramine	Sedative[b]	Marked	Moderate	High
Amoxapine	Sedative[c]	Moderate	Moderate	Moderate
Maprotiline	Sedative	Moderate	Moderate to high	Moderate
SEROTONIN UPTAKE BLOCKERS				
Fluoxetine	Stimulant[d]	None	None	None/Low
Sertraline	Stimulant[d]	None	None	None/Low
Paroxetine	Stimulant[d]	Low	Low	None/Low
OTHER CYCLIC ANTIDEPRESSANTS				
Trazodone	Sedative[b]	None/Low	Low	Low
Bupropion	Stimulant	None	None	None/Low
MONOAMINE OXIDASE INHIBITORS				
Phenelzine	Neither	None	High	None
Tranylcypromine	Stimulant	None	High	None

[a] At usual therapeutic doses, drug-induced conduction disturbances are unlikely to be clinically significant in patients without preexisting cardiac disease. The entries in the table indicate the likelihood that a given drug will produce clinically significant disturbances in either high dosages or in patients with preexisting cardiac disease.

[b] High incidence.

[c] Low incidence.

[d] Some patients experience sedation.

to be due to a direct action on the heart in that these drugs produce changes in the electrophysiologic profile similar to those produced by Group I antiarrhythmic drugs such as quinidine. These drugs can increase the PR interval and produce atrioventricular (AV) blockade and flattening or inversion of the T wave on the electrocardiogram.

Pharmacokinetics

Following oral administration, the tricyclic antidepressants are absorbed relatively rapidly with peak plasma levels generally occurring within 2 to 4 h. Although absorption of tricyclic antidepressants from the gastrointestinal tract is complete, these drugs are not 100 percent bioavailable because the amount of drug is reduced by the hepatic "first pass" effect. There is considerable inter-subject and inter-drug variability in the magnitude of the first pass effect owing mainly to differences in the activity of the hepatic microsomal drug-metabolizing enzymes. This appears to be of major importance in determining the steady state concentration of drug for an individual. The tricyclic antidepressants are highly lipid-soluble drugs and are, therefore, widely distributed in the body. They are strongly bound to plasma proteins and to tissues. Blood levels are low (generally in the 20 to 300 ng/mL range), leading to large apparent volumes of distribution, typically 10 to 50 L/kg.

Tricyclic antidepressants are metabolized extensively by hepatic microsomal enzymes. Only small quantities of the tricyclics are excreted intact. A major pathway for the tertiary amine tricyclics is demethylation to the corresponding secondary amine; e.g., imipramine is demethylated to desipramine, amitriptyline to nortriptyline, and doxepin to desmethyldoxepin. Thus, patients treated with tertiary amine tricyclics will be exposed, in addition, to the corresponding secondary amine metabolites, which themselves have antidepressant activity. (Desmethyldoxepin has antidepressant activity although it is not marketed as a separate drug, in contrast to desipramine and nortriptyline). In some subjects, the extent of demethylation is so great that the predominant pharmacologically active compound present in the body of patients taking a tertiary amine tricyclic is the secondary amine metabolite. Since the demethylation reaction is not reversible, patients treated with a secondary amine tricyclic are exposed only to the parent compound and not to the corresponding tertiary amine. Thus, patients treated with desipramine or nortriptyline are not exposed to imipramine or amitriptyline.

Hydroxylation on the ring structure is another important metabolic pathway for these drugs. The hydroxylated metabolites are excreted in urine, mainly in the form of their glucuronides. Other relatively minor metabolic pathways for the tricyclics include loss of the side chain, oxidation of the amine group to form N-oxides and demethylation of the secondary amine to form primary amines. With the possible exception of the N-oxides, these pathways lead to inactive metabolites.

The half-lives of the different tricyclics vary widely among themselves. Some estimates of these half-lives are shown in Table 21-3. In general, the half-lives of the secondary amine tricyclics are longer than those of the tertiary amine drugs. For the tertiary tricyclics, it is, however, important to consider not only the half-life of the parent compound but also that of the secondary amine metabolite. The rates of metabolism of tricyclic antidepressants also varies widely among the individuals receiving them. Differences in plasma levels of three-fold and greater have been found among groups of patients treated with the same dose of tricyclic drug, and variations of five- to ten-fold are relatively common. This variability arises primarily from genetic differences in the activity of the hepatic microsomal drug metabolizing enzymes. Individual differences in volume of distribution of drug also contribute to these variations. Additional factors may involve concurrent administration of other drugs and, possibly, smoking.

Adverse Effects

These drugs do produce prominent side effects. Most common are their antimuscarinic effects, which may be evident in over 50 percent of patients. Clinically, the antimuscarinic effects may manifest as dry mouth, blurred vision (due to loss of accommodation), constipation, tachycardia or palpitations, dizziness, and urinary retention. Such side effects may be nothing more than bothersome in young, depressed adults who are otherwise healthy, but can be intolerable in the elderly. The anticholinergic properties of the tricyclic antidepressants can precipitate an acute confusional state in the elderly. Also, constipation can lead to fecal impaction, and acute glaucoma may be precipitated in the presence of a narrow-angle glaucoma. As depression is one of the most common psychiatric disorders in the elderly, with

TABLE 21-3 Usual doses and elimination half-lives of antidepressant drugs

Drug	Usual daily dose[a], mg	Maximal daily dose, mg	Plasma elimination half-life
TRICYCLIC ANTIDEPRESSANTS			
Amitriptyline	75 to 150	300	10 to 25 h
Desipramine	75 to 150	300	7 to 60 h
Doxepin	50 to 150	300	8 to 25 h
Imipramine	50 to 200	300	4 to 18 h
Nortriptyline	75 to 100	150	13 to 90 h
Protriptyline	15 to 40	60	2 to 5 days
Trimipramine	50 to 150	300	Similar to imipramine?
Amoxapine	200 to 300	600	7 to 8 h
Maprotiline	75 to 150	225	1.5 to 4.5 days
SEROTONIN UPTAKE BLOCKERS			
Fluoxetine	20 to 40	80	1 to 3 days
Sertraline	50 to 100	200	26 h
Paroxetine	20	50	21 h
OTHER CYCLIC ANTIDEPRESSANTS			
Trazodone	150 to 400	600	2 to 11 h
Bupropion	200 to 400	450	8 to 24 h
MONOAMINE OXIDASE INHIBITORS			
Phenelzine	45 to 60	90	1.5 to 4 h
Tranylcypromine	20 to 30	60	1.5 to 3 h

[a] Usual dosage range for depressed patients without other serious medical diseases. Adolescent, brain-injured, or elderly patients generally require lower doses.

prevalence rates of from 2 to 18 percent, antidepressants with minimal anticholinergic effects may be of particular use in this patient population (see Table 21-1).

In addition to antimuscarinic effects, the tricyclic antidepressants can cause cardiovascular side effects. In otherwise healthy individuals, perhaps the most clinically significant cardiovascular effect is orthostatic hypotension, due, at least partly, to the α_1-adrenergic blocking properties of these drugs (see Tables 21-1 and 21-2). There is some evidence that nortriptyline may causes less orthostatic hypotension than imipramine. Changes in myocardial conduction are caused also by the tricyclics. At "therapeutic" plasma concentrations, these drugs usually do not cause changes in the electrocardiogram (EKG). However, at plasma concentrations only moderately higher than the usual "therapeutic" ones, these drugs will increase the PR interval because of an increase in intraventricular conduction time (i.e., the AV interval). These drugs also cause an inversion or flattening of the T wave. In depressed patients with normal cardiac conduction, the changes in cardiac conduction caused by the tricyclics are, in the main, not clinically significant. However, there is an increased tendency for patients with preexisting cardiac conduction disease to develop AV block when treated with a tricyclic antidepressant (Table 21-2).

The direct cardiac effects of the tricyclic antidepressants are important in overdosage, as death from these agents can result from heart block and/or arrhythmias. Unfortunately, overdosage is not an uncommon event, since these drugs are prescribed for depressed patients, some of whom may be suicidal. The third most common cause of drug-related death is alcohol-drug combinations and heroin. Symptoms of tricyclic antidepressant overdosage include slurred speech, confusion, coma, tachycardia, hypotension, respiratory distress, conduction delays, and seizures. Such symptoms may persist for days, given the relatively long half-lives of these drugs. Treatment should be directed at removal of the drug from the stomach and support of vital functions.

There are a number of CNS side effects produced by the tricyclic antidepressants that are clinically significant. These drugs lower the seizure threshold and can increase the risk of tonic-clonic seizures. Other CNS effects may include confusion or delirium, and a fine tremor may be produced in some patients, especially the elderly. Many of the tricyclics are sedative, presumably because of either their strong antihistaminic and/or α_1-adrenergic antagonist properties (see Tables 21-1 and 21-2). In depressives with the diagnosis of bipolar illness, tricyclics can precipitate the transition from depression into mania or hypomania, the so-called "switch process". Because of this, caution should be exercised in prescribing tricyclic antidepressants to bipolar patients not taking lithium carbonate or to first-time depressives with a strong family history of mania or hypomania. Although not a side effect, it should be noted that these drugs cause changes in the characteristic stages of sleep, in particular an increase in stage 4 sleep and a very marked decrease in time spent in paradoxical, or rapid-eye movement (REM), sleep.

Finally, the safety of these drugs during pregnancy or in the treatment of young children is not well established. Although there are no convincing data linking tricyclic antidepressants with teratogenic effects, it is advisable to avoid the use of these drugs in the first trimester of pregnancy.

Drug Interactions

A number of drug-drug interactions involving the tricyclic antidepressants are of potential importance. Tricyclic antidepressants block the antihypertensive effects of guanethidine and similarly acting agents by blocking their uptake into adrenergic neurons. They also block the centrally-mediated antihypertensive effect of clonidine. The tricyclic antidepressants potentiate the effects of sympathomimetic agents such as norepinephrine and epinephrine which are normally inactivated by neuronal uptake; these effects can be severe. In contrast, they block the effects of indirectly acting sympathomimetic agents, such as tyramine, which must be taken up into neurons to cause release of norepinephrine. Tricyclic antidepressants may potentiate the effects of CNS depressants such as alcohol, sedatives, or hypnotics. Barbiturates stimulate the metabolism of the tricyclic antidepressants and hence reduce plasma levels. The clinical importance of this effect has not been demonstrated. Benzodiazepines do not appear to affect the metabolism of the tricyclic antidepressants. Concurrent administration of amitriptyline and ethchlorvynol has been reported to produce transient delirium.

Although monoamine oxidase inhibitors and tricyclic antidepressants can be administered together safely in patients, these drugs, when administered together, have been occasionally reported to produce severe CNS toxicity, including hyperpyrexia, convulsions, and coma. It is generally recommended that these drugs not be given together and that at least 2 weeks separate the initiation of the administration of tricyclic antidepressants following termination of monoamine oxidase inhibitor therapy. Conversely, it is generally recommended that monoamine oxidase inhibitors not be administered until 7 to 10 days following termination of tricyclic antidepressant therapy.

The anticholinergic effects of the tricyclic antidepressants may delay gastric emptying; this can result in substantial inactivation in the stomach of drugs such as levodopa and phenylbutazone, which are absorbed from the intestine. A number of drugs increase plasma levels of the tricyclic antidepressants by inhibiting the activity of the hepatic microsomal drug metabolizing enzymes. Most neuroleptics increase plasma levels of tricyclic antidepressants, and this has occasionally been associated with ECG changes (AV block or changes associated with myocardial ischemia). Other drugs which have been demonstrated to increase plasma levels of these drugs are methylphenidate and cimetidine. Whereas the clinical significance of these effects has not been demonstrated conclusively, it would be expected that drugs that inhibit the metabolism of tricyclics would decrease the dose of the antidepressant necessary for beneficial therapeutic effect.

Amoxapine and Maprotiline

These two drugs are classified as tricyclic antidepressants because of somewhat similar chemical structure and their pharmacological profile. Maprotiline is actually a tetracyclic compound. Both of these antidepressants primarily block the reuptake of norepinephrine into adrenergic neuronal terminals, and thereby bring about a down-regulation of adrenergic receptors on the postsynaptic membranes.

The pharmacokinetics of these compounds are similar to the aforementioned tricyclic antidepressants. Amoxapine is biotransformed to active hydroxylated products in the liver.

These drugs have antimuscarinic properties and cause sedation. Maprotiline seems to cause similar cardiac effects as do the tricyclic antidepressants, whereas the cardiac effects of amoxapine may be slightly less than those of the tricyclic antidepressants. There does seem to be an increased risk for seizure development in patients treated with maprotiline; however, there is a greater incidence of seizures after overdosage with maprotiline than with tricyclic antidepressants. The incidence of seizures after overdosage with amoxapine is also relatively high.

Amoxapine is unique in having neuroleptic activity, presumably because of its structural relationship to the antipsychotic drug, loxapine. Consequently, this drug is also a potent antagonist of dopamine at dopamine (D_2) receptors. Treatment with amoxapine can produce many of the movement disorders, e.g., dystonia, akathesia, akinesia, and parkinsonism, that can be associated with neuroleptic treatment. Amoxapine can also cause galactorrhea.

SEROTONIN UPTAKE INHIBITORS

The first member of this class of antidepressants was fluoxetine which was introduced in 1988 in the United States. Since then, two other serotonin uptake inhibitors were introduced: sertraline and paroxetine. All these compounds have been demonstrated to be effective antidepressants. Fluoxetine in the most widely prescribed drug of this group at the present time.

Chemistry

Fluoxetine is a phenylpropylamine derivative, sertraline is a naphthalenamine derivative, and paroxetine is a phenylpiperidine derivative. All are secondary amines, but are chemically unrelated to the other antidepressants.

Mechanism of Action

These antidepressants appear to alleviate depression by blocking the reuptake of serotonin from the synaptic space (Table 21-1). The increased amount of serotonin that is chronically maintained at the postsynaptic membrane brings about a down-regulation of serotonin receptors. It is noteworthy that primary action on either norepinephrine or serotonin uptake mechanism can result in an antidepressant effect.

Pharmacokinetics

Fluoxetine is absorbed almost completely following oral administration, although the rate of absorption is relatively slow with maximal blood levels generally not seen until 4 to 8 h after dosing. Bioavailability is close to 100 percent, since the first pass effect is small. Fluoxetine is a lipophilic compound which, like the tricyclics, is highly bound to plasma proteins and has a large apparent volume of distribution (averaging approximately 30 L/kg). Fluoxetine is demethylated in the liver to an active compound, norfluoxetine. The half-lives of fluoxetine and norfluoxetine are long, with values reported in the range of 1 to 3 days for fluoxetine and 3 to 15 days for norfluoxetine. There is also some preliminary evidence that the half-life of fluoxetine increases on repeated administration of the drug, although the half-life of the metabolite does not appear to be affected. The long half-lives of fluoxetine and norfluoxetine are consistent with the clinical practice of prescribing this drug on a once-a-day dosing schedule. Only small amounts of fluoxetine and its demethylated metabolite are excreted intact; most are excreted in the form of conjugated metabolites whose identities have not yet been determined. Plasma levels of fluoxetine and norfluoxetine vary widely among individuals, but it is not known whether these levels correlate with the clinical response.

Sertraline reaches its peak plasma level between 4 and 8 hours after dosing and has an elimination half-life of approximately 26 hours. The presence of food in the stomach appears to enhance slightly the bioavailability of this antidepressant. Sertraline is highly bound to plasma proteins. Following single dose administration of sertraline, it takes about one week to reach steady state plasma levels of the drug. The drug is biotransformed in the liver first by an N-demethylation reaction which forms N-desmethylsertraline. This metabolite is less active than the parent compound. Further biotransformation of sertraline and its N-desmethyl derivative occurs by oxidative deamination, reduction, hydroxylation, and then conjugation with glucuronic acid. The metabolites of sertraline are excreted in the urine and feces. Unchanged sertraline is found only in feces.

Paroxetine is well absorbed following oral administration. The drug is widely distributed in the body. Its protein binding in plasma is greater than 90 percent. At the steady state, the elimination half-life of paroxetine is about 21 hours. This antidepressant is biotransformed by oxidation and methylation followed by conjugation with either sulfate or glucuronic acid. Elimination from the body is by excretion in the urine and feces.

Adverse Reactions

The serotonin uptake blockers appear to be better tolerated by many patients than the tricyclic antidepressants. These drug do not produce significant sedation, adrenergic receptor blockade or weight gain. Side effects reported with these antidepressants include dizziness, CNS stimulation, insomnia (although somnolence has occurred in some patients), anxiety, restlessness (especially with fluoxetine), gastrointestinal upset, dry mouth, tremors, and anorgasmia in women and ejaculatory delay in men. These drugs cause less toxicities in overdosage, particularly of a cardiovascular nature, when compared with the tricyclic compounds. Although rare, the serotonin uptake blockers may cause seizures and extrapyramidal effects.

Drug Interactions

Fluoxetine is contraindicated with monoamine oxidase inhibitors and after stopping a monoamine oxidase inhibitor up to 5 weeks should pass before using fluoxetine. When fluoxetine was administered with other antidepressants, it increased plasma levels of other antidepressants by approximately two-fold. Patients receiving lithium should have their plasma levels monitored if fluoxetine is administered. This antidepressant also prolongs the half-life of diazepam. Caution should be exercised if other CNS active drugs are given together with fluoxetine. Drugs that are highly bound to plasma proteins (e.g., warfarin and digitoxin) may have their effects enhanced if fluoxetine is administered.

Sertraline also may potentiate the effects of drugs that are highly bound to plasma proteins and may potentiate the effects of diazepam and tolbutamide. Monoamine oxidase inhibitors should be discontinued for at least 2 weeks before sertraline is given. Other CNS active drugs should be used with caution in the presence of this compound.

Paroxetine should be administered only after a monoamine oxidase inhibitor has been stopped for at least 2 weeks. The effects of drugs that exhibit high protein binding may be enhanced with the administration of paroxetine. Phenobarbital may reduce the effectiveness of this antidepressant. It is suggest that plasma levels of lithium, digoxin, warfarin, and phenytoin should be monitored when paroxetine is administered. The dosage of procyclidine should be decreased in the presence of paroxetine.

In addition, alcohol and tryptophan should be avoided when serotonin uptake blockers are administered.

OTHER CYCLIC AGENTS

Trazodone and Bupropion

The two antidepressants in this group are trazodone and bupropion. Trazodone has weak activity in blocking the reuptake of serotonin and norepinephrine and it appears that other mechanisms are involved in its antidepressant action such as antagonism of serotonin at its receptor sites. Bupropion is a blocker of dopamine reuptake in the CNS.

Trazodone causes little or no antimuscarinic effects; however, it can produce sedation similar to the tricyclic antidepressants. Lightheadedness, orthostatic hypotension, and confusion can occur. Of serious concern with trazodone is the fact that it can cause priapism, a number of cases of which have required corrective surgery or caused permanent loss of erectile function.

Adverse reactions with bupropion may include agitation, insomnia, confusion, activation of psychosis or mania, and fewer antimuscarinic and cardiac effects than the tricyclic antidepressants. Experience with bupropion overdosage has been limited; however, seizures are prominent, occurring in a significant number of patients. Bupropion overdosage is treated supportively, with most patients recovering without serious sequelae. Few deaths have been reported and only occurred with massive doses.

MONOAMINE OXIDASE INHIBITORS

These drugs appear to act by combining irreversibly with the enzyme monoamine oxidase (MAO), thereby inactivating it. Phenelzine and tranylcypromine are the only two monoamine oxidase inhibitors available in the United States.

Chemistry

Phenelzine is the hydrazide analog of phenylethylamine. Tranylcypromine is *trans*-2-phenylcyclopropylamine, a cyclopropyl analog of phenylethylamine and amphetamine; it consists of a racemic mixture (see Fig. 21-1).

Mechanism of Action

Phenelzine and tranylcypromine inhibit MAO by forming covalent bonds at the active site of the enzyme. Phenelzine inactivates MAO by reacting with the flavin prosthetic group of the enzyme. Inactivation of MAO by tranylcypromine appears to involve the reaction of an activated intermediate with a group (probably a sulfhydryl group) in the active site of the enzyme itself.

The monoamine oxidase inhibitors increase the availability of endogenous amines such as norepinephrine and serotonin in the CNS by inhibiting intracellular deamination of these amines; their antidepressant effect might result from this inhibitory action. Although these antidepressants inactivate MAO almost immediately and their maximum effect on the enzyme occurs within 24 to 48 h, the therapeutic effect derived from administration of these drugs is not observed for about 2 to 3 weeks. As in the case of the tricyclic antidepressants, one hypothesis for the mechanism of action of the monoamine oxidase inhibitors suggests that chronic administration of these drugs increases the concentration of biogenic amines in the synapse and eventually causes a down-regulation of the β-adrenergic and serotonin receptors in the postsynaptic membrane. Although down-regulation of biogenic amine receptors might play a role in the antidepressant effect of monoamine oxidase inhibitors, it appears that their mechanism of action is complex and not completely understood at the present time.

Tranylcypromine possesses two modes of action. The first is due to its potent inhibition of MAO, and the second is the result of an amphetamine-like action. The latter effect has been attributed to the release of norepinephrine from central neurons.

The more rapid onset of action of tranylcypromine may be a consequence of its amphetamine-like action and its sustained antidepressant effects may be related to the biochemical events produced by the inhibition of MAO. Thus, this nonhydrazide drug has sometimes has been referred to as a "bimodal" antidepressant.

Pharmacokinetics

Surprisingly little is known about the metabolism and pharmacokinetics of the monoamine oxidase inhibitors due, in part, to the fact that these drugs received FDA approval before 1962, a time when such detailed studies were not required. Despite extensive clinical use for over 20 years, the metabolism of phenelzine is poorly understood. Although the effects of phenelzine on MAO are long-term, the drug itself is rapidly absorbed following oral administration and is rapidly cleared from plasma (half-life, 1.5 to 4 h) (see Table 21-3). Until recently, it had been thought that acetylation represented the major pathway for drug inactivation. However, more recent studies have failed to find the acetylated derivative in plasma or urine and it appears now that oxidation rather than acetylation is the major metabolic pathway for this drug. The major metabolic products are phenylacetic acid and *para*-hydroxyphenylacetic acid. The drug may inhibit its own metabolism somewhat, since steady-state plasma concentrations gradually increase over the initial 5 to 8 weeks of chronic treatment.

Tranylcypromine is absorbed rapidly with peak levels occurring 40 min to 3.5 h after each dose. Elimination is also rapid with a half-life of from 1.5 to 3 h.

Adverse Effects

Some of the side effects caused by monoamine oxidase inhibitors are similar to those produced by the tricyclic antidepressants. For example, orthostatic hypotension is produced by monoamine oxidase inhibitors. The hypotensive effect has been attributed to either (1) heightened stimulation of central α-adrenoceptors due to the buildup of norepinephrine in brain, which can lead to a reduction in sympathetic outflow from the CNS or (2) the accumulation of the "false transmitter", octopamine, in peripheral sympathetic nerve terminals, with the displacement of norepinephrine from the same terminals. Octopamine has much less of an effect at α-adrenoceptors than does norepinephrine, and consequently sympathetic tone is diminished. In addition, the monoamine oxidase inhibitors may also precipitate hypomanic or manic episodes in bipolar depressives. Again similar to the tricyclics, inhibitors of MAO produce very marked reductions in the time spent in REM sleep.

Other clinically significant side effects caused by these drugs include excessive weight gain, sexual dysfunction, insomnia, and bipedal edema. As opposed to tricyclic antidepressants, inhibitors of MAO do not seem to have any important direct cardiac effects or prominent anticholinergic effects. Because of this, their use is increasing in the treatment of the elderly depressive.

Monoamine oxidase inhibitors can elicit a hypertensive crisis, and this has, perhaps unduly, led practitioners to avoid their use. Often times, the high blood pressure elicits a headache which may be associated with sweating, pallor, nausea, and vomiting. These painful, frightening attacks usually end in several hours. However, more serious and even fatal syndromes, such as intracranial hemorrhage, can develop. The drug-induced hypertensive crises result from the ingestion of foodstuffs containing agents that can cause the release of stored norepinephrine, i.e., indirectly acting sympathomimetic amines such as tyramine. Tyramine is normally metabolized by MAO in the gastrointestinal tract and does not enter into the circulation in appreciable amounts. However, when MAO is inhibited, tyramine enters the circulation to release greater than normal amounts of norepinephrine stored in sympathetic nerve terminals and the adrenal medulla. Foodstuffs such as aged and overripe cheeses, certain prepared meats such as chicken liver pâté, smoked meats such as sausages, preserved foods such as pickled herring, broad bean pods, and certain yeast products contain a variety of indirectly acting sympathomimetic amines. For this reason, patients treated with monoamine oxidase inhibitors are placed on diets which either eliminate entirely or reduce substantially such foodstuffs. Perhaps even more problematic for patients on these drugs are sympathomimetic drugs contained in over-the-counter medications (see "Drug Interactions," below).

Documented deaths due to overdosage with monoamine oxidase inhibitors have been infrequent. However, overdosage with these drugs can cause a toxic syndrome characterized by altered mental status, hyperpyrexia, and hyperreflexia, which may progress to metabolic acidosis, seizures, and cardiovascular collapse. Treatment of this state is primarily supportive in nature and should include procedures to reduce or retard further drug absorption.

Drug Interactions

The hypertensive effects of sympathomimetic agents during monoamine oxidase inhibitor therapy can be potentiated. This effect is greater with indirectly acting amines than with directly acting amines. Significant interactions have been observed with both centrally and peripherally acting sympathomimetics including nonprescription or prescription cold remedies that contain pressor agents. Parenteral administration of guanethidine with a monoamine oxidase inhibitor may cause a severe pressor response as a result of a sudden release of accumulated catecholamines. It is generally recommended that monoamine oxidase inhibitors not be administered concurrently with levodopa, since agitation and hypertension can result. It is also recommended that CNS depressants be administered cautiously to patients receiving monoamine oxidase inhibitors to avoid excessive sedation and acute hypotension. The hypotensive and CNS depressant effects of general and local anesthetics may also be enhanced in patients taking these drugs. Meperidine should not be given to patients on monoamine oxidase inhibitors, since a rapid hyperpyrexia reaction, which appears to be mediated via serotonin release, can occur. Finally, a period of a least 2 weeks is recommended when switching from one monoamine oxidase inhibitor to another.

THERAPEUTIC USES OF ANTIDEPRESSANTS

Depression

As stated previously, the use of these drugs should be restricted to patients having a psychiatric diagnosis of depression rather than a transient dysphoric mood.

The physician is faced with a choice from a number of drugs. The choice between monoamine oxidase inhibitors and other antidepressants would weigh in favor of the other drugs because of the risk of hypertensive crises with the inhibitors of MAO. However, clinical trials indicate that monoamine oxidase inhibitors may be more effective in patients presenting with "atypical" depression.

When starting treatment with a tricyclic antidepressant, it is better to start with a lower dose and gradually to increase the dose until good clinical results are obtained in the absence of serious side effects. The tricyclic antidepressants have a sedative effect, so the dose is generally given at bedtime.

Serotonin uptake blockers are effective antidepressants and may be considered for initial therapy in the treatment of depression or they may be used in patients who are not receiving adequate relief from their depression with tricyclic antidepressants. In addition, for patients who cannot tolerate tricyclic antidepressants, these newer agents should be considered. Serotonin uptake blockers do offer certain advantages over the tricyclic antidepressants, notably an absence of or relatively less anticholinergic activity and less potential to cause orthostatic hypotension or cardiac arrhythmias.

Other Uses

Panic disorder responds to treatment with tricyclic antidepressants and monoamine oxidase inhibitors. Imipramine has been most extensively used for this purpose. Akin to panic disorder are the *phobic disorders*. Agarophobia has been most commonly treated with imipramine or phenelzine while fluoxetine shows great promise in the treatment of global social phobias which has also been treated effectively with phenelzine.

Enuresis, or bed-wetting in children over six years old, is responsive to treatment with imipramine, which is a drug of choice for this condition.

Chronic pain syndromes, whether or not they are a part of the overall major depressive state, are often managed with antidepressants, all of which have some analgesic properties in addition to their antidepressant effects. In general, doses lower than those employed to treat major depression are used.

The binge eating of *bulimia nervosa* has been controlled by treatment with tricyclic antidepressants, monoamine oxidase inhibitors, and fluoxetine. Of the tricyclics, desipramine, which is less likely to stimulate appetite and weight gain, is preferred. At present, this condition is a contraindication to the use of bupropion since bulimic patients were reported to have an increased incidence of seizures when they were treated for depression with bupropion.

Obsessive compulsive disorder responds well to treatment with fluoxetine, which is a drug of choice for this condition. Three months of treatment may be required for maximum therapeutic benefit.

Sleep disorders of two types have been found to respond to treatment with tricyclic antidepressants. Protriptyline, the tricyclic with some stimulant properties, has become the drug of choice for cataplexy. Obstructive sleep apnea has been effectively treated with both protriptyline and imipramine.

BIBLIOGRAPHY

Baldessarini, R.J.: "Current Status of Antidepressants: Clinical Pharmacology and Therapy," *J. Clin. Psychiatry* **50**: 117-126 (1989).

Blackwell, B.: "Newer Antidepressant Drugs," in H.Y. Meltzer (ed.), *Psychopharmacology. The Third Generation of Progress*, Raven Press, New York, 1987, pp. 1041-1049.

Blier, P., C. de Montigny, and Y. Chaput: "Modifications of the Serotonin System by Antidepressant Treatments: Implications or the Therapeutic Response in Major Depression," *J. Clin. Psychopharmacol.* **7**: 24S-25S (1987).

Brotman, A.W., W.E. Falk, and A.J. Gelenberg: "Pharmacologic Treatment of Acute Depressive Subtypes," in H.Y. Meltzer (ed.), *Psychopharmacology. The Third Generation of Progress*, Raven Press, New York, 1987, pp. 1031-1040.

Fisher, S., S.G., Bryant, and T.A. Kent: "Postmarketing Surveillance by Patient Self-monitoring: Trazadone versus Fluoxetine", *J. Clin. Psychopharmacol.* **13**: 235-242 (1993).

Glassman, A.H., S.P. Roose, and J.T. Bigger, Jr.: "The Safety of Tricyclic Antidepressants in Cardiac Patients", *J. Am. Med. Assoc.* **269**: 2673-2675 (1993).

Glassman, A.H., S.P. Roose, E.G.V. Giardina, and J.T. Bigger, Jr.: "Cardiovascular Effects of Tricyclic Antidepressants," in H.Y. Meltzer (ed.), *Psychopharmacology. The Third Generation of Progress*, Raven Press, New York, 1987, pp. 1437-1442.

Herringer, G.R., and D.S. Charney: "Mechanism of Action of Antidepressant Treatments: Implications for the Etiology and Treatment of Depressive Disorders," in H.Y. Meltzer (ed.), *Psychopharmacology. The Third Generation of Progress*, Raven Press, New York, 1987, pp. 535-544.

Katz, M.M., S.H. Koslow, J.W. Maas, A. Frazer, C.L. Bowden, R. Casper, J. Croughan, J. Kocsis, and E. Redmond, Jr.: "The Timing, Specificity and Clinical Prediction of Tricyclic Drug Effects in Depression," *Psychol. Med.* **17**: 297-309 (1987).

Murphy, D.L., C.S. Aulakh, N.A. Garrick, and T. Sunderland: "Monamine Oxidase Inhibitors as Antidepressants: Implications for the Mechanism of Action of Antidepressants and the Psychobiology of the Affective Disorders and Some Related Disorders," in H.Y. Meltzer (ed.), *Psychopharmacology. The Third Generation of Progress*, Raven Press, New York, 1987, pp. 545-552.

Piridsky, D.M. and J.S. Cohn: *Clinical Primer of Psychopharmacology. A Practical Guide*, McGraw-Hill, Inc., New York, 1992, pp. 33-71.

Plotkin, D.A., C. Gerson, and L.F. Jarvik: "Antidepressant Drug Treatment in the Elderly," in H.Y. Meltzer (ed.), *Psychopharmacology. The Third Generation of Progress*, Raven Press, New York, 1987, pp. 1149-1158.

Wander, T.J., A. Nelson, H. Okazaki, and E. Richelson: "Antagonism by Antidepressants of Serotonin S_1 and S_2 Receptors of Normal Human Brain in Vitro," *Eur. J. Pharmacol.* **132**: 115-121 (1986).

Warrington, S.J.: "Clinical Implications of the Pharmacology of Serotonin Reuptake Inhibitors", *Internat. Clin. Psychopharmacol.* **7 (Suppl. 2)**: 13-19 (1992).

CHAPTER 22

Antiepileptic and Antiparkinsonian Drugs

Arthur Raines

EPILEPSY

Epilepsy is a syndrome characterized by recurrent seizures, i.e., paroxysmal alterations in behavior caused by abnormal cerebral electrical discharges. The seizures may manifest as abnormal motor and/or sensory function as well as changes in affect or consciousness. Seizures are usually brief events lasting from a few seconds to several minutes, but can, at times, go on for protracted periods and, when of the generalized tonic-clonic type, can be life-threatening as in status epilepticus. Epilepsy was described in ancient times and is a common illness estimated to affect 0.5 to 1 percent of the population. Known causes of epilepsy include head trauma, neoplasms or other space-occupying lesions in the brain, vascular abnormalities, scarring, and infectious processes. The single most common etiology however, occurring in perhaps 70 to 75 percent of patients, is "idiopathic" (cause unknown). A familial tendency to inherit a low seizure threshold is well recognized and epilepsy often occurs in relatives of persons with idiopathic epilepsy. Approximately 75 percent of patients with epilepsy can have their seizure frequency substantially reduced by drug therapy. In those cases not adequately controlled by medication, surgical therapy may be an option to either extirpate a triggering focus or interrupt the spread of a seizure by sectioning neural pathways.

The time during which a seizure occurs is referred to as the *ictal period*, the time between seizures, the *inter-ictal period* and the time immediately after the seizure as the *post-ictal period*. The latter is a period of recovery from excessive neural discharges and symptoms range from none, to headache, to confusion, to profound exhaustion depending on the intensity and duration of the ictal phase.

A large number of seizure types can occur; they may be convulsive, involving massive motor manifestations or they may be non-convulsive, involving loss of some function (postural tone, control of movement, consciousness). An overview of the international classification of seizures helps in the communication among health care workers and between health care workers and patients. A proper characterization of the seizure is necessary to increase the probability that drug selection will prove successful. That is, e.g., the agents phenytoin and carbamazepine, although quite effective in generalized tonic-clonic seizures and complex partial seizures, are not effective in generalized absence seizures. The classification which follows is a simplified version suitable for a rational approach to drug therapy.

I. Partial seizures (these involve limited areas of the brain)

   A. Simple partial seizures — motor or sensory (focal seizures)
   B. Complex partial seizures (formerly *psychomotor* or *temporal lobe*)
   C. Partial seizures which become secondarily generalized

II. Generalized seizures (these involve extensive areas of the brain)

   A. Tonic-clonic seizures (formerly *grand mal*)
   B. Absence seizures (formerly *petit mal*)
   C. Tonic seizures
   D. Clonic seizures
   E. Atonic seizures ("drop attacks")
   F. Akinetic seizures (arrested movement)

Partial Seizures

Partial seizures arise from one area of the brain (often referred to as an epileptogenic focus). They may remain localized to that area (simple partial) or they may spread (secondarily generalized). The initial symptomatology is usually functionally related to the locus of the focus. For instance, if seizures start in the motor strip, clonic movements of the opposite limb, face, or tongue often occur initially. The abnormal, electrical discharges can then spread along the motor strip and elsewhere to involve the entire brain, producing a secondarily generalized tonic-clonic seizure (formerly called *Jacksonian epilepsy*). If the focus is in a functionally sensory area, sensations (e.g., visceral, visual, olfactory, *deja vu*) may accompany the seizure. Many patients can recognize the preliminary symptoms of an impending seizure (the "aura") and are able to avoid harm; if the focus of the seizure is in the occipital lobe, visual hallucinations may occur. These are examples of simple partial seizures. During a simple partial seizure, consciousness is usually well preserved.

A seizure focus in the temporal lobe in the region of the hippocampus or amygdala (mesial surface) or frontal lobe can produce complex partial seizures (formerly psychomotor or temporal lobe seizures); there is loss of awareness. A person in a complex partial seizure can wander about in a dazed state, picking at clothing, lip smacking, or having other stereotyped and usually inappropriate behaviors.

Generalized Seizures

These seizures involve most or all of the cerebrum and consciousness is lost. These seizures may occur abruptly with little or no warning; although these seizures do not appear to have a focal origin, a focus deep in the brain-stem or thalamus projecting to widespread areas of the cerebrum could produce what appears to be a generalized seizure without focal origin.

Tonic-Clonic Seizures Tonic-clonic seizures, are convulsive and have two phases. The tonic phase (which is the most severe) is associated with sustained cerebral discharge observable in EEG leads and results in sustained contractures of the muscles (tonic contractions) with the stronger muscle groups of antagonists determining body configuration; the patient becomes stiff with stretched out arms and legs, ventilation is arrested as the respiratory muscles become fixed and the jaw is tightly closed. Bone breakage can occur, particularly in vertebrae and most particularly when bone loss (osteoporosis, osteomalacia) is present; tongue biting often occurs. During this (and other) generalized seizures, consciousness is lost. Urinary or fecal incontinence may occur at this time but more usually occurs after the seizure is over and sphincter tone relaxes (i.e., in the post-ictal period). The person may fall and become injured and the first intervention is usually to protect the person against injury and protect the airway. The tonic phase passes into a less intense phase when the person enters the clonic phase, which consists of alternating relaxation and contraction of the skeletal muscles. The EEG shows bursting behavior with major muscle jerkings correlating with the cerebral discharges. The duration of the seizure is quite variable and when sustained requires immediate intervention with intravenous medication, lest respiratory and cardiovascular collapse ensue. Speedy intervention may also prevent bone breakage, acid-base and electrolyte derangements, renal injury, and other complications. As noted above, seizures may also be either tonic only or clonic only.

Absence Seizures Absence seizures are an example of non-convulsive seizures and usually emerge in childhood and may persist into adulthood; occasionally they may begin after the age of 20. The attacks are characterized by sudden, brief lapses in consciousness which may be accompanied by eyelid flutter. Postural tone is preserved. The attack is usually brief (lasting 5 to 30 sec) but absence *status epilepticus* can occur lasting many hours. After the usual short episodes, the patient is alert and able to resume normal activity. These seizures can often be precipitated by hyperventilation. Absence seizures can occur with great frequency many times per day and hence can be quite debilitating. The EEG is normal between attacks and shows a characteristic 3 per sec spike and wave abnormality in all EEG leads during the attack.

Status Epilepticus Although most seizures last seconds to several minutes, at times seizure activity is sustained for protracted periods. The term *status epilepticus* is generally applied when seizure activity reaches or exceeds 30 minutes, regardless of the type of seizure at hand. Clearly the implications for survival and serious complications are quite different in convulsive and non-convulsive forms of *status epilepticus*. Termination of the seizure is attempted with intravenous medication and if that proves ineffective, general anesthesia may be required.

ANTIEPILEPTIC DRUGS

The modern and responsible use of antiepileptic medication requires an understanding of the pharmacokinetics of these agents, the periodic monitoring of serum levels and the awareness of potential drug interactions. For each antiepileptic drug, a therapeutic serum level is recognized and serves as a guide to therapy and dosage adjustment (see Table 22-1). Presently, therapy with a single agent is the goal, as keeping the drug taking regimen simple avoids confusion by the patient and the people caring for the patient; it also minimizes drug interactions which may be deleterious or unpredictable. Only after one has satisfied oneself that one drug cannot provide adequate seizure control, or by itself produces an unacceptable degree of adverse effect, that more than one drug should be used. Another justification for the use of more than one agent is the co-existence of more than one seizure type, each needing a separate drug for management.

Experience has shown that each antiepileptic medication has a serum level range within which most patients responsive to the drug will fall. Above the therapeutic range, the incidence of toxicity rises; some patients will require maximal tolerated doses and these may exceed the upper limit of the therapeutic range. Similarly some patients will be well controlled with serum levels somewhat lower than the lower limit of the usual therapeutic range. The serum levels thus serve as a valuable guide in understanding response or lack of response to medication.

These agents are used orally for the prevention (as prophylaxis) of seizures in persons who have epilepsy and are used intravenously to arrest status epilepticus.

As a first approximation, the antiepileptic drugs fall into basically two categories: those that are effective against absence seizures and those effective against both tonic-clonic seizures and complex partial seizures.

Those antiepileptic drugs effective against the latter conditions include the hydantoin derivatives (phenytoin, mephenytoin, and ethotoin), carbamazepine, some barbiturates (phenobarbital and mephobarbital), and primidone. Felbamate and

TABLE 22-1 Selected antiepileptic drugs

Drug	Usual plasma levels, μg/mL	Plasma protein binding, %	Elimination half-life, h
DRUGS FOR TONIC-CLONIC AND PARTIAL SEIZURES			
Phenytoin	10 to 20	89	6 to 24
Carbamazepine	10 to 25	74	10 to 20
Phenobarbital	15 to 40	51	90 to 100
Primidone	5 to 12	19	20 to 23
DRUGS FOR ABSENCE SEIZURES			
Ethosuximide	40 to 120	0	40 to 50
Valproic acid[a]	50 to 150	93	12 to 18
Clonazepam	15 to 70	86	20 to 25
Trimethadione	10 to 40	0	16 to 24

[a] in multiple seizures which include absence seizures

gabapentin are effective in the treatment of partial seizures. In the treatment of absence seizures, succinamides (ethosuximide, methsuximide, and phensuximide), valproic acid, certain benzodiazepines (e.g., clonazepam), acetazolamide, and the oxazolidinediones (paramethadione and trimethadione) are useful. In addition, valproic acid is considered to be a secondary drug for focal and tonic-clonic seizures. Only occasionally are drugs helpful in both categories.

Hydantoin Derivatives

The chemical structures of the hydantoin derivatives are shown in Table 22-2. They have five-membered rings and are cyclic derivatives of glycollyl urea, in contrast to the six-membered ring of the barbiturates (see below) which are cyclized derivatives of malonyl urea (Table 22-3).

Phenytoin

Originally discovered to have anticonvulsant properties in 1937 in the first experimental investigations targeted at identifying a drug for use in epilepsy, phenytoin was shown to be an effective antiepileptic agent in generalized tonic-clonic seizures in epileptic patients. In its overall effect on the central nervous system (CNS) this drug comes close to being an ideal antiepileptic drug, since unlike other agents used in the management of epilepsy, in full antiepileptic doses it has only minor sedative effects. Even in large doses it does not cause hypnosis.

TABLE 22-2 Hydantoin derivatives

Drug	R_1	R_2	R_3
Phenytoin	[benzene ring]	[benzene ring]	$-H$
Mephenytoin	[benzene ring]	$-C_2H_5$	$-CH_3$
Ethotoin	[benzene ring]	$-H$	$-C_2H_5$

Mechanism of Action The drug appears to have little effect on the initial focal discharge as patients adequately controlled by phenytoin still often experience the aura. Furthermore the initial focal discharge can often be detected, although the ensuing convulsion does not develop (i.e., it is aborted). The action of the drug thus appears to be on suppression of the spread of the discharge from an initiating site to adjacent (presumably normal) and subsequently remote brain areas. A hallmark of seizure discharge and its propagation through nervous tissue is the capacity of large numbers of neurons to discharge at exceedingly high frequencies (up to and occasionally in excess of 1000 Hz) more or less synchronously. The drug curtails the capacity of neurons to fire at very high frequencies and thus diminishes the ability of the brain to be driven into a seizure state. As high frequency discharges are needed to greatly facilitate synaptic transmission, as for example in the case of post-tetanic potentiation (PTP, a condition in which subsequent to high frequency conditioning, synapses transmit greatly augmented responses), phenytoin by preventing the high frequency discharges prevents the synaptic conditioning and hence, blocks the augmented responses and the resultant spread of seizure activity.

The mechanism whereby phenytoin suppresses high frequency discharges involves a frequency dependent blockade of voltage dependent sodium and calcium channels in nerve membranes. The drug appears to bind with axonal sodium channels in the activated or inactivated state (but seemingly not in the resting state) so that the drug binding with channel constituents is actually enhanced by nerve discharges. The drug thus has minimal effect when neurons are discharging at low frequency levels and has substantial effects at high frequencies, where the drug can find channels in a state conducive for binding and blockade. Thus at a membrane level, the actions of phenytoin are not unlike those of lidocaine and other local anesthetics. Perhaps the property of being more effective in a setting of high frequency discharge is what confers on the drug the apparent selectivity for suppression of convulsive activity, where nerve discharges are known to be exceedingly high and seemingly little effect during non-convulsive states. Phenytoin exerts analogous frequency dependent effects on calcium channels in nerve terminal structures and thus presumably limits neurotransmitter release. The alteration in these ionic fluxes appears to inhibit spread of excitation throughout the brain.

Pharmacokinetics Phenytoin is a weak acid (pK_a = 8.4) which is administered either as the acid or the sodium salt. It is absorbed primarily from the small intestine; solubility of the drug in the stomach is very low and hence little drug is available for absorption; only after moving into the small intestine where the pH rises substantially, does appreciable dissolution of the drug take place. Peak plasma levels occur from 2 to 8 hours after oral dosing and (as expected from a poorly water soluble material), larger doses lead to later peak levels. Rate and extent of absorption are subject to several factors: (1) some individuals are simply poor at absorbing the drug (malabsorbers); (2) gastrointestinal contents can inhibit absorption; calcium from dietary sources or antacids (containing calcium, aluminum or magnesium) can bind phenytoin and impair absorption, as can cholestyramine; (3) pharmaceutical formulation can be important as the poorly soluble material is even less soluble if the particle size of the drug in the dosage form is large, thus providing a reduced surface area for dissolution. Calcium salts in the dosage form can retard or prevent absorption. The volume of distribution approximates total body water. Plasma protein binding is approximately 90 percent in patients with normal amounts of circulating plasma proteins; cerebrospinal fluid and saliva contain about 10 percent of the prevailing serum concentration. Hypoproteinemia (e.g., produced by cirrhosis, malnutrition, and renal disease) requires reduced dosing due to the higher free fraction which occurs; under these conditions, determinations of free fraction are required. Hypoproteinemic patients whose doses are not reduced are at risk of drug toxicity. The high degree of plasma protein binding makes phenytoin an agent to be concerned with as regards drug interactions based on mutual displacement of protein-bound drug. Although the mean plasma half-life is about 22 h, individual differences are very large and have been reported to range from 6 to 42 h; additionally a group of genetically determined slow metabolizers have been identified who exhibit plasma half-lives in the order of 75 h.

Unlike most drugs (but like ethanol and in the case of poisoning with aspirin) phenytoin, at elevated serum levels saturates the cytochrome P-450 enzyme system which biotransforms the drug. This shift from first-order elimination to zero-order elimination creates a paradoxical situation in which the half-life of the drug appears to be longer when the serum levels are higher. Another consequence of this phenomenon is that serum levels can rise out of proportion to an increase in dose. Thus whereas a daily dose of 200 mg may produce a serum level of 3 to 7 μg/mL, and a dose of 300 mg may yield a level of 8 to 12 μg/mL, a dose of 400 mg may produce a level close to or in excess of 20 μg/mL. Clearly, daily doses that exceed the daily capacity to eliminate the drug (in humans this ranges from about 300 to 1200 mg) will lead to continuing accumulation, not a steady state level.

With usual doses, steady state levels are achieved in 4 to 5 half-lives and thus can occur in as little as a few days up to about 2 weeks; this is important as premature sampling of serum in slow metabolizers for drug determinations can be misleading. Phenytoin is biotransformed by hydroxylation in the microsomal system in the liver. Biotransformation can be increased by drugs such as phenobarbital, which induces increased activity of hepatic microsomal enzymes, but the extent of this is unpredictable. Phenytoin itself can induce microsomal enzymes. Several drugs can decrease phenytoin biotransformation; these include cimetidine, dicumarol, disulfiram, chloramphenicol, and isoniazid.

The principal metabolite of phenytoin is the parahydroxy derivative, hydroxyphenyl-phenyl hydantoin with subsequent conjugation with glucuronic acid and renal excretion. The urinary output of this compound may account for 50 to 70 percent of the total amount of drug given, with the unchanged drug accounting for less than 5 percent. Some patients have been subject to adverse effects on ordinary doses of the drug as a result of a defect in parahydroxylation or because of drug interactions mentioned above. Other hydroxylated metabolites have been identified, as well as epoxide intermediates which are thought by some to form adducts with proteins and/or nucleic acids and cause toxicity.

Therapeutic Uses The major clinical uses of phenytoin are in the treatment of tonic-clonic seizures which are or become generalized and complex partial seizures. The drug is not useful in absence seizures. Clinical response is the major determinant of dose; however measurements of serum levels are essential in the management of patients, particularly in establishing a dosing regimen in those who fail to respond to usual doses of medication or experience untoward effects. The usual therapeutic serum level of phenytoin is 10 to 20 μg/mL. Other uses of phenytoin are in paroxysmal pain syndromes such as trigeminal neuralgia, phantom limb, or peripheral nerve damage.

Adverse Reactions Adverse effects can occur in a patient at plasma levels of phenytoin less than 20 μg/mL, but are far more common at doses above this level. The most common dose-related toxicity is a motor disturbance resembling cerebellar impairment: patients experience ataxia, lack of coordination, diplopia, tremor, and a horizontal nystagmus. Some obtundation of higher function may occur, but drowsiness is uncommon. A skin rash is fairly common in as much as 5 percent of the patients and can result in serious morbidity and occasional mortality due to extensive exfoliative dermatitis; the drug should be stopped if a rash occurs, and another medication (preferably chemically unrelated) should be prescribed. Use of phenytoin can lead to hyperplasia of the gums; this is apparently due to an effect on protein metabolism and the primary gum overgrowth does not show signs of pain or inflammation; a secondary inflammatory process often develops due to entrapment of foreign material in the teeth and gums; this latter problem can be minimized with conscientious brushing and flossing of the teeth. Although the mechanism for this adverse drug effect is not entirely clear, it is known that drug, bacteria, and teeth are necessary for the hyperplasia to develop. Interestingly, other drugs with calcium ion blocking capacity (diltiazem, dihydropyridines) can also induce gingival hyperplasia. Improvement may or may not occur after drug removal and corrective surgery may be needed. Hirsutism (particularly bothersome in women and children) is another effect which is seen occasionally with this drug. Phenytoin has been associated with numerous other adverse reactions including osteomalacia, pseudolymphoma (reversible on drug cessation), hepatitis, megaloblastic anemia (due to folate reduction), and other blood dyscrasias.

Teratogenicity has been alleged to be produced by phenytoin (as has been the case for all antiepileptic drugs), but this remains controversial and the teratogenicity may be related to the underlying genetic predisposition to epilepsy and congenital malformations. Trimethadione or paramethadione, are regarded as human teratogens (mental retardation, microcephaly, characteristic facial features), as is valproic acid which increases the incidence of neural tube defects (anencephaly, spina bifida); folic acid supplementation is recommended and may be beneficial in preventing these latter effects.

Mephenytoin and Ethotoin

As seen in Table 22-2, mephenytoin differs chemically from phenytoin in two respects. At position 5 an ethyl group is substituted for one of the phenyl rings; at position 3 a methyl group is added. This latter group is readily removed in the liver, leaving phenyl-ethylhydantoin. This latter compound was used many years ago for the treatment of chorea and choreoathetosis (neurological disorders characterized by writhing movements) but the drug was abandoned due to the production of occasional fatal blood dyscrasias due to bone marrow depression, drug fever and serious dermatological effects. Thus mephenytoin is used only in patients who have not exhibited a favorable response to safer agents; these patients must have frequent blood counts.

Ethotoin is the third antiepileptic hydantoin derivative. It is less potent than phenytoin and also less toxic. It is occasionally used when a patient is allergic to phenytoin. Because the half-life is 4 h, it must be given 4 to 6 times a day.

Carbamazepine

Carbamazepine is an iminostilbene carboximide; it has a tricyclic structure like several antidepressants and cyclobenzaprine.

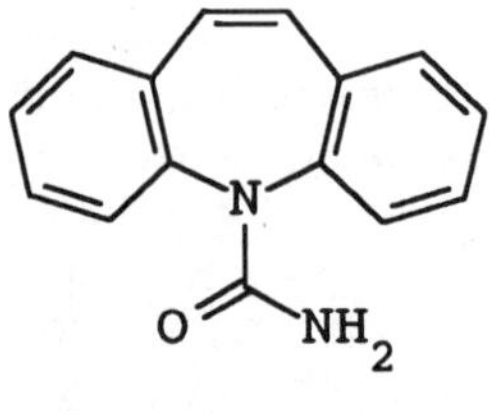

N

O NH$_2$

Carbamazepine is indicated in the treatment of tonic-clonic seizures, complex partial seizures, and mixed seizures. Although carbamazepine has not enjoyed as much investigative attention as phenytoin, the mechanism of action of the drug appears to be similar to the neuronal effects of phenytoin. With the exception of seemingly rare blood dyscrasias, it is the well tolerated and produces the least cognitive impairments as measured by neuropsychologic tests. Carbamazepine is also used for paroxysmal pain disorders such as trigeminal neuralgia and in bipolar manic-type disorders.

Pharmacokinetics Carbamazepine is reasonably well absorbed after oral dosing. Peak serum levels are usually observed 6 to 8 h after administration. Whereas its half-life initially ranges from about 12 to 30 h, in chronically treated epileptic patients the range is about 7 to 12 h due to enzyme induction. Volume of distribution of the drug is 1 L/kg. It is bound 70 percent to plasma proteins. The drug is oxidized in the liver where one metabolic product of carbamazepine, the 10,11-epoxide derivative, also possesses antiepileptic activity. This compound is inactivated by conjugation.

Adverse Reactions In high doses, carbamazepine causes a reduction of granulocytes, almost invariably to blood levels of approximately 1000 granulocytes/mm^3. The granulocytes rarely go below that level, and it is a dose-dependent phenomenon. Aplastic anemia has also been reported with carbamazepine, but the number of cases is small and thus difficult to evaluate as regards risk. However, frequent blood counts are necessary to identify hematologic changes promptly. Other adverse reactions are urinary retention, impotence, and elevated blood pressure. Dose-related side effects are similar to those of phenytoin, involving motor coordination and blurred vision. Skin allergies to carbamazepine occur, but are less frequent than with phenytoin. Like all other antiepileptic agents, this drug has also been alleged to be a human teratogen.

Barbiturates

Phenobarbital

Phenobarbital was the first antiepileptic agent and is still regarded to be a primary antiepileptic agent. The drug is regarded as the prototype barbiturate antiepileptic (Table 21-3). This drug is indicated in the treatment of generalized seizures and partial seizures.

As with other barbiturates and benzodiazepines, the efficacy of phenobarbital as an antiepileptic agent appears, at least in part, to be related to its effects on GABAergic transmission in the CNS, in which the drug enhances the capacity of GABA to open chloride channels and thus inhibit neurons. In addition, phenobarbital and other

TABLE 22-3 Barbiturates derivatives effective in epilepsy

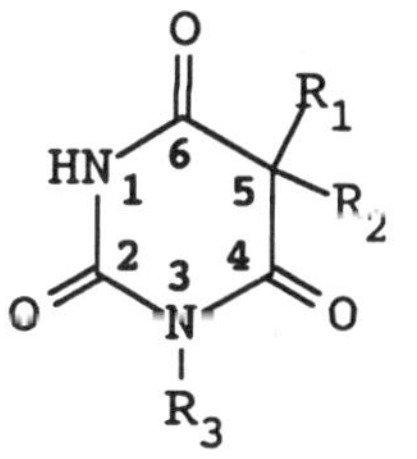

Drug	R_1	R_2	R_3
Phenobarbital	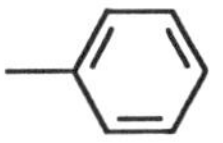	$-C_2H_5$	$-H$
Mephobarbital	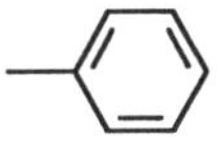	$-C_2H_5$	$-CH_3$

barbiturates seems to exert CNS depressant effects at synapses by other mechanisms such as reducing the effect of the excitatory amino acid, glutamic acid.

Pharmacokinetics Phenobarbital is slowly but essentially completely absorbed from the gastrointestinal tract with peak plasma levels occurring about 4 to 8 hours after oral dosing. The drug is approximately 50 percent protein bound and distributes itself in total body water. Phenobarbital is eliminated to the extent of about 75 percent oxidized in the liver and the balance via the kidney in a pH-dependent manner (more drug is eliminated at elevated pH due to ion-trapping). In the treatment of epilepsy the dosage of phenobarbital is approximately 2 to 3 mg/kg with a usual therapeutic blood level of between 20 and 40 μg/mL. The half-life is approximately 4 days and thus steady state levels occur in about 2 to 3 weeks if patients are receiving a maintenance dose; the use of a loading procedure may be necessary to more rapidly effect a therapeutic serum level. The long half-life of the drug proves to be very convenient as the drug can usually be taken only once a day, and blood level fluctuations vary only about 15 to 20 percent over the course of the day.

Phenobarbital is a powerful inducer of microsomal enzymes and this can lead to increased clearance of other drugs. As this is a variable and unpredictable event, serum levels of phenobarbital must be measured periodically as well as the blood levels of concomitantly administered agents.

Adverse Reactions The most common adverse effect of phenobarbital is sleepiness; this can be minimized by gradual escalation of the dose so that tolerance to the soporific effects of the drug develops. There is no evidence that tolerance develops to the antiepileptic effects of the drug. Skin rashes may occur even after the drug has been used for years but more usually after a latency of a few weeks. This requires withdrawal of the drug, for there is always the possibility of exfoliative dermatitis with a potentially fatal outcome.

Sudden withdrawal of this or any other antiepileptic drug from epileptic patients may precipitate seizures and occasionally leads to status epilepticus. For this reason, unless one has to deal with a potentially life-threatening adverse reaction, barbiturates or other antiepileptic medications should be withdrawn slowly and replaced by other drugs to prevent this complication. Rarely do the usual doses employed in epileptic therapy lead to dependence or barbiturate "inebriation". Further information on phenobarbital is presented in Chapter 16.

Mephobarbital

Mephobarbital is the 3-methyl derivative of phenobarbital (Table 22-3). This structural change makes the compound more lipid-soluble and less water-soluble.

The potency of mephobarbital is somewhat less than that of phenobarbital, but its actions on the CNS are quite similar to those of phenobarbital. Gastrointestinal absorption of mephobarbital is less complete than that of phenobarbital. In the liver, demethylation occurs; about 75 percent of an oral dose of mephobarbital is converted to phenobarbital within 24 hours. Chronic administration of the drug leads to accumulation of therapeutic concentrations of phenobarbital. It is very likely that the derived phenobarbital is responsible for most of the clinical efficacy of mephobarbital.

Primidone

The chemical structure of primidone has a close resemblance to that of the barbiturates (it is often referred to as a deoxy-barbiturate); the only difference lies in the replacement of the C=O group in position 2 by CH_2.

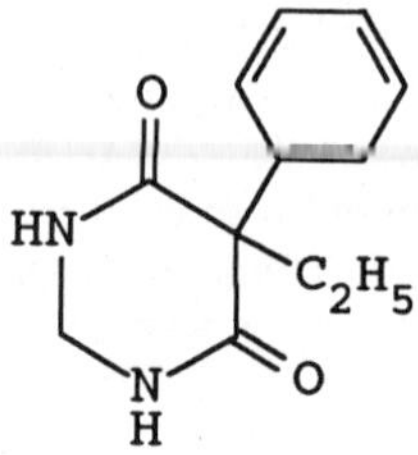

O HN C_2H_5 N H O

Approximately 15 to 25 percent of administered primidone is oxidized in the liver to phenobarbital, leading to therapeutic levels of phenobarbital which gradually accumulate. Primidone is also biotransformed to phenylethylmalonamide, the major metabolite, which has anticonvulsant activity in animals, but has not been evaluated in humans. Phenylethylmalonamide also will accumulate during chronic use of primidone. See Table 22-1 for some of the pharmacokinetics of this drug.

Primidone is useful in the treatment of tonic-clonic seizures and simple and complex partial seizures. The mechanism for the antiepileptic action of primidone appears to be similar to that of phenytoin.

Side effects such as ataxia and sedation are quite marked, even in minimal anticonvulsant doses. Because of the high incidence of drowsiness, the drug can seldom be used alone. The somnolence tends to decrease as the drug is continued (i.e., tolerance develops). Other side effects common to barbiturates, such as skin rashes, also occur. Rare instances of megaloblastic anemia have been reported.

Felbamate

This agent is one of the more recent addition to the antiepileptic drug armamentarium. Structurally it is related to meprobamate, an antianxiety agent. The drug is effective in partial seizures (with and without generalization).

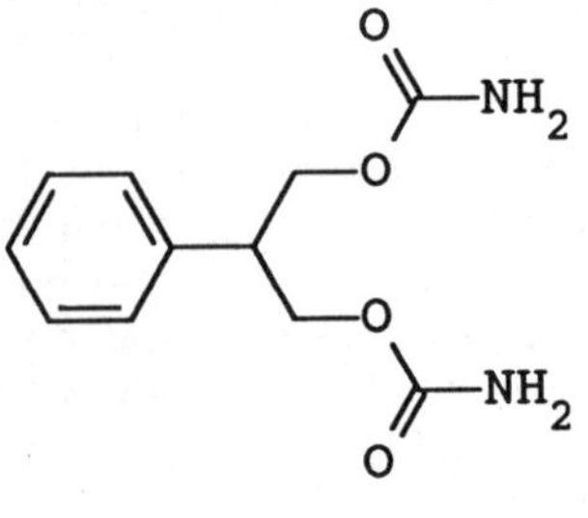

O NH_2 O O NH_2 O

Mechanism of Action The mechanism through which felbamate exerts its antiepileptic activity is unknown. *In vitro* receptor binding studies show that it has weak inhibitory activity on both GABA receptor and benzodiazepine receptor binding. It also has some antagonistic activity on the strychnine-insensitive modulatory glycine binding site on the N-methyl-D-aspartate (NMDA) receptor (see Chapter 3).

Pharmacokinetics The drug is well absorbed after oral dosing and exhibits a terminal half-life of about 22 h and does not appear to change on repeated dosing. It is only bound to plasma proteins to the extent of about 20 to 25 percent. Approximately half of the absorbed dose appears unchanged in urine. About 15 percent appears in urine as parahydroxyfelbamate, 2-hydroxyfelbamate, and felbamate monocarbamate; about 40 percent is excreted as yet to be identified metabolites.

Felbamate appears to raise phenytoin and valproate serum concentrations and a reduction in those other agents dose may be necessary when these agents are co-administered. Felbamate can reduce serum levels of carbamazepine and raise levels of the carbamazepine epoxide, effects that should also be monitored with timely serum level determinations.

Adverse Reactions Anorexia, nausea, vomiting, constipation, dizziness, headache, insomnia, somnolence, and fatigue have been observed in adults and children receiving felbamate.

Gabapentin

This drug is structurally related to γ-aminobutyric acid (GABA). However, gabapentin does not have affinity for GABA receptors, is not biotransformed to GABA or to a GABA receptor agonist, and does not alter GABA reuptake or the metabolic inactivation of GABA. Thus the mechanism of action is presently unknown. The drug is indicated as an adjunct in the therapy of partial seizures with and without secondary generalization. Presently it is being used in combination with other antiepileptic drugs.

Gabapentin is an orally active antiepileptic drug with a bioavailability of about 60 percent. Plasma protein binding is insignificant (less than 3 percent) and the drug is not biotransformed to any appreciable extent. Elimination is by the kidney; the elimination half-life is 5 to 7 h.

Common adverse reactions associated with gabapentin include somnolence, dizziness, ataxia, nystagmus, minor motor tremors, diplopia, and blurred vision. At present, hematologic abnormalities (e.g., anemia, thrombocytopenia, and elevated white cell counts) are rare.

Succinimides

A group of five-membered ring structures effective in absence seizures are the succinimides. The most important drug in this category is **ethosuximide** (or 2-ethyl-2-methylsuccinimide) which has the following structure:

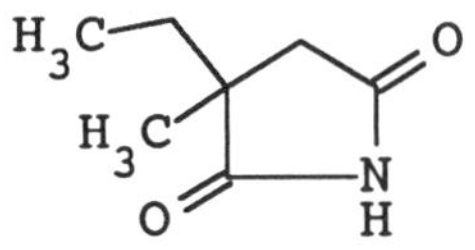

H_3C H_3C O N H O

The compound is absorbed well from the gastrointestinal tract. Peak blood levels occur between 3 and 7 h after oral administration. The volume of distribution approximates total body water. Ethosuximide is almost completely metabolized by hydroxylation in the liver, which is then followed by conjugation. The elimination half-life is approximately 30 h in children and may be as long as 60 h in adults. The therapeutic plasma levels appear in Table 22-1.

Ethosuximide is used in the treatment uncomplicated absence seizures. If a particular patient has both absence seizures and tonic-clonic seizures, then the addition of either carbamazepine or phenytoin is required because ethosuximide will not prevent tonic-clonic seizures. The mechanism of action is not clear but the drug has been shown to prolong synaptic refractoriness and to block a subclass of calcium channels (type T).

Phensuximide and **methsuximide** are two other drugs in this class that are less well tolerated than ethosuximide and probably less effective as well. There are reports in the literature that methsuximide may also be effective in complex partial seizures.

The succinimides cause sedation and drowsiness, particularly when they are given in large doses. Ethosuximide causes the least sedation in this group of antiepileptic drugs. Minor side effects are headaches, nausea, vomiting, and disequilibrium. Severe blood dyscrasias have been reported with ethosuximide but are quite rare. There are other reports of hepatic and renal dysfunction associated with these drugs.

Valproic Acid

Valproic acid is a simple eight-carbon branched-chain fatty acid (dipropylacetic acid). Valproic acid is as effective as ethosuximide in absence seizures. It is also effective for myoclonic epilepsy and somewhat effective for atypical absence seizures. This drug is considered to be helpful as adjunctive therapy with complex partial seizures and is used as an adjunct in patients with multiple seizures which include absence seizures.

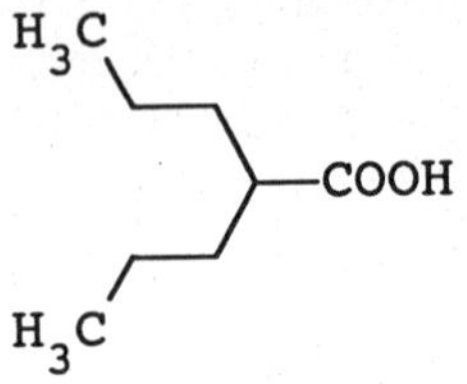

H_3C

COOH

H_3C

Mechanism of Action The mechanism of action of valproic acid may be related to an increase in brain levels of GABA that are produced by the competitive inhibition of GABA transaminase and succinic semialdehyde dehydrogenase by the drug. In addition, this antiepileptic agent reduces rapid repetitive discharges of neuronal cells by sodium channel blockade. This action of valproic acid on high-frequency repetitive neuronal firing is similar to the action of phenytoin and may explain the effectiveness of valproic acid in other types of seizures that may occur with absence seizures. These effects of valproic acid to inhibit the degradation of GABA and to block sodium channels have been proposed as possible explanations for its antiepileptic action in the CNS.

Pharmacokinetics Valproic acid is well absorbed by the oral route, and peak plasma concentrations of valproic acid are reached in 0.5 to 4 h. Its volume of distribution is 0.15 to 0.40 L/kg of body weight. Circulating valproic acid is 90 to 95 percent bound to plasma proteins. The major biotransformation pathways are beta and omega oxidations followed by conjugation. The elimination half-life is 12 to 18 h, and the therapeutic plasma level is at least 50 μg/mL and can be as high as 150 μg/mL.

Adverse Reactions Anorexia, nausea, and vomiting occur in 20 percent of patients receiving valproic acid, but these effects occur much less frequently with patients who are administered the coated tablet (divalproex) or receive smaller doses. When valproic acid is given in combination with phenobarbital, it raises the phenobarbital levels by 25 percent because of the decreased rate in the biotransformation of phenobarbital. Valproic acid can also increase the appetite in some patients and occasionally causes some sedation and produces alopecia. In high doses, valproic acid can cause delirium and hallucinations. A common side effect is an action tremor of the hands, which can be severe enough to alter handwriting and make drinking from a cup almost impossible. This is a dose-related phenomenon.

There are dose-related effects of valproic acid which produce (1) an increase in liver enzymes to 2 to 3 times the baseline level, (2) a thrombocytopenia, and (3) a decrease of fibrinogen with an associated increased bleeding time. An interaction with aspirin to induce bleeding disorders has been described. Reduction in dosage of the drug improves these side effects. An idiosyncratic hepatic failure can occur, which usually improves upon stopping the drug. Rarely does pancreatitis occur. However, there have been reported deaths from hepatic failure and pancreatitis with the use of valproic acid. This may present as Reye's syndrome. Carnitine is reported to be beneficial in counteracting this valproic acid toxicity.

Benzodiazepines

These drugs, represented by diazepam and clorazepate, are used mainly by the oral route as antianxiety agents. They have mild sedative effects along with anticonvulsant and skeletal muscle relaxant properties. The pharmacology of these agents is presented in Chapter 17. Diazepam is also used by the intravenous route in the treatment of status epilepticus. Diazepam may also have some value as a secondary drug in myoclonic spasms and atonic seizures. Another benzodiazepine derivative reported to be effective in status epilepticus is lorazepam, although at this time this is not an FDA-approved indication. The drug, clorazepate, which is used in the management of anxiety, is also indicated as an adjunct in the treatment of partial seizures. A fourth benzodiazepine derivative is clonazepam, which is described below.

Clonazepam

Clonazepam is a chlorinated benzodiazepine that is not used as an antianxiety drug but in the treatment of absence seizures, myoclonic seizures, and atonic seizures. It is quite sedating and tolerance has been shown to develop to its antiepileptic effects limiting its utility; therefore, it is not a primary antiepileptic agent.

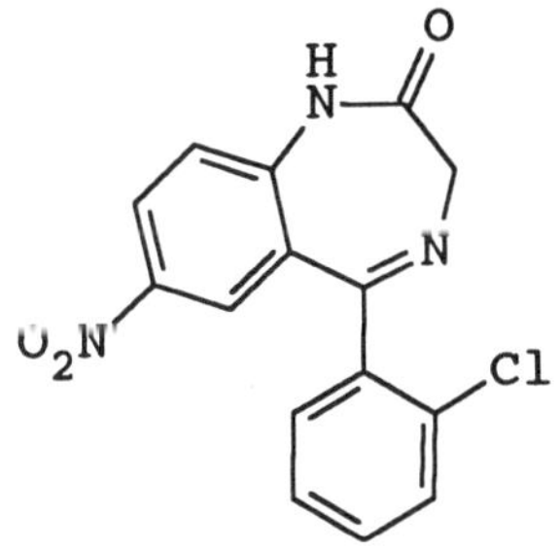

Pharmacokinetics Between 80 and 100 percent of clonazepam is absorbed via the oral route. Biotransformation involves reduction, acetylation, and hydroxylation with the formation of inactive metabolites. Protein binding is approximately 50 percent, and the elimination half-life is approximately 20 to 25 h. The therapeutic plasma level is 15 to 70 μg/mL. Because of its extreme sedation, the drug should be started at a very low dosage such as 0.5 mg/day and increased slowly.

Adverse Reactions Ataxia, drowsiness, and dysarthria are commonly seen. Exacerbation of preexisting or new seizures has been reported in 2 to 10 percent of patients. Excessive salivation and bronchial secretion, elevated liver enzymes, and blood dyscrasias are rare toxic effects.

Acetazolamide

The carbonic anhydrase inhibitor, acetazolamide, has been found clinically useful in absence seizures. However, it is regarded to be only an adjunctive agent with primary antiepileptic drugs. The adverse reactions are drowsiness, anorexia, and paresthesias of the hands and feet. Skin rashes and blood dyscrasias have been rarely reported. Further information on the pharmacology of acetazolamide is presented in Chapter 31.

Phenacemide

Phenacemide is a monoureide, resembling many older hypnotic agents. The drug is very well absorbed from the gastrointestinal tract. It is biotransformed in the liver, and its metabolites are excreted in the urine. Phenacemide is probably as efficacious as carbamazepine or phenytoin as an antiepileptic drug but is very toxic. It should be used only in the most severe forms of complex partial seizures refractory to other agents. The major adverse effects are hepatotoxicity and bone marrow depression, and in approximately one-third of the patients taking this medication a toxic psychosis occurs, appearing as a major depression. The drug has very little use today.

Oxazolidinediones

In this group there are two drugs which are closely related and both of which, **trimethadione** and **paramethadione** are used in absence seizures. These drugs have a five-membered ring structure similar to the hydantoin derivatives except that oxygen replaces the nitrogen in the 1 position. Some of the pharmacokinetics of trimethadione are listed in Table 22-1.

Large doses are required for the antiepileptic effect of these drugs, and their therapeutic indices are small; hence, frequent side effects occur such as ataxia and sedation. The most common complaints are minor skin allergies, photosensitivity, and gastric irritation. About 25 percent of patients complain of a visual disturbance, called *hemeralopia*, in which there is a visual aberration with diminished visual acuity and objects appearing whitish and, at times, dazzling as if seeing objects through snow. No optic nerve damage has been documented. Liver, kidney, and bone marrow damage have been reported.

Prior to the availability of the succinamides and valproic acid, these agents were frequently used for absence seizures; presently they are rarely used except when other agents prove unsatisfactory.

Drugs Used for the Management of Status Epilepticus

As status epilepticus represent a serious threat to life or serious morbidity, rapid intervention is often necessary to arrest the seizure; life-support equipment and trained personnel are required. The intravenous route is usually the preferred route of drug administration, as it affords a rapid and controllable means of drug administration.

Diazepam This agent can be thought of as a "broad spectrum" anti-epileptic agent, having efficacy in most types of status epilepticus. The drug is administered intravenously in doses depending on age and body size, and at a rate so that apnea is not produced or such that the infusion is so slow as to fail to achieve a sufficiently high serum level so as to yield effective brain levels for seizure termination. Diazepam is highly lipid-soluble and enters and emerges from the brain during the redistribution phase of the drug. Thus, the duration of effect may be relatively brief and other agents having greater persistence (e.g., phenobarbital or phenytoin) may need to be administered. Great caution needs to be exercised in administration, as inadvertent intraarterial injection of the poorly soluble drug dissolved in organic solvents can cause injury to the intima of small blood vessels with resultant occlusion of vessels and gangrene.

Lorazepam This benzodiazepine has been shown to be an effective agent in the treatment of status epilepticus in various studies, although not officially approved for this purpose. Upon intravenous administration lorazepam produces a quick onset of action and a duration of action that is much longer than diazepam. The effect of lorazepam may last as long as 12 to 14 h. Caution should be exercised in the rate of intravenous drug administration and the amount of drug given because lorazepam can cause a reduction in blood pressure and suppression of respiration. The other drugs that are given to treat status epilepticus can also produce similar adverse reactions.

Phenytoin Phenytoin may be used for seizures which are susceptible to control with the drug (e.g., it is not effective in *absence status epilepticus* or drug withdrawal, including alcohol withdrawal seizures). The drug is given intravenously as a full loading dose and thus establishes a serum level initially above the usual therapeutic range. The infusion rate is limited primarily by cardiovascular depression which may manifest as hypotension, bradycardia, and atrio-ventricular conduction abnormalities. Advantages of the drug include the lack of prominent hypnotic actions, which makes neurological evaluation easier and the fact that one need not add a second agent due to a brief anticonvulsant effect, since phenytoin serum levels fall as a result of biotransformation (not redistribution) and hence exhibit appreciable duration. The intramuscular route is not recommended, as rate of absorption of the drug, which precipitates in the muscle at physiologic pH, is slow and yields very low serum levels.

Barbiturates Phenobarbital may be used to terminate seizures; it is usually administered intravenously. Due to its polarity, it penetrates the blood-brain barrier more slowly than other barbiturates and may not achieve peak effect for 20 to 30 minutes after intravenous injection. As with other agents of this class, respiratory depression is a prominent adverse effect.

Pentobarbital is more rapid in onset and has been used to terminate seizures; it is also used to deeply depress (anesthetize) patients with seizures which are not responsive to more usual measures.

PARKINSONISM

Parkinsonism is a movement disorder characterized by muscle rigidity, akinesia or bradykinesia, and tremor at rest. Usually the face lacks expression and a simian posture with shuffling gait are observed. A few causes have been identified (viral encephalitis, manganese poisoning, carbon monoxide, the designer drug MPTP) but most cases are idiopathic. The latter form of the disease usually manifests itself in the 5th decade of life and progresses. A reversible form of Parkinson's disease is often produced by neuroleptic antipsychotic drugs such as chlorpromazine and haloperidol, which are dopamine receptor antagonists.

The underlying pathophysiology involves the progressive degeneration of dopaminergic neurons which project from the substantia nigra to the caudate-putamen and participate in the regulation of motor output. Thus this is a disorder of the basal ganglia. Parkinsonian features may be among the symptoms of cerebral vascular disease and other degenerations of the CNS. Furthermore, Parkinson's disease may be pure or accompanied by more diffuse neuronal degeneration; when relatively pure, intellectual functions are normal despite what may be considerable physical debilitation. It appears that symptoms do not appear until about 85 percent of the dopamine neurons have disappeared, there being an appreciable safety factor in neurotransmission. The function of the dopamine, according to presently entertained hypotheses, is that of an inhibitory neurotransmitter on cholinergic neurons in the corpus striatum. Thus the loss of dopamine influence is presumed to result in a release from inhibition of cholinergic neurons.

ANTIPARKINSONIAN AGENTS

For more than a century, the treatment of Parkinsonism was empirical and rested primarily on the use of centrally active anticholinergic agents which provided some relief of symptoms, particularly in the early disease stages. Initially, various crude preparations of the belladonna alkaloids were used, including belladonna leaf, stramonium, atropine, and hyoscine. Recognition of the neurotransmitter function of acetylcholine in the brain led to the suggestion that the clinical efficacy of anticholinergic agents in Parkinsonism might be due to their antagonism of acetylcholine at central muscarinic cholinergic receptors.

The fact that cholinergic agents such as physostigmine exacerbate the Parkinsonian state, whereas centrally active anticholinergic agents reduce its intensity, suggests that the symptomatology reflects the disinhibited activity of striatal cholinergic systems. According to this hypothesis, a beneficial action could be exerted in Parkinsonism either by blocking the excessive stimulation of the cholinergic system or restoring the normal function of the inhibitory dopaminergic system by restoration of its deficient neurohumor.

More recently, with a greater understanding of the pathophysiology of the disease, therapy has centered on attempting to restore dopaminergic influences in the basal ganglia.

Levodopa

This drug is identical to the natural L-amino acid DOPA, formed as an intermediate in the biosynthesis of the catecholamines, norepinephrine and epinephrine (see Chapter 7). Presently levodopa (combined with a peripheral aromatic L-amino acid decarboxylase inhibitor, i.e., carbidopa) is the most effective therapy available for the treatment of Parkinson's disease.

Mechanism of Action Levodopa raises dopamine levels in the basal ganglia. The simplest approach to replenishing the deficient neurotransmitter might appear to be to administer dopamine itself. However, this is not done since (1) the dopamine is too highly charged at physiologic pH and does not enter the brain through the blood-brain barrier, and (2) peripheral cardiovascular effects of dopamine preclude such an approach. On the other hand, the precursor, levodopa readily crosses the blood-brain barrier (through the neutral amino acid transport system) and is converted to dopamine within the brain. It is believed that the therapeutic effect of levodopa reflects the partial replenishment of striatal dopamine stores. The drug seems effective even in advanced Parkinsonism and presumably does not need to be taken up into dopaminergic neurons (as there may no longer be any available), but may be converted by the ubiquitous and relatively non-specific enzyme, aromatic L-amino acid decarboxylase, so as to raise dopamine concentrations in the brain (Fig. 22-1).

As the disease progresses, control usually becomes more difficult to achieve as the reserve capacity to store dopamine diminishes and disappears. The interval between doses of levodopa is progressively shortened and periods of overdosing leading to adventitious choreiform movements and under-dosing leads to a return of Parkinsonian symptoms. Foods containing proteins interfere with the uptake of levodopa into the brain and may have to be avoided until late in the day, lest they block the effects of levodopa.

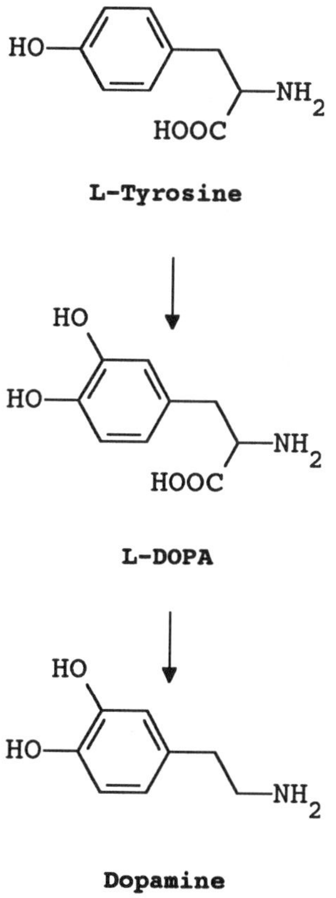

HO
NH_2
HOOC
L-Tyrosine

HO
HO
NH_2
HOOC
L-DOPA

HO
HO
NH_2
Dopamine

FIGURE 22-1 *Schematic pathway of the synthesis of dopamine from tyrosine in dopaminergic neurons. Presumably, by increasing the supply of L-DOPA (levodopa), the production of dopamine will increase.*

Pharmacokinetics Levodopa is administered orally. Peak plasma levels occur within 0.5 to 2 h. Food may delay the absorption. Enzymes of the gastric mucosa can reduce absorption by degradation. Levodopa is extensively metabolized in the gastrointestinal tract and the liver. Less than 1 percent of the unmetabolized drug passes to the CNS. The elimination half-life is brief, lasting only 1 to 3 h. The major urinary metabolites are dihydroxyphenylacetic acid and homovanillic acid.

Adverse Reactions Anorexia, nausea, and vomiting are the chief dose-limiting side effects in the initial period of treatment. This was particularly the case with large doses prior to the availability of carbidopa. Other adverse reactions include tachycardia, palpitations, orthostatic hypotension, insomnia, agitation, and occasionally more severe mental disturbances with delusions and hallucinations. Cardiac arrhythmias can be quite severe. These effects diminish with lowering the daily dosage or increasing the frequency of dosing while maintaining effective total daily dose. Choreiform involuntary movements may develop in patients receiving long-term treatment for the reasons alluded to. If the movements are severe and interfere with function, the dose should be adjusted as to size and frequency of administration in an effort to optimize treatment.

Drug Interactions The dosage requirement of levodopa can be reduced without altering clinical effectiveness by combining it with the decarboxylase inhibitor carbidopa. This compound does not penetrate the blood-brain barrier to inhibit central decarboxylase. As a result, levodopa is not degraded in the peripheral blood and more levodopa can enter the brain, thus permitting the dosage to be reduced without reducing the striatal dopamine effect. Furthermore, by reducing total levodopa dose, peripheral side effects attributable to levodopa or derived dopamine are reduced. Adverse effects attributable to CNS effects, as expected, are not diminished. For these reasons, a combination of carbidopa and levodopa is the drug product of choice in the United States. It is well tolerated by most patients. Many patients benefit from the combination of levodopa and carbidopa with one of the anticholinergic agents.

Pyridoxine markedly reduces or completely blocks the effect of levodopa administration. Pyridoxine appears to accelerate the biotransformation of the drug in extra-cerebral tissues by increasing decarboxylation, thereby preventing levodopa from gaining access to the CNS. Phenothiazines such as chlorpromazine antagonize the effect of levodopa and are best avoided. The therapeutic effect of levodopa is reduced by methyldopa and reserpine and enhanced by the tricyclic antidepressants. Concurrent administration of levodopa and a monoamine oxidase inhibitor will result in a hypertensive crisis. Levodopa is contraindicated in narrow-angle glaucoma and malignant melanoma.

Anticholinergic Agents

The belladonna alkaloids have been replaced in the treatment of Parkinsonism by the synthetic anticholinergic antiparkinsonian drugs. The drugs include biperiden, benztropine, orphenadrine, procyclidine, and trihexyphenidyl; diphenhydramine, an antihistamine with high anticholinergic activity, is also used occasionally. Although less potent than the natural alkaloids, these synthetic agents possess similar pharmacologic properties. Their advantage over older drugs is unproven. The goal in drug development has been to synthesize drugs with greater selectivity towards central rather than peripheral muscarinic sites and hence agents with fewer or less severe anticholinergic side effects; this has never been convincingly demonstrated to have been achieved.

Mechanism of Action The wide distribution of cholinergic neurons in the CNS makes it difficult to identify the specific structure involved in the beneficial effect of the anticholinergic drugs, but it has been suggested that the cholinergic neurons are in the striatum and are normally inhibited by the dopamine neurons from the substantia nigra. Thus a prevailing hypothesis (though perhaps overly simplistic) is that the loss of dopamine neurons release a set of cholinergic neurons which, freed from inhibition, discharge excessively; this excessive cholinergic activity is presumed to be blocked by antimuscarinic agents.

Therapeutic Uses There is little reason for preferring one of the anticholinergic antiparkinsonian drugs over another. In general, treatment is begun with small doses which may be increased gradually based on tolerance and effect. The benefits obtained are limited to a modest reduction in the intensity of the parkinsonian state. A decrease in muscular resistance to passive movement, i.e., rigidity, is the most striking effect observed. There is also a general improvement in motor function and posture. Tremor may be reduced but is rarely abolished and is generally the least responsive feature of the parkinsonian syndrome.

These drugs are also of value in reducing the extrapyramidal (parkinson-like) effects of antipsychotic drugs (see Chapter 20).

Adverse Reactions Side effects attributable to the anticholinergic activity of these drugs are encountered in nearly all patients, and usually some compromise must be made in adjusting the dosage between levels that produce therapeutic effects and those that induce the side effects common to all anticholinergic drugs. Bladder emptying in older males can be a problem as can the precipitation of a glaucoma attack in narrow-angle glaucoma.

Amantadine

This antiviral agent was accidentally discovered to relieve Parkinsonism when used prophylactically against A_2 influenza viral infection in patients suffering with Parkinsonism. The antiparkinsonian action of amantadine has been associated with the release of dopamine from storage sites and with the blockade of reuptake. Additionally, increases in the concentration of GABA in the striatum and substantia nigra have been reported.

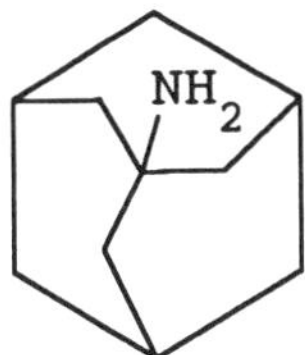

Amantadine has a peculiar chemical structure consisting of four fused cyclohexane rings substituted with a single amine group. It is well absorbed from the gastrointestinal tract. Among the numerous reactions are hyperexcitability, tremors, ataxia, slurred speech, psychic depression, insomnia, lethargy, and, in high doses, convulsions. Other side effects are dry mouth, gastrointestinal symptoms, skin eruptions, polyuria, and nocturia.

The treatment of Parkinsonism by combining levodopa, anticholinergic agents, and amantadine has produced better results than are seen with any of these drugs alone. This combined therapeutic program is of particular importance in those individuals who cannot tolerate higher doses of levodopa because of toxicity. Amantadine may be used as initial therapy for Parkinsonism.

Bromocriptine

This dopamine receptor agonist can be used in Parkinson's disease (Fig. 22-2), often adjunctively with levodopa. Bromocriptine mimics the action of dopamine in the brain but is not destroyed as readily as dopamine. It apparently causes fewer abnormal involuntary movements than levodopa but more mental aberrations, including hallucinations, possibly because of chemical similarity to lysergic acid diethylamide (LSD); both compounds are derived from ergot. Since bromocriptine does not require enzymatic transformation in the brain to have a therapeutic effort (unlike levodopa), it is useful for patients not responding to levodopa.

About 28 percent of an oral dose of bromocriptine is absorbed from the gastrointestinal tract and a high first pass hepatic metabolism results in only 6 percent reaching the systemic circulation unchanged. The drug is 90 to 96 percent bound to serum albumin. Bromocriptine undergoes rather complete biotransformation, and the major route of excretion is biliary; approximately 85 percent of the administered dose is excreted in the feces in 120 h.

In addition to its use in Parkinson's disease, bromocriptine is also indicated for short-term treatment of amenorrhea and galactorrhea associated with excessive secretion of prolactin. Bromocriptine is also useful in the treatment of some pituitary tumors, female infertility associated with hyperprolactinemia, and acromegaly.

The major adverse effects of bromocriptine are nausea, nasal congestion, and orthostatic hypotension. Other less common side effects include constipation, headaches, fatigue, and hallucinations.

FIGURE 22-2 *The chemical structure of bromocriptine (the heavy lines represent the dopamine moiety).*

Pergolide

This compound is a direct-acting dopaminergic agonist at both D_1 and D_2 receptors. Pergolide is as effective as bromocriptine in the treatment of Parkinson's disease but has a longer duration of action. This drug, like bromocriptine, is used in combination with levodopa/carbidopa for parkinsonism.

About 50 percent is absorbed after oral administration. Plasma protein binding is about 90 percent. Biotransformation of pergolide is extensive; at least ten metabolites have been identified, some of which have dopaminergic activity in animals. The major route of excretion is through the kidney.

The adverse reactions that may occur from pergolide are similar to those of bromocriptine.

Selegilene

This drug (also known as L-deprenyl) is an inhibitor of monoamine oxidase (MAO) type B, one of the isoenzymes of MAO. It inhibits the intracerebral enzymatic degradation of dopamine and thus spares the neurotransmitter from degradation. Unlike nonspecific inhibitors of MAO, selegilene does not cause hypertensive episodes when tyramine-containing food or drink are consumed, as the MAO type A is not inhibited.

Selegilene is rapidly and well absorbed after oral dosing. Hepatic biotransformation results in the production of three products: N-desmethyldeprenyl (the major metabolite), amphetamine, and methamphetamine. These products are eliminated in the urine; little unchanged selegilene is found in the urine.

Common adverse reactions to this drug include nausea, abdominal pain, dizziness, lightheadedness, confusion, and hallucinations. A large number of less common untoward effects have been reported involving the CNS, cardiovascular, genitourinary, and dermatologic systems.

Some investigators have suggested that selegilene may slow the progression of Parkinson's disease, but this is yet to be shown convincingly. The drug is often used as an adjunct to levodopa or levodopa/carbidopa where it is regarded as a useful agent.

BIBLIOGRAPHY

Bergmann, K.J., M.R. Mendoza, M.D. Yahr: "Parkinson's Disease and Long Term Levodopa Therapy," in K.J. Bergmann and M.D. Yahr (eds.), *Parkinson's Disease, Advances in Neurology*, Raven Press, New York, **45**: 463-468 (1987).

Borowski, G.D., and L.I. Rose: "Bromocriptine Update," *Am. Fam. Physician* **30**: 218-219 (1984).

Commission on Classification and Terminology of the International League Against Epilepsy: "Proposal for Revised Clinical and Electroencephalographic Classification of Epileptic Seizures," *Epilepsia* **22**: 489-501 (1981).

Delorenzo, R.J.: "Mechanisms of Action of Anticonvulsant Drugs," *Epilepsia* **29**: 535-547 (1988).

Guelen, P.J.M., and E. Vanderklein: "Practical Pharmacokinetics," in D.M. Woodbury, J.K. Penry, and C.E. Pippenger (eds.), *Antiepileptic Drugs*, Raven Press, New York, 1982, pp. 57-72.

Macdonald, R.L., and K.M. Kelly: "Antiepileptic Drug Mechanisms of Action," *Epilepsia* **34 (Suppl. 5)**: S1-S8 (1993).

Marsden, C.D., and S. Fahn: "Problems in Parkinson's Disease and Other Akinetic Rigid Syndromes," in C.D. Marsden and S. Fahn (eds.), *Movement Disorders II*, Butterworth, Boston, 1987, pp. 65-72.

Ragowski, M.A., and R.J. Porter: "Antiepileptic Drugs: Pharmacological Mechanisms and Clinical Efficacy with Consideration of Promising Developmental Stage Compounds," *Pharm. Rev.* **42**: 223-286 (1990).

Ramsey, R.E.: "Advances in the Pharmacotherapy of Epilepsy," *Epilepsia* **34 (Suppl. 5)**: S9-S16 (1993).

Treiman, D.M.: "Efficacy and Safety of Antiepileptic Drugs: A Review of Controlled Trials," *Epilepsia* **28**: 51-58 (1987).

Wotten, G.F.: "Progress in Understanding the Pathophysiology of Treatment Related Fluctuations in Parkinson's Disease," *Ann. Neurology* **24**: 263-365 (1988).

Yaari, Y., M.E. Selzer, and J.H. Pincus: "Phenytoin: Mechanisms of its Anticonvulsant Action," *Ann. Neurol.* **20**: 171-184 (1986).

CHAPTER 23

Opioid Analgesics

Anthony J. Triolo

The opioids, also known as *narcotic analgesics*, are also referred to as any naturally occurring or synthetic drug that has morphine-like pharmacologic actions. The term *narcotic* refers to the ability of these agents to produce stupor or sleep, and *analgesia* refers to their capacity to relieve pain. Morphine is the prototype opioid: it is a naturally occurring alkaloid present in *opium* which is obtained from the poppy plant, *Papaver somniferum*. This plant grows to a height of approximately 4 feet and is a capsule-containing plant indigenous to Asia; it is grown in abundance in India and Turkey, and also in Mexico. Cutting the unripe fruit capsule of the plant yields a milky white exudate, which when air-dried, becomes a resinous brown mass called opium.

Opium is a term derived from the Greek word for juice. Opium has been used medicinally since 4000 BC. In 1803 Friedrich Serturner, a German pharmacist, isolated the alkaloid morphine from opium and proposed to name it after Morpheus, the Greek god of dreams. Of the 20 alkaloids present in opium, morphine is the most important as well as the most abundant. The term *opiate* applies only to those alkaloids obtained from opium (e.g., morphine and codeine) and the semisynthetic and synthetic congeners of these alkaloids. A group of naturally occurring peptides with opioid-like activity, the enkephalins, are normally present in the central nervous system (CNS) as well as in many other tissues. *Opioid* is a broader term than opiates and includes both opiates and these endogenous peptides.

The opioid drugs are the most effective compounds available for the relief of severe pain. An understanding of the nociceptive (pain-transmitting) pathways and the mechanisms involved in opioid action, especially the interaction between drug and receptor, are essential for the rational use of these agents.

THE SENSATION OF PAIN

An important distinction exists between pain and nociception. Nociception refers to an increased activity in the afferent nervous system induced by a noxious stimulus (e.g., mechanical, thermal or chemical) which depolarizes specialized sensory receptors (nociceptors or pain receptors) in the periphery and provides the brain with information about tissue injury. Pain, however, is a perception, the consequence of the filtering, modulating, and distorting of this afferent nerve activity through the affective and cognitive processes unique to the patient. In essence, pain like suffering is highly subjective, pain depends on the intensity of the noxious stimulus, the sensitivity of the individual, and the environmental and emotional context in which the noxious stimulus induces tissue injury.

Following injury or inflammation, primary afferent axons conduct nociceptive stimuli from the periphery (e.g., skin or viscera) to the spinal cord where they terminate in the laminae of the dorsal horn. Sharp well-localized pain stimuli are transmitted by the fast conducting myelinated A-delta fibers which terminate in lamina I (the marginal zone) and V, whereas poorly localized, dull pain stimuli are transmitted by the unmyelinated C fibers which terminate mostly in lamina II (substantia gelatinosa). The subsequent excitation of secondary spinal cord neurons (projection neurons) in the dorsal horn then conveys nociceptive information along several ascending pathways that project to the thalamus, reticular formation of the medulla and pons, and the periaqueductal gray (PAG) region of the midbrain.

Pathways that descend from the brain to the spinal cord mediate antinociception or analgesia. One descending antinociceptive pathway arising in the PAG region is connected with the hypothala-

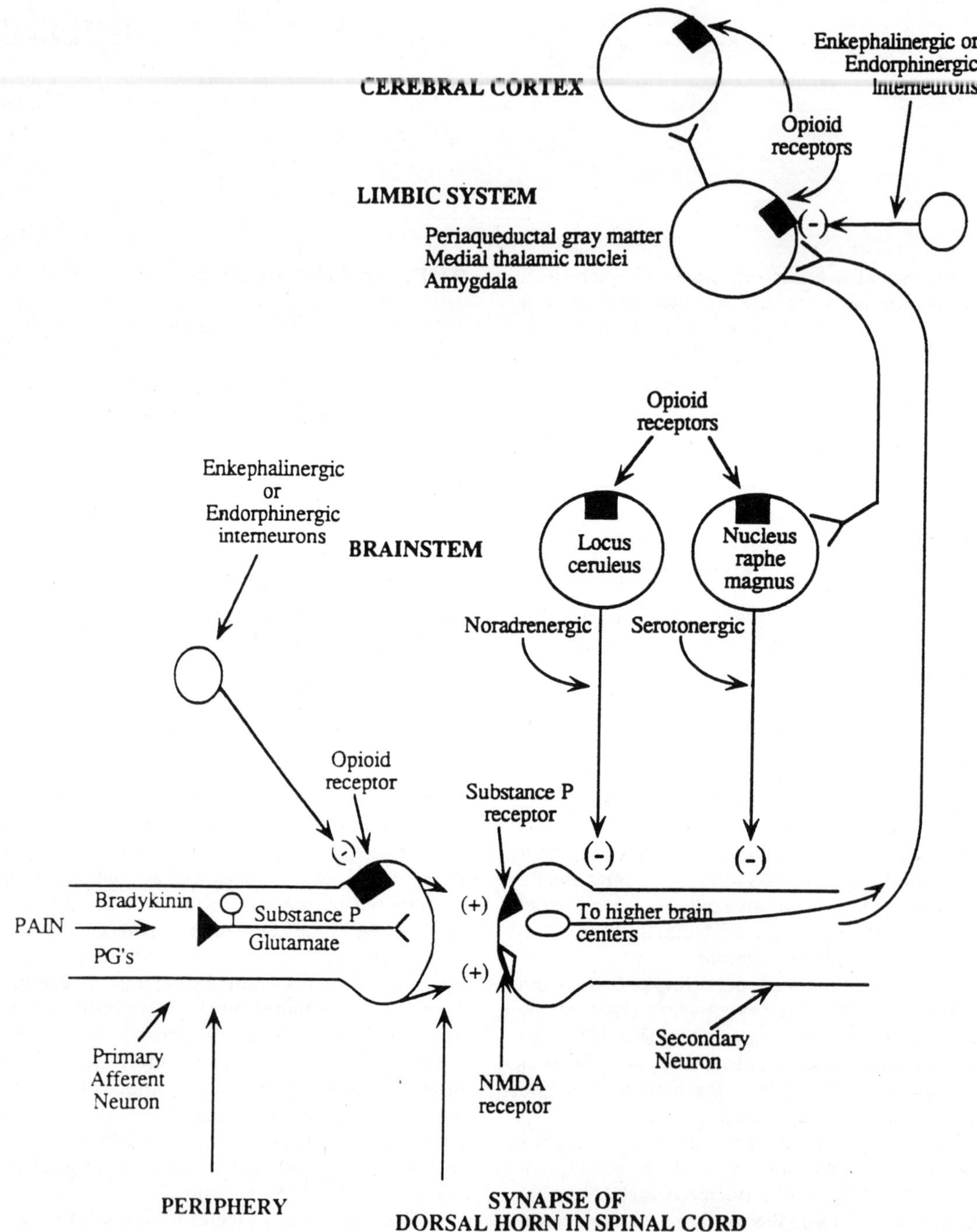

FIGURE 23-1 *Simplified scheme showing nociceptive (pain) and antinociceptive (or pain reducing) pathways. Pain is mediated by the release of the neurotransmitters substance P and glutamate from presynaptic neurons which then interact with their individual receptors to activate postsynaptic neurons.*

mus and acts on the spinal cord to inhibit second order neurons at laminae I, II, and V of the dorsal horn. Before descending, this pathway synapses first in the nucleus raphae magnus of the medulla from which serotonergic fibers project to the spinal cord to selectively inhibit dorsal horn neurons receiving nociceptive impulses. There is also a noradrenergic descending fiber tract with its cell body in the locus ceruleus which inhibits nociceptive transmission in the dorsal horn cells of the spinal cord. This descending system can be blocked by lesions at any of the sites along the pathway, thus promoting hyperalgesia. It can also be activated by pain, psychological factors (e.g., stress), and therapeutic agents such as the opioid drugs or clonidine, resulting in an antinociceptive or analgesic effect. A simple scheme showing the opioid receptors and the nociceptive pathways of importance at spinal cord and supraspinal sites of the CNS is shown in Fig. 23-1.

Finally, third and higher order neuronal connections from the midbrain, reticular formation, thalamus, hypothalamus, and other limbic structures ultimately reach the somatosensory cortices of the brain, where pain perception occurs.

A. POMC

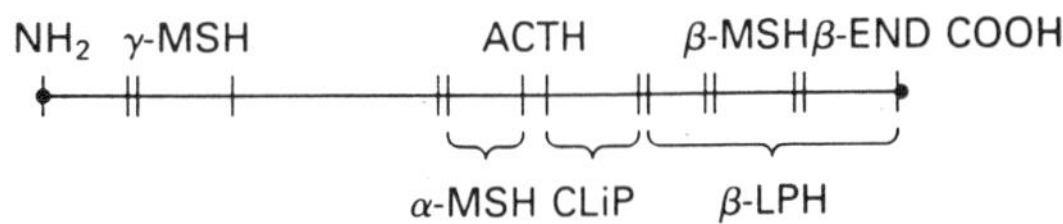

B. Proenkephalin

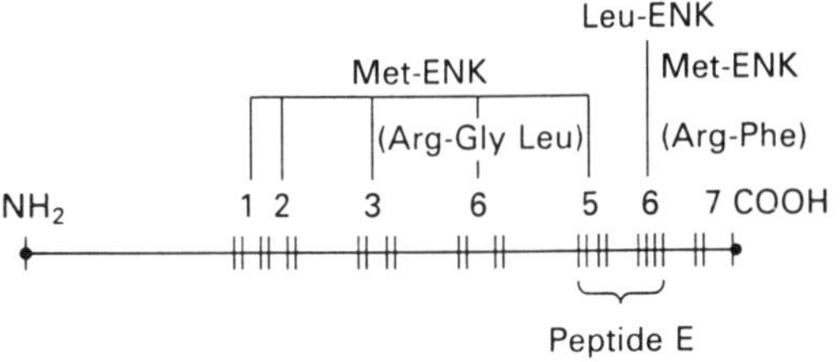

C. Prodynorphin

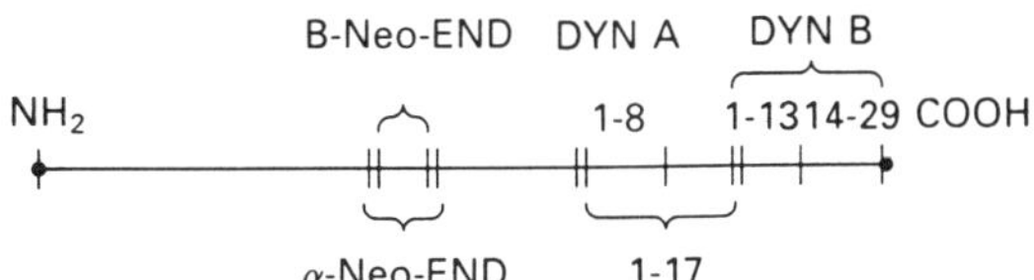

FIGURE 23-2 *Schematic representation of the protein precursor structures of three opioid peptide families. POMC = proopiomelanocortin. [From: Akil, H., et al.: Annu. Rev. Neurosci. 7: 223 (1984).]*

MOLECULAR BASIS OF ACTION

Endogenous Opioid Peptides

In 1975, two endogenous pentapeptides, Met- and Leu-enkephalin were isolated from pig brain. They were called *enkephalins* from the Greek word for "in the head". Later, a number of other endogenous opioid peptides were identified, the most prominent of which are beta-endorphin and dynorphin.

Like many other peptides present in the nervous system, the endogenous opioid peptides are not synthesized individually. Instead, a single gene encodes a large inactive polypeptide that contains within its structure the sequences of several small active molecules that are subsequently split from the precursor. Three families of endogenous opioid peptides arise from precursor or prehormone molecules: proopiomelanocortin (POMC), proenkephalin and prodynorphin (Fig. 23-2). These precursors and their products are widely distributed in the CNS, the pituitary gland, and some peripheral tissues. Discrete tissue localization of these peptides has been established by fluorescent immunohistochemical techniques.

POMC, the first of the precursors to be identified, is produced in the pituitary gland, the hypothalamus, and in several peripheral tissues, including the placenta, gastrointestinal tract, and lungs. Beta-endorphin is the 61-91 amino acid sequence in the beta-lipoprotein portion of POMC and is the predominant active opioid peptide product. POMC also gives rise to non-opioid peptides of great importance, including adrenocorticotropic hormone (ACTH) and α-, β- and γ-melanocyte stimulating hormones (MSH). Although the 61-65 amino acid sequence of beta-endorphin contains the pentapeptide Met-enkephalin, POMC is not the source of Met-enkephalin in the brain.

The endogenous source of Met-enkephalin is proenkephalin, initially discovered in bovine adrenal cortex where enkephalin biosynthesis was first demonstrated. Proenkephalin cleavage also gives rise to Leu-enkephalin and other extended enkephalins containing additional amino acids and peptide E. The smallest endogenous peptides with opioid activity are the two pentapeptides Met- and Leu-enkephalin: each of these analgesic peptides contains the amino acid sequence Tyr^1-Gly^2-Gly^3-Phe^4 and either a Met^5 or Leu^5 terminal amino acid.

Prodynorphin is a precursor peptide isolated from brain, spinal cord, anterior pituitary, adrenal gland, and reproductive organs. Prodynorphin is the source of various dynorphins having the Leu-enkephalin sequence attached to other peptide fragments. Dynorphin A is a peptide having either 8 or 17 amino acids and dynorphin B may have either 13 or 29 amino acids.

These endogenous opioid peptides are believed to be the body's own natural analgesics and are released in response to pain, stress, and other noxious stimuli. Endogenous opioid peptides mimic many of the pharmacologic effects of plant-derived, synthetic, and semi-synthetic opiates to be covered in this chapter. The opioid peptides are localized at sites in the CNS associated with the processing or modulation of nociceptive (pain) stimuli.

Enkephalin- and dynorphin-containing neuronal cell bodies and nerve terminals have been found in the PAG, the nucleus raphae magnus of the rostroventral medulla, and in laminae I, II, IV and V of the dorsal horn of the spinal cord. The most intense fluorescence identifying the opioid peptides is seen in nerve terminals. In the spinal cord, enkephalin- and dynorphin-containing interneurons are found in close proximity to the terminals of the nociceptive primary afferent neurons and the dendrites of the secondary dorsal horn projection neurons. The endogenous opioid peptides can modulate nociceptive transmission to higher centers of the CNS from this site in the spinal cord by a combination of presynaptic (e.g., neurotransmitter release) and postsynaptic actions.

A type of contact called an "axo-axonic synapse" results when an enkephalin-containing interneuron contacts nerve terminals of the primary afferent neuron that conducts nociceptive input to the CNS. These synapses are important for understanding the analgesic actions of opioids at the spinal cord level. In the case of dynorphin-containing interneurons, no "axo-axonic synapse" has been seen in the dorsal horn of the spinal cord. Endogenous opioid peptides are also found in tissues other than the brain. Enkephalin-containing neurons are present in the myenteric plexuses of the intestine, a site where opioid drugs inhibit motility of the gastrointestinal tract. Enkephalins are the most widely distributed endogenous opioid peptides, the level of Met-enkephalin always being higher than that of Leu-enkephalin. Dynorphins have their highest concentrations in the posterior pituitary and the hypothalamus; they are also present in the PAG region and the dorsal horn of the spinal cord. Staining for beta-endorphins shows that these are found in separate neurons from those containing either enkephalin or dynorphin. Neurons containing beta-endorphin have a more restricted distribution than those containing enkephalins and are present in high concentration in the arcuate nucleus of the hypothalamus and the nucleus of the solitary tract. In the descending nociceptive pathway, beta-endorphin-containing interneurons are present in the PAG region and the dorsal horn; these interneurons play an important role in pain-modulation.

In addition to analgesia, the endogenous opioid peptides depress respiration, reduce intestinal motility, decrease release of prolactin and growth hormone, alter body temperature, modify learning and memory, change immune system responsiveness, and with repeated administration, induce tolerance and physical dependence. Thus, these endogenous opioids have profiles of effects similar to those of the plant opiates like morphine.

Synthetic Opioid Peptides

Beta-endorphin not only has analgesic activity but it also exhibits an antidepressant effect when administered intravenously to some depressed patients. Its main disadvantage as an analgesic is a short duration of action due to rapid metabolism by tissue enzymes. The analgesic action of the enkephalins is even more fleeting than that of beta-endorphin due to the enzymatic removal of the N-terminal tyrosine by tissue peptidases. No synthetic opioid peptide is commercially available for clinical use.

Opioid analgesic drugs given for prolonged periods of time produce tolerance to their pharmacologic effects. The development of synthetic peptide drugs having analgesic efficacy when given orally, but without such typical side effects as constipation, tolerance, and physical dependence would be clinically desirable and may become available in the future.

Opioid Receptors

Opioid drugs produce their pharmacologic effects by interacting with receptors located at synaptic membrane surfaces. The endogenous opioid peptides are thought to be the physiologic ligands that bind to these receptors. These opioid receptors consist of four major classes as follows: mu, kappa, delta, and sigma. With the exception of the sigma receptor, the other three opioid receptors modulate pain both at the supraspinal and spinal cord level. Sigma receptors are not exclusively opioid, since non-opioid drugs (e.g., the hallucinogen phencyclidine and some antipsychotic drugs) will also bind to this receptor. Some authorities do not consider the sigma receptor to be a true opioid receptor and refer to it as the "sigma site." Each of the receptor classes has been further divided into subtypes (e.g., mu_1 mediates supraspinal and mu_2 mediates spinal analgesia). The binding of a radiolabeled opioid agonist or antagonist to these opioid receptors is stereospecific, occurring with high affinity for only the levo(-) isomer.

The mu opioid receptors were named after morphine; thus, the effects associated with the interaction of a ligand and the mu receptor are those typically seen with morphine. Beta-endorphin is the endogenous ligand that appears to interact primarily with the mu receptor. The CNS sites containing high concentrations of mu receptors include the PAG region, the dorsal horn of the spinal cord, the medial thalamus, and the nucleus raphe magnus. In the dorsal horn, the mu receptors are located both on terminals of nociceptive afferent fibers and on dendrites of postsynaptic neurons. The effects associated with agonist binding to mu receptors include analgesia, sedation, respiratory depression, constipation, nausea and vomiting, pruritus, growth hormone and prolactin release, euphoria, tolerance, and physical dependence.

The distribution of kappa opioid receptors in the CNS is similar to that of the mu receptors, except that kappa receptors are also highly concentrated in limbic structures including the locus ceruleus. Dynorphins are endogenous agonists for kappa receptors; these receptors are involved in opioid-induced analgesia, sedation, dysphoria and psychotomimetic effects, tolerance, and a mild degree of physical dependence.

Enkephalins exert their primary effects on the delta receptors: agonist actions at this receptor mediate analgesia and cardiovascular effects.

Finally, the sigma receptor (a different receptor than the "PCP" receptor) has been implicated in dysphoria and other undesirable psychotomimetic effects associated with the use of opioid agonists and mixed agonist-antagonists. Sigma receptor actions are not reversed by the opioid antagonist naloxone which binds with higher affinity than opioid agonists to opioid receptors but fails to activate them. Opioid antagonists can prevent or reverse the pharmacologic actions of opioid agonists. Naloxone antagonizes the effects of opioid agonists on the three major opioid receptors with a rank order of potency for antagonism as follows: mu > delta > kappa. Opioid receptors are thought to undergo conformational changes in the presence of sodium ions which affect drug binding to the receptors. Sodium increases antagonist binding and decreases agonist binding to the opioid receptor.

Molecular Mechanisms of the Opioid Agonists

Painful stimuli initiate the firing of primary afferent fibers which synapse in various laminae of the spinal cord and release a number of peptides (e.g., substance P, calcitonin gene-related peptide, somatostatin, cholecystokinin-like peptide, vasoactive intestinal peptide, and bradykinin), adenosine and excitatory acidic amino acids (e.g., glutamate, aspartate, and homocysteate), all of which are potential mediators of nociceptive transmission. Substance P and glutamate are suggested most often as the major mediators of nociception transmission at synapses located both in the spinal cord and brain.

Substance P is an 11-amino acid neuropeptide which interacts with postsynaptic neurokinin (NK-1 and NK-2) receptors to excite the nerve cell and make it more responsive to other endogenous peptides. Its release from primary afferent terminals is Ca^{2+}-dependent and produces excitatory postsynaptic potentials that provide slow nociceptive signals to the CNS (Fig. 23-1). The release of substance P enhances postsynaptic neuronal electrical activity by closing K^+ channels through an unidentified pertussis toxin-insensitive G_x-protein. When substance P is administered spinally, it releases aspartate and glutamate, suggesting that substance P acts on presynaptic receptors to modulate the release of glutamate from primary afferent fibers. The similarity in distribution of opioid receptors, enkephalin-containing inter-neurons, and substance P has led to the hypothesis that opioid drugs cause many of their pharmacologic effects by reducing substance P release.

Glutamate is an excitatory amino acid that transmits nociceptive stimuli by producing fast excitatory postsynaptic potentials in neurons. The postsynaptic inotropic receptors for glutamate are of two types: (a) the NMDA receptor complex, which, although selective for N-methyl D-aspartate, is also activated by glutamate, and (b) the non-NMDA receptor which binds glutamate, but is selective for the agonists kainate and AMPA (α-amino-3-hydroxy-4-methyl-4-isoxazole propionic acid). When glutamate is released from primary afferent neurons in the spinal cord, it combines with non-NMDA receptors to depolarize the neuronal membrane by promoting Na^+ entry into the cell through an intrinsic ion channel. Depolarization in turn releases Mg^{2+} ions from an intrinsic cationic channel and activates the NMDA receptor. NMDA receptor activation causes an influx of both Na^+ and Ca^{2+} ions into the postsynaptic neuron. Glutamate receptors have been found in the PAG region, the thalamus, and the lateral reticular formation. In summary, it is thought that noxious stimuli release substance P which in turn enhances NMDA-elicited responses so that these two receptor systems operate in concert to prolong and amplify pain signals to the CNS. These same brain areas contain a high density of opioid receptors and are important sites in the pathway for modulating both ascending and descending nociceptive (pain) transmission.

Morphine induces analgesia directly by inhibiting synaptic transmission in the spinal cord and brain and indirectly by increasing the descending inhibitory control of noxious stimuli to the dorsal horn cells of the spinal cord. In brain and spinal cord, morphine and/or the endogenous opioid peptides can activate presynaptic mu and delta opioid receptors. Activation of these receptors hyperpolarizes the neuron by increasing K^+ conductance (open K^+ channels) which then blocks Ca^{2+} entry into nerve terminals via voltage-dependent Ca^{2+} channels. This mechanism blocks the release of substance P and glutamate.

At the molecular level, the mu and delta opioid receptors are linked to an inhibitory G_i-protein that can either directly open the K^+ ion-gated channel or acts indirectly by inhibiting the effector enzyme adenylate cyclase to decrease the intracellular concentration of the second messenger cyclic AMP. The binding of morphine or endogenous dynorphin to kappa opioid receptors inhibits Ca^{2+} conductance (closes Ca^{2+} channels), thus blocking Ca^{2+} influx and preventing neurotransmitter release. The kappa receptor is also linked to an inhibitory G_i-protein which in turn can act directly on the Ca^{2+} ion-gated channel or indirectly via the second messenger cyclic AMP.

Opioid drugs or endogenous opioid peptides from interneurons may also act postsynaptically on all three types of specific opioid receptors (mu, kappa, and delta) by a similar mechanism involving G-proteins which inhibit ascending pathways that convey nociceptive information to the higher brain centers. Morphine can also act indirectly on higher brain centers to increase descending inhibitory control of the dorsal horn cells in the spinal cord. Agonist interaction with opioid receptors in the PAG region and the nucleus raphae magnus activates serotonergic fiber tracts that inhibit nerve cells in the dorsal horn. Opioid receptors in the locus ceruleus also activate descending noradrenergic fiber tracts which form inhibitory synapses with dorsal horn cells. Serotonin and/or norepinephrine released from these fiber traces increase K^+ conductance (open K^+ channels), thus hyperpolarizing second-order neurons at these synapses and thus inhibit nociceptive input from the periphery (Fig. 23-1).

Classification

The opioids are classified into three major subgroups according to their activities at opioid receptors: (1) agonists, (2) mixed agonist-antagonists, and (3) antagonists. Table 23-1 lists the various drugs according to their classification and divides the opioid agonists chemically into four major groups.

The opioid agonists have both affinity for and intrinsic activity at all opioid receptors, thus mimicking the activity of the endogenous opioid peptides. The mixed agonist-antagonists have agonistic activity at some opioid receptors but antagonistic activity at others (see Table 23-2). Antagonists bind to opioid receptors without activating them and also block activation of these receptors by agonists. Therapeutically, opioid antagonists are mainly used as antidotes to reverse the adverse effects associated with acute overdose of opioid drugs and for the diagnosis of addiction due to the prolonged use of opioids.

AGONISTS

The opioid agonists act primarily at mu receptors to produce analgesia but also have varying activities at kappa, delta, and sigma receptors. The analgesic activity of these opioids resides in the levo(-) isomer. The analgesic activity of opium is due largely to the alkaloid morphine. Morphine is the oldest and most thoroughly studied opioid. It remains the standard by which all other analgesics are compared.

TABLE 23-1 Selected opioid agonists, agonist-antagonists, and antagonists

Classification and drugs
OPIOID AGONISTS
Phenanthrene Derivatives
Morphine
Codeine
Hydromorphone
Oxymorphone
Oxycodone
Morphinan Derivative
Levorphanol
Phenylpiperidine Derivatives
Meperidine
Fentanyl
Sufentanil
Alfentanil
Diphenoxylate
Difenoxin
Loperamide
Diphenylheptylamine Derivatives
Methadone
Propoxyphene
OPIOID AGONIST-ANTAGONISTS
Pentazocine
Nalbuphine
Butorphanol
Dezocine
Buprenorphine
OPIOID ANTAGONISTS
Naloxone
Naltrexone

Morphine

Source and Chemistry Opium, prepared from the poppy plant, contains a number of alkaloids that are classified into two chemical groups: the benzoisoquinolines and the phenanthrenes. The benzoisoquinolines are not analgesic and are not considered opioids; they include papaverine, which has vasodilator properties, and noscapine, which has antitussive (cough suppressing) properties. The alkaloids of the phenanthrene group have analgesic actions and are considered opioids; the two most important phenanthrene alkaloids are morphine (about 10 percent by weight of opium) and codeine (about 0.5 to 1.0 percent).

Structure-Activity Relationship The chemical structure of morphine, a substituted phenanthrene, is shown below.

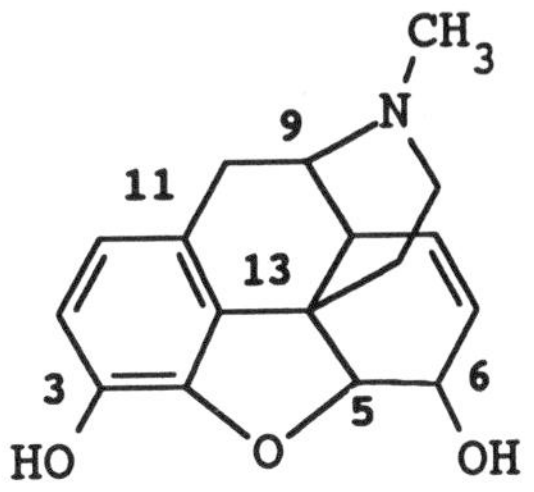

CH_3 N 9 11 13 3 6 5 HO O OH

Morphine is a polycyclic aromatic hydrocarbon containing an N-methyl piperidine ring and an oxygen bridge. The piperidine ring is essential for opioid activity. Reacting morphine with a strong mineral acid removes the oxygen bridge and forms apomorphine, an agent which lacks analgesic activity but has emetic properties. Other key features of the molecule include a phenolic hydroxy at position 3, an alcohol hydroxy at position 6 and chiral carbons at positions 5, 6, 9, 11, and 13. Among the chiral carbons, the center of optical asymmetry is at carbon 13. Only the levo (-) asymmetry in the racemic mixture of morphine binds to the opioid receptors with high affinity and has opioid activity. Since the nitrogen atom in the piperidine ring is approximately 80 percent cationic at physiologic pH (morphine pK_a = 7.9), it is presumed that the opioid receptor has an anionic site with which morphine forms an ionic bond. A second reactive site on the opioid receptor is believed to bind the oxygen atom present in the phenolic hydroxy group at position 3 on the morphine phenanthrene nucleus, since substitutions made on this oxygen atom, like that in codeine, reduce the binding affinity of such morphine derivatives and their analgesic activity. Replacing the methyl group on the nitrogen of the piperidine ring with allyl, propyl or cyclopropylmethyl groups produces derivatives having opioid antagonistic actions. Some antagonists like nalorphine retain some of their analgesic actions (mixed agonist-antagonist), while others, like naloxone and naltrexone, are pure antagonists with no detectable opioid agonistic actions (see Table 23-1).

TABLE 23-2 Opioid receptor binding of representative opioid agonists, antagonists, and agonist-antagonists

Drug	Opioid receptor types		
	Mu	Delta	Kappa
OPIOID AGONISTS			
Morphine[a]	Agonist	Agonist	Agonist
OPIOID ANTAGONISTS			
Naloxone	Antagonist	Antagonist	Antagonist
Naltrexone	Antagonist	Antagonist	Antagonist
OPIOID AGONIST-ANTAGONISTS			
Pentazocine	Antagonist	--------[b]	Agonist
Nalbuphine	Antagonist	---------	Agonist
Butorphanol	Antagonist	---------	Agonist
Buprenorphine	Partial Agonist	---------	Antagonist

a All of the opioids of the agonist type listed in Table 23-1 bind to and activate mu, delta, and kappa receptors similar to morphine. However, differences exist with respect to the degree of activity at each opioid receptor with a rank order of potency as follows: mu > delta > kappa.

b ------- indicates that no significant activity has been observed or the experimental data are inadequate to define the receptor binding activity.

[Modified from: Digregorio, G.J., E.J. Barbieri, A.P. Ferko, G.H. Sterling, J.F. Camp, and M.F. Prout: Handbook of Pain Management, Fourth Edition, Medical Surveillance Inc., West Chester, 1994.]

Relatively simple modifications of morphine's phenanthrene nucleus significantly alter its lipid solubility and its pharmacokinetics, resulting in compounds with varying analgesic potency. Codeine is formed when a methyl group is added to the oxygen atom (methoxyether linkage) at position 3 of morphine; this increases the lipid solubility of the product and enhances its absorption from the gastrointestinal tract. Although the methyl group also protects codeine from first pass metabolic inactivation, codeine has a lower binding affinity for opioid receptors than morphine and thus is less potent as an analgesic agent. Morphine is about 12 times more potent than codeine. Differences in the ability to induce analgesia among the opioids vary greatly (see Table 23-3). Heroin (3,6-diacetylmorphine), which is made by acetylating the two hydroxy groups at positions 3 and 6 of morphine, also has a greater lipid solubility than morphine and allows greater quantities of drug to penetrate the blood-brain barrier, thus increasing its ability to produce analgesia and euphoria. This is especially true when heroin is administered intravenously, as is frequently done by drug abusers. If heroin is taken orally, its analgesic potency is drastically reduced to that of oral morphine, since it is rapidly hydrolyzed by intestinal and liver esterases to form morphine.

Pharmacokinetics *Absorption* Morphine can be administered either orally or parenterally. The absorption and distribution of opioids to various

TABLE 23-3 Potency comparisons of selected opioid agonists and agonist-antagonists

Drug	Equianalgesic doses (mg)[a]		Oral : Parenteral Dose Ratio
	PO	IM	
OPIOID AGONISTS			
Morphine	60.0	10.0	6.0
Codeine	200.0	120.0	1.7
Fentanyl	--------[b]	0.1	--------
Hydromorphone	7.5	1.5	5.0
Levorphanol	4.0	2.0	2.0
Meperidine	300.0	75.0	4.0
Methadone	20.0	10.0	2.0
Oxycodone	30.0	--------[b]	--------
Oxymorphone	6.0	1.0	6.0
Propoxyphene	130.0	--------[b]	--------
Sufentanil	--------[b]	0.02	--------
OPIOID AGONIST-ANTAGONISTS			
Pentazocine	150.0	30.0	5.0
Nalbuphine	--------[b]	10.0	--------
Butorphanol	--------[b]	2.0	--------
Buprenorphine	--------[b]	0.3	--------
Dezocine	--------[b]	10.0	--------

[a] A 10 mg intramuscular dose and a 60 mg oral dose of morphine are considered reference standards against which the other opioids and mixed agonist-antagonist drugs are compared for analgesic effectiveness. The equianalgesic doses of the various agents represents a medical consensus. Since variability occurs among patients, these values should be used only as a guide.

[b] Not used by this route.

[Modified from: Digregorio, G.J., E.J. Barbieri, A.P. Ferko, G.H. Sterling, J.F. Camp, and M.F. Prout: Handbook of Pain Management, Fourth Edition, Medical Surveillance Inc., West Chester, 1994.]

tissues is primarily a function of their lipid solubility. The preferred parenteral route is the intramuscular one, which provides an onset of action of approximately 30 min (see Table 23-4). Peak effects occur between 30 and 90 min, with a 3 to 7 h duration of action and a plasma half-life of 2 to 3 h. When morphine is given orally, its bioavailability is poor (10 to 20 percent) due to a high first pass metabolism by glucuronide conjugating enzymes in the intestine and liver. Higher doses of morphine must therefore be given orally than parenterally. The ratio for producing equal analgesic effects when morphine is given as a single dose orally is approximately 6 times that given intramuscularly (Table 23-3); this ratio is reduced to 2 to 3 with chronic morphine dosing. Oral morphine preparations are commercially available either as hydroalcoholic solutions with an approximate duration of 4 h or as sustained release tablets with a duration of 8 to 12 h.

TABLE 23-4 Pharmacokinetic data of opioid agonists and agonist-antagonists

Drug	Onset of effect[a] (minutes)	Peak effect[a] (minutes)	Duration of effect (hours)	Plasma half-life (hours)
OPIOID AGONISTS				
Morphine	30	30 to 90	3 to 7	2 to 3
Alfentanil	------[b]	-------------[b]	0.5 to 1	1 to 2
Codeine	30	45 to 90	4 to 6	3 to 4
Fentanyl	10	20 to 30	1 to 2	3 to 4
Hydromorphone	30	30 to 90	4 to 5	2 to 4
Levorphanol	30	60 to 90	4 to 8	10 to 12
Meperidine	15	30 to 60	2 to 4	3 to 4
Methadone	15	60 to 120	4 to 6	21 to 25
Oxycodone[c]	15	45 to 60	4 to 6	------------[b]
Oxymorphone	10	30 to 90	3 to 6	------------[b]
Propoxyphene[c]	60	60 to 90	4 to 6	6 to 12
Sufentanil	5	-------------[b]	-------------[b]	2 to 3
OPIOID AGONIST-ANTAGONISTS				
Buprenorphine	15	45 to 60	4 to 6	2 to 3
Butorphanol	10	30 to 60	3 to 4	2 to 4
Dezocine	30	30 to 150	2 to 4	----------[b]
Nalbuphine	15	45 to 60	3 to 6	4 to 6
Pentazocine	15	30 to 60	2 to 3	2 to 3

[a] Based on intramuscular administration.

[b] No data available.

[c] Based on oral administration.

[Modified from: Digregorio, G.J., E.J. Barbieri, A.P. Ferko, G.H. Sterling, J.F. Camp, and M.F. Prout: Handbook of Pain Management, Fourth Edition, Medical Surveillance Inc., West Chester, 1994.]

Distribution Following its absorption, about one-third of the plasma level of morphine is bound to plasma proteins. Higher concentrations of the drug are taken up by the lung, liver, and kidney than by the CNS, the primary site of morphine's analgesic action. During pregnancy, opioids readily cross the placenta and the fetal blood-brain barrier, which is not fully developed. Therefore, immediately following delivery, infants born to addicted mothers must be treated with oral opioids to prevent serious and life-threatening opioid withdrawal symptoms. The use of opioids in obstetrics during delivery can also result in the delivery of an infant with respiratory depression.

Biotransformation Morphine is converted in the liver to polar metabolites, which are then excreted, primarily by the kidney. The major pathway of biotransformation involves hepatic glucuronidation of the free hydroxyl groups at both the 3 and 6 positions in a 2:1 ratio. While the 3-glucuronide is inactive, it is now known that the morphine-6-glucuronide is active and a more potent analgesic than morphine, particularly when injected intrathecally. The analgesic activity of morphine during chronic therapy may be due primarily to morphine-6-glucuronide. In patients with severely impaired renal function, the dosage of morphine should be decreased to prevent the cumulative toxicity that results from the impaired ability to excrete this active metabolite. Whereas morphine-6-glucuronide binds readily to opioid receptors and activates them, morphine-3-glucuronide does neither, thus explaining the analgesic activity of the 6-glucuronide. A minor pathway in the biotransformation of morphine involves enzymatic N-demethylation of the methyl group on the piperidine ring by hepatic enzymes to form normorphine. While normorphine has little analgesic activity, it possesses greater excitatory and convulsant effects than morphine.

Excretion The polar glucuronide metabolites of morphine are excreted mostly in urine with very little unchanged morphine detectable in urine. Metabolites of morphine may also be found in saliva. About 10 percent of morphine in the form of its metabolites are normally excreted in the feces as a result of their excretion into bile and their enterohepatic circulation.

Effects on Organ Systems While morphine generally depresses the CNS, certain sites in the CNS are stimulated, although this latter effect is generally masked by general depressant effects. Morphine also has a distinct effect in the periphery on the smooth muscles in the lung and in the intestinal, biliary, and urinary tracts.

Central Nervous System Effects Morphine is very effective for relieving, dull chronic-type pain, and its use is restricted for the treatment of moderate to severe pain. Morphine and other opioids are useful for treating the pain referred from smooth muscles such as those found in ureteral and intestinal colic. Morphine is also the preferred drug for treating the pain associated with acute myocardial ischemia. When morphine is administered parenterally to a patient in pain, the patient experiences euphoria after a period of 30 min; euphoria is an exaggerated feeling of well-being in which the person is less anxious and concerned about their pain. Higher doses of morphine produce sedation, but the level of sedation produced is not as deep as that produced by the sedative-hypnotic barbiturates; the patient may sleep but can be readily aroused. Not all individuals given morphine are made euphoric. Some individuals, such as those without pain, may experience an ill and unpleasant feeling, or dysphoria, along with nausea and vomiting on initial exposure to morphine. These individuals also include those who may eventually become dependent on opioids. With continued chronic use, the dysphoria is diminished and euphoria develops. It is this euphoria that is the driving force for the compulsive behavior of individuals to continue using these drugs. An individual may still feel the pain after opioid administration, but the fear and worry associated with the cause of the pain is considerably reduced. An example of the importance of the effect of morphine in reducing the psychic component of pain is the finding that some antipsychotic drugs potentiate the analgesic effects of morphine.

The effects of morphine on spinal cord reflexes are complex. Spinal cord stimulation is always present but is masked by the CNS depressant effects. The excitatory effects observed in some species or physiologic systems cannot be correlated with the metabolism of morphine to normorphine, which is known to have convulsant properties. It has been suggested that the excitation and convulsant effects of opioids result from inhibition of inhibitory neuronal pathways mediated by the neurotransmitters such as γ-aminobutyric acid (GABA) or glycine. Due to the underlying excitatory activity of morphine, caution is urged for its use in patients with seizure disorders.

Respiration Morphine and other opioids depress all phases of respiration (respiratory rate, tidal volume, and minute volume) in a dose-dependent manner by decreasing the sensitivity of the medullary chemoreceptors to the carbon dioxide tension (pCO_2) in blood. The degree of respiratory depression is also influenced by pain stimuli which stimulate the respiratory center and tend to counterbalance the respiratory depressant effect of the opioid. When the pain is relieved by the administration of an opioid, failure to reduce the dose of the opioid may lead to severe respiratory depression. Thus, opioids produce more respiratory depression in pain-free individuals than in patients with pain. Therefore, the dose of opioids must be titrated against the pain to avoid subsequent respiratory depression. The major side effect of opioids is respiratory depression and the cause of death in opioid overdose is respiratory arrest. Following parenteral administration of morphine, impaired respiration will increase blood pCO_2. The increased pCO_2 can then override the reduced sensitivity of the chemoreceptors in the medulla and the respiratory rate may return to normal.

High blood pCO_2 also dilates the cerebral vessels which then results in an increase in cerebrospinal fluid pressure. Because morphine tends to elevate cerebrospinal fluid pressure, it should be used with great caution when treating patients who have head injuries in which elevated cerebrospinal fluid pressures already exist.

Emetic and Antiemetic Effects Initial therapy with morphine may induce nausea and vomiting (emesis) by stimulating the chemoreceptor trigger zone (CTZ) in the area postrema at the base of the fourth ventricle. Vestibular stimulation may be responsible for the nausea and vomiting often seen in ambulatory pain-free individuals who abuse the opioid drugs. Although morphine initially acts as an emetic by stimulating the CTZ, continued therapy with morphine can directly depress the emetic center, causing an antiemetic effect. Therefore, chronic administration of morphine blocks the nausea and vomiting induced by chemical agents like the antineoplastics, which stimulate the CTZ.

Antitussive Effect The cough center consists of a cluster of neurons adjacent to the vomiting (emetic) center in the medulla. Irritation of various parts of the tracheobronchial tree by foreign matter or excessive secretions stimulate sensory stretch receptors and activate vagal afferent nerves that terminate in the cough center and initiate the cough reflex. Opioids, in general, act directly on the cough center to suppress the cough reflex, producing its antitussive action. Opioids raise the threshold required for activating the medullary cough center. The prototype opioid commonly used as an antitussive agent is codeine. The dose of codeine required for antitussive activity is less than that required to produce analgesia. For treating mild to moderate pain, codeine is generally given orally in doses of 60 mg or less. However, only 15 mg is required for an antitussive action. The interactions of codeine with receptors in the cough center that mediate antitussive activity are different from the opioid receptors previously described which mediate the other actions of opioids. Drugs that interact with the receptors in the cough center and have antitussive properties lack stereospecificity and seem to be less sensitive to the opioid antagonist naloxone. Whereas only the levo(-) isomers of opioid drugs have analgesic activity, both the levo(-) and dextro(-) isomers of the opioids depress the cough center. The opioid isomer dextromethorphan has selective antitussive properties and is commercially available alone or with other ingredients in several over-the-counter preparations. This centrally-acting antitussive agent does not produce many of the side effects associated with codeine.

Miosis Small doses of morphine and most opioids given systemically constrict the pupils (miosis) by stimulating the neurons located rostral to the oculomotor nuclear complex. Morphine increases neuronal firing in the Edinger-Westphal nucleus of the oculomotor nerve (3rd cranial nerve) which enhances parasympathetic tone input to the sphincter muscle of the iris. This central pupillo-constricting action of morphine can be blocked by locally applied anticholinergic drugs like atropine, but not by adrenergic drugs like phenylephrine. Tolerance does not develop to the miotic effects of the opioids.

Orthostatic Hypotension The cardiovascular system is generally resistant to the effects of morphine. However, in large doses, especially when morphine is given intravenously, orthostatic hypotension may develop. The hypotensive effect of morphine has two components: a peripheral component due to local release of histamine, a vasodilator, and a central component due to depression of the medullary vasomotor center which decreases sympathetic tone to blood vessels. Histamine release may occur after low or therapeutic doses of morphine. The decreased sympathetic outflow to blood vessels along with the vasodilation induced by histamine thus produce hypotension.

Endocrine Morphine and other opioid drugs interact with the opioid receptors in the hypothalamus and posterior pituitary to increase the release of antidiuretic hormone, growth hormone, prolactin, and ACTH; they also decrease the circulating levels of thyrotropin, luteinizing hormone, and follicle-stimulating hormone.

Peripheral Effects *Gastrointestinal System* Morphine and opioid drugs, in lower than analgesic doses, have a constipating effect by reducing the activity of the entire gastrointestinal tract. Opium was used for treating diarrhea and dysentery many years before it was used for the relief of pain. The actions of morphine on the intestine include depression of longitudinal muscle contractions with a resultant decrease in propulsive peristaltic activity, increased tone of the circular muscles (spasmogenic), and increased contraction of all sphincters. These effects delay gastric emptying and produce a dehydrated fecal mass. Higher doses of morphine reduce pancreatic and biliary secretions which hinder digestion. Cortical depression in the CNS also blocks afferent sensory input from the lower bowel to inhibit the defecation reflex. All of these actions in combination produce constipation as a major side effect when opioids are used as analgesics. Substance P, present in the myenteric plexuses, is thought to play an important role in regulating intestinal peristalsis, whereas 5-hydroxytryptamine (serotonin) release may be important for increasing the tone (spasmogenic) of intestinal circular smooth muscle. Opioids are thought to decrease the release of substance P in the myenteric plexuses, which then decrease peristaltic contractions of the longitudinal smooth muscle in the intestine. Tolerance does not develop to the constipating effects of opioids.

Biliary System Morphine causes spasm and an increase in biliary pressure by increasing the tone of smooth muscle in the bile duct and by constricting the sphincter of Oddi in the common bile duct. Biliary stasis and increased biliary pressure build-up may cause epigastric distress or biliary colic. Meperidine, a synthetic opioid agonist, or certain mixed agonist-antagonist drugs may be used for treating biliary colic, since these agents are less spasmogenic to the biliary tract.

Genitourinary System Morphine decreases urine volume by increasing the release of antidiuretic hormone. As in the intestine, morphine can also induce smooth muscle spasm in the ureters and the detrusor muscle, as well as contracting the sphincter. Morphine also inhibits the micturition reflex by its CNS cortical depressant action. In postoperative patients and in elderly males with benign prostatic hypertrophy, morphine may cause acute urinary retention or oliguria.

Bronchial System While morphine directly constricts bronchi, part of its action is also mediated by the local release of histamine from mast cells. Morphine can be life-threatening in asthmatics due to its central effect in depressing respiration and its peripheral effects in inducing severe bronchial constriction. Systemically, morphine can precipitate an asthmatic attack.

Skin Morphine liberates histamine both at the site of injection and at other sites following systemic absorption. This may cause urticaria, sweating, dermatitis, pruritus, and redness of the skin and the eyes.

Adverse Reactions and Acute Poisoning Most of the known adverse reactions of morphine are the result of the pharmacologic actions noted above. These include nausea, vomiting, dizziness, pruritus, constipation, and CNS depression. Urticaria and other allergic phenomena due to histamine release may also occur occasionally. Deaths from opioid overdosage are almost always due to respiratory depression. Opioids are CNS depressants, and synergism with or potentiation of other CNS depressants may occur. Respiratory depression may pose an even greater risk in the fetus than in the adult, since the relative absence of a blood-brain barrier allows larger amounts of morphine to enter the brain.

The triad of coma, pinpoint pupils, and markedly depressed respiration strongly suggests opioid poisoning. The treatment of choice is the administration of small doses of naloxone intravenously, repeated every few minutes as needed. Naloxone will restore the respiratory rate and total volume to normal, thereby normalizing blood pCO_2. It will also reverse the miotic effects on the pupils, spasm in the gastrointestinal tract, and the euphoria induced by opioids. It may also be necessary in opioid poisoning to support respiration mechanically to achieve adequate ventilation. After the respiration recovers following naloxone administration, the patient should not be left unattended because the duration of action of naloxone is much shorter than that of the agonist. Particular care should be exercised in using the antagonist in an opioid-dependent individual because naloxone may precipitate a severe abstinence syndrome.

The use of naloxone is particularly beneficial when the cause of poisoning is unknown or when a mixture of drugs is involved. Naloxone will antagonize all the opioids, including the mixed agonist-antagonist group.

Tolerance and Physical Dependence When the opioid agonists are administered chronically, both tolerance and physical dependence may be observed. Tolerance is said to occur when the usual dose of a drug shows a decreased effectiveness or when very high doses are required to maintain the desired effect. Physical dependence is an addictive state that results from continued administration of the opioid and leads to a pattern of use that alters the normal biochemical and psychologic state in an individual. One of the cardinal signs of physical dependence is the characteristic withdrawal or "abstinence syndrome" which occurs when opioid administration is stopped abruptly. The time required to produce physical dependence may be as short as 1 to 2 weeks if large quantities of the drug are used. Opioid withdrawal is characterized initially by restlessness and an intense craving for the drug, followed by lacrimation, chills, fever, vomiting, insomnia, hypertension, anorexia, and weight loss. The pupils become dilated. Hyperthermia, hyperventilation, diarrhea, and anxiety develop, and pilomotor stimulation produces a gooseflesh appearance in the skin.

Tolerance occurs to many but not all of the effects of morphine. Most commonly, patients become tolerant to the following effects: analgesia, sedation, respiratory depression, nausea, vomiting, euphoria, and cough suppression. Minimal or no tolerance occurs to the constipating or miotic effects of morphine. Tolerance is closely associated with physical dependence on morphine and both characteristics are dose and time dependent. Large doses of morphine given at short time intervals will produce tolerance more rapidly and a higher degree of physical dependence than small doses administered at longer intervals. Tolerance to morphine does not become important until 2 or 3 weeks after its continued administration.

The severity and duration of the withdrawal syndrome is a function of both the onset and the duration of action of the specific opioid used. Since morphine has a shorter onset and duration of action than methadone, the signs and symptoms of withdrawal develop more quickly after withdrawal from morphine than from methadone withdrawal. However, the severity of symptoms is greater at its peak and the total withdrawal period is shorter for morphine than for methadone. Because cross-dependence within the opioid group is common, methadone, which has the advantages of oral effectiveness and a long duration of action, may substitute for other opioids as a strategy to wean addicts through the withdrawal period with minimal discomfort. Since clonidine reduces the severity of some withdrawal effects, the treatment period of addicts going through withdrawal may be shortened by precipitating the withdrawal syndrome with naloxone while using clonidine to provide symptomatic relief.

Therapeutic Uses The most important use of opioids is to relieve pain. Differences among the various agonists relate primarily to oral efficacy, duration of action, and specific side effects. These potent agents, with their liabilities for respiratory depression and physical dependence, should never be used when less hazardous measures will suffice. On the other hand, no patient should be denied the use of opioids when other forms of pain relief are inadequate, particularly in chronic pain states such as cancer. To delay the progress of tolerance to opioids, dosage should be advanced only to the point of pain relief. Since cross-tolerance among opioid agonists is common, switching to another opioid does not avoid or delay the development of tolerance.

The traditional method of opioid administration on a fixed "by the clock" schedule frequently provides inadequate pain relief due to "peaks and valleys" in opioid blood levels obtained on such fixed dosage schedule. In addition, it has been well established that many physicians prescribe opioids in smaller doses at longer intervals than what is required for the relief of pain, fearing either that the patient would become dependent on the drug or that respiration would be severely impaired by the opioid. An alternative approach for pain management is to use patient-controlled analgesia (PCA) in which the patient titrates the dose of the analgesic according to his or her needs by pressing a button. With the PCA system, a microprocessor-driven infusion pump is required to prevent misuse or overdose. The physician chooses the parenteral opioid and the dose; the decision is also made if the drug is to be given by continuous infusion or as a bolus, and the lock-out interval (i.e., the least amount of time before the next dose may be given) is determined. PCA may be used to administer opioids intravenously or intraspinally (i.e., intrathecally or epidurally). Studies show that patients using PCA are the best judges of their own analgesic needs, achieving maximum effects with minimum doses. Experience also shows that PCA patients develop tolerance at a slower rate and that they do not abuse opioids to experience the euphoric effects. However, PCA is not recommended for individuals who have a history of drug abuse. By inserting catheters epidurally or intrathecally, selected opioids can be injected into various areas of the spinal cord to act on specific opioid receptors in these areas. Small doses of morphine (0.5 to 1.0 mg) intrathecally (subarachnoid) administered as a bolus may thus provide long-lasting analgesia for up to 24 h. Small doses of morphine given spinally produce analgesia equal to larger doses given orally or intramuscularly. Epidurally, higher doses of morphine (2 to 10 mg) must be given than intrathecally, since the drug must cross the dura to interact with opioid receptors in the spinal cord. Morphine administered epidurally as a continuous infusion or as a bolus can also provide long-lasting analgesic effects up to 24 h.

Opioids have proven to be beneficial in relieving some forms of diarrhea. In myocardial infarction, when not only pain but apprehension is often intense, morphine relieves the pain, calms the patient and may decrease oxygen consumption and cardiac work. Morphine is valuable in treating the dyspnea and acute pulmonary edema which is secondary to left ventricular failure. Morphine is given intravenously for this purpose and produces dramatic effects in correcting the arrhythmia and increasing cardiac output as well as decreasing peripheral resistance and clearing fluid from the lungs. Morphine probably corrects the cardiac abnormality in part by reducing the patient's apprehension about his impaired respiration. Another very common use of opioids is as part of premedication for surgery. The opioids can reduce the apprehension of the patient before induction of general anesthesia, as well as reduce the amount of anesthetic drug necessary. Some opioid agonists can be used by themselves or combined with a neuroleptic agent to produce a state termed "neuroleptanalgesia" in which surgery can be performed. Some opioids, especially codeine, are useful as antitussives, although morphine is not employed for this purpose.

Paregoric

Paregoric is prepared from opium as a hydroalcoholic solution and contains about 2 mg of morphine in an adult oral dose of 5 mL. When given orally for the treatment of diarrhea, it has a local action on the intestine to reduce intestinal motility. Also it is used orally for its systemic effects in the early postpartum period to prevent withdrawal symptoms in neonates who have become physically dependent *in utero* because of chronic maternal use of opioids during pregnancy.

Codeine

Like morphine, codeine is a naturally occurring alkaloid found in the poppy plant. It differs from morphine structurally only in that a methoxy group is substituted for the 3-hydroxy group of morphine.

About 10 percent of orally administered codeine is O-demethylated to morphine, which is about 12 times more potent as an analgesic than codeine. A significant amount of codeine is also N-demethylated to norcodeine, a metabolite that has stimulant properties. After a 15 mg oral dose of codeine, the peak blood level of codeine is approximately equal to the level of norcodeine. The formation of significant quantities of the metabolite norcodeine helps to explain why toxic effects of codeine include seizures, especially in children, and why codeine has greater central stimulatory effects and less sedative properties than morphine. Small quantities of free codeine, norcodeine, and morphine, along with larger quantities of their conjugated forms, are excreted primarily in the urine. Although the pharmacodynamic actions of codeine are similar to those of morphine, there are also significant differences between the two opioids. Codeine is more effective orally, is used as an antitussive, and is more widely used as an analgesic for the treatment of mild to moderate degrees of pain. The maximum oral dose commonly used for analgesia is 60 mg, while the antitussive dose is much lower, usually about 15 mg. The antitussive action of codeine has been postulated to result from interactions with receptors in the cough center that differ from the typical opioid receptors, as discussed earlier. Because codeine acts centrally, and aspirin (a non-opioid) works mainly in the periphery, to produce analgesia, there are many preparations available combining both drugs. Combining codeine with aspirin or acetaminophen produces additive analgesic effects. As with morphine, tolerance and physical dependence can develop to codeine, but the incidence for codeine is lower than for morphine.

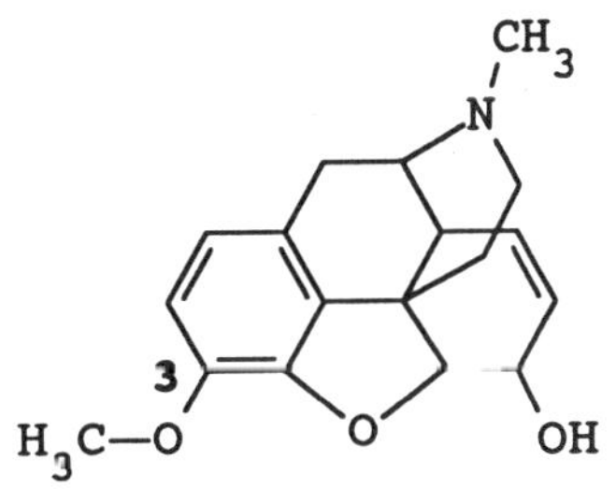

Heroin

Heroin, or diacetylmorphine, is a synthetic opioid and a classical prodrug.

Heroin differs from morphine in that heroin has acetyl groups at positions 3 and 6 whereas morphine has hydroxyl groups. The presence of acetyl groups in heroin increases its lipid solubility about 10-fold over morphine, which accounts for the rapid passage of heroin through the blood-brain barrier. Heroin is converted to the active metabolites 6-monoacetylmorphine, morphine-6-glucuronide, and morphine to produce analgesia. After intravenous dosing, plasma and tissue esterases remove the 3-acetyl group, forming the 6-monoacetylmorphine. Heroin and 6-monoacetylmorphine each penetrate the blood-brain barrier more quickly than morphine. Present also in brain is the active morphine-6-glucuronide; however, it is not known whether this metabolite is formed locally in brain, or whether it enters the brain following hepatic glucuronidation. The two active biotransformation products 6-monoacetylmorphine and morphine-6-glucuronide contribute substantially to the analgesic activity of heroin. Other evidence indicating that heroin is really a prodrug comes from studies which show that the metabolites of heroin, 6-monoacetylmorphine, morphine-6-glucuronide, and morphine bind to opioid receptors, whereas heroin does not. Although heroin is 2 to 3 times more potent than morphine, controlled clinical studies show that no therapeutic advantages are obtained by using heroin in place of other opioid drugs. Possession and use of heroin is illegal in the Unites States as the compound is classified as a Schedule I drug, a classification reserved for those agents having a high abuse potential.

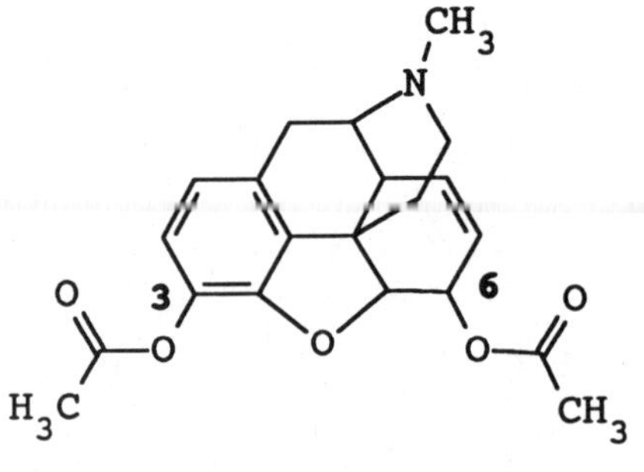

Hydromorphone and Oxymorphone

These agents are congeners of morphine. Hydromorphone is approximately 8 times more potent than morphine by the intramuscular route (Table 23-3). Its absorption following oral administration is somewhat better than that of morphine. Although commonly use orally and by subcutaneous or intramuscular injection, hydromorphone can be used by slow intravenous administration. In addition, rectal suppositories are available that may be useful in some patients. The drug is an effective oral antitussive; however, the high dependence liability makes it less useful for this purpose than other drugs.

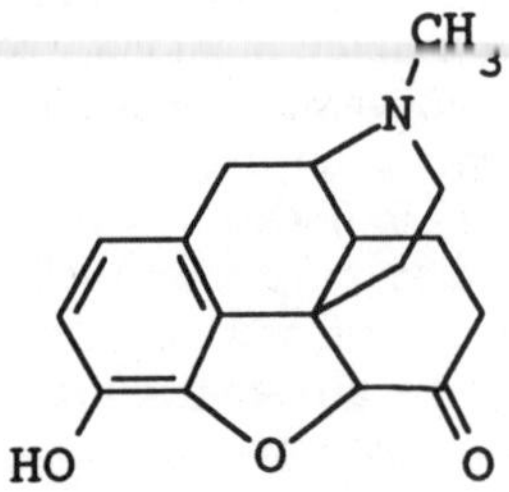

Hydromorphone

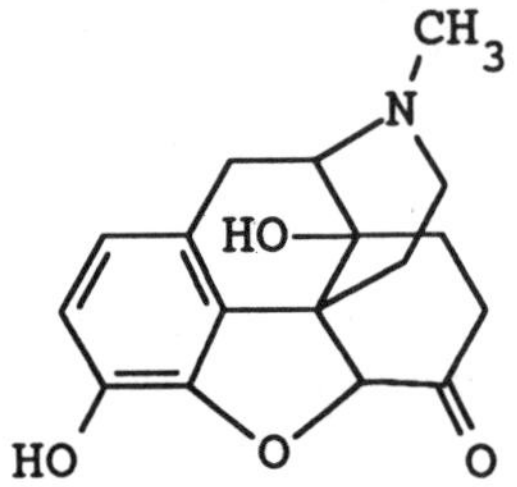

Oxymorphone

Oxymorphone is about 10 times more potent and has a shorter onset of action than morphine when given intramuscularly. It can be given by the same routes as hydromorphone. It is also used for the relief of pain.

Except as noted above, the pharmacologic effects, the latencies to peak effects, and the durations of action for both of these drugs are about the same as that of morphine (Table 23-4).

Hydrocodone and Oxycodone

These two drugs are chemically related to codeine and morphine. Both are absorbed quite well from the gastrointestinal tract, both are analgesics and good antitussives. Hydrocodone is used primarily as an antitussive; its potency for this use when given orally is about twice that of codeine. When used as an analgesic, the compound is commonly combined with acetaminophen. Oxycodone is used as an analgesic in many oral proprietary preparations in combination with aspirin or acetaminophen. Oxycodone has two-thirds the analgesic potency of morphine when compared by the intramuscular route (Table 23-3).

Levorphanol

This drug is structurally different than the aforementioned compounds in that it lacks the oxygen bridge, making it a morphinan derivative.

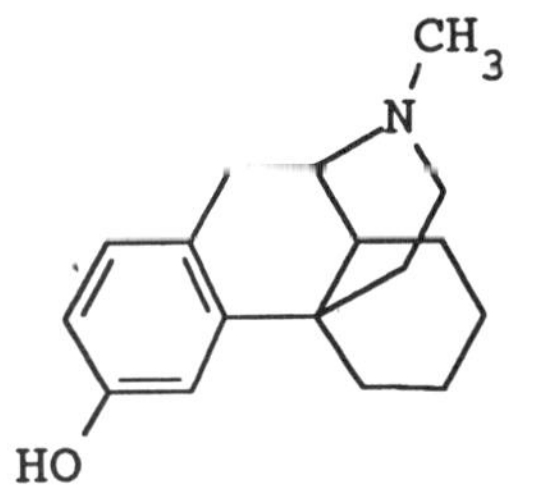

The pharmacologic effects of levorphanol are similar to those of morphine except that the incidence of nausea, vomiting, and constipation are reported to be less than with morphine. When injected intramuscularly, levorphanol is about 5 times more potent than morphine, and like codeine, it is effective orally, having a very low oral to parenteral dose ratio of 2 (Table 23-3). The onset and peak analgesic effects are comparable to those of morphine; however, the duration of the analgesia is much longer, since levorphanol is slowly metabolized, resulting in a longer plasma half-life (Table 23-4).

Methorphan

Methorphan is a methylated derivative of levorphanol. The levo(-) isomer, levomethorphan, produces opioid-like effects, it can be substituted for morphine, and it is fully addictive. On the other hand, the dextro(+) isomer, dextromethorphan, is not analgesic, will not substitute for morphine, and is not addicting. However, dextromethorphan has antitussive properties and is available for this use as an over-the-counter product.

Meperidine

Meperidine is a prototype phenylpiperidine compound which is made synthetically and differs markedly in its structure from morphine and the other opioid agonists discussed above. Fentanyl, alfentanil, sufentanil, diphenoxylate, difenoxin, and loperamide are all opioid agonists chemically related to meperidine.

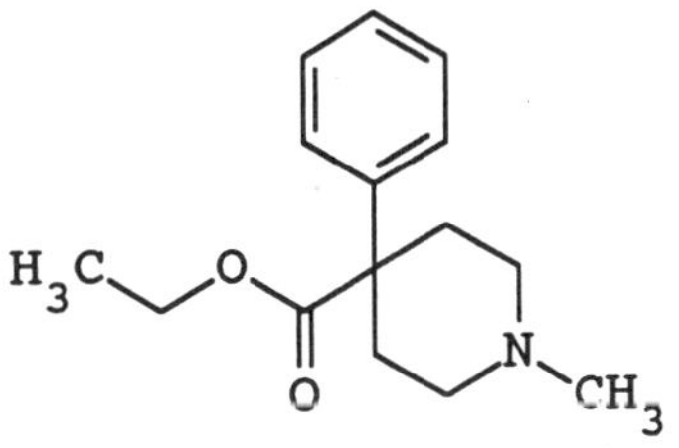

Meperidine is only about one-tenth as potent as morphine for inducing analgesia, sedation, euphoria, and respiratory depression. The pharmacologic effects of meperidine are similar to those of morphine with the following exceptions. (1) Meperidine in toxic doses causes CNS excitation and convulsions due to hepatic N-demethylation forming the metabolite, normeperidine, which is a stimulant. (2) Unlike morphine, meperidine causes mydriasis, tachycardia, and dry mouth due to its inherent anticholinergic properties. (3) Meperidine is less constipating than morphine. (4) This drug is less likely than morphine to raise intrabiliary pressure. (5) Meperidine is not an effective antitussive.

The pharmacology of meperidine shows both opioid and atropine-like (anticholinergic) characteristics, but only the opioid effects are reversed by the opioid antagonist, naloxone. Meperidine is shorter-acting (2 to 3 h) than morphine, and contrary to popular belief, is not particularly useful when administered orally. Approximately 4 times the parenteral dose is needed for equivalent oral efficacy (Table 23-3). Because meperidine has a short duration of action with a half-life of about 3 h, it is widely used as an analgesic during diagnostic procedures such as cystoscopy, endoscopy, and retrograde pyelography. It is also used as a preanesthetic medication and as an obstetrical analgesic. Because it is less spasmogenic than morphine, it is also useful in treating the pain of biliary colic. The half-life of the metabolite normeperidine is long and has been estimated to be between 15 and 20 h; therefore, impaired renal or hepatic function increases the likelihood of developing CNS stimulatory effects due to accumulation of this compound.

The dependence liability of meperidine is similar to that of morphine, although signs of abstinence differ somewhat due to its anticholinergic properties. Administration of meperidine to a patient also being treated with a monoamine oxidase inhibitor may produce excitation, delirium, and convulsions due to a decreased metabolism of the convulsant metabolite normeperidine.

Fentanyl

Fentanyl is a chemical relative of meperidine that is nearly 100 times more potent than morphine, and about 750 times more potent than meperidine when compared by intramuscular injection (Table 23-3).

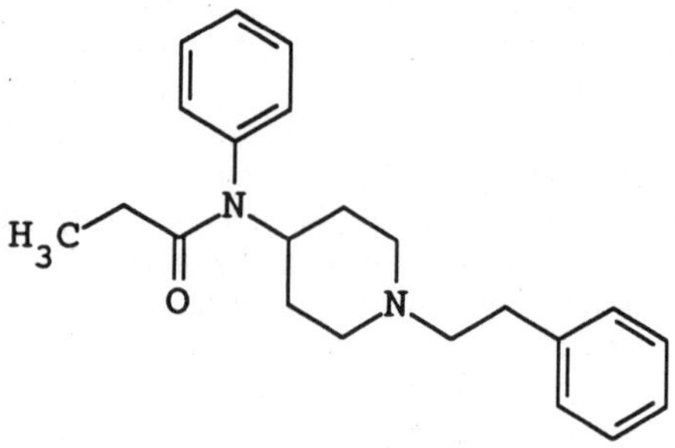

The duration of action of fentanyl is shorter than that of meperidine, usually between 30 and 60 min after intravenous administration, and 1 to 2 h after intramuscular injection. Fentanyl citrate is available for parenteral administration. Used in combination with droperidol, a butyrophenone antipsychotic, the analgesia is potentiated by the combined use of these two drugs. Droperidol, the antipsychotic, is thought to reduce the individual's reactions (psychic component) to noxious stimuli, whereas fentanyl as an opioid inhibits the afferent sensory nociceptive input (threshold component). Fentanyl is combined with droperidol and is frequently used by anesthesiologists for treating postoperative pain, a use called "neuroleptanalgesia". When the combined drugs are used to supplement general anesthetics during surgery, this practice is termed "neuroleptanesthesia".

A new transdermal therapeutic system (in which patches containing four different sizes and strengths of fentanyl) are available for chronic pain management. Systemic absorption of fentanyl through the skin avoids the discomfort of injections and provides a continuous supply of fentanyl for about 72 h after application. After several sequential 72 h applications, patients reach a steady state plasma concentration of fentanyl.

Synthetic drugs of abuse, the so-called "designer drugs", which are derivatives of fentanyl, are very potent opioids made illegally in makeshift laboratories by underground chemists. These analogs, which are more lipid soluble than fentanyl itself, include α-methylfentanyl, para-fluorofentanyl, α-methylacetylfentanyl, and 3-methylfentanyl. Most of these dangerous drugs have now been placed in Schedule I. High lipid solubility increases their permeability through the blood-brain barrier and makes 3-methylfentanyl, for example, about 2000 times more potent than meperidine. Due to its extreme potency, 3-methylfentanyl alone was responsible for more than 100 overdose deaths in California.

Alfentanil

Alfentanil is a synthetic tertiary amine derivative of fentanyl. Alfentanil is for intravenous use, and it is about 1/10th as potent as fentanyl and has a shorter duration of action (from 15 to 60 min). The quick onset of action and the short duration of action makes alfentanil useful in anesthesiology as a supplement to anesthetics for out-patient surgical procedures; it is given by infusion for maintenance of anesthesia during surgery and as an inducing agent prior to surgery.

Sufentanil

Sufentanil is a substituted derivative of fentanyl marketed for intravenous use. Sufentanil is 5 to 10 times more potent than fentanyl. Its onset of action is more rapid than that of fentanyl because of higher lipid solubility, while its duration of action (about 30 to 60 min) is about the same as that of fentanyl. Among the congeners of fentanyl, sufentanil has less cardiovascular side effects than the others, making it useful in patients undergoing long cardiovascular or neurosurgical procedures. It is used intravenously as an adjunct to other general anesthetics and as a primary anesthetic agent.

Diphenoxylate and Difenoxin

Diphenoxylate is a synthetic phenylpiperidine derivative structurally similar to meperidine. Difenoxin is the major, active biotransformation product of diphenoxylate.

Following high doses (40 mg) given orally, diphenoxylate is absorbed and produces typical systemic opioid effects. When given orally in lower therapeutic doses (2.5 to 5 mg), its effects are limited to the gastrointestinal tract, reducing motility to exert an antidiarrheal effect.

Ester hydrolysis rapidly and extensively converts diphenoxylate to diphenoxylic acid (difenoxin), the pharmacologically active and major biotransformation product. Difenoxin is metabo-

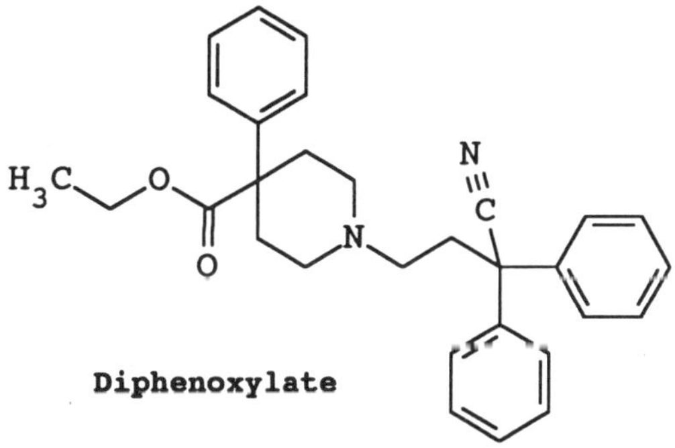

Diphenoxylate

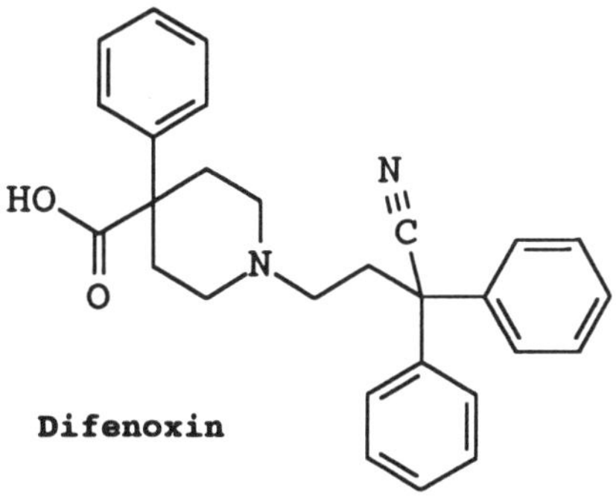

Difenoxin

lized to an inactive hydroxylated product. Most of diphenoxylate and difenoxin are eliminated through the feces; inactive metabolites are excreted, primarily as glucuronide conjugates, in the urine.

Both diphenoxylate and difenoxin are indicated in the management of diarrhea. Both compounds are marketed combined with 0.025 mg of atropine sulfate (a subtherapeutic amount) so as not to divert the use of this product from its intended purpose.

Loperamide

Loperamide is another synthetic phenylpiperidine derivative used exclusively as an antidiarrheal.

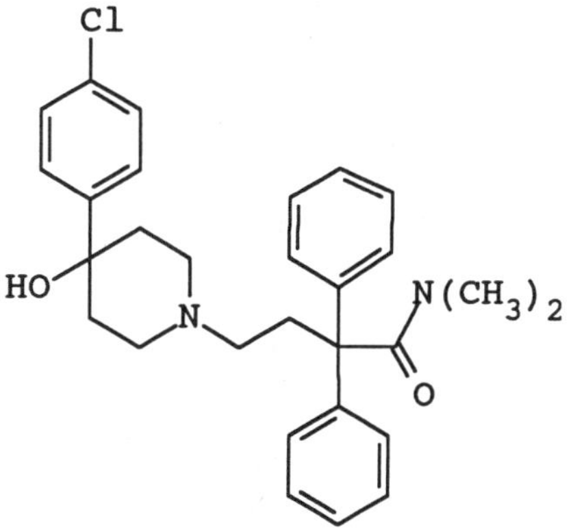

When given orally, loperamide is poorly absorbed. The minute amount of loperamide that is absorbed does not penetrate the blood-brain barrier readily. This makes loperamide an ineffective CNS opioid; however, this drug is useful for treating diarrhea because of its local effect in reducing motility of the gastrointestinal tract. Loperamide is not combined with atropine as are diphenoxylate and difenoxin, since even at high doses, the abuse potential is very low. The drug has a low incidence of systemic adverse effects and is also available as an over-the-counter product.

Methadone

Methadone is a synthetic, diphenylheptylamine derivative, not structurally related to morphine. It exists as a racemic mixture and it is primarily the levo-enantiomer in the racemic mixture that has opioid activity.

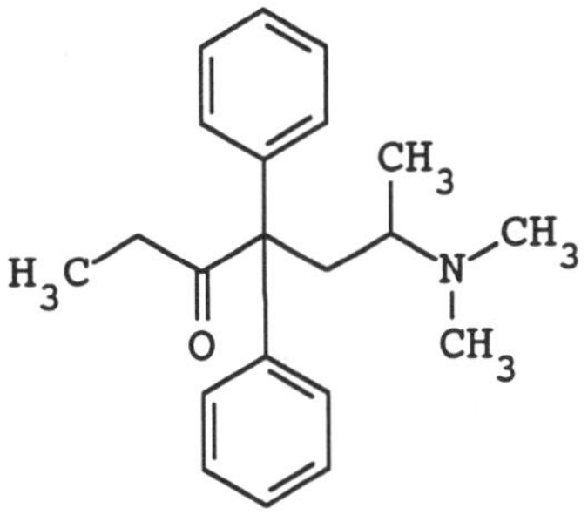

Methadone is effective orally and parenterally with analgesic potency which equals that of morphine when given intramuscularly (Table 23-3). It also has other opioid agonistic effects such as respiratory depression, nausea and vomiting, spasmogenic effects on smooth muscle, and cough suppression. Orally, methadone has greater bioavailability (over 90 percent) than morphine and is only slowly biotransformed by the liver (biological half-life = 24 to 36 h) to inactive products before excretion in bile and urine. Its principal difference from morphine lies in its greater oral efficacy and its longer duration of action. Another advantage over morphine is that methadone does not liberate histamine to cause allergic side effects. Because it is slowly biotransformed by the liver, patients with reduced renal or hepatic function should be monitored carefully for signs of drug accumulation or toxicity. For analgesia, methadone is administered at intervals of 6 to 8 h to prevent accumulation.

Methadone is also used to treat individuals with opioid-dependence in so-called "methadone maintenance" or "substitution" programs. Withdrawal signs and symptoms occurring after abrupt discontinuation of methadone are milder, but more prolonged, than with morphine because of the long duration of action of the compound. Due to cross-tolerance and cross-dependency that exist between opioid agonists, methadone can allay the withdrawal effects of individuals dependent on heroin or other opioid agonists. These properties make methadone a useful drug both for detoxification in methadone substitution programs and for minimizing withdrawal symptoms in methadone maintenance programs. For detoxification, a dose of methadone equivalent to that of the substituted opioid is given. The individual is then weaned from methadone by gradually decreasing its daily dose. The opioid user experiences a mild and more endurable withdrawal syndrome. In methadone maintenance programs, the individual is stabilized by being given a fixed daily oral dose (50 to 100 mg) of methadone. In such maintenance programs, the opioid-dependent person no longer has to engage in criminal activity to obtain money for illegal purchase of drugs. Ideally, the individual may also then be more receptive to psychological counseling while he or she is receiving methadone on a daily basis.

Levomethadyl acetate is an opioid agonist that is indicated for the treatment of opioid addiction similar to the use of methadone in the management of opioid dependence. This compound is not to be used outside of an approved drug treatment program. Levomethadyl acetate is has a long duration of action and doses for initial treatment and for maintenance may be given every 2 or 3 days. Caution should be exercised when determining the required dosage to prevent overdosage. Levomethadyl acetate has the same pharmacological effects as do other opioids such as sedation, respiratory depression, and reduction of cardiovascular function. Since cross-dependence exists with opioid agonists, patients can be converted from methadone to levomethadyl acetate without significant difficulty.

Propoxyphene

Propoxyphene, which is chemically similar to methadone, has four isomers. Dextropropoxyphene is an isomer with an oral analgesic potency about two-thirds that of codeine and is considered to be a weak analgesic.

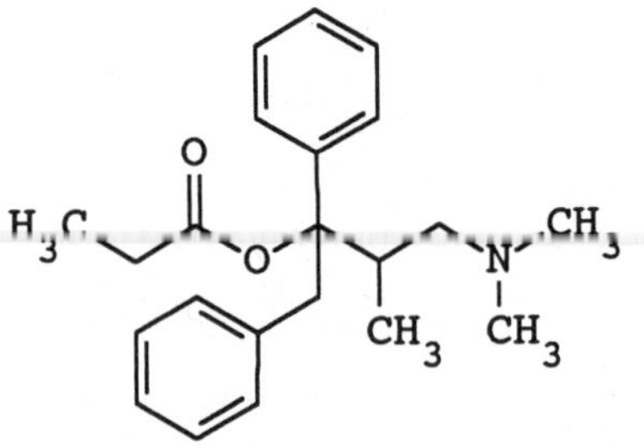

Although it is frequently compared with codeine for its analgesic effects, dextropropoxyphene does not have the antitussive properties of codeine. Several commercial products are available (some containing caffeine) which combine dextropropoxyphene with either aspirin or acetaminophen. In large doses, dextropropoxyphene can produce respiratory and CNS depression, and sometimes convulsions. Chronic use of large doses of dextropropoxyphene can produce tolerance and physical dependency similar to other opioids.

MIXED AGONIST-ANTAGONISTS

Drugs in this group possess both agonist and antagonist activity at various opioid receptors (see Table 23-2). In general, with the exception of buprenorphine, the analgesic effects of pentazocine, nalbuphine, butorphanol, and dezocine occur through their interaction with specific subtypes of kappa receptors. These four drugs are weak agonists at sigma receptors, and at high doses produce dysphoria and psychotomimetic effects mediated through this receptor interaction. However, their interaction with kappa receptors also contributes to their psychotomimetic effects.

The antagonistic actions of these drugs are mediated primarily at the mu receptors. When administered to individuals physically dependent on mu receptor agonists, these drugs may precipitate an abstinence syndrome through their antagonist actions on mu opioid receptors. They can also antagonize the respiratory depression associated with overdosage from opioid agonists. However, if the respiratory depression is due to sedative-hypnotics or other CNS depressants, the patient may be made worse since the mixed agonist-antagonists depress respiration as part of their agonist profile.

Buprenorphine differs from the other drugs in this class since it is a partial agonist at mu receptors and an antagonist at kappa receptors. Analgesia produced by buprenorphine is mediated through the stimulation of mu receptor sites.

Tolerance develops to the agonist actions of this group of drugs, but no tolerance develops to the antagonist properties. Although dependence liability to this group of drugs is relatively low, dependence can develop from their continued use. The abstinence syndrome that may result differs considerably from that associated with the dependence on the mu agonists such as morphine or heroin.

Mixed agonist-antagonist drugs may be used for analgesia against moderate and even severe forms of pain. However, it is generally agreed that these agents are less effective than morphine in treating severe pain. These drugs are less spasmogenic to the biliary tree and less constipating than morphine. Thus, some drugs in this group are used to treat pain from biliary colic; some are also used to supplement anesthesia because their respiratory depressant effects are more limited than pure agonists like morphine.

Pentazocine

Structurally, pentazocine is a benzomorphan derivative shown below.

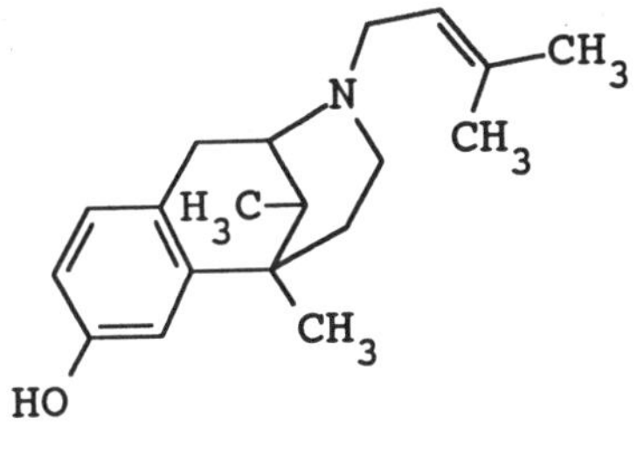

The effect of pentazocine in producing analgesia is largely through its agonistic activity on kappa receptors (see Table 23-2).

Intramuscularly, the drug is about one-third as potent an analgesic as morphine. When administered orally, its analgesic potency is about equal to that of codeine (Table 23-3). Although the analgesic use of pentazocine is primarily by the oral route, its effective oral dose is 5 times higher than the parenteral dose. Pentazocine is well absorbed from the gastrointestinal tract; however, its first pass metabolism limits its oral bioavailability to approximately 20 percent. The half-life in plasma is 2 to 3 h.

Large doses produce tachycardia, hypertension, dysphoria, and psychotomimetic effects. These adverse effects, which limit the clinical uses of pentazocine as an analgesic, are due primarily to interactions with sigma receptors and secondarily to agonist effects on kappa receptors. Other untoward effects commonly seen with pentazocine therapy include dizziness, sweating, nausea, and vomiting. As a weak antagonist at mu receptors, pentazocine will thus precipitate an abstinence syndrome in an opioid dependent individual, but it will not antagonize a morphine-induced respiratory depression. The fact that pentazocine cannot suppress withdrawal symptoms associated with abstinence from morphine or other mu agonists, indicates that its analgesic actions are not mediated through mu receptors. Respiratory depression from pentazocine is limited and can be antagonized with naloxone.

Tolerance to the actions of pentazocine may be slower and less complete than that seen with morphine. Although originally touted as a compound essentially devoid of abuse liability, psychological and physical dependence on pentazocine have been reported after parenteral administration. As the hydrochloride salt, pentazocine is used by the oral route. When combined with naloxone, its potential for parenteral use and for abuse of the oral tablets is reduced. Because of its opioid antagonistic effects and its unpleasant dysphoric and psychotomimetic effects, the risk of drug dependence with pentazocine is lower than that with full agonists such as morphine. Pentazocine is an orally effective analgesic that is especially useful for pain due to biliary colic, since it elevates intrabiliary pressure less than morphine.

Nalbuphine

Nalbuphine is a phenanthrene derivative, structurally similar to the analgesic oxymorphone and the opioid antagonist naloxone.

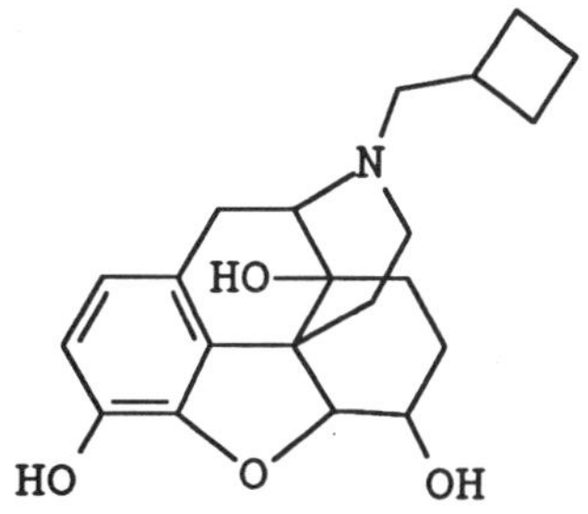

By intramuscular injection, nalbuphine is equivalent in potency to morphine as an analgesic (Table 23-3). However, unlike morphine, the analgesic actions of nalbuphine are mediated through kappa receptors (Table 23-2). Qualitatively, nalbuphine is similar to pentazocine with regard to receptor interactions. Quantitatively, nalbuphine is a weaker agonist at kappa receptors than pentazocine, but a stronger antagonist at mu receptors. Because nalbuphine has a "ceiling for respiratory depression", it has an advantage over morphine that makes it useful as a supplement to anesthetics during surgery. Given parenterally in 10 mg doses morphine and nalbuphine depress respiration equally. At 30 mg and higher doses, however, the respiratory depression with nalbuphine plateaus, whereas with morphine the respiratory depression increases progressively with increasing doses.

Nalbuphine-induced respiratory depression may be reversed by the opioid antagonist naloxone. Nalbuphine produces a lower incidence of postoperative nausea and vomiting than morphine and is widely used to supplement anesthesia during surgery. Nalbuphine is also indicated for the relief of moderate to severe pain in obstetrics during labor and delivery as well as postoperatively. It is only available for parenteral administration.

Butorphanol

This drug is similar in structure to nalbuphine except that it lacks an oxygen bridge and a hydroxy group at the 6 position on the phenanthrene ring.

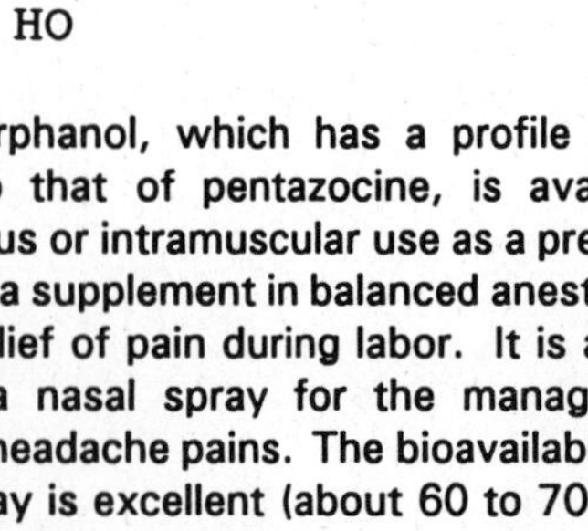

Butorphanol, which has a profile of action similar to that of pentazocine, is available for intravenous or intramuscular use as a preoperative agent, as a supplement in balanced anesthesia and for the relief of pain during labor. It is also available as a nasal spray for the management of migraine headache pains. The bioavailability of the nasal spray is excellent (about 60 to 70 percent), with peak blood levels occurring 30 to 60 min after application. Butorphanol is about 5 times more potent than morphine when given by intramuscular injection. Its analgesic effects are mediated by kappa receptors; it also has agonistic activity at sigma receptors and weak antagonistic activity at mu receptors (Table 23-2). Butorphanol does not seem to precipitate the abstinence syndrome as readily as pentazocine, and in contrast to most other opioids, has a low dependence liability.

Dezocine

This drug is a synthetic opioid agonist-antagonist that is structurally unique from all of the other opioids, belonging to a class of drugs known as amino-tetralins.

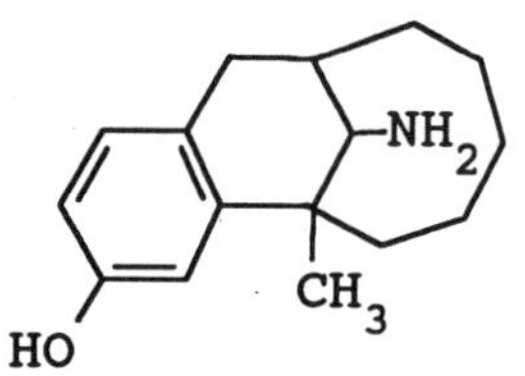

Dezocine appears to have greater affinity for mu receptors than kappa receptors and its antagonistic activity at mu receptors it greater than that of pentazocine. The analgesic activity of dezocine is believed to reside in its ability to activate kappa receptors.

The analgesic potency and the pharmacokinetics of dezocine are comparable to morphine. The drug is used only by the intramuscular and intravenous routes. Most of the compound is biotransformed by glucuronide conjugation and these inactive metabolites are excreted in the urine. In patients with kidney or liver impairment the dosage of dezocine should be decreased. The pharmacologic effects of dezocine are similar to other agonist-antagonist opioids and although respiratory depression has been observed, a ceiling effect occurs rapidly in the degree of respiratory depression produced. Like butorphanol, dezocine appears to have a very low potential for abuse; consequently it is not regulated under the Controlled Substances Act.

Buprenorphine

Buprenorphine is a derivative of thebaine, which is a phenanthrene alkaloid occurring naturally in the poppy plant.

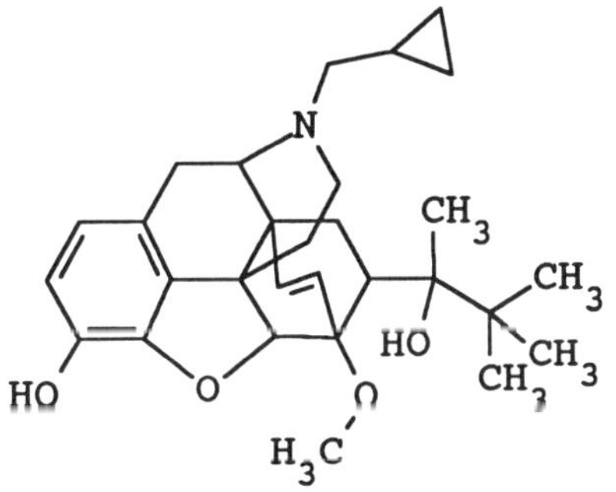

Buprenorphine is 25 to 50 times more potent intramuscularly than morphine as an analgesic (Table 23-3); it has a high affinity for the mu receptor through which it produces its analgesic effects. Therefore, its mu receptor specificity differs from other drugs in this mixed agonist-antagonist group. Buprenorphine also acts as a partial agonist at mu receptors. The response plateau for a partial agonist is below that of a full agonist, so that increasing drug concentrations does not produce a greater response. Furthermore, when a full agonist occupies the opioid receptors, a partial agonist will mimic the actions of an antagonist, with the effects of the full agonist being reduced or reversed. Therefore, buprenorphine given to an opioid-dependent individual may produce withdrawal symptoms due to its antagonist-like effects in the presence of a full opioid agonist. The high affinity and slow dissociation of buprenorphine from the mu receptor provides a longer duration of action (about 6 h) than that of other drugs in this group.

Due to the high affinity at mu receptors, naloxone may fail to antagonize respiratory depression caused by buprenorphine. Therefore, adequate ventilation with mechanical assistance should also be provided in treating overdose with this drug. Buprenorphine abstinence symptoms are milder and much longer in duration than those seen with morphine. In addition, some reports suggest that buprenorphine may be as effective as methadone in the detoxification and maintenance of heroin abusers. Buprenorphine is available only for injection and for the treatment of moderate to severe pain.

OPIOID ANTAGONISTS

The first agent found to be efficacious in the treatment of heroin overdose was nalorphine, a compound formed by substituting an allyl group in place of the methyl group on the nitrogen of morphine. Nalorphine reversed the adverse effects of respiratory depression, coma, nausea, and vomiting produced by overdoses of opioid agonists. In addition, nalorphine also precipitated the withdrawal syndrome when given to an individual physically dependent on opioids, making this drug useful for diagnosing opioid dependency. However, using nalorphine as an antidote to respiratory depression due to CNS depressant drugs other than opioids further compromised respiratory function, since nalorphine itself depressed respiration because it was a partial agonist. In addition, when given in high doses for treating severe pain, nalorphine often produced dysphoria, confusion, and psychotomimetic effects, the latter being mediated by its partial agonist action on kappa and sigma receptors. The psychotomimetic effects associated with its use as an analgesic in addition to its ability to depress respiratory function further in cases where CNS depressants other than the opioids were used, made the use of nalorphine undesirable and unnecessary, since pure antagonists are now widely available in the U.S.

The opioid antagonists, naloxone and naltrexone, unlike the partial agonist nalorphine, have no agonist activity and are described as pure opioid antagonists. They are effective in blocking or reversing the effects of full agonist opioids such as morphine. They combine with opioid receptors with greater affinity than morphine, but do not activate these receptors. Naloxone and naltrexone compete with agonists at opioid receptors, but their effectiveness as antagonists decreases at specific opioid receptors in the following order: mu > delta > kappa.

Questions have arisen as to whether these so called pure opioid antagonists are totally devoid of any agonist activity. What seems apparent is that any effects associated with low to moderate doses of the drugs are most likely due to the antagonism of the effects of endogenous opioid peptides. Very high doses of the antagonists can produce other effects, but these may not be related to the activity at the opioid receptors. In clinical practice, these effects can be largely ignored. They can precipitate the abstinence syndrome and they can also antagonize the actions of opioid agonists and the mixed agonist-antagonists.

Naloxone

Chemically, naloxone is N-allyl noroxymorphone. In general, the N-allyl substitution leads to antagonist properties at opioid receptors.

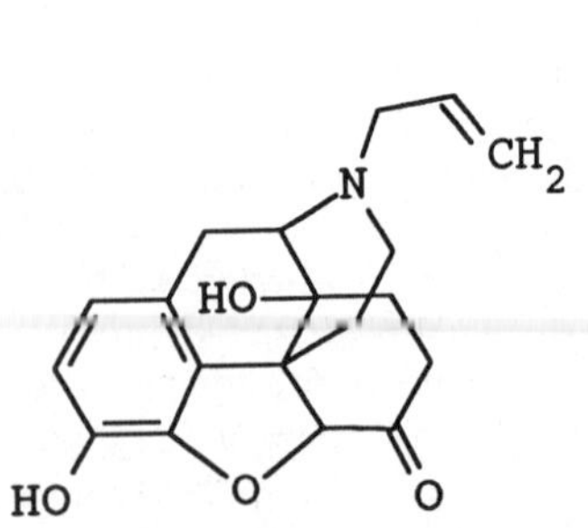

Naloxone is much more potent as an antagonist than nalorphine, and is the drug of choice for treating respiratory depression caused by opioid overdose. In poisoning by opioids, it will quickly increase the respiratory rate and reverse coma. Because this drug has no agonist action, it will not cause respiratory depression, nor will it enhance respiratory depression caused by other CNS depressants (e.g., alcohol, sedative-hypnotics, and benzodiazepines). Therefore, naloxone is safe to use for all cases of unknown drug-induced respiratory depression. If naloxone reverses the impaired respiration, then the suspected drug is probably an opioid. If naloxone does not correct the decreased respiratory rate, then the suspected drug is probably not an opioid but some other CNS depressant. Naloxone can also reverse other actions of opioids such as analgesia, gastrointestinal effects, biliary duct spasms, pupillary constriction, and the release of antidiuretic hormone. In addition, naloxone reverses and/or terminates the psychotomimetic and dysphoric effects induced by such mixed agonist-antagonists as pentazocine and the convulsions associated with large doses of meperidine or dextropropoxyphene in drug abusers. Naloxone is used to diagnose opioid addiction, but small doses must be given cautiously to avoid precipitating a severe withdrawal syndrome. Small doses of naloxone will immediately dilate the constricted pupil in an opioid-dependent individual, a positive diagnostic sign. Similarly, only carefully administered small doses should be used in treating respiratory depression of newborns from mothers suspected of opioid depression in order to avoid severe withdrawal effects.

Naloxone must be given parenterally because it is subject to extensive first pass biotransformation mediated by tissue enzymes in the intestine and liver. The intravenous route is preferred for treating opioid-induced respiratory depression. For adults, doses are given as a bolus. Because of its short duration of action (1 to 2 h), additional doses of naloxone may be required at 2 to 3 min intervals if the initial dose fails to reverse symptoms in suspected opioid overdosage. If no response is noted after a total dose of 10 mg has been administered, the offending agent is probably not an opioid. In patients with suspected opioid dependence, 0.1 to 0.2 mg increments may be given initially by the subcutaneous route to avoid an abrupt opioid withdrawal syndrome.

Morphine-like drugs administered to the mother during labor and delivery may cause neonatal respiratory depression. For respiratory depression in the infant, naloxone may be administered into the umbilical artery or given either subcutaneously or intravenously.

Other potential uses of naloxone derived from studies include protection against the ischemic effects of spinal cord injury and stroke, and the reversal of opioid-induced constipation. Studies in several animal species show that naloxone reduces the ischemic area, improves the electrical activity, and survival rate in spinal cord injury or in animal stroke models. Clinical trials are in progress to evaluate these other potential uses for the pure opioid antagonists.

Naltrexone

Naltrexone is a cyclopropylmethyl derivative of oxymorphone as shown below. It differs from naloxone only by the substitution on the nitrogen.

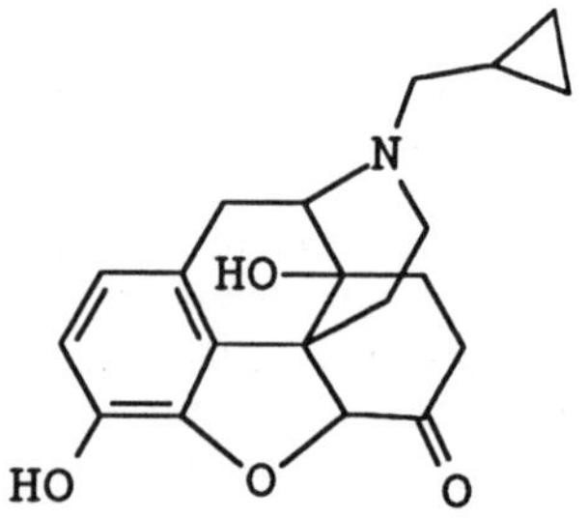

Naltrexone resembles naloxone in that it is a pure opioid antagonist and can competitively antagonize opioid drugs. It differs from naloxone in two important ways: (1) it is effective orally and (2) it has a long duration of action, on the order of 1 to 2 days. It is subject to extensive first pass biotransformation, and only about 5 percent of a given oral dose reaches the systemic circulation. One of its principal metabolic products, 6-β-naltrexol, exhibits some minor opioid antagonistic activity. Despite its longer elimination half-life, the metabolite does not contribute much to the clinical effects of naltrexone.

The principal use of naltrexone is as an adjunct in maintaining detoxified opioid users in an opioid-free state. The individual should be free of opioids for 7 to 10 days before starting maintenance therapy with naltrexone. If used in an individual still taking opioids, an abstinence syndrome will be precipitated. However, once the person has been weaned from opioids, the use of naltrexone will prevent the effects expected of opioid agonists. Steady state blood levels achieved after continued oral dosing with naltrexone will block the psychological and physical effects of administered opioids for 2 to 3 days. Naltrexone given every 24 h in doses of 50 mg has been shown to block the effects of 25 mg of heroin given intravenously. Drug therapy as well as psychological counseling may be required during initial therapy with naltrexone to reduce anxiety, depression, and insomnia associated with maintenance therapy.

Naltrexone is potentially hepatotoxic. The hepatoxicity, which seems to be readily reversible, is most common in obese patients. Patients should be carefully monitored for hepatic function by measuring serum transaminases before initiating therapy with naltrexone and periodically thereafter.

Dosage schedules of naltrexone may be tailored to the probable compliance of the patient (e.g., 100 mg on Monday and Wednesday and 150 mg on Friday). Because of difficulties in compliance using the oral route, studies are in progress utilizing a monthly subcutaneous biodegradable matrix containing naltrexone; the drug is slowly released from the matrix and absorbed to give a prolonged effect. Naltrexone also shows promise in alcohol detoxification programs. Following withdrawal from alcohol, naltrexone appears to inhibit the craving for alcohol, thereby reducing the incidence of relapses.

DRUG INTERACTIONS AND CONTRAINDICATIONS

Opioid drug interactions occur with sedative-hypnotics as well as other CNS depressants which increase respiratory depression. Monoamine oxidase inhibitors followed by the administration of meperidine may result in serious excitatory and depressant effects on the CNS; the combination of these drugs may cause severe respiratory depression, cyanosis, and hypotension, and have resembled acute opioid overdosage. It some cases, deep coma and death have occurred.

The opioid drugs are contraindicated in various clinical situations as follows:

1. Avoid the use of opioid agonists with mixed agonist-antagonist drugs because of the possibility of inhibiting the analgesic activity. In addition, the possibility may exist of producing a state of opioid withdrawal.

2. Avoid the use of opioids in patients with poor liver function, since the major metabolic pathways of the opioids are via the liver.

3. Avoid the use of opioids in patients with poor respiratory function because of the respiratory depressant effects of these analgesics.

4. Avoid chronic use of opioids in pregnant women because they may cause dependence *in utero* and produce withdrawal symptoms in the newborn after birth.

BIBLIOGRAPHY

Akil, H, S.J. Watson, E. Young, M.E. Lewis, H. Khachaturian, and J.M. Walker: "Endogenous Opioids: Biology and Function," *Annu. Rev. Neurosci.* 7: 223-255 (1984).

DeBiasi, S., and A. Rustioni: "Glutamate and Substance P Coexist in Primary Afferent Terminals in the Superficial Laminae of Spinal Cord," *Proc. Natl. Acad. Sci.* **85**: 7820-7824 (1988).

Dickenson, A.H.: "Mechanism of the Analgesic Actions of Opiates and Opioids," *Brit. Med. J.* **47**: 691-702 (1991).

DiGregorio, G.J., E.J. Barbieri, A.P. Ferko, G.H. Sterling, J.F. Camp, and M.F. Prout: *Handbook of Pain Management, Fourth Edition*, Medical Surveillance Inc., West Chester, 1994.

Jessell, T.M., and D.D. Kelly: "Pain and Analgesia," in Kandel, E.R., J.H. Schwartz, and T.M. Jessell (eds.): *Principles of Neural Science*, Chapter 27, Elsevier, New York, 1991.

Junien, J.L., and B.E. Leonard: "Drugs Acting on Sigma and Phencyclidine Receptors: A Review of Their Nature, Function and Possible Therapeutic Importance," *Clin. Neuropharmacol.* **12**: 353-374 (1989).

Klepstad, P., A. Maurset, E.R. Moberg, and I. Oye: "Evidence of a Role for NMDA Receptors in Pain Perception," *Eur. J. Pharmacol.* **187**: 513-518 (1990).

Loh, H.H., and A.P. Smith: "Molecular Characterization of Opioid Receptors", *Annu. Rev. Pharmacol.* **30**: 123-147 (1990).

Nakajima, Y., S. Nakajima, and M. Inque: "Substance P Induced Inhibition of Potassium Channels Via a Pertussin Toxin-Insensitive G Protein," in Leeman, S.E., J.E. Krause, and F. Lembeck (eds.): Substance P and Related Peptides: Cellular and Molecular Physiology, *Ann. N.Y. Acad. Sci.* **632**: 103-111 (1991).

Pastenak, G.W.: "Multiple Morphine and Enkephalin Receptors and the Relief of Pain," *J. Am. Med. Assoc.* **259**: 1362-1367 (1988).

Pastenak, G.W.: "Pharmacological Mechanisms of Opioid Analgesics," *Clin. Neuropharmacol.* **16**: 1-18 (1993).

Sato, T., S. Sakurada, T., Sakurada, S. Furata, K. Chaki, K. Kisara, Y. Sasaki, and K. Suzuki: "Opioid Activities of D-Arg^2-Substituted Tetrapeptides," *J. Pharmacol. Exp. Therap.* **242**: 654-659 (1987).

Simon, E.J., and J.M. Hiller: "Opioid Peptides and Opioid Receptors," in Siegal, G.J., B.W. Agranoff, R.W. Albers, and P.B. Molinoff (eds.): *Basic Neurochemistry, Molecular Cellular and Medical Aspects*, Chapter 13, Raven Press, New York, 1989.

Wilcox, G.L.: "Excitatory Neurotransmitters and Pain," in Bond, M.R., J.E. Charlton, and C.F. Woolf (eds.): *Proceedings of the VIth World Congress on Pain*, Chapter 12, Elsevier, New York, 1991.

CHAPTER 24

Nonsteroidal Anti-Inflammatory Drugs and Drugs Used in the Treatment of Gout

Joan Y. Summy Long

This chapter is divided into two major sections which will detail the pharmacology of two groups of medications. The first section discusses those drugs that are utilized for the treatment of pain and a variety of acute and chronic inflammatory diseases and are commonly referred to as *nonsteroidal anti-inflammatory drugs (NSAIDs)*. The second section deals with the drugs that are specifically used for the treatment of acute and chronic gouty arthritis, some of which are included in the first section.

NONSTEROIDAL ANTI-INFLAMMATORY DRUGS

Analgesic drugs which are not related to opioids have a different spectrum of pharmacologic action than do the opioid analgesics discussed in the preceding chapter. Because these drugs do not interact at opioid receptors, tolerance does not develop to their analgesic effect nor do they produce physical or psychological dependence with chronic use. Most non-opioid analgesic drugs are also antipyretic and have anti-inflammatory properties. Since they are structurally and pharmacologically different from the anti-inflammatory steroids, this class of drugs is referred to as *nonsteroidal anti-inflammatory drugs (NSAIDs)*.

Although many NSAIDs are dissimilar in chemical structure, they exhibit similar therapeutic responses and adverse effects indicative of a common mechanism of action. NSAIDs interfere with the synthesis of prostaglandins and other eicosanoids by inhibiting cyclooxygenases.

Because prostaglandins are not stored in the cell, but are released as they are synthesized, inhibition of cyclooxygenases by NSAIDs can dramatically alter tissue responses or disease processes dependent upon these eicosanoids. In general, NSAIDs effectively alleviate pain associated with inflammation such as occurs in arthritis; lower body temperature during fever; and inhibit platelet aggregation to provide secondary prevention of myocardial infarction, unstable angina, stroke, and occlusion of grafts after coronary artery bypass surgery. Aspirin and several other NSAIDs increase uric acid excretion and can be used in the treatment of gout. Adverse effects of NSAIDs include gastrointestinal irritation with ulceration, renal (large doses, chronic use) and liver toxicity, blood dyscrasias, and hypersensitivity-allergic reactions.

Aspirin and Salicylates

Aspirin, the prototype NSAID, is an acetyl derivative of salicylic acid. Salicylic acid was first synthesized by Piria in 1838 from salicin found in extracts of willow bark. Although the medicinal property of willow bark to relieve fever was known for several centuries, the first pharmacologic data on aspirin appeared in the late 1800s when its antipyretic and analgesic properties were recognized. Aspirin and a number of structurally related salicylates possess analgesic, antipyretic, and anti-inflammatory effects, many of which are prescribed chronically in the treatment of rheumatic conditions (Table 24-1). Aspirin (acetylsalicylic acid) itself is active, but it is also deacylated to form a pharmacologically active metabolite, salicylic acid. Although other NSAIDs have not proven more effective than high doses (over 1 g/day) of aspirin in the treatment of several rheumatic conditions, gastrointestinal side effects frequently limit their use. Moreover, in patients who have low circulating blood volume (e.g., hemorrhage, cirrhosis of the liver, congestive heart failure, hypertension with treatment by diuretics), the

TABLE 24-1 Classification and half-lives of some nonsteroidal anti-inflammatory drugs

Drug	Half-life, h
SALICYLIC ACID DERIVATIVES	
Aspirin (acetylsalicylic acid)	0.3
Salicylic acid	2 to 3
Choline magnesium trisalicylate	9 to 18
Diflunisal	8 to 12
Magnesium salicylate	2 to 15
Salsalate	2 to 15
PROPIONIC ACID DERIVATIVES	
Fenoprofen calcium	3
Flurbiprofen	3 to 9
Ibuprofen	2
Ketoprofen	2
Naproxen, naproxen sodium	12 to 15
Oxaprozin	50
INDOLE DERIVATIVES	
Etodolac	7 to 8
Indomethacin	2 to 3
Sulindac	7 to 18
OXICAM DERIVATIVE	
Piroxicam	30 to 80
PYRAZOLON DERIVATIVES	
Phenylbutazone	60 to 100
Oxyphenbutazone	55 to 90
ANTHRANILIC ACID DERIVATIVES	
Meclofenamate sodium	2
Mefenamic acid	2
NAPHTHYLALKANONE DERIVATIVE	
Nabumetone	24
PHENYLACETIC ACID DERIVATIVES	
Diclofenac sodium	2
Diclofenac potassium	2
PYRROLE DERIVATIVES	
Ketorolac tromethamine	4 to 6
Tolmetin sodium	1 to 2

salicylates and certain other NSAIDs can precipitate acute renal failure which is usually reversed by removal of the drug.

Chemistry Aspirin and other salicylates are weak organic acids, derivatives of salicylic acid. The structures of salicylic acid, methyl salicylate, and aspirin are shown below.

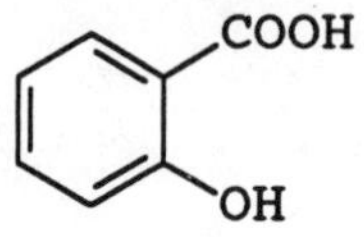

COOH, OH

Salicylic acid

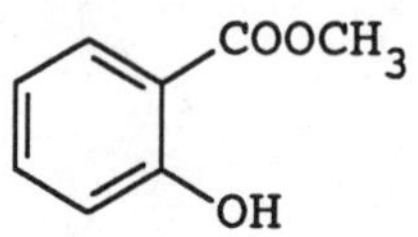

$COOCH_3$, OH

Methyl salicylate

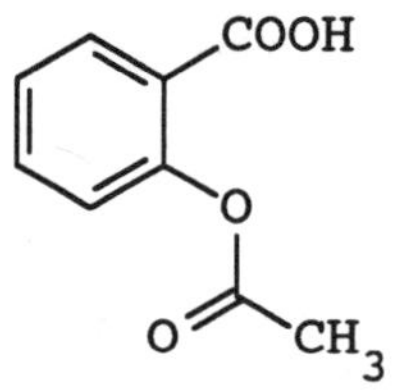

COOH, O, O, CH_3

Aspirin
(Acetylsalicylic acid)

Aspirin has a pK_a of 3.5, making it less ionized and more readily absorbed from the stomach (pH 1.5 to 3.0). In contrast, to promote excretion through the kidney when overdosed, alkalinization with sodium bicarbonate will raise the pH of the urine resulting in a greater proportion of ionized salicylate which is less readily reabsorbed and more easily excreted.

Mechanism of Action According to present concepts, the mechanism of action by which aspirin and the other NSAIDs are analgesic, antipyretic, and anti-inflammatory results from their ability to decrease prostaglandin (PG) formation by inhibiting cyclooxygenases, i.e., cyclooxygenase-1 and cyclooxygenase-2. A simplified scheme for the production of prostaglandins is given in Fig. 24-1. Arachidonic acid bound to phospholipids is present in cell membranes. In response to various stimuli including injury to the cell, arachidonic acid is hydrolyzed from the phospholipids by phospholipase A_2, then rapidly oxygenated by cyclooxygenases (part of an enzyme complex known as *prostaglandin endoperoxide synthase* or *prostaglandin synthetase*) to form the cyclic endoperoxides PGG_2 and PGH_2. These cyclic endoperoxides, which produce pain and vasoconstriction, may be

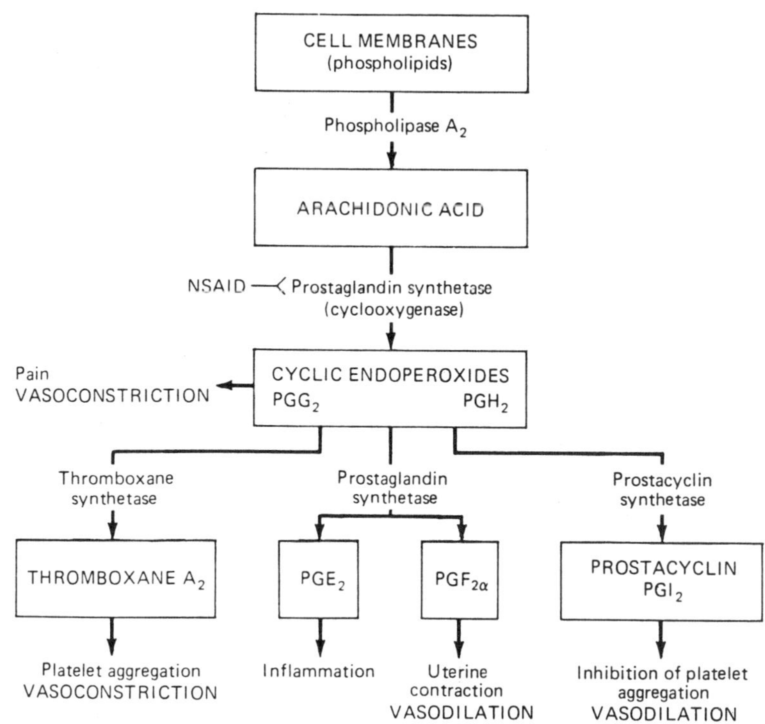

FIGURE 24-1 *Schematic representation of the production of some prostaglandins and thromboxane A_2. [Adapted from Nickander, R., F.G. McMahon, and A.S. Rudolfo: Annu. Rev. Pharmacol. Toxicol.* ***19****: 469 (1979).]*

further metabolized by different enzymes in the prostaglandin synthetase complex to form other eicosanoids (e.g., PGE_2 and $PGF2_{2\alpha}$), thromboxanes, or prostacyclin. These end-products are not stored in the body; they are produced as required, exert their various physiologic or pathologic effects, and are quickly metabolized to inactive products. In addition, arachidonic acid can be converted to leukotrienes by the lipoxygenase pathway (see Chapter 14, Fig. 14-2). Aspirin has been shown to inhibit the conversion of arachidonic acid to cyclic endoperoxides by irreversible acetylation of cyclooxygenases. Other NSAIDs, in contrast, are reversible inhibitors of cyclooxygenases. Other mechanisms of action of the NSAIDs have been suggested, but the effect on the cyclooxygenases appears the best explanation for the common actions of these drugs. Importantly, these drugs do not inhibit the lipoxygenases, thromboxane synthetase, or prostacyclin synthetase nor are they antagonists at prostaglandin receptors. Further information on the eicosanoids is presented in Chapter 14.

Anti-Inflammatory Effect Numerous autacoids are released in response to tissue injury and acute or chronic inflammation. These include histamine, serotonin, bradykinin, prostaglandins, thromboxanes, prostacyclin, leukotrienes, platelet-activating factor (PAF) and interleukin-1 (endogenous pyrogen). The release of prostaglandins, especially PGE_2, during an inflammatory reaction causes vasodilation, localized edema, erythema, and heat, and may potentiate the action of bradykinin resulting in pain. NSAIDs prevent these symptoms of inflammation and are, therefore, useful in the treatment of arthritis (inflammation of a joint). Several NSAIDs (e.g., aspirin, indomethacin, others) are used clinically to treat the inflammatory response associated with various forms of arthritis (e.g., rheumatoid arthritis, osteoarthritis, ankylosing spondylitis, and psoriatic arthritis). Importantly, NSAIDs alleviate the symptoms but do not cure the disease. In rheumatoid arthritis, for example, these drugs do not affect proliferation of the synovium nor do they prevent the progression of the disease.

Analgesic Effect Local prostaglandin formation intensifies the pain-producing properties of bradykinin, lowering the threshold to pain and producing a hyperalgesic state. Thus, combined with other autacoids released at the site of inflammation, prostaglandins potentiate pain transmission. Aspirin and the other NSAIDs act as analgesics by decreasing the synthesis of prostaglandins and indirectly affecting the algesic effect of bradykinin. Clinically the NSAIDs are most effective in relieving pain associated with inflammation by a mechanism (inhibition of cyclooxygenases) and at a site (peripheral) different than that of centrally-acting opioid analgesics such as morphine.

Antipyretic Effect Fever involves a resetting of the thermoregulatory system in the preoptic region of the forebrain allowing a controlled elevation in body temperature. This response is mediated by the production and release of interleukin-1 (endogenous pyrogen) from leukocytes activated by invading viruses and bacteria (i.e., exogenous pyrogens). Prostaglandin E_1 is a potent fever-producing agent known to be synthesized in the brain and present in cerebrospinal fluid during fever. It is believed to mediate the resetting of the thermoregulatory neurons to produce fever. The NSAIDs inhibit the synthesis of prostaglandins in the brain and thereby produce their antipyretic effect. Aspirin and other NSAIDs lower an elevated body temperature during fever, but they have no effect on normal body temperature or on hyperpyrexia associated with exercise (heat stroke), drugs (atropine, inhalation anesthetics, skeletal muscle relaxants), hypothalamic lesions, disturbances in monoamine metabolism in the central nervous system or metabolic disorders.

Effects on Organ Systems *Central Nervous System* It has been suggested that aspirin has a slight calming action and may be synergistic with the hypnotic effect of barbiturates. Central nervous system (CNS) disturbances such as delirium and occasionally psychoses may develop in patients after high doses of aspirin. These symptoms in their mild form are so common that the term *salicylism* is generally applied to them (see Adverse Reactions below). Other NSAIDs can cause confusion, delirium, dizziness, drowsiness, depression, and headaches. These effects are especially prominent in the elderly.

Gastrointestinal Tract Nausea, vomiting, and gastric irritation are common; nausea and vomiting are produced partially by CNS stimulation. PGE_2 plays a significant role in the production of gastric mucus and maintains the integrity of the gastric mucosal barrier. In addition, prostaglandins decrease gastric acid secretion and promote vasodilation. Aspirin produces gastrointestinal irritation directly by an effect of the drug itself and indirectly by inhibiting the synthesis of PGE_2 resulting in diminished gastric cytoprotection. NSAID therapy, especially at doses needed to treat inflammation, is associated with a variety of gastrointestinal disorders, including gastritis, peptic ulcer disease (with perforation), and upper gastrointestinal bleeding. These effects are independent of the route of administration and can be life-threatening. Thus, NSAIDs are nonselective in their anti-inflammatory effect such that doses needed to reduce the symptoms of inflammation also produce side effects, such as gastrointestinal irritation and bleeding in a large number of patients. For these reasons, therapy needs to be individualized for patients with arthritis, i.e., different NSAIDs should be tried until one is effective and can be tolerated. However, these drugs should not be used in persons with a history of peptic ulcers or bleeding disorders and these drugs should be used cautiously in the elderly who appear more susceptible to their toxicity (see below). Misoprostol, a prostaglandin analog, has been approved for the prevention of gastric ulcers in patients on chronic NSAID therapy (see Chapters 14 and 37). NSAIDs can produce hepatotoxicity which is manifested by hepatitis or a mild elevation of hepatic enzymes.

Respiratory System and Acid-Base Balance The average analgesic dose of aspirin (325 mg) does not affect respiration or acid-base balance. Frequently however, after larger doses of aspirin or other salicylates used in the treatment of arthritis, respiration is increased in rate and depth. This occurs by both direct and indirect mechanisms. Increased oxygen consumption and the production of CO_2 occurs predominately in skeletal muscle where salicylates uncouple oxidative phosphorylation. The elevation in blood CO_2 stimulates respiration indirectly via a chemoreceptor mechanism. Salicylates, when they reach the medulla in adequate concentration, also directly stimulate neurons in the respiratory center to increase respiration. Changes in acid-base balance result. Initially, there is an intra- and extra-cellular respiratory alkalosis (increased pH); compensation quickly occurs by renal excretion of bicarbonate ion accompanied by increased loss of sodium and potassium and a return of plasma pH to normal.

Subsequent changes in acid-base balance generally occur only when toxic overdoses of salicylates are ingested by children or adults. As greater amounts of salicylate are absorbed, respiratory depression ensues, compounding these changes with respiratory and metabolic acidosis (see Salicylate Overdose).

Hematologic System In susceptible individuals, large doses of aspirin produce a degree of hypoprothrombinemia, probably by antagonizing vitamin K and thereby decreasing the synthesis of certain blood coagulation factors in the liver. Changes in sedimentation rate are common after aspirin ingestion and occur by an unknown mechanism. Sedimentation rates are inversely related to the fibrinogen concentration in both normal subjects and patients with rheumatic fever or rheumatoid arthritis.

Aggregation of platelets can be regulated by substances interacting with membrane receptors on platelets (e.g., catecholamines, collagen, thrombin, and prostacyclin) and cellular products from within the platelet that are either released and interact with membrane receptors on the platelet (e.g., adenosine diphosphate, PGE_2, PGD_2, 5-hydroxytryptamine) or act at intracellular sites (the cyclic endoperoxides, thromboxane A_2, cyclic AMP, cyclic GMP, and ionic calcium). Thromboxane A_2, synthesized in and released from platelets, causes these cells to change their shape, release their granules, and aggregate. In contrast, prostacyclin, synthesized in and released from endothelial cells, inhibits platelet aggregation and causes vasodilation. When tissue injury occurs, platelets are exposed to thromboxane A_2 and aggregation occurs. Aspirin and other NSAIDs produce their antiplatelet action by inhibiting cyclooxygenases in the platelet and reducing the production and release of thromboxane A_2.

As mentioned, aspirin can irreversibly inhibit cyclooxygenases (acetylating a serine moiety) whereas salicylates without an acetyl group (i.e., choline magnesium trisalicylate, diflunisal, magnesium salicylate, and salsalate) are less effective. This property of aspirin at low doses (40 mg/day) is especially evident in platelets, since without a nucleus platelets cannot resynthesize thromboxane A_2 for the life of the cell. This is the presumed mechanism by which aspirin prevents secondary recurrence of strokes, myocardial infarction, and episodes of unstable angina.

Kidney There are several clinical renal syndromes associated with NSAID use, including papillary necrosis, acute interstitial nephritis, nephrotic syndrome, hyperkalemia, and acute renal failure. Prostaglandins synthesized and released within the kidney maintain renal blood flow and glomerular filtration rate (GFR) under conditions of decreased intravascular volume or existing renal disease. In patients whose renal function is dependent upon prostaglandins, treatment with NSAIDs may precipitate a marked reduction in GFR and acute renal failure. Risk factors for NSAID-induced renal failure include cirrhosis, chronic renal disease, congestive heart failure, use of diuretics, and possibly advanced age. It is important to monitor kidney function in patients having these problems and taking NSAIDs since, if recognized early, acute renal failure has been reversed by removing the drug.

Analgesic nephropathy characterized as a primary renal papillary necrosis and secondary chronic interstitial nephritis has been associated with chronic use of tablets containing aspirin, phenacetin, and caffeine (APC tablets). Although these are no longer marketed in the United States, the causative agent or agents were not clearly identified. Another form of renal injury related to NSAIDs is an idiosyncratic acute interstitial nephritis. This has been seen more frequently in women, particularly in the elderly, and after the long-term use of fenoprofen calcium for myalgia. NSAIDs (especially phenylbutazone and oxyphenbutazone) may also cause sodium and water retention and certain NSAIDs (primarily indomethacin) have been shown to interfere with diuretic therapy in hypertensive patients.

Uric Acid Excretion Drugs which enhance the excretion of uric acid are termed *uricosuric agents*. There seems to be no doubt that aspirin can lower the urate level in the blood and the drug was used in the past to treat acute and chronic gout. Presumably because aspirin is an organic acid, it competes with uric acid for both secretion and reabsorption by the organic acid transport system in the renal proximal tubule. The uricosuric action of aspirin, however, is markedly dependent on the dose administered. Doses of 1 to 2 g/day may actually decrease uric acid excretion (and elevate blood urate levels), intermediate doses of 2 to 3 g/day usually do not change urate excretion, whereas higher doses of aspirin (over 5 g/day) lower plasma urate levels by a uricosuric effect. Moreover, even at high doses, aspirin will antagonize the uricosuric effect of sulfinpyrazone and probenecid, since these drugs are more potent inhibitors of the organic acid transport systems.

Skin Free salicylic acid and methyl salicylate (Oil of Wintergreen) irritate the skin and should never be ingested. Topical application of salicylic acid produces a slow and painless destruction of the epithelium (keratolytic effect), which is useful for the removal of corns and warts. While salicylic acid may have some direct activity against certain fungi, it is more likely that its effectiveness in this area is due chiefly to its keratolytic action. Methyl salicylate is used as a counterirritant in liniment or ointment form for the relief of painful muscles or joints. Because of its pleasant odor and taste, methyl salicylate is occasionally involved in poisoning in children.

Uterus Prostaglandins, especially $PGF_{2\alpha}$, are potent stimulants of uterine contraction and are known to be released from the endometrium in primary and secondary dysmenorrhea. By inhibiting the synthesis of prostaglandins, NSAIDs can reduce the pain and menstrual cramping associated with dysmenorrhea. Ibuprofen is more effective than aspirin. Treatment should begin only after menstrual flow has begun to avoid exposure of a developing embryo to the drug.

Ductus Arteriosus The ductus arteriosus is the distal segment of the sixth aortic arch connecting the pulmonary artery with the descending aorta. During fetal life, it shunts blood flow from the nonfunctional lungs. Prostacyclin and PGE_2 act to keep the ductus arteriosus patent *in utero* and in some infants born prematurely. In the neonatal period, if the ductus arteriosus does not close, the NSAIDs, notably indomethacin, may induce closure by inhibiting the synthesis of these eicosanoids.

Indomethacin should be used only after medical therapy (fluid restriction, diuretics with or without digoxin) has failed. Treatment with the NSAID is preferred over surgery. Early diagnosis is necessary as the ductus becomes less sensitive to NSAIDs after 14 days. It is important to correctly diagnose whether the newborn has a patent ductus arteriosus or a congenital abnormality such as pulmonary atresia or stenosis, tricuspid atresia, coarctation of the aorta, or tetralogy of Fallot. In the latter, the intravenous infusion of PGE_1 (generic name alprostadil) is essential for survival to keep the ductus arteriosus patent after birth until surgery can be performed.

Pharmacokinetics After oral administration, aspirin is rapidly absorbed from the upper gastrointestinal tract. The presence of food or antacid delays its absorption. Aspirin rapidly distributes into cerebrospinal fluid, saliva, peritoneal and synovial fluid, and crosses the placental barrier by pH-dependent processes. In plasma, 50 to 80 percent of aspirin is bound to protein and will compete with other drugs (e.g., hydantoins, sulfonylureas, sulfonamides) for these binding sites, displacing them and increasing their toxicity.

Once absorbed, aspirin is rapidly deacetylated in plasma and the liver to form the pharmacologically active metabolite, salicylic acid. Salicylic acid is then biotransformed in the liver by conjugation with glycine, resulting in the formation of salicyluric acid, or by conjugation with glucuronic acid, forming either the acyl (ester) or phenolic (ether) glucuronide metabolites. A slower oxidation of salicylate results in the formation of small amounts of gentisic acid.

Importantly, the metabolism of salicylic acid follows either first-order or zero-order kinetics depending on the dose. At low doses of aspirin (325 to 650 mg), the enzymes that mediate the metabolic reactions are not saturated and the clearance of salicylate from plasma follows first-order kinetics, i.e., a constant fraction of the drug is removed per unit of time. As long as first-order kinetics apply, and when this low dose of aspirin is administered repeatedly at time intervals equal to the plasma half-life, there will not be an accumulation of plasma salicylate. However, as the dose of aspirin is increased, the salicylate concentration saturates the enzymes that are involved in either glycine or glucuronic acid conjugation to the salicylate to the phenolic group. When this occurs, salicylate begins to increase in plasma since its clearance has now changed from first-order kinetics to zero-order kinetics, i.e., a constant amount of the drug is removed per unit of time. This explains the prolonged time during which the drug can be metabolically cleared from plasma after repetitive high doses of aspirin used in the treatment of arthritis.

Since the plasma half-life of a drug is defined using only first-order rate processes, the half-life of aspirin is 15 to 20 min and that of salicylic acid is 3 h after the administration of 325 mg of aspirin. However, as the dose of aspirin increases, the time it takes to clear 50 percent of the plasma concentration of salicylate increases from 3 h (with 325 mg of aspirin), to 5 to 6 h (with 1 g of aspirin) to 20 h after toxic overdose of the drug (20 g of aspirin). Failure to lower the dose or lengthen the dosing interval in patients with arthritis taking high doses of aspirin may result in salicylism, more severe toxicity, and possibly death.

The biotransformation products of aspirin as well as the free drug are excreted by the kidney by passive, pH-dependent processes. Rates of excretion can be altered by changes in urinary pH and volume as well as by the presence of organic acids (competition for transport sites). Administration of a soluble antacid, such as sodium bicarbonate, elevates the urinary pH and thereby increases the amount of ionized drug, promoting excretion and reducing reabsorption of unchanged aspirin by the kidney. For example, at a urine pH of 4.0, 10 percent of salicylic acid is excreted unchanged, whereas at pH 8.0, 80 percent is excreted.

Therapeutic Uses Analgesia constitutes the major use of aspirin. The general public employs aspirin mainly in the treatment of simple headache or neuralgic pain in doses of 325 to 650 mg. Aspirin is especially useful in pain of low intensity associated with inflammation.

Aspirin is an antipyretic and is commonly used for this purpose, i.e., to reduce or prevent fever and to relieve the discomfort associated with elevated body temperature.

An important application of aspirin is in the treatment of rheumatoid arthritis. In order to achieve an anti-inflammatory effect it must be administered chronically in doses greater than 1 to 4 g/day. At these doses, objective changes such as decrease of joint size, increase in grip strength, reduction of erythrocyte sedimentation rate, and decrease in morning stiffness are seen in addition to relief of pain. It is important to stress that for the anti-inflammatory effect to be optimal, aspirin must be administered at a dose higher than that used for simple analgesia and over prolonged periods of time. Preferably, therapy should be monitored by measuring salicylate blood levels, and a level of 20 to 25 mg per 100 mL is considered the therapeutic range.

Acute rheumatic fever, an inflammatory disease following infection with β-hemolytic streptococci, manifests itself in arthritis, carditis, chorea, and skin rash. In combination with penicillin G and erythromycin, large doses of aspirin are of value in the symptomatic therapy of the disease. Aspirin, however, cannot alter the progression of the disease, i.e., cardiac complications, or encephalopathy.

The clinical use of aspirin's ability to inhibit platelet aggregation and reduce mortality and morbidity associated with cardiovascular diseases involving thrombosis and injury to the vascular endothelial cell has been and is currently being pursued. Aspirin therapy (0.3 g to 1.5 g/day) has been shown to reduce the risk of myocardial infarction and strokes in patients with a history of myocardial infarction, unstable angina, transient ischemic attacks, and stroke (i.e., secondary prevention). Aspirin alone, or in combination with dipyridamole, has also been shown to be effective in decreasing the incidence of early graft occlusion, but not re-stenosis, following coronary artery bypass surgery. Moreover, aspirin therapy (combined with streptokinase), administered within 24 h of experiencing symptoms to patients having an evolving myocardial infarction, provided the greatest reduction in risks of re-infarction, stroke, and vascular mortality.

Aspirin has also been evaluated in two large, randomized clinical trials of healthy American and British physicians for the ability to prevent a first myocardial infarction (i.e., primary prevention). Although the American study showed that aspirin treatment (325 mg every other day) lowered the incidence of non-fatal myocardial infarctions, both studies showed no reduction in overall cardiac and cerebral vascular mortality. There was, however, a significant increase in serious stroke, peptic ulcer disease, and gastrointestinal bleeding (in the British study in which 500 mg/day was used) as well as hemorrhagic stroke (in the American study) related to aspirin treatment. Although the Food and Drug Administration (FDA) has approved the use of aspirin (325 mg/day) for primary prophylaxis of myocardial infarction, its use should be limited to those patients with a family history of heart disease and the presence of other risk factors because of the increased incidence of serious hemorrhagic side effects with chronic use.

Adverse Reactions Gastric irritation, which may lead to gastric ulceration, perforation and bleeding, is a principal adverse reaction seen with aspirin and other NSAIDs. Bleeding problems associated with chronic use also can occur.

Salicylism is a series of responses frequently recurring when the therapeutic dose of aspirin is high, such as that used in rheumatic fever and rheumatoid arthritis. These symptoms, which may be manifest at plasma levels in excess of 25 mg per 100 mL, consist of nausea and vomiting, tinnitus (ringing in the ears), deafness, severe headache, mental dullness and confusion, quickened pulse, and increased respiration. The condition resembles cinchonism (which occurs with quinidine and quinine) and may be quite troublesome, but it disappears completely on stopping or reducing the drug.

Hypersensitivity reactions manifested by

bronchoconstriction, urticaria, angioneurotic edema, or anaphylactic shock may develop from the administration of relatively small doses of aspirin. The cause of this hypersensitivity is unknown but is commonly seen in asthmatics with nasal polyps and may be due to an airway response to a decrease in prostaglandins. Another hypothesis is that inhibition of cyclooxygenase results in shunting of arachidonic acid metabolism to the lipoxygenase pathway, increasing certain mediators of the allergic response (e.g., leukotrienes C_4, D_4, and E_4 cause bronchoconstriction). In very sensitive patients, the reaction may be fatal. Cross-sensitivity occurs with all other NSAIDs as well as with tartrazines, yellow dyes used in pharmaceutical preparations. Therefore the use of all NSAIDs is contraindicated in patients with hypersensitivity to aspirin.

There is evidence linking Reye's syndrome to aspirin intake during viral illnesses. Reye's syndrome is an illness which is directly related to viral epidemics and can result in hepatic failure, severe neurologic symptoms, and death. Most cases occur in children 4 to 12 years of age. Therefore, it is recommended that aspirin not be used in children and teenagers with influenza or viral illnesses.

Salicylate Overdose Despite its relatively low toxicity, aspirin is responsible for many accidental poisonings as well as poisoning with suicidal intent. It also ranks very high as a cause of poisoning in children under 5 years of age. Because of its pleasant odor, methyl salicylate (Oil of Wintergreen) may be ingested by children and may cause salicylate intoxication. Fatalities have occurred after the ingestion of 4 mL of methyl salicylate and from 10 g to 30 g of sodium salicylate or aspirin. There is a greater frequency of deaths in fever-ridden children after therapeutic misuse of aspirin or other salicylates, apparently because of their lesser ability to withstand acid-base changes and dehydration.

As discussed previously, the initial effects of salicylate overdose are those of respiratory stimulation caused both by a rise in CO_2 resulting from the uncoupling of oxidative phosphorylation primarily in skeletal muscle and by a direct stimulatory action on neurons in the respiratory center of the medulla. When this occurs, plasma P_{CO2} falls and respiratory alkalosis (elevation in blood pH) ensues. Compensatory mechanisms then promote increased renal excretion of bicarbonate accompanied by sodium and potassium, returning blood pH toward normal. This stage of compensated respiratory alkalosis is most often seen in adults given intensive salicylate therapy.

When toxic doses are ingested, however, further complications ensue resulting in a combined respiratory acidosis and metabolic acidosis (Fig 24-2). These are caused by a direct effect of the drug causing depression of the respiratory center in the medulla after high doses or prolonged exposure to salicylate. This permits the increased production of CO_2 (from the uncoupling of oxidative phosphorylation primarily in skeletal muscle) to decrease blood pH. Since the bicarbonate concentration in blood is already low due to increased renal excretion, this respiratory acidosis cannot be compensated. Superimposed on these changes is a true metabolic acidosis caused by the accumulation in plasma of salicylic acid, strong acids of metabolic origin (sulfuric and phosphoric acids) resulting from impaired renal function and organic acids (pyruvic, lactic and acetoacetic acids) from the altered carbohydrate metabolism. Coincident with these changes, dehydration progresses as water is lost by salicylate-induced sweating and by insensible loss through the lungs

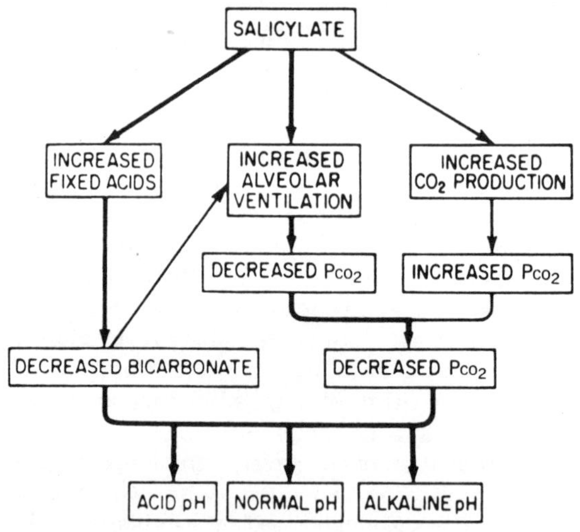

FIGURE 24-2 *Summary of the pathogenesis of mixed disturbances of acid-base equilibrium in salicylate intoxication. From the above downward are depicted the basic actions of salicylate, the separate effects of these actions on acid-base equilibrium, and the interaction of these effects in dictating the final pH. The line connecting "decreased bicarbonate" and "increased alveolar ventilation" is meant to imply that low blood pH may augment the primary effect of the drug upon respiration.*

during hyperventilation. Plasma sodium concentration becomes elevated and potassium concentration depleted.

Salicylism is characterized by nausea, vomiting, tinnitus, deafness, confusion, rapid pulse rate and increased respiration and is frequently experienced by patients taking high doses of salicylates (plasma levels above 30 to 40 mg/100 mL) for arthritis. As plasma levels of salicylate continue to rise (above 50 mg/100 mL plasma) fever, dehydration, electrolyte disturbances and metabolic acidosis ensue and are compounded by vasomotor collapse, delirium, coma, and ultimately renal and respiratory failure leading to death. Therefore, overdose with salicylates needs to be treated immediately and aggressively. Salicylate plasma levels above 90 mg per 100 mL are frequently lethal. Treatment of acute poisoning should be aimed at preventing absorption and increasing elimination of the drug and treating the complicated acid-base and electrolyte imbalances. Activated charcoal may be of considerable value in reducing absorption and in severe cases hemodialysis may be needed to lower plasma levels of salicylate. The clinical profile of salicylate toxicity, such as hyperpnea, hyperglycemia, ketosis, acidosis, polyuria, and dehydration, may be similar to that seen in diabetic acidosis. These can be distinguished by a history of salicylate ingestion, the presence of tinnitus, muscle irritability, petechiae, and plasma levels of salicylate.

Pregnancy During pregnancy, salicylates may reach substantial levels in the fetus since they cross the placental barrier. Women who used aspirin habitually have been shown to have children with smaller birth weights, but birth defects are not more common. Aspirin taken near parturition may delay the onset of labor and is associated with bruising of the newborn child. It can also promote closure of the ductus arteriosus *in utero*.

NSAID Therapy in the Elderly Many patients taking NSAIDs are elderly, since this population has an increased prevalence of arthritic conditions. The elderly also frequently have coexisting medical problems or are receiving concurrent medical therapy which may predispose them to adverse effects of NSAID therapy. Renal, gastrointestinal, and CNS toxicities are of particular concern in the elderly. The metabolic and renal clearance of salicylates and other NSAIDs may be altered in the aged due to organ or cardiovascular disease. Therefore these patients should be monitored closely while on aspirin or other NSAIDs. Use of nonacetylated salicylates is preferred, since these agents are weak cyclooxygenase inhibitors and therefore may hold less risk for adverse effects.

Drug Interactions Aspirin may be involved in a number of interactions with other drugs. Since it is not a prescription item and is widely used by the general public, patients receiving certain medications should be warned against the use of aspirin. Competition for protein binding sites occurs between aspirin and oral anticoagulant drugs such as warfarin. Moreover, since both drugs reduce the ability of the blood to clot (by different mechanisms), major hemorrhage problems can result. For these reasons, aspirin should not be administered to patients taking oral anticoagulants. Aspirin may increase the hypoglycemic effect of insulin and oral hypoglycemic agents. Its action on uric acid clearance by the kidney causes it to interfere with the uricosuric effect of probenecid and sulfinpyrazone. Aspirin can also increase serum levels and the toxicity of methotrexate.

Nonacetylated Salicylates

The nonacetylated salicylates available in the United States are diflunisal, choline magnesium trisalicylate, magnesium salicylate, and salsalate (Table 24-1). These drugs have been shown to be effective in rheumatic conditions because of their anti-inflammatory and analgesic effects. Choline magnesium trisalicylate, magnesium salicylate, and salsalate are metabolized to salicylic acid. The serum salicylate levels that are achieved show a wide variability. Careful titration is required to produce therapeutic levels, since at or near therapeutic (anti-inflammatory) levels a small increment in dose may cause large increases in plasma salicylate levels due to saturation of enzymes (zero-order kinetics) involved in the metabolic clearance of salicylic acid.

Diflunisal Diflunisal is a derivative of salicylic acid but is not metabolized to salicylic acid.

COOH
F OH
F

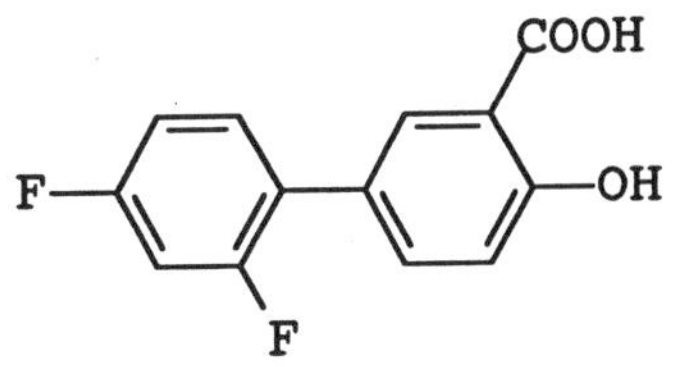

This drug is a reversible inhibitor of cyclooxygenases. It has analgesic and anti-inflammatory activity, but is only weakly antipyretic. Diflunisal has weak uricosuric activity and also has a mild, dose-related effect on platelet function. The drug is well absorbed orally, is highly bound to plasma proteins, and has an elimination half-life of 8 to 12 h. Ninety percent is excreted in the urine as a soluble glucuronide conjugate. Adverse reactions include nausea, vomiting, gastrointestinal toxicity, renal insufficiency, headache, and tinnitus. It is used for the treatment of arthritis and pain.

Choline Magnesium Trisalicylate and Magnesium Salicylate Choline magnesium trisalicylate is a combination of choline salicylate and magnesium salicylate. These compounds are weak inhibitors of cyclooxygenases. They are metabolized to salicylic acid and provide effective anti-inflammatory activity when salicylate levels are maintained in the therapeutic range. Glycine and glucuronide metabolites are excreted through the renal system. Adverse reactions include symptoms of salicylism. Choline magnesium trisalicylate does not affect platelet aggregation, and it produces minimal gastrointestinal and renal toxicity. Magnesium salicylate is indicated for pain and choline magnesium salicylate is used for pain and, on occasion, for the treatment of some arthritides.

Salsalate Chemically, salsalate is salicylsalicylic acid, a dimer of salicylic acid. Some of the drug is hydrolyzed in the small intestine to two molecules of salicylic acid, but most is absorbed unchanged and hydrolyzed in the plasma. This drug is weak cyclooxygenase inhibitor and exhibits similar therapeutic and adverse effects to those seen with choline magnesium trisalicylate. It is indicated only for the treatment of arthritis; during therapy, salicylate levels should be monitored.

OTHER NONSTEROIDAL ANTI-INFLAMMATORY AGENTS

In general, like aspirin and salicylates, these drugs have anti-inflammatory, antipyretic, and analgesic activity resulting from their ability to inhibit cyclooxygenases. Because many of these agents can produce more serious side effects than aspirin at analgesic and antipyretic doses, these NSAIDs are used more frequently for their anti-inflammatory properties in the treatment of rheumatoid arthritis, osteoarthritis, acute attacks of gout or pseudogout, ankylosing spondylitis, and other seronegative spondyloarthropathies. Aspirin, however, remains the drug of choice in the treatment of rheumatoid arthritis when its side effects can be tolerated.

A few of the newer NSAIDs, however, are also used in the treatment of dysmenorrhea and for mild to moderate pain. There is considerable variation in response to these drugs, making it necessary to individualize therapy until a drug is found that is both efficacious and tolerated by the arthritic patient.

Many of these NSAIDs have a high degree of plasma protein binding with the potential to displace highly bound drugs such as warfarin, phenytoin, sulfonylureas, and sulfonamides and increase their pharmacologic effects. All NSAIDs show cross-sensitivity with aspirin and therefore are contraindicated in patients hypersensitive to this salicylate. NSAIDs are metabolized principally through hepatic mechanisms, and metabolites are primarily excreted by the kidney. These drugs may be classified chemically as listed in Table 24-1. Specific characteristics of the agents are discussed under each chemical group.

Propionic Acid Derivatives

The propionic acid derivatives include fenoprofen calcium, flurbiprofen, ibuprofen, ketoprofen, naproxen and its sodium salt, and oxaprozin. The chemical structures of these drugs are shown in Fig. 24-3.

Ibuprofen Ibuprofen was the first of the propionic acid derivatives, to be available without prescription and approved for clinical use as an anti-inflammatory drug. Ibuprofen is well absorbed orally; peak serum concentrations are attained in 1 to 2 h after oral administration. In the presence of food there is a decrease in the rate but not in the extent of absorption. Ibuprofen is rapidly biotransformed by hydroxylation and carboxylation with a plasma half-life of the parent drug of 1.8 to 2 h. There is no evidence of drug accumulation. In general, the overall incidence of adverse reactions with ibuprofen is lower than for aspirin, indomethacin or phenylbutazone. The principal adverse reaction of ibuprofen is gastrointestinal irritation. Epigastric distress occurs in 14 to 16 percent of patients. Skin rashes, dizziness, tinnitus, renal failure, and edema may occur. Aseptic meningitis has been observed rarely and has occurred most commonly in individuals with systemic lupus erythematosus. Renal failure and aseptic meningitis have also been seen with over-the-counter preparations of ibuprofen. Although some studies have failed to show a drug interaction between ibuprofen and warfarin, because of its high protein binding ibuprofen should be used with caution, if at all, in patients receiving oral anticoagulants. As mentioned above, patients with hypersensitivity to aspirin manifested by nasal polyps, angioneurotic edema, and bronchospasm will show hypersensitivity to ibuprofen as well as the other NSAIDs.

Naproxen Naproxen is completely absorbed from the gastrointestinal tract. Naproxen sodium is also available and is more rapidly absorbed than naproxen. Peak plasma levels of these drugs are attained in 2 to 4 h. The plasma half-life is 12 to 15 h. Naproxen is 99 percent bound to plasma proteins and can displace other drugs bound to albumin resulting in potentially toxic drug interactions. Approximately 95 percent is excreted in the urine in a conjugated form. As with ibuprofen, the principal toxicity is gastrointestinal irritation, which may lead to ulceration and hemorrhage. Rare cases of bone marrow depression have occurred. The drug is contraindicated in aspirin hypersensitivity and should be used cautiously in patients with a history of peptic ulcer. Naproxen readily crosses the placenta in pregnant women and is excreted in the milk during lactation and therefore should not be used in pregnancy. These compounds are used in the treatment of rheumatoid arthritis, ankylosing spondylitis, osteoarthritis, and juvenile rheumatoid arthritis. They also provide pain relief within 1 h and are useful in the management of acute and chronic pain.

Fenoprofen Calcium A third propionic acid derivative, fenoprofen, is related chemically and pharmacologically to ibuprofen and naproxen. Fenoprofen is rapidly absorbed from the fasting stomach, reaching peak plasma levels within 90 min. The plasma half-life is approximately 3 h. Fenoprofen is 99 percent bound to plasma protein; 90 percent of the drug is eliminated within 24 h as fenoprofen glucuronide and hydroxyfenoprofen glucuronide. The major adverse reaction is gastrointestinal irritation. Skin rashes, somnolence, palpitations, headache, and tinnitus have been reported.

Flurbiprofen Flurbiprofen is well absorbed from the gastrointestinal tract and produces peak plasma levels in approximately 1.5 h. The compound is extensively biotransformed by the liver with an elimination half-life of 3 to 9 h. Excretion of the drug occurs primarily through the kidney,

Fenoprofen

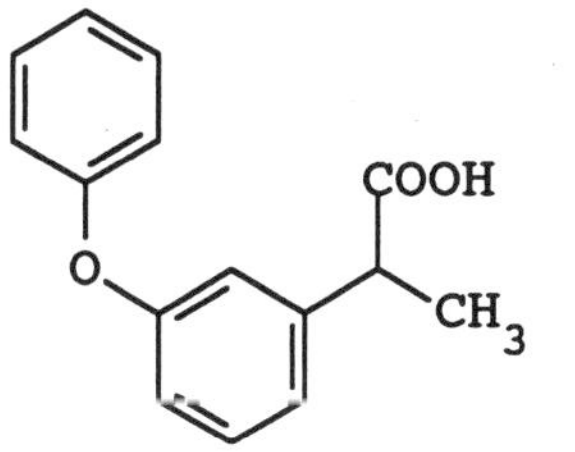

Flurbiprofen

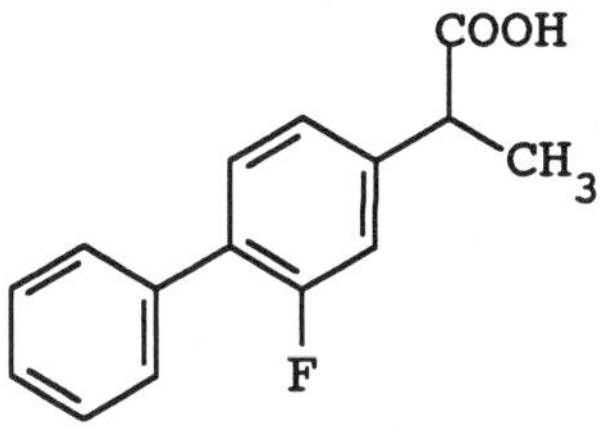

Ibuprofen

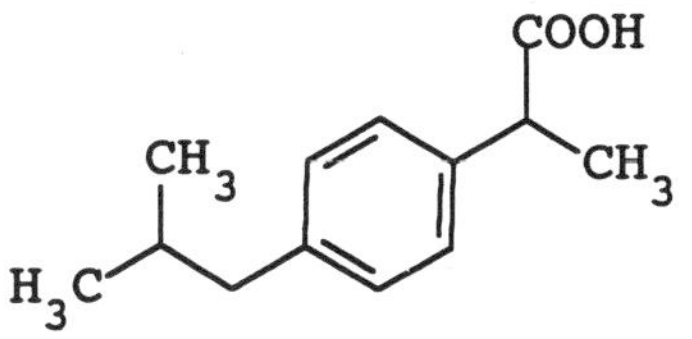

Ketoprofen

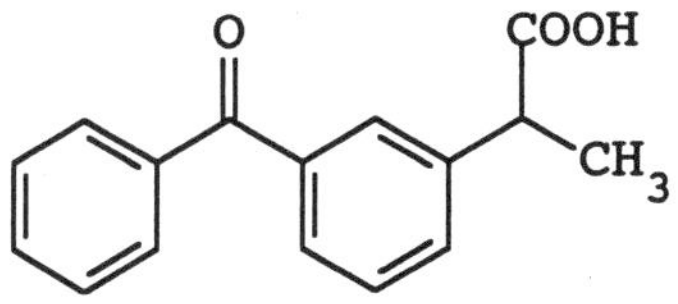

Naproxen

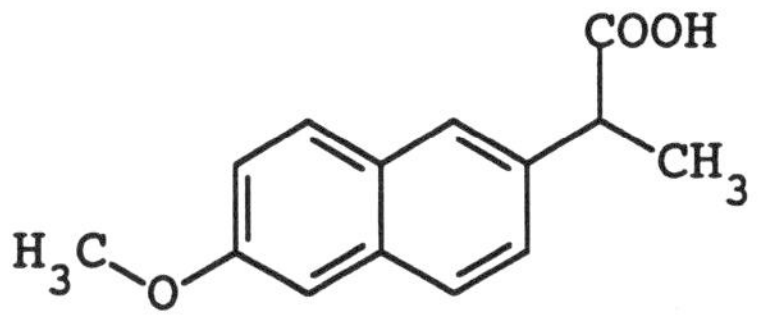

Oxaprozin

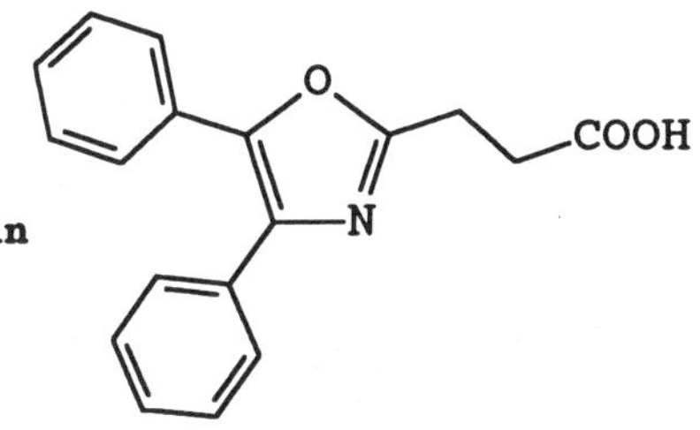

FIGURE 24-3 ***Structures of some propionic acid derivatives.***

and in the urine are found parent drug as well as conjugated and hydroxylated metabolites. Flurbiprofen exhibits a very high degree of plasma protein binding (99 percent). The adverse reactions reported for flurbiprofen are similar to those of the other NSAIDs. Dyspepsia, gastrointestinal bleeding, abdominal pain, diarrhea, edema, and tinnitus are some reactions that can occur. The drug is used in acute and chronic conditions of rheumatoid arthritis and osteoarthritis. A topical preparation is available for inhibition of intraoperative miosis.

Ketoprofen This compound is a propionic acid derivative which is rapidly and completely absorbed from the gastrointestinal tract. Ketoprofen attains peak plasma levels in 0.5 to 2 h and has a mean plasma half-life of 2 h. Sixty percent of the glucuronide metabolite is excreted in the urine. Some adverse reactions reported for ketoprofen include renal and gastrointestinal toxicities, edema, fluid retention, and abnormalities in liver function tests. The drug is indicated for the treatment of mild to moderate pain of unknown origin and the pain associated with various arthritides.

Oxaprozin This compound has a long duration of action due to low hepatic and renal clearance. Oxaprozin may be used once daily for the treatment of osteoarthritis and rheumatoid arthritis. Like other NSAIDs, it has analgesic, anti-inflammatory, and antipyretic activity. The drug is well absorbed following oral administration and has a bioavailability greater than 95 percent. The drug primarily undergoes hepatic biotransformation with a resultant glucuronide derivative that is secreted into the bile and excreted in the feces. Adverse reactions reported for oxaprozin are similar to those found with other NSAIDs.

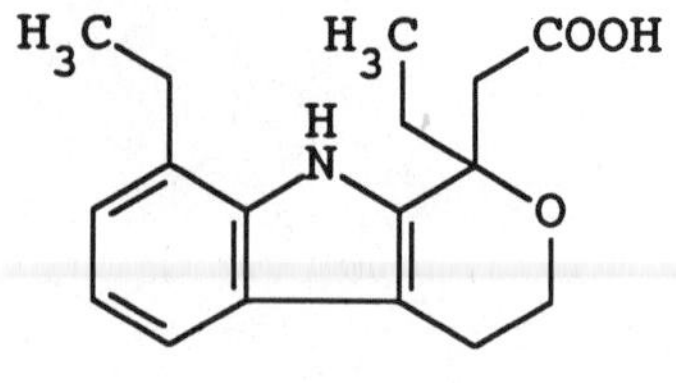

Indole Derivatives

As shown in Fig. 24-4, there are three NSAIDs that are related structurally and called indole derivatives: etodolac, indomethacin, and sulindac. The latter compound is strictly not an indole, but is usually included with this group.

Indomethacin This drug is an indole acetic acid derivative and is a very potent cyclooxygenase inhibitor. It also inhibits phosphodiesterase and thereby can increase intracellular concentrations of cyclic AMP. Indomethacin is rapidly and completely absorbed from the gastrointestinal tract,

Etodolac

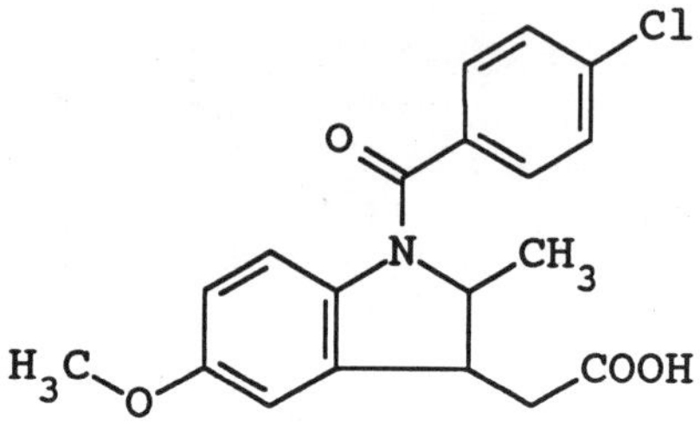

Indomethacin

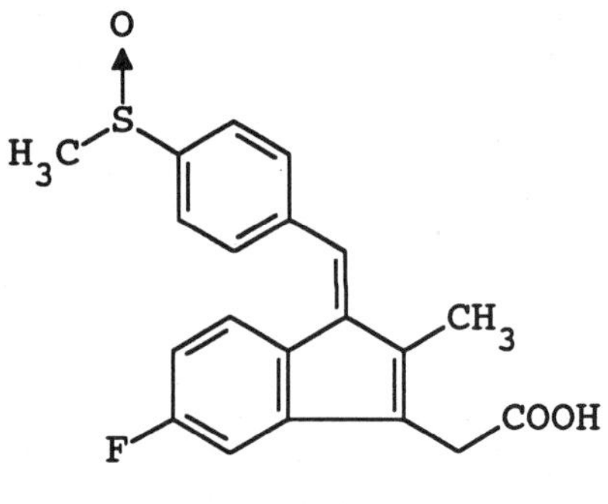

Sulindac

FIGURE 24-4 *Structures of the indole derivatives.*

attaining peak plasma concentrations in 1 to 2 h. The half-life is about 2 to 3 h. Indomethacin is 90 percent bound to plasma proteins. The drug is biotransformed by demethylation and deacetylation. Both the parent drug and the biotransformation products undergo enterohepatic circulation. Thirty-three percent is eliminated in the feces and the remainder in the urine. Indomethacin causes a significant amount of gastrointestinal toxicity. Other adverse reactions include headaches, dizziness, tinnitus, vertigo, and nephrotoxicity. Occasionally, convulsions, peripheral neuropathy, syncope, confusion, and behavioral disturbances have been reported. Corneal deposits and retinal changes have also been associated with prolonged use of the drug. Blood dyscrasias (leukopenia, hemolytic or aplastic anemia, agranulocytosis and thrombocytopenia) are observed rarely but fatalities have resulted from hepatitis (with jaundice). The use of indomethacin is contraindicated in pregnant women, nursing mothers, children 14 years old and younger, and in patients with a history of gastrointestinal disease. It should be used cautiously in the elderly and in those with parkinsonism, epilepsy, or psychiatric problems since it may aggravate those conditions. Because of its potentially serious adverse effects, indomethacin is only indicated to treat moderate to severe inflammatory conditions. It is usually used orally, but rectal suppositories are available for those who cannot tolerate the oral dosage forms. In addition, indomethacin sodium trihydrate is used by intravenous injection to close a patent ductus arteriosus in premature infants.

Etodolac Like other NSAIDs, this indole derivative inhibits cyclooxygenases and has analgesic, anti-inflammatory, and antipyretic activity. The drug has a high oral bioavailability and attains peak plasma concentrations in 1 to 2 h following oral administration. The plasma protein binding is high (99 percent). Approximately 70 percent of an administered dose is eliminated in the urine, mainly as metabolic products. Adverse effects are typical of the NSAIDs. Etodolac is used in the treatment of osteoarthritis and for the management of pain.

Sulindac This drug is an indene acetic acid derivative of indomethacin. It has the same pharmacology as the other members of this group. Sulindac is well absorbed after oral administration, with peak plasma levels appearing in about 2 h. The parent drug sulindac, a sulfoxide, is inactive until it is reduced (reversibly) to the sulfide derivative that has anti-inflammatory, antipyretic, and analgesic activity. The active sulfide has a plasma half-life of 7 to 18 h and is oxidized to an inactive sulfone metabolite. Sulindac and the sulfide and sulfone analogs undergo extensive enterohepatic circulation. This effect appears to account for the long duration of action of the drug. Both sulindac and its sulfide are highly bound to plasma proteins (95 percent). About 25 percent of the drug and its biotransformation products are excreted in the feces and the remainder in the urine. As with other NSAIDs, gastrointestinal toxicity is the main side effect of sulindac. Skin rash, tinnitus, dizziness, headaches, edema, and renal toxicity have been reported. As with all NSAIDS, sulindac is contraindicated in patients with hypersensitivity to aspirin.

Oxicam Derivative

Piroxicam Piroxicam is the only oxicam derivative available in the United States. It is widely used in the treatment of osteoarthritis and rheumatoid arthritis due to its convenience of dosing (long plasma half-life), efficacy, and relative safety.

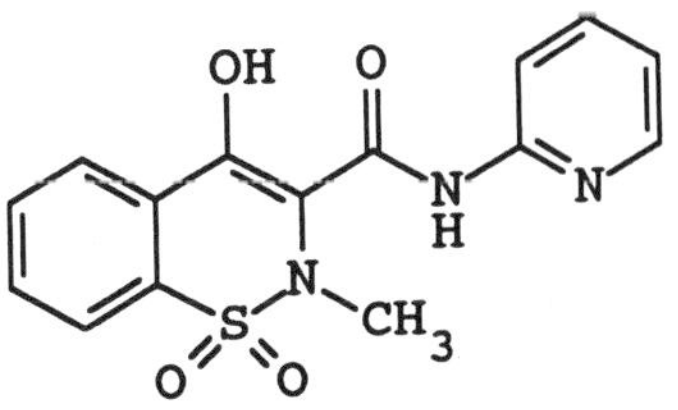

Piroxicam has a similar mechanism of action and pharmacology when compared with other NSAIDs. Peak oral absorption occurs in 3 to 5 h, and piroxicam has an half-life of 30 to 80 h; it is highly bound to plasma protein. The drug is metabolized by hydroxylation on the pyridyl side chain followed by conjugation. The compound also undergoes a sequence of reactions involving hydrolysis of the amide linkage, decarboxylation, ring contraction, and N-demethylation. Two-thirds of piroxicam and its metabolites are excreted in the urine and one-third in the feces; less than 5 percent is excreted unchanged. Adverse reactions include gastrointestinal toxicity, renal insufficiency, papillary necrosis, edema, and abnormalities in liver function tests. Interactions with warfarin have been reported.

Pyrazolon Derivatives

Phenylbutazone and oxyphenbutazone are the two compounds that are available in this group. Phenylbutazone and oxyphenbutazone have similar pharmacologic properties.

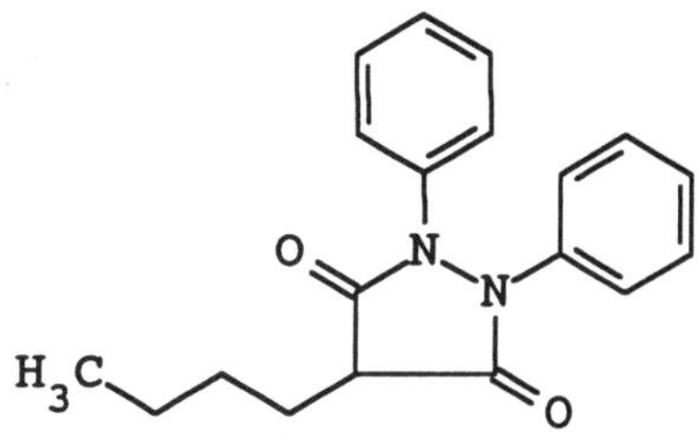

Phenylbutazone

Phenylbutazone and Oxyphenbutazone Phenylbutazone is partially biotransformed to oxyphenbutazone, which is an active product. The mechanism of action and pharmacology of these drugs are similar to those of other NSAIDs, but their use is limited due to adverse effects. These drugs should not be given for periods over one week, except in highly selected cases of severe ankylosing spondylitis where less toxic NSAIDs such as indomethacin have not proven effective, and should only be used for severe inflammatory conditions. The most serious adverse reactions seen with phenylbutazone and oxyphenbutazone is agranulocytosis. Two types of agranulocytosis are found: one is idiosyncratic and irreversible, while the other is dose-related and reversible with discontinuation of the drug. Agranulocytosis may appear at any time following administration and severely limits the use of these drugs. Serious gastrointestinal toxicity leading to ulceration and bleeding may be caused by the drugs. Liver function tests and histologic studies show evidence of toxic hepatitis in some patients and a cholangiolitic change in others. Jaundice and increased prothrombin time with purpura have been observed, and toxic cirrhosis has led to death. Kidney damage has been caused by hematuria, anuria, and uremia, with severe destruction of the convoluted tubules. Sodium retention due to increased reabsorption of sodium has been observed regularly and is frequently associated with water and chloride retention and edema. For this reason, neither of these drugs should be used in patients with borderline or overt congestive heart failure. Skin irritation in the form of a drug rash with an occasional fatal exfoliative dermatitis is not uncommon after administration of these drugs. The elderly are more susceptible to the toxic effects of these compounds and their use is contraindicated in children under 15 years of age and in the very elderly.

Anthranilic Acid Derivatives

The two NSAIDs that compose this group are meclofenamate sodium and mefenamic acid. The structures of these drugs are shown in Fig. 24-5.

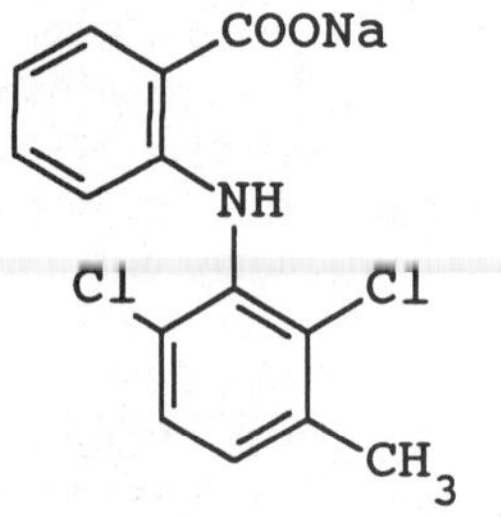

Meclofenamate Sodium Meclofenamate sodium has a mechanism of action similar to that of the other NSAIDs and has been shown to inhibit 5-lipoxygenase activity *in vitro*. The drug is a potent anti-inflammatory compound. Meclofenamate is rapidly absorbed following oral administration and blood levels peak in 30 to 60 min. The compound is biotransformed partially to a weakly active hydroxymethyl derivative and an inactive carboxyl derivative, both of which are conjugated with glucuronic acid prior to elimination in the urine. The mean plasma half-life is 2 h. Adverse reactions are similar to those of the other NSAIDs, except that diarrhea is a frequent side effect that is dose-related and subsides with dosage reduction. In addition, the effect of the oral anticoagulant warfarin is enhanced by meclofenamate. Meclofenamate sodium is used to treat mild to moderate pain, rheumatoid arthritis, and osteoarthritis.

COONa NH Cl Cl CH_3

Meclofenamate sodium

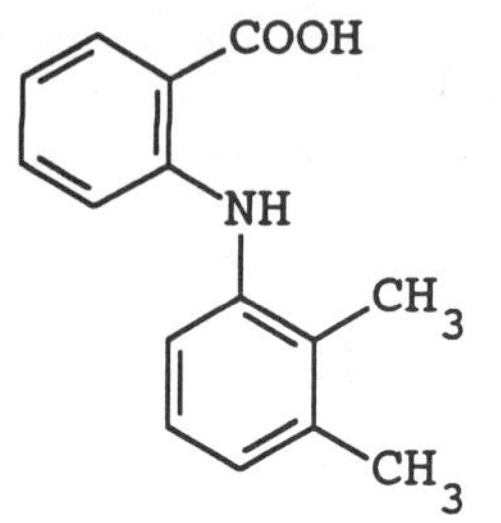

COOH NH CH_3 CH_3

Mefenamic acid

FIGURE 24-5 *Structures of the anthranilic acid derivatives.*

Mefenamic Acid In addition to inhibition of cyclooxygenases, mefenamic acid has been shown to compete for binding at the prostaglandin receptor site. This oral drug is indicated for use in dysmenorrhea and moderate pain for no more than 1 week. The use of mefenamic acid for greater than 1 week is not recommended because of the development of possible serious gastrointestinal toxicity, nephrotoxicity, hemolytic anemia, and bone marrow hypoplasia. Autoimmune hemolytic anemia is associated with continuous administration of the drug for more than 12 months. Little is known concerning its pharmacokinetics, except that it is metabolized and excreted in the urine.

Naphthylalkanone Derivative

Nabumetone This compound is a prodrug that is biotransformed in the liver to its active product, 6-methoxy-2-naphthylacetic acid (MNA).

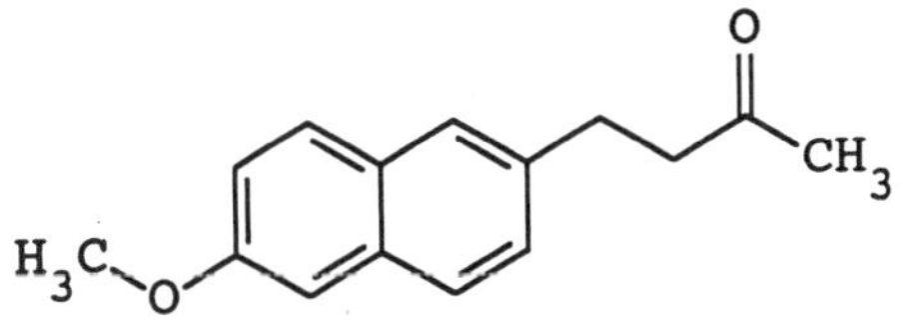

MNA is a potent inhibitor of prostaglandin synthesis. This metabolite has analgesic, antipyretic, and anti-inflammatory activity. Nabumetone is well absorbed from the gastrointestinal tract; food appears to increase the rate of oral absorption. About 35 percent of a dose is rapidly converted to MNA with 50 percent metabolized to a number of unidentified products. Over 99 percent of MNA is bound to plasma proteins. Most of the metabolites of nabumetone are excreted in the urine. Adverse reactions associated with nabumetone are similar to those of other NSAIDs. The drug is indicated for the treatment of acute and chronic osteoarthritis and rheumatoid arthritis.

Phenylacetic Acid Derivatives

Diclofenac Sodium and Potassium Diclofenac is a phenylacetic acid derivative that is available as the sodium salt and the potassium salt.

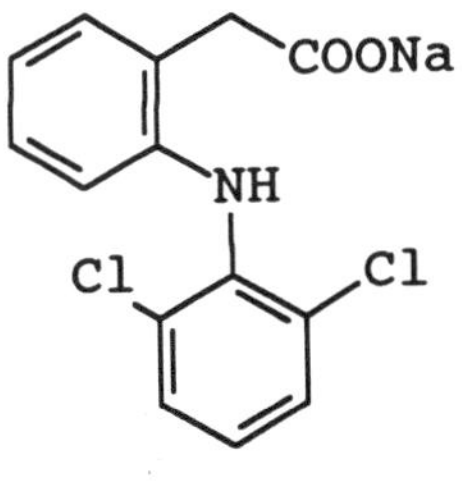

Diclofenac Sodium

The sodium salt is administered as an enteric-coated tablet, which is completely absorbed from the gastrointestinal tract. First pass metabolism occurs, and only 50 percent of the dose is bioavailable. The mean plasma half-life is 2 h. Adverse reactions include gastrointestinal, renal, and hepatic toxicity; edema; dizziness; and tinnitus. It is contraindicated in individuals with porphyria. Diclofenac sodium is indicated for the treatment of rheumatoid arthritis, osteoarthritis, and ankylosing spondylitis; diclofenac potassium is used for the management of pain and for dysmenorrhea.

Pyrrole Derivatives

Tolmetin sodium and ketorolac tromethamine are NSAIDs that make up the pyrrole derivatives. Their structures are shown in Fig. 24-6.

Tolmetin Sodium This drug is rapidly and almost completely absorbed from the gastrointestinal tract; peak plasma levels are reached within 30 to 60 min and the plasma half-life is biphasic with the first phase being approximately 1 to 2 h and the second phase about 5 h. The drug is eliminated within 24 h in the urine as conjugated tolmetin and an inactive product of oxidative biotransformation. The toxicities of tolmetin are similar to those of the other NSAIDs. Unlike aspirin, however, tolmetin has minimal effects on platelet aggregation. In addition, although plasma protein binding of tolmetin is high (99 percent) it does not appear to affect the anticoagulant activity of warfarin or the hypoglycemic response to sulfonylureas. This drug is approved for the treatment of juvenile rheumatoid arthritis, adult rheumatoid arthritis, and osteoarthritis.

Ketorolac Tromethamine Ketorolac is a substituted pyrrole derivative that is structurally related to tolmetin. Like most other NSAIDs, ketorolac acts by inhibition of prostaglandin synthesis and has

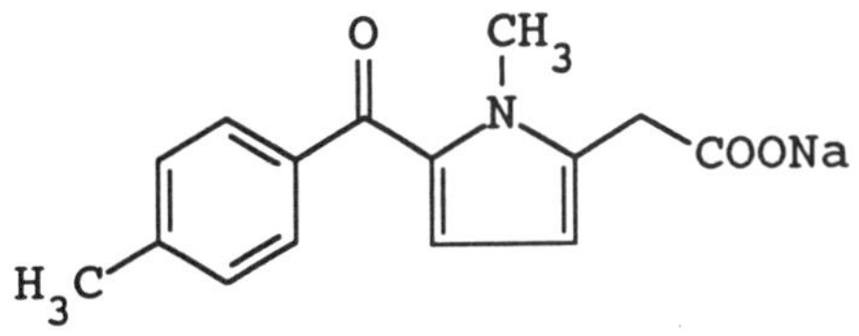

Tolmetin sodium

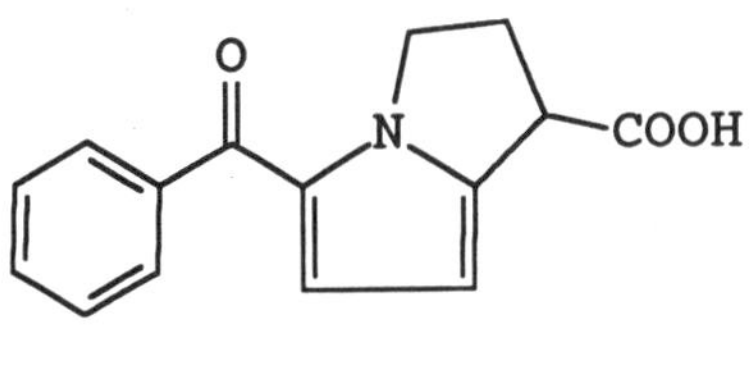

Ketorolac

FIGURE 24-6 *Structures of the pyrrole derivatives.*

analgesic, anti-inflammatory and antipyretic activities; however, it appears that the analgesic activity of this compound is greater than its anti-inflammatory potency. The compound is unique in that it is the only drug of this type available for intramuscular as well as oral administration for the short-term management of moderate to severe pain; clinical studies indicate that this drug is at least as effective, if not superior to morphine, meperidine, or pentazocine for the treatment of moderate to severe postoperative pain. Ketorolac tromethamine is completely absorbed following intramuscular administration; mean peak plasma concentrations occur within 1 h. Similar to most other NSAIDs, ketorolac tromethamine is highly bound to plasma proteins resulting in a low apparent volume of distribution. The drug is biotransformed by hydroxylation and conjugation reactions in the liver and most of the parent compound is eliminated in the urine. The mean elimination half-life is approximately 4.5 h in young adults and 7 h in the elderly. Adverse reactions, warnings, precautions, and contraindications of ketorolac tromethamine are similar to other NSAIDs.

Topical ophthalmic administration of this compound is used to relieve ocular itching in seasonal allergic conjunctivitis. It has been shown to reduce the concentration of prostaglandins in the eye, which are believed to be associated with the itching.

AN ANALGESIC AND ANTIPYRETIC DRUG

Acetaminophen

Acetaminophen is employed for its analgesic and antipyretic effects. It is a metabolite of phenacetin, a drug no longer used in the United States because of its toxicity. Acetaminophen relieves pain and lowers fever but has no significant anti-inflammatory or uricosuric effects, nor does it inhibit platelet aggregation or cause gastric irritation.

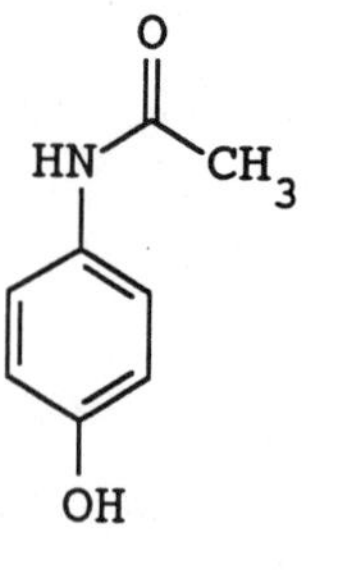

O
HN CH$_3$
OH

Mechanism of Action Since it has been demonstrated that acetaminophen inhibits brain cyclooxygenase even more effectively than does aspirin, it is probable that both drugs are antipyretic by an effect on heat regulatory centers. On the other hand, the mechanism of the analgesic action of acetaminophen is uncertain because this drug is only a weak inhibitor of peripheral cyclooxygenases.

Pharmacokinetics Acetaminophen is totally absorbed from the gastrointestinal tract, attaining a peak plasma level in 1 to 1.5. Acetaminophen is metabolized into a number of metabolites, and these, together with free drug, are excreted in the urine.

Therapeutic Uses Acetaminophen is widely used as an analgesic and antipyretic in the treatment of mild pain and fever. It has not been associated with Reye's syndrome and, therefore, can be used to reduce fever in children with influenza and other viral infections. In contrast to the NSAIDs, acetaminophen is devoid of anti-inflammatory activity and is not used to treat inflammatory conditions.

Adverse Reactions Because of the widespread use of acetaminophen as an alternative to aspirin in the treatment of mild pain and fever, there has been an increased incidence of toxicity due to overdose of drug with suicidal intent or by accident. Ingestion of over 7.5 g of acetaminophen at one time has been associated with severe hepatic toxicity. After ingestion, nausea, vomiting, and lethargy develop within 12 h. These symptoms resolve, and then liver damage occurs 48 h after ingestion, often resulting in death from hepatic failure if untreated. The hepatotoxicity is due to the formation of an N-hydroxylated biotransformation product, N-acetylbenzoquinoneimine. This metabolite reacts with sulfhydryl groups on glutathione and when the hepatic stores of glutathione are depleted, N-acetylbenzoquinoneimine reacts with sulfhydryl groups on cellular proteins to produce hepatotoxicity.

Treatment consists of gastric lavage followed by the administration of N-acetylcysteine within 12 h of acetaminophen ingestion. N-Acetylcysteine provides sulfhydryl groups for the toxic metabolite and can reduce liver toxicity. Following recovery from overdose, there appears to be complete resolution of hepatic damage. Dialysis is not recommended in the treatment of acetaminophen overdose.

As mentioned above, acetaminophen does not

cause gastrointestinal irritation or inhibit platelet aggregation as do other NSAIDs. For this reason, it would be a drug of choice for pain relief or treatment of fever in patients with gastrointestinal disease or bleeding disorders.

DRUGS USED IN THE TREATMENT OF GOUT AND HYPERURICEMIA

Acute gout is caused by precipitation of sodium urate crystals in a synovial joint. It is a classic example of acute inflammation. Hyperuricemia (serum urate levels above 7 mg per 100 mL) may be caused by a variety of secondary etiologies or may be idiopathic. If idiopathic, it may be caused by the over-production of uric acid or by the reduced excretion by an otherwise normal kidney. The defects causing idiopathic hyperuricemia are unknown. The disorder may be asymptomatic, requiring no treatment. When present for many years, it may cause acute gouty arthritis, tophi (precipitation of sodium urate crystals in interstitial tissues), or uric acid stones in the urinary system.

Drugs used in the treatment of gout may be divided into two groups. The first group includes drugs used to treat the inflammation of an acute attack of gouty arthritis occurring in a synovial joint. Most of the NSAIDs are effective for this purpose. Colchicine, as described below, is also effective in acute attacks of gout. The second group includes drugs to treat hyperuricemia if such treatment is indicated.

Colchicine

Chemistry Colchicine is an alkaloid found in *Colchicum autumnale* (autumn crocus or meadow saffron). Aside from its use in the therapy of acute gouty arthritis for about 1500 years, colchicine is of considerable biologic interest because of its ability to arrest cell division in metaphase when given in larger doses.

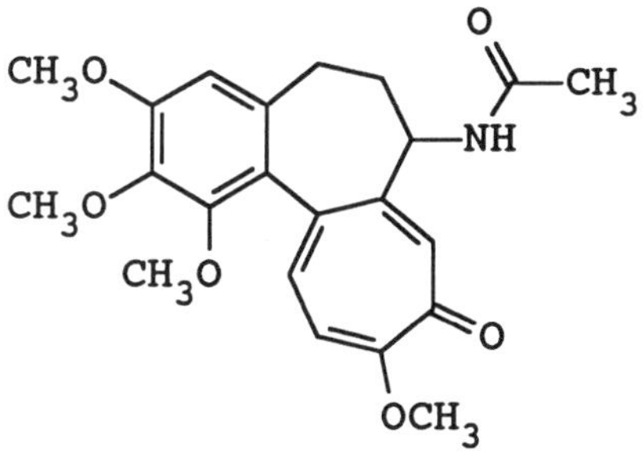

CH_3O CH_3O CH_3O NH CH_3 O O OCH_3

Mechanism of Action Colchicine has the ability to penetrate the cell and migrate into the microtubular system. By an unknown mechanism it stabilizes the intracellular membranes, and inflammatory cells lose their ability to respond to the inflammatory reaction caused by sodium urate crystals. Colchicine has no effect on the urinary excretion of uric acid or its biosynthesis and therefore is of no value in the treatment of hyperuricemia. There is little evidence that it acts primarily as an analgesic and is usually ineffective in arthritis other than that caused by sodium urate deposition. Colchicine does provide rapid relief of pain associated with acute gout and can also be used prophylactically to prevent recurrent exacerbations of this disease.

Therapeutic Use Administration of colchicine should begin at the earliest possible moment after the appearance of one or more symptoms suggestive of acute gouty arthritis, since it may be ineffective if administration is delayed for more than 24 h. Treatment of an acute attack of gout requires the ingestion of one tablet (0.6 mg) every hour until there is an unmistakable subsidence of articular symptoms or until the patient develops severe nausea, vomiting, or diarrhea. Usually the total amount of drug required is between 1.8 and 3 mg administered over several hours. The drug may also be given intravenously, and by this route 1 or 2 mg is administered as one dose, which may be repeated once in 2 to 4 h. In case of renal impairment, the dose of colchicine should be reduced and should not be used in presence of simultaneous hepatic and renal disease. Adverse reactions include nausea, vomiting, diarrhea, and severe neutropenia, while an acute overdose of 7 mg may be fatal.

Probenecid

Chemistry Probenecid is a sulfonamide with the following chemical structure:

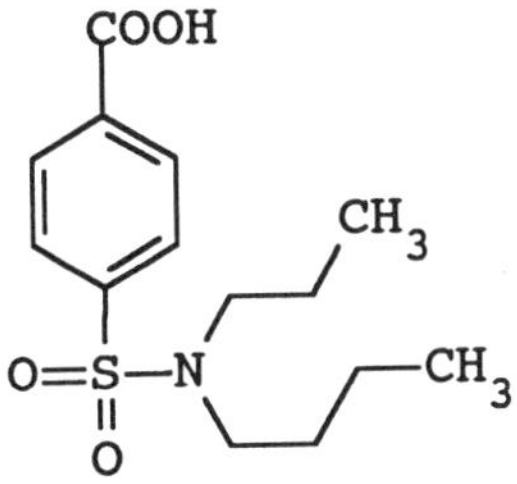

COOH CH_3 O=S—N CH_3 O

Mechanism of Action Uric acid is derived chiefly from the catabolism of nucleic acids. In a person on a low purine diet, about 700 mg of uric acid is excreted daily, two-thirds of it via the kidney. Uric acid is filtered in the glomerulus and secreted into and reabsorbed from the proximal tubule. There is some evidence that there may be further reabsorption in the distal tubule. Probenecid inhibits renal tubular secretion and reabsorption of a variety of organic acids, including uric acid.

Pharmacokinetics Probenecid is totally absorbed on oral administration, reaching a peak in 1 to 5 h. The drug is almost totally metabolized and is excreted by the kidney.

Therapeutic Uses Probenecid produces a large negative balance of uric acid when first administered particularly at a time when the uric acid concentration in the plasma is high. Probenecid and other uricosuric agents are of no value in relieving the pain and inflammation in acute attacks of gout, since they are not anti-inflammatory. In fact by altering the serum uric acid level, acute attacks of gout may be precipitated. Probenecid is used in the presence of reduced excretion of uric acid with normal renal function. When probenecid does not lower the uric acid blood level sufficiently or in the presence of severely impaired renal function, allopurinol may be used.

Adverse Reactions Probenecid is well tolerated by most patients. Gastrointestinal irritation and hypersensitivity causing nausea and vomiting or skin rashes may occur.

Aspirin, even at uricosuric doses, should not be administered with probenecid, since the actions of the two drugs are antagonistic. If an analgesic agent is needed, acetaminophen may be used. Probenecid decreases the renal clearance of penicillin, indomethacin, certain cephalosporins, and thiazide diuretics. When administered in conjunction with these drugs, increased blood levels will occur, and if not corrected may cause toxicity. Probenecid, by altering the excretion of penicillins or cephalosporins, may be used as a therapeutic modality to increase the blood level of these antimicrobial agents.

Sulfinpyrazone

Sulfinpyrazone is a pyrazolon derivative closely related chemically to phenylbutazone. The drug is a uricosuric agent which acts by inhibiting tubular secretion of uric acid as well as its reabsorption. This results in an increased uric acid excretion and decreased serum urate concentration. In addition, the drug inhibits platelet aggregation. Sulfinpyrazone is used as a uricosuric agent in the treatment of hyperuricemia.

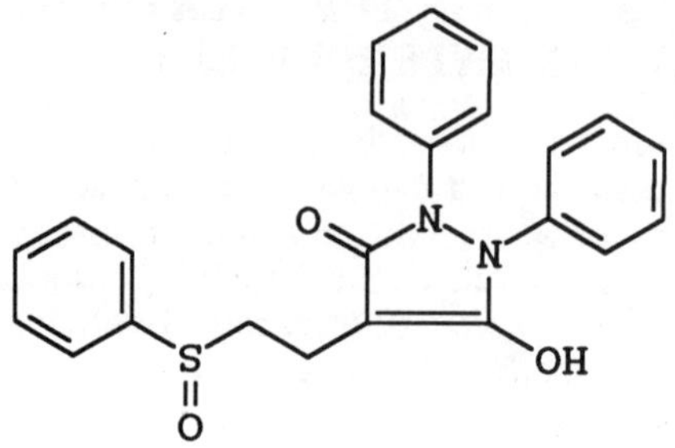

O N N S O OH

The drug is completely absorbed from the gastrointestinal tract following oral administration, obtaining a peak level in 1 h. It is highly bound to plasma proteins and is excreted 50 percent unchanged and 50 percent as the parahydroxy metabolite which is also uricosuric.

The common adverse effects of sulfinpyrazone are similar to that seen with phenylbutazone, namely, gastrointestinal irritation, which may lead to ulceration and bleeding. Agranulocytosis, however, is much less frequent than that reported with phenylbutazone. Sulfinpyrazone may exacerbate hypoglycemia by decreasing the excretion of the sulfonylurea oral hypoglycemic agents.

Salicylates at any dose will block the uricosuric effect of sulfinpyrazone. Probenecid will have a synergistic effect on the uricosuric effect of sulfinpyrazone but will increase the plasma level of the drug.

Allopurinol

Like the uricosuric agents, allopurinol has no analgesic or anti-inflammatory activity and is therefore of no value in the treatment of acute gouty arthritis.

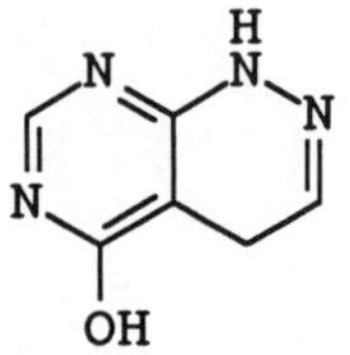

H N N N N OH

Mechanism of Action Allopurinol is an antimetabolite of xanthine and hypoxanthine and inhibits the enzyme xanthine oxidase; thus the conversion of hypoxanthine and xanthine to uric acid is reduced. Since the solubility of hypoxanthine and xanthine is considerably greater than that of uric acid, there is a net loss of urate from the total body pool. Despite the fact that allopurinol inhibits an enzyme and is an antimetabolite, it is relatively free of severe effects on organ systems.

Pharmacokinetics Allopurinol is about 80 percent bioavailable, reaching a maximum blood level in 2 to 6 h. It is oxidized by xanthine oxidase to alloxanthine (oxypurinol). Both allopurinol and alloxanthine inhibit xanthine oxidase. The half-life of allopurinol is 2 to 3 h and that of alloxanthine is 18 to 30 h. Both drugs are excreted entirely in the urine.

Therapeutic Uses Allopurinol is indicated for treatment of patients with symptoms of gout. It is not used for asymptomatic hyperuricemia. Because the half-life of its metabolite alloxanthine is long, following continued dosing with allopurinol to the steady state, the drug may be used once daily during maintenance therapy.

In addition to its use in gout, allopurinol is used in patients with leukemia, lymphomas, and other malignancies who are receiving antineoplastic drugs which cause elevated blood urate levels (see Chapter 43).

Adverse Reactions Mild reactions to allopurinol include fever, skin rash, headache, vertigo, and nausea. The most common adverse effects of allopurinol are hypersensitivity reactions. Severe reactions, frequently fatal, may occur in hypersensitive individuals. Severe skin involvement causing exfoliative dermatitis with Stevens-Johnson syndrome may be seen. Severe renal damage with eosinophilia, frequently associated with skin rash of a severe degree, has been recorded and is frequently fatal. Hepatitis may occur in mild form or may go on to hepatic insufficiency.

Since allopurinol is a xanthine oxidase inhibitor, it will interfere with the biotransformation of azathioprine and 6-mercaptopurine. If allopurinol must be administered concurrently with these drugs, such as in the treatment of acute leukemia, the dose of the cytotoxic agent must be reduced by one-third to one-half. The dose should also be reduced in the presence of renal insufficiency.

BIBLIOGRAPHY

_______ "Secondary Prevention of Vascular Disease by Prolonged Antiplatelet Treatment. Antiplatelet Trialists' Collaboration," *Br. Med. J. (Clin. Res. Ed.)*: **296**: 320-331 (1988).

Clive, D.M., and J.S. Stoff: "Renal Syndromes Associated with Nonsteroidal Anti-inflammatory Drugs," *N. Engl. J. Med.* **310**: 563-572 (1984).

Hennekens, C.H., R. Peto, G.B. Hutchison, and R. Doll: "An Overview of the British and American Aspirin Studies," *N. Engl. J. Med.* **318**: 923-924 (1988).

Huskisson, E.C. (ed.): *Anti-Rheumatic Drugs*, Praeger Publishers, New York, 1983.

Lanza, F.L.: "Gastrointestinal Toxicity of the Newer NSAIDs", *Am. J. Gastroenterol.* **88**: 1318-1323 (1993).

Nickander, R., F.G. McMahon, and A.S. Rudolfo: "Nonsteroidal Anti-inflammatory Agents," *Annu. Rev. Pharmacol. Toxicol.* **19**: 469-490 (1979).

Oates, J.A., G.A. FitzGerald, R.A. Branch, E.K. Jackson, H.R. Knapp, and L.J. Roberts, 2nd: "Clinical Implications of Prostaglandin and Thromboxane A2 Formation," *N. Engl. J. Med.* **319**: 689-698, 761-767 (1988).

Peto, R., R. Gray, R. Collins, et al.: "Randomized Trial of Prophylactic Daily Aspirin in British Male Doctors," *Br. Med. J.* **296**: 313-316 (1988).

Rainsford, K.D.: "Mechanisms of Gastrointestinal Damage by NSAIDS", *Agents Actions Suppl.* **44**: 59-64 (1993).

Relman, A.S.: "Aspirin for the Primary Prevention of Myocardial Infarction," *N. Engl. J. Med.* **318**: 245-246 (1988).

Roberts, W.N., M.H. Liang, and S.H. Stern: "Colchicine in Acute Gout. Reassessment of Risks and Benefits," *J. Am. Med. Assoc.* **257**: 1920-1922 (1987).

Robinson, D.R.: "Eicosanoids, Inflammation, and Anti-inflammatory Drugs," *Clin. Exper. Rheumat.* **7 (Suppl. 3)**: S155-S161 (1989).

Shirota, H., M. Goto, and K. Katayama: "Application of Adjuvant-Induced Local Hyperthermia for Evaluation of Anti-inflammatory Drugs," *J. Pharmacol. Exp. Ther.* **247**: 1158-1163 (1988).

Smith, W.L., L.J. Marnett, and D.L. DeWitt: "Prostaglandin and Thromboxane Biosynthesis," *Pharmacol. Ther.* **49**: 153-179 (1991).

Stevenson, D.D.: "Diagnosis, Prevention and Treatment of Adverse Reactions to Aspirin and Nonsteroidal Anti-inflammatory Drugs," *J. Allergy Clin. Immunology* **74**: 617-622 (1984).

Vane, J., and R. Botting. "Inflammation and the Mechanism of Action of Anti-inflammatory Drugs," *FASEB J.*. 1: 89-96 (1987).

Young, F.E., S.L. Nightingale, and R.A. Temple: "The Preliminary Report of the Findings of the Aspirin Component of the Ongoing Physicians' Health Study. The FDA Perspective on Aspirin For the Primary Prevention of Myocardial Infarction," *N. Engl. J. Med.* **318**: 3158-3160 (1988).

CHAPTER 25

Local Anesthetics

Jonathan T. Abrams and Jerry D. Levitt

Local anesthetics are drugs which reversibly block nerve conduction in therapeutic concentrations. Although these agents are used primarily to block conduction in nerves (peripheral, spinal cord), they also affect other excitable tissues such as cardiac, skeletal, and smooth muscle and brain tissue. Local anesthetics are usually administered near the desired nerves to be affected. They can be administered topically, subcutaneously, near nerve roots (spinal or epidural), or near nerve plexuses to achieve analgesia or, at higher concentrations, anesthesia.

Complete reversibility is basic to the definition of local anesthetics because many substances including ethanol and phenol can block nerve conduction permanently and therefore are not useful as local anesthetics. A wide variety of substances exhibit mild local anesthetic activity such as volatile general anesthetic agents, α- and β-adrenergic receptor blocking agents, alcohols, opioids, barbiturates, antihistamines, anticonvulsants, tranquilizers, and plant and animal toxins. However these agents are not used clinically for this activity.

Peruvian natives first noticed the anesthetic and central nervous system (CNS) stimulating effects of cocaine when they chewed the leaves of the *Erythroxylon coca* plant. Isolated in 1860, cocaine was first used clinically in 1884 as a topical anesthetic for ophthalmologic surgery. Procaine, the first synthetic local anesthetic, was introduced into clinical practice in 1905. However, like cocaine, it was an ester and had a relatively short duration of action due to enzymatic hydrolysis, and a risk of allergic reactions. The next significant era in the development of local anesthetics occurred in Sweden between 1930 and 1940, with the development of the amide local anesthetics. The prototype aminoamide, lidocaine, was introduced into clinical practice in 1947, followed by the long-lasting amide bupivacaine in 1963. Many agents have been introduced since; however, scientists continue to search for longer-acting and safer local anesthetic agents.

CHEMISTRY AND STRUCTURE-ACTIVITY RELATIONSHIPS

Local anesthetics are composed of three parts: a lipophilic aromatic ring, an intermediate chain, and a hydrophilic amino group (see Fig. 25-1). These agents are classified as either esters or amides according to the structure of the intermediate chain. This classification is of more than academic interest, as the metabolism, allergic potential, stability, and systemic toxicity is determined by this intermediate chain.

In its tertiary form, local anesthetics are poorly soluble in water, but because they are weak bases, they combine readily with acids to form water-soluble salts. Thus commercially available local anesthetics are often prepared in their hydrochloride salt form. The hydrochloride salt ionizes in aqueous solution to form a cationic ion and a chloride anion. The charged form is in equilibrium with the uncharged tertiary amine form (Fig. 25-2). The exact fraction in each form depends upon the pK_a or dissociation constant of the specific local anesthetic and the pH of the surrounding tissue or solution.

Clearly, the higher the pK_a of a drug, the less will be in the free-base form at physiologic pH. The penetration of a local anesthetic to its site of action is largely dependent on its ability to cross lipid membranes. The free-base form has a high lipid-to-water partition coefficient and can therefore penetrate such membranes easily. Cationic forms, because of their charge, are unable to penetrate lipid membranes. In general, local

	Lipophilic Group	Intermediate Chain	Amine Substituents
Esters			
Cocaine	C_6H_5–C(=O)–O–	CH_3–O–C(=O)–	N–CH_3
Procaine	H_2N–C_6H_4–	–C(=O)–O–CH_2–CH_2–	–N(C_2H_5)(C_2H_5)
Tetracaine	C_4H_9–HN–C_6H_4–	–C(=O)–O–CH_2–CH_2–	–N(CH_3)(CH_3)
Chloroprocaine	H_2N–C_6H_3(Cl)–	–$COOCH_2CH_2$–	–N(C_2H_5)(C_2H_5)
Amides			
Lidocaine	C_6H_3(CH_3)(CH_3)–	–NH–C(=O)–CH_2–	–N(C_2H_5)(C_2H_5)
Mepivacaine	C_6H_3(CH_3)(CH_3)–	–NH–C(=O)–	piperidine ring, N–CH_3
Bupivacaine	C_6H_3(CH_3)(CH_3)–	–NH–C(=O)–	piperidine ring, N–C_4H_9
Etidocaine	C_6H_3(CH_3)(CH_3)–	–NH–C(=O)–CH(C_2H_5)–	–N(C_2H_5)(C_3H_7)
Prilocaine	C_6H_4(CH_3)–	–NH–C(=O)–CH(CH_3)–	–NHC_3H_7

FIGURE 25-1 *Chemical structures of some local anesthetics.*

$$R\text{-}CH_2\text{-}NH^+(C_2H_5)_2 \rightleftharpoons R\text{-}CH_2\text{-}N(C_2H_5)_2 + H^+$$

Quaternary amine | Tertiary amine

FIGURE 25-2 *The dissociation equilibrium of charged quaternary amine and uncharged tertiary amine local anesthetic molecules in an aqueous milieu. [From Carpenter, R.L., and D.C. Mackey: "Local Anesthetics," In Barash, P.G., B.F. Cullen, and R.K. Stoelting (eds.): Clinical Anesthesia, Second Edition, J.B. Lippincott, Philadelphia, 1992, p. 510.]*

anesthetics with lower pK_a's exhibit faster onset than drugs with high pK_a's.

Manipulation of the local anesthetic structure can change the physical properties of these drugs (Fig. 25-1). Alterations in the intermediate chain determine whether these compounds undergo hydrolysis in the blood (esters) or liver metabolism (aminoamides). Substitutions on the aromatic ring and on the amino group change the lipid solubility and the degree to which the local anesthetic binds to protein. As with the volatile general anesthetic agents, lipid solubility of the local anesthetic correlates with potency. Protein binding correlates with the duration of action. Bupivacaine (95 percent bound) and etidocaine (94 percent bound) are the most protein bound of the local anesthetics and provide the longest duration of action because they stay in the protein acceptor site for a longer time. The dissociation constant correlates with onset of action, because local anesthetics with pK_a's closer to physiologic pH, have more local anesthetic available in the lipid-soluble tertiary form. The ability of a local anesthetic to cause vasodilation correlates inversely with the drug's duration and apparent potency. Drugs which cause greater vasodilation lead to increased rapidity of their absorption into the systemic circulation and early termination of neural blockade.

MECHANISM OF ACTION

In the resting state, the axoplasm is at about −90 mV with respect to the outside of the cell. This "resting potential" is maintained by the relative concentrations and permeabilities of sodium and potassium ions across the nerve membrane. In the resting state, the membrane is highly impermeable to sodium ions, but relatively more permeable to potassium ions through the potassium channels. When the nerve is stimulated, the transmembrane potential becomes less negative (depolarizes), some sodium channels in the region of the depolarization open, and sodium moves inward along its concentration gradient. At the peak of depolarization, the axoplasm is +20 mV with respect to the exterior of the cell. Near this peak, potassium channels open, potassium ions leave the cell, and the cell repolarizes. The propagated sequence of depolarization and repolarization takes 1 to 2 ms and is called an action potential. Only a small proportion of the available sodium and potassium ions move during a single action potential. After repolarization, the sodium-potassium pump reestablishes the ion gradients.

Local anesthetics have been shown to (1) increase the threshold for electrical excitation in the nerve, (2) slow propagation of the depolarization, (3) reduce the rate of rise of the action potential, and (4) eventually block conduction of the action potential. Local anesthetics have no effect on the resting membrane potential. Experiments have demonstrated that local anesthetics cause a dose-related decrease in sodium conductance and that the block of sodium channels is sufficient to account for the action of these drugs.

The sodium channels pass through at least three states: closed, open, and inactivated. From the closed state depolarization opens the "gate," allowing sodium ions and local anesthetics to enter the channel. Upon entering the open sodium channel, the local anesthetics interfere with sodium influx and subsequently change the gate to become more refractory to depolarization. Local anesthetics block nerve fibers more strongly when the fiber is stimulated at higher frequency. This phenomenon, termed frequency-dependent block, may occur because the sodium channel is in the open state more when stimulated at higher frequencies and this may permit more access for the local anesthetic. In the inactive state the channel is refractory to depolarization. Local anesthetics likely increase the time the sodium channel is in the inactive state.

The following is a likely sequence for the production of clinical local anesthesia (Fig. 25-3). After injection, the uncharged (free-base) and cationic forms of the local anesthetic are in equilibrium in the extracellular space in proportion determined by the pK_a of the local anesthetic solution and the pH of the surrounding tissue. The uncharged lipid-soluble form diffuses through the

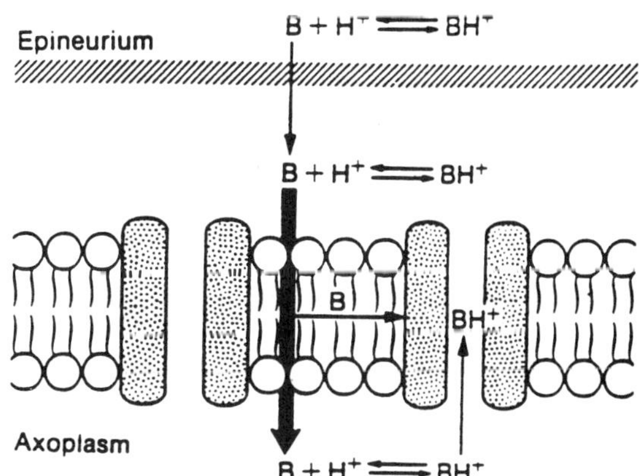

FIGURE 25-3 *Local anesthetic access to the sodium channel. The uncharged molecule diffuses most easily across lipid barriers and interacts with the channel through axolemma interior. The charged species formed in the axoplasm gains access to a specific receptor via the sodium channel pore. [From Carpenter, R.L., and D.C. Mackey: "Local Anesthetics," In Barash, P.G., B.F. Cullen, and R.K. Stoelting (eds.): Clinical Anesthesia, Second Edition, J.B. Lippincott, Philadelphia, 1992, p. 510.]*

connective tissue surrounding the nerve fiber and through the phospholipid layer of the nerve cell membrane to reach the axoplasm. Here the cationic form attaches to the intracellular opening of the sodium channel decreasing sodium conductance and blocking depolarization. The process is reversed by diffusion of the local anesthetic into the vasculature and systemic circulation.

Benzocaine is a permanently uncharged local anesthetic whose mechanism of action differs from that of other agents. It seems to work by dissolving into and expanding the phospholipid membrane. This expansion deforms the sodium channel to reduce sodium conductance. Membrane expansion has also been proposed as a mechanism of action of inhalation general anesthetic agents.

PHARMACOKINETICS

Table 25-1 shows some of the pharmacokinetic properties of various local anesthetics. Local anesthetics are usually administered in close proximity to the nerves to be blocked. As a result local physical factors are much more important than pharmacokinetic factors for predicting the

TABLE 25-1 Pharmacokinetic comparisons of various local anesthetics[a]

Drug	Potency[b]	Lipid solubility	Plasma protein binding, %	Site of metabolism	Elimination half-life, min	Duration of action
Esters						
Procaine	1	Low	6	Plasma	—	Short
Chloroprocaine	4	—	—	Plasma	—	Short
Tetracaine	16	Moderate	76	Plasma	—	Long
Amides						
Lidocaine	4	Low	70	Liver	96	Moderate
Mepivacaine	2	Low	77	Liver	114	Mod.-long
Bupivacaine	16	Moderate	95	Liver	210	Long
Etidocaine	16	High	94	Liver	156	Long
Prilocaine	3	Low	55	Liver[c]	—	Moderate

[a] Surface anesthetics such as benzocaine, butamben, dyclonine, and pramoxine are used for topical or surface anesthesia and are not significantly absorbed.
[b] Potency comparison is based on procaine = 1.
[c] Also metabolized to some extent b extrahepatic tissues.

desired effect. In contrast, for most other drugs, initial uptake and distribution moves the drug from the site of administration to the target organ(s). But for local anesthetics, pharmacokinetics determines only the rate of drug removal from the site of action. Uptake into the systemic circulation begins the process of biotransformation and elimination and can lead to systemic toxicity. The blood level of a local anesthetic depends on the total dose, the vascularity at the site of administration, the drug clearance, and whether or not vasoconstrictor drugs were added. If the local anesthetic agent is injected directly into a vein, the uptake is instantaneous and a small dose may produce toxic blood levels. Local anesthetics are absorbed from different sites at markedly different rates, so that for the same dose of a given local anesthetic, the peak blood level is a function of what type of nerve block has been performed. The relative rate of absorption in decreasing order, for various nerve blocks are as follows: intercostal > caudal > epidural > brachial plexus > subcutaneous infiltration. Thus one can find the highest serum concentrations of local anesthetics following multiple intercostal nerve blocks.

Vasoconstrictors, such as epinephrine or occasionally phenylephrine, may be added to local anesthetic solutions to slow absorption of the anesthetic from the site of injection. These drugs prolong the duration of the block, reduce the peak blood concentration of the anesthetic, intensify the block, and reduce the surgical bleeding in local infiltration anesthesia. It may also permit a larger dose of anesthetic to be injected without systemic toxicity. The effect of a vasoconstrictor is greater when used with local anesthetics which are intrinsically strong vasodilators and not highly lipid-soluble such as procaine and lidocaine. When used in epidural anesthesia, epinephrine increases the duration of lidocaine by about 50 percent; in contrast, the duration of bupivacaine is increased by only 15 percent. Local anesthetics containing vasoconstrictors should not be used for infiltration of structures supplied by end arteries such as fingers, toes, and penis because of the possibility of causing ischemia. The vasoconstrictor itself may cause systemic toxicity if injected directly into a blood vessel or in an excessive dose. Contraindications to the use of epinephrine include severe hypertension, cardiac arrhythmias, and unstable angina.

The initial step in the metabolism of the ester local anesthetics is hydrolysis by plasma (pseudocholinesterase) and liver cholinesterases. The ester linkage is cleaved by plasma cholinesterase, forming para-aminobenzoic acid (PABA) and an amino alcohol. A small proportion of the population is allergic to PABA and this is the basis of allergic reactions to the ester local anesthetics. Conversely, the risk of an allergic reaction to an amide local anesthetic is very low. Plasma metabolism of most ester local anesthetics (procaine and chloroprocaine) occurs so rapidly (7 to 20 sec) that serum levels remain low and toxic reactions (as distinguished from allergic reactions) are rare. Tetracaine, on the other hand, is more slowly hydrolyzed. It is, therefore, used almost exclusively for spinal anesthesia, where the low dose and slow systemic uptake results in very low blood levels. Genetic variations in the activity of pseudocholinesterase may affect the rates of hydrolysis of these drugs. Thus, patients with abnormal or deficient plasma cholinesterases can exhibit evidence of toxicity at usual clinical doses of these drugs.

The amide local anesthetics are not hydrolyzed by esterases and are more stable in solution during storage and heat sterilization than are the esters. They are cleared from the circulation by liver metabolism, except for prilocaine which exhibits extrahepatic metabolism. Lidocaine is biotransformed by several pathways. The primary route involves the removal of one of the ethyl groups on the terminal tertiary nitrogen followed by hydrolysis of the amide linkage to form 2,6-xylidine and monoethylglycine. Oxidation occurs prior to sulfate conjugation. Both free and conjugated forms are excreted in the urine with less than 3 percent of the total administered dose excreted unchanged. The elimination half-life of lidocaine is about 90 min. However, one of its metabolite, glycinexylide, has a half-life of 10 h. Several of the metabolites of lidocaine have local anesthetic, antiarrhythmic, and convulsant properties. These may contribute to the systemic toxicity of lidocaine administered by infusion or repeated doses, especially in patients with renal insufficiency. The elimination half-lives of mepivacaine, bupivacaine, and etidocaine like lidocaine are considerably longer than that of the esters.

EFFECTS ON NERVES

The small nonmyelinated nerve fibers, which transmit pain and autonomic impulses, seem to be more susceptible to local anesthetic action than the larger myelinated fibers. In spinal anesthesia, the order of blockade by local anesthetics occurs initially with sympathetic fibers (hypotension) followed by the sensations of pain, cold, warmth, touch, deep pressure, proprioception, and motor activity. Recovery usually proceeds in the reverse order. However, etidocaine does not seem to follow this pattern and motor blockade may be more intense than sensory blockade. In addition, the arrangement of neural structures may influence the order of blockade. In the brachial plexus the large motor fibers are located in the periphery of the nerve bundles and the sensory fibers are centrally located. The local anesthetics will block the motor fibers first. Clinically, arm weakness occurs before onset of sensory anesthesia following a brachial plexus block.

ADVERSE EFFECTS

In addition to their local anesthetic activity, these drugs may produce effects on other organ systems. The CNS and the heart are the most likely areas of toxicity. Allergic and hypersensitivity reactions are most likely with the ester agents. Certain local anesthetics and their preservatives may cause damage to nerves and surrounding tissues.

Blood levels of local anesthetics sufficient to cause systemic toxicity may result from accidental intravascular injection or absorption of a toxic dose of anesthetic from the injection site. Factors which predispose to systemic toxicity include (1) injection of high concentrations and volumes of local anesthetics, (2) highly vascular site of injection, (3) diseases causing decreased clearance of amide local anesthetics such as hepatic failure and congestive heart failure, (4) drugs that decrease liver blood flow like propranolol, cimetidine, and halothane, and (5) plasma pseudocholinesterase deficiency which will increase the toxicity of ester local anesthetics.

Central Nervous System

Local anesthetic agents initially produce CNS excitation followed by generalized CNS depression. This seemingly biphasic effect is due to early selective blockade of inhibitory pathways in the cerebral cortex. Consequently, facilitatory neurons function unopposed, causing increased excitatory activity which can progress to grand mal seizures. Generalized CNS depression follows, as all neural conduction is blocked by local anesthetics. Only cocaine is a true CNS stimulant.

Following intravenous injection of local anesthetics, sedation, lightheadedness, and dizziness are followed by visual and auditory disturbances such as diplopia and tinnitus. Additional symptoms include drowsiness, circumoral paresthesias, and numbness of the tongue. More observable signs of CNS toxicity include muscular twitching, shivering, and tremors which can progress to generalized tonic-clonic seizures. The seizure activity seems to originate in subcortical brain structures, probably in the amygdala. Very high blood levels of local anesthetics can cause depression of the brain stem resulting in severe respiratory depression, apnea, and coma.

The CNS toxicity of local anesthetics is related primarily to the intrinsic anesthetic potencies. The speed at which blood levels are obtained is important as the rapid infusion of local anesthetics will produce toxicity at lower doses. Severe CNS toxic reactions have occurred during anesthesia of the nerves in the neck when very small quantities of local anesthetic were injected directly into an artery supplying the brain (carotid or vertebral artery).

Hypoxemia develops rapidly in a patient with local anesthetic-induced seizure activity because of respiratory depression and increased oxygen consumption from muscle activity. The rapid initiation of basic life support include effective ventilation with 100% oxygen which will prevent any permanent neurologic damage. Usually bag and mask ventilation is adequate until the return of spontaneous respiration. Occasionally a short-acting neuromuscular blocking drug (e.g., succinylcholine) is used to facilitate ventilation and the placement of an endotracheal tube. Low doses of a benzodiazepine or ultrashort-acting barbiturate can be administered to terminate the seizure activity.

Cardiovascular System

Local anesthetic-induced toxicity of the cardiovascular system is manifest by hypotension and arrhythmias secondary to depressed electrical conduction and cardiac contractility as well as vasodilation of the peripheral vasculature. As with CNS toxicity, there is a close relationship between intrinsic local anesthetic potency and the dose required to produce cardiovascular effects. However, the cardiovascular system is more resistant to toxicity than the CNS. The dose of local anesthetic required to produce cardiovascular collapse is 4 to 7 times greater than that which will cause seizures. However, it is much more difficult to treat local anesthetic-induced cardiovascular collapse.

The electrophysiologic effects of local anesthetics include decreased electrical excitability and conduction. High blood levels can cause bradycardia progressing to sinus arrest as a result of sinoatrial pacemaker depression. Additionally, partial or complete atrioventricular dissociation may result from depressed atrioventricular node conduction.

High blood levels of local anesthetics impair the mechanical activity of cardiac muscle in a dose-dependent manner. There is evidence that local anesthetics with greater potency, lipid solubility, and protein binding (specifically bupivacaine and to a lesser extent etidocaine) are relatively more cardiotoxic than other agents. Resuscitation from bupivacaine-induced cardiovascular collapse is much more difficult than that following other local anesthetics. Severe cardiac arrhythmias including ventricular tachycardia and ventricular fibrillation occur following rapid infusion of bupivacaine but not following the administration of lidocaine or mepivacaine.

Hypersensitivity

True hypersensitivity or allergic-type reactions to local anesthetics are more likely to occur with the esters than with the amides. The metabolic breakdown product of ester local anesthetics, para-aminobenzoic acid (PABA), is a common allergen. It is also found in many commercially available sunscreens. Allergic-type reactions with amide local anesthetics are extremely rare. The preservative methylparaben, structurally similar to PABA, can be found in multiple-dose vials of amides and is thought to be responsible for some hypersensitivity reactions.

A meticulous history can be helpful in distinguishing possible allergic reactions from other local anesthetic reactions. Many sensitivities to these drugs are actually due to inadvertent intravascular injection of the local anesthetic or to systemic effects of additives such as epinephrine. Skin testing may be of value in determining if a patient has a true local anesthetic allergy.

Local Tissue Reactions

Local anesthetic-induced tissue toxicity is extremely rare when approved agents in appropriate concentrations are administered. However, local neurotoxicity may result from injection of large volumes or high concentrations of local anesthetics.

In the past, the accidental subarachnoid injection of chloroprocaine was associated with the production of permanent neurologic deficits. The toxicity was linked to the combination of the preservative sodium bisulfite and a low pH. The new bisulfite-free formulation of chloroprocaine does not appear to cause this neurotoxicity.

CLINICAL APPLICATIONS OF LOCAL ANESTHETICS

Local anesthetics are used clinically for both their local effects (local and regional anesthesia) and systemic effects.

Local anesthetics permit those skilled in their administration to render various regions of the body insensitive to pain. In contrast to general anesthesia, regional and local anesthesia causes loss of sensation without loss of consciousness. General anesthetics alter many centrally-mediated controls of body function including respiration and circulation. Barring systemic toxicity, the effect of local anesthetics is limited to that part of the body which is anesthetized.

Neural blockade is established at terminal nerve endings and receptors (surface and infiltration anesthesia), at the peripheral nervous system (discrete nerve blocks and plexus blocks) and at the level of the CNS (spinal and epidural anesthesia). The following section reviews these techniques.

Surface Anesthesia

Topical application of local anesthetics to mucous membranes of the nasopharynx, oropharynx, larynx, tracheobronchial tree, eyes, tympanic membrane, urinary tract, and gastrointestinal tract induces surface anesthesia. However, to be effective topically, relatively high concentrations of local anesthetics are required. Following such application, local anesthetics are absorbed rapidly into the circulation (5 to 10 minutes) and thus carry the risk of systemic toxicity. Cocaine is the only local anesthetic agent with vasoconstrictive properties. It is ideally suited for surface anesthesia because it decreases its own absorption through vasoconstriction and improves surgical conditions through shrinkage of mucous membranes and decreased local bleeding. Phenylephrine in dilute concentrations can be added to other local anesthetics to produce similar vasoconstrictive effects. Epinephrine is not effective in producing topical vasoconstriction. EMLA cream is a recently introduced eutectic mixture of lidocaine and prilocaine in a 1:1 ratio which provides excellent skin penetration. Following one hour of skin contact, EMLA provides superficial skin anesthesia sufficient for intravenous catheter placement and minor surgical procedures.

Surface anesthetic agents include drugs for application to the skin and/or mucous membranes. Dibucaine, lidocaine, tetracaine, pramoxine, benzocaine, and butamben are used as topical anesthetics for various skin disorders. Tetracaine and proparacaine are used in ophthalmology to produce corneal anesthesia. Benzocaine and lidocaine can be applied to the tissues of the mouth and throat. Cocaine is used for its local anesthetic properties in nasal surgery.

Infiltration Anesthesia

The direct injection of local anesthetics into skin or deeper structures to produce surgical anesthesia is called *infiltration anesthesia*. This technique is used most commonly for superficial procedures such as skin or breast biopsies and to suture superficial wounds. However, in the absence of other anesthetic options infiltration anesthesia can be used to facilitate emergency procedures such as appendectomy or cesarean delivery. As previously mentioned, the addition of vasoconstrictors to local anesthetics for infiltration anesthesia has several desirable features including decreased systemic absorption, decreased bleeding, and prolonged duration of anesthesia.

Field block anesthesia is a technique of infiltrating local anesthetics so as to produce a wall of anesthesia around an operative field. A clinical example of this would be field block anesthesia for inguinal herniorrhaphy. Local anesthetic agents commonly used for infiltration or field block anesthesia include lidocaine, mepivacaine, bupivacaine, etidocaine, and chloroprocaine.

Peripheral Nerve Block

Interruption of neural pathways of the peripheral nervous system is accomplished by depositing local anesthetics in the vicinity of individual nerves or plexuses. These techniques as well as spinal and epidural anesthesia are referred to as *regional anesthesia*. At appropriate local anesthetic concentrations they result in anesthesia of all nerve fibers and therefore block sensory, motor, and autonomic pathways.

Many surgical procedures are performed under regional anesthesia. Examples include brachial plexus blocks for shoulder, arm, and hand procedures; cervical plexus blocks for surgery of the neck; intercostal blocks for abdominal and thoracic wall procedures; and blocks of individual nerves at the wrist or ankle for hand and foot procedures. The most commonly used local anesthetic agents for peripheral nerve blocks are lidocaine, mepivacaine, and bupivacaine.

Spinal Anesthesia

Spinal anesthesia, also called *intrathecal* or *subarachnoid block*, is performed by injecting local anesthetics into the cerebrospinal fluid (CSF) in the subarachnoid space. The injection of local anesthetic is most commonly made below the termination of the spinal cord, which correlates with the 2nd lumbar vertebra. Spinal anesthesia, including sympathetic, sensory, and motor block, is due primarily to the action of local anesthetics at the spinal nerve roots and in the dorsal root ganglia. The extent of neural blockade is determined by the distribution of local anesthetics in the CSF. Factors governing local anesthetic spread in the subarachnoid space include the density of the anesthetic solution relative to the CSF, the position of the patient, and the total dose administered. *Baricity* is the ratio of anesthetic solution density to the CSF density. Spinal anesthetic solutions can be hypo-, iso-, or hyperbaric. Hyperbaric solutions are the most commonly used clinically because they have a predictable and controllable degree of cephalad spread.

The onset of spinal anesthesia is very rapid, with detectable analgesia within 1 to 2 minutes and progression to desired levels of sensory and motor blockade by 5 to 10 minutes. Factors such as total dose of agent, baricity, use of vasoconstrictors, and lipid solubility determine the intensity and duration of spinal anesthesia.

In addition to blocking motor and sensory pathways, spinal anesthesia may cause profound physiologic alterations due to the interruption of the sympathetic nervous system. The preganglionic sympathetic fibers leave the spinal cord between T-1 and L-2 and travel in the corresponding anterior roots across the subarachnoid and epidural spaces. Because of the increased sensitivity of the preganglionic autonomic fibers to local anesthetics, the level of sympathetic nervous system blockade will extend higher than the sensory and motor blockade. Physiologic effects of this blockade include venous (capacitance vessels) and arterial (resistance vessels) dilatation, causing decreased venous return and cardiac output leading to hypotension.

Preservative-free solutions of lidocaine, bupivacaine, and tetracaine the most frequently used agents for spinal anesthesia.

Epidural Anesthesia

Epidural or peridural anesthesia is produced by injection of local anesthetic into the space surrounding the dura mater, within the bony cavity of the spinal canal. Spinal nerves with their dural cuffs pass through the epidural space on their way to the intervertebral foramina. Following epidural injection, local anesthetics gain access to their site of action by diffusing through the dural cuffs to the nerve roots, through the dura into the CSF, and through the intervertebral foramina to the paravertebral area. Larger doses of local anesthetic (approximately ten-fold greater than spinal anesthesia) are required for epidural anesthesia, because of greater distance to the neural tissues and necessity of diffusion through tissue barriers (dura, arachnoid). As a consequence there is a greater potential for local anesthetic-induced systemic toxicity. Another concern is the risk of injecting large doses of local anesthetic intended for epidural anesthesia into the subarachnoid space. A high or "total" spinal can occur which may be accompanied by hypotension, bradycardia, and respiratory arrest secondary to complete sympathetic blockade and diaphragmatic paralysis.

Epidural anesthesia induced by administration of anesthetic solution into the sacral canal through the sacral hiatus is referred to as *caudal anesthesia*. It has applications in obstetric, perineal, and lower extremity procedures. Agents used for epidural anesthesia include lidocaine, mepivacaine, bupivacaine, etidocaine, and chloroprocaine.

Both epidural and spinal anesthesia may be administered and maintained via a catheter placed in the proper anatomic location. Anesthesia can then be maintained and closely titrated for indefinite periods of time.

Other Uses of Local Anesthetics

In addition to their use in neural blockade, local anesthetics have beneficial systemic effects. The antiarrhythmic effects of lidocaine are well known (see Chapter 28). It is useful in situations where rapid control of ventricular arrhythmias is necessary. The effect is maintained by intravenous infusion and then rapidly dissipates when discontinued. Lidocaine has been used extensively intravenously or topically on the larynx and trachea to blunt the hemodynamic response to endotracheal intubation. It may also prevent the rise in intraocular and intracranial pressure during intubation. Intravenous lidocaine can be used to suppress coughing and prevent bronchospasm. Low serum levels of lidocaine provide systemic analgesia and decrease the minimum alveolar concentration (MAC) for inhalation anesthetics. They have also been shown to augment the effect of neuromuscular blocking agents. Local anesthetics have been used extensively for the treatment of acute and chronic pain syndromes.

THERAPEUTIC USES OF LOCAL ANESTHETICS

Amide Agents

Lidocaine Lidocaine is the most versatile of all local anesthetic agents. It has a rapid onset, a moderate duration of action, and can be used for all types of neural blockade.

Mepivacaine Mepivacaine has similar properties to lidocaine, but its duration of action is somewhat longer. This agent is not used in obstetric anesthesia due to its prolonged metabolism in the fetus and neonate, leading to an increased possibility of toxicity.

Bupivacaine Bupivacaine is characterized by slow onset, long duration of action, and intense analgesia. Most notable is the separation of sensory analgesia and motor blockade. At lower concentrations, bupivacaine can provide analgesia with minimal motor block. As discussed above, bupivacaine exhibits more serious cardiovascular toxicity owing to its high affinity for the sodium channels of myocardial conduction fibers.

Dibucaine Dibucaine is very potent and has a long duration of action. It is used primarily for spinal anesthesia and is similar to tetracaine in this application.

Etidocaine Etidocaine is distinguished by the profound motor blockade it produces. It is similar to bupivacaine with respect to duration of action and analgesia but etidocaine has a more rapid onset of action.

Prilocaine Prilocaine is comparable to lidocaine in clinical profile, yet it has a lower potential for systemic toxic reactions. However, because of the formation of methemoglobinemia at high doses, this drug is not commonly used.

Ester Agents

Procaine Procaine is an agent of low potency and short duration of action. Allergic reactions are more common with this agent due to its metabolism to para-aminobenzoic acid. Its primary clinical use is for spinal anesthesia.

Chloroprocaine Chloroprocaine is notable for rapid onset of action and low systemic toxicity due to rapid serum hydrolysis. It is popular for epidural anesthesia in obstetrics because of its low fetal and maternal toxicity.

Tetracaine Tetracaine has a long duration of action. In contrast to chloroprocaine, tetracaine undergoes slow plasma hydrolysis. Potential for systemic toxicity at large doses has deterred its use in many regional anesthetic techniques. It is most commonly used for spinal anesthesia and for topical anesthesia of the airway.

Cocaine Cocaine is used primarily as a surface anesthetic because of its intrinsic vasoconstrictor properties. Its widespread abuse as a CNS stimulant is discussed elsewhere (see Chapter 19).

Surface Anesthetics

A few compounds, because of poor water solubility or other chemical properties which limit their diffusion capabilities, are not useful for regional or local anesthesia upon injection, but demonstrate excellent therapeutic qualities when applied to the skin or mucous membranes. It should be noted that most of the compounds in this classification do not conform to the structure previously described for classic local anesthetics. The following drugs are representative of those utilized as surface anesthetics.

Benzocaine and Butamben Benzocaine and its close relative butamben are esters of para-aminobenzoic acid, yet differ from the parent procaine-type esters in that they do not contain the terminal hydrophilic amine group. It is thus an uncharged local anesthetic.

Benzocaine

Benzocaine is very slightly soluble in water and is slowly absorbed, with a prolonged duration of action. Sensitization may occur with these compounds in susceptible patients, when applied over extensive areas, and when utilized repeatedly. Benzocaine produces a sustained and effective local anesthetic action when applied to abraded skin. These drugs are employed as topical anesthetics on intact or abraded skin, as antipruritics, and for various dermatologic conditions.

Ethyl Chloride Ethyl Chloride is a highly flammable and volatile liquid which is used in the form of a spray to obtain brief periods of skin surface local anesthesia. Its anesthetic action is based on the principle of rapid evaporation, which produces superficial freezing of the tissue, promoting loss of peripheral sensory function. Fluorocarbons, because of similar physical properties, also exhibit this action. Ethyl chloride is useful for the temporary relief of pain in inflamed areas and for muscle spasms.

BIBLIOGRAPHY

Arpey, C.J., and W.S. Lynch: "Advances in Local Anesthesia," *Clinics Dermatol.* **10**: 275-283 (1992).

Ayoub, S.T., and A.E. Coleman: "A Review of Local Anesthetics," *Gen. Dentistry* **40**: 285-287 (1992).

Carpenter, R.L. and D.C. Mackey: "Local Anesthetics," In Barash, P.G., B.F. Cullen, and R.K. Stoelting (eds.): *Clinical Anesthesia*, J.B. Lippincott Co., Philadelphia, 1992, pp. 509-541.

Covino, B.G.: "Pharmacology of Local Anaesthetic Agents," *Br. J. Anaesth.* **58**: 701-716 (1986).

Covino, B.G.: "Clinical Pharmacology of Local Anesthetic Agents," In Cousins, M.J., and P.O. Bridenbaugh (eds.), *Neural Blockade in Clinical Anesthesia and Management of Pain, 2nd Ed.*, J.B. Lippincott Co, Philadelphia, 1988.

McCaughey, W.: "Adverse Effects of Local Anaesthetics," *Drug Safety* **7**: 178-179 (1992).

Mulroy, M.F.: *Regional Anesthesia*, Little, Brown & Company, Boston, 1989, pp. 1-29.

Reiz, S., and S. Nath: "Cardiotoxicity of Local Anaesthetic Agents," *Br. J Anaesth.* **58**: 736-746 (1986).

Tucker, G.T.: "Pharmacokinetics of Local Anaesthetics," *Br. J. Anaesth.* **58**: 713-717 (1986).

CHAPTER 26

Drug Dependence

Charles P. O'Brien

Drug dependence is a problem with important medical and social ramifications. From the medical perspective, it is important that physicians understand the dependence and abuse potential of the medications that they prescribe. Physicians must also understand the medical complications of street drugs that are used by some of the patients presenting in hospitals and clinics. Social complications are also important because abuse of street drugs is associated with crime, violence, unemployment, homelessness, and the spread of disease. Various drugs have risen to prominence at different times. In the 1980s, the United States was faced with a cocaine epidemic. In the 1990s, cocaine is still widely available in spite of billions of dollars spent on efforts to keep it out of the country. However, the number of new cocaine users decreased during the late 1980s and early 1990s while heroin availability and use went up. Then the 1993 survey of high school seniors found sharp increases in the use of illegal drugs, indicating that the general decline in illegal drug use had ended. This chapter will focus on pharmacological principles, but for the clinician, the problem of drug dependence must be considered in its social context.

TERMS CONCERNED WITH DRUG DEPENDENCE AND ABUSE

Modern scientific approaches have shed a great deal of light on the mechanisms involved in drug dependence and on improving treatment approaches. In the past there was great focus on tolerance and physical dependence. *Tolerance* refers to the reduced effect that occurs with repeated doses of the same drug or repeated doses of several drugs within the same class. The reduced effect is the result of homeostatic processes in which organ systems adapt to the effects of the drug. This adaptation tends to oppose the pharmacological changes produced by the drug, thus resisting changes from the status quo with the result that higher doses are required to achieve the same effect which could be produced initially by a lower dose of the drug. Mechanisms involved in tolerance may be classified in three categories: (1) *metabolic tolerance*, which involves more efficient disposition of the drug; (2) *pharmacodynamic tolerance*, which includes synaptic adaptations such as changes in numbers or sensitivity of receptors so as to counteract the effects of a drug at the synapse; and (3) *behavioral tolerance*, which involves learning to function in the presence of drug impairment or conditioned reflex changes which counteract the changes produced by the drug. With regular dosing, tolerance increases and a state of physical dependence follows. When tolerance develops very rapidly, following either a single dose or a few doses given over a short period of time, it is called *acute tolerance*, or *tachyphylaxis*. When the drug must be administered over a long period of time to induce tolerance, it is called *chronic tolerance*. Cross-tolerance exists when tolerance to one drug confers tolerance to another. For example, methadone produces opioid tolerance that produces cross-tolerance to heroin and thus prevents heroin injections from producing their usual rewarding effects.

Physical dependence is defined by the appearance of a rebound known as a *withdrawal syndrome* that follows cessation of drug taking. The withdrawal syndrome includes bodily changes that tend to be opposite to the effects of the drug which produced the dependence. Thus a drug that produces stimulation such as cocaine, is followed by weakness and depression during withdrawal. And a drug that produces sedation such as alcohol leads to hyperreflexia, anxiety, and irritability during withdrawal.

Drug dependence, also referred to as *addiction*, consists of a loss of control over drug use, compulsion to use the drug in spite of medical, family, social, or occupational problems caused by the drug. Tolerance and physical dependence is usually present, but it is not required by the definition. The term *drug abuse* is officially considered to be a degree of problematic drug use that is not severe enough to be classified as dependence.

Drugs vary in their liability to be abused and in their likelihood of producing dependence. The Drug Enforcement Administration (DEA) of the U.S. Department of Justice has classified drugs known to have potential for abuse into schedules according to their abuse potential and their clinical usefulness. The DEA schedules are as follows.

Schedule I Drugs in this schedule have a high potential for abuse and no currently accepted medical use in the United States. Examples of such drugs include heroin, marijuana, peyote, mescaline, some tetrahydrocannabinol derivatives, and various opioid derivatives. Substances listed in this schedule are not for prescription use; they may be obtained for chemical analysis or research instruction by submitting an application and a protocol of the proposed use to the DEA.

Schedule II The drugs in this schedule have a high abuse potential with severe psychological or physical dependence liability. Schedule II substances consist of certain opioid drugs, preparations containing amphetamines or methamphetamine as the single active ingredient or in combination with each other, and certain sedatives. Examples of opioids included in this schedule are opium, morphine, codeine, hydromorphone, methadone, meperidine, cocaine, oxycodone, and oxymorphone. Also included are stimulants, e.g., dextroamphetamine, methamphetamine, methylphenidate, and depressants, e.g., amobarbital, pentobarbital, secobarbital, and glutethimide.

Schedule III The drugs in this schedule have a potential for abuse that is less than that for those drugs in Schedules I and II. The use of these drugs may lead to low or moderate physical dependence or high psychological dependence. Included in this schedule, for example, are methyprylon, phendimetrazine, maxindol, and paregoric.

Schedule IV The drugs in this category have the potential for limited physical or psychological dependence and include barbital, phenobarbital, paraldehyde, chloral hydrate, ethchlorvynol, zolpidem, meprobamate, chlordiazepoxide, diazepam, clorazepate, flurazepam, oxazepam, clonazepam, prazepam, lorazepam, and propoxyphene.

Schedule V Schedule V drugs have a potential for abuse that is less than that for those listed in Schedule IV. These consist of preparations containing moderate quantities of certain opioids for use in pain (e.g., buprenorphine), as antidiarrheals (e.g., diphenoxylate), or as antitussives (such as codeine-containing cough mixtures). They may be dispensed without a prescription order in some States, provided that specified dispensing criteria are met by the pharmacist. Physicians should be clearly aware of the abuse potential of drugs: (1) their capacity to induce compulsive drug-seeking behavior, (2) their toxicity, and (3) the social consequences of abusing drugs as well as the attitude of society toward drug abuse.

The drugs of abuse can be divided into four major categories: (1) *depressants*, including opioids, benzodiazepines, and alcohol; (2) *stimulants*, including cocaine and the amphetamines; (3) *hallucinogens*, including lysergic acid diethylamide (LSD) and phencyclidine (PCP); and (4) *miscellaneous*, including marijuana and nicotine.

DEPRESSANTS

Opioid Dependence

There are two major clinical patterns of opioid abuse. The first occurs in individuals who receive prescription analgesic medication because of chronic pain. Tolerance to opioids begins with the first dose, and when patients receive these drugs chronically, tolerance and physical dependence are inevitable. This is why such drugs generally should not be used in the treatment of chronic pain unless the pain is associated with a terminal illness or unless the pain is so severe that the opioids must be used as a last resort (See Chapter 23 for pharmacological details). Problems such as chronic headaches, back pain, or neuritis should rarely be treated with opioids.

On the other hand, acute pain is often undertreated by physicians because of the fear of producing addiction. If pain is caused by a known source such as surgery or myocardial infarction, opioids can be prescribed on a short-term basis. It is important to be sure that the patient has adequate pain relief. There should be a clear distinction between the tolerance and physical dependence, which are expected occurrences when opioids are used repeatedly, and the opioid dependence syndrome, which involves drug-seeking behavior and the intention to use the drug in order to "get high" rather than simply to relieve pain.

The second type of opioid abuse pattern is that seen in street heroin addicts. These are most commonly young men who begin the use of heroin between 14 and 18 years of age and typically increase their dose over time so that within several years they are using the drug 3 to 6 times per day. The actual dose of heroin obtained in purchases on the streets of the United States is actually small. Perhaps 4 to 6 percent of the material in each heroin bag is actually heroin; the other 96 percent contains fillers such as quinine, maltose, sodium bicarbonate, or worse. Thus even a person injecting as often as 6 times per day is not usually receiving a large amount of opioid.

The opioid dependence syndrome is associated with many medical problems, in addition to preoccupation with drug-seeking behavior. Street heroin addicts tend to have multiple infections because of contaminated substances injected into their veins. These produce abscesses, sclerosed veins, lung lesions (because of contaminants filtered in the pulmonary circulation), cardiac lesions (such as bacterial endocarditis), and hepatitis (as many as 70 percent of street heroin addicts have some type of hepatitis). Street addicts are also often malnourished and suffering from associated psychiatric disorders, especially depression and anxiety.

In recent years, intravenous drug abuse has become a major risk factor for acquired immunodeficiency syndrome (AIDS). Not only does the virus spread because of addicts habit of sharing dirty needles, but it is also possible that some of the drugs used and the deteriorated condition of the addicts may make the drug abuser more susceptible to infection with human immunodeficiency virus (HIV).

Tolerance and Dependence Tolerance develops very rapidly to repeated use of opioids, but it develops in different systems at different rates. Thus a chronic user who no longer gets a "high" from a given dose may still continue to suffer from constipation and endocrine suppressant effects. Cross-tolerance refers to tolerance to all opioids produced by repeated dosing with a single opioid. The phenomenon of cross-tolerance forms the basis of the most widely used treatment for heroin dependence, methadone maintenance. Methadone is a long-acting opioid, given orally, which blocks opioid withdrawal and produces a level of tolerance such that the effects of the usual dose of street heroin can barely be perceived. Since there is little or no reward in taking heroin, properly maintained patients stop or at least greatly diminish their use of street opiates. They are required to come to a clinic daily or at least three times a week, and thus they are available for psychotherapy, counseling, and other treatment which might be indicated. In 1993, the Food and Drug Administration (FDA) approved levo-α-acetyl methadol (LAAM, generic name: levomethadyl) for the treatment of opioid dependence. LAAM is similar to methadone, but because of its long half-life and active metabolites, it blocks opioid withdrawal for 72 hours. This means that patients need to come to the clinic only three times a week, thus interfering less with their occupational activities.

When a chronic user stops taking opioids, a withdrawal syndrome develops, which consists of signs opposite to the effects seen when opioids are administered. For example, opioids produce pupillary constriction, and during withdrawal there is pupillary dilatation. Opioids produce calming, and in withdrawal extreme anxiety is common. The severity of the withdrawal syndrome depends on the dose of the opioid. Most cases of opioid withdrawal require little medication, and some patients can stop on their own without assistance, although relapse under those circumstances is almost universal. Short-acting drugs such as heroin have a brief, severe withdrawal syndrome, which peaks at 36 to 48 h and lasts up to 7 to 10 days. Long-acting drugs such as methadone have significantly longer withdrawal syndromes, which are just beginning at 36 to 48 h. In addition to the acute withdrawal syndrome, all opioids produce a protracted withdrawal syndrome, which consists of subtle but measurable signs and symptoms for at least 6 months. Most of the signs and symptoms of opioid withdrawal are related to rebound hyperactivity of central adrenergic pathways. Clonidine, a drug used in the treatment of hypertension, will reduce most of the symptoms of opioid withdrawal. The action of clonidine that is believed to be key in the blocking of withdrawal is the stimulation of α-adrenergic auto-receptors in the locus coeruleus of the brainstem. This results in reduced adrenergic outflow and therefore reduced symptoms of opioid withdrawal. Unfortunately, there are non-adrenergic symptoms that are not affected by clonidine and patients are, therefore, not as comfortable as when they are treated with an opioid such as methadone. Also, patients often become hypotensive when treated with clonidine; still, it is very useful in treating withdrawal in those institutions where methadone is not available on the formulary.

Opioid Antagonists Because opioids act at specific receptor sites, their effects can be blocked by other drugs which can occupy those receptors. Naloxone is such an antagonist, and it represents one of the few true antidotes in medicine. Persons suffering from an acute overdose of an opioid will be immediately awakened by the intravenous administration of naloxone because it competes with opioid molecules at receptor sites.

In addition to the treatment of overdose, there are two other uses of opioid antagonists in the treatment of dependence. Antagonists can be used to diagnose dependence because, when injected, they will displace opioids from receptors and will produce an acute withdrawal syndrome. The prevention of relapse is yet another use of opioid antagonists. When given to a drug-free, formerly dependent person, the antagonist will occupy opioid receptors and prevent the user from experiencing opioid effects. For this relapse/prevention function, a long-acting antagonist, naltrexone, is used. The completeness of the blockade depends on the dose of naltrexone, the time since the last dose of naltrexone, and the dose of the opioid used in the attempt to override the blockade. Naltrexone is effective in antagonizing typical doses of street opioids for 48 to 72 h. In practice, most patients do not test the blockade, and the treatment is effective for well-motivated patients when combined with a comprehensive rehabilitation program.

SEDATIVE DEPENDENCE

The most important sedative is alcohol, which is covered in Chapter 18. However, it should be noted that alcohol, while it has sedating effects, also has general anesthetic effects and is often used in combination with other sedatives to be described here. The subjective effects of all sedatives are somewhat similar to alcohol (see Chapters 16 and 17 for pharmacological details). In low doses they cause a suppression of inhibition, which produces a feeling of relaxation, even euphoria, although not as intense as that produced by stimulants. At higher doses, the sedation is more intense and the subject goes to sleep. The balance between euphoria and sedation is a function of dose, speed of entry into the central nervous system, and the prior experience of the user. Benzodiazepine dependence is the most common type of sedative dependence apart from alcoholism, and thus it will be discussed in more detail.

Benzodiazepine Abuse and Dependence

Benzodiazepines are used mainly in the treatment of anxiety disorders. The abuse liability of the benzodiazepines is a controversial subject because they are so widely prescribed and there is uncertainty over what level of usage constitutes abuse. About 15 percent of the population of the United States takes a benzodiazepine at least once during a given year. About a third of these users take the drug chronically. Most, if not all, chronic users develop some degree of physical dependence, and they will experience withdrawal symptoms when the drug is terminated. This does not necessarily mean, however, that these patients are abusing benzodiazepines, providing that they are taking them in accordance with a doctor's prescription.

Many cases can be cited of individuals who were unable to function because of chronic anxiety, but with the use of low and continual doses of benzodiazepines they are able to lead normal lives. When the drug is withdrawn, such long-term users experience typical withdrawal symptoms, and later they may experience symptoms of the return of the anxiety disorder which were present prior to the original prescription of the benzodiazepine. Such a patient would be physically dependent on benzodiazepines.

Iatrogenic or inadvertent dependence on benzodiazepines can still be a clinical problem when benzodiazepines are prescribed by a physician. Some patients tend to gradually increase their dose of benzodiazepines as their tolerance to the antianxiety and sedating effects of the drug increase. This may be more common with those benzodiazepines that have a relatively rapid onset of action such as alprazolam. There is another problem with very potent benzodiazepines such as alprazolam where doctors may be willing to prescribe doses of 5 to 10 mg/day because this seems like a low dose. However, when translated to diazepam equivalents, this is 50 to 100 mg/day.

There is also a significant problem with deliberate abuse of benzodiazepines. These drugs have a street value, and they are sold on the black market. Drug abusers use them to "get high" or to ameliorate the withdrawal symptoms from opioids, alcohol, or other sedatives. Because of the capacity to develop tolerance to the sedating effects of benzodiazepines, huge doses are sometimes taken by drug abusers.

Tolerance Benzodiazepines exhibit an excellent example of the phenomenon of differential tolerance. That is, tolerance develops within different systems for different functions at different rates. It is very clear that a large degree of tolerance can develop for the sedative effects of the benzodiazepines. However, it is equally clear that the memory impairment effects of benzodiazepines do not diminish with repeated use. Benzodiazepines have significant disruptive effects on short-term memory as demonstrated by tests of recall and speech fluency. These effects are relatively greater than those caused by barbiturates or alcohol. Memory impairment after a dose of a benzodiazepine is found in subjects who have taken low or moderate doses of these compounds consistently for 10 years.

A very important clinical question is whether tolerance develops to the antianxiety effects of benzodiazepines. This question is difficult to answer in clinical studies because benzodiazepine withdrawal resembles the symptoms of anxiety. Only one double-blind study has clearly addressed this issue, and it suggests that while tolerance develops to the sedating effects of the drugs, tolerance does not develop to the antianxiety effects, and thus it is rational to continue to medicate patients with chronic anxiety. Another argument in this direction by inference is the lack of tolerance to the memory disrupting effects. Since there is clearly lack of tolerance for these effects of benzodiazepines, there may also be lack of tolerance for the antianxiety effect.

Benzodiazepine Withdrawal The benzodiazepine withdrawal syndrome depends on the dose, duration, and half-life of the benzodiazepine used. Those taking even a moderate dose of a benzodiazepine may show withdrawal symptoms if the drug is abruptly discontinued after about 4 months of chronic use. The severity of the withdrawal syndrome and the time of onset depend on the above variables. The symptoms include irritability, tremors, dysphoria, sweating, headache, unpleasant dreams, insomnia, anorexia, dizziness, muscle twitches, and paresthesias. After higher doses, generalized seizures, panic, paranoia, and delirium have been observed. It should also be noted that mild but definite withdrawal symptoms have been documented after as little as 15 mg of diazepam per day.

Treatment Benzodiazepine withdrawal should be suspected in all alcoholics and other sedative abusers at the time of detoxification. Symptoms may occur unexpectedly, especially in individuals taking long-acting benzodiazepines such as diazepam where the syndrome may occur 5 to 7 days after the patient is admitted to the hospital and the diazepam discontinued. The standard detoxification regimen consists of placing the patient on a long-acting benzodiazepine and gradually reducing the dose over 7 to 10 days, but sometimes a much longer treatment is required. The particular treatment circumstances may require an even longer term outpatient detoxification.

When deliberately abused, benzodiazepines are usually taken in combination with other drugs, and the dangers of accidental overdose are increased markedly. This is particularly true when benzodiazepines are combined with alcohol. After the acute detoxification, the treatment for prevention of relapse is aimed at the overall drug-dependence syndrome. This involves psychotherapy, possibly living in a therapeutic community, group therapy, and behavioral relapse prevention techniques. Benzodiazepines should rarely, if ever, be prescribed for people with a history of alcoholism or other forms of drug abuse. If an antianxiety agent is found to be absolutely necessary, physicians should consider a benzodiazepine with a low abuse potential.

Barbiturate and Other Nonbenzodiazepine Sedative Abuse

Barbiturates tend to have a greater abuse potential than benzodiazepines, but they are prescribed less often since the benzodiazepine era. Slow-onset, long-acting barbiturates such as phenobarbital are very rarely abused despite widespread use in the treatment of seizure disorders. Accidental overdose is a danger with barbiturates and other nonbenzodiazepines because tolerance to the "high" effects occurs more rapidly and extensively than tolerance to the brainstem depressant effects. Sleeping pills such as glutethimide or ethchlorvynol are notorious in this regard. The abuser who keeps increasing the dose to obtain a "high" may unexpectedly suffer cardiorespiratory arrest as the toxic range for the brainstem is reached. In general, barbiturates and other nonbenzodiazepine sedatives are far more dangerous than benzodiazepines from the perspective of abuse potential and overdose risk.

The withdrawal syndrome from sedative dependence is more dangerous than opioid or stimulant withdrawal. All patients being detoxified from sedative dependence require at least a medical evaluation to determine whether hospitalization and treatment with medication to assist the withdrawal is necessary.

STIMULANTS

Cocaine and Amphetamine Dependence

Oral cocaine has been used for centuries by Indians of the Andes who chew coca leaves with an alkaline material which facilitates absorption of the alkaloid base through oral mucous membranes. This technique produces relatively mild stimulation which results in increased endurance but no known abuse. The hydrochloride salt of cocaine can be produced from coca leaves and placed in the nose for absorption through the nasal mucous membranes ("snorting"). By this route, the local vasoconstricting effects of the drug slow absorption and prolong the effect. The hydrochloride salt can also be taken intravenously, and this produces a much more rapid effect which is difficult to regulate and may result in seizures. Cocaine hydrochloride cannot be smoked because it will be volatilized only at temperatures which degrade it. However, the alkaloidal cocaine, called *free-base*, or "crack", is readily volatilized undegraded at much lower temperatures. Simply heating crack enables a person to smoke it and absorb the cocaine through the lungs, where it is rapidly absorbed into the pulmonary circulation and carried to the left side of the heart. It then reaches the brain in seconds and produces an intense euphoric effect. The smoking of crack cocaine thus produces rapid and strong effects, and dependence can occur within days to weeks of initial use.

With the next use, perhaps one to several days later, the tolerance is no longer present and the original effects are again present. Under certain conditions, reverse tolerance or sensitization occurs. This phenomenon has not been studied systematically in humans, but it may be the explanation for some of the cases of seizures or cardiac arrhythmias which have been seen in people who have previously taken the same dose of cocaine without significant toxicity.

Cocaine is an effective topical local anesthetic and vasoconstrictor of mucous membranes. Stimulants do reduce appetite, but significant tolerance to this effect develops. When stimulants are discontinued, a rebound increase in weight can leave the person heavier than before the drug was taken (See Chapter 19 for a discussion of the pharmacology of cocaine).

Amphetamine has a longer duration of action than cocaine, but many of the effects are similar. Amphetamine has been prescribed by physicians for a variety of conditions, including weight reduction, narcolepsy, and attention-deficit disorder. Amphetamine has not been shown to be of value in weight reduction programs, and the use of stimulants has been curtailed by legal restrictions.

Methylphenidate has a much lower abuse potential than either cocaine or amphetamine. It has been useful in the treatment of attention-deficit disorder in children and in narcolepsy.

Detoxification The withdrawal syndrome from cocaine dependence consists of fatigue, lack of energy, and a depressed mood. There is also intense craving for the drug. The withdrawal syndrome is thought to represent a dopamine depletion syndrome because the blockage of dopamine reuptake results in lack of dopamine conservation and eventual depletion of available dopamine stores. During acute intoxication, stimulants can also produce a paranoid syndrome which resembles an acute paranoid schizophrenic episode. After a binge, the withdrawal syndrome is often referred to as a *crash* because of the severe depression and desire for sleep.

Toxic Effects The most likely complication of cocaine use is dependence. Another common consequence is the development of a psychiatric disorder such as paranoid symptoms or a depressive syndrome. While sexual drive and sexual appreciation may be increased during early cocaine use, subsequently there is often loss of interest in sex and difficulty with sexual performance.

There are also important toxic effects on the cardiovascular system. There is evidence that cocaine is capable of causing acute myocardial infarction even in patients with normal coronary arteries. There is also evidence that cases of sudden death may be due to cocaine-induced ventricular arrhythmia. The arrhythmia may be the result of the direct effect of cocaine on the cardiac conduction system or an indirect effect that is mediated via cocaine on the central nervous system. There is also evidence that cocaine can produce myocarditis.

Treatment Cocaine withdrawal usually does not require pharmacological intervention although there is some evidence that a drug such as amantadine will ease withdrawal and increase the likelihood of the patient becoming cocaine free. The major clinical problem is the prevention of relapse of compulsive cocaine use. There are reports that tricyclic antidepressants, especially desipramine, can reduce some of the effects of cocaine craving and thus reduce the rate of relapse.

HALLUCINOGENS

Lysergic Acid Diethylamide (LSD) and Phencyclidine (PCP) Dependence

There are many mechanisms for producing hallucinations, and drugs which act on the serotonergic, cholinergic, and adrenergic systems can produce such effects by various mechanisms. The drug which is currently the greatest problem is phencyclidine, which has pharmacological effects similar to those of certain anesthetics, and it produces amphetamine-like stimulation. Phencyclidine is easily synthesized, however, and it is found in many street samples misrepresented as other drugs, for example as LSD or as tetrahydrocannabinol (THC) (See Chapter 19).

Phencyclidine produces a rapid stimulant effect similar to that seen with amphetamine, and it may produce a feeling of euphoria. Numbness, clumsiness, slurred speech, and nystagmus are common. Phencyclidine also produces frightening hallucinations, especially visual and tactile hallucinations. There may be assaultive and hostile behavior, and the person has amnesia for these actions. Occasionally individuals inadvertently take a large dose of phencyclidine which can produce catatonia and coma. Phencyclidine overdose should always be considered in a comatose patient with dilated pupils and elevated blood pressure.

LSD is effective at doses as low as 20 μg; however, the usual street dose is around 200 μg. The drug produces central sympathomimetic stimulation characterized by dilatation of the pupils, hyperthermia, rapid heartbeat, elevated blood pressure, piloerection, and increased alertness. Nausea and vomiting occasionally occur. The psychological effects of LSD depend on the expectations of the user, the setting, the dose, and the previous experiences. Individuals with a preexisting psychiatric disorder often have a very frightening response to the hallucinations produced by LSD. Typical reactions include a feeling that insights are enhanced and that ordinary sights and sounds seem louder and clearer. Perceptual distortions commonly occur, causing an individual, for example, to see his or her hand suddenly grow large or the hairs on the hand look like snakes. Usually visual distortions or hallucinations occur, and they may occur in vivid colors. The reaction to LSD persists for about 10 h, but fatigue and tension may continue for an additional 24 h. Other hallucinogenic drugs such as mescaline and dimethyltryptamine are shorter in duration.

Tolerance and Dependence Tolerance develops to some of the effects of hallucinogens after several administrations. Thus experienced users may require a somewhat higher dose in order to get the effects that they are seeking. A withdrawal syndrome has not been described for these drugs in human subjects although signs of withdrawal in animals after high, chronic doses of phencyclidine have been reported.

Toxic Effects Significant toxic problems can occur with the use of hallucinogens after only one administration. Individuals may have a "bad trip," which involves terror, anxiety, and a prolonged psychotic reaction. Occasionally individuals have harmed themselves or others when having a bad trip. Phencyclidine appears the most toxic of the hallucinogens, with severe reactions being more common than mild reactions. Several studies have indicated a high frequency of phencyclidine abuse in individuals admitted to psychiatric hospitals with a diagnosis of acute psychotic reaction and no diagnosis of drug abuse on admission. Phencyclidine appears to be capable of producing a psychosis which can be indistinguishable from an acute schizophrenic disorder. Patients being treated for chronic schizophrenic disorders in mental health clinics often give a history of hallucinogen abuse in the past, but it is not possible to determine whether the hallucinogen caused chronic schizophreniform disorder or whether hallucinogen abuse was merely associated with the onset of schizophrenia which would have occurred even in the absence of drug abuse.

Frequent hallucinogen users may report the occurrence of flashbacks after stopping hallucinogen use. These flashbacks consist of brief periods of hallucinations resembling the acute effects of the drug but occurring days, weeks, or months after last ingestion of the drug.

MISCELLANEOUS

Marijuana Dependence

Cannabis is called *marijuana, hashish*, or *hemp*, depending on the part of the world and the part of the marijuana plant prepared. Actually, cannabis is not a single drug, but a complex preparation containing many biologically active chemicals. Studies have shown that Δ^9-tetrahydrocannabinol (THC) produces most of the pharmacological effects of the complex (see Chapter 19 for additional information). Throughout the 1970s the use of marijuana increased dramatically among young people so that in 1979 more than 60 percent of high school seniors reported trying it and 9 percent were using it daily. During this time period, the potency of marijuana also increased dramatically so that some cigarettes were found to contain up to 14 percent THC, which is more than has been found in potent forms such as hemp seen in other parts of the world.

In the United States, marijuana is usually taken by inhalation. This route is 3 to 4 times more potent than the oral route, and it permits users to more accurately titrate their dose. The effects of inhaled marijuana begin within minutes and subjectively persist for 2 to 3 h, depending on the dose and the experience of the user. However, psychomotor impairment has been demonstrated for up to 11 h after taking a single dose even though the subjects reported that they felt normal at the time of the testing.

Marijuana, of course, is taken for its psychoactive effects, and these include relaxation, giddiness, a feeling of enhanced perceptions, and a feeling that time is passing slowly. Attention and learning are impaired. Anxiety reactions are occasionally reported, and sometimes there is acute pain which causes the user to be brought to an emergency room. There are also increases in heart rate, conjunctival vascular reaction ("red eyes"), decreases in intraocular pressure, peripheral vasodilatation, bronchodilation, and an increase in airway conductance. Ataxia, nystagmus, fine tremors, and dryness of the mouth may occur.

Cannabis has been found to be an effective antiemetic for some patients receiving chemotherapy for cancer. The antinausea effect is not seen without the psychoactive changes which prevent normal daily functions. Thus, the antinausea effect has not been found to be useful for many patients who do not like the psychoactive side offooto.

It is important to note that the operation of a motor vehicle is definitely impaired by cannabis, and the impairment may persist for hours after the user feels normal and confident about driving ability.

The compound, Δ^9THC, and other cannabinols have unusually high lipid solubility, and thus they persist in brain tissue for long periods of time. In regular users who terminate their use, the metabolites remain detectable in the urine for several weeks. The biologic significance of low levels is unknown. Cannabis metabolites can also be detected in the urine of individuals who have sat for several hours in a room filled with marijuana smoke but who have not smoked marijuana cigarettes themselves. Under ordinary circumstances, however, the levels produced by such passive inhalation do not reach the usual threshold for calling a test positive.

In recent years, specific receptors for cannabinoids have been identified and cloned. They are widely distributed in the brain, suggesting an important physiologic function. Recently, an endogenous substance named anadamide was discovered that has affinity for these receptors and cannabinoid-like effects. This research may lead to a new class of endogenous substances that activate the cannabinoid system of receptors.

Tolerance and Dependence Tolerance to the sedating and cardiovascular effects of marijuana has been observed in experimental subjects given marijuana at regular intervals on a research unit. When the drug was stopped, a definite withdrawal syndrome was noted. In clinical situations, however, most patients do not take marijuana in high enough doses and at regular intervals so as to produce clinically significant dependence and a noticeable syndrome. Also, when present, the withdrawal syndrome is usually mild and does not require treatment with medication. While compulsive marijuana use is seen in some patients, the marijuana-seeking behavior does not resemble the frantic drug-craving and drug-seeking behavior seen among cocaine addicts and heroin addicts.

Toxic Effects Regular marijuana use by adolescents is associated with impairment of psychological maturation and poor social and scholastic adjustment. There has been no experimental demonstration that marijuana is the cause of such deterioration in social behavior, but there is general agreement that the drug is at least a contributing factor. Young people who exhibit the so-called "amotivational syndrome" also have many other problems besides marijuana use. Successful treatment of this syndrome requires that the individual cease marijuana use as well as become engaged in psychotherapy, often family psychotherapy.

Occasional users of marijuana have fewer problems, but even intermittent users report episodes of acute panic, paranoid reactions, and frightening distortions of body images at times. These reactions seem to occur more frequently with higher doses and in individuals who take large doses by the oral route, where the dose cannot be readily controlled, instead of smoking the drug. Certain individuals seem to be extremely sensitive to the toxic effects of marijuana, and they often include individuals who are recovering from a psychotic episode or who suffer from a chronic psychiatric disorder.

Since cannabis stimulates the cardiovascular system, it may pose a problem for individuals with heart disease. There is also clear evidence that marijuana cigarettes cause inflammatory changes in the bronchi and in the mucosa of the sinuses. In experimental tests, cannabis products are found to produce carcinoma, but it is difficult to find cases of this phenomenon clinically because it is rare to find a marijuana smoker who does not also use tobacco cigarettes.

NICOTINE DEPENDENCE

Nicotine is the dependence-producing component of tobacco and as such it results in the most severe mortality of any drug of abuse (See Chapter 10 for pharmacological details). Nicotine in the typical smoker produces relaxation of skeletal muscle and a reduction in deep tendon reflexes. There is also an increase in hand tremor and a desynchronization of the electroencephalogram, a pattern associated with increased alertness. Subjects report a sense of alertness with relaxed muscles and a facilitation of memory and attention. There is also a reduction of appetite. The mechanisms by which nicotine produces these effects are multiple, and they include changes in the release of acetylcholine depending on the dose and facilitation of the release of dopamine and norepinephrine.

The net effect of these changes is to produce something which smokers describe as pleasant. Each puff on a cigarette produces a small bolus of nicotine which is absorbed by the lungs and delivered rapidly to the brain via the arterial circulation. Since each cigarette takes approximately 10 puffs, one-pack-a-day smokers deliver approximately 200 reinforcements to their brains each day. This establishes a very strong habit.

Tolerance and Dependence With repeated use, the unpleasant side effects of cigarettes including nausea, vomiting, and dizziness no longer occur. The other effects of nicotine also show tolerance, but some of the tolerance is lost each morning, since cigarettes are not ordinarily used during the night. Thus, the first cigarette in the morning seems to have a greater effect than cigarettes later in the day. Also, experienced smokers show tolerance to the effects of intravenous nicotine as compared with nonsmokers.

Sudden cessation of smoking usually produces a withdrawal syndrome. While this is not seen in all smokers, it can be very unpleasant, lasting for at least several days and in some cases for several weeks. The signs and symptoms of nicotine withdrawal consist of irritability, restlessness, anxiety, shortened attention span, drowsiness, increased appetite, insomnia, headaches, and upset stomach. The withdrawal symptoms respond to doses of nicotine, including nicotine chewing gum and the nicotine patch. There is also evidence that the antihypertensive drug clonidine, which reduces opioid withdrawal symptoms, is also effective in nicotine withdrawal. This suggests that many of the symptoms of nicotine withdrawal are related to sympathetic nervous system rebound hyperactivity.

Toxicity The significant toxic effects of smoking are related to the tars found in tobacco. Carcinomas, emphysema, and other diseases have been related to carbon monoxide produced by burning tobacco. The cardiovascular effects of nicotine may be harmful to individuals with heart disease.

DESIGNER DRUGS

In an attempt to synthesize derivatives of meperidine, two derivatives were developed that have gained popularity as street drugs as new heroin compounds. These compounds are commonly known as "designer drugs." The two most popular ones are MPPP (1-methyl-4-phenylproprionoxypiperidine) and MPTP (1-methyl-4-phenyl-1,2,5,6-tetrahydropyridine).

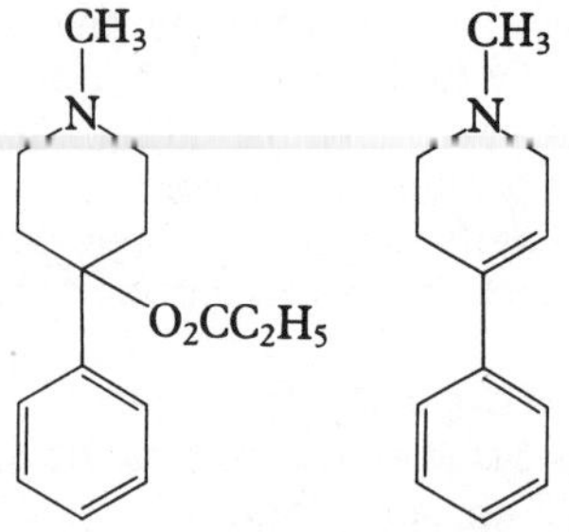

CH_3 CH_3

N   N

$O_2CC_2H_5$

MPPP   MPTP

These compounds are administered by injection and produce a syndrome of muscle rigidity, weakness, and tremulousness which resembles idiopathic Parkinson's disease. A significant number of individuals who abused these chemicals have developed permanent damage to their central nervous system. Because of their severe toxic effects, the illicit use of these so-called designer drugs has decreased drastically, so they play only a small part in the overall dependence area.

CONCLUDING COMMENTS

Drug abuse is a complicated disorder that results from the interaction of a number of variables. These include the availability of the drug, the characteristics of the user, and the setting in which the drug is used. Virtually any drug described in this book can be abused by some people at some time. However, certain drugs, because of their pharmacological characteristics carry a much higher potential for abuse. While pharmacology is very important in understanding the phenomenon of drug abuse, the problem actually goes far beyond pharmacology; the problem is at the interface of behavior, pharmacology, sociology, psychology, and clinical medicine.

BIBLIOGRAPHY

Alterman, A.I., M. Droba, R.E. Antelo, J.W. Cornish, K.K. Sweeney, G.A. Parikh, and C.P. O'Brien: "Amantadine May Facilitate Detoxification of Cocaine Addicts," *Drug and Alcohol Dependence* **31**: 19-29 (1992).

Chiang, C.N., and R.S. Rapaka: "Pharmacokinetics and Disposition of Cannabinoids," *Natl. Inst. Drug Abuse Res. Mang. Ser.* **79**: 173-188 (1987).

DiGregorio, G.J., and M.A. Bukovinsky: "Clonidine for Narcotic Withdrawal," *Am. Family Physician* **33**: 203 (1981).

Gawin, F.H., and E.H. Ellinwood: "Cocaine and Other Stimulant Actions, Abuse and Treatment," *N. Engl. J. Med.* **318**: 1173-1182 (1988).

O'Brien, C.P.: "Opioid Addiction," *Handbook of Experimental Pharmacology, Vol. 104/II, Opioids II*, A. Herz, (ed.), Berlin Heidelberg: Springer-Verlag, 1992, pp 803-823.

Schuster, C.R.: "The United States Drug Abuse Scene: An Overview," *Clin. Chem.* **33**: 7B-12B (1987).

Semlitz, L. and M.S. Gold: "Diagnosis and Treatment of Adolescent Substance Abuse," *Psychiatric Med* **3**: 321-323 (1985).

PART V

The Cardiovascular and Renal and Respiratory Systems

SECTION EDITOR

Joseph R. DiPalma

CHAPTER 27

Congestive Heart Failure: Cardiac Glycosides and Other Inotropic Agents and Vasodilator Therapy

Joseph R. DiPalma

Heart failure is a very common disorder. It may be defined simply as a failure of the heart to pump enough blood to supply the oxygen and nutritive demands of peripheral tissues. Heart failure may present clinically in two major forms: (1) forward failure, which is acute and represents a dramatic decrease in cardiac output and is manifest by the symptoms of circulatory failure, i.e., low blood pressure, fast pulse, cold clammy skin, and collapsed veins, and (2) congestive heart failure, which presents clinically as either with severe dyspnea (left-sided heart failure) or peripheral edema (right-sided heart failure). More often the two are combined and really represent a form of chronic failure of the heart as a pump that has been compensated for by a number of adjusting mechanisms. Consequently the output of the heart is not severely compromised. Indeed, it may be high as in high output failure, and shock does not result, but the individual is embarrassed by a number of distressing symptoms brought on by the inefficiency of the heart pumping function. The treatment of this syndrome, commonly called *congestive heart failure (CHF)*, is the focus of this chapter.

CAUSES OF CONGESTIVE FAILURE

There are numerous disorders which can precipitate CHF, and these are shown in Table 27-1. By far the most common cause is ischemia of cardiac muscle caused by atherosclerotic disease of the coronaries. Other causes are less common. CHF secondary to other causes is best treated by alleviating the cause. Beriberi heart failure is cured by thiamine, and thyrotoxicosis by antithyroid drugs and surgery. Valvular disease is cured by surgery, and even ischemic heart disease is amenable to bypass coronary repair. The emphasis in this chapter is on those cases not amenable to therapy for the primary disease which need to have therapy for the CHF. Three groups of drugs have great utility in CHF. These are the diuretics (Chapter 31); the inotropic agents comprising mainly digitalis glycosides, sympathomimetic agents (Chapter 8), nonsympathomimetic drugs including amrinone and milrinone; and vasodilators such as nitrates, sodium nitroprusside, angiotensin converting enzyme (ACE) inhibitors, and calcium-channel blockers (Chapters 29 and 32).

To understand drug therapy for CHF, it is necessary to appreciate the mechanisms by which the body attempts to compensate for the heart with an inadequate output.

MECHANISMS OF COMPENSATION

As the heart fails to pump enough blood to answer the demands of peripheral tissues, certain neuronal and endocrine reflexes become activated. These are

1. *Neuronal* The afferent arcs involve the baroreceptors of the atrium and mediastinum, the great vessels in the mediastinum, and the carotid sinus. Sensory afferent neurons from these areas terminate in the solitary tract nucleus in the brain stem; neurons from the solitary tract nucleus relay information concerning the activity of the peripheral baroreceptors to the vasomotor center. Reinforcement of the afferent arc occurs from somatic sensations from skin and muscle and from the cerebral cortex as the individual experiences apprehension over his or her condition. The vasomotor center adjusts the

TABLE 27-1 Some common causes of congestive heart failure

Coronary artery disease (ischemia)
Metabolic muscle disease
Lipodystrophy
Amyloidosis
Hemochromatosis
Sarcoidosis
Thyrotoxicosis
Vitamin deficiency (thiamine: beriberi)
Infections
Viral cardiomyopathy
Subacute bacterial endocarditis
Elevated afterload
Hypertension
Aortic stenosis
Hypertrophic cardiomyopathy
Elevated preload (increased venous pressure)
Aortic insufficiency
Mitral insufficiency
Tricuspid insufficiency
Congenital left to right
AV fistula

activity of the sympathetic nervous system to peripheral cardiovascular structures (the efferent arc) expressed as increased release of norepinephrine and other catecholamines. The result is an increase in heart rate and a moderate rise in blood pressure; but more significant is a redistribution of blood flow to the most vital organs. The blood vessels of the brain and the heart do not constrict under sympathomimetic stimulation; the arterioles to the kidney do and consequently the ability to excrete and control water balance is compromised and sodium and water are retained.

2. *Neuroendocrine* The main reaction is stimulation of the renin-angiotensin-aldosterone system. As a result of anoxemia, the kidneys secrete more renin, which results in the formation of angiotensin, a powerful vasoconstrictor and a stimulant for aldosterone secretion by the adrenal cortex (see Chapter 32). The progression of these events is manifested by a rise in blood pressure, redistribution of blood flow, and retention of sodium and water. In addition, anoxemia of the kidney leads to the increased production of erythropoietin (a peptide similar in structure to angiotensin) which stimulates red blood cell production. The patient with chronic heart failure may have an increased blood volume not only because of fluid retention but also due to an increased red blood cell volume.

3. *Autoregulatory* The heart, particularly the ventricles, is very rich in neuronal structures capable of secreting catecholamines. Due to this, there are apparently local reflexes, perhaps due to anoxemia, which cause self-stimulation of the heart—the so-called catecholamine heart drive. This self-stimulatory effect works well in the normal heart but is less effective in the heart with CHF, and, indeed, it is thought to wear out in the later stages.

   An even more intriguing self-regulatory mechanism involves atrial natriuretic factor (ANF), or atriopeptin. As the name suggests, this is a peptide produced by the atrium, which has natriuretic and vasodilating properties. The normal level of ANF is 10 to 70 ng/mL. It rises in response to volume expansion and atrial tachycardia, both factors in increasing atrial pressure. ANF, acting on the kidneys, causes natriuresis and diuresis. Furthermore, it suppresses vasopressin release and aldosterone secretion and has a direct action in the relaxation of blood vessels. Apparently ANF is the major hormone whose function is to modulate the compensatory mechanisms which lead to CHF.

4. *Mechanical factors* The Frank-Starling law is often used to explain some of the features of CHF. It states that an increase in the length of ventricular muscle fibers is related to an increase in work output, i.e., increased filling pressure (increased atrial pressure) will cause an increase in cardiac output. This law works nicely in the isolated heart and the heart-lung preparation. However *in vivo*, changes in heart rate, inotropism, and peripheral resistance complicate the picture. Nevertheless, the law is useful particularly in its extreme extent for there is a point beyond which increased filling pressure and excessive distention of the ventricular muscle result in decreased rather than increased cardiac output.

The increased filling pressure (increased preload) brought about by the mechanisms described above has more important consequences than the Frank-Starling law. The ventricles dilate, the diastolic size is larger; the heart does not empty itself as completely of blood (ejection fraction reduced), the ventricular wall is thinner, contraction is more isotonic than isometric, the velocity of ejection is reduced (*dv/dp* reduced), and, most importantly, at the price of an increased cardiac output, the efficiency of the heart as a pump is reduced. The heart in CHF uses more oxygen per unit of work than the normal heart. Moreover, because of the consequences of anoxemia, the heart depends on a less efficient carbohydrate rather than fat metabolism to produce the energy for muscle contraction.

In summary, the pathophysiology of CHF consists of a precipitating cause which results in a decrease in contractile capacity of the heart. This is followed by a complex series of compensatory measures, which include fluid volume, heart rate, blood pressure, and redistribution of blood flow to vital organs. Eventually the heart dilates and hypertrophies. Initially, the compensatory measures allow the heart to function marginally, but gradually the compensatory measures become excessive and fluid collects in the lungs and periphery. Increases in heart rate and peripheral resistance can no longer cope with an inadequate pumping action.

The therapy of CHF, therefore, consists of correction and modulation of the compensatory responses of the body which have become excessive and self-destructive. By far the most important measure is the reduction of fluid volume by the induction of diuresis. The various diuretics are described in Chapter 31 and are not further discussed here. The aim is to approach the dry weight of the individual but not to cause hyponatremia. This measure reduces preload by diminishing venous filling pressure.

The second most important measure is to improve the pumping action of the heart. The ideal heart rate is about 60 beats per minute. If there is any arrhythmia such as atrial fibrillation or flutter with a rapid ventricular response, this may be corrected by agents which produce block at the atrioventricular (AV) node. Similarly bradycardia (less than 40 beats per minute) should be treated with chronotropic drugs or a pacemaker. Inotropic drugs such as the digitalis glycosides, which do not exhaust the energy production of the heart, are ideal. In some instances inotropic drugs such as amrinone may be preferable.

Finally an attempt is made to adjust the peripheral circulation so that *preload* and *afterload* of the heart are at ideal levels. *Preload* refers to atrial filling pressure, which is determined by blood volume and venous tone. *Afterload* refers to the peripheral resistance. The ventricle performs less work when pumping a given volume of blood at a blood pressure of 120/70 mmHg than at a pressure of 150/90 mmHg. Preload and afterload are decreased by agents which decrease venous tone and arteriolar tone, respectively. Such therapy is collectively called *vasodilation therapy* and is usually applied in the later stages of therapy but may be used initially in selected cases.

DIGITALIS GLYCOSIDES

Chemistry

Digitalis is a generic name that applies to a group of glycosides which are found in a large group of plants and even some animals. Most of these glycosides have cardiotonic properties. Today only the glycosides digoxin and digitoxin are preponderantly used clinically. They are extracted from *Digitalis purpurea* and *Digitalis lanata*.

The structure of the most used digitalis glycoside, digoxin, is shown in Fig. 27-1. As can be seen, a typical digitalis glycosides consists of a central steroid nucleus called an aglycone or genin. An unsaturated lactone at position 17 is essential for cardiotonic activity. Three residues of digitoxose, a plant sugar, attached at position 3 complete the structure. Both digoxin and digitoxin have a hydroxyl substituted at position 14, but only digoxin has a hydroxyl at position 12.

All attempts to alter the structure of digitalis glycosides so as to enhance their cardiotonic properties have failed. However, structural changes do change the pharmacokinetic properties of the drugs. Digoxin appears to have the most desirable pharmacokinetic properties both for oral and parenteral therapy. Refer to older editions of this text for a more complete description of the glycosides which have been available in the past.

Mechanism of Action: Inotropic Effect

Exquisite proof that the action of digitalis is associated with a transient calcium increase has been obtained by using *aequorin*, a photoprotein which undergoes luminescence on exposure to calcium.

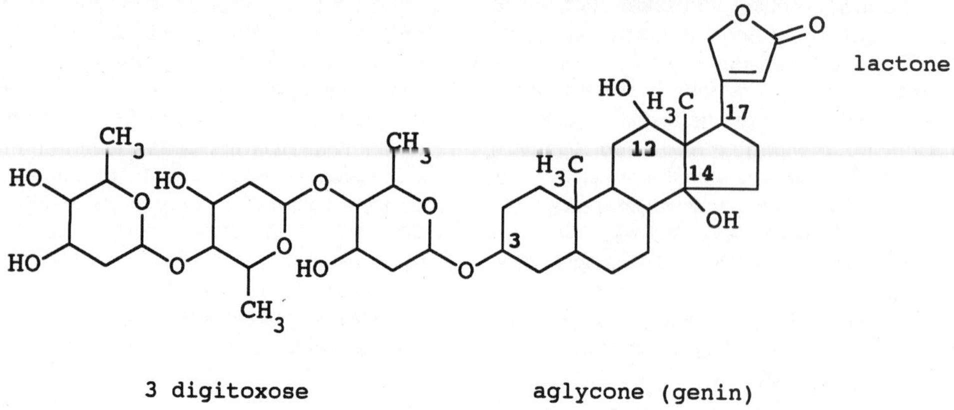

lactone

3 digitoxose aglycone (genin)

FIGURE 27-1 *Structure of digoxin with its component parts: aglycone, lactone, and 3 digitoxose residues*

Using direct recordings from a canine Purkinje fiber, a close coupling can be demonstrated between depolarization, free calcium level and contraction. Digoxin causes an increase in calcium and increased muscle tension. At toxic levels of digoxin there is an abnormal increase of calcium during diastole, accompanied by depolarization and muscle contraction.

There is also good experimental evidence that digoxin acts at a specific receptor in the sarcolemma and the transverse tubular of the myocyte. This receptor is Na^+,K^+-ATPase, whose function it is to pump 3 Na^+ out of the myocyte against a concentration gradient, while allowing 2 K^+ to enter the myocyte, thus maintaining the normal electrical potential of the cell. At same time, another mechanism is operative which exchanges 4 Na^+ for 1 Ca^{2+}, thus maintaining homeostasis of Ca^{2+} in the myocyte. Ordinarily this mechanism is secondary to the Na^+,K^+-ATPase pump. When excitation occurs, the myocyte membrane becomes extremely permeable to Na^+ and depolarizes. During the plateau period of the activation potential (phase 2), Ca^{2+} also enters the myocyte. This trigger Ca^{2+} causes the release of Ca^{2+} stores in the sarcoplasmic reticulum. The sudden increase in intracellular Ca^{2+} initiates contraction by attaching to troponin on the actin filaments, removing the barrier to the actin-myosin interaction. Normally, the troponin-tropomyosin complex inhibits the actin-myosin interaction during diastole. Potassium ions, flowing out of the myocyte repolarizes the membrane, restoring its electrical potential. Ca^{2+} is, therefore, the messenger which couples electrical excitation with contraction in heart muscle.

A secondary sodium-calcium exchange mechanism also functions to remove intracellular Ca^{2+} following repolarization. However, when digoxin inhibits Na^+,K^+-ATPase, some intracellular Na^+ remains and reduces the exchange that involves an influx of Na^+ and an efflux of Ca^{2+}. This slight increase in cytoplasmic Ca^{2+}, which results from the reduced Na^+-Ca^{2+} exchange, is then sequestered by the sarcoplasmic reticulum. On the next stimulus to the ventricular muscle cell, a normal amount of Ca^{2+} is released from the sarcoplasmic reticulum along with this extra Ca^{2+}. Therefore, more Ca^{2+} is available to the myofibrils and a positive inotropic effect is manifested during systole.

The great advantage of digoxin as compared to other inotropic agents is that it achieves its inotropic action at no expense to energy metabolism. Other inotropic agents also achieve their effects by altering Ca^{2+} movement. For example, epinephrine stimulates the formation of intracellular cyclic AMP and this second messenger increases tubular stores of calcium. This increases the energy expenditure of the heart and is, therefore, not as efficient a mechanism as that exerted by digoxin.

The electrical effects of digoxin, including the increase of the refractory period of the AV node, are also believed to be due to the inhibition of Na^+,K^+-ATPase. In this case, it is the changes in Na^+, K^+ and Ca^{2+} which bring about the changes in electrical events.

Interactions between digoxin and Ca^{2+} and K^+ at a membrane level have important clinical and toxicologic implications. There is a synergistic action between Ca^{2+} and digoxin, increases in serum calcium may result in arrhythmias in the digitalized patient. On the other hand, digoxin and K^+ are antagonistic. Hypokalemic patients have a decreased tolerance to digitalis. In patients with digitalis toxicity, raising the serum levels of K^+ tends to alleviate the toxic effects.

In occasional cases, magnesium seems to play an interactive role with digoxin which is similar to that of potassium. It must be recalled that vigorous diuresis results in depletion of magnesium as well as potassium.

Electrophysiologic Effects

The changes that occur following the administration of digoxin are best described by an analysis of the monophasic action potential of a Purkinje fiber (Fig. 27-2) (for a complete description of this recording, see Chapter 28). Moreover, comparison of the monophasic action potential with the ECG allows a further analysis.

The intrinsic deflection of the R wave of an ECG coincides in time with phase 0, the ST segment with phase 2, and the T wave with phase 3. In contrast to this ventricular record, the transmembrane potential recorded from a pacemaker fiber (i.e., sinoatrial (SA) node, AV node, or His-Purkinje fibers) does not remain constant after repolarization but exhibits slow diastolic depolarization during phase 4. If this slow depolarization carries the membrane potential to the threshold potential, firing occurs. Many fibers develop this phase, but the one that first attains the threshold potential usually acts as the dominant pacemaker, and the others, with slower rates of depolarization during phase 4, are latent pacemakers. Digoxin affects this slow diastolic depolarization of Purkinje fibers by increasing the rate of diastolic depolarization, i.e., it increases the slope of phase 4 and, therefore, ultimately enhances automaticity with resultant ventricular ectopic beats and ventricular tachycardia.

In the AV node, the cardiac glycosides slow phase 0 (depolarization), thereby diminishing conduction velocity and possibly leading to various degrees of heart block. On the surface ECG this effect is manifested as a lengthening of the PR interval. A direct effect of digoxin on repolarization of cardiac tissue is an alteration of phases 1, 2, and 3, resulting in a shortening of the duration of the intracellular action potential and a subsequent decrease in refractoriness. On the ECG this is seen as a shortening of the QT interval. Furthermore, the quickening of phases 1 and 2 of repolarization is reflected as an ST segment depression on the ECG, sometimes referred to as the *boot heel depression*.

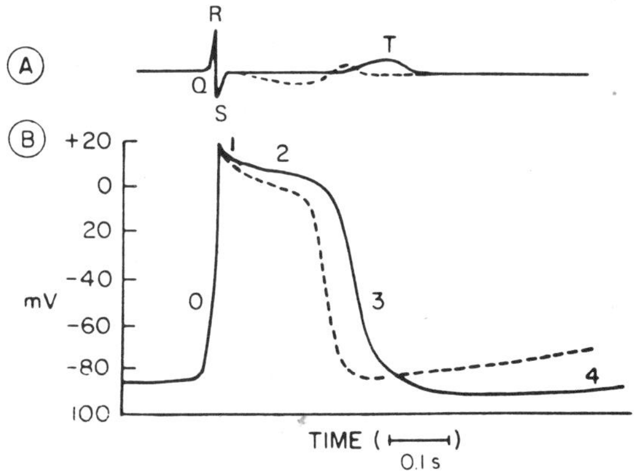

FIGURE 27-2 *Representation of (A) an electrocardiogram (ECG) and (B) ventricular intracellular action potential before (solid line) and after (broken line) digoxin administration. Note the depression of the ST segment of the ECG related to a more rapid decline of phase 2 of the action potential. In addition, the QT duration is shortened, correlating with a shorter action potential duration.*

Effects on Organ Systems

Cardiac Effects At therapeutic dose levels, digoxin acts primarily by increasing the force of myocardial contraction. In the failing heart, this results in an increase in cardiac output and, usually, a decrease in heart size because of an increase in the ejection fraction. In the AV node and bundle of His, the refractory period is lengthened and conduction is slowed by heightened reflex vagal activity (and possibly by reduced adrenergic activity) as well as by direct effects. This increased refractoriness is particularly beneficial in atrial fibrillation, since the number and irregularity of ventricular contractions are reduced as a result of A-V block.

Digoxin directly increases contractility of the myocardium in both the failing heart and the normal heart. In the failing, dilated heart, digoxin has been shown to double the stroke volume or cardiac output. The heightened contractility causes more complete ejection with less residual systolic volume. In this manner, the drug corrects the depressed contractility which is responsible for ventricular failure. When digoxin is used alone, its most dramatic manifestation is diuresis. This diuresis is believed to be due to improved renal circulation, although when digoxin is injected directly into the renal artery it causes diuresis. At therapeutic doses administered systemically, the direct diuretic effect is considered to be minimal.

The cardiac output in normal subjects who are given digoxin generally remains unchanged (although occasionally it decreases), since these individuals have a normal blood volume, and no diuresis occurs. In addition to exerting a positive inotropic action on the normal (nonfailing) heart, the cardiac glycosides also produce a direct contraction of peripheral arterial and venous smooth muscle. This increased peripheral resistance, along with increased contractility, generally results in unchanged cardiac output. However, in CHF, there is already increased peripheral resistance (a compensatory mechanism), resulting in increased redistribution of blood flow that favors the kidney and promotes diuresis. It is this effect, rather than the increased contractility, which causes a decrease in the diastolic size of the heart. These latter changes are not attributed to digoxin today because diuretics are administered first or simultaneously with the glycoside.

The improved cardiac efficiency which occurs with digoxin suggests a relationship to some direct effect on energy production. However, extensive studies have demonstrated no direct action of this sort. Even the feature of increased energy utilization has been questioned, since oxygen consumption, which is considered an ultimate measure of this variable, reportedly does not change in proportion to cardiac work. This implies an increase in efficiency which is interpreted on the basis of the important mechanical advantage which comes from the decrease in heart size during diastole, typically caused by digoxin.

Vagal Effects Vagal effects occur early in therapy or with minimal therapeutic dose levels, and increase with higher dosages. Pacemaker activity is slowed at the SA and AV nodes, conduction rate is decreased, and refractory intervals of the conduction tissue are increased. Vagal effects decrease contractility in the atria but have no pronounced effects on the ventricles, and apparently the direct positive inotropic effects of digoxin overshadow these negative inotropic effects. The heightened vagal activity has been attributed to an action on afferent nerves in the nodose ganglion and the carotid sinus, as well as to effects at peripheral sites and central vagal nuclei.

Early effects on conduction and refractoriness at the AV node and the bundle of His are now generally thought to be mediated almost entirely through the vagal action, except for a component which is antiadrenergic and which can be relatively more important under conditions of heightened sympathetic nervous system activity, as in heart failure.

Digoxin-induced vagal influences on automaticity are complicated by the marked difference in responsiveness of pacemaker cells, on the one hand, and muscle fibers of the atria and ventricles, on the other, which do not generate spontaneous action potentials. The pacemaker cells of the SA node (and possibly other specialized atrial cells) respond to vagal simulation by a decrease in the ascending slope of the diastolic phase (phase 4) and an increase in transmembrane negativity. These effects, acting to maintain the subthreshold state, result in a pronounced reduction in heart rate, and with more intense vagal stimulation, there may be arrest of automatic activity of these cells. Under these conditions, pacemaker activity of the bundle of His and the Purkinje system may assume dominance, since automaticity in these conduction systems is not as responsive to vagal activity. This type of "vagal escape" is enhanced by adrenergic influences and by decreased levels of intracellular potassium. Release from the control of higher pacemakers and increased automaticity correspond to the later stages of digoxin-induced arrhythmias, such as induced nodal rhythms, ventricular ectopic beats, and ventricular tachycardia.

Peripheral Vascular Effects Rapid intravenous injection of a cardiac glycoside leads to increased arterial pressure and increased total peripheral resistance, usually of moderate degree. When administered more slowly, as by oral ingestion, digitalis glycosides do not have significant effects on arterial pressure, although venous constriction may be observed. In patients with heart failure, the existing sympathetic influences are more pronounced and the relief of failure may act to reduce the sympathetic effects. This may be because the improved renal blood flow may reduce the renal production of renin, and hence angiotensin II, a potent vasoconstrictor.

Effects on Other Organs The frequent gastrointestinal effects of digoxin (nausea and vomiting) are attributable to direct effects, as well as to stimulation of the chemoreceptor trigger-zone. With the use of pure glycosides, as compared with that of older crude preparations, these effects are minimal.

In the elderly, disorientation and hallucinations may occur. It is difficult to ascribe these changes to the drug or to the rapid diuresis and occasional dehydration which may occur. Yellow vision is a fairly frequent phenomenon which may not be noticed by some patients.

Gynecomastia and galactorrhea are rarely reported. These may be the result of a direct effect (recall the steroid structure of digoxin) or, more likely, hypothalamic stimulation.

Pharmacokinetics

Some of the pharmacokinetic parameters determined for digoxin and digitoxin are shown in Table 27-2. Digoxin is effective both orally and parenterally. Gastrointestinal absorption of digoxin is a passive process and the absolute oral bioavailability ranges from 60 to 100 percent depending on the preparation used. Oral bioavailability is almost complete with an encapsulated hydro-alcoholic preparation (90 to 100 percent), followed by a hydro-alcoholic elixir preparation (70 to 85 percent), with tablets being the lowest (60 to 80 percent) and dependant on many factors. For example, food slows absorption and intestinal bacteria (*Eubacterium lentum*) can convert digoxin into inactive products, e.g., dihydrodigoxin. Digitoxin is only used by the oral route and tablets of this more lipophilic drug have a more complete oral bioavailability (90 to 100 percent) than tablets of digoxin. It is wise to adhere to a single commercial source of either drug which experience shows to have consistent absorption.

Due to the large volume of distribution, the glycosides slowly spread throughout the body. With digoxin given orally, for example, a distribution phase of 6 to 8 hours is common; time to onset of effect ranges from 5 to 30 minutes for IV injection and up to 2 hours after oral use. As a result of protein binding, the plasma half-life of the glycosides, especially digitoxin, is long and results in slow accumulation. Digoxin, given in an appropriate daily maintenance dose, will reach therapeutic levels in 6 to 7 days; thereafter a steady-state ensues. Digitoxin, given in the same manner, might take weeks to reach a steady-state. Therefore, it is customary to give the entire loading dose (or digitalizing dose), in one initial dose and thereafter, continue with a daily maintenance dose.

For digoxin, the kidney is the chief route of elimination. The drug is excreted unchanged mainly by glomerular filtration, and with some eliminated by tubular secretion. Seriously depressed kidney function can result in accumulation of the drug. This is considered a major factor contributing to its toxicity. The time course of elimination is slower in elderly patients and in individuals with decreased kidney function.

Digitoxin is biotransformed in the liver by the drug-metabolizing microsomal system, predominantly to inactive products; a small portion (8 percent) of digitoxin is hydroxylated to digoxin. Most biotransformed products are excreted in the urine, while approximately 25 percent of these are excreted into the bile and appear in feces.

Following the administration of digoxin or digitoxin, plasma concentrations of these drugs can be measured in the ng/mL range by radioimmunoassay. Typical therapeutic plasma levels for digoxin and digitoxin are given in Table 27-2.

TABLE 27-2 Pharmacokinetics of digoxin and digitoxin

Drug	Oral bioavailability, %	Plasma protein binding, %	Apparent volume of distribution, L/kg	Elimination half-life	Therapeutic plasma concentration, ng/mL
Digoxin	60 - 100[a]	20 - 25	6 - 10	33 - 51 hours	0.8 - 2.0
Digitoxin	90 - 100	90 - 95	0.5 - 1	7 - 9 days	15 - 25

[a] Variable depending on the oral preparation used (see text).

Therapeutic Uses

Congestive Heart Failure The main indication for a digitalis glycoside is heart failure, regardless of the cause. Although not so effective in high-output failure of the type seen in cor pulmonale and thyrotoxicosis, digoxin or digitoxin may be used here together with other measures. The response to these drugs is less in conditions associated with mechanical obstruction or insufficiency, such as in valvular lesions or constrictive pericarditis, although a sufficient improvement warrants their use. In heart failure associated with acute rheumatic fever or myocarditis, a digitalis glycoside should be used concomitantly with other drugs. Thus clinical improvement may be expected in congestive failure regardless of cause, level of cardiac output, or type of cardiac rhythm.

Left-sided heart failure may develop quite precipitously as acute pulmonary edema with widely distributed rales and frothy sputum. In these cases, digoxin may be given intravenously.

A practical view of the treatment of CHF is that diuretics provide the best management of congestive heart failure and edema and that digitalis is an auxiliary measure to be used only in certain cases, especially in patients with atrial flutter or fibrillation.

Diuretics administered to a digitalized, but still edematous patient, often bring on copious diuresis, but concurrently may bring on the typical arrhythmias of digitalis overdose. The explanation for this phenomenon is that the diuretic lowers intracellular potassium levels, which increases the sensitivity to digitalis-induced arrhythmias. For this reason, some clinicians are wary of giving digitalis first, or even simultaneously with the initial period of diuresis. The diuretics are so effective in relieving CHF that digitalis is often considered unnecessary in the early stages of therapy. Once stabilized with respect to fluid and electrolyte balance, the patient is given digitalis for what added benefit it may contribute in improvement of exercise tolerance.

Arrhythmias In atrial fibrillation, digoxin and digitoxin reduce the ventricular rate by increasing the refractory period of the conduction tissue. The rapid, irregular atrial impulses showered on the AV node are extinguished in greater numbers as the refractory period is increased by the glycoside. The refractory period of the atria, on the other hand, may be shortened; this favors perpetuation of atrial fibrillation and increased atrial rate. Similarly, atrial flutter may be altered to reach the state of atrial fibrillation. The vagal effect of the digitalis glycosides is responsible for the early shortened refractory period of the atrium. General improvement in myocardial function, measured as increased contractile force, and relief of ischemia may have the later effect of converting the arrhythmias into normal sinus rhythm.

This has been a most satisfactory action of digitalis and effectively cures CHF that is due to this cause. With the advent of the calcium-channel blockers, namely, verapamil and diltiazem, AV blockade can be produced just as effectively, and with less toxicity, than with digitalis. Today many clinicians will use calcium-channels blockers alone or in combination with digitalis for this purpose.

Similarly, digoxin or digitoxin are often used to control paroxysmal atrial tachycardia (not caused by digitalis). The calcium-channel blockers and adenosine have gained ascendancy for this purpose.

Myocardial Infarction with Failure Digitalis is one of the inotropic agents considered effective in myocardial infarction associated with heart failure, and here it has an advantage over adrenergic agents in that its effects are better sustained and are associated with less of an imposed load due to pressor effects.

Adverse Reactions

The prime danger with these glycosides is the dose-related, progressively severe cardiac arrhythmias that may terminate in ventricular fibrillation. The common predisposing influence is a decrease in intracellular potassium, which may develop following the use of potassium-excreting diuretics or any condition causing vomiting or diarrhea. Other predisposing situations occur in the elderly with decreased kidney function and correspondingly decreased renal excretion of the drug; in premature infants deficient in the usual excretory and metabolic processes; in conditions such as hypothyroidism, with decreased biotransformation; in any condition of decreased kidney function; and during variabilities in absorption from the alimentary tract. Additionally, hyperthyroidism is associated with a faster rate of elimination of digoxin and hypothyroidism with a slower rate, as compared with the euthyroid state.

Digitalis toxicity is relatively common. Some estimates indicate that 5 to 20 percent of patients on a digitalis glycoside develop some adverse effects, with 15 to 20 percent of these being considered serious. Cardiac effects may include the various stages of AV block, premature systoles and tachycardia (especially when ventricular in origin), paroxysmal atrial tachycardia with AV block, AV dissociation with nonparoxysmal nodal tachycardia, and ventricular fibrillation. The most common arrhythmia produced in digitalis toxicity is paroxysmal atrial tachycardia with AV block.

Other adverse reactions are observed on the gastrointestinal tract (nausea, vomiting, anorexia) and central nervous system (blurred or yellow vision, headache, weakness, dizziness, apathy, or psychosis).

As a result of all the toxicities of digoxin and digitoxin, there has been more conservative use. Reliance on other agents such as vasodilators, newer inotropic agents, calcium-channel blockers, and angiotensin-converting enzyme inhibitors is increasing the scope of therapy of CHF.

Drug Interactions

Adverse interactions between digitalis glycosides and other drugs have been reported. Concurrent administration of digoxin and oral antacids or kaolin-pectin products decreases the pharmacologic effect of digoxin by interfering with its absorption from the gastrointestinal tract. Cholestyramine, which can bind digitoxin and digoxin in the intestine, may reduce their effectiveness. Propantheline and diphenoxylate reduce gastrointestinal motility and may increase the absorption of digoxin.

It is known that diuretics which produce hypokalemia may augment digitalis toxicities. Spironolactone has also been implicated in increasing the effects of digoxin; the probable mechanism of this interaction is a reduction in renal digoxin excretion caused by spironolactone. Also quinidine has been implicated in increasing plasma digoxin concentration. The exact mechanism of this interaction is unknown, although it has been suggested that quinidine displaces digoxin from tissue binding sites.

The cardiac effects of digitoxin may be decreased by barbiturates or rifampin, both of which induce the hepatic microsomal enzymes. In addition, when sympathomimetic amines are administered in the presence of digitalis compounds, there may be an increased predisposition to cardiac arrhythmias. Calcium administered by the IV route increases the intensity of digitalis action and the combination may cause serious arrhythmias.

Contraindications

Ventricular fibrillation and ventricular tachycardia are considered in the majority of cases to be absolute contraindications to digitalis. Patients with hypersensitivity to digitalis and those with a hypersensitive carotid sinus syndrome should not receive digitalis. Allergy rarely occurs following the use of digoxin or digitoxin.

Warnings

There are several other conditions where the use of a digitalis glycoside is unwise. These include subacute aortic stenosis, cardioversion, partial heart block, Wolff-Parkinson-White Syndrome, sick sinus syndrome and amyloid disease or constrictive cardiomyopathies.

Treatment of Digitalis Toxicity

When digitalis toxicity occurs, discontinuation of the drug may be the only treatment necessary if toxicity is not severe. Correction of factors such as electrolyte disturbances, hypoxia, and acid-base disturbances also should be considered. The use of potassium salts for treating hypokalemia and digitalis-induced arrhythmias may be warranted. Potassium chloride may be administered orally or by intravenous infusion.

There is broad agreement that increased extracellular potassium decreases automaticity and suppresses the ectopic beats induced by digitalis by forcing potassium into the cell. Conversely, lowered potassium levels are associated with the appearance of arrhythmias in the presence of even small doses of cardiac glycosides, and this may occur with potassium-excreting diuretics or hemodialysis. Depressed conduction due to digitalis is further depressed by increasing potassium levels or, again, by rapidly rising potassium levels. Abnormally low potassium levels also may act to depress conduction. Some cases of digitalis toxicity are due to low magnesium tissue levels and are helped by relieving this deficiency.

Antiarrhythmic drugs, such as lidocaine, propranolol, procainamide, or phenytoin, have been used to correct disturbances in cardiac rhythm caused by digitalis. In advanced heart block with sinus bradycardia, atropine and/or temporary ventricular pacing may be helpful.

Direct-current shock may be indicated and used in certain arrhythmias such as ventricular tachycardia and fibrillation secondary to the cardiac glycosides. However, if cardioversion must be employed, an initial small energy of countershock should be used and the patient should be pretreated with lidocaine. Also electrical conversion of arrhythmias may require that digitalis be discontinued before the countershock is applied.

In accidental massive overdoses or suicidal attempts with digitalis, the above measures are usually unsuccessful. Such extreme toxicity is best treated with antibodies that consist of immune Fab fragments for digoxin. The immune Fab fragments have a very high affinity for the glycoside binding it, thus reducing the concentration available to the heart. The Fab-digitalis combination is readily excreted in the urine.

Patients with massive digitalis overdose should be treated with large amounts of activated charcoal to reduce the oral absorption and to bind drug in the intestine that undergoes enterohepatic recirculation.

OTHER INOTROPIC AGENTS

There is no doubt that digoxin is still the most satisfactory cardiac inotropic agent. However, there is a subset of patients who have a slow sinus rhythm for whom digoxin seems to add no benefit and only toxicity. In all patients afflicted with CHF, eventually there comes a time when digitalis and diuretics no longer are able to restore compensation. There is, therefore, a desire to find an inotropic agent which can rescue the heart in intractable heart failure.

Many agents have been tested including the sympathomimetic agents. A wide variety of these drugs is available, which have agonistic activity on α-adrenergic, β-adrenergic, or dopaminergic receptors (see Chapter 8 for more detail about these drugs). The β-adrenergic agonists (e.g., dobutamine, epinephrine, isoproterenol, and dopamine) increase cardiac output, but they also may increase heart rate, which is disadvantageous. Dobutamine (by IV administration) is indicated for short-term use in patients with cardiac decompensation due to heart disease or cardiac surgery. Epinephrine (by IV administration) and isoproterenol (by intra-cardiac injection) are used as inotropic agents only in acute ventricular standstill. Dopamine (by IV infusion) may be used in patients with refractory CHF. Thus the sympathomimetic agents have a usefulness in short-term support of the heart. The development of tolerance or unacceptable adverse effects, e.g., arrhythmias, further limits the usefulness of these agents.

A large number of nonsympathomimetic drugs have also been explored, and all appear to function by augmenting or stimulating the action of cyclic AMP. Theophylline, a methylxanthine derivative, was extensively studied many years ago as an inotropic agent but was found unsatisfactory for long-term use. Other methylxanthines have been tried, but none have proven to be useful as inotropic agents. On the other hand, some related bipyridine derivatives, i.e., amrinone and milrinone, have been successful.

Amrinone and Milrinone

These bipyridine derivatives have gained acceptance as useful inotropic agents for short-term use. They are used postoperatively in surgical operations where the heart is compromised and requires some aid to restore normal function. They are also indicated in CHF where there has been an inadequate response to diuretics, digitalis and vasodilators. Their chemical structures are:

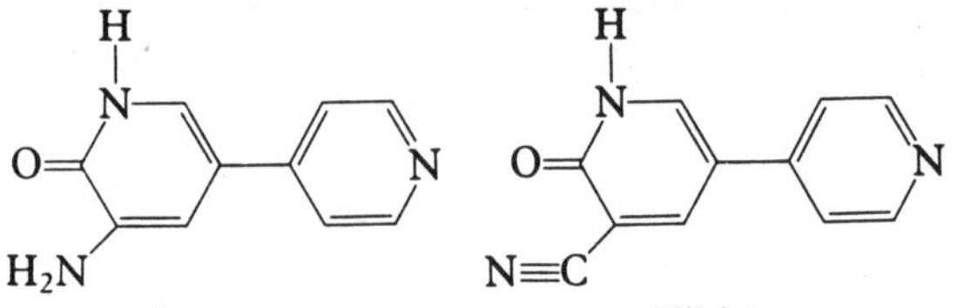

Amrinone Milrinone

The mechanism of action of the these drugs is inhibition of the phosphodiesterase III isoenzyme both in cardiac and vascular smooth muscle. This enzyme metabolizes cyclic AMP to the inactive 5'-AMP. Inhibition of the enzyme results in prolongation of cyclic AMP activity, increased protein kinase activity, and increased accumulation of intracellular Ca^{2+}, resulting in an increase in cardiac contractile force and increased arteriolar vasodilation.

Acutely, these drug cause an increase in cardiac output, decreased peripheral vascular resistance, and improvement in pulmonary capillary wedge pressure in patients with CHF. During prolonged use, deterioration in cardiac function may occur, limiting the use of these drugs to short-term therapy.

Although amrinone and milrinone have been used both orally and intravenously, the intravenous route is preferred since the drugs are mainly used

TABLE 27-3 Some pharmacokinetics of amrinone and milrinone in patients with congestive heart failure

Drug	Plasma protein binding, %	Apparent volume of distribution, L/kg	Elimination half-life, h	Therapeutic plasma concentration, μg/mL
Amrinone	10 - 50	1.2 - 1.6	5.5 - 6.0	2.4
Milrinone	65 - 70	0.33 - 0.47	1.7 - 2.7	0.2

in acute situations in a hospital setting where monitoring of vital signs is available.

Some of the pharmacokinetic parameters of these compounds are shown in Table 27-3. Amrinone is converted in the body to a variety of metabolites including N-glycolyl, N-acetate, and N- and O-glucuronide derivatives. Approximately 80 percent of an administered dose is eliminated in the urine as amrinone and amrinone metabolites; the remained is excreted via the feces. The major biotransformation product of milrinone is the O-glucuronide; excretion is primarily via the urine.

Cardiac arrhythmias and hypotension are the most common adverse reactions of both amrinone and milrinone and hence drug administration should be accompanied by cardiac monitoring. Amrinone can cause a rather high incidence of dose-related thrombocytopenia (about 2.4 percent) especially during chronic use. A metabolite, N-acetylamrinone, is believed to be at least partly responsible; the condition is reversible. Milrinone induces a much smaller incidence of thrombocytopenia. Other adverse effects of these drugs include headache, abdominal distress, nausea and emesis. Hypersensitivity after 2 weeks of therapy has been manifested by pericarditis, pleuritis, and ascites. Liver enzymes may be elevated and even bilirubin elevation may eventuate in long-term therapy.

In selected cases, amrinone and milrinone are important additions to the management of intractable heart failure of an acute nature, especially in patients who fail to respond to usual therapy. While improvement in cardiac function has been documented, there is no evidence that these bipyridine derivatives reduce mortality.

VASODILATOR DRUGS

As reviewed previously, when the heart fails compensatory mechanisms are activated. The major compensatory mechanisms include an increase in sympathetic tone and activation of the renin-angiotensin-aldosterone system to maintain cardiac filling, perfusion pressure, and intravascular volume. Vasoconstriction and fluid overload become excessive and eventually represent an additional burden on the failing heart.

Vasodilators have established themselves as primary agents in the therapy of CHF since they will lower excessive vasoconstriction. As shown in Table 27-4, a number of drugs are available. They differ based on their relative ability to relax venous smooth muscle (capacitance vessels) and arteriolar smooth muscle (resistance vessels). Thus, compounds such as nitroglycerin is mainly a venodilator and reduces ventricular filling pressure or cardiac preload; while hydralazine acts almost exclusively on arteriolar tone and thus primarily lessen aortic impedance or afterload. Other drugs are more balanced in their effects on vascular smooth muscle.

Intravenous nitroglycerin is indicated for short-term therapy of CHF associated with myocardial infarction. The development of tolerance is a major source of difficulty with nitroglycerin (see Chapter 29). Short-term intravenous administration of sodium nitroprusside, alone or in combination with dopamine, has been used successfully for severe refractory CHF.

Angiotensin converting enzyme (ACE) inhibitors such as captopril, enalapril, and lisinopril are indicated for chronic use in the treatment of CHF and are especially suitable for CHF therapy where presumably the renin-angiotensin-aldosterone system is overactive and benefit is to be obtained by its modulation. Although these three antihypertensive compounds are the only drugs officially indicated as vasodilators for the treatment of CHF, other drugs (listed in Table 27-4) are commonly used and, at present, their use should be considered as "unlabeled" or investigational for this purpose.

TABLE 27-4 Vasodilators commonly employed in congestive heart failure

Drug	Dilation of vascular beds	
	Venous (reduced preload)	Arteriolar (reduced afterload)
Nitroglycerin	+ + + +	+ +
ACE Inhibitors		
Captopril	+ + +	+ +
Enalapril	+ + +	+ +
Lisinopril	+ + +	+ +
Quinapril	+ + +	+ +
Ramipril	+ + +	+ +
Calcium-channel Blockers		
Nifedipine	+	+ + +
Nicardipine	+	+ + +
Direct-acting Vasodilators		
Nitroprusside	+ + +	+ + +
Hydralazine	–	+ + +
α-Adrenergic Blockers		
Prazosin	+ + +	+ +
Doxazosin	+ + +	+ +

MANAGEMENT OF CHF

CHF may present as an acute event which is dramatic and life-threatening. Pulmonary edema and consequent anoxemia and dyspnea, along with signs of hypervolemia such as dilated veins, dominate the picture. Required are hospitalization and intravenous therapy, along with airway and oxygen support. However, the principles of therapy are the same as in chronic CHF and follow the same stepwise therapeutic modalities. In Table 27-5 these steps are outlined. All these steps may be applied at once or progressively as required. In chronic CHF it is wise to move slowly. For example, overenthusiastic use of diuretics may lead to hyponatremia, which may precipitate circulatory failure and renal shutdown.

TABLE 27-5 Major steps in the management of CHF

Principal	Therapy
Reduce heart work	Bed rest, limit activity Control hypertension Weight reduction Sedation (as needed)
Reduce blood volume	Diuretics Sodium restriction Fluid restriction (seldom required)
Improve cardiac efficiency	Digitalis glycoside Correct arrhythmias
Modulate the circulation	Vasodilators Nondigitalis inotropes

BIBLIOGRAPHY

Abrams, J.: "Vasodilator Therapy for Chronic Congestive Heart Failure," *J. Am. Med. Assoc.* **254**: 3070 (1985).

Cody, R.J., D.W. Franklin, and J.H. Laragh: "Combined Vasodilator Therapy for Chronic Congestive Heart Failure," *Am. Heart J.* **105**: 575-580 (1983).

Cohn, J.N.: "Marriage of the Heart and the Peripheral Circulation," *Prog. Cardiovac. Dis.* **24**: 189-190 (1981).

Cohn, J.N., et al.: "Effect of Vasodilator Therapy on Mortality in Chronic Congestive Heart Failure: Results of a Veteran Administration Cooperative Study," *N. Eng. J. Med.* **314**: 1547 (1986).

Colucci, W.S.: "The Cardiovascular Actions of Milrinone" *Am. Heart J.* **121**: 1945-1947 (1991).

DiPalma, J.R.: "The Digitalis Controversy," *Am. Fam. Physician* **26**: 217-218 (1982).

DiPalma, J.R.: "Vasodilator and inotropic Therapy for Heart Failure," *Am. Fam. Physician* **31**: 177-180 (1985).

DiPalma, J.R.: "Atrial Natruretic Factor," *Am. Fam. Physician* **34**: 174-176 (1986).

Hamer, J.: "The Modern Management of Congestive Heart Failure", in D.S. Rowlands (ed.), *Recent Advances in Cardiology-9*, Churchill-Livingstone, Edinburgh, 1984, pp. 275-288.

Hayward, R.: "Digitalis the Present Position," in J. Hamer (ed.), *Drugs for Heart Disease, 2nd ed.*, Chapman and Hall, London, 1987, p. 145.

LeJemtel, T.H., E. Keung, E.H. Sonnenblick: "Amrinone: A New Non-glycosidic, Non-adrenergic Cardiotonic Agent Effective in the Treatment of Intractable Myocardial Failure in Man," *Circulation* **59**: 1098-1104 (1979).

Notterman, D.A.: "Inotropic Agents: Catecholamines, Digoxin, and Amrinone," *Crit. Care Clin.* **7**: 583-613 (1991)

Needleman, P.: "Atriopeptin Biochemical Pharmacology," *Fed. Proc.* **45**: 2096-2100 (1986).

Schocken, D.D. and J.D. Holloway: "Vasodilators in the Management of Congestive Heart Failure," *Rational Drug Therapy* **22**: 1-7 (1988).

Schwartz, K., C. Chassagne, and K.R. Boheler: "The Molecular Biology of Heart Failure," *J. Am. Coll. Cardiol.* **22 (4-S)**: 30A-33A (1993).

Smith, T.W., et al.: "Treatment of Life-Threatening Digitalis Intoxication with Digoxin Specific Fab Antibody Fragments," *N. Engl. J. Med.* **307**: 1357-1362 (1982).

Smith, T.W.: "Digitalis, Mechanisms of Action and Clinical Use," *N. Engl. J. Med.* **318**: 358-365 (1988).

Sonnenblick, E.H., and T.H. LeJemtel: "Heart Failure: Its Progression and Its Therapy," *Hosp. Pract.* **28**: 121-130 (1993).

Tzivoni, D., and A, Keren: "Suppression of Ventricular Arrhythmias by Magnesium," *Am. J. Cardiol.* **65**: 1397-1399 (1990).

Weber, K.T., et al.: "Amrinone and Exercise Performance in Patients with Chronic Heart Failure," *Am. J. Cardiol.* **48**: 164-169 (1981).

CHAPTER 28

Drugs for Tachyarrhythmias

Joanne I. Moore

The realization that sudden death due to cardiovascular disease has reached epidemic proportions in the western world has led to efforts to stem this seemingly avoidable tragedy. The cause is believed to be the sudden and sometimes unprovoked onset of ventricular fibrillation, which can occur even in young persons and quite often without obvious coronary artery disease. In cases which have occurred in fortuitous circumstances where cardioversion and resuscitative measures could be immediately applied, patients have gone on to live normal lives, and this lends credence to the idea that prophylactic measures could be successful. Of course, heart disease, depending on its severity, proportionally increases the risk of sudden death from ventricular fibrillation. Often it is preceded by lesser arrhythmias such as frequent ventricular premature beats and runs of ventricular tachycardia. Prevention of these premonitory arrhythmias is felt by most cardiologists to be useful prophylactically beyond the immediate relief of symptoms. Consequently there has been a much greater use of antiarrhythmic drugs in the last 10 years, and the demand for new and better ones has increased. This chapter covers those tachyarrhythmias (atrial flutter and fibrillation and ventricular tachycardia and fibrillation) which are most responsible for causing severe symptoms and sudden death. The few bradyarrhythmias which cause symptoms are handled in other chapters.

Meanwhile the comprehension of the mechanisms of action of antiarrhythmic drugs has greatly advanced and has permitted an orderly classification. As shown in Table 28-1, the drugs are arranged according to their actions on the excitable membrane of the cardiac myocyte. In order to understand the reasoning which led to this classification, it is necessary to review the excitation and recovery cycle of the various contractile and conducting cells of the heart. As in nervous tissue, excitation and conduction are phenomena which are related to the influx and efflux of sodium, calcium, and potassium with some contribution of chloride and magnesium. These are best studied by the technology of recording monophasic action currents in individual cardiac myocytes. In addition, it is necessary to have an appreciation of the gating mechanisms by which the channels in the membrane of the myocyte conduct these ions into and out of the cell.

REVIEW OF CARDIAC ELECTROPHYSIOLOGY

When a cardiac cell is quiescent, its transmembrane potential varies from −80 to −90 mV (inside negative) and is called the *transmembrane resting potential*. On excitation, the transmembrane potential reverses and the inside of the membrane rapidly becomes positive with respect to the outside. On recovery from excitation, the resting potential is restored. The changes in potential following excitation are summarily referred to as the *transmembrane action potential*. These changes have been divided into five phases: depolarization and reversal of transmembrane potential, designated phase 0; three phases of repolarization, designated phases 1, 2, and 3; and the resting potential, designated phase 4. However not all cardiac action potentials show a clear separation between phases 1, 2, and 3. Also, there are quantitative differences between transmembrane potentials recorded from different types of cardiac fibers and between their responses to depolarization (Fig. 28-1).

Fibers displaying two distinct types of responses have been identified; they have been named *slow-response fibers* and *fast-response fibers*. Fibers which normally display only slow-

TABLE 28-1 Classification of antiarrhythmic drugs based on their mechanism of action

Group	Drugs	Major mechanism of action	Dominant electrophysiologic effects
IA	Quinidine Procainamide Disopyramide	Sodium-channel blockade	Depolarization depressed Repolarization prolonged Conduction slowed
IB	Lidocaine Tocainide Mexiletine Phenytoin	Sodium-channel blockade	Depolarization slightly depressed Repolarization shortened Conduction slowed
IC	Flecainide Propafenone Moricizine	Sodium-channel blockade	Depolarization markedly depressed Repolarization slight effects Conduction slowed
II	Propranolol, others	Beta-adrenergic blockade	Action mainly on slow-response fibers to suppress automaticity and delay conduction
III	Amiodarone Bretylium Sotalol	Sodium-, calcium-, and probably potassium-channel blockade	Repolarization prolonged
IV	Verapamil Diltiazem	Calcium-channel blockade	Action mainly on slow-response fibers to suppress automaticity and delay conduction
—	Adenosine	Purinergic receptor agonist	Depressed AV nodal activity

response characteristics include normal sinoatrial (SA) and atrioventricular (AV) nodal tissue and injured or partially depolarized fast-response fibers. Slow-response tissues have low resting membrane potentials (between −40 and −70 mV) and exhibit slower conduction of impulses than that seen in fast-response fibers. The slow response is dependent on the extracellular concentration of calcium ions and is initiated when membrane permeability to calcium is increased during membrane depolarization (phase 0). During this time, calcium ions, and possibly sodium ions, enter the cell, elevating the transmembrane potential to approximately +10 mV. Because all cardiac cells possess slow-response characteristics and because nodal tissue is exclusively slow-response in nature, it has been suggested that the property of automaticity (see below), which is fundamental to all cardiac conduction tissue, may be linked to, among other factors, the slow response. An example of the monophasic action potential typical of slow-response tissue is illustrated in Fig. 28-1a.

Fibers which exhibit a fast response in addition to the slow response are found in normal atrial and ventricular muscle and specialized ventricular conduction tissue such as Purkinje fibers. The monophasic action potential of fast-response fibers is characterized by a very steep slope for phase 0 upstroke (also referred to as the *sodium spike*) resulting from a rapid inward movement of extracellular sodium ions (See Fig. 28-1). These tissues have high resting membrane potentials (−80 to −95 mV) which must be maintained for maximum upstroke velocity, i.e., maximum responsiveness. Consequently, impulse propagation through such tissues is sodium-dependent and rapid. The following is a description of events which occur during the monophasic action potential of fast-response fibers: As the wave of excitation spreads from neighboring cells, the permeability for sodium ions increases and sodium rapidly enters the cell, causing it to become depolarized, i.e., electrically positive relative to the exterior (phase 0). This ionic shift creates an electrochemical and concentration gradient which reduces the rate of sodium influx, but favors the influx of

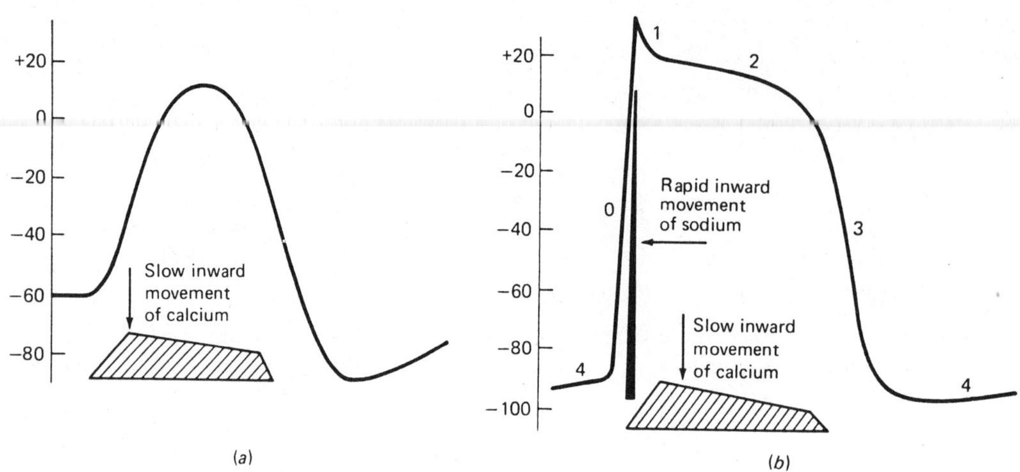

FIGURE 28-1 ***(a)*** *Monophasic action potential recorded from a slow-response fiber (SA node) showing the relationship of calcium influx to depolarization in the absence of sodium influx. The ordinate is in millivolts.* ***(b)*** *Diagrammatic representation of a monophasic action potential recorded from a fast-response fiber showing the relationship between ionic movements and the phases of depolarization (0), repolarization (1, 2, 3), and the resting membrane potential (4). The ordinate is in millivolts.*

chloride and the efflux of potassium (phase 1). Rapid sodium influx triggers the slow inward movement of calcium, which balances potassium leakage and holds the membrane potential fairly steady (phase 2 plateau). When calcium influx slows, the continued efflux of potassium restores the membrane potential to predepolarization levels. Finally, active pumping mechanisms restore the all of the ions to their proper local concentrations (phase 4).

During injury or ischemia in fast-response fibers, the rapid influx of sodium is believed to be lost or inhibited. This results in an action potential which closely resembles that of a slow-response fiber exhibiting slowed impulse conduction, which may favor the development of certain arrhythmias (see below).

The Gating Mechanisms

Recent work indicates that the movement of the ions across the cell membrane is not simply a question of the size of the ion versus the size of a hole in the membrane. Rather there is a complex system of channels for each ion which is composed of highly structured proteins capable of acting as valves or gates to allow or to prevent the passage of ions. The gating mechanism (opening and closing) of ion-specific channels that control the transmembrane flow of current is both voltage-dependent and time-dependent.

The sodium channel, which has been most studied in the electric eel *Electrophorus electricus*, is voltage-gated and consists of a single polypeptide of 26 to 30 kDa. The polypeptide is composed of some 1800 amino acid residues and has four repeating homologous units so oriented that they form a channel and a gating mechanism. Some variation exists in different species and organs, but it appears that the essential structure and design are the same. In mammalian counterparts the unit also contains 2 or 3 smaller polypeptides of 37 to 45 kDa. DNA recombinant techniques have permitted cloning of DNA sequences complementary to the messenger RNA coding for the channel protein of the electroplax of *E. electricus*.

By use of binding assays using specific neurotoxins, such as tetrodotoxin, similar channels have been identified in rat brain and skeletal muscles as well as in chick cardiac muscle. In addition, specific neurotoxins have enabled an analysis of the mechanisms of the functioning sodium channel. Three states are described: (1) resting, but available for activation; (2) activated, channel open and conducting; (3) inactivated, channel closed and not available (see Fig. 28-2).

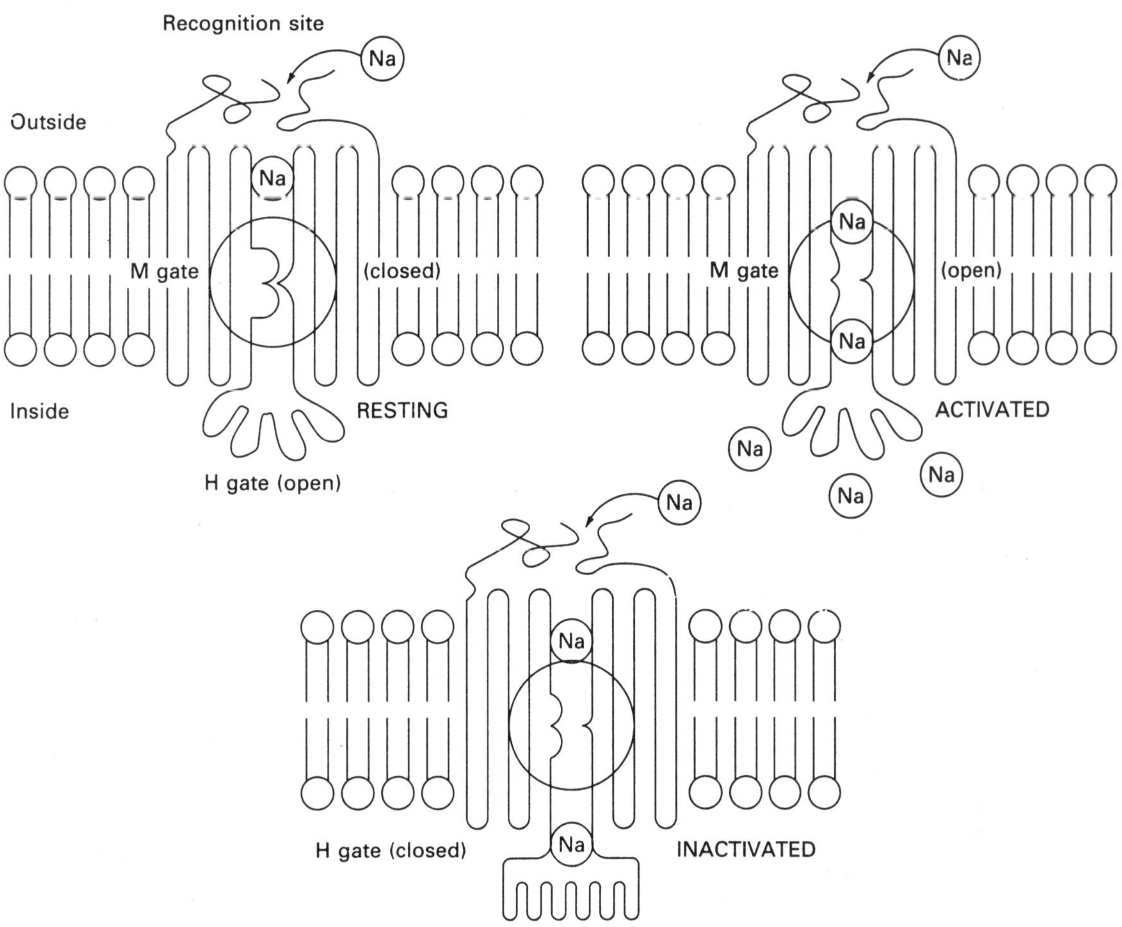

FIGURE 28-2 *A highly schematic diagram of the sodium channel of a cardiac myocyte. The channel is composed of a large protein which is folded in the bimolecular lipid membrane in such a manner as to form four homologous units which in turn form a channel or pore. On the outside of the membrane, the ends of the protein chain form a recognition site, or specificity gate, which identifies ionic sodium. In the channel itself, there is an area which is sensitive to stimuli and, presumably by an allosteric mechanism, can open or close the pore. This is the M gate. Inside the membrane, a portion of the protein forms an additional gate which can also block the passage of sodium (H gate). The channel is thought to exist in three states. In the fully polarized membrane, the channel is at rest with the M gate closed and the H gate open. Upon stimulation, the M gate opens and sodium can enter the myocyte (activated state). A millisecond later the H gate closes, inactivating the channel and blocking the entrance of sodium into the myocyte. The area in the vicinity of the M gate is thought to be the receptor site for local anesthetics (circled). It is thought that the local anesthetic cannot easily reach this sensitive area when the M gate is closed. When the M gate in open, the local anesthetic can reach the receptor area both in the disassociated and undisassociated forms. Thus in most instances, these agents are generally more effective on activated channels. On the other hand, highly lipid-soluble drugs such as lidocaine can reach the M gate receptor area through the membrane or even the cytosol, and thus such drugs are effective on both activated and inactivated channels.*

A postulated mechanism for the functioning of the sodium channel is as follows (review Fig. 28-2): the complex protein has at least three sensitive components which handle only sodium. Outside the membrane there is a free portion which identifies and allows only this ion to enter the channel (recognition site). The middle portion of the channel has an area which is *voltage-sensitive* and serves as a gate to keep the channel closed at rest or diastole (M gate). Apparently the M gate is kept closed by the negativity of the electronic membrane potential. Any slight change toward positivity may trigger the M gate to open (a stimulus); this is known as a *threshold potential*. Inside the cell membrane a portion of the protein is apparently sensitive to the concentration of sodium (H gate). Normally in the resting state the H gate is open. Thus when the membrane is stimulated, sodium enters the channel and rapidly flows freely into the cytosol. Realize that there is a very large pressure behind the sodium because of the large differential concentration between the intercellular fluid and the cytosol. As the sodium rushes in, the membrane becomes completely depolarized and the potential rises toward positivity, causing the M gate to stay open (phase 0 of action potential). Meanwhile, as the concentration of sodium builds up in the cytosol, the H gate closes, preventing further inflow. This whole phase of the depolarization takes only 1 ms or less in the case of nerve and only several milliseconds in the case of heart, so that the inward flow of sodium, although fast, is very small in amount. This allows many excitations or depolarizations to take place without exhausting the system and the Na^+,K^+-ATPase system gradually pumps out the accumulated sodium. Once the H gate closes, the channel is inactivated and must return to the resting state before it can again allow sodium to enter the cell. It should be pointed out that all changes in the configuration of the sodium channel from resting to open to closed and back to the resting state not only are voltage-dependent but also are time or rate-dependent. The shift from the resting to the open state follows first-order kinetics and is very fast but not instantaneous. Inactivation of the open channel to the closed state also is quite rapid. However, there is a relatively slow recovery of an inactivated (closed) channel to the resting state. In normal tissue during diastole, recovery to the resting state is easily accomplished, and thus there are many channels available for the next excitation. In ischemic or damaged cells, recovery is difficult and fewer channels are readied for the next cycle.

Voltage-activated calcium ion channels are controlled by the same processes that control sodium ion channels. They differ from sodium channels, however, in the voltage range of activation and inactivation and the slower rate constants required for the changes in the configuration of the calcium channel from activation to inactivation and recovery to the resting state.

It is important to point out that drugs which owe their antiarrhythmic properties to a blocking action in the sodium channel have differential effects because they have diverse physicochemical properties. For example, the M gate region can be affected by drugs which enter the channel like sodium (more hydrophilic) or by drugs which dissolve in the membrane and enter the cytosol (more lipophilic). When the M gate is closed or in the resting state in normal tissues, hydrophilic drugs cannot affect the H gate. Nor can they be completely effective in the M gate, since the receptor area in the protein may be below the M gate and they must wait for the gate to open (activated state) to act. Therefore they will be most active in cases of fast rhythms where the ratio of open to closed channels is higher. Drugs which are more lipophilic will tend to be active on resting as well as inactivated channels. In ischemic myocytes, such drugs are more effective, since the number of inactivated channels is greater than in normal tissues. For these reasons local anesthetics, i.e., group IB drugs in Table 28-1, have diverse actions on the sodium channel and are therefore useful in differing clinical situations.

It follows that the quality, number, physical state, and distribution of channels for sodium, potassium, and calcium mainly determine the contour and functional characteristics of the monophasic action potential of various myocytes in the heart. Thus the pacemaker regions of the heart (SA and AV nodes) have a monophasic action potential which has relatively slow depolarization (phase 0), a small plateau (phase 2), while repolarization (phase 3) is comparable to that in other myocytes. However, the most remarkable difference is in the resting potential (phase 4). Instead of being isoelectric, it rises in a gentle slope, seemingly triggering the next depolarization (see Fig. 28-3). In fact, experimental conditions which favor and increase this slope cause tachycardia and conditions which flatten the slope cause bradycardia. Indeed, when an atrial or ventricular myocyte "takes over" pacemaker activity, the normal flat resting potential now becomes sloped, resembling that of pacemaker myocytes.

As shown in Fig. 28-3, atrial and ventricular myocytes have essentially the same contour of action potential except that the atrial potential is of smaller amplitude and shorter in duration. Atrial and Purkinje fibers have more overshoot (phase 1), which may be indicative of their conductive properties.

PATHOPHYSIOLOGY OF CARDIAC ARRHYTHMIAS

Many factors influence the normal rhythm of electrical activity in the heart, including automaticity, refractoriness, conduction velocity, excitability, and impulse conduction through the AV node. In general, however, all arrhythmias can be shown to result from defects in automaticity, which cause abnormal impulse formation, or defects in conduction, which allow abnormal impulse propagation, or both.

Automaticity

The term *automaticity* is used to describe the behavior by which cardiac fibers spontaneously generate action potentials. The property of automaticity is a feature common to all cardiac conduction tissue, and in some cells, e.g., nodal tissue, it is believed to be related to the slow inward movement of calcium ions.

Under normal circumstances, the task of impulse generation in the heart is under control of specialized cells that spontaneously depolarize during phase 4 (the resting phase). Once such depolarizations reach the threshold potential, an action potential is initiated which subsequently propagates throughout the myocardium. These specialized cells, by virtue of their rapid rate of spontaneous discharge, control impulse formation for the entire heart and are consequently known as *pacemaker cells*.

Other cells with a high degree of automaticity exist which discharge more slowly than the pacemaker cells. Normally, such cells are depolarized before they attain threshold potential by impulses originating in the pacemaker area (SA node). Pacemaker control of the heart, therefore, resides in those cells whose rate of spontaneous depolarization is most rapid. This rate of discharge can be increased by a number of mechanisms either singly or in combination: (1) increasing the slope of phase 4 of the myocardial action potential, (2) decreasing (making less negative) the resting membrane potential, and (3) increasing (making more negative) the threshold potential. Conversely, the rate of spontaneous depolarization can be decreased by changing these variables in the opposite direction. The relative decrease in the rate of spontaneous depolarization of the SA node or the relative increase in spontaneous depolarization rate of cells outside the SA node favors the loss of pacemaker control by the SA node to a new area of pacemaker activity called an *ectopic focus*. Ectopic foci typically arise in circumstances under activity of other automatic cells, for example, during vagal overtone or in the presence of drugs which depress the SA node. Ectopic foci can also assume pacemaker activity when the automaticity of nonnodal cells is stimulated, as occurs in ischemia, acidosis, digitalis toxicity, ionic imbalance, and catecholamine excess. Arrhythmias which appear to result from an increase in the automaticity of SA nodal tissue or ectopic pacemaker tissue include sinus tachycardia and atrial tachycardia. Arrhythmias produced by reductions in automaticity of these tissues include premature ventricular beats and AV junctional rhythm.

Conduction

The progressive movement of an action potential from one area of the myocardium to another is termed *conduction*. It is a property of excitable tissue which allows an impulse to pass from cell to cell, that is, to be propagated.

Disturbances in conduction also contribute to the development of arrhythmias. Slowing or loss of impulse propagation from the atria to the ventricles results in various degrees of AV block with subsequent dissociation of pacemaker control. Conduction is influenced by several factors: the *excitability* of cells which lie in the path of a propagated impulse, the *responsiveness* of these cells, and the *refractoriness* and response characteristics of the tissue which a propagated impulse encounters.

Excitability is defined as the reciprocal of the magnitude of an electric impulse required to change the resting membrane potential to the threshold potential at which an action potential is propagated. *Responsiveness* is the maximum rate of depolarization during phase 0 of the action potential, i.e., the slope of phase 0, and is influenced by the value of the transmembrane potential at the time of excitation. Higher resting membrane potentials increase responsiveness; conversely, lower (less negative) potentials reduce it.

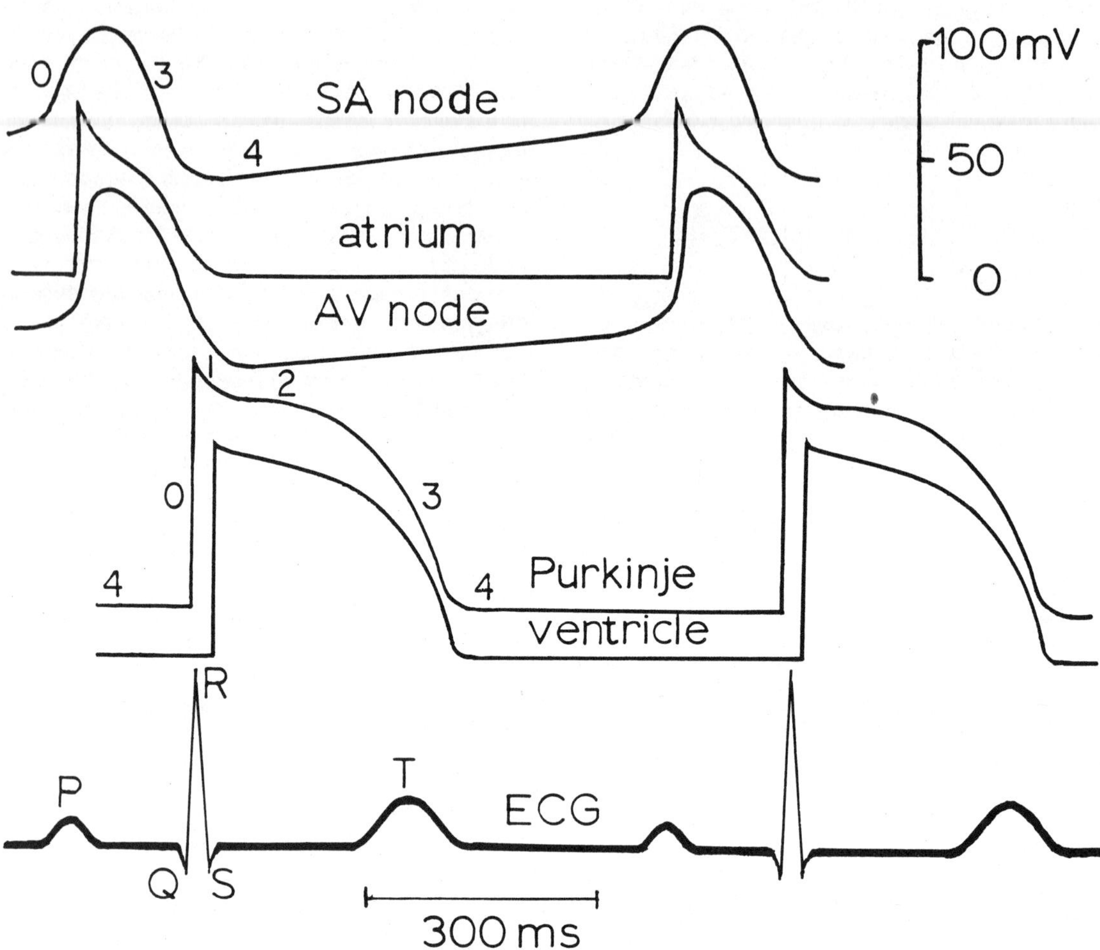

FIGURE 28-3 *Schematic reconstruction of the monophasic action potentials of selected myocytes of the heart arranged in temporal sequence for two complete cycles. The clinical ECG is included to illustrate the relationship of this diphasic recording to the cyclic events which are occurring in pertinent parts of the heart. Note that the amplitude of the ECG has no relationship to that of the monophasic action potentials. The latter potentials have five phases: phase 0 = depolarization; phase 1 = early and brief repolarization; phase 2 = plateau; phase 3 = rapid repolarization; phase 4 = resting, or the diastolic, potential. The potentials of the SA node and the AV node myocytes differ from those of the atrium, Purkinje, and ventricle myocytes by having slow depolarization and no phases 1 and 2. In addition, the resting potential slopes upward (becomes more positive) during diastole, characteristic of pacemaker myocytes. The Purkinje and ventricular myocytes have potentials of greater amplitude and duration than the nodal and atrial myocytes. The SA node, because of its anatomic location, innervation, and inherently greater automaticity, sets the rhythm of the heart. The ECG reflects the temporal events of the cycle. Thus, the P wave is related to atrial depolarization; the QRS complex to ventricular depolarization; the T wave to ventricular repolarization. It follows that the PR interval measures atrial-ventricular conduction time; the QRS ventricular activation (depolarization plus conduction); the QT interval mainly the duration of the ventricular action potential. The ECG is a surface reflection of the electrical activity of the heart; but as indicated, it can serve as an accurate diagnostic tool for changes brought about in rhythm and in the effects of antiarrhythmic agents.*

Refractoriness is defined as the inability to respond to a stimulus. For the most part, we restrict our consideration of refractoriness to the duration of the *effective refractory period* (ERP). The ERP is the period during which a premature stimulus, regardless of strength, will fail to propagate an impulse (Fig. 28-4).

These factors influence conduction in a number of ways. Generally, if an ectopic focus develops, the relatively more rapid rate of diastolic depolarization of the SA node will prevent impulses propagated by the ectopic focus from encountering any but refractory tissue. During the *relative refractory period* (RRP), a premature stimulus may, depending on strength, propagate an impulse but at a slower rate than when the stimulus occurs outside the refractory periods (Fig. 28-4).

Decreasing the ERP favors the propagation of premature impulses because the chances of encountering excitable tissue are increased. Conversely, lengthening the ERP decreases the chances that impulses from ectopic foci will be propagated. Since the ERP constitutes a portion of the action potential duration (APD), it is sometimes useful to determine its change relative to that of the APD. The ERP/APD ratio serves to express the relationship between these intervals and has been employed as an index of refractoriness.

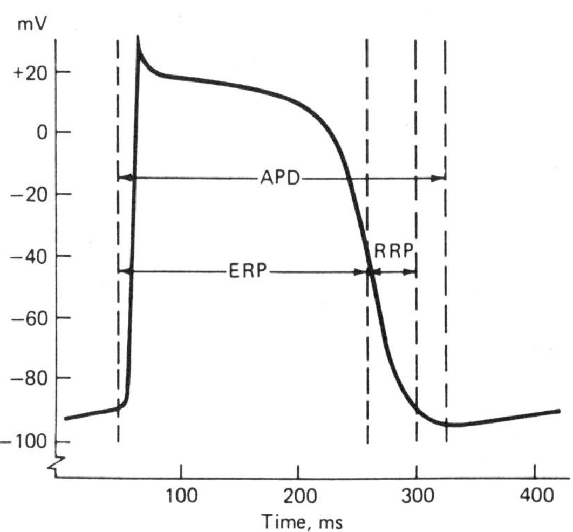

FIGURE 28-4 *Diagrammatic representation of a monophasic action potential recorded from a Purkinje myocyte showing the durations of the effective refractory period (ERP), the relative refractory period (RRP), and the action potential (APD).*

Interference with conduction of propagated impulses may produce serious dysfunctions of the heart, including AV block, bundle branch block, and various tachyarrhythmias. Cardiac stretch and local tissue hypoxia may reduce the speed of impulse conduction through segments of the myocardium, resulting in the reexcitation of recently depolarized, but no longer refractory, tissue. This phenomenon, known as *reentry*, is often responsible for coupled beats, called *bigeminy*, and AV nodal and ventricular tachycardias.

Conduction of propagated impulses is also influenced by the response characteristics of the tissue which an impulse encounters. This is particularly true for slow-response tissues like SA and AV nodal tissue, which have long, time-dependent refractory periods. In these tissues, impulse conduction is very slow, and this can result in the unidirectional block of an impulse and subsequent reentrant arrhythmias.

TYPES OF CARDIAC ARRHYTHMIAS

Cardiac arrhythmias can arise at practically every level of the heart. Arrhythmias which develop at or above the level of the AV node are classified as *supraventricular arrhythmias*, whereas those which develop in the His-Purkinje system or the ventricles are called *ventricular arrhythmias*.

Supraventricular Arrhythmias

Paroxysmal Atrial Tachycardia Paroxysmal atrial tachycardia (PAT) is characterized by atrial rates of 150 to 250 beats per minute and most often 180 to 200 beats per minute. This rhythm often occurs in the absence of demonstrable heart disease. In the absence of heart disease and drug therapy, it is common to see each atrial depolarization conduct to ventricles so that the atrial and ventricular rates are identical. Paroxysms often spontaneously terminate but also may be tenaciously persistent and cause severe anxiety and palpitations or induce heart failure even in otherwise normal hearts.

Atrial Flutter Atrial flutter is characterized by regular beating of the atria at rates between 250 and 300 beats per minute; most commonly the atrial rate is precisely 300 beats per minute. In adults who have not been treated, every other atrial depolarization is usually conducted to the ventricles, producing a ventricular rate of 150 beats per minute. Unlike atrial fibrillation, atrial flutter produces effective contraction of the atria with less thrombosis in the atria. Subsequent embolization is consequently much less common.

Atrial Fibrillation Atrial fibrillation is a rhythm characterized by irregular, disorganized depolarization of the atrium at rates of 350 to 600 beats per minute. These rapid depolarizations do not produce effective atrial contractions. The rapid atrial rate exceeds the ability of even the normal AV conducting system to transmit impulses; therefore, the ventricular rate is much slower, 130 to 170 beats per minute in untreated cases, and is characteristically irregular. This rhythm diminishes the "cardiac reserve," produces palpitations, and is associated with an increased incidence of thromboembolization of the pulmonary or systemic arterial systems. The decrease in cardiac reserve commonly leads to the onset or aggravation of congestive heart failure, angina pectoris, or symptoms of cerebrovascular insufficiency.

Ventricular Arrhythmias

Premature Ventricular Contractions Premature ventricular contractions (PVCs), or extrasystoles, originate in the ventricles and travel in unorthodox pathways, and the QRS complexes are thus wide and bizarre in configuration, prematurely interrupting the dominant rhythm. Premature ventricular contractions are very common both in individuals with normal hearts and in those with heart disease. Most of these cases require no treatment. If premature depolarizations are frequent or cause troublesome symptoms or signs, treatment should be considered. The decision to treat PVCs also may be based on the condition associated with the arrhythmia. For instance, digitalis in excessive doses may lead to frequent premature ventricular beats. If digitalis is continued, ventricular tachycardia or ventricular fibrillation may occur and can prove fatal. Another example is the occurrence of PVCs during acute myocardial infarction, where PVCs may presage ventricular tachycardia or fibrillation.

Ventricular Tachycardia Ventricular tachycardia is a rapid rhythm (150 to 200 beats per minute) originating in the ventricles. This site of origin produces QRS complexes in the ECG which are slurred and widened. The configuration of the QRS complexes during ventricular tachycardia is the same as that of PVCs originating in either the right or left ventricle. The cycle length between beats is slightly irregular, and the QRS complexes are independent of the P waves. The etiologic factors and therapeutic goals are similar to those discussed under PVCs. However, ventricular tachycardia is much more likely to produce circulatory impairment than even frequent PVCs, and congestive cardiac failure or severe hypotension may ensue. When such catastrophic events are precipitated by ventricular tachycardia, it should be terminated immediately using appropriate drugs or electric countershock.

Ventricular Fibrillation This tachyarrhythmia is exactly analogous to atrial fibrillation. However, while in the atrium the arrhythmia has relatively little consequence with respect to the pumping function of the heart, fibrillation in the ventricle results in an instantaneous drop in blood pressure to zero because of absence of cardiac output. Death is inevitable in a few minutes unless the arrhythmia is converted and the normal heart beat restored. No drug therapy is practical. The remedy is cardiac massage to restore some circulation, artificial respiration, and dc countershock (cardioversion). *The aim of drug therapy is to prevent this most common cause of sudden death by lessening the chance of its development.*

Unusual Tachyarrhythmias

Wolff-Parkinson-White (WPW) Syndrome A reexcitation syndrome is one in which the impulse from the atrium reaches the ventricle by an abnormal route without the usual delay built into the normal conduction pathway. Hence the ventricle is "preexcited." Patients with this syndrome are subject to paroxysmal attacks of atrial tachycardia, flutter, and fibrillation. These are, of course, attended by rapid ventricular rates, even as rapid as 250 to 300 beats per minute which are life-threatening, especially if the individual does not have adequate cardiac reserve.

Torsade de Pointes This literally means turning of the points (QRS complexes). It occurs in situations where the QT interval is prolonged (long action potential duration) and consists of ventricular tachycardia which undulates around the ECG isoelectric base. It usually begins with a single premature contraction superimposed on the T wave of the previous normal beat.

There are many causes including congenital long QT interval; drugs with quinidine-like properties such as type IA antiarrhythmics, tricyclic antidepressants and others; electrolyte imbalance, especially hyperkalemia and hypomagnesemia;

liquid protein diets; CNS lesions; myocarditis and myocardial ischemia; marked bradycardia; and mitral valve prolapse syndromes.

Fortunately torsade de pointes usually terminates spontaneously. However, it easily converts to ventricular fibrillation, and thus it must be recognized and treated properly to avoid sudden death.

ANTIARRHYTHMIC DRUGS

Few groups of drugs have been so well studied and understood from the viewpoint of the molecular, as well as the physiologic, mechanism of action. This has permitted a useful and logical classification based upon accurate data (review Table 28-1). Based upon the exquisite understanding of the mechanism of tachyarrhythmias and the knowledge of how the drugs affect these mechanisms, it is possible to prescribe with considerable accuracy a particular drug for a particular arrhythmia. In difficult cases it is necessary to actually invasively study the patient's electrophysiologic disturbance. In advanced cardiac clinics, the patient who is subject to a tachyarrhythmia is sedated, electrodes are placed in the heart, and by electrical pacing the tachyarrhythmia is induced. Then by giving one drug after another intravenously, the threshold for inducing the arrhythmia is measured. By this method the best available drug is determined which presumably will increase the chance that the arrhythmia will not occur spontaneously and hence prevent sudden death. Selection of a specific drug by this method is believed to yield better results than empirical prescribing.

Such electrophysiologic testing in humans is possible only because cardioversion can rescue the patient in case a fatal type of arrhythmia, such as ventricular fibrillation, is induced. In fact, cardioversion is so effective that it has replaced antiarrhythmic drugs in many instances in the conversion of tachyarrhythmias to sinus rhythm. Thus the role of antiarrhythmic drugs has changed to become more prophylactic—that is, to prevent recurrence of an arrhythmia once sinus rhythm has been established by cardioversion. *Thus the ultimate proof of clinical efficacy of an antiarrhythmic drug must be not only in that it relieves signs and symptoms but also in that it prolongs life.*

There is no doubt that the central nervous system exerts some control over the rhythm of the heart. This is expressed by impulses over the autonomic nervous system. Therefore, the arrhythmogenic action of catecholamines and cholinomimetic substances on the heart is most important.

Catecholamines

It is certain that sympathetic stimulation of the heart, either by nerve impulse or endogenous and exogenous catecholamines, initiates and perpetuates both atrial and ventricular tachyarrhythmias. Particularly in prophylaxis therapy, beta-adrenergic blockade seems effective, and actually this is the only group of drugs which has proven ability to reduce mortality and prolong life. It is to be noted that drugs in groups IA and III also enhance blockade of the sympathetics, but this is mainly an alpha-adrenergic type block.

Cholinomimetic Action

Cholinergic stimulation of the atrium can lead to atrial tachycardia and even flutter and fibrillation. Innervation of the ventricle by parasympathetic fibers is absent, and so ventricular arrhythmias are not produced by excessive parasympathomimetic activity. Drugs with anticholinergic action are used particularly in the prophylaxis of atrial arrhythmias. This seems to be especially true during anesthesia and surgery.

GROUP I DRUGS

All these drugs have local anesthetic properties and have a common major mechanism of action in blocking the sodium channel. Depending on which stage of sodium channel activity is most severely blocked, the change in physiology of the myocyte is variously affected (see Table 28-1). All the drugs in this group have unequal actions on the physiologic properties described above. Table 28-2 provides a summary of these effects.

Group IA

Quinidine

Quinidine is the dextro stereoisomer of quinine; it exerts all the pharmacologic actions of quinine, including antimalarial, antipyretic, and oxytocic effects. The actions of quinidine on cardiac

TABLE 28-2 Effects of antiarrhythmic drugs on the physiologic functions of heart muscle and the conduction system; comparison to the effects of digitalis

Function	Drugs in Groups IA	IB	IC	II	III	IV	Digitalis
Automaticity							
SA node	+/−	+/−	+/−	− − −	− − −	− − −	− − −
Ectopic foci	− − −	− − −	− − −	− − −	− − −	− − −	+ + +
Conduction velocity							
Atrium	− − −	0	− − −	+/−	− − −	0	+/−
AV node	− − −	0	− − −	− − −	− − −	− − −	− − −
His – Purkinje	− − −	0	− − −	+/−	− − −	0	+/−
Refractory period							
Atrium	+ + +	+/−	+/−	+/−	+ + +	0	− −
AV node	+ +	+/−	+/−	+ + +	+ + +	+ + +	+ + +
His-Purkinje	+ + +	+/−	+ + +	0	+ + +	0	0
Ventricle	+ + +	+/−	+ + +	0	+ + +	0	− − −
Accessory pathways	+ + +	+ + +	+ + +	+/−	+ + +	0	+/−
Action-potential duration	+ + +	− − −	0	0	+ + +	0	− − −
Responsiveness (rate of depolarization)	− − −	0	− − −	0	− −	0	+ +
Catecholamine blockade	+ +	0	0	+ + +	+ +	0	0
Anticholinergic activity	+ + +	0	0	0	0	0	0
Local anesthetic activity	+ +	+ + +	+ +	+	+	+	0
Sodium-channel blockade	+ + +	+ + +	+ + +	+	+ + +	0	0
Calcium-channel blockade	0	0	0	0	+	+ + +	0

Increase = + to + + +
Decrease = − to − − −
Effect varies with the dose and circumstances = +/−
Unknown or indefinite = 0

muscle are relatively more intense than those of quinine. Conversely, quinidine, although less effective against malaria than quinine, can be used for this purpose.

Source and Chemistry Quinidine is one of the four most important alkaloids isolated from cinchona bark. Quinidine consists of a quinoline group attached by a secondary carbinol to a quinuclidine ring. There is a methoxy group on the quinoline ring and a vinyl group on the quinuclidine ring. Quinidine differs from quinine only in the configuration of the carbinol grouping (*).

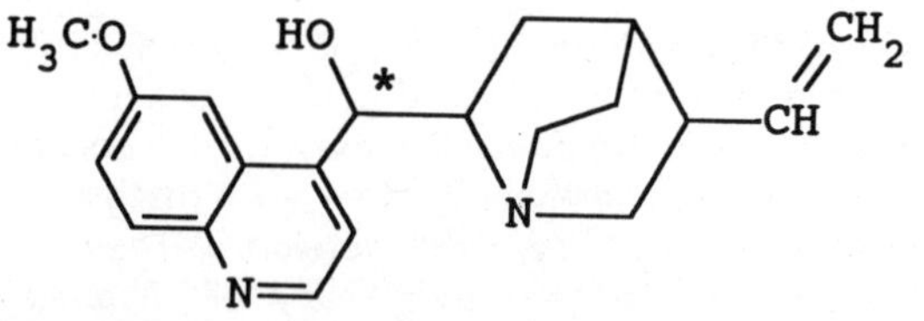

$H_3C{\cdot}O$ HO * CH_2 CH N N

Pharmacodynamics *Cardiovascular system* The major effects of quinidine on the electrical activity of the heart have been described above. In addition, quinidine depresses contractility, especially in toxic doses. In therapeutic usage, however, it may actually increase cardiac output because of its vasodilator properties. The depressant effect on contractility may be of real importance when myocardial disease is present. Large oral doses of quinidine reduce arterial pressure in humans. Considerably smaller intravenous doses have the same effect. Rapid intravenous injection may cause a precipitous decrease in blood pressure and cardiac output.

Many of the effects of quinidine on the electrical activity of the heart can be appreciated from the ECG. Patients in sinus rhythm may show an increase in sinus rate, which presumably is caused by anticholinergic action, a reflex increase in sympathetic activity, or both. High doses, particularly in patients with atrial disease, may produce sinus arrest or SA nodal block. Because of its effects on conduction in the His-Purkinje system and ventricle, quinidine causes a progressive prolongation of the QRS complex. Prolongation of the QRS complex and serious conduction disturbances are more likely when abnormality of the conduction system is present before quinidine administration. Quinidine increases the QT interval corrected for rate. This effect, at low doses, is due primarily to the effects of quinidine on repolarization of ventricular muscle. At higher doses, changes in the QT interval and in the configuration of the T wave result also from the quinidine-induced disturbances of conduction. In usual therapeutic doses quinidine has little effect on the PR interval. This may be due to the fact that an anticholinergic action is balanced by a direct depressant effect on AV conduction. In sufficiently high concentrations quinidine can produce heart block of any degree.

Central Nervous System Quinidine initially stimulates and then depresses the higher nerve centers. Intravenous administration of quinidine may produce a sensation of warmth, profuse diaphoresis, and nausea and vomiting. Rarely, it may produce psychosis-like symptoms.

Autonomic Nervous System Quinidine appears to interfere with the effects of the parasympathetic nervous system on the heart. A vagal blocking action would be expected to increase the heart rate. However, this is opposed by the direct action of quinidine on pacemaker and conduction tissue, which is to slow the heart rate. For this reason, variable effects are noted on heart rate dependent on the initial vagal tone (see Table 28-2). Note that the drug also causes some degree of catecholamine blockade.

Skeletal Muscle Quinidine, like the other cinchona alkaloids, increases the maximum tension developed by skeletal muscle in response to direct electrical stimulation. This action contrasts with its negative inotropic effect on cardiac muscle. Quinidine increases refractoriness of skeletal muscle. Quinidine also decreases the effectiveness of transmission across the neuromuscular junction and diminishes the response of skeletal muscle to intraarterial injections of acetylcholine. This had led to the use of quinidine (actually quinine) for "night cramps" or spasm of the leg skeletal muscle.

Pharmacokinetics The oral bioavailability of quinidine is approximately 70 to 80 percent depending on the salt form used. A single oral dose produces a peak plasma concentration within 1 to 2 h. Therapeutic plasma levels vary from 2 to 6 μg/mL.

Quinidine disappears from plasma with a half-life between 6 and 7 h. The drug is biotransformed in the liver to an active derivative, dihydroquinidine, and inactive hydroxylated products. Approximately 85 percent of plasma quinidine is bound to plasma proteins. The amount of quinidine excreted unchanged varies from 20 to 50 percent. About 95 percent of an administered dose can be recovered from the urine as the sum of quinidine and its biotransformation products.

Therapeutic Uses Quinidine is commonly used to abolish atrial and premature ventricular contractions and to prevent paroxysmal supraventricular or ventricular tachycardia. Quinidine is also useful in converting atrial fibrillation to normal sinus rhythm. In the absence of a digitalis-induced AV block, quinidine can precipitate a 1:1 heart block and a dangerously rapid ventricular rate in about 10 percent of patients. When used to eliminate atrial flutter, some clinicians feel that quinidine administration should not precede that of digitalis. Although available for intravenous use, quinidine is not frequently administered parenterally because of adverse reactions such as hypotension.

Adverse Reactions One of the major problems in the effective use of quinidine is its toxicity. Few patients find quinidine tolerable in chronic use, particularly in higher dosage ranges.

Cinchonism Quinidine, like the other cinchona alkaloids, can induce cinchonism. Symptoms of mild cinchonism may include tinnitus, impaired hearing, headache, mild diarrhea, or slight blurring of vision. Symptoms of severe toxicity include severe tinnitus and hearing loss, blurred vision, diplopia, photophobia, and altered perception of color. Severe cerebral signs, such as confusion, delirium, or psychosis, may accompany the headache. Nausea, vomiting, and diarrhea may be severe and accompanied by abdominal pain. The skin is often hot and flushed.

Gastrointestinal Effects Nausea, vomiting, and diarrhea each occur alone or in varying combinations and often in the absence of symptoms involving other systems. Quinidine administration is often continued even with mild gastrointestinal symptoms; more severe reactions may force discontinuing the drug.

Blood Pressure Effects When given intravenously, and to a lesser extent intramuscularly, quinidine may cause significant and even profound arterial hypotension. In most instances this pressure drop is primarily due to a decrease in arteriolar resistance without marked reduction in cardiac output. Severe, protracted hypotension may be treated with pressor agents.

Cardiac Effects Quinidine in concentrations above 2 μg/mL causes a progressive linear increase in duration of the QRS and QT intervals of the ECG; the change in the QRS has a higher correlation with plasma drug concentration. This relationship is useful in monitoring the cardiac effects of quinidine; the dose administered should be reduced if a normal QRS duration increases by 50 percent over the control value. The QT interval is also a useful measurement to follow, and changes in this interval are easy to detect at ordinary ECG recording speeds. At plasma concentrations that may be toxic (8 μg/mL), complete SA block, high-grade AV block, or total asystole may occur. Ventricular ectopic depolarizations may become frequent and occur repetitively; ventricular tachycardia or fibrillation may ensue. Although such severe myocardial toxicity may diminish as plasma concentration declines after withholding quinidine, the ECG and hemodynamic parameters of each patient should be closely monitored. In cases which require more active intervention, metaraminol or norepinephrine may be used to counteract the hypotension, lidocaine or phenytoin may be given to reduce tachydysrhythmias, and sodium lactate may be useful to counteract quinidine toxicity.

A frequently mentioned complication of quinidine therapy for atrial fibrillation is the so-called paradoxical increase in ventricular rate. In many cases of atrial fibrillation, when quinidine is used alone for conversion, the atrial rate slows markedly before the change to sinus rhythm occurs. However, in a few of these cases the ventricular rate may suddenly rise as atrial rate falls because of a decrease in concealed conduction of atrial impulses in the AV junction. Even though this event is uncommon in patients treated with quinidine alone, many physicians use an AV nodal blocking agent such as digoxin, verapamil or a β-adrenergic blocker in their patients prior to using quinidine to avoid this eventuality. Hypersensitivity reactions, including fever, thrombocytopenic purpura, and hepatitis, are not uncommon complications of quinidine therapy.

Drug Interactions Quinidine can have additive effects when administered together with digoxin, phenytoin, procainamide, propranolol, phenothiazines, and other agents, and caution should be exercised when using such combination therapy. Quinidine potentiates the neuromuscular blockade produced by curariform drugs. Barbiturates and anticonvulsants which induce the drug-metabolizing microsomal system shorten the half-life of quinidine, and therapy with agents in these classes should be started and stopped with great caution in patients receiving quinidine. Anticonvulsants and antacids containing aluminum hydroxide may reduce or delay quinidine absorption from the gastrointestinal tract. Other antacid agents which indirectly alkalinize the urine may potentiate quinidine via increased tubular reabsorption. Quinidine is known to increase serum digoxin concentrations. It has been suggested that quinidine displaces digoxin from tissue binding sites; interference with renal digoxin excretion by quinidine has also been proposed. Quinidine may inhibit the formation of prothrombin and of other vitamin K-dependent clotting factors, heightening the effect of oral anticoagulants. Quinidine toxicity may be exaggerated by simultaneous use of pyrimethamine, quinine, and reserpine. Because of its anticholinergic nature, quinidine may antagonize the effects of cholinergic agents.

Procainamide

The actions of procainamide are qualitatively similar to those of procaine. Its effects on the electrical activity of the heart are almost identical to those of quinidine. Procainamide is superior to procaine as an antiarrhythmic agent because, in contrast to procaine, (1) it is well absorbed after oral administration, (2) it has a long duration of action because it resists hydrolysis by plasma esterases, and (3) its effects on the heart are relatively strong, while its effects on the central nervous system are relatively weak.

Chemistry Procainamide differs from procaine in that the ester linkage has been replaced by an amide bond.

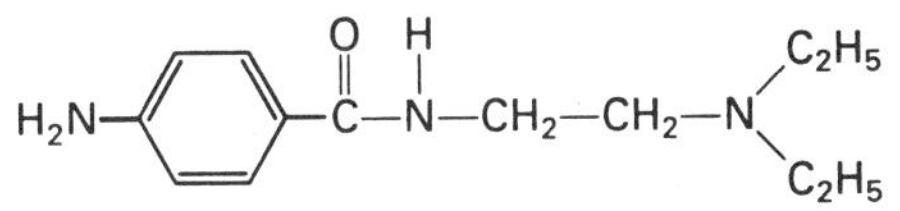

$$H_2N-C_6H_4-\overset{O}{\overset{\|}{C}}-\overset{H}{\overset{|}{N}}-CH_2-CH_2-N(C_2H_5)_2$$

Pharmacodynamics The effects of procainamide on the electrical activity of the heart are qualitatively the same as those of quinidine. In comparison to quinidine, procainamide has weaker vagal blocking activity, has a less intense negative inotropic effect, and does not induce adrenergic blockade. Procainamide causes a decrease in systemic arterial pressure, which is particularly prominent with intravenous administration. Peripheral vasodilation and depression of cardiac contractility contribute to the hypotensive action.

The changes in the ECG produced by procainamide are similar to those caused by quinidine. Prolongation of the QRS complex is a most consistent change. Prolongation of the corrected QT interval (QT_c), changes in the morphology of the T wave, and at high doses, prolongation of the PR interval or production of heart block are less frequent. As in the case of quinidine, changes in the ECG may provide some guide to the doses of procainamide to be employed. The presence of abnormalities of conduction increases the likelihood that the drug will cause further conduction delay or block.

Pharmacokinetics Procainamide can be given orally, intramuscularly, or intravenously. Absorption is approximately 85 percent complete following oral administration, and peak plasma concentrations are reached in 90 to 120 min. Intramuscular injections produce peak levels within 15 to 60 min, but values are more variable than after oral or intravenous doses. Procainamide is only sparingly bound to plasma proteins (approximately 15 percent). However, it is bound in various body tissues in concentrations in excess of the plasma concentrations. Disappearance of procainamide from the plasma approximates a first-order process with a half-life of 3 to 4 h. Unlike its homolog procaine (an ester), procainamide (an amide) is highly resistant to esterases, but is hydrolyzed by amidases in the liver. The major product is N-acetylprocainamide (NAPA), which appears as 16 to 21 percent of a single dose in slow acetylators and 25 to 33 percent in rapid acetylators. This product is pharmacologically active and equal to procainamide in antiarrhythmic potency. Nearly 90 percent of procainamide and its biotransformation products are excreted in the urine by glomerular filtration and tubular secretion. Approximately 50 to 60 percent is excreted unchanged.

Therapeutic Uses Procainamide is indicated for the treatment of premature ventricular contractions, and ventricular tachycardia. Therapeutic plasma concentrations range from 3 to 8 μg/mL. Intravenous and oral dosage schedules may require adjustment upward in dialysis patients and downward in undialyzed individuals with renal failure. For rapid establishment of therapeutic concentrations, parenteral procainamide is superior to quinidine.

Adverse Reactions Many of the undesirable effects of procainamide are related to the plasma concentrations, the rate of change of plasma concentration, and the route of administration. The intravenous route of administration is more often associated with hypotension and cardiac toxicity (widening of the QRS complex, ventricular ectopic beats, ventricular tachycardia and fibrillation, or asystole) than is oral administration. High doses of procainamide may diminish myocardial contractility or worsen cardiac failure.

A syndrome resembling systemic lupus erythematosus (SLE) may be produced by procainamide after chronic use. Prolonged drug administration often leads to the development of a positive antinuclear antibody (ANA, or anti-DNA antibody) titer (estimates are up to 30 percent of patients). Clinically, these patients may remain asymptomatic; however, those who exhibit symptoms resembling SLE more often than not are slow acetylators and thus the condition is believed to associated with procainamide and not NAPA. Arthralgia is the most prevalent symptom, and fever, pleuropneumonia, and hepatomegaly are all common. This syndrome possesses features distinct from idiopathic SLE in that there is no predilection for females and renal and cerebral involvements are not observed.

Agranulocytosis has occurred after repeated use of the drug; it may be severe and responsible for fatal infections. Neutropenia, thrombocytopenia, and hemolytic anemia are only rarely seen.

Drug Interactions Procainamide may potentiate the hypotensive effect of antihypertensive drugs and thiazide diuretics. Like quinidine and other antiarrhythmic drugs, procainamide may potentiate the neuromuscular blockade produced by skeletal muscle relaxants, magnesium salts, and certain antibiotics. Also, like quinidine, procainamide has anticholinergic properties which antagonize cholinergic drugs and enhance the effects of other drugs with anticholinergic activity.

Individuals sensitive to procainamide will exhibit cross-sensitivity to lidocaine and other local anesthetic agents. Because of additive effects, procainamide should be combined with other antiarrhythmic agents cautiously. Although occasionally useful in treating digitalis-induced tachyarrhythmias, procainamide should be administered with care to prevent the development of ventricular fibrillation or cardiac depression.

Disopyramide

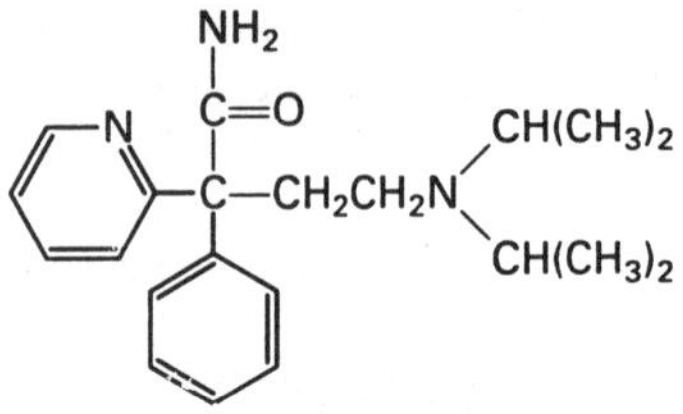

Pharmacodynamics *Cardiovascular System* The ERP of the atrium and the ERP of the ventricle are prolonged with therapeutic doses of disopyramide. Unlike quinidine, disopyramide has little effect on impulse conduction through the AV node, bundle of His, and Purkinje fibers and consequently little effect on PR or QT intervals or on QRS duration. However, prolongation of conduction occurs in accessary pathways. In addition, recommended oral doses of the drug rarely produce significant reductions in blood pressure in patients without congestive heart failure.

Autonomic Nervous System Disopyramide has relatively more anticholinergic activity than quinidine. Oral disopyramide has no effect on resting sinus rhythm, but it is likely that the anticholinergic actions have a role in the activity of this drug at the AV node. These anticholinergic actions are also responsible for the gastrointestinal and urogenital side effects cited below.

Pharmacokinetics Orally administered disopyramide is rapidly and almost completely absorbed from the gastrointestinal tract. Peak plasma levels are attained within 2 h of a single oral dose. Therapeutic plasma levels are approximately 2 to 4 μg/mL.

Approximately 50 to 65 percent of the drug is bound to plasma proteins. The average half-life of disopyramide is about 7 h, with an apparent volume of distribution of about 0.8 L/kg. In patients with impaired renal function, the serum half-life is prolonged, ranging from 8 to 18 h. About one-half of a disopyramide dose is excreted unchanged in the urine, about 25 percent appears as the mono-N-dealkylated product, and the remainder appears as other products. The major biotransformation product of disopyramide is approximately 25 percent as active biologically as the parent compound and is present in the blood at about 10 percent of the concentration of the parent compound. Excretion is via the urine.

Therapeutic Uses Oral disopyramide is indicated for the treatment of documented ventricular arrhythmias that are considered life-threatening; the drug is not recommended for use in lesser arrhythmias. Due to the proarrhythmic activity of the drug, treatment should be initiated in the hospital. Because of the large contribution of renal excretion to the termination of the drug's action, patients with reduced renal function must be monitored carefully to avoid the adverse effects listed below, and dosing intervals must be adjusted accordingly. This drug is freely dialyzable and presents no elimination problems for the chronic hemodialysis patient.

Adverse Reactions Most often these effects are related to the anticholinergic activity of the drug and include xerostomia, urinary retention, constipation, blurred vision, and reduction in nasal and lacrimal secretions. Other more serious adverse effects, including acute psychoses, cholestatic jaundice, hypoglycemia, and agranulocytosis, are less frequent and reversible upon removal of the drug.

Because disopyramide elevates intraocular pressure, caution should be exercised in patients with narrow angle glaucoma who are using this drug. Likewise, urinary retention may make the drug unsuitable for use in patients with prostatic hypertrophy. Careful attention should be paid to individuals with congestive heart failure who are treated with this drug, since disopyramide may worsen this condition.

Group IB

With the exception of phenytoin, the drugs in this group are chemically related to lidocaine. Actually, they represent oral forms of this primarily parenteral drug.

Lidocaine

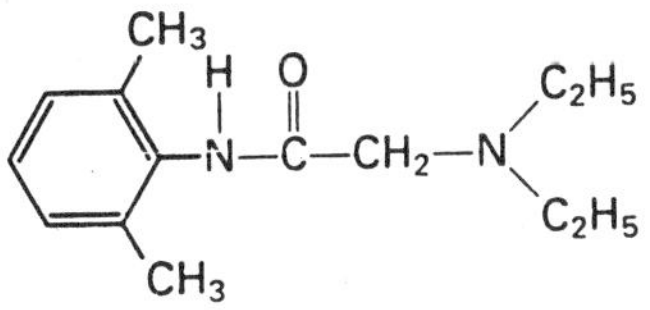

CH_3 H O C_2H_5
—N—C—CH_2—N
C_2H_5
CH_3

Like procainamide, lidocaine is an amide with a local anesthetic effect. The chemistry of lidocaine and its effects on most organ systems are discussed in Chapter 25 ("Local Anesthetics").

Pharmacodynamics Lidocaine and its oral congeners differ substantially from the group IA drugs with respect to action on the sodium channel. Lidocaine is a true local anesthetic with a pK_a and lipophilic quality to penetrate membranes easily. Furthermore, its action is more easily reversible than quinidine and other group IA drugs. Consequently, its ability to affect inactivated blocked sodium channels is greater than that of the group IA drugs (see explanation above, under "Gating Mechanisms"). Since in ischemic myocytes the proportion of blocked to unblocked sodium channels is greater than in nonischemic myocytes, lidocaine and its relatives have a greater effect in myocytes deprived of oxygen. This makes lidocaine and other group IB antiarrhythmic drugs most suitable in cases of acute myocardial infarction and in the recovery period following such injury. Furthermore, lidocaine does not lengthen repolarization and thus is inherently less apt to cause torsade de pointes. This fits in nicely with the fact that lidocaine is of most utility in ventricular tachyarrhythmias associated with myocardial infarction (ischemia) and those of digitalis toxicity.

Although it is the least arrhythmogenic of all drugs used for this purpose, lidocaine is still toxic to the circulation because it depresses contractility and may cause excessive vasodilation. Attention to proper dosage and blood levels is important.

Pharmacokinetics Because of its extensive (70 percent) first-pass biotransformation, lidocaine is not given by the oral route. When used as an antiarrhythmic drug, lidocaine is administered almost exclusively via the intravenous route by intermittent bolus or continuous infusion. In emergencies it may be given intramuscularly. The half-life of lidocaine in plasma ranges from 1 to 2 h, but the actual duration of action is shorter (approximately 0.25 h) because the parent compound is redistributed rapidly out of the plasma to other tissues. Lidocaine is well distributed despite the fact that its binding to plasma proteins is in the range of 60 percent. It is concentrated in many tissues relative to the plasma, including heart muscle. Rapid biotransformation and redistribution of the drug cause the concentration in tissues to fall rapidly after a single dose. The liver is the primary site of biotransformation; the hepatic microsomal enzyme system produces at least two active products: monoethylglycinexylidide and glycinexylidide, which have antiarrhythmic and convulsant activities. Only about 5 to 10 percent of a dose is excreted in the urine without undergoing biotransformation. Plasma concentrations higher than expected can occur when usual doses are given to individuals with severe impairment of hepatic function.

Therapeutic Uses Lidocaine disappears rapidly from the plasma compartment as it is redistributed to other tissues. A steady-state plasma concentration is quickly reached, however, using a continuous, constant rate of infusion, and this is the mode of administration most frequently employed. It is imperative that the infusion rate be meticulously controlled to avoid ineffective or toxic concentrations. Therapeutic plasma concentrations range from 1 to 5 μg/mL. Lidocaine is usually administered intravenously for the short-term therapy of life-threatening ventricular arrhythmias such as those which may accompany myocardial infarction, and for ventricular arrhythmias which may arise during surgical manipulation of the heart.

Adverse Reactions Most untoward effects of lidocaine are related to the central nervous system and are believed to be due to the two active biotransformation products noted above. The undesirable effects can be seen at plasma lidocaine concentrations of above 6 μg/mL. They include dizziness, excitement, drowsiness, psychosis, confusion, euphoria, and seizures. Respiratory acidosis and alkalosis, nausea, and vomiting may also occur. In normal therapeutic doses, hypotension, heart block, and sinoatrial arrest have been reported.

Drug Interactions The half-life of lidocaine is prolonged when used simultaneously with β-adrenergic blocking drugs probably as a result of altered hepatic blood flow reducing the biotransformation of lidocaine. Cimetidine decreases the clearance of lidocaine and enhances its activity. Like quinidine and procainamide, lidocaine interacts with certain neuromuscular blocking agents, enhancing their activity. Procainamide and lidocaine have an additive effect on the cardiovascular system and the central nervous system.

Tocainide and Mexiletine

Both of these drugs are close chemical congeners of lidocaine. Both compounds have electrophysiologic properties and cardiac effects that are qualitatively similar to lidocaine. They differ from lidocaine in that they are orally active.

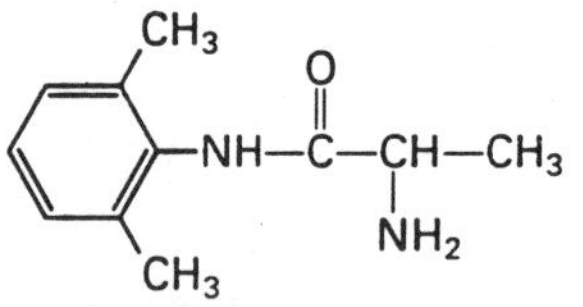

CH3, CH3 — NH—C(=O)—CH(NH2)—CH3

Tocainide

CH3, CH3 — O—CH2—CH(NH2)—CH3

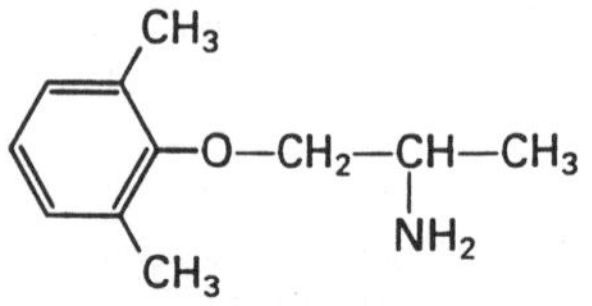

Mexiletine

Pharmacokinetics The oral bioavailability of both drugs is excellent (90 to 95 percent), and both avoid the first-pass effect that occurs with lidocaine. Tocainide is only 10 percent bound to plasma proteins and has a half-life of 11 to 15 h. Plasma protein binding of mexiletine is 50 to 60 percent and its half-life is 10 to 12 h. Therapeutic plasma levels of tocainide and mexiletine are 4 to 10 μg/mL and 0.5 to 2 μg/mL, respectively. Tocainide has no cardioactive metabolites, whereas mexiletine is converted to several products with minimal antiarrhythmic activity; 25 to 55 percent of tocainide and only 10 percent of mexiletine is excreted unchanged in the urine.

Clinical Use Both drugs are indicated for life-threatening ventricular arrhythmias such as sustained ventricular tachycardia. They are ineffective in supraventricular arrhythmias. In practice, these drugs find the most usage as replacements to IV lidocaine therapy with oral therapy in patients with post-myocardial infarction accompanied by symptomatic ventricular arrhythmias.

Adverse Reactions Both drugs have all the cardiovascular toxicities of lidocaine, including worsening of arrhythmias, conduction disturbances, hypotension, and cardiogenic shock. Gastrointestinal adverse effects include nausea, vomiting, heartburn, and diarrhea; CNS effects include dizziness, tremor, nervousness, and paresthesias. Skin rash, arthralgia, and blood dyscrasias (e.g., leukopenia, neutropenia, agranulocytosis, bone marrow depression) have also been reported with both compounds. Tocainide has also been associated with pulmonary toxicity (e.g., fibrosis, interstitial pneumonitis, and pulmonary edema) and increased ANA titers (much less than with procainamide). Due to the toxicity profile, it is doubtful that these drugs are actually more tolerable than quinidine or procainamide in long-term usage.

Phenytoin

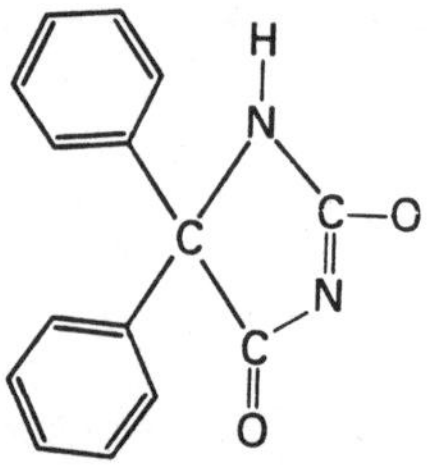

H, N, C—O, N, C, O, C

The chemistry of phenytoin and effects on most organ systems are discussed in Chapter 22. The major effects of phenytoin on the heart are similar to those of lidocaine. Actually its activity is limited, and it has been useful only because oral substitutes for lidocaine have not been available until recently. Its many adverse reactions do not favor its use in preference to the lidocaine substitutes which are orally bioavailable. Phenytoin has been useful in digitalis-induced arrhythmias, however, the more intelligent use of digitalis has supplanted even this use.

Group IC

This subset of sodium-channel blockers is the most powerful of the series presumably because they have a more marked effect on depolarization (see Table 28-1).

Flecainide

Chemically flecainide is a fluorinated congener of procainamide; it is created by insertion of trifluoroethoxy groups on positions 2 and 5 of the benzene ring. The side chain ends in a piperidine ring. These changes alter the pharmacologic effects of procainamide considerably, but flecainide retains its local anesthetic and sodium-channel blocking activity.

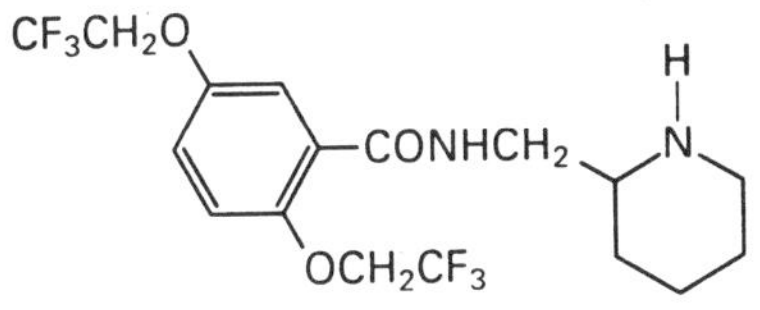

CF_3CH_2O — CONHCH$_2$ — N(H) piperidine — OCH_2CF_3

Electrophysiology Depolarization is markedly slowed, whereas repolarization is only slightly affected; consequently, responsiveness is reduced and conduction is slowed. The greatest effect occurs on the His-Purkinje system. The refractory period of normal myocytes is not significantly affected, except in the ventricle where the drug modestly increases the refractory period. High doses of flecainide may produce conduction defects such as prolonged atrial-His and His-ventricular intervals, i.e., various degrees of heart block. Generally, PR and QRS intervals are increased even with therapeutic doses. The J-T interval (measured from the end of the QRS complex to the end of T wave and equivalent to the QT interval), is insignificantly prolonged as might be expected from the mild effects on repolarization. As with other local anesthetics, these changes in membrane actions are more marked in ischemic myocytes, as compared to normal tissue. Thus we have the picture of a powerful antiarrhythmic agent, but one which also is potentially quite toxic.

Cardiovascular Effects Cardiac performance is depressed as shown by increases in pulmonary capillary wedge pressure and left ventricular end-systolic volume. Heart rate, blood pressure, and pulmonary vascular resistance ordinarily do not change. Where there is a reduced left ventricular ejection fraction, further depression must be expected. Consequent to the depressive actions, new or worsened heart failure occurs in 5 percent of patients receiving flecainide. In patients who already have considerable heart failure, flecainide therapy can be safely administered only in the hospital, with continuous cardiac monitoring.

Pharmacokinetics Oral bioavailability of the drug is 95 percent with peak plasma levels in 2 to 4 h. The plasma half-life is about 20 h. Plasma protein binding is 30 to 40 percent. A significant fraction of a single dose is biotransformed to weakly active or inactive products; about 95 percent is excreted in urine as flecainide and metabolites. Dosage must be reduced in patients with renal disease. Therapeutic plasma levels are from 0.2 to 1.0 μg/mL, which is associated with a 90 percent suppression of PVCs. Plasma levels above 0.7 μg/mL are associated with a greater rate of cardiac adverse effects and these show a good correlation with adverse ECG changes.

Therapeutic Uses Flecainide is used primarily for severe ventricular arrhythmias, such as sustained ventricular tachycardia. The drug is also indicated for the prevention paroxysmal atrial fibrillation or flutter and a variety of supraventricular tachycardias with disabling symptoms. Due to a number of severe adverse effects, flecainide is not recommended for use in patients with less severe ventricular arrhythmias.

Adverse Reactions As with most local anesthetics, CNS symptoms such as dizziness, tremor, fatigue, and paresthesias can occur. Dyspnea, blurred vision, headache, and nausea are common adverse effects.

The provocation of congestive heart failure is uncommon. Ventricular proarrhythmic effects (e.g., PVCs, ventricular tachycardia, ventricular fibrillation) are highest in patients with atrial fibrillation or flutter. In addition, an increase in mortality was reported in patients who had a myocardial infarction and were later treated with flecainide for asymptomatic non-life-threatening ventricular arrhythmias.

Propafenone

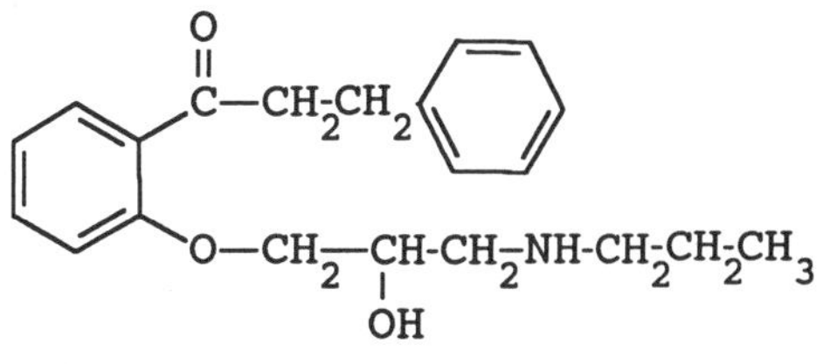

C(=O)—CH_2CH_2—phenyl; O—CH_2—CH(OH)—CH_2—NH—$CH_2CH_2CH_3$

Electrophysiology The spectrum of activity of this antiarrhythmic drug resembles that of the other IC agents. Propafenone exerts its effect primarily on the fast inward sodium channel, but it also has weak β-adrenergic blocking and calcium channel blocking properties. Conduction time through the AV node and the His-Purkinje system is prolonged. The ERP of the AV node is prolonged, but atrial refractory periods are not affected. Effects on the ECG are manifested as a prolongation of the PR interval and of the QRS complex; however, QT_c interval does not change. In patients with Wolff-Parkinson-White (WPW) syndrome, conduction in accessory pathways in both directions is slowed and ERP is prolonged.

Pharmacokinetics Propafenone is well absorbed after oral administration and reaches peak plasma levels in about 3.5 h. The drug undergoes first-past metabolism in the liver and therapeutic plasma concentrations are highly variable, from 0.2 to 3.0 μg/mL. Propafenone is extensively biotransformed and two active products have been identified: 5-hydroxypropafenone and N-depropylpropafenone. Due to genetic differences in metabolism (slow and fast hydroxylators), doses must be individualized. Steady state levels of the parent drug and metabolites are approached in 4 to 5 days.

Therapeutic Uses The approved use of this compound is only for life-threatening ventricular arrhythmias, such as sustained ventricular tachycardia, but it suppresses ventricular and supraventricular arrhythmias, including those of the WPW syndrome.

Adverse Reactions Proarrhythmiac effects of propafenone may not be as frequent as with flecainide. Propafenone has a negative inotropic effect and may increase peripheral vascular resistance. Other common adverse effects are chiefly gastrointestinal, including nausea and vomiting, abdominal discomfort, constipation, dyspepsia, and alteration in taste or smell. Dizziness, headache, blurred vision and dyspnea are also common untoward effects. Because of its negative inotropic effect, propafenone is contraindicated in patients with a history of congestive heart failure. Depressed left ventricular cardiac function and bronchial asthma are relative contraindications to its use.

Drug interactions include substantial increases in serum digoxin levels, increased plasma levels and effects of β-adrenergic blockers, and increased plasma levels and anticoagulant effects of warfarin. Cimetidine and quinidine may increase the plasma concentration of propafenone, possibly enhancing its pharmacologic effects.

Moricizine

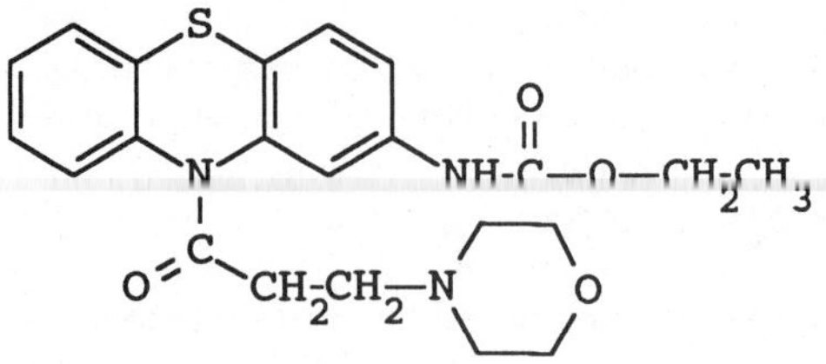

S
O
N NH-C—O—CH_2CH_3
C
O CH$_2$CH$_2$—N O

Chemically, moricizine is a phenothiazine derivative originally developed in the Soviet Union; it has no central or peripheral dopaminergic activity. The drug is effective for the treatment of both ventricular and supraventricular arrhythmias, but the recently approved clinical use in the USA is only for the management of ventricular arrhythmias that are judged to be life-threatening. It has electrophysiologic effects in common with lidocaine-like Class IB agents, but it also prolongs the PR and QRS intervals, while leaving the QT interval relatively unchanged. It blocks the fast inward sodium channel but does not prolong action potential duration. Therefore, moricizine may represent a "mixed" Class IB/IC agent.

After oral administration, there is significant first-pass metabolism in the liver. The compound induces its own biotransformation, which is extensive, but active metabolites are not important for its action. Plasma protein binding is approximately 95 percent. The plasma half-life is between 1.5 and 3.5 h. About 60 percent is excreted in the feces and the remainder in the urine; some enterohepatic recirculation occurs.

Generally, during oral therapy, side effects are mild and include dizziness, fatigue, headache, nausea, cardiac palpitations, and dyspnea. Similar to other drugs, moricizine has proarrhythmic effects. It has only mildly depressant effects on left ventricular function, thus may be less likely to worsen congestive heart failure. More information on adverse effects are required to determine whether this drug really is better tolerated than flecainide and propafenone.

GROUP II DRUGS

Beta-Adrenergic Blockers

In that all β-adrenergic blocking agents decrease stimulatory sympathetic nervous impulses and endogenous catecholamine influences on the heart, they are inhibitory of both supraventricular and ventricular tachyarrhythmias. However, only propranolol, esmolol, and acebutolol have FDA approval for use as antiarrhythmic drugs. The complete pharmacology of β-adrenergic blocking agents blockers is covered in Chapter 9 and only the features that relate to their antiarrhythmic activity is discussed here.

Propranolol has been studied most extensively both experimentally and clinically. Unlike the majority of β-adrenergic blocking agents available, propranolol has considerable membrane stabilizing activity (MSA). Although once believed to be responsible for the antiarrhythmic actions of these drugs, MSA appears to occur only at high doses that exceed those used clinically. Thus responsiveness and conduction velocity of most cardiac tissues are not greatly affected by propranolol. Some effect on potassium efflux is evident even at low doses.

Suppression of automaticity at the SA and AV nodes is a major action of these drugs. Sinus heart rate is decreased when sympathetic stimulation is high as in emotional states or in exercise. Suppression of automaticity of Purkinje fibers can also be demonstrated. Although the β-adrenergic blockers have little effect on the ERP and APD of most cardiac tissues, the increased ERP of the AV node is the basis for the use of these drugs as antiarrhythmics.

It must be emphasized also that propranolol and other β-adrenergic blockers can control arrhythmias by the relief of ischemia by lessening oxygen demand of the heart.

As might be expected, propranolol finds most utility for the control of supraventricular arrhythmias. Atrial premature beats are usually controlled by propranolol alone. In combination with digitalis, propranolol has been used for the control of atrial flutter and fibrillation. Here, however, the end object is not the conversion of the arrhythmia but the slowing of the ventricular rate. In cases refractory to digitalis alone, the addition of propranolol permits sufficient slowing of the ventricular rate apparently by further increasing the refractory period of AV conduction.

In perioperative, postoperative, and other emergency situations, esmolol, a short-acting β-adrenergic blocker that is only administered intravenously, can be used for the rapid control of ventricular rate in patients with atrial fibrillation or atrial flutter. Esmolol is also indicated for noncompensatory sinus tachycardia where rapid heart rate demands intercession.

The combination of quinidine and propranolol to convert atrial fibrillation to sinus rhythm may work when quinidine alone fails. Similarly, control of WPW syndrome may be achieved by this combination. In this case, not only is supraventricular tachyarrhythmia suppressed, but also the increase in refractory period of the AV nodal area prevents ventricular tachyarrhythmias by suppressing reentry pathways.

Ventricular tachyarrhythmias usually do not respond to propranolol alone. Premature ventricular contractions which occur in the absence of demonstrated heart disease are well controlled and often, even if not suppressed, become asymptomatic. Indeed, acebutolol is only approved for the management of PVCs. Tachyarrhythmias as a result of hyperthyroidism and sympathetic stimulation of the heart are usually well controlled by propranolol, and digitalis-induced tachyarrhythmias can be treated with this drug.

Beta-adrenergic blockers are often prescribed in ischemic heart disease for they have been proven to decrease mortality especially post-myocardial infarction. They are not a contraindication to the use of other antiarrhythmic agents.

GROUP III DRUGS

Amiodarone

Chemically, amiodarone is quite different from other antiarrhythmics. It has a benzofuranyl cyclic ring with a hydrocarbon chain in addition to the usual benzene ring. The latter with iodine substitutes and chain structure is faintly reminiscent of a thyroxine-like molecule.

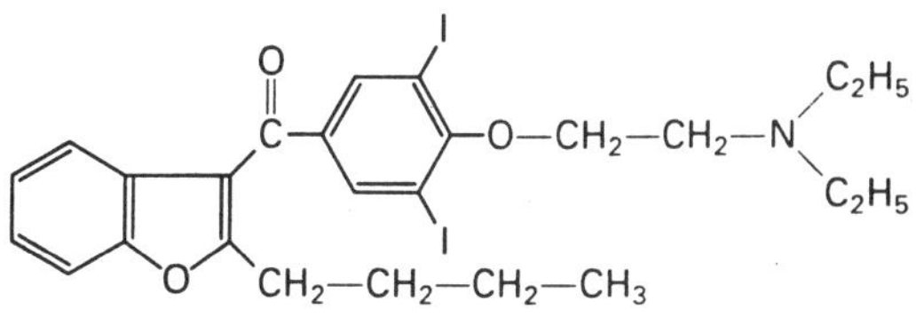

Electrophysiology The electrophysiologic effects of amiodarone are unique and complex. The drug is a powerful blocker of sodium channels and it differs from quinidine in being most effective in the channels which are in the inactivated state. Thus, it primarily affects tissues with long action potentials. The main result is a prolongation of APD and ERP in all cardiac tissues, including the bypass tracts. The prolongation of the APD is much greater than that seen with the Class IA drugs. Automaticity is depressed, and conduction through all tissues is moderately slowed. These are ancillary effects that probably relate to other properties of the drug. In addition to its primary action to block sodium channels, amiodarone has a β-adrenergic blocking effect, weak calcium-channel blocking activity, and may also block potassium channels. As a consequence of these complex actions the ECG may show a decrease of sinus rate, slowing of AV conduction, and slight increases of PR and QRS duration; however, the most marked action is prolongation of the QT interval.

Pharmacokinetics The complex pharmacokinetics of amiodarone contribute to the difficulty of its use. The orally administered drug is absorbed slowly and variably, averaging about a 50 percent bioavailability. Peak plasma concentrations are observed 3 to 7 h after a single dose. The onset of action may occur in 2 to 3 days; more commonly, a 1 to 3 week lag occurs between the achievement of an adequate blood level of 1 to 2 μg/mL and observable clinical effects. The volume of distribution is very large, averaging 60 L/kg, due to accumulation in adipose tissue and in those tissues with a high rate of perfusion (liver, lung, and spleen). The drug is biotransformed in the liver; one major metabolite exists: desmethylamiodarone. The contribution of the metabolite to the antiarrhythmic action of the parent drug is not known. Amiodarone has a very long plasma half-life, averaging more than 50 days, which fits in with its tissue accumulation. Elimination is mainly by biliary excretion, with negligible removal by the urine. After discontinuance of the drug, the antiarrhythmic effects may persist for weeks or months.

Because of these unusual pharmacokinetic parameters, amiodarone requires large loading doses (500 to 1600 mg for 1 to 3 weeks), which are then gradually adjusted to a maintenance daily dose of 400 mg.

Therapeutic Uses Both supraventricular and ventricular arrhythmias often respond to this compound when other antiarrhythmic drugs fail. The drug has been used in a variety of arrhythmias including WPW syndrome. However, the clinical use of amiodarone is limited because of its cardiac and extracardiac toxicities and most authorities believe that the drug is too toxic to treat most supraventricular arrhythmias. Amiodarone is indicated only for the therapy of very serious tachyarrhythmias such as recurrent ventricular fibrillation and hemodynamically unstable ventricular tachycardia. Therapy is usually started in a hospital where monitoring and resuscitation facilities are available.

Adverse Reactions Cardiac toxicity consists of bradycardia, heart block, and induction of heart failure. As with other antiarrhythmics, proarrhythmia can be produced. It is the extracardiac effects which actually limit the use of this drug. Potentially fatal toxicities have occurred involving the lung. Cough and progressive dyspnea leading to interstitial/alveolar pneumonitis have occurred in 10 to 15 percent of patients with ventricular arrhythmias; about 10 percent of these cases have resulted in deaths. Hepatic toxicity is generally mild (asymptomatic increase in liver enzymes), but fatalities due to hepatocellular necrosis have occurred.

Amiodarone induces lipofuscin deposits as microcrystals in various tissues. These are visible in the cornea as yellow brown granules which rarely cause visual disturbances, except as a halo effect at night in peripheral vision. On discontinuation of the drug, they slowly resolve over weeks to months. The deposition of crystals also occurs in the skin resulting in a grayish-blue skin discoloration. This causes photosensitivity, and the sun must be avoided.

Less serious adverse reactions are constipation and peripheral neuropathy. Paradoxically amiodarone may cause either hyperthyroidism (possibly due to iodine overload when the drug is metabolized) or hypothyroidism (which probably results from amiodarone's ability to inhibit the conversion of T_4 to T_3. The thyroid function must be monitored, particularly in patients with previous history of thyroid dysfunction.

Drug Interactions Amiodarone interacts with many other cardiac drugs. When administered together with either warfarin, digoxin, quinidine, procainamide, or phenytoin, the activity of these drugs is increased.

Bretylium

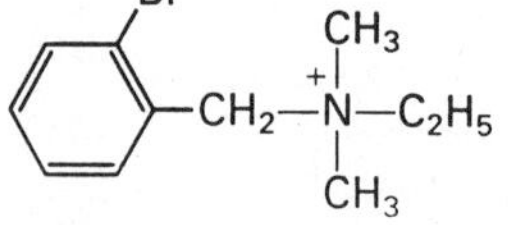

Br

CH_3

$-CH_2-N^{+}-C_2H_5$

CH_3

This agent is unique in being a quaternary amine. As such it is poorly absorbed orally and is used only as an intravenous or intramuscular agent.

Like many quaternary amines, bretylium first initiates release of neuronal catecholamines, then inhibits it. This, however, is not its main antiarrhythmic action. In fact, the initial release of catecholamines can increase heart rate and blood pressure and may precipitate arrhythmias. Bretylium has a direct action, especially on ischemic myocytes, where the APD and ERP are lengthened. Conduction and responsiveness are not affected. Automaticity of the SA node and of ectopic foci is suppressed. The ECG shows decreased sinus rate and slightly increased PR and QT intervals.

Oral bioavailability of bretylium is poor. Peak plasma concentrations are seen within 1 h of intramuscular administration. However, suppression of premature beats may not be seen until 6 to 9 h after drug administration. Intravenous administration results in immediate antiarrhythmic effects, but generally suppression of ventricular tachycardia may take 20 min to several hours to be clearly manifested. The elimination half-life is usually between 7 and 8 h. The drug is not biotransformed; elimination of the unchanged drug is mainly via the kidney.

Bretylium is an emergency drug which is used in situations where other procedures and drugs have failed. It is clearly of utility only in life-threatening ventricular tachyarrhythmias and there on an emergency basis.

Adverse reactions to bretylium may consist of transient hypertension with tachycardia, followed by postural hypotension. Dizziness, lightheadedness, and syncope may occur. Nausea and vomiting are commonly induced by rapid intravenous infusion. Initial worsening of arrhythmias may occur, and precipitation of anginal pain is a possibility.

Sotalol

Sotalol is a β-adrenergic blocking agent that is placed into the Group III category because it increases the duration of the action potential and prolongs the ERP by a mechanism unrelated to its nonselective β-adrenergic receptor blocking action. Sotalol inhibits repolarizing potassium currents. On the ECG, sotalol prolongs the PR and QT intervals without QRS prolongation.

Sotalol is rapidly and completely absorbed after oral administration and does not undergo first-pass metabolism. The plasma half-life is about 12 to 18 h after long term therapy. The drug is not extensively metabolized and is excreted unchanged in the urine. Thus, in the presence of renal disease, dosage should be lowered.

Sotalol is used to prevent the reoccurrence of arrhythmias in patients with life-threatening ventricular arrhythmias. It is reported to be as effective as procainamide in suppressing PVCs. Since sotalol recently was approved by the FDA for the same therapeutic indications as amiodarone, and because it is less toxic, it may become a drug of choice for life-threatening arrhythmias.

The adverse effects related to β-adrenergic blockade are similar to those observed with other β-blockers (tiredness, lassitude, impotence, depression and headache) but because of poor lipid solubility, the drug does not enter the CNS readily and CNS effects are less. Adverse effects related to its Group III properties include AV block, bradycardia, hypotension and worsening of heart failure. The incidence of proarrhythmias with sotalol appears low.

GROUP IV DRUGS

Verapamil and Diltiazem

The calcium-channel blockers are of greater utility in supraventricular tachyarrhythmias where the slow calcium current has a greater influence on the action potential of nodal myocytes as compared with that of ventricular myocytes. The sinus rate is slowed, and the ERP of atrial myocytes and the AV node is prolonged. Thus calcium-channel blockers can effectively suppress atrial tachycardia. Also, by increasing AV nodal conduction time and refractoriness, they can very effectively suppress the ventricular rate in atrial flutter and fibrillation. For these purposes the calcium-channel blockers have either supplemented or replaced digoxin, propranolol, and even cardioversion for these arrhythmias. Furthermore, except in patients with congestive heart failure or in those receiving other myocardial depressants, the negative inotropic effect of these compounds is not pronounced at therapeutic doses.

Verapamil has been the preferred agent in this category, but diltiazem is also effective. Although large oral doses of verapamil have been effective in reducing AV nodal reentrant tachycardia, both drugs are only approved for use in treating tachyarrhythmias by the intravenous route. Other calcium-channel blockers have little or no antiarrhythmic activity. The complete pharmacology of these agents is discussed in Chapter 29.

MISCELLANEOUS GROUP

Adenosine

This endogenous nucleoside does not fit the classification of antiarrhythmic drugs thus far presented.

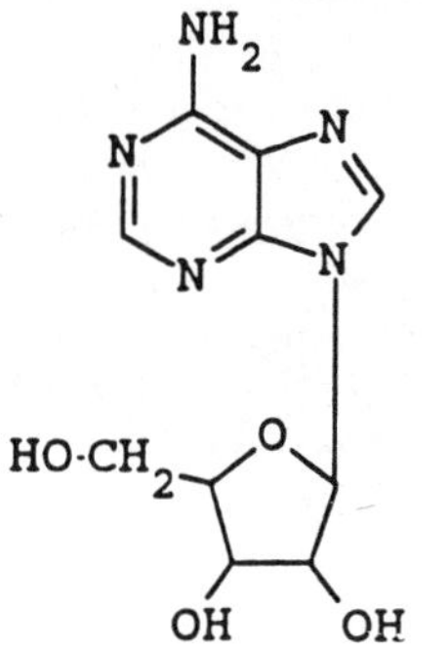

Pharmacodynamics Adenosine has very specific actions and is clearly not a β-adrenergic blocking agent, calcium-channel or sodium-channel blocker. The mechanism of its antiarrhythmic action is not completely understood. Specific receptors for adenosine exist throughout the body (subtypes: A_1 and A_2, also called P_1-purinergic receptors). Upon combination with these receptors, adenosine acts as a agonist with the response dependant on the receptor subtype and tissue involved. Other drugs which interact with adenosine receptors, such as caffeine and theophylline, are competitive antagonists of adenosine.

A potent coronary and peripheral vasodilator, adenosine has also other systemic actions including bronchoconstriction, decreased glomerular filtration rate and decreased renal blood flow, increased steroidogenesis, and effects on the CNS such as depressed neurotransmission and neuronal firing. Some investigators consider adenosine to have a hormonal function in the body.

Adenosine depresses the upstroke of the action potential of AV node "N" cells, depresses sinus node automaticity, and prolongs AV nodal conduction time resulting in bradycardia. There is no major effect on ventricular conduction or excitation.

Pharmacokinetics Following an intravenous bolus injection, adenosine is rapidly taken up by erythrocytes and vascular endothelial cells resulting in a plasma half-life of less than 10 seconds. The compound is metabolized to inosine and adenosine monophosphate through the normal pathways of nucleoside metabolism.

Therapeutic Use At the proper dose, adenosine has actions restricted to the heart and blood vessels. The advantage of adenosine is its rapid onset of action combined with a remarkably short plasma half-life. This allows for rapid treatment of an arrhythmia while any adverse reactions of the drug are dispelled in a very brief time. The short duration of effect also permits additional doses to be given, if necessary, without drug accumulation.

The only indication for adenosine is conversion of paroxysmal supraventricular tachycardia including that associated with WPW syndrome to sinus rhythm. The efficiency of adenosine in arresting supraventricular tachycardia is 90 to 100%. Adenosine has no effect on atrial flutter or fibrillation (in fact, it may precipitate them) or ventricular arrhythmias. As a prophylactic antiarrhythmic drug, adenosine has no value because of its short plasma half-life and because it must be given by intravenous administration. Other uses for adenosine are being intensively investigated.

Adverse Effects Adverse reactions are generally mild. Common adverse effects include facial flushing, dyspnea, chest pressure, headache, lightheadedness, and nausea. More severe, but less common, untoward events include various degrees of heart block and several types of arrhythmias.

CLINICAL ASPECTS OF ANTIARRHYTHMIC THERAPY

Very few therapies match antiarrhythmic drug therapy with respect to the capacity to accurately pinpoint physiologic and anatomic defects and to select specific agents or devices for correction. Unfortunately, all antiarrhythmic drug therapy treats symptoms and not the cause of the membrane aberration which precipitates the arrhythmia. Therefore, the first guiding principle is to treat the cause rather than the symptoms. Since a great majority of arrhythmias are the result of ischemia, oxygen therapy, heart failure therapy, and attention to respiratory difficulties are the first line of attack. Ultimately surgical correction (coronary angioplasty, bypass surgery, etc.) may be needed. Drugs which aid the coronary circulation such as β-adrenergic blockers and nitrites have been shown to reduce mortality, and none of the many antiarrhythmic drugs have this distinction.

A patient with a tachyarrhythmia will surely die unless the arrhythmia stops spontaneously or is arrested by medical or surgical interventions.

TABLE 28-3 Therapy of Tachyarrhythmias

Arrhythmia	Drug or other therapy
Tachyarrhythmias requiring immediate therapy to prevent sudden death (in ascending order of urgency)	
Atrial tachycardia	Verapamil, digitalis, β-blockers, adenosine
Atrial flutter	Verapamil, digitalis, β-blockers, sodium-channel blockers
Wolff-Parkinson-White with ventricular tachycardia	Sodium-channel blockers, especially group IC; in desperate cases amiodarone, ablation of accessory pathway by catheter cautery
Ventricular tachycardia	Sodium-channel blockers, sotalol, bretylium, cardioversion, surgical removal of ectopic focus
Ventricular fibrillation	Cardioversion with or without the prior use of drugs followed by prophylactic drug therapy, usually sodium-channel blockers and, in refractory cases, amiodarone
Tachyarrhythmias which are treated for the relief of symptoms and with the expectation that sudden death will be prevented	
Wolff-Parkinson-White without ventricular tachycardia	Any group IA drugs such as quinidine or disopyramide
Frequent atrial premature beats	Propranolol or other β-blockers and verapamil or diltiazem
Ventricular premature beats Frequent with symptoms	Any of group I drugs Quinidine, disopyramide, tocainide, and flecainide. With myocardial infarction, group IB drugs are favored, lidocaine and congeners.
Ventricular tachycardia (unsustained)	Any of group I drugs which can be tolerated and which significantly reduce incidence. Group IC drugs are the most effective but also the most toxic.

The tachyarrhythmias which require immediate intervention in ascending order of urgency are shown in Table 28-3. Those arrhythmias which are frequently treated because they cause symptoms or because it is felt that therapy will be prophylactic against sudden death are also shown in Table 28-3.

The currently available technology has refined antiarrhythmic therapy so that selection of the proper drug or procedure may depend on sophisticated diagnostic procedures such as clinical electrophysiologic testing. At the least, the minimal requirement to effectively prescribe antiarrhythmic therapy requires ECG rhythm monitoring both in and out of the hospital. In addition, most antiarrhythmic drugs have a narrow therapeutic range, and, in many cases, maintenance of plasma levels spells the difference between success, failure, and toxicity. This assumes that qualified laboratories are available. In addition, the fragile nature of rhythm maintenance in sick hearts requires that resuscitative measures be accessible at all times. Devices which are worn by the patient and continuously monitor the rhythm of the heart and diagnose the onset of a dangerous tachyarrhythmia, as well as immediately apply cardioversion, have been devised. The efficacy of these devices in preventing sudden death is being compared to that of drugs.

BIBLIOGRAPHY

Anderson, G.J.: "Antiarrhythmic Actions of Amiodarone," *Am. Fam. Physician* **25**: 178-180 (1982).

Anderson, J.L.: "Effectiveness of Sotalol for Therapy of Complex, Ventricular Arrhythmias and Comparisons with Placebo and Class I Antiarrhythmic Drugs," *Am. J. Cardiol.* **65**: 37A-42A (1990).

DiPalma, J.R., and J. Schultz: "Antifibrillatory Drugs," *Medicine* **29**: 123-168 (1950).

DiPalma, J.R., and G.J. Anderson: "Premature Beats", in R.E. Rakel (ed.), *Conn's Current Therapy*, Saunders, Philadelphia, 1984.

DiPalma, J.R.: "Adenosine for Paroxysmal Supraventricular Tachycardia," *Am. Fam. Phys.* **44**: 929-931 (1991).

Fagbemi, S.O, L. Chi, and B.R. Luchesi: "Antifibrillatory and Profibrillatory Actions of Selected Class I Antiarrhythmic Agents," *J. Cardiovasc. Pharmacol.* **21**: 709-718 (1993).

Grant, A.O.: "On the Mechanism of Action of Antiarrhythmic Agents," *Am. Heart J.* **123**: 1130-1136 (1992).

Grubb, B.P.: "Moricizine: A New Agent for the Treatment of Ventricular Arrhythmias," *Am. J. Med. Sci.* **301**: 398-401 (1991).

Hamer, J.: "Antiarrhythmic Drugs," in J. Hamer (ed.), *Drugs for Heart Diseases, 3rd ed.*, Chapman and Hall, London, 1987, pp. 1-28.

Hearse, D.J., A.S. Manning, and M.J. James: *Life-Threatening Arrhythmias During Ischemia and Infarction*, Raven Press, New York, 1987.

Miller, R.H., and J.C. Scherer: "Ventricular Arrhythmias: Assessment of Risk for Sudden Cardiac Death and Current Treatment Options," *Hosp. Formul.* **27**: 617-635 (1992).

Morganroth, J.: "Proarrhythmic Effects of Antiarrhythmic Drugs: Evolving Concepts," *Am. Heart J.* **123**: 1137-1139 (1992).

Muhiddin, K.A., and P. Turner: "Is There an Ideal Antiarrhythmic Drug? A Review—With Particular Reference to Class I Antiarrhythmic Agents," *Postgrad. Med. J.* **61**: 665-678 (1985).

Nestico, P.F., and J. Morganroth: "Flecainide: A New Antiarrhythmic Agent," *Am. Fam. Physician* **34**: 197-200 (1986).

Noda, M., et al.: "Primary Structure of *Electrophorus electricus* Sodium Channel Deduced from cDNA Sequence", *Nature* **312**: 121-127 (1984).

Noda, M., K. Ikeda, T. Kayano, H. Suzuki, H. Takeshima, M. Kuraski, H. Takahashi, and S. Numa: "Existence of Distinct Sodium Channel Messenger RNAs in Rat Brain," *Nature* **320**: 188-192 (1986).

Pritchett, E.L.C.: "Management of Atrial Fibrillation," *New Engl. J. Med.* **326**: 1264-1271 (1992).

Salkoff, L.B., and M.A. Tanouye: "Genetics of Ion Channels," *Physiol. Rev.* **66**: 301-320 (1986).

Scholtysik, G., and U. Quast: "Sodium Channel Pharmacology in Mammalian Cardiac Cells: Extension by DPI 201-106," *Triangle* **25**: 105-116 (1986).

Singh, B.N.: "Is Class III Antiarrhythmic Activity Important?," *Cardiovasc. Drugs and Ther.* **3 (Suppl)**: 597-602 (1990).

Summitt, J., F. Morady, and A. Kadish: "A Comparison of Standard and High-Dose Regimens for the Initiation of Amiodarone Therapy," *Am. Heart J.* **124**: 366-373 (1992).

Tomaselli, G.F., P.H. Backx, and E. Marban: "Molecular Basis of Permeation in Voltage-Gated Ion Channels," *Circ. Res.* **72**: 491-496 (1993).

Vanerio, G., and J.D. Maloney: "Moricizine: Pharmacodynamic, Pharmacokinetic, and Therapeutic Profile of a New Antiarrhythmic," *Cleve. Clin. J. Med.* **59**: 79-86 (1992).

Vaughan Williams, E.M.: "A Classification of Antiarrhythmic Actions Reassessed after a Decade of New Drugs," *J. Clin. Pharmacol.* **24**: 129-147 (1984).

Vaughan Williams, E.M.: *Antiarrhythmic Action and the Puzzle of Perhexiline*, Academic Press, New York, 1980.

Volosin, K.J., and A.J. Greenspon: "Tocainide: A New Drug for Ventricular Arrhythmias," *Am. Fam. Physician* **33**: 233-235 (1986).

Woosley, R.L., A.J.J. Wood, and D.M. Roden: "Encainide," *N. Engl. J. Med.* **318**: 1107-1115 (1988).

Woosley, R.A.: "Antiarrhythmic Drugs," *Annu. Rev. Pharmacol. Toxicol.* **31**: 427-455 (1991).

CHAPTER 29

Antianginal Drugs

Joanne I. Moore

Angina pectoris, or pain in the chest, is a characteristic painful sensation which is reflective of ischemia of the myocardium. Usually it is precipitated by exercise, excitement, or a heavy meal. It is relieved by rest. This type of angina is classified as fixed, or stable angina, because it occurs under predictable circumstances. The cause is an obstruction in one or more of the major coronary arteries, and the lesion is usually arteriosclerotic. Generally, narrowing of the vessel must be 50 percent or more before any appreciable ischemia occurs.

A second type of angina (so-called variant, or Prinzmetal, angina) is believed to be due to vasospasm. It occurs at rest or even during sleep and is unpredictable or unstable. An individual may have a mixture of both stable and unstable angina.

The heart has no pain fibers. Angina is, therefore, a referred type of pain mediated probably over autonomic nervous system fibers segmentally to the upper thoracic spinal segments. It is usually felt in the left shoulder and arm, the neck, and rarely in the right shoulder. Resection of the cervical sympathetic ganglia relieves the pain. So does any chest operation which disturbs the autonomic innervation of the heart. Sedatives, alcohol, opioids, and various CNS drugs also relieve the pain, but obviously do nothing for the ischemia. The physician must recognize this and treat the ischemia primarily and not simply make the patient more comfortable. In fact, ischemia of the myocardium may occur without pain or any symptoms—so-called *silent ischemia*. It is even more important for the physician to recognize the existence of this type of ischemia by appropriate diagnostic methods and to treat it in order to prevent myocardial infarction and possible sudden death.

The major drugs which have been found useful in the therapy of myocardial ischemia and the relief of the pain of angina pectoris are peripheral vascular and coronary vessel vasodilators. These include the nitrates and nitrites, β-adrenergic blockers and calcium-channel antagonists.

THE NITRATES AND NITRITES

Pharmacologic Classification

This group includes both organic nitrites and organic nitrates. The names and structures of four antianginal compounds are shown in Fig. 29-1. It is believed that all the compounds in this class have a similar mechanism of action. As antianginal agents, the nitrates may be classified into (1) rapidly acting agents used to terminate an attack of angina and (2) agents with prolonged action, which are employed to prevent attacks of angina. Nitroglycerin (glycerol trinitrate) and amyl nitrite are rapidly acting agents with a short duration of action. Other organic nitrates used for prolonged action are erythrityl tetranitrate, isosorbide mononitrate, isosorbide dinitrate, and pentaerythritol tetranitrate. These agents are administered orally to prevent angina attacks. However, isosorbide dinitrate and erythrityl tetranitrate have been administered sublingually to terminate acute attacks and obtain a more prolonged effect.

Mechanism of Action

The consensus today is that organic nitrates are prodrugs which must undergo biotransformation in smooth muscle cells to exert their therapeutic actions (Fig. 29-2). When they react with tissue sulfhydryl groups, inorganic nitrite is released and this then undergoes denitration to form nitric oxide

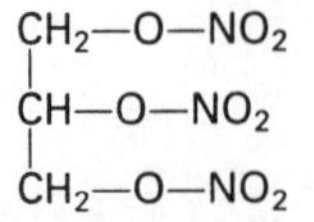

$CH_2—O—NO_2$
$CH—O—NO_2$
$CH_2—O—NO_2$

Nitroglycerin

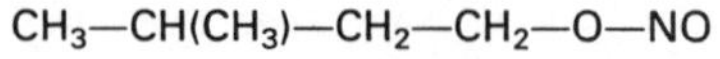

$CH_3—CH(CH_3)—CH_2—CH_2—O—NO$

Amyl nitrite

$O_2N—O—CH_2$ $CH_2—O—NO_2$
C
$O_2N—O—CH_2$ $CH_2—O—NO_2$

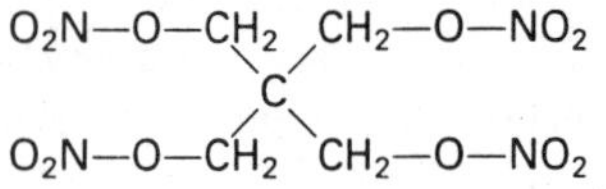

Pentaerythrityl tetranitrate

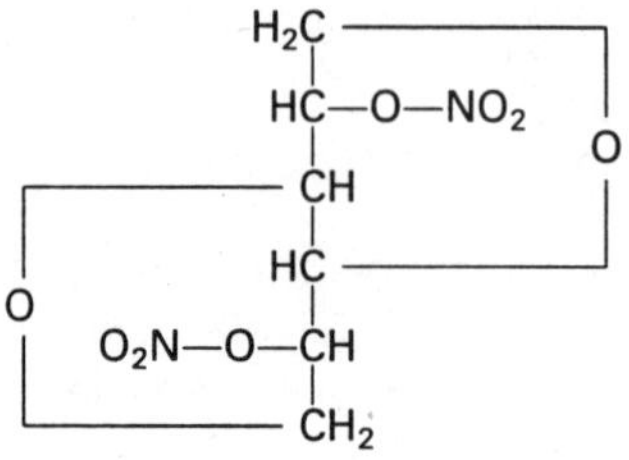

H_2C
$HC—O—NO_2$
O
CH
HC
O
$O_2N—O—CH$
CH_2

Isosorbide dinitrate

FIGURE 29-1 *Chemical structures of some nitrates and amyl nitrite.*

(NO) and a reactive S-nitrosothiol. These short lived, reactive intermediates are capable of activating a cytosolic form of the enzyme guanylate cyclase. Activation of this enzyme stimulates the formation of the intracellular second messenger cyclic guanosine 3′5′-monophosphate (cyclic GMP), proposed to be the mediator of the vascular smooth muscle relaxation produced by organic nitrates. As a result, cyclic GMP-dependent protein kinase is activated, which may lower cytosolic free calcium, resulting in less phosphorylation of muscle protein. Dephosphorylated muscle protein has less capacity to contract. In this manner, nitrates relax all smooth muscle, including that of the biliary system, ureters and bronchioles. However the relaxing action is most active in blood vessels. It is of interest that an endogenous relaxing factor has been identified in endothelial cells lining vascular smooth muscle. This endothelium-derived relaxing factor (EDRF) is thought to play a pivotal role in the regulation of vascular tone and the maintenance of coronary blood flow during increased metabolic demand. EDRF, proposed to be either NO or a closely related nitrosothiol intermediate, diffuses from endothelial cells to vascular smooth muscle cells where it activates guanylate cyclase, generates cyclic GMP, and relaxes vascular smooth muscle. Thus, the effects of the naturally occurring vasodilator, EDRF, are mimicked by the organic nitrates and this mechanism of action is shared with sodium nitroprusside which also releases NO (see Chapter 32).

Dilating the coronary vessels selectively cannot completely explain the beneficial actions of vasodilators. In the stable form of angina, this does not work because the lesion in the vessel forms a rigid structure which is incapable of dilation. Moreover, the coronary circulation always operates under conditions of maximum dilation and responds to ischemia itself as a most powerful stimulus to dilate. Also the vessels not involved with the atherosclerotic lesion, which are capable of dilating, increase the blood flow to normal myocardium, thus relatively decreasing the flow to the ischemic area. This is commonly called *coronary steal* and is actually harmful rather than beneficial. There is one exception. In variant angina the atherosclerotic lesion is only partially developed, and the vessel is capable of spasm. This has been proven by the injection of small amounts of ergonovine into the involved coronary artery under direct visualization during catheterization. This produces spasm in sensitized vessels. Coronary vasodilators relieve this spasm and do benefit the ischemic area.

The consensus of most cardiologists is that it is mainly the effects of vasodilators on the peripheral circulation which produce the beneficial action in angina. This is best considered in terms of the oxygen supply/demand ratio. At each level of work, the heart requires a definite amount of oxygen. Vasodilators reduce peripheral arterial resistance and thus afterload; they also dilate veins and reduce venous return, hence preload. The resulting decrease in left ventricular volume

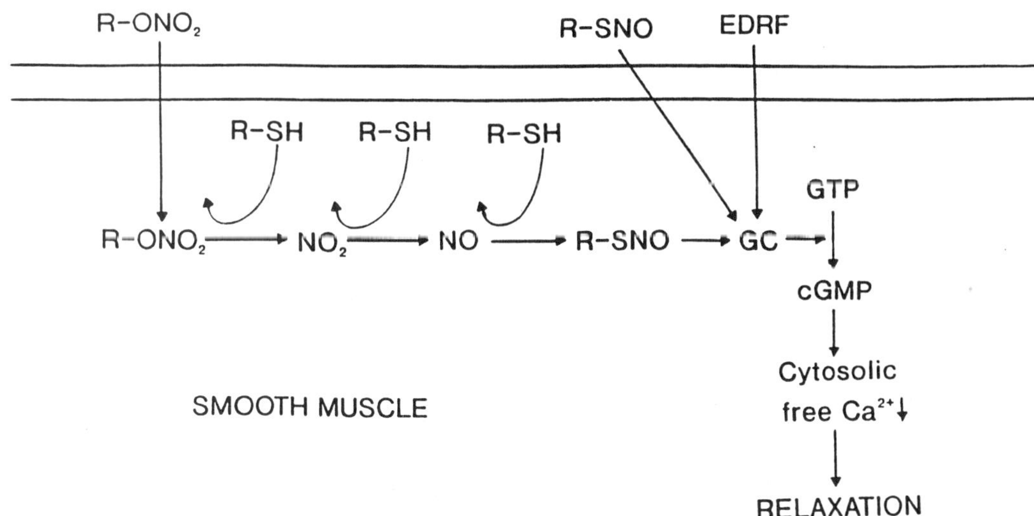

FIGURE 29-2 *Organic nitrates (R-ONO$_2$) undergo denitration to nitric oxide (NO) in vascular and other smooth muscle. Nitric oxide activates the enzyme guanylate cyclase (GC), which induces the formation of cyclic GMP (cGMP). Endothelium-derived relaxing factor (EDRF), which is thought to be NO itself, also activates guanylate cyclase. Thus, this is thought to be the final common pathway for initiating the cellular events leading to smooth muscle relaxation and vasodilation by lowering intracellular Ca^{2+} concentration. Sulfhydryl groups (R-SH) supplied by tissue thiols (e.g., cysteine, glutathione) are required for denitration of the parent compound to nitric oxide. Nitrate tolerance may be related to insufficient tissue supplies of sulfhydryl compounds. It is uncertain if formation of short-lived S-nitrosothiols (R-SNO) are required for activation of guanylate cyclase or if they are formed extracellularly and permeate the membrane to stimulate guanylate cyclase directly.*

makes the heart more efficient. The demand for oxygen is thus reduced at a given level of cardiac output. It may also be said that the vasodilator agents used to relieve angina increase the tolerance of the individual to exercise. As will be seen when other agents are discussed, other factors such as heart rate enter into the equation, but it is important to appreciate that the main thrust in the drug therapy of angina is to reduce the work of the heart to the point where the diseased coronary vessels are still able to supply the required oxygen.

There is, however, considerable evidence that some vasodilator drugs, e.g., the nitrates, directly affect the coronary circulation beneficially. They are particularly effective in vasospastic angina, and there is no doubt about their ability to dilate coronaries as observed by angiography. In animal models, nitrates also increase circulation in the ischemic zone. Nitrates appear to favor the development of collateral circulation and also improve the ratio of endocardial to epicardial flow. The latter is important, since most ischemic areas are more severe in the endocardial zone as compared with the epicardial zone. The direct cardiac effects of nitrates, or indeed any vascular dilator, undoubtedly depend also on individual differences. The number of coronary vessels involved, the degree of development of collateral circulation, and the nature of the arteriosclerotic lesion are all important factors.

Pharmacodynamics

Nitrates have been shown to have a general vasodilator effect. Their action is generally more prominent in the postcapillary vessels, which favors pooling of blood in the systemic peripheral circulation. Venous return is thus consistently decreased and becomes more dependent on positional changes. Nitrates produce relaxation of all vascular smooth muscle, but the magnitude of their effect varies in different vascular beds. In the skin, nitrates produce vasodilation often associated with "flushing" of the skin of the neck and face. This effect is more prominent with amyl nitrite than with the longer-acting compounds.

Nitrates tend to produce tachycardia and reflex increase in contractility, which increases the work of the heart and may reduce its efficiency. In those patients in whom tachycardia is a problem, it is wise to use other antianginal drugs such as β-adrenergic blocking agents and calcium-channel blockers, which slow heart rate.

In the cerebral vessels, nitrates produce vasodilation and an increase in intracerebral pressure. This, coupled with the decrease in systemic pressure, results in a decrease in blood flow through the brain, which may account for the headaches that are usually associated with nitrate therapy.

Retinal vessels dilate following use of nitrates; this can be directly observed through the ophthalmoscope. As may be expected, intraocular tension is also increased, but with the short-acting compounds, this effect is not considered to be significant in relation to the drainage of the anterior chamber. However, caution in the use of short-acting compounds is recommended in glaucoma.

The relaxation of the smooth muscle of the ureter, bile duct, and intestine requires high doses. Attempts to utilize nitrates as antispasmodics have met with little success.

Pharmacokinetics

Most of the nitrates used therapeutically are absorbed through the mucous membranes, and many are absorbed through the skin. Gastrointestinal absorption, however, is variable. Amyl nitrite, a highly volatile liquid, is rapidly absorbed from the lungs as well as through mucous membranes. Its onset of action is 0.5 min and duration is 3 to 5 min. It is partially eliminated from the lungs and partially hydrolyzed to nitrite ion. Amyl nitrite is little used in medical practice. It has become a drug of abuse imagined to increase sexual pleasure and prowess.

Nitroglycerin is absorbed through mucous membranes, the lungs, and the skin. It is less effective following oral administration than sublingual administration. It is biotransformed in the liver by action of a glutathione-organic nitrate reductase. The products are 1,3- and 1,2-dinitroglycerol, which are weakly active compared with nitroglycerin. Excretion is urinary after inactivation to mononitrates. The oral dose is 20 times the sublingual dose because of the inactivation by gastric juice and an extensive hepatic first-pass effect.

Although most other organic nitrates are administered orally, absorption through the mucous membranes has been demonstrated in most cases. Isosorbide dinitrate and erythrityl tetranitrate, for example, are also available for sublingual administration. Oral preparations of organic nitrates are absorbed slowly from the gastrointestinal tract. The exact fate of these compounds is not entirely known, although most appear to be biotransformed and excreted in the form of various nitrites and nitrates. The half-life for isosorbide dinitrate is 1 h and 4 h following sublingual and oral administration, respectively; why there is a dependence of half-life on the route of administration for this drug is not understood. The half-life for pentaerythritol tetranitrate is 2 h. Unlike other organic nitrate compounds, isosorbide mononitrate does not undergo first-pass metabolism and has a half-life of about 5 hours.

There are now many forms of nitroglycerin available, from intravenous to transdermal (see Table 29-1). The translingual spray is the most recent addition, with a spectrum of activity similar to that of sublingual tablets but somewhat more convenient to use. Transdermal patches have become a most popular method of administration.

TABLE 29-1 Available dosage forms of nitroglycerin with estimates of onset and duration of action

Dosage form	Onset	Duration
Intravenous	Immediate	3 - 5 min
Sublingual tablet	1 - 3 min	0.5 - 1 h
Translingual spray	2 min	0.5 - 1 h
Transmucosal tablet	1 - 2 min	3 - 5 h
Oral, sustained release	30 min	4 - 8 h
Topical ointment	0.5 - 1 h	2 - 12 h
Transdermal	0.5 - 1 h	18 - 24 h

Tolerance

Repeated administration of nitrates leads to the development of tolerance manifested by the need for higher doses to produce the same effect. There is cross-tolerance among the various compounds of this class. The mechanism of nitrite tolerance may be associated with the inability to convert NO_2 to NO by sulfhydryl groups; experimental evidence lends support to the sulfhydryl depletion hypothesis of nitrate tolerance. Decreases in the tissue content of sulfhydryl groups correlate with tolerance to nitroglycerin after prolonged exposure. In addition, tolerance may be reversed by the administration of dithiothreitol, or N-acetylcysteine, sulfhydryl regenerating agents. In general, tolerance develops quickly, within 2 to 3 weeks, but also disappears quickly, so that lack of exposure to nitrates for several days reestablishes the original sensitivity. Tolerance to nitrate-induced headache appears to develop more quickly than other nitrate effects. Headache symptoms may disappear within a few days after onset of therapy. Some cardiologists use intermittent administration to avoid tolerance.

Therapeutic Use

The short-acting nitrates are the most potent agents known for terminating an acute attack of angina. Nitroglycerin is the most frequently used agent. Pain is relieved within 1 to 3 min after sublingual administration of nitroglycerin. A similar effect can be produced with inhalation of amyl nitrite, but side effects are usually more prominent. Sublingual preparations of long-acting nitrates (isosorbide dinitrate, erythrityl tetranitrate) are effective within 3 to 5 min, and their effect may last for 1 to 2 h. Orally administered nitrates require a longer period (up to 30 min) to produce an effect which may last from 4 to 8 h (see Table 29-1). In general, oral preparations of organic nitrates are used prophylactically to reduce the frequency of attacks of angina, especially prior to activities known to precipitate angina attacks in a patient (e.g., physical exertion or emotional stress). The value of such prophylactic use of nitrates apparently varies and has not been conclusively demonstrated.

Various other drugs have been combined for the treatment of angina. It is not unusual to combine nitrates, β-adrenergic blockers, and calcium-channel blockers. Antianxiety agents may overcome the apprehension of heart disease and the resulting enforcement of pain sensation. In general, the use of various mild sedatives and tranquilizers is considered a valuable adjuvant therapy in the treatment of angina pectoris. Similarly, therapeutic management includes the exclusion of stimulants (e.g., tobacco products), reassurance by the physician, and avoidance of excessive emotional or physical stress. Moderate exercise, however, is considered by many to be an important part of long-term treatment.

Adverse Reactions

Certain undesirable effects of nitrates are related to their effects on the cardiovascular system. Throbbing headaches, flushing of the face, and dizziness are common, especially at the beginning of treatment. Headache is particularly common with some of the longer-acting compounds. Usually its severity decreases with continued use, but occasionally it may be so severe as to preclude further treatment. Postural hypotension is another common reaction which is apparently due to pooling of blood in the veins of the dependent parts of the body. The hypotensive effect of nitrates is potentially dangerous in patients with renal insufficiency, since it can aggravate renal ischemia. The use of nitrates is also contraindicated in acute myocardial infarction. Similarly, administration of nitrates in patients who also receive potent antihypertensive agents requires particular caution. Marked hypotension has also been reported in patients under nitrate treatment following ingestion of alcoholic beverages.

Gastrointestinal disturbances, including nausea and vomiting, are not uncommon following orally administered nitrates. The inorganic nitrites may lead to the development of methemoglobinemia. This is due to oxidation of hemoglobin by the nitrite ion and is useful in cyanide poisoning because of the high affinity of CN^- for methemoglobin (see Chapter 53).

Acute nitrate poisoning in humans is manifest by flushing of the face, marked fall in blood pressure, vomiting, cyanosis, and collapse. Death may occur from circulatory collapse or from respiratory failure.

BETA-ADRENERGIC BLOCKING DRUGS

A considerable advance in the therapy of angina has been the use of β-adrenergic blocking agents (Chapter 9). The hemodynamic effects of these drugs are decreased heart rate, reduced blood pressure and cardiac contractility, without appreciable reduction in cardiac output. These effects are most evident at rest but also persist during exercise. There is, in brief, a modulating effect on the heart with a buffering action against sympathetic stimulation and the cardiac autoregulatory mechanism. The reduced heart rate improves efficiency, while the longer diastolic interval allows improved coronary blood perfusion. The decrease in contractility is the cause of the reduced blood pressure. The *β*-adrenergic blocking agents do not directly cause a decrease in peripheral resistance.

Blockade of the adrenergic drive of the heart may account for the moderation of blood pressure and the decrease in heart work. Patients complain of fatigue and lack of drive and not being able to perform heavy exercise. Also patients with poor cardiac reserve are susceptible to the induction of congestive heart failure. Attempts to correct this by producing antagonists with some *β*-adrenergic receptor agonist activity, such as pindolol, have not been entirely successful. Although only propranolol, nadolol, atenolol and metoprolol have been approved by the FDA for the therapy of angina, the other *β*-adrenergic blockers that are available appear to be equally effective.

Acute attacks of angina are best treated with nitroglycerin. *β*-Adrenergic blockers are suitable for chronic therapy and are especially useful in the angina which sometimes develops post-myocardial infarction. Indeed the *β*-adrenergic blockers are complementary to nitrate therapy because they correct the tendency of these drugs to increase heart rate. They also allow the nitrates to be used intermittently, thus minimizing the development of tolerance to nitrates. On the other hand, nitrates can be said to counteract some undesirable effects of *β*-adrenergic blockers.

While it does not seem to matter which *β*-adrenergic blocker is selected to treat angina, the question of dosage is an important one. It is wise to start with minimal effective doses and gradually build up the dosage to a satisfactory level, balancing beneficial actions against side effects. As a guide, the resting heart rate should be 50 to 60 beats per minute. Exercise should increase the heart rate to no more than 100 to 120 heartbeats per minute.

CALCIUM-CHANNEL BLOCKERS

The membranes of most cells, but especially those of smooth muscle, cardiac muscle, and nerve, contain channels for the conduct of calcium ions into the cell. These channels are of two major types; one is *voltage-dependent* or *voltage-gated* (like that of the sodium channel) while other channels exist which are not voltage-sensitive and are activated by ligands such as neurotransmitters, hormones, etc. (termed *receptor-operated* or *ligand-gated*). The voltage-gated calcium channels have been further divided into subtypes (L, N, P, and T). The calcium channels, in contrast to sodium channels, are slowly conducting, and hence the term *slow calcium channel* is used to describe these structures (see Chapter 28 for their relationship to cardiac action potentials). As with sodium, ionic calcium must be pumped out of the cell against a gradient and this is accomplished by a calcium-sensitive ATPase. In addition, recall that there is a sodium-calcium exchange mechanism which further regulates the available amount of free calcium in the cytosol; this mechanism comes into play with the action of digitalis glycosides in heart muscle (see Chapter 27). Ionic calcium is involved in a variety of other important cellular metabolic processes, not the least of which is the formation of bone. In this chapter, the focus is the role of calcium in the control of the tone of smooth muscle (especially that of the vasculature) and cardiac muscle.

Originally this group of drugs was developed as coronary vasodilators, and they were used as such in Europe for some years before it was found that they inhibited the contractile action of calcium on smooth muscle and cardiac muscle. Originally known as *calcium antagonists*, their main action is on membrane calcium channels that are voltage-gated; they have little effect on the ligand-gated calcium channels. Presently these drugs are indicated for use in the treatment of angina, hypertension, and arrhythmias.

Chemistry

The calcium-channel blockers have a very diverse chemistry, and this may indicate that there are different receptor sites in calcium channels on the cell membrane and within the cell. These compounds are usually classified by structure: *verapamil* is a diphenylalkylamine derivative and is the oldest of the currently available agents, *diltiazem* is a benzothiazepine derivative, *bepridil* is a pyrrolidineethanamine derivative, and *nifedipine* and all of the others are dihydropyridines. Structural formulas of representative drugs are shown in Fig. 29-3.

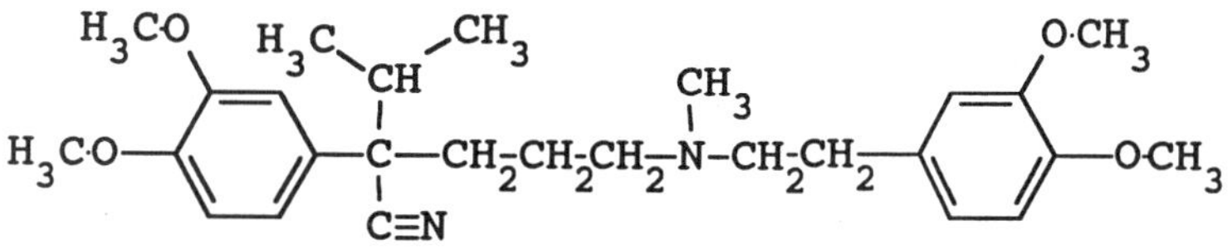

Verapamil

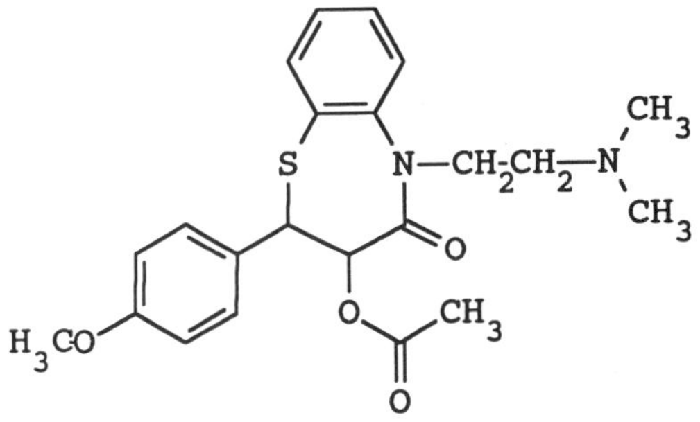

Diltiazem

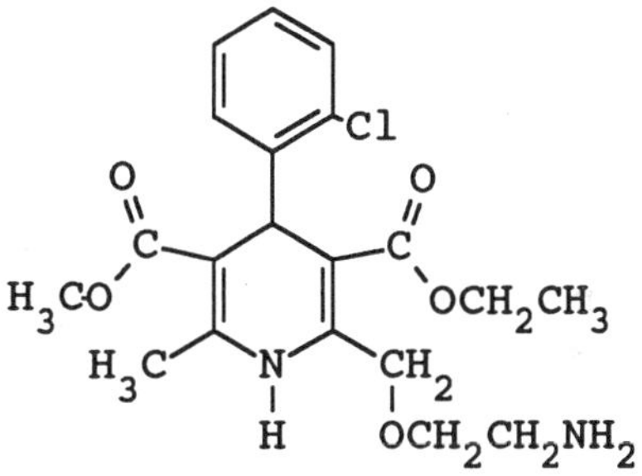

Amlodipine

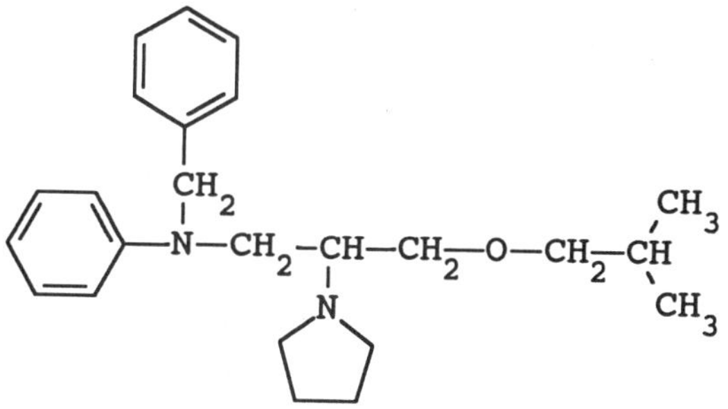

Bepridil

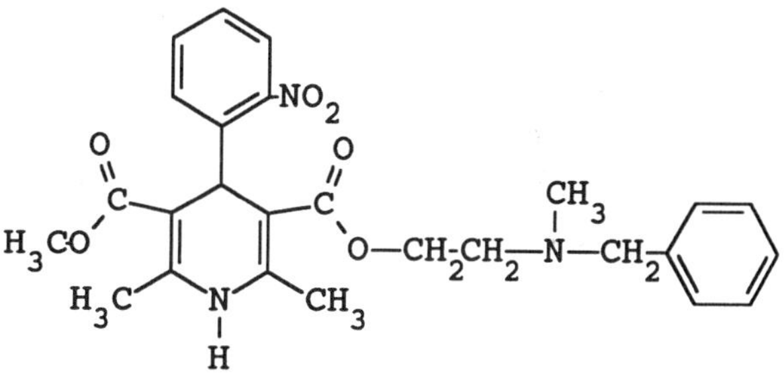

Nicardipine

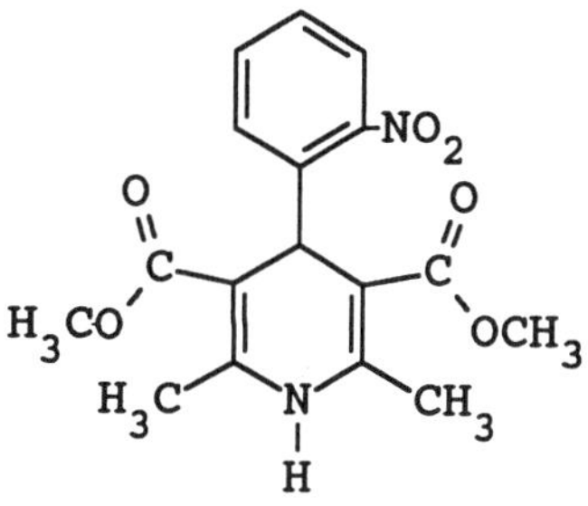

Nifedipine

FIGURE 29-3 *Structures of representative calcium-channel blockers used in angina.*

Mechanism of Action

Major advances in the past few years have improved our understanding of the key role played by transmembrane calcium ion movement in controlling many different physiological processes, such as muscle contraction, neurotransmitter release, secretion and platelet function. There is now ample evidence that contraction of vascular smooth muscle is controlled by the cytoplasmic concentration of calcium. Two main mechanisms regulate the cytosolic calcium concentration. The first of these involves voltage-gated calcium channels which open when the cell membrane is depolarized. Extracellular calcium moves into the cells as a result. This mechanism is known as *electromechanical coupling*. The second mechanism, sodium-calcium exchange, is independent of membrane polarization. In addition, some calcium channels may be ligand-gated, which open in response to the binding of a ligand to the receptor. This involves the release of calcium from the sarcoplasmic reticulum, which secondarily causes an influx of extracellular calcium through non-voltage-linked calcium channels. Cardiac muscle is dependent on sarcoplasmic reticulum storage and release of calcium ions for contraction. This is a less important mechanism for controlling cytosolic calcium concentration in vascular smooth muscle and other smooth muscle because the sarcoplasmic reticulum is less well developed.

Transduction of the increased ionic calcium concentration, by any of these mechanisms, occurs by binding of calcium to calmodulin. In turn, the calcium-calmodulin complex initiates phosphorylation of the light chain of myosin by activation of light-chain kinase. Contraction of smooth muscle results from the interaction of phosphorylated light-chain myosin and actin (see Fig. 29-4).

The channel that is most responsive to the calcium-channel blockers is the so-called L-type voltage channel located in vascular smooth muscle and the heart; diverse forms of L-type channels allow for tissue selectivity and diversity of function (skeletal muscle L-type channels, for example, are unresponsive to calcium-channel blockers). L-type calcium channels consist of 5 subunits. The α_1 subunit appears to contain distinct receptors for each of the four chemical classes of blockers and is responsible for voltage-gating and channel opening. Voltage-dependent channels respond to a lower concentrations of calcium than the non-voltage-dependent channels. It thus appears that the ratio of voltage-sensitive to non-voltage-sensitive channels determines the selectivity of response of veins and arteries. At the doses used clinically, calcium-channel blockers relax arterial smooth muscle with little action on veins.

It will be recalled that excitation-contraction coupling in cardiac myocytes depends more on sodium ion than calcium ion influx. Consequently calcium-channel blockers have relatively little effect on contractility at doses which relax smooth muscle. However, the cardiac myocytes at the sinoatrial (SA) and atrioventricular (AV) nodes are more dependent on movement of calcium through slow channels. The calcium-channel blockers (especially verapamil and also diltiazem, but not nifedipine) impede recovery of the cardiac slow calcium channels. Consequently heart rate is slowed and conduction from atrium to ventricle is blocked (see Chapter 28).

Pharmacodynamics

The calcium-channel blockers tend to relax and reduce the tone of all smooth muscle. This has led to attempts to use such agents as antispasmodics in gastrointestinal disorders and asthma. Clearly the relaxing action is most marked on vascular smooth muscle. Arterioles are much more affected than veins. Thus calcium-channel blockers lower blood pressure and reduce afterload without an appreciable effect on preload. In this regard, nifedipine and most other dihydropyridines, are the most effective, followed by verapamil and then diltiazem and bepridil (Table 29-2). Benefit in angina consists not only of the vasodilator action on coronary vessels, especially vasospastic ones, but also in the reduction of afterload, hence oxygen requirements of the heart.

Both the action potential and muscle contraction of the heart are calcium-related. A reduction in calcium entry into the myocyte, especially those of the SA and AV nodes, results in slowing of the rate of the SA node and slowing of conduction in the AV node. Actual contractility of the ventricular muscle is usually not affected at therapeutic dose levels, and cardiac output may actually increase as a result of the decrease in peripheral resistance. With toxic doses or in hearts already in failure, myocardial contractility may be severely compromised. The cardiac effects are useful. Verapamil and diltiazem are effective in blocking the numerous impulses to the ventricle in atrial flutter and fibrillation by effectively slowing the ventricular rate to an effective level. In this regard these calcium-channel blockers can be used

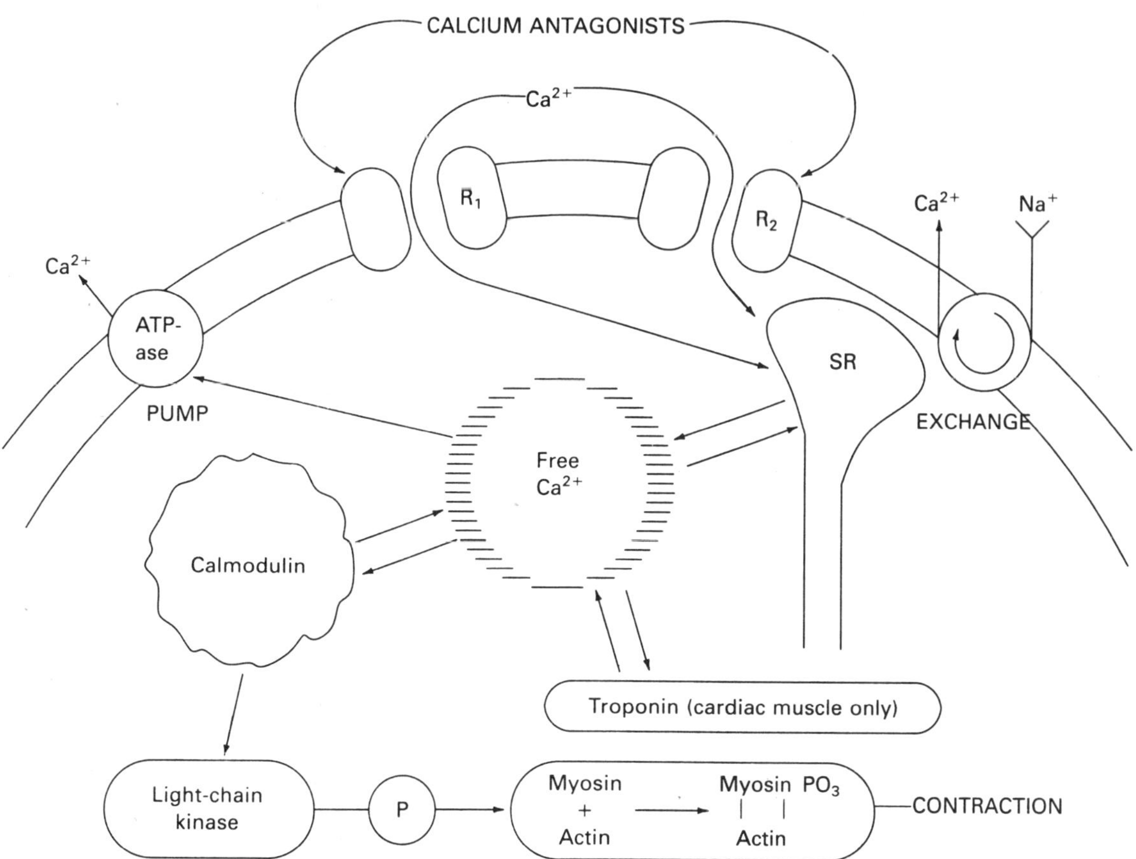

FIGURE 29-4 *Schematic diagram of the mechanism of action of calcium-channel blockers. A section of cell membrane is shown with calcium channels R_1 (voltage-dependent) and R_2 (non-voltage-dependent). Calcium (Ca^{2+}) influx occurs through both channels and calcium is stored in the sarcoplasmic reticulum (SR). There is a small pool of free calcium, which is a second messenger. It is in equilibrium with the calcium in the SR and also with calcium bound to calmodulin. The level of free calcium is crucial to muscle tone and contraction. In heart muscle which has troponin, the action of calcium is direct, i.e., to remove the barrier between the interaction of myosin and actin to cause contraction. In smooth muscle, free calcium attaches to a small protein, calmodulin, which in turn activates light-chain kinase which promotes the phosphorylation (P) of myosin, which again permits the myosin-actin interaction and muscle contraction. (It might be recalled that nitrates, through cyclic GMP, and β-adrenergic receptor antagonists, through cyclic AMP, inhibit light-chain kinase). Calmodulin-calcium stimulates, and it is in this manner that the level of cytosolic free calcium controls the tonus of smooth muscle. It must also be mentioned that calcium is pumped out of the cell by an ATPase system in the membrane similar to that of sodium. There is also a sodium-calcium exchange during depolarization: with sodium influx some calcium leaves the cell. Thus the receptors for calcium antagonists are the calcium influx channels. These have gates and have activated and resting states similar to the sodium channels, but their workings are less well understood. [Modified from Opie, L.H., and U. Thadani: in J. Hamer (ed.): Antianginal Vasodilators in Drugs for Heart Disease, 2nd ed., Chapman and Hall, London, 1987, pp. 103-143.]*

TABLE 29-2 Comparative indications and cardiovascular actions of calcium-channel blockers

Drug	FDA indications	Reduction of peripheral vascular resistance	Slowing of AV nodal conduction	Reduction of cardiac contractility
Verapamil	Vasospastic angina Chronic stable angina Atrial flutter and fibrillation Paroxysmal atrial tachycardia Essential hypertension	+ + +	+ +	+ +
Diltiazem	Vasospastic angina Chronic stable angina Essential hypertension	+ +	+ +	+
Bepridil	Chronic stable angina	+ +	+ +	+ +
Amlodipine	Vasospastic angina Chronic stable angina	+ + + +	0	0
Felodipine	Essential hypertension	+ + + +	0	0
Isradipine	Essential hypertension	+ + + +	0	0
Nicardipine	Chronic stable angina Essential hypertension	+ + + +	0	0
Nifedipine	Vasospastic angina Chronic stable angina Essential hypertension	+ + + +	0	+

Slight to pronounced effect = + to + + + +
No effect = 0

instead of, or in combination with, digitalis to control the ventricular rate in atrial flutter or fibrillation. They are also effective in arresting atrial tachycardia (see Chapter 28).

Skeletal muscle is not affected by calcium-channel blockers. Fortunately, there is a large intracellular pool of calcium in the skeletal muscle fiber so that dependence on transmembrane calcium influx is not required.

The excitation-contraction coupling mechanism involving calcium also is operative in other tissues such as glands and the functioning of nerve endings. Experimentally, inhibition of peptide hormone secretion by the pituitary gland and pancreas, inhibition of insulin secretion, and depression of the release of neurotransmitters from synaptosomes by calcium-channel blockers have been shown. Generally, the dose is higher for these glandular and neuronal effects than is required in the management of angina.

Pharmacokinetics

The pharmacokinetics of the calcium-channel blockers may vary widely (see Table 29-3). These drugs are orally effective drugs that are well absorbed through the gastrointestinal mucosa (85 to 100 percent); however, their oral bioavailability tends to be depressed due to high first-pass biotransformation. The onset of action differs depending on the compound and ranges from 20 min to a few hours; likewise, the peak effect may occur as quickly as 30 min or as long as 12 hours following a single dose. Plasma protein binding varies from 70 to 99 percent. Biotransformation of all the available compounds is extensive. Verapamil is biotransformed to norverapamil and diltiazem to desacetyldiltiazem, both pharmacologically active (approximately 25 percent of parent compound); the other drugs are converted to inactive products. Elimination half-lives range

TABLE 29-3 Some pharmacokinetic parameters of calcium-channel blockers

Drug	Absolute oral bioavailability, %	Onset of action, min	Peak effect, h	Plasma protein binding, %	Half-life, h
Verapamil	20 - 35	30	1 - 2	80 - 90	3 - 7
Diltiazem	40 - 65	30 - 60	2 - 3	70 - 80	3 - 6
Bepridil	60	60	2 - 3	99	24
Amlodipine	65	—[a]	6 - 12	90 - 95	30 - 50
Felodipine	20	120 - 300	2.5 - 5	99	11 - 16
Isradipine	15 - 25	—	1.5	95	8
Nicardipine	35	20	0.5 - 2	95 - 99	2 - 4
Nifedipine	45 - 70	20	0.5	90 - 99	2 - 5

—[a] No data are available

from 2 to 36 h. Excretion is through both the urine and feces, the extent of which depends on the compound.

Clinical Use

The most intensive use of calcium-channel blockers has been for angina and particularly the vasospastic variety. The FDA-approved uses are listed in Table 29-2. Most of these drugs are also used for hypertension (see Chapter 32). As antiarrhythmic drugs, verapamil and diltiazem are superior, especially when used by the intravenous route (see Chapter 28).

Adverse Reactions

The most serious toxic effects of calcium-channel blockers stem from their pharmacologic actions. With higher doses, or in especially sensitive cardiac muscle, reduction in calcium influx can cause severe reduction in contractility with consequent abrupt fall in cardiac output. In addition, excessive cardiac slowing and heart block can also precipitate heart failure. Actually severe and fatal episodes have been rarely reported; nevertheless, as shown in Table 29-4, the most frequent adverse reactions are cardiovascular. These include episodes of hypotension due to excessive vasodilation.

The central nervous system adverse effects may be due to the hypotensive effects but are more likely the result of a direct action. They are more frequent with the dihydropyridine derivatives, which have the greatest effect on vascular resistance. Adverse reactions are summarized in Table 29-4.

Drug Interactions

As might be expected from a drug group that affects so vital a mechanism as calcium control of cellular functions, there are many drug interactions which have clinical significance. Some of the most important may be listed as follows:

1. Physiologic-Pharmacologic basis

   a. β-Adrenergic blockers have negative inotropic and chronotropic cardiac effects. These are additive to similar actions of calcium-channel blockers. While both groups of drugs can be used together, caution is required to prevent excessive depression of myocardial function.

   b. Simultaneous administration of calcium salts and vitamin D may lower the effectiveness of calcium-channel blockers. Calcium can be used to treat verapamil overdose.

TABLE 29-4 Adverse reactions generally encountered with the use of calcium-channel blockers

Adverse reaction	Verapamil	Diltiazem	Bepridil	Dihydropyridine derivatives
Cardiovascular				
Peripheral edema	+	+ + +	+	+ + + + +
Hypotension	+ +	+/−	−	+ + +
Bradycardia	+	+ +	+	−
Congestive heart failure	+	+/−	−	+ +
Pulmonary edema	+	−	−	+ +
Central nervous system				
Dizziness	+ +	+ +	+ + + + +	+ + + + +
Lightheadedness	+ +	+ +	+ + + + +	+ + + + +
Headache	+ +	+ +	+ + + +	+ + + + +
Weakness, shakiness	+/−	+ +	−	+ + + +
Gastrointestinal				
Nausea	+ +	+ +	+ + + +	+ + + +
Dermatologic				
Rash	+/−	+	+	+
Pruritis	+/−	+/−	−	+
Hair loss	+/−	−	−	+/−
Photosensitivity	−	+/−	−	−

+ + + + + = 15 - 25%
+ + + + = 10 - 15%
+ + + = 5 - 10%
+ + = 2 - 5%
+ = < 2%
+/− = ≤ 1%
− = no data

c. Antihypertensive drugs (e.g., prazosin, methyldopa, clonidine) can add to the hypotensive effects of calcium-channel blockers to cause dangerous hypotensive effects.

d. Nondepolarizing skeletal muscle relaxants may have increased action due to the ability of calcium-channel blockers to block pre- and postjunctional channels. Caution is to be exercised in using these agents together.

2. Metabolic effects

a. Verapamil, and possibly diltiazem, inhibit hepatic biotransformation of carbamazepine, increasing the effects of this drug.

b. Cimetidine decreases the first-pass metabolism of calcium-channel blockers. This may require a lower dose of these agents.

c. Lithium plasma levels are decreased by verapamil. Monitoring of lithium levels is necessary to maintain therapeutic effects of lithium.

3. Plasma protein binding

a. Calcium-channel blockers are highly bound to plasma proteins. They may displace other drugs such as warfarin and oral hypoglycemic drugs.

MISCELLANEOUS DRUGS

Angina pectoris is so common a disease syndrome that over the years many different remedies have been used. Unfortunately, verification that seems to work most comes from anecdotal evidence. Modern techniques of measuring vascular dynamics have weeded out the less effective drugs. There is only one that merits mention.

Dipyridamole

This is a compound which has had more than 20 years of use, especially in Europe, as a coronary vasodilator. At usual doses there is little change in blood pressure or peripheral blood flow. It does increase coronary flow, but mainly in normal myocardium, and the benefit in this regard is considered minimal. Dipyridamole has been recommended as prophylaxis for angina pectoris, but there is no substantial evidence that this goal is accomplished. The FDA presently allows the indications to read "possibly effective" for long term treatment of chronic angina, but is currently considering withdrawal of approval of this drug.

Because it can produce *coronary steal* in patients with coronary disease, dipyridamole is used with thallium for imagining of the heart to detect the presence and severity of the coronary artery disease.

Due to its antiplatelet effects, dipyridamole has been widely used in conjunction with warfarin to prevent embolization from prosthetic heart valves. In combination with aspirin, dipyridamole prolongs the survival of platelets in thrombotic disease. By itself dipyridamole has little effect. The mechanism of its antiplatelet effect may be inhibition of cyclic nucleotide phosphodiesterase activity. Concerning prevention of coronary thrombosis, several large studies have shown that aspirin alone is as effective as the combination of dipyridamole and aspirin.

BIBLIOGRAPHY

Abshagen, U.: "Pharmacokinetics of Isosorbide Mononitrate," *Am. J. Cardiol.* **70**: 61G-66G (1992).

Ahlner, J., R.G. Andersson, K. Torfgard, and K.L. Axelsson: "Organic Nitrate Esters: Clinical Use and Mechanisms of Actions," *Pharm. Rev.* **43**: 351-423 (1991).

Braunwald, E.: "Mechanism of Action of Calcium Channel Blocking Agents," *N. Engl. J. Med.* **307**: 1618 (1982).

Busse, R., A. Muloch, I. Fleming, and M. Hecker: "Mechanisms of Nitric Oxide Release From the Vascular Endothelium," *Circ.* **Suppl. 87**: V18-V25 (1993).

Cavin, C., R. Loutzenbieser, and C. Van Breeman: "Mechanisms of Calcium Antagonist Induced Vasodilation," *Annu. Rev. Pharmacol. Toxicol.* **23**: 373-396 (1983).

Cohn, P.F.: "Mechanisms of Myocardial Ishemia," *Am. J. Cardiol.* **70**: 14G-19G (1992).

Frishman, W.H., and M. Teicher: "Antianginal Drug Therapy for Silent Myocardial Ischemia," *Med. Clin. North Am.* **72**: 185-196 (1988).

Gerstenblith, G.: "Treatment of Unstable Angina Pectoris," *Am. J. Cardiol.* **70**: 32G-37G (1992).

Gerthoffer, W.T., M.A. Trevethick, and R.A. Murphy: "Myosin Phosphorylation and Cyclic Adenosine 3',5'-Monophosphate in Relaxation of Arterial Smooth Muscle by Vasodilators," *Circ. Res.* **54**: 839 (1984).

Gorlin, R.: "Treatment of Chronic Stable Angina Pectoris," *Am. J. Cardiol.* **70**: 26G-31G (1992).

Janis, R.I., and A. Scriabine: "Commentary: Sites of Action of Calcium Channel Inhibitors," *Biochem. Pharmacol.* **32**: 3499-3507 (1983).

Lüscher, T.F.: "Interactions Between Endothelium-Derived Relaxing and Contracting Factors in Health and Cardiovascular Disease," *Circ.* **Suppl. 87**: V36-V44 (1993).

Moncada, S., R.M. Palmer, and E.A. Higgs: "Nitric Oxide: Physiology, Pathophysiology, and Pharmacology," *Pharm. Rev.* **43**: 109-142 (1991).

Meredith, I.T.: "Role of Impaired Endothelium-Dependent Vasodilation in Ischemic Manifestations of Coronary Artery Disease," *Circ.* **Suppl. 87**: V56-V66 (1993).

Nordlander, R.: "Use of Nitrates in the Treatment of Unstable and Variant Angina," *Drugs* **33, Suppl. 4**: 131-139 (1987).

O'Hara, M.J., et al.: "Diltiazem and Propranolol Combination for the Treatment of Chronic Stable Angina Pectoris," *Clin. Cardiol.* **10**: 115-123 (1987).

Opie, L.H.: *The Heart, Physiology, Metabolism, Pharmacology and Therapy*, Grune and Stratton, London, 1986.

Opie, L.H., and U. Thadani: in J. Hamer (ed.): *Antianginal Vasodilators in Drugs for Heart Disease, 2nd ed.*, Chapman and Hall, London, 1987, pp. 103-143.

Parker, J.O.: "Nitrate Therapy in Stable Angina Pectoris," *N. Engl. J. Med.* **316**: 1635-1642 (1987).

Pepine, C.J., and C.R. Lambert: "Usefulness of Nicardipine for Angina Pectoris," *Am. J. Cardiol.* **59**: 13J- 19J (1987).

Rodrigues, E.A., A. Lahiri, and E.B. Raftery: "Improvement in Left Ventricular Diastolic Function in Patients with Stable Angina after Chronic Treatment with Verapamil and Nicardipine," *Br. J. Clin. Pract.* **60**: 27-32 (1988).

Samuelsson, O., L. Wilhelmsen, K. Pennert, and G. Bergland: "Angina Pectoris, Intermittent Claudication and Congestive Heart Failure in Middle-Aged Male Hypertensives. Development and Predictive Factors during Long-Term Antihypertensive Care," The Primary Preventive Trial, Goteborg, Sweden, *Acta Med. Scand.* **221**: 23-32 (1987).

Shub, C.: "Stable Angina Pectoris: 3. Medical Treatment," *Mayo Clin. Proc.* **65**: 256-273 (1990).

Schwartz, A.: "Molecular and Cellular Aspects of Calcium Channel Antagonism," *Am. J. Cardiol.* **70**: 6F-8F (1992).

Thompson, R.H.: "The Clinical Use of Transdermal Delivery Devices with Nitroglycerine" *Angiology* **34**: 23-31 (1983).

CHAPTER 30

Agents Used in Hyperlipoproteinemia

Evangelos T. Angelakos and G. John DiGregorio

The relationship between plasma cholesterol and atherosclerotic disease has been established over the past decade through large scale studies. Cholesterol levels above 200 mg/dL are considered to be elevated and require evaluation. A strong statistical relationship exists between elevated cholesterol levels and the development of coronary artery disease. It is further established that the atherogenic potential of cholesterol is dependent on the type of lipoprotein which carries it in the plasma. Specifically, high levels of low-density lipoprotein (LDL) cholesterol have a strong and direct correlation with the development of atherosclerosis. A lesser relationship was found with very-low-density lipoprotein (VLDL) cholesterol while high-density lipoprotein (HDL) cholesterol shows an inverse relationship. Therefore the desired therapeutic goal is to decrease primarily LDL cholesterol and secondarily VLDL cholesterol and total cholesterol without affecting, or preferable increasing, HDL cholesterol.

Studies on the specific role of LDL in the formation of atherosclerotic lesions over many years have led to the development of changing concepts. There is evidence of hereditary predisposition to hypercholesterolemia which is expressed when combined with other dietary or "stress" factors. However, there are some individuals with consistently elevated levels of cholesterol with no detectable vessel disease and, more commonly, there are those with moderate elevations and extensive vessel disease. Some individuals have predominantly coronary or cerebral vessel disease while others develop primarily peripheral vessel disease. Both are usually found with advancing age.

It is generally believed that the formation of atherosclerotic plaques is somehow related to prolonged "injury" of the vessel with an initial accumulation of platelets and LDL. This concept is supported by the close (although not consistent) association between arteriosclerotic and atherosclerotic lesions and the common association between hypertension and atherosclerosis.

Of particular interest to the physician is the developing evidence that reduction of plasma lipids have often a more pronounced effect on future morbidity and mortality in patients with coronary artery disease than would be expected from a simple relationship between plasma lipid concentrations and their accumulation on critical blood vessels. More recent information has begun to clarify the complex role of hyperlipidemia in the development of atherosclerosis and the beneficial effects of treatment. In the presence of hereditary predisposition, arteriosclerotic "injury", and other factors, elevated plasma levels of LDL favor its accumulation in tissue monocytes (macrophages) by active uptake through LDL receptors. LDL accumulation in monocytes leads to the formation of the large "foam" cells found in atherosclerotic plaques. Release of local kinins provide chemotactic factors for the further accumulation of monocytes as well as stimulation of myocyte and connective tissue proliferation resulting in the characteristic microscopic picture of the atheromatous plaque.

In the coronary arteries (as well as in other vessels) narrowing of the blood vessel lumen as a result of the protrusion of the atherosclerotic plaque may be initially asymptomatic due to the ability of the microcirculation to autoregulate flow in the presence of moderate reductions in arterial pressure. If the narrowing is more severe it may and does produce the classical syndrome of angina pectoris. However, infarction does not necessarily result from complete occlusion of the vessel lumen by the plaque. More commonly (or almost invariably) coronary occlusion and myocardial infarction (MI) result from rupture of the atheromatous lesion followed by thrombosis. This accounts for the generally abrupt onset of MI. Thus small lesions that produce no significant occlusion can precipitate MI. Therefore, the critical element in the development of MI, especially in young previously asymptomatic patients, is not the size of the atheromatous lesion but the rate of development of that lesion. Slowly developing atheromatous plaques may reach large size producing severe angina for many years before an ultimate rupture and thrombotic occlusion. By contrast, small rapidly developing lesions may rupture at an early age producing MIs and/or sudden death from the arrhythmic consequences of MI.

These more recent concepts are of critical importance in the evaluation of the benefits provided by treatment. Antilipidemic treatment producing even a modest decrease in plasma LDL (or in LDL deposition on vessel walls) can have a significant effect in reducing the incidence of lesion rupture by delaying the rate of development of the lesion. This is believed to account for the recent observations in clinical trials where a modest decrease in plasma cholesterol levels achieved by antilipidemic drug treatment had very significant effects in reducing the incidence of myocardial infarction and mortality.

As indicated above, accumulation of LDL in monocytes is the first step in the formation of the atherosclerotic plaque. This accumulation seems to depend on prior oxidative modification of the LDL particle. Monocyte receptors for oxidized LDL (sometimes referred to as "scavenger" receptors) do not exhibit feed-back regulation to limit the progressive accumulation of lipoproteins in monocytes.

A close and consistent association has also been found between low levels of HDL and atherogenesis. This apparently relates to the role of HDL to remove cholesterol from peripheral tissues and transport it to the liver (Figure 30-1). High levels of VLDL, as are found in certain types of hyperlipidemia, may also contribute to the development of atherogenesis. Subfractions of smaller (more dense) VLDLs are believed to be more atherogenic than larger (less dense) VLDL particles. Furthermore, high levels of VLDL provide a source for the atherogenic LDL particles (Figure 30-1).

As indicated above, the therapeutic goal is a reduction of primarily LDL and possibly VLDL cholesterol without altering, or preferably, with an elevation of the HDL cholesterol.

In general, the lipoproteins which carry the cholesterol are the critical factors for atherogenesis since they determine the uptake or removal of cholesterol to or from the tissues. The specific lipoproteins that are found in the particles identified by their density (such as VLDL, LDL, and HDL) are critical in determining receptor binding and will most likely serve as the targets for future therapeutic approaches to treatment of the clinical sequence of hyperlipoproteinemia. The major components of the various lipoproteins are listed in Table 30-1.

Other recent advances involve various subtypes of the major lipoproteins. A variant of LDL has been identified and termed lipoprotein(a) or Lp(a). It contains both apo(B) the major apoprotein of LDL as well as another apoprotein, apo(A). Lp(a) is highly atherogenic and has been found to be an independent risk factor in coronary artery disease.

On another front, HDL has been subfractioned into a less dense HDL_2 fraction and a heavier HDL_3 fraction. HDL_2 is considered to be the specific fraction involved in the removal of cholesterol from the tissues. Therefore, an increase in the HDL_2/HDL_3 ratio is considered beneficial. Based on these recent advances, desirable therapeutic goals, in addition to those listed above, include a decrease in Lp(a) and an increase in the HDL_2/HDL_3 ratio.

CHOLESTEROL TRANSPORT

Cholesterol is transported as various size particles composed of triglycerides, proteins, cholesterol esters, and phospholipids. In Table 30-1 are listed the major blood particles whose function is to carry fats from one tissue to another. The chylomicrons are the largest particles, composed mostly of triglycerides, and their function is to transport fat from the intestine to the liver. Chylomicrons contain little cholesterol and are not involved in the arteriosclerotic process. In contrast, LDL particles contain the most cholesterol, and they are the source of this steroid for synthesis of bile salts and adrenal and sex hormones, and also for the atherosclerotic lesion. HDL particles contain less cholesterol and little triglyceride and a large amount of protein. They are involved in the removal of excess cholesterol from the tissues, a process termed *reverse cholesterol transport*. Recent studies indicate that protection from atherogenesis is associated with a specific lipoprotein fraction of HDL (i.e., HDL_2).

The amount of cholesterol in the blood as represented by the above particles is determined by many factors. The crucial element appears to

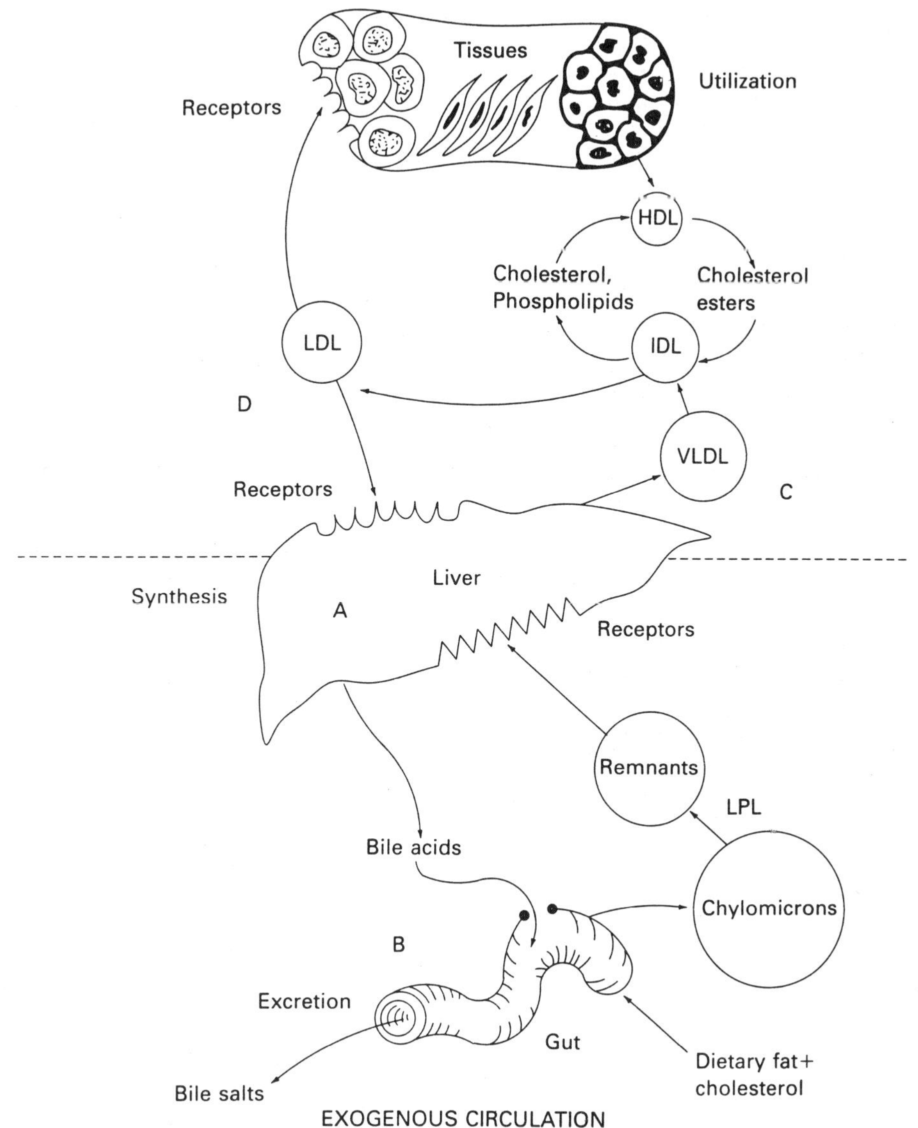

FIGURE 30-1 *Schematic diagram of lipid, lipoprotein, and cholesterol circulation. Dietary fat and cholesterol are ingested. From the gut, fatty acids and cholesterol are absorbed to enter the portal circulation as chylomicrons composed mostly of triglycerides but also containing protein and cholesterol. These break up into smaller remnants, due to the action of lipoprotein lipase, which are handled by the liver at various receptor sites. The liver synthesizes bile acids as well as cholesterol de novo. The bile acids are secreted into the intestine; most are reabsorbed, and only a small amount is excreted. From the liver, triglycerides and cholesterol enter the systemic circulation and form very-low-density lipoproteins (VLDL). This particle breaks up into intermediate-density lipoprotein (IDL) particles, which further form low-density lipoproteins (LDL) and are contributed to by high-density lipoproteins (HDL) from the tissues. Special receptors are present in the tissues and the liver for LDL, which contains the largest amount of cholesterol.*

Sites of action of cholesterol-lowering drugs are as follows: (A) inhibition of synthesis by lovastatin in the liver by blocking HMG-CoA reductase; (b) increased excretion of bile salts by blocking reabsorption by bile acid sequestering drugs; (C) decreased production of VLDL by the liver caused by nicotinic acid; and (D) probucol-induced increased degradation of LDL cholesterol.

TABLE 30-1 Composition of the human plasma lipoproteins[a,b]

Lipoprotein macromolecules	Size, Å	% TG	% Chol	% PL	% Prot	Major apoproteins	Predominant function
Chylomicrons	2000 to 5000	85	7	6	3	A1, A4, B, C, E	Transport of fat from intestine to liver
Very-low-density (VLDL)	500 to 800	60	16	14	9	B, C1, E	Transport of lipoprotein lipids to adipose tissue and muscle from the liver
Low-density (LDL)	200	11	46	22	21	B	Transport of cholesterol to the liver for bile acid synthesis and to the adrenals and the ovaries
High-density (HDL)	80	8	20	22	50	A1, A2	Transport of cholesterol from tissues to the liver for excretion

[a] Partially adapted from Weis, S., and A.G. Lacko: "Role of Lipoproteins in Hypercholesterolemia," *Practical Cardiology* (special issue), May 1988, p 12.

[b] TG = triglycerides; Chol = cholesterol; PL = phospholipids; Prot = protein.

be the kind and quantity of receptors present in the various organs and tissues. This is genetically determined. The lipid particles which are produced by the body are composed of specific proteins (see Table 30-1). These serve as ligands for the receptors which are also proteins and also genetically determined. The function of LDL is to carry cholesterol to the tissues. Its role in the atherosclerotic lesion was described above.

VLDL is a large particle produced by the liver, which has a high concentration of triglyceride and considerable cholesterol. Its main function is to transport fat and be a source of the other particles in the bloodstream (Table 30-1).

The amount of LDL in the blood is determined by (1) the level of VLDL, (2) the rate of removal of LDL by the liver cellular LDL receptors, and (3) the rate of utilization of LDL by the tissues. There is an up- or down-regulation of the liver LDL receptors which is dependant on the level of cholesterol in the liver. When liver cholesterol synthesis is inhibited, there is an up-regulation of liver LDL receptors and an increased rate of removal of LDL by the liver. Conversely a high level of cholesterol in the liver results in down-regulation of the LDL receptors and increased levels of LDL in the bloodstream. Extremely high levels of LDL cholesterol occur in rare individuals having a genetic reduction or absence of liver LDL receptors.

Since HDL is responsible for removing cholesterol from the tissues, a high blood level is perceived to be favorable and vice versa.

The formation and disposition of the various lipoproteins are imperfectly understood. Empiric observations have established some other parameters which must be taken into consideration in the diagnosis and therapy of hyperlipoproteinemias:

1. *Dietary intake of fat and cholesterol.* The high caloric content of fat contributes to high caloric intake relative to caloric expenditure leading to the accumulation of body fat. Excess body weight appears to be a more significant factor than dietary cholesterol.

2. *Ratio of saturated to unsaturated fatty acids in the diet.* A well-established observation is that a diet high in saturated fats (meats) is associated with high levels of plasma cholesterol; similarly, a diet high in unsaturated fats (vegetable oils) is associated with low levels of plasma cholesterol. However, unsaturated fat intake decreases both LDL and HDL cholesterol. Mono-unsaturated fats (olive oil) decrease LDL without affecting HDL cholesterol.

3. *Rate of utilization of cholesterol.* Exercise, for example, increases the burning of fats for energy and also decreases plasma cholesterol. Growth increases and senescence decreases utilization of fats and cholesterol.

4. *Endocrine diseases.* Diabetes or insulin insufficiency leads to poor utilization of fat and early arteriosclerosis. Hyperthyroidism decreases and hypothyroidism increases the level of plasma cholesterol and atherogenic tendency. Changes in growth and adrenal and sex hormones are more tenuous factors but still important.

There are many other causes of secondary hyperlipoproteinemia. These are listed in Table 30-2. On the whole, the diagnosis and treatment of hyperlipoproteinemias are based upon an accurate estimation of the level of plasma cholesterol, the ratio of LDL and HDL in the plasma, and the plasma triglyceride level.

CLASSIFICATION OF THE HYPERLIPOPROTEINEMIAS

Based upon electrophoretic patterns of the plasma of persons with clinical disease, it has been possible to separate the hyperlipoproteinemias into categories which represent genetic phenotypes (see Table 30-3). The familial hyperlipoproteinemias are usually severe and are represented by obvious clinical diseases such as xanthomas of various types and early atherogenesis (before age 40). In the general population of middle-aged persons, about 15 percent have elevated blood cholesterol levels. Of these, only 2 percent are of a familial type. The metabolic basis of the rest (polygenic, type II) remains unexplained, except for those which are secondary to severe alcoholism, endocrine disease, or uremia.

CHOLESTEROL METABOLISM

Very briefly, the pathway of synthesis of cholesterol is as follows:

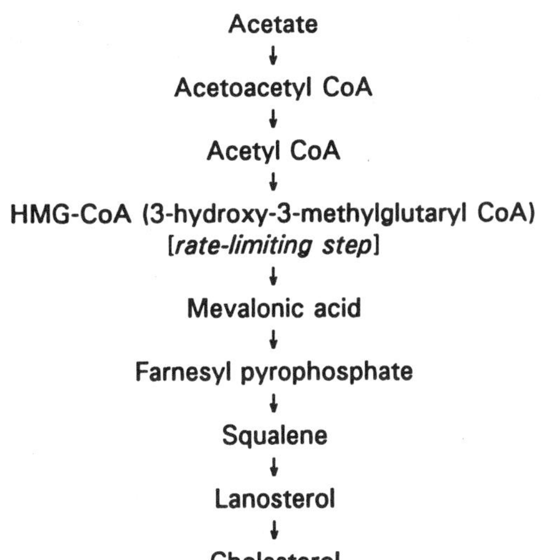

TABLE 39-2 Causes of secondary hyperlipoproteinemia

Hypercholesterolemia	Hypertriglyceridemia
Nephrosis	Obesity
Biliary cirrhosis	Diabetes mellitus
Hypothyroidism	Alcoholism
Hypopituitarism	Estrogens
Extreme starvation	Uremia
Immunoglobulin-lipoprotein disorders	Corticosteroids
	Thiazide diuretics
	Isotretinoin

TABLE 30-3 Classification of the hyperlipoproteinemias

Type	Prevalence	Cholesterol	Triglycerides	Elevated lipoproteins	Risk of atherogenesis
I	Rare	Normal	Normally elevated	Chylomicrons	None
IIa	Relatively common	Increased	Normal	LDL	High
IIb	Common	Increased	Increased	LDL, VLDL	High
III	Uncommon	Increased	Increased	IDL	High
IV	Common	Moderately elevated	Increased	VLDL	Moderately high
V	Uncommon	Moderately elevated	Markedly elevated	Chylomicrons, VLDL	Low

Cholesterol can be synthesized by many cells in the body, but the largest source is the liver. Dietary cholesterol contributes significantly to the body pool. The average American diet contains 1500 mg of daily cholesterol. It is important to point out that the rate-limiting step in the cascade of cholesterol synthesis involves the enzyme 3-hydroxy-3-methylglutaryl-coenzyme A (HMG-CoA) reductase. High levels of liver cholesterol inhibit this enzyme; this serves as a negative feed-back control of liver cholesterol synthesis. This enzyme is also the target of a class of compounds ("reductase inhibitors") introduced for reducing cholesterol synthesis. The only available excretion pathway for cholesterol is via the intestine as bile salts. Some cholesterol is utilized for conversion to adrenal and sex hormones and vitamin D. The endogenous and exogenous pathways of circulating cholesterol are shown in Fig. 30-1. There are obviously many points where disturbance of synthesis, circulation, or excretion may result in a decrease of blood cholesterol levels. Measures which have proven most feasible and effective are enhancement of excretion (as with the resins that sequester bile salts) and reduction of synthesis (at the rate-limiting step involving HMG-CoA reductase inhibitors). Now that more is known about tissue and liver receptors for cholesterol and the specific protein content of the various cholesterol particles, new opportunities exist for the creation of drugs which might be particularly effective to prevent atherogenesis.

HYPERTRIGLYCERIDEMIA

Some epidemiologic studies have suggested an inverse correlation between plasma triglyceride levels and coronary heart disease. However, clinical trials have not confirm this relationship. Although VLDL particles (which carry most of the triglycerides), are not considered to be atherogenic, there is some evidence that a subtype of smaller denser VLDL may be atherogenic. In any event VLDLs are the source of LDLs and, therefore in combined hyperlipidemias, reduction of VLDL is often accompanied by a reduction of LDL.

As shown in Table 30-3, which classifies the hyperlipoproteinemias, elevated levels of triglycerides occur in phenotypes I, IIb, III, IV, and V and sometimes in IIa. In phenotype I, or familial lipoprotein lipase deficiency, the cholesterol is normal and only the triglycerides are elevated. It is of interest that there is no increased risk of atherogenesis in these patients. In the other cases of hypertriglyceridemia, the cholesterol is also elevated. Therapy aims to lower both cholesterol and triglycerides. Very high triglyceride levels (over 1000 mg/dL) can precipitate acute pancreatitis and require treatment.

DIAGNOSIS

Establishment of clinically significant hyperlipoproteinemia is based on the plasma levels of total cholesterol, the LDL/HDL ratio, and triglycerides. The LDL/HDL ratio is important because the risk of atherogenesis is higher the greater the amount of LDL as compared to HDL. Recall that HDL carries cholesterol from tissues, while LDL is the main particle bringing cholesterol to organs. In addition, there are instances where the elevated total cholesterol is composed mainly of increased HDL. Such individuals are not at risk of atherogenesis and need not be treated.

Other risk factors must be considered. These are hypertension, smoking, alcohol, age, obesity, and most important, family history of early onset of atherosclerosis.

Evidence from large epidemiologic and controlled clinical studies indicate that the approach to the treatment of hyperlipidemia should be somewhat different for patients without evidence of vascular disease and/or risk factors from those with established vascular disease. For patients with coronary heart disease the effects of antihyperlipidemic treatment in reducing morbidity and mortality are now well established. However, the findings from primary prevention trials of treating hypercholesterolemic subjects that have no evidence of vascular disease or other risk factors are less impressive and require evaluation of the risk/benefit ratio.

According to the 1993 recommendations of the National Cholesterol Education Program, Adult Treatment Panel (NCEP-ATP II), total plasma cholesterol levels below 200 mg/dL are considered to be a low risk for vascular disease. Levels above 240 mg/dL are considered distinctly elevated with the in-between range identified as borderline. Individuals with levels greater than 200 mg/dL should be evaluated further by lipoprotein analysis. Patients with LDL cholesterol levels between 130 and 160 mg/dL are considered to be at moderate risk while those with greater than 160 mg/dL are at high risk. The risk for atherosclerosis is also higher for those with HDL cholesterol levels less than 35 mg/dL. By contrast patients with HDL levels higher than 60 mg/dL are at a distinctly lower risk. Fasting levels of plasma triglycerides of 200 to 400 mg/dL are considered "borderline high", above 400 mg/dL are "high" and above 1,000 mg/dL are termed "very high" and have the added risk of pancreatitis.

Treatment (diet and/or drugs) is recommended for patients with LDL cholesterol levels greater than 160 mg/dL if they have one or no other risk factors and for levels greater than 130 mg/dL for those with two or more other risk factors, and at above 100 mg/dL for patients with established coronary artery disease. Lowering the LDL cholesterol to below these levels for each group are the goals of the treatment.

Postmenopausal women and all older individuals with risk factors and/or atherosclerotic disease should be treated similarly as younger patients. However, epidemiologic studies indicate that the risk of cardiovascular death associated with high LDL cholesterol levels is highest between 40 and 50 years of age and decreases between the ages of 50 and 80 years. Over 60 years of age the risk becomes progressively smaller and above 80 the LDL cholesterol is negatively correlated with mortality. This may reflect the higher mortality of susceptible individuals at younger ages.

An association between low cholesterol and overall mortality from all causes has been reported for younger individuals and it was related to an increased incidence of traumatic deaths and suicides. However, recent reports suggest that the increased mortality was secondary to a high incidence of depression and alcoholism in this group.

DIETARY MANAGEMENT

Therapy is always initiated first with dietary measures. A diet of restricted caloric intake fat and cholesterol should be the first step in the management of hyperlipidemia. Some mild cases may need no further therapy, but dietary measures at the least will diminish the dose of required drug medication.

The aim of therapy is to reduce saturated fatty acid intake. The National Cholesterol Education Project has recommend two-step low fat diets. Step I diet is to reduce fat intake to 30 percent and saturated fat to approximately 10 percent or less of total calories. Step II diet reduces fat to 20 percent and saturated fat to approximately 7 percent. Foods such as fish, fruit, vegetables, grain, chicken, and legumes are recommended to reduce saturated fat intake. The daily dietary intake of cholesterol should be restricted to less than 300 mg. Control diet, weight control, and exercise should be initiated for at least 6 months before drug therapy is begun. It must be emphasized that reduction in body weight to an optimal level by diet and exercise should be the primary goal since this can provide a significant decrease in plasma cholesterol. Furthermore exercise has been shown to increase HDL cholesterol. A program which combined a vegetarian diet, no smoking, exercise, and alleviation of stress demonstrated a regression of coronary artery atherosclerosis. A decrease in the rate of progressive of vascular lesions has been achieved with low fat diets.

DRUG MANAGEMENT

The decision to use drugs to control cholesterol levels should not be taken lightly. Therapy must be continued for the rest of the individual's life. None of the drugs is without toxicity, and all incur considerable expense. Selection of a specific drug depends on the nature of the hyperlipidemia. It is not logical to use a drug designed to lower cholesterol when the patient's disease is hypertriglyceridemia. Selection of patients for drug therapy depends on the total blood cholesterol level; increased LDL, VLDL, LDL/VLDL cholesterol levels, and low HDL cholesterol; family history of atherosclerotic disease; presence of arteriosclerosis (coronary heart disease for example); and other risk factors such as hypertension and an unwillingness to give up smoking and alcohol.

SPECIFIC DRUGS

The drugs are classified into three major therapeutic categories depending on the type of lipid disorder. The drugs recommended for hypercholesterolemia (an increase in LDL) are niacin, bile acid binding resins, HMG-CoA inhibitors, and probucol. The drugs recommended for hypertriglyceridemia (an increase in VLDL) include niacin, gemfibrozil, and fish oils. Those drugs recommended for use in patients with combined increase in both LDL cholesterol and triglycerides are niacin and HMG-CoA reductase inhibitors. A new class of compounds, anti-oxidants (e.g., vitamin E, probucol), are currently under evaluation for their effect in preventing the oxidation of LDL which is necessary for the accumulation of LDL by macrophages leading to the formation of the atheroma in blood vessels.

Bile Acid Binding Resins

At the present time, two drugs are available which bind bile acids in the intestinal tract. These are colestipol and cholestyramine, and although they differ chemically, they have essentially the same actions. Both are large molecules acting as cationic exchange resins. Being insoluble in water, they are not absorbed. They bind bile acids in the intestinal lumen at their quaternary ammonium binding sites, releasing chloride in exchange for the bile acids. Since the complexed bile acids cannot be reabsorbed, they are excreted along with the resin in the feces.

Mechanism of Action Bile acids are byproducts of cholesterol and are ordinarily almost completely reabsorbed in the small intestine. Thus the essential structure of cholesterol is preserved for reuse by conversion of bile acids back to cholesterol in the liver. The bile acid sequestrants increase greatly the excretion of cholesterol (as bile acids), and thus the body must rely on increased synthesis to maintain cholesterol levels (see Fig. 30-1). The overall effect is a decrease in the body pool of cholesterol resulting in about a 10 to 20 percent decrease in total cholesterol mostly reflected in decreased LDL. VLDL and triglycerides may actually increase as does HDL. The decrease in LDL, which is responsible for the therapeutic effect, is achieved indirectly by feed-back regulation of the LDL liver receptors. Increased loss of cholesterol leads to increased cholesterol synthesis by the liver as well as an up-regulation of liver LDL receptors; thus enhancing the uptake of LDL and reducing plasma LDL levels. However, this is somewhat limited by an increase in VLDL synthesis. The resins are not effective in patients who have homozygous familial hypercholesterolemia, because they do not have functioning receptors for LDL.

Triglyceride levels may actually increase during the early course of resin therapy, but tend to return to normal with continued use. In some cases (especially in patients with type IIb disease) the elevation of triglycerides may be high enough to limit the use of these compounds. Resins should not be taken by patients with triglyceride levels in excess of 250 mg/dL. Combined treatment with HMG-CoA reductase inhibitors can reduce the elevation of triglycerides induced by resins.

Adverse Effects Since colestipol and cholestyramine are not absorbed or significantly metabolized, they have little systemic toxicity. However, by binding bile acids, they affect the normal digestive process, and the most common complaints are constipation and a bloating sensation. Bran and a high fiber diet offer relief. Some patients with sensitive bowels or cholestasis may have steatorrhea. At best, many patients find the resins unpleasant to take because of poor palatability and the many gastrointestinal side effects, and compliance is often inadequate.

Drug Interactions Since these resins may bind to many essential nutrients and other drugs, vitamin deficiencies and drug interactions are frequent and must be taken into account for each patient. Malabsorption of vitamin K may occur, and great care is required in patients taking both a resin and an oral anticoagulant. Due to the potential for drug interactions, it is recommended that medications be taken 1 h before or 4 h after taking the resins. Among the drugs whose absorption may be impaired by these resins are digitalis glycosides, thiazide diuretics, β-adrenergic receptor blockers, oral anticoagulants, oral hypoglycemic drugs, thyroxine, iron salts, and folic acid. Colestipol and cholestyramine also impair the bioavailability of HMG-CoA reductase inhibitors and fibric acid derivatives.

Therapeutic Uses The bile acid sequestrants are indicated in patients with primary hypercholesterolemia who have not responded adequately to diet. Patients who also have hypertriglyceridemia in addition to cholesterol elevation, may also respond, but the resins are not indicated when the triglycerides alone are elevated. The long-term effectiveness of bile acid sequestrants and their safety have been established. Treatment with resins alone produces modest 15 to 20 percent decreases in plasma cholesterol. However, when combined with HMG-CoA inhibitors, it is possible to obtain up to 50 percent reductions in plasma cholesterol levels.

The resins may also be used to reduce pruritus in partial biliary obstruction. Other uses are to bind the bacterial toxin in pseudomembranous colitis. Cholestyramine has also been used to bind the pesticide chlordecone (Kepone) in cases of poisoning. In this manner, recirculation through the liver and bile is prevented and fecal excretion is increased.

Nicotinic Acid

Large doses of niacin, or vitamin B_3, in the form of nicotinic acid, lowers both plasma cholesterol and triglycerides. Despite its troublesome side effects, it has had a long and successful history as a drug. The actions of nicotinic acid in reducing plasma lipids is not related to the action of niacin as a vitamin. In the body, nicotinic acid is converted to nicotinamide and is used in the nicotinamide adenine nucleotide (NAD) cycle. Therefore, both compounds satisfy the vitamin needs. However, nicotinamide has no antilipidemic activity. Furthermore, large amounts of nicotinic acid (several grams) are necessary for lowering plasma lipids. Nicotinic acid is well absorbed in the gastrointestinal tract and is excreted as such along with smaller quantities of other metabolites.

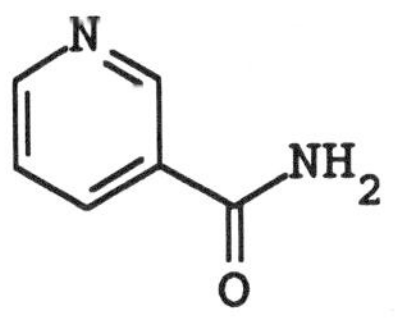

Nicotinamide 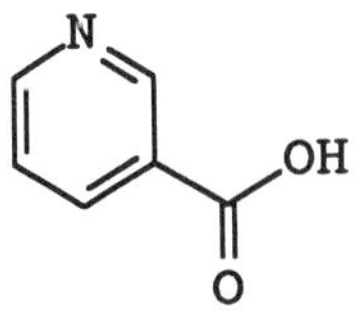 **Nicotinic acid**

Mechanism of Action The locus of action is a reduction of the production of VLDL by the liver, which in turn results in lower amounts of IDL, and LDL and raised HDL levels. The reduction in VLDL production is thought to be related to inhibition of lipolysis in adipose tissue, decreased esterification of triglycerides in the liver, and increased activity of lipoprotein lipase. Recent studies indicate that the decrease in VLDL synthesis is related to a decrease in the synthesis of apo(B) a major component of VLDL. Apo(B) is also a component of Lp(a) whose synthesis is also decreased by nicotinic acid. Other currently used antilipidemic agents have no effect or may increase Lp(a). As indicated above, Lp(a) is highly atherogenic and an independent risk factor for coronary artery disease. The increase in HDL produced by nicotinic acid involves primarily the HDL_2 fraction (the anti-atherogenic form of HDL) resulting in an increase in the HDL_2/HDL_3 ratio. There is also some evidence that nicotinic acid may inhibit the synthesis of cholesterol in the liver.

Adverse Effects At the high doses necessary for an antilipidemic effect, nicotinic acid produces an intense cutaneous flush. The cutaneous vasodilation involves mainly the face, neck, and upper trunk and resembles the "flush" experienced by women in menopause. It is often accompanied by pruritus and may develop into a skin rash. It is related to a local release of prostaglandins and it is blocked by prostaglandin synthesis inhibitors. It is therefore largely relieved by the administration of aspirin 30 min before nicotinic acid is taken. This symptom is also minimized by gradually increasing the dosage over several days to the desirable therapeutic level.

Various gastrointestinal dysfunctions such as vomiting, diarrhea, dyspepsia, and increased acidity are common, and even peptic ulceration has been reported. Rarely there have been instances of hyperpigmentation of the skin and the formation of acanthosis nigricans. The most serious toxicity is confined to the liver. Elevations of plasma transaminase may be severe, and jaundice has occurred. Liver toxicity and gastric acidity are dose-related and occur more frequently with sustained-release preparations. In addition, hyperglycemia and decreased glucose tolerance can occur in nondiabetic individuals. Plasma uric acid can increase, and gouty arthritis has been reported. Consequently, nicotinic acid should not be used in individuals with liver disease, diabetes, or gout.

Sustained-release preparations of nicotinic acid reduce or eliminate the "flush", but they exhibit greater hepatotoxicity (with increased levels of aminotransferase) which could lead to acute hepatitis and death. These preparations also have a higher incidence of gastrointestinal symptoms including increased gastric acidity and are therefore less safe than the immediate release forms. These side effects are dose-related and are more frequent at the higher dose levels (greater than 1 to 5 g/day). Both types of preparations are equally effective in lowering cholesterol and triglycerides in moderate doses (up to 1.5 g/day) although the sustained-release forms are more effective in reducing cholesterol (but not triglycerides) in the highest doses (2 to 3 g/day).

Therapeutic Uses Nicotinic acid alone or in combination with bile acid binding resins can lower both cholesterol and triglycerides from 10 to 30 percent. As one of the drugs compared in the Coronary Drug Project, it was successful in reducing the overall incidence of recurrent myocardial infarction. However, there was no effect on overall cardiovascular mortality. Compliance is a major difficulty, and the drug is reserved for patients who do not respond to other measures.

Clofibrate

This derivative of aryloxylisobutyric acid was the most active of a series of compounds which were found in the early 1960s to be capable of reducing plasma concentrations of total lipids and cholesterol. Although widely used in hypercholesterolemia and as a test drug in the Coronary Drug Project, at the present time the use of clofibrate is mainly restricted to familial dysbetalipoproteinemia (type III hyperlipidemia).

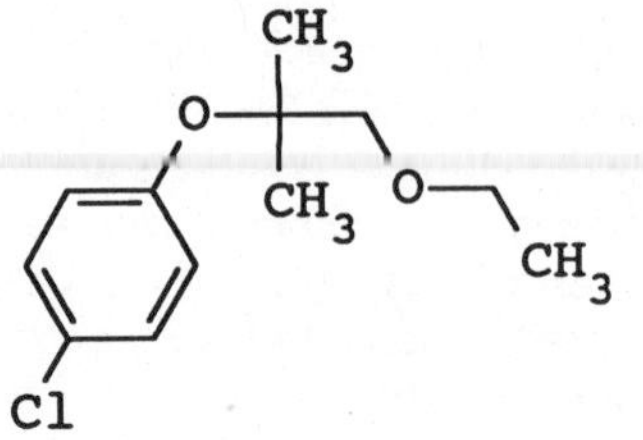

Mechanism of Action The site of action of clofibrate is uncertain. It does increase the activity of lipoprotein lipase, which enhances the rate of conversion of VLDL to IDL and LDL within the vascular lumen. It also inhibits the release of lipoproteins (especially VLDL) from the liver.

Clofibrate decreases plasma triglyceride concentrations by reducing levels of VLDL. Most patients also have a fall in levels of LDL and plasma cholesterol. Unfortunately, a large fall in VLDL can also result in an increase in LDL, but the net effect on cholesterol is reduced. This increase in LDL is often referred to as "beta shift" referring to the old designation of LDL as "beta" lipoproteins. It is a common experience that only modest reductions in levels of cholesterol (5 to 10 percent) occur. In contrast, triglyceride levels are reduced by about 20 to 25 percent. HDL levels are not affected. An exception is familial dysbetalipoproteinemia where cholesterol may be lowered by as much as 50 percent.

Pharmacokinetics The oral absorption of clofibrate is almost total. The drug is hydrolyzed to clofibric acid (p-chlorophenoxyisobutyric acid), which is the active compound. Clofibric acid is highly protein-bound (95 to 97 percent). Over 95 percent of clofibric acid appears in the urine as free and conjugated clofibric acid. The mean elimination half-life is about 20 h, but can vary considerably among patients.

Adverse Effects Clofibrate is deceptively well tolerated by most patients in the initiation of therapy. With long-term use there may occur weight gain (increased appetite), skin rash, alopecia, weakness, impotence, breast tenderness, and loss of libido. A disturbing action is a flu-like syndrome of muscle aches, cramps, stiffness, and weakness, which is associated with elevations of creatinine phosphokinase activity in the plasma. Patients who have elevation of this enzyme and other enzymes (transaminase) of liver and muscle origin should not receive clofibrate. With long-term use the incidence of gallstones and cholecystitis increases.

Clofibrate may cause an increased risk of malignancy and cholelithiasis and the use of the drug should be limited and discontinued if an adequate response is not obtained.

Therapeutic Uses Clofibrate is indicated for primary dysbetalipoproteinemia that does not respond to dietary measures. The drug may be considered for use in patients with type IV or V hyperlipoproteinemia where plasma triglyceride levels are very high (over 1000 mg/dL) who have pancreatitis or abdominal pain suggestive of pancreatitis, and who have not responded adequately to dietary control.

Gemfibrozil

Related to clofibrate chemically, gemfibrozil has similar pharmacologic activity, toxicologic effects, and clinical usefulness.

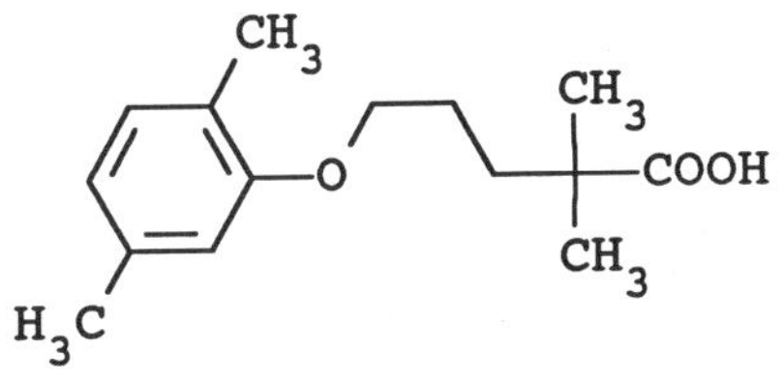

The mechanism of action is unknown and the changes in plasma lipid levels are similar to clofibrate, with the greatest effect being a reduction of elevated triglyceride levels. Plasma VLDL levels are decreased; only modest decreases in LDL levels occur, while HDL is elevated moderately. Clofibrate does not elevate HDL levels and this may be an important difference between clofibrate and gemfibrozil.

Pharmacokinetics Absorption from the intestinal tract is excellent. Peak plasma levels occur in 1 to 2 hours following a single dose. Gemfibrozil is biotransformed by conversion of a methyl group on the phenyl ring to a hydroxymethyl, and then to a carboxymethyl moiety. Excretion is urinary with about 70 percent eliminated as a glucuronide conjugate of the metabolites.

Adverse Effects The adverse reactions associated with gemfibrozil are similar to those observed with clofibrate; however, the latter drug appear somewhat safer on long-term use. Common adverse reactions that patients may experience include gastrointestinal upset, blurred vision, impotence, or gallstones.

Unlike niacin, gemfibrozil does not affect the diabetic or insulin-resistant patient. It is also has little or no effect on uric acid and can be used in the hypertriglyceride gouty patient.

Therapeutic Uses Gemfibrozil has an indication for hypertriglyceridemia in adults with plasma triglyceride levels greater than 1000 mg/dL (types IV and V hyperlipoproteinemia) who are at risk of pancreatitis and who do not respond to dietary therapy.

Probucol

Probucol differs chemically from the other agents. Chemically probucol is a *bis*-phenol containing sulfur and many methyl groups. It is highly lipophilic and distributes into adipose tissue, where it persists with as much as 20 percent of peak blood levels remaining after 6 months.

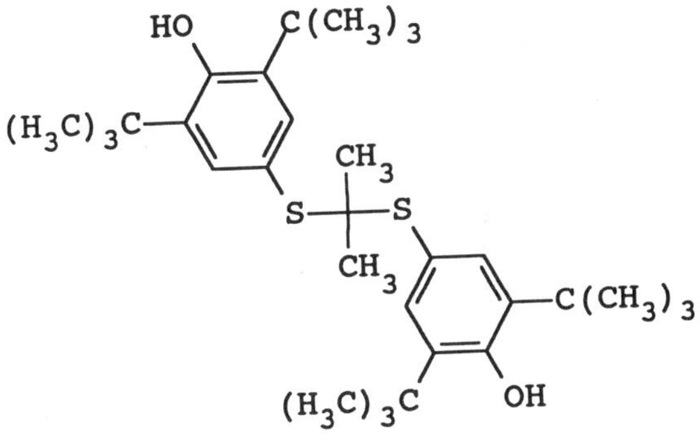

Mechanism of Action Probucol lowers plasma cholesterol with little or no effect on triglycerides. The LDL fraction is decreased, but there is a proportionally greater decremental effect on the HDL fraction. From an epidemiologic viewpoint, this is harmful because a decrease in HDL signifies less removal of cholesterol from the tissues, and patients who respond favorably to anticholesterolemic therapy generally have a decrease in LDL and a rise in HDL fractions. In any event, the fall in plasma total cholesterol is a modest 10 to 15 percent when probucol is used alone.

The mechanism of action of probucol on lipoprotein metabolism is obscure. It appears that the LDL fraction is more rapidly degraded, but there is no increase in LDL receptors in the liver. An increase in the excretion of bile acids is observed, which may be related to the effect on LDL. Probucol decreases the synthesis of apoproteins A1 and A2, which may account for the decrease in HDL. Probucol is a potent anti-oxidant and it has been suggested that its beneficial clinical effects are related to the prevention of LDL oxidation which is necessary for its binding to the scavenger monocytes receptors and the formation of foam cells. This action is similar to that suggested for vitamin E and β-carotene (see below).

Pharmacokinetics The gastrointestinal absorption of probucol is limited (less than 10 percent) and variable; food appears to enhance absorption. With daily use, blood levels slowly increase over the first 3 to 4 months, at which time steady state blood concentrations occur. Since the drug is very lipid-soluble, it accumulates slowly in adipose tissue and will persist in fat and blood for as long as 6 months after the last dose (the effects on plasma lipids dissipate long before the drug disappears from the body. Most of the compound is eliminated via the bile and feces.

Therapeutic Uses The indications for probucol therapy include types IIa and IIb hyperlipoproteinemia in patients who have not responded adequately to diet and weight reduction. There have been limited large-scale studies which have compared probucol with other agents. The best results are reported when probucol is used in conjunction with the bile acid sequestrants. An advantage of the combined use is that probucol antagonizes the constipating action of the resins. The decrease in HDL fraction is considered a risk factor for atherogenesis, and thus probucol is usually reserved for patients who do not respond or cannot tolerate the other agents. However, this limitation may be less significant if it is demonstrated that the beneficial effects of probucol are related primarily to its anti-oxidant properties.

Adverse Effects Adverse reactions to probucol include prolongation of the QT interval. In animals probucol is cardiac arrhythmogenic, and this limits probucol use to patients who have no evidence of heart disease. Diarrhea and loose stools are a common complaint. Other gastrointestinal complaints such as nausea, abdominal pain, vomiting, and flatulence disappear with continued use. Less frequent adverse effects are skin rashes, thrombocytopenia, peripheral neuritis, and angioneurotic edema. Probucol does not appear to be toxic to the liver, but mild elevations of serum transaminase have been seen.

HMG-CoA Reductase Inhibitors

There are three hydroxy-methylglutaryl-coenzyme A (HMG-CoA) reductase inhibitors available in the United States: lovastatin, simvastatin, and pravastatin. Collectively these compounds are often referred to as "reductase inhibitors". These agents are potent, competitive inhibitors of HMG-CoA reductase, which is the rate-limiting step in cholesterol synthesis. When properly used they are the most effective agents for lowering plasma cholesterol.

The chemical structures of lovastatin, simvastatin, and pravastatin are shown in Figure 30-2. Lovastatin and its chemical derivative simvastatin are lactones and serve as prodrugs. They must be biotransformed by the liver to the active β-hydroxyacid form. Pravastatin is in the active form.

Mechanism of Action Inhibition of HMG-CoA reductase by these drugs is competitive and reversible. The decrease in the hepatic synthesis of cholesterol leads to a compensatory increase of liver LDL receptors and LDL uptake. Thus plasma LDL levels are diminished, and there is a shift in the utilization of body cholesterol by the liver to the formation of bile acids. However, overall bile secretion is reduced. It follows that if dietary intake of cholesterol is not restricted, the liver will use exogenous cholesterol to make up for the deficit in synthesis (see Fig. 30-1). There is a corresponding increase in HDL levels in the blood. This is favorable and interpreted to signify an increased movement of cholesterol from the tissues to the liver. The blood levels of apo(B) also fall which indicates that these compounds reduce the concentration of LDL particles. Triglyceride blood levels are also lowered reflecting a decrease in VLDL. The magnitude of the effect of the HMG-CoA reductase inhibitors in reducing blood cholesterol is greater than that of all other agents.

Pharmacokinetics The bioavailability of lovastatin and pravastatin is approximately 35 percent of the oral dose. Simvastatin has a higher oral bioavailability of approximately 85 percent. All three compounds have a high first pass extraction by the liver and only small percentages of the original drugs and their metabolites reach the general circulation. Liver metabolism is through the P-450 system which accounts for several drug interactions. Major metabolites of lovastatin include the β-hydroxyacid, a 6′-hydroxy derivative (both active) and two additional metabolites.

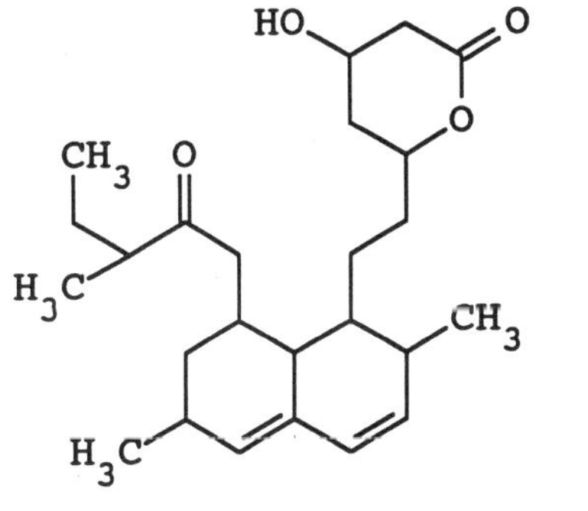

Lovastatin

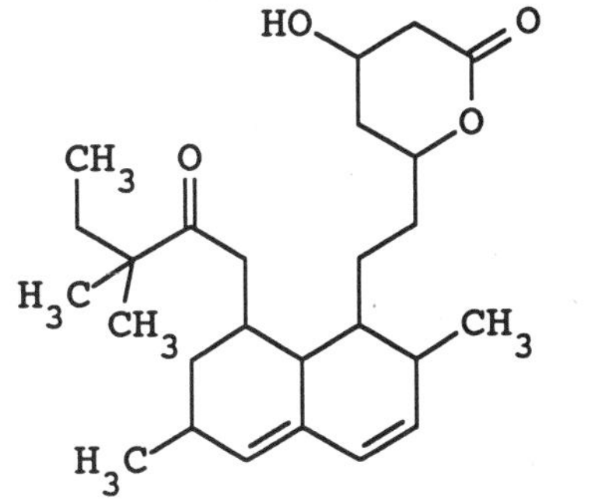

Simvastatin

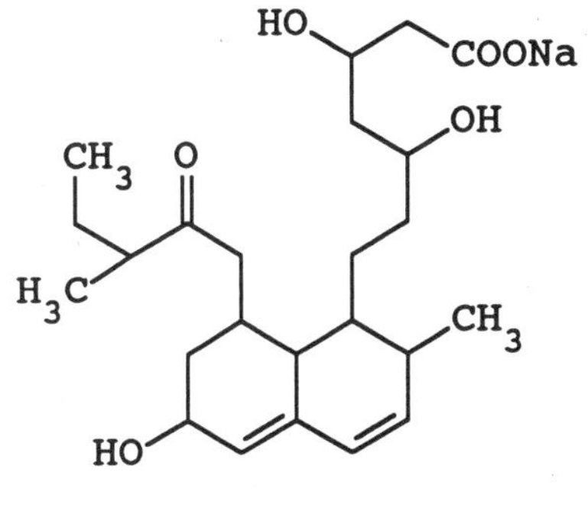

Pravastatin

FIGURE 30-2 *Structures of the HMG-CoA reductase inhibitors.*

Pravastatin is biotransformed to a 3α-hydroxy derivative (which has one-tenth to one-fortieth the activity of the parent compound) and a number of other inactive products. Simvastatin is metabolized to the active β-hydroxyacid and to 6′-hydroxy and 6′-hydroxymethyl derivatives. Excretion of all of these metabolites is primarily through the bile and feces with smaller amounts eliminated in the urine. There is some enterohepatic recirculation which accounts in part for the relatively long elimination half-lives of these drugs.

Peak inhibition of HMG-CoA reductase occurs 2 to 4 hours after drug administration. A single evening dose is effective; in this connection, it has been determined that the peak in the synthesis of cholesterol occurs around midnight. Lovastatin has been found to be highly effective when given with the evening meal, whereas the pravastatin and simvastatin are not affected when given with or without food. In plasma, the active metabolites of lovastatin and simvastatin are highly protein bound (95 percent) whereas pravastatin is bound only 50 percent to plasma proteins. The lactones (lovastatin and simvastatin) can cross the blood-brain barrier while pravastatin does not. However, all three compounds have very low arterial blood levels due to their high first pass extraction by the liver.

Therapeutic Uses These reductase inhibitors are indicated in types IIa and IIb hyperlipoproteinemias. They should be used only after diet and other non-drug measures have failed to achieve a satisfactory lowering of total cholesterol blood level. In addition, other correctable causes of hypercholesterolemia such as hyperthyroidism, diabetes mellitus, and the nephrotic syndrome should be managed. It is important to determine the actual LDL and HDL levels, as there is a subset of patients with high total cholesterol who do not have elevated LDL. Instead, they apparently have non-LDL fractions, which do not involve an increased risk for atherogenesis.

With diet and drug therapy with an HMG-CoA reductase inhibitor, as much as 30 percent lowering of total blood cholesterol may be achieved. Combined with cholestyramine or colestipol, the lowering may be as much as 50 to 60 percent. A dose-response relationship has been found. On a mg basis, simvastatin is twice as potent as lovastatin or pravastatin. However, no significant differences have been demonstrated for the lipid-lowering effectiveness among the three compounds when each is used in the recommended dosage regimens.

Adverse Effects In about 2 percent of patients receiving reductase inhibitors for a year or more, elevations of serum transaminase may occur. When the drug is removed, the levels gradually return to normal. Patients receiving one of these compounds should have liver function tests performed before initiating therapy, every 6 to 8 weeks for the next year, and every 6 months thereafter. Liver disease of any kind and alcoholism are contraindications to the use of these drugs.

Myalgia is a relatively common complaint. About 0.5 percent of patients develop myositis which is associated with elevated levels of creatinine phosphokinase. Elevated levels of this enzyme or active clinical myositis require termination of therapy. In fact, therapy should be withheld in any patient at risk from renal failure as a result of rhabdomyolysis (severe infection, shock, trauma, electrolyte disturbances, and uncontrolled seizures). The risk for rhabdomyolysis is increased with co-administration of cyclosporine, erythromycin, gemfibrozil, nicotinic acid, and possibly other compounds which can produce myositis. The elevation of serum transaminase and creatine phosphatase are dose-dependant and are rare in low doses. Higher doses of reductase inhibitors are also progressively less effective, therefore, lower doses with combination therapy (e.g., with a bile acid binding resin) is preferable. Pravastatin shows less drug interactions with gemfibrozil, cyclosporine, and oral anticoagulants presumably due to differences in liver biotransformation.

Because of an increased prevalence of baseline lenticular opacities and the appearance of new opacities, it has been suggested that reductase inhibitors may cause this defect. Slit lamp studies should be done before therapy is started and at yearly intervals thereafter. At present there is no conclusive evidence that these drug favor the development of cataract formations in humans.

Dextrothyroxine

It has been known for many years that hyperthyroidism is associated with hypocholesterolemia. Although thyroid hormones enhance cholesterol biosynthesis, they reduce LDL concentrations and have a greater effect on catabolism; the end result is a reduction of plasma cholesterol levels. Dextrothyroxine has substantially less calorigenic activity than the natural hormone, levothyroxine.

Dextrothyroxine has been recommended in hyperlipoproteinemia, types II and III, as an adjunct to dietary measures. Its mechanism of action is to increase the degradation of cholesterol and lipoproteins, resulting in a lowering of plasma cholesterol.

The adverse effects observed with dextrothyroxine therapy are generally related to increased metabolism and cardiotoxicity. These include palpitations, loss of weight, nervousness, insomnia, excessive sweating, glucose intolerance, and diarrhea. As can be expected, this drug is contraindicated in patients with organic heart disease or cardiac arrhythmias and with advanced liver or kidney disease. In addition, dextrothyroxine may potentiate the effect of oral anticoagulants.

Estrogens

It is well-known that females, during their reproductive years, have a very low incidence of atherosclerosis which is related to a low LDL/HDL ratio. The risk increases in females to that of males a few years after menopause as the ratio of LDL/HDL increases. In fact, postmenopausal women have higher levels of LDL cholesterol than men of the same age. They also have a high LDL cholesterol/apo(B) ratio which indicates more cholesterol per LDL particle than men. Hypercholesterolemia in postmenopausal women is found to be associated with a decrease in LDL liver receptors and responds to treatment with any of the agents that act by increasing the activity of these receptors (e.g., reductase inhibitors and bile acid binding resins).

Administration of estrogens increases the number of liver LDL receptors and decreases LDL cholesterol. Such treatment is appropriate only for females and especially after menopause. In postmenopausal women, estrogen treatment can reduce the risk of coronary disease by 50 percent.

Neomycin

Many drugs have had a trial in an attempt to lower blood cholesterol. Among them is neomycin, an aminoglycoside which, when combined with a bile acid binding resin or with nicotinic acid, has had some degree of success. Apparently neomycin is able to block the absorption of cholesterol as well as bile acids. Studies have shown that when administered alone, by the oral route, neomycin can reduce LDL by about 20 percent; when used with niacin the effect was greater. Although not officially indicated for this purpose, some physicians consider neomycin as an alternative for patients who tolerate the resins poorly. Like nicotinic acid, neomycin also reduces the levels of the atherogenic lipoprotein Lp(a).

Antioxidants

Several recent epidemiologic observations and retrospective studies have suggested that the antioxidants α-tocopherol (vitamin E) and β-carotene (a precursor of vitamin A) are associated with lower risk of coronary artery disease and its sequelae. Large doses of these compounds, much in excess of the vitamin requirements, over long periods are necessary for a significant effect. *In vitro* and *in vivo* experimental studies with these compounds indicate that they inhibit the oxidative modification of LDL which is necessary for its binding on scavenger monocyte receptors leading to the accumulation of lipids in foam cells of the blood vessel wall and formation of atheromatous plaques. The oxidative modification of Lp(a) is also inhibited by antioxidants.

Epidemiologic and clinical studies which showed significant protection from large doses of vitamin E and β-carotene did not indicate a similar effect with the water-soluble antioxidant vitamin C. It is, therefore, suggested that the effects of vitamins E and β-carotene are also related to their lipid-solubility (for additional information on these vitamins, see Chapter 36). The beneficial effects observed with probucol in clinical trials are now believed by some to be due to its antioxidant properties especially since its effects on plasma lipid profiles is marginally beneficial.

These observations require confirmation by long-term prospective controlled clinical trials and although no serious adverse effects have been reported from the large doses of the vitamins needed, potential long-term adverse effects need to be evaluated.

Antioxidants and other compounds which inhibit the deposition of lipids on blood vessels could provide a different therapeutic approach and possible development of new therapeutic agents for the control of the cardiovascular effects of the hyperlipidemia.

BIBLIOGRAPHY

-------- "Expert Panel on Detection, Evaluation and Treatment of High Blood Cholesterol in Adults. Report of the National Cholesterol Education Program (NCEP), Adult Treatment Panel II," *J. Am. Med. Assoc.* **269**: 3015-3023, (1993).

-------- "Lovastatin Study Group II: "Therapeutic Response to Lovastatin (Mevinolin) in Non-familial Hypercholesterolemia," *J. Am. Med. Assoc.* **256**: 29-34 (1986).

-------- "The Lipid Research Clinic Coronary Primary Prevention Trial, Results 1. Reduction in Incidence of Coronary Disease," *J. Am. Med. Assoc.* **251**: 351 364 (1984).

Brown, M.S., P.T. Kovaneu, and J.L. Goldstein: "Regulation of Plasma Cholesterol by Lipoprotein Receptors," *Science* **212**: 628-635 (1981).

Brown, M.S., and A. Goldstein: "Receptor-Mediated Pathway for Cholesterol Homeostasis," *Science* **232**: 34-47 (1986).

Canner, P.L.: "Fifteen Year Mortality in Coronary Drug Project Patients. Long Term Benefits with Niacin," *J. Am. Coll. Cardiol.* **8**: 1245-1255 (1986).

Connor, W.E., and S.L. Connor: "Dietary Treatment of Hyperlipidemia: Rationale and Benefit," *Endocrinologist* **1**: 33-44 (1991).

Consensus Conference: "Lowering Blood Cholesterol to Prevent Heart Disease," *J. Am. Med. Assoc.* **253**: 2080-2086 (1985).

Davidson, M.H., R.S. Rosenson, and T. Mazzone: "From Diagnosis to Treatment: Focus on Costs, Safety, and Efficacy of Antihyperlipidemic Agents," *Hospital Formulary* **28**: 262-282 (1993).

DiPalma, J.R.: "Lovastatin: Cholesterol-Lowering Agent," *Am. Fam. Physician* **36**: 189-192 (1988).

Goldstein, J.L., T. Kita, and M.S. Brown: "Defective Lipoprotein Receptors and Atherosclerosis: Lessons from an Animal Counterpart of Familial Hypercholesterolemia," *N. Engl. J. Med.* **309**: 288-296 (1983).

Grady, D., S.M. Rubin, and D.B. Petitti: "Hormone Therapy To Prevent Disease and Prolong Life in Postmenopausal Women," *Arch. Int. Med.* **117**: 1016-1037 (1992).

Manninen, V., L. Tenkanen, and P. Koskinen: "Joint Effects of Serum Triglyceride and LDL Cholesterol and HDL Cholesterol Concentrations on Coronary Heart Disease Risk in the Helsinki Heart Study: Implications for Treatment," *Circulation* **85**: 37-45 (1992).

McKennedy, J.M., and J.D. Proctor: "A Comparison of the Efficacy and Toxic Effects of Sustained vs. Immediate Release Niacin in Hypercholesterolemia," *J. Am. Med. Assoc.* **271**: 672-677 (1994).

Repka, F.J., and R.F. Leighton: "Step Management of Hypercholesterolemia," *Am. Fam. Physician* **36**: 236-248 (1987).

Rimm, E.B., E.L. Gioannucci, and W.C. Willet: Prospective Study of Alcohol Consumption and Risk of Coronary Disease in Men," *Lancet* **338**: 464-468 (1991).

Steinberg, D.: "Antioxidants, Vitamins and Coronary Heart Disease," *New Engl. J. Med.* **328**: 1487-1489 (1993).

Tyroler, H.A.: "Review of Lipid Lowering Clinical Trials in Relation to Observational Chemical Studies," *Circulation* **76**: 515-522 (1987).

Vega, G.L., and S.M. Grundy: "Mechanisms of Primary Hypercholesterolemia in Humans," *Am. Heart J.* **113**: 493-502 (1987).

Weis, S., and A.G. Lacko: "Role of Lipoproteins in Hypercholesterolemia," *Practical Cardiology* (special issue), May 1988, p 12.

CHAPTER 31

Diuretics

Charles T. Stier, Jr.

The development of effective oral diuretic agents began in the 1950's with the introduction of chlorothiazide. Diuretics are a widely prescribed group of drugs used primarily in the management of edema and hypertension. They are drugs which increase urine flow (diuresis) by promoting urinary excretion of sodium ions (natriuresis) and water from the body by interfering with ionic transport. The principal site of action for the diuretics in the removal of edematous fluid from the body is the nephron unit of the kidney. These agents are classified according to their proposed mechanism of action in the nephron (Table 31-1).

RENAL PHYSIOLOGY

In the kidney, regulation of water and electrolyte reabsorption occurs at several sites along the nephron: the proximal tubule, loop of Henle, distal tubule, and collecting duct (Fig. 31-1). The glomerulus permits filtration of most of the essential constituents of the extracellular fluid and waste products. However, it prevents passage of plasma proteins, lipids, and substances bound to proteins.

The nephron normally reabsorbs 99 percent of the glomerular filtrate. In the first segment of the nephron, the proximal tubule, 50 to 60 percent of ions and water are reabsorbed. Sodium is reabsorbed along the lumen-to-cell sodium gradient maintained by Na^+,K^+-ATPase in the basolateral cell membrane; chloride and water diffuse passively. Also, most of the filtered bicarbonate is reabsorbed in this portion of the nephron and is mediated by the enzyme carbonic anhydrase. The fluid in the proximal tubule is similar in osmolality (300 mOsm) to that of the interstitial fluid and plasma.

The proximal tubule contains the secretory processes for organic acids and bases by which these compounds enter the renal tubular fluid from the blood. This secretory system provides not only a means for the renal elimination of certain diuretics but it also allows these diuretics (e.g., furosemide, triamterene) to gain access to their site of action on the luminal side of tubular cells.

As the remaining portion of the glomerular filtrate, approximately 40 percent, enters the descending limb of the loop of Henle, a concentrating mechanism operates. Water is removed passively, and the tubular fluid becomes hypertonic as it approaches the curvature.

In the thick ascending limb of the loop of Henle, the tubular fluid becomes hypotonic. This area is divided into medullary and cortical portions.

TABLE 31-1 Classification of diuretic drugs

I. Agents which increase renal solute excretion
   - A. Inhibit sodium/chloride symporter
     - Thiazides, chlorthalidone, indapamide, metolazone
   - B. Inhibit sodium/chloride/potassium cotransport
     - Furosemide, ethacrynic acid, bumetanide, torsemide
   - C. Potassium-sparing diuretics
     - Amiloride, spironolactone, triamterene
   - D. Inhibit carbonic anhydrase
     - Acetazolamide

II. Agents used as osmotic nonelectrolytes
   - Mannitol

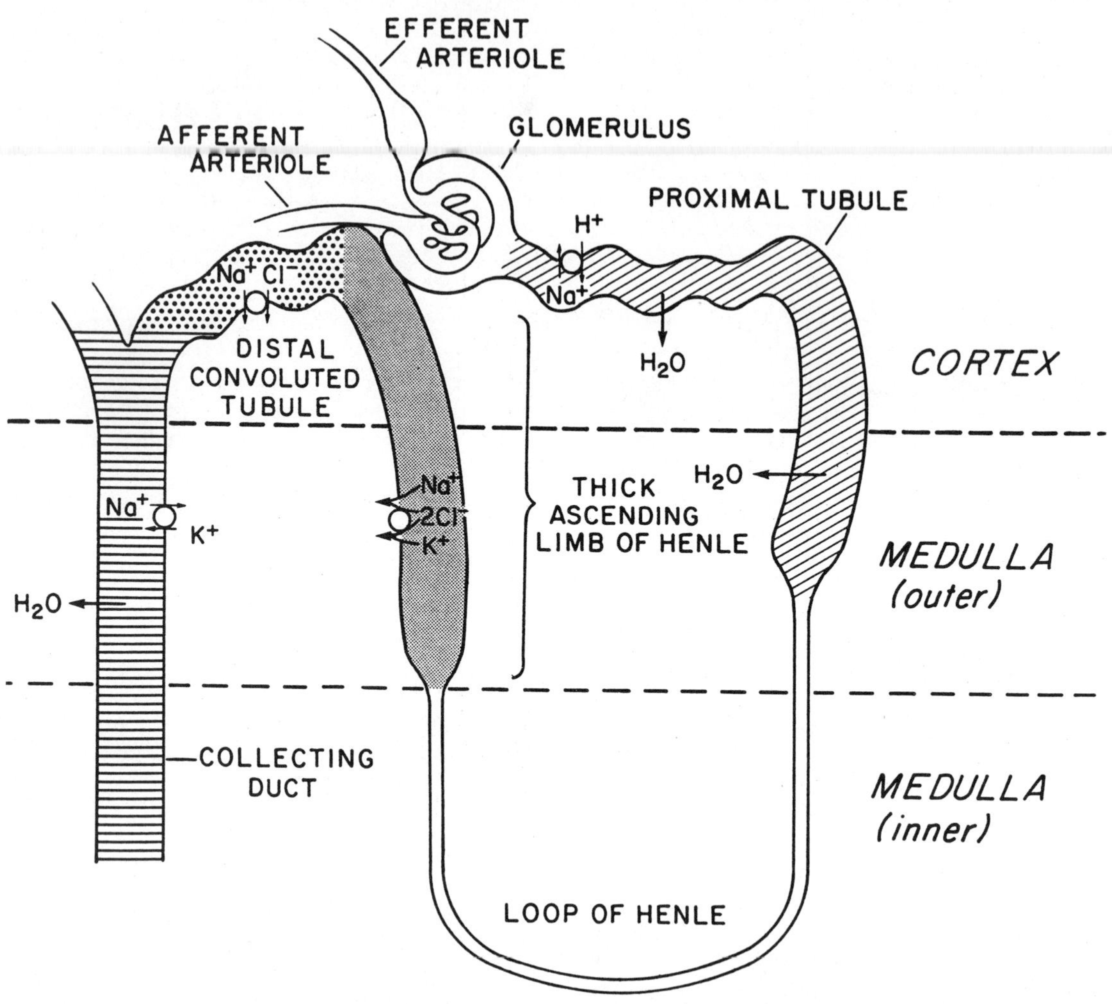

FIGURE 31-1 *Diagrammatic representation of the nephron unit showing sites of electrolyte and water reabsorption.*

In the thick ascending limb it appears that a Na^+-K^+-$2Cl^-$ cotransporter located on the luminal side is responsible for the reabsorption of sodium and chloride. In this region magnesium and calcium ions are also removed from the tubular luminal fluid. However, water does not follow sodium and chloride, since the entire ascending limb is impermeable to water. The sodium entering the medullary interstitium, along with urea, maintains the hypertonicity of this tissue and is responsible for the free-water reabsorption from the collecting duct. Since sodium is removed and water remains in the lumen, the tubular fluid becomes hypotonic. For didactic purposes, the hypotonic fluid formed may be said to consist of two hypothetical compartments: one isosmotic with plasma and the other free of solute, or so-called free water.

In the cortical segment of the ascending limb, more sodium and chloride are reabsorbed from the lumen by a sodium-chloride cotransport mechanism, and further formation of free water occurs. The sodium chloride reabsorbed from the cortical area, however, does not contribute to the hypertonicity of the interstitium. In total, about 20 to 30 percent of filtered sodium chloride is reabsorbed in the ascending limb of the loop of Henle.

The tubular fluid entering the distal convoluted segment is hypotonic. Sodium chloride is reabsorbed out of this region. Calcium reabsorption is secondarily active, being driven by Na^+,K^+-ATPase. This active sodium extrusion sets up a gradient for sodium/calcium exchange at the basolateral membrane which favors calcium reabsorption. Parathyroid hormone stimulates calcium reabsorption in this segment of the nephron.

When fluid enters the last segment of the nephron unit, the collecting duct, sodium is actively reabsorbed. This active transport mechanism is facilitated by the mineralocorticoid aldosterone. Potassium and hydrogen ions are secreted passively in response to the removal of sodium. Water movement out of the collecting duct is controlled by antidiuretic hormone (ADH), which increases the permeability of the collecting duct to water. The concentrations of ADH are highest in states of dehydration or water deprivation. Free water which is formed in the ascending limb of the loop of Henle can be reabsorbed in this area. The amount of reabsorption depends on the concentration of ADH and the degree of hypertonicity of the medullary interstitium.

The hypertonicity of the medullary interstitium plays an important part in the hypothesis of the countercurrent multiplier mechanism. According to this theory, sodium, actively transported from the ascending limb of Henle's loop into the medullary interstitium, moves passively down its electrochemical gradient into the descending limbs of neighboring loops. This establishes a small concentration gradient between the fluid contents of the ascending and descending limbs at successive levels along the course of the loop. Tubular fluid sodium concentration and osmolality increase progressively down the descending limb because of countercurrent flow, and become maximally concentrated at the hairpin turn of the loop of Henle in the inner medulla. This process establishes the medullary hypertonicity, which provides the osmotic gradient necessary to abstract water from the lumen of the collecting duct in the final concentration of urine.

The high concentration of solute in the medulla is maintained by the vasa recta acting as a countercurrent exchanger. This process, which depends on the slow rate of medullary blood flow, maintains the 300/1200 mOsm/kg concentration differential between the cortex and the tip of the medulla. Only the water and sodium necessary to maintain the normal electrolyte concentrations of the body pass into the systemic circulation. The countercurrent exchange system thus prevents excessive loss of sodium from the medulla and papilla(e).

THIAZIDE DIURETICS

The thiazides are sulfonamide derivatives which (1) promote the renal excretion of sodium and chloride, (2) remain effective in the presence of acidosis or alkalosis, (3) inhibit carbonic anhydrase *in vitro*, and (4) lower arterial blood pressure in hypertensive patients. Qualitatively, the thiazide diuretics are the same. The structures of chlorothiazide and other thiazide diuretics are presented in Table 31-2.

Hydrochlorothiazide causes less inhibition of carbonic anhydrase but produces 5 to 10 times more sodium diuresis than does chlorothiazide at equal milligram doses. The hydrogenated ring of hydrochlorothiazide permits many possible substitutions, and the structure-activity relationships for this series of compounds have been extensively studied.

Mechanism of Action

Thiazides promote urinary excretion of sodium, chloride, potassium, water, and, in the case of chlorothiazide, bicarbonate. Urinary loss of bicarbonate, when it occurs, is due to a weak inhibition of carbonic anhydrase by the thiazides in the proximal convoluted tubule. This effect of chlorothiazide is insignificant at usual dose levels. The thiazide diuretics cause sodium excretion even in the presence of systemic alkalosis or acidosis and, therefore, do not exhibit the phenomenon of refractoriness.

The principal site of action for the diuretic effect of the thiazides is the early distal convoluted tubule of the nephron. The mechanism of action is thought to be inhibition of the luminal electroneutral NaCl symporter. As a result of inhibition of sodium and chloride reabsorption in the distal nephron, the thiazides diminish the capacity of the kidney to produce a dilute urine. In addition, the thiazides enhance the reabsorption of calcium ion in the distal tubule. Microperfusion studies have localized this effect to predominantly the early portion of the distal convoluted tubule. When the increased load of sodium in the renal tubular fluid reaches the collecting duct, some sodium is actively reabsorbed and potassium is secreted, resulting in an increased urinary potassium concentration. If thiazides evoke sufficient potassium excretion, hypokalemia is produced. The thiazides may also promote the loss of magnesium from the body.

TABLE 31-2 Structure and therapeutic dose of some thiazide diuretics

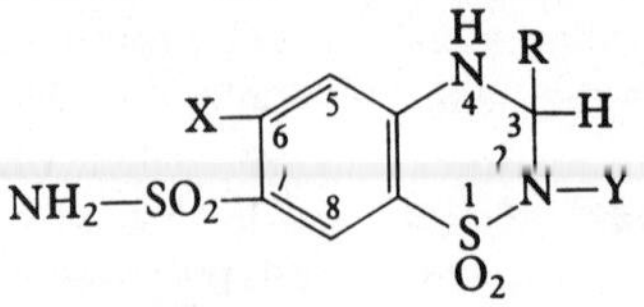

Generic name	X	Y	R	Δ 3,4	Oral dose, mg/day
Chlorothiazide	Cl	H	H	Yes	500 - 1000
Hydrochlorothiazide	Cl	H	H	No	50 - 150
Bendroflumethiazide	CF_3	H	CH_2–C₆H₅ (phenyl) 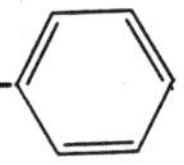	No	5 - 15
Polythiazide	Cl	CH_3	$CH_2SCH_2CF_3$	No	2 - 4

In addition to the action of removing edematous fluid from the body, the thiazides are used clinically to reduce elevated blood pressure. This antihypertensive effect of the thiazides is not entirely explained by their diuretic effect and the consequent decrease in circulating blood volume. It appears that relaxation of the peripheral vascular smooth muscle may also be involved in the antihypertensive effect of the thiazides, particularly when they are used for longer than 2 weeks.

Pharmacokinetics

These drugs are well absorbed from the gastrointestinal tract, except for chlorothiazide. The thiazides appear in the bloodstream and remain there in active concentrations for several hours, the exact length of time depending on the derivative. After intravenous injection, diuresis begins promptly but lasts only about 2 h. These drugs, therefore, are more suitable for oral rather than intravenous administration. After oral administration of chlorothiazide and hydrochlorothiazide, diuresis begins in 2 h and lasts about 6 to 12 h.

The half-life for chlorothiazide is 1 to 2 h, whereas the half-life for hydrochlorothiazide is 6 to 15 h. Bendroflumethiazide and polythiazide have durations of action of 6 to 12 h and 24 to 48 h, respectively. The thiazides are highly bound to plasma proteins (>90 percent) and are excreted primarily by the kidney and, to lesser extent, by the liver. These diuretics are excreted into the urine both as a consequence of glomerular filtration and secretion by the proximal tubule.

Adverse Reactions

Most adverse effects which develop during thiazide therapy are due to hypotension or electrolyte abnormalities such as hyponatremia, hypokalemia, and hypomagnesemia. Lassitude, weakness, and vertigo occur with large doses of thiazides. Anorexia, heartburn, nausea, vomiting, cramps, diarrhea, and constipation have all been reported, but they usually disappear when the dose is lowered and plasma electrolyte abnormalities are corrected.

A common toxic reaction to thiazide diuretics is a maculopapular skin rash. This occurs in about 1 percent of patients treated with chlorothiazide. Blood dyscrasias from chlorothiazide are rare. The drugs may also cause photosensitivity.

Thiazide diuretics tend to precipitate digitalis intoxication in patients receiving any of the cardiac glycosides. The development of digitalis toxicity under these conditions is attributable to hypokalemia which is caused by enhanced excretion of potassium. The development of hypokalemia seems to enhance the binding of digitalis glycosides to Na^+,K^+-ATPase. Restoration of normal serum potassium levels usually eliminates the toxicity. Also, individuals with ischemic heart disease may be predisposed to serious arrhythmias if hypokalemia occurs while on thiazides.

A gradual increase in blood uric acid level is commonly recorded during thiazide therapy. Hyperuricemia is the result of competition between uric acid and the diuretic for secretion by the organic acid pathway and volume depletion. Acute attacks of thiazide-induced gout, however, are less common. This effect, which is caused by the thiazides as a class, is apparently due to an inhibition of renal tubular secretion of uric acid and an increased urate reabsorption in the distal tubule as a result of the diuretic-induced volume depletion. These drugs do not increase the rate of production of uric acid. Thiazide administration causes an increase in urinary excretion of phosphate and a reduction in calcium excretion.

Hyperglycemia may develop occasionally from the thiazide diuretics and may be due to interference with the release of insulin from the pancreas. However, this effect should not prevent the use of these compounds in patients with diabetes mellitus if therapy is carefully monitored. Also, thiazides may produce pancreatitis and elevation of blood lipids (hyperlipidemia).

It has been shown that this group of diuretic agents reduces the hypertensive action of pressor amines and increases the skeletal muscle paralysis caused by tubocurarine and other antidepolarizing agents. The latter interaction may be related to the hypokalemic effect of the thiazides. Additionally, increased lithium intoxication has been noted with diuretic therapy, since the diuretic agents reduce renal lithium clearance from the body.

The thiazides should be used with caution in pregnancy, since they may produce adverse reactions such as jaundice, thrombocytopenia, and possibly other adverse effects, as mentioned above, on the fetus and newborn infant.

Clinical Uses

The thiazide drugs are used extensively in treating hypertension, either alone, or as baseline drugs to which are added the more potent antihypertensive agents. For further information, see Chapter 32.

The thiazide diuretics can be used in the day-to-day management of chronic congestive heart failure when renal function is normal. However, their use does not reduce the importance of other factors in the management of congestive heart failure, such as bed rest and controlled salt and fluid intake. Digitalis therapy may be continued in patients with cardiac failure who are receiving thiazide drugs. However, the serum potassium level should be monitored, since low serum potassium concentration potentiates digitalis toxicity. Use of potassium supplements may be necessary.

Thiazide may cause a diuretic response in patients with nephrosis and other types of renal disease. In general, the efficiency of a thiazide is directly related to the remaining functional properties of the kidney. In such circumstances, the therapeutic efficacy of thiazide diuretics is less than that of a loop diuretic. Surprisingly, thiazides are also effective for palliative treatment of the polyuria of nephrogenic and neurohypophyseal diabetes insipidus. The mechanism by which diuretic agents exert this antidiuretic action is not completely known, but it is postulated that they indirectly decrease urinary volume by depleting body sodium and thus may enhance the action of antidiuretic hormone.

Other conditions which may respond to thiazide therapy include liver disease with ascites, premenstrual fluid retention, and the positive salt balance associated with glucocorticoids and some estrogens. Thiazide diuretics have been shown to reduce both calcium excretion and the incidence of renal stone formation in hypercalciuric patients.

It has been suggested that the use of thiazide diuretics in pregnancy should be limited. In pregnancy, edema is common and usually needs no treatment. However, thiazides are recommended in pregnancy when edema is due to pathologic causes. The use of thiazides in pregnant women necessitates that the expected benefit be weighed against possible risks to the fetus.

THIAZIDE-RELATED COMPOUNDS

Metolazone and *chlorthalidone* are classified as diuretic and antihypertensive drugs. Chemically they resemble the thiazides in that both are sulfonamide derivatives. The mechanism of action of these compounds is similar to that of the thiazides; however, they do not inhibit carbonic anhydrase.

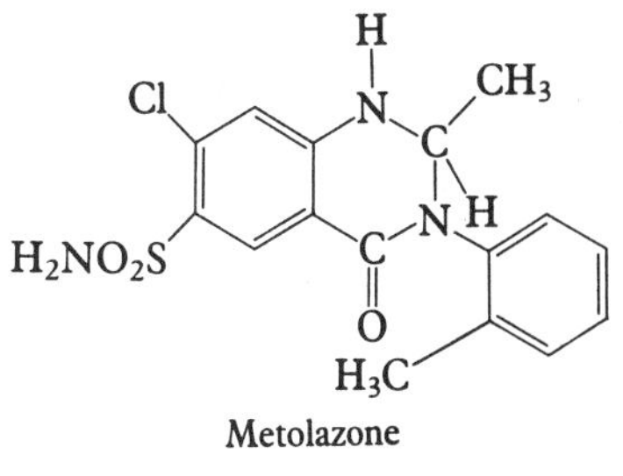

H
Cl N CH_3
C
N H
H_2NO_2S C
O
H_3C

Metolazone

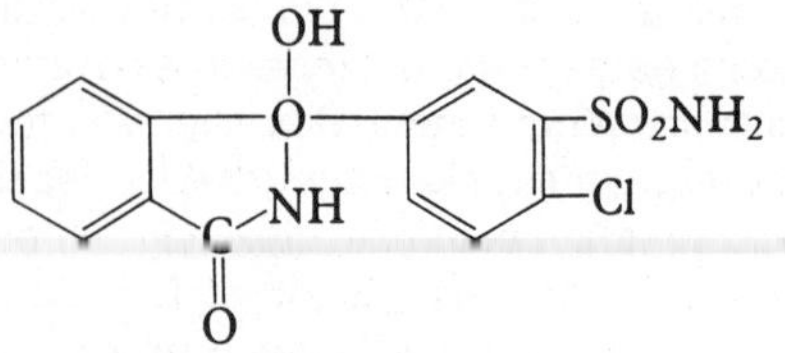

Chlorthalidone

Following oral administration of metolazone, the onset of diuresis occurs in about 1 h and lasts from 12 to 24 h. Chlorthalidone is orally effective with an onset of action at 2 h and a duration of action from 24 to 72 h. Its long duration of action is attributed to a high degree of protein binding and enterohepatic recirculation of the drug. Both diuretics are excreted by the kidney through glomerular filtration and proximal renal tubular secretion.

Indapamide is chemically a benzene-sulfonamide derivative, and its mechanism of action for the diuretic response appears to be similar to that of the thiazides.

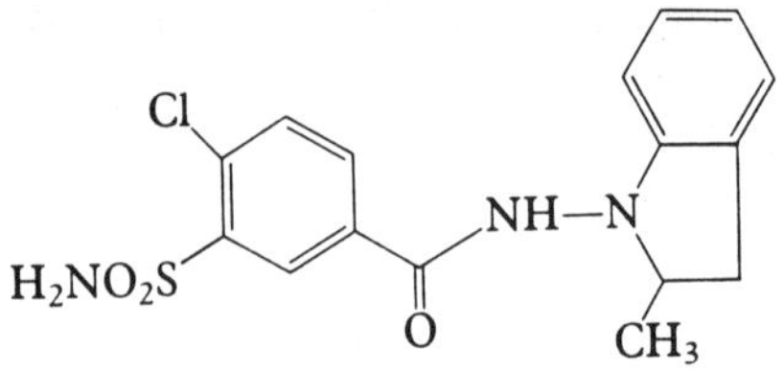

Indapamide

The drug is well absorbed (>90 percent) following oral administration and attains peak plasma concentration at 1 to 2 h. A duration of action of up to 36 h has been reported. Plasma protein binding is approximately 75 percent. Indapamide is extensively biotransformed in the liver, and about 7 percent appears in urine as the parent drug. The half-life of indapamide is 14 h.

The ability of indapamide, metolazone, and chlorthalidone to remove edematous fluids is equivalent to that of the thiazide diuretics but less than that of furosemide. These agents are useful in the management of edema associated with liver, kidney, or heart disease and in the treatment of essential hypertension, either alone, or in combination with other antihypertensive drugs.

Adverse reactions encountered with indapamide, metolazone, and chlorthalidone are similar to those of the thiazides as described previously.

LOOP DIURETICS

Bumetanide (a monosulfamoyl metanilamide derivative), ethacrynic acid (an aryloxyacetic acid derivative), furosemide (a monosulfamoylanthranilic acid derivative), and torsemide (a pyridine sulfonylurea derivative) are representative of this group of diuretics. The structures of these drugs are shown in Fig. 31-2. These agents have greater diuretic efficacy than the thiazides when used at maximal therapeutic doses since they inhibit transport at a site in the nephron where the amounts of sodium reabsorbed (20 to 30 percent) are larger than at the distal tubular site of action of the thiazides (5 to 8 percent). Administered orally or intravenously, these diuretics produce a prompt increase in renal sodium and chloride excretion and urine volume.

Mechanism of Action

Loop diuretics cause their potent diuretic response primarily by inhibiting the Na^+-K^+-$2Cl^-$ cotransporter that is localized to the luminal membrane of the cortical and medullary portions of the thick ascending limb of the loop of Henle. Along with the increased urinary sodium and chloride excretion, there is an increase in the excretion of potassium, hydrogen, magnesium, and calcium ions. Renal chloride and potassium excretion is greater than that of sodium. Urinary titratable acidity increases after administration of a loop diuretic and ammonium concentration and pH fall. Hypochloremic alkalosis can be produced.

Since the loop diuretics decrease the reabsorption of sodium and chloride in the medullary portion of the loop of Henle, there occurs a reduction in the hypertonicity of the medullary interstitium. In addition, inhibition of sodium and chloride reabsorption in the cortical portion of the loop of Henle results in diminished ability to form a dilute urine. These diuretic agents cause urinary osmolality to approach that of plasma under conditions of water overload or water deprivation. As a result, loop diuretics can decrease either free-water production or free-water reabsorption.

Pharmacokinetics

When given orally, the loop diuretics have an onset of action in about 30 min to 1 h, and the diuretic response may last for 6 to 8 hours; with intravenous or intramuscular injection, the effect

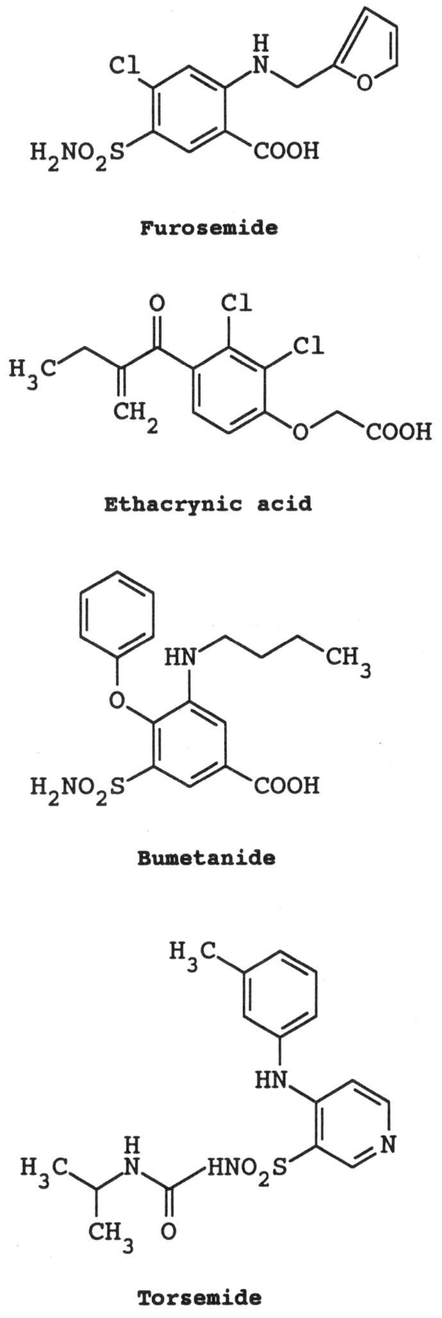

Furosemide

Ethacrynic acid

Bumetanide

Torsemide

FIGURE 31-2 *Structures of the loop diuretics.*

is almost immediate with a duration of 2 h. The duration of action of torsemide is 6 to 8 hours following intravenous administration. Some other pharmacokinetic data are presented in Table 31-3.

About 90 percent of the administered dose of furosemide is excreted by the kidney as unchanged drug and as a glucuronide metabolite. The remainder of the dose is present in the feces. Furosemide is extensively bound (95 percent) to plasma proteins, mainly to albumin. Although filtration through the glomerulus is limited, furosemide readily gains access to its luminal site of action in the loop of Henle via secretion by the organic acid pathway in cells of the proximal convoluted tubule. By administering probenecid, tubular secretion of furosemide can be blocked and the diuretic response blunted.

Approximately 60 percent of an intravenous dose of ethacrynic acid is excreted in the urine by filtration and active proximal tubular secretion. The remaining portion of the drug is eliminated in the bile. In both the urine and bile, ethacrynic acid is excreted unchanged and in a conjugated form (e.g., with cysteine).

Bumetanide is mainly eliminated from the body in the urine as unchanged drug (45 percent) and oxidative metabolites. The metabolism of bumetanide contrasts with that of furosemide where only glucuronidation occurs.

Torsemide undergoes biotransformation and urinary excretion. It is biotransformed to several metabolites; the major one is a carboxylic acid derivative. Urinary excretion mainly occurs by proximal tubular secretion.

Adverse Reactions

Bumetanide, ethacrynic acid, furosemide, and torsemide produce adverse reactions that are largely the same and are usually related to excessive fluid and electrolyte loss. Side effects include thirst, urinary frequency, nocturia, muscle weakness and cramps, headache, and mental confusion. Sudden alterations of fluid and electrolyte balance in patients with cirrhosis may precipitate hepatic coma. Hypokalemia, hypotension, hyperuricemia, hyperglycemia, blood dyscrasias, and shock have been reported.

In the presence of hypokalemia the toxicities of digitalis glycosides may be increased. The development of hyperuricemia is due to the interference of the active secretion of uric acid in the proximal tubule by the loop diuretic. The elevation of blood glucose, glucosuria, or alteration in glucose tolerance tests may be related to a decreased release of insulin from the pancreas by the loop diuretics.

TABLE 31-3 Pharmacokinetic data of the loop diuretics

Drug	Duration of action, h	Half-life, h	Percent oral absorption	Protein binding
Bumetanide	3 to 6	1 to 1.5	70 to 95	95
Ethacrynic acid	6 to 8	1.0	100	95
Furosemide	6 to 8	1.0	65	97
Torsemide	6 to 8	3.5	80	> 90

Other adverse reactions are transient hearing loss, tinnitus, irreversible hearing impairment, jaundice, and gastrointestinal disturbances such as anorexia, nausea, vomiting, abdominal pains, and diarrhea. In addition, lowering of serum calcium and magnesium concentrations have been observed. Individuals sensitive to sulfonamides may show similar allergic reactions to furosemide and bumetanide.

Drug Interactions

The loop diuretics can exhibit drug-drug interactions when they are administered concomitantly with other therapeutic agents. Bumetanide, ethacrynic acid, furosemide, and torsemide may increase the toxicities of lithium because they reduce the renal clearance of lithium. These diuretics may enhance the ototoxic potential of aminoglycoside antibiotics and may increase the nephrotoxicity of other drugs that possess potential nephrotoxicity. The loop diuretics augment the therapeutic effect of antihypertensive agents. It has been shown that nonsteroidal anti-inflammatory agents, e.g., indomethacin, can decrease the natriuretic and antihypertensive effect of these diuretics. This action of the nonsteroidal anti-inflammatory agents is related to inhibition of prostaglandin formation, which appear to have a role in sodium excretion.

In addition, furosemide may increase the toxicities of high doses of prescribed salicylates because of competition at renal excretory sites. Furosemide may decrease the hypertensive response of pressor amines, e.g., norepinephrine. The drug should be stopped prior to surgery. This diuretic also attenuates the neuromuscular blockade of tubocurarine and may potentiate the effect of succinylcholine.

Clinical Uses

The loop diuretics are recommended in the treatment of fluid retention because of their high therapeutic efficacy. Maximum therapeutic doses produce a greater diuretic response than the thiazide diuretics. Bumetanide, ethacrynic acid, furosemide, and torsemide are useful in treating edema associated with congestive heart failure, cirrhosis of the liver, nephrotic syndrome, chronic heart failure, and renal failure. These diuretics are frequently employed in patients who do not respond to thiazides, e.g., in patients who show evidence of hypervolemia and decreased glomerular filtration rates, manifested by elevated serum creatinine or blood urea nitrogen (BUN) concentrations. Furosemide and ethacrynic acid are used in the therapy of acute pulmonary edema when a rapid onset of diuresis is desired. They also decrease left ventricular filling pressure by increasing venous capacitance. This hemodynamic action together with a rapid reduction in extracellular fluid volume are beneficial in reducing pulmonary congestion. Furosemide and torsemide are also indicated for the treatment of chronic hypertension alone or with other antihypertensive drugs. The safety and efficacy of ethacrynic acid and bumetanide for the treatment of chronic hypertension have not been established. It is reported that the loop diuretics are effective in the acute treatment of hypercalcemia due to their ability to enhance urinary calcium excretion. Administration of furosemide and volume replacement with saline has been used to reduce plasma calcium concentration acutely.

POTASSIUM-SPARING DIURETICS

Spironolactone

Spironolactone is an aldosterone receptor antagonist and thus interferes with the action of the hormone at the target organ and is most effective when circulating aldosterone levels are high.

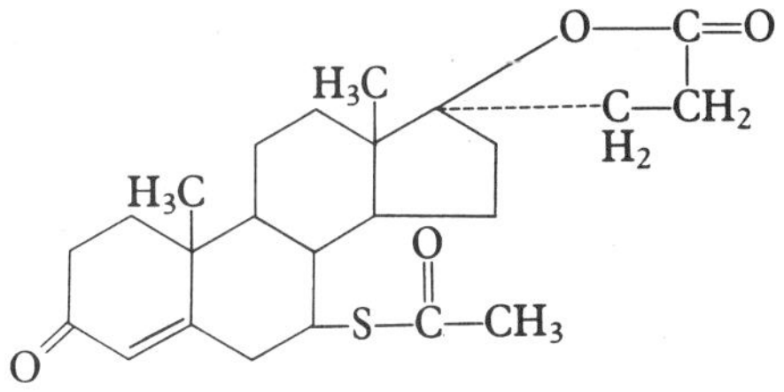

Spironolactone

Mechanism of Action Spironolactone exerts its diuretic effect by interfering with the aldosterone-mediated sodium reabsorption in the collecting duct, thereby increasing sodium loss in the urine and allowing for retention of potassium in the body. Spironolactone acts presumably by binding to the cytoplasmic aldosterone receptor complex in a competitive manner. The binding of spironolactone prevents the conversion of the receptor complex to its active form, and this eventually leads to a reduction in the synthesis of a transport protein that is required for the reabsorption of sodium in the collecting duct.

Canrenone, an active biotransformation product of spironolactone, has the same mechanism of action as spironolactone and, therefore, adds to the pharmacologic effect of spironolactone. Both compounds are competitive antagonists of aldosterone.

Pharmacokinetics Spironolactone is well absorbed from the gastrointestinal tract (Table 31-4). Its onset of action is delayed, and the maximum effect may not be observed for several days after initiating therapy. The drug is biotransformed by the liver to an active metabolite, canrenone. Canrenone and other metabolites are excreted by the kidney and bile.

Adverse Reactions Spironolactone is contraindicated in the presence of hyperkalemia, since it may cause further elevation of plasma potassium concentrations. Potassium supplements should not be used during spironolactone therapy. When angiotensin-converting enzyme inhibitors (ACE inhibitors) are administered with spironolactone, extreme caution should be used since the combination can cause severe hyperkalemia.

Lethargy, drowsiness, ataxia, headache, and mental confusion have been observed during spironolactone therapy, and a few patients have developed a transient maculopapular or erythematous rash while receiving the drug. These eruptions usually disappear within 48 h after discontinuing the drug. Diarrhea and other gastrointestinal disturbances, such as gastritis and ulceration, may occur during spironolactone therapy. Spironolactone may produce metabolic acidosis. Androgenic adverse effects of the drug include hirsutism, irregular menses, and deepening of the voice. It is reported that spironolactone may induce gynecomastia, which appears to be related to dose and duration of therapy. Generally, this effect is reversible on discontinuation of therapy. Spironolactone may increase the effects of digoxin, since it decreases the renal excretion of the cardiac glycosides. In addition, this diuretic may increase the blood levels of lithium and decrease the effects of pressor amines.

Clinical Uses Spironolactone increases renal sodium excretion when prescribed alone or in combination with hydrochlorothiazide and may amplify the antihypertensive effect of hydralazine. The drug diminishes the kaliuresis induced by thiazide

TABLE 31-4 Pharmacokinetic data of the potassium-sparing diuretics

Drug	Duration of action, h	Half-life, h	Percent oral absorption	Protein binding
Amiloride	24	6 - 9	15 - 20	23
Spironolactone	48 - 72	20	90	98
Triamterene	12 - 16	3	30 - 70	50 - 70

diuretics. Spironolactone is therefore a useful adjunct in the management of patients with intractable edema in whom hypokalemia is a frequent complication. It is also indicated for the treatment of primary hyperaldosteronism, hypertension, and edematous conditions associated with cirrhosis of the liver, nephrotic syndrome, and congestive heart failure. Most patients with chronic congestive heart failure, however, are satisfactorily maintained with the proper use of thiazides or a loop diuretic.

Triamterene

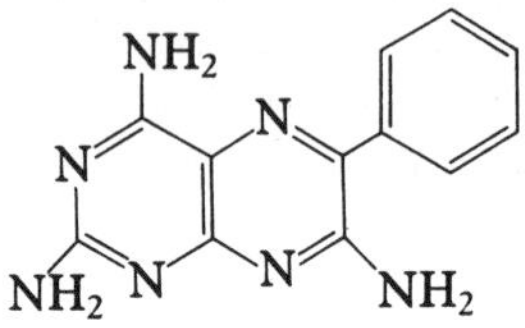

Triamterene is a pyrazine derivative which inhibits sodium reabsorption and, consequently, prevents potassium secretion in the collecting duct. Such a potassium-sparing diuretic causes a moderate increase in sodium and bicarbonate excretions in the urine and decreases urinary potassium and ammonia. It has little effect on urine volume, but when combined with a thiazide or loop diuretic, it enhances the diuretic response without increasing the output of potassium in the urine.

Its principal effects appear to be on the collecting duct, where, as mentioned above, it inhibits sodium reabsorption and potassium secretion. Although triamterene behaves like an aldosterone antagonist, its action is due to a direct effect on the collecting duct and is not due to competitive inhibition of aldosterone.

Pharmacokinetics Triamterene is absorbed from the gastrointestinal tract and has an onset of action in 2 to 4 h. The drug is eliminated from the body by the liver and kidney. In the liver, triamterene is biotransformed by hydroxylation and then conjugated to a sulfate. In the kidney, the drug is excreted by proximal tubular secretion. Other pharmacokinetic data are presented in Table 31-4.

Adverse Reactions Triamterene either alone or with a thiazide diuretic may cause hyperkalemia, electrocardiographic changes, and death. Renal function must be known before the drug is administered, and it should not be used in the presence of renal insufficiency. Triamterene has also been reported to decrease glomerular filtration rate and to increase blood urea concentrations. This diuretic is contraindicated in hyperkalemia and for use in combination with cyclooxygenase inhibitors. The latter has been reported to result in renal failure.

Clinical Uses Triamterene causes a moderate increase in sodium and bicarbonate excretion and a decrease in urinary potassium and ammonia. It is a weak diuretic when used alone, but when combined with a thiazide diuretics, the combination is more effective than either drug alone. Triamterene is usually recommended in combination with other diuretics for the treatment of edema due to congestive heart failure, cirrhosis of the liver, and nephrotic syndrome. When used with hydrochlorothiazide in treating hypertension, triamterene produces a positive potassium balance and a rise in plasma potassium concentrations.

Amiloride

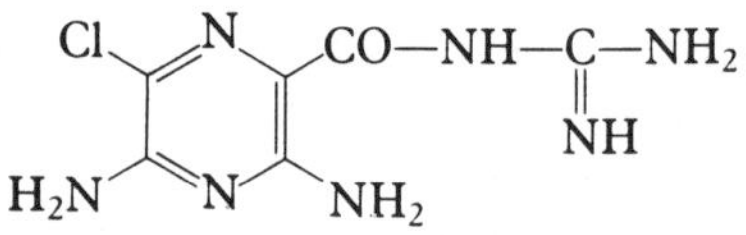

Mechanism of Action Amiloride is a potassium-sparing (antikaliuretic) diuretic that exhibits mild diuretic and natriuretic activity. Amiloride has its site of action in the distal convoluted tubule, cortical collecting tubule and collecting duct of the nephron. The drug appears to directly inhibit the reabsorption of sodium and reduce the tubular secretion of potassium and hydrogen ions. This potassium-sparing diuretic is not a direct aldosterone antagonist.

Pharmacokinetics The drug is adequately absorbed from the gastrointestinal tract but shows low bioavailability (Table 31-4). The onset of action is approximately 2 h. Unlike spironolactone and triamterene, this diuretic is not biotransformed by the liver. It is excreted unchanged by the kidney and undergoes active secretion in the proximal tubule of the nephron.

Adverse Reactions Adverse reactions of this drug include headache, weakness, fatigability, muscle cramps, dizziness, and hyperkalemia. Gastrointestinal effects such as nausea, vomiting, anorexia, and diarrhea have been reported. Less frequently there are occurrences of orthostatic hypotension, dry mouth, paresthesia, mental confusion, and insomnia. Amiloride is contraindicated in hyperkalemia and should not be administered together with potassium supplements or other potassium conserving agent (i.e., spironolactone, triamterene). An increased risk of hyperkalemia can occur when amiloride is used with an ACE inhibitor.

Clinical Uses Amiloride is rarely used alone, and its main indication is in combination with the thiazide or loop diuretics in congestive heart failure or hypertension. Amiloride is incorporated into the treatment of these patients to prevent or correct the condition of hypokalemia. Amiloride, as well as thiazide diuretics, may correct the nephrogenic diabetes insipidus caused by lithium; however, this therapy is still experimental.

CARBONIC ANHYDRASE INHIBITOR

Acetazolamide

Acetazolamide, an aromatic sulfonamide with a free sulfamyl group ($-SO_2NH_2$), is a carbonic anhydrase inhibitor. The drug produces an alkaline urine with increased excretion of sodium, potassium, bicarbonate, and phosphate. Patients may exhibit refractoriness to the diuretic response of acetazolamide.

Mechanism of Action The diuretic action of acetazolamide is due to inhibition of carbonic anhydrase in the renal tubule, mainly in the proximal tubule. Following administration of the drug, reabsorption of sodium ions in exchange for hydrogen ions is depressed, sodium bicarbonate excretion is increased, and chloride output is decreased. Inhibition of proximal tubular reabsorption of sodium is compensated by the high reabsorptive rate in the thick ascending limb of the loop of Henle. Bicarbonate excretion is increased because of the lack of hydrogen ions to neutralize urinary bicarbonate. Since phosphate ions are poorly reabsorbed beyond the proximal tubule, their excretion leads to an increased loss of sodium and water.

Chloride ions are retained by the kidney to offset the loss of bicarbonate and maintain ionic balance. Due to decreased availability of hydrogen ions, potassium is excreted in exchange for sodium, and urinary potassium output increases.

The renal electrolyte excretion pattern of patients receiving a carbonic anhydrase inhibitor is characterized by increased amounts of sodium, potassium, bicarbonate, and phosphate output, with only moderate increases in water output. The urine becomes alkaline, and the plasma bicarbonate concentration decreases. If therapy is continued, the patient develops a metabolic acidosis. Plasma chloride levels increase. Urinary ammonia concentrations drop when hydrogen ions present in the tubule are insufficient to convert ammonia to ammonium ions.

Pharmacokinetics Acetazolamide is absorbed rapidly from the gastrointestinal tract; peak plasma levels are reached within 2 h after oral administration. Acetazolamide is excreted unchanged in the urine by proximal tubular secretion, about 80 percent of a single oral dose appearing in the urine within 8 to 12 h.

Adverse Reactions Acetazolamide produces reversible side effects, which include flushing, headache, drowsiness, dizziness, fatigue, irritability, and excitability. Instances of polydipsia and polyuria, paresthesias, ataxia, hyperpnea, anorexia, vomiting, and gastrointestinal distress have been reported during therapy with carbonic anhydrase inhibitors. Such manifestations disappear when the dosage is reduced.

Like antibacterial sulfonamides, acetazolamide may cause fever and blood dyscrasias such as leukopenia, agranulocytosis, thrombocytopenia, and aplastic anemia. Allergic skin reactions, including exfoliative dermatitis, may develop during acetazolamide administration. Genitourinary complications of acetazolamide therapy include crystalluria, calculus formation (chiefly calcium phosphate and citrate) with renal colic, and secondary renal lesions.

Clinical Uses Acetazolamide is a weak diuretic with limited use since the introduction of the thiazides. However, there are five indications for a carbonic anhydrase inhibitor: (1) in edema, to promote a diuretic response, (2) in glaucoma, (3) in absence seizures, (4) in premenstrual tension, and (5) in altitude sickness. Of these indications, the most common usage of acetazolamide is in the treatment of glaucoma. Acetazolamide decreases the formation of aqueous humor and thereby reduces the intraocular pressure of the eye.

SUMMARY

The comparative effects of the various diuretic agents are listed in Table 31-5. A relative comparison of urinary excretion patterns, urinary pH, alteration in the blood acid-base balance, and refractoriness is indicated.

OSMOTIC NONELECTROLYTES

Mannitol

Mannitol is the most clinically used member of this drug category. In the presence of normal cardiac and renal function, mannitol causes a decrease in water reabsorption by the nephron and promotes an osmotic diuresis, generally without significant sodium excretion. Mannitol is ineffective when given orally and requires parenteral administration. This agent is freely filterable at the glomerulus and is not metabolized or reabsorbed by the tubular cells; it is excreted by the glomeruli and, being osmotically active, retains water in the tubular fluid to increase urine volume. Loss of therapeutic effectiveness is associated with increased solute permeability of the nephron.

Adverse Reactions Mannitol does not penetrate the cells, and its only method of excretion is via the glomerular filtrate. Intravenous infusions of mannitol, therefore, increase blood volume. Expansion of blood volume in patients with congestive heart failure may cause further decompensation and may precipitate acute pulmonary edema. When given to patients with renal failure, mannitol produces vascular overfilling with hyperosmolality and hyponatremia. Clinically, there is a picture of tissue dehydration accompanied by signs of congestive heart failure. Hyperosmolality has been reported after mannitol infusions in patients with cirrhosis and ascites. Peritoneal dialysis may correct the overhydration produced by mannitol infusions, but deaths due to vascular overfilling, hyperosmolality, and hyponatremia have also been reported.

Clinical Uses Mannitol is used as an adjunct in the prevention or treatment of oliguria and anuria. It may also be employed to reduce intraocular pressure pre- and post-operatively in ophthalmic procedures, and it is also used in the treatment of brain edema.

TABLE 31-5 A comparison of various diuretic drugs: Urinary excretion patterns, pH, acid-base alterations, and refractoriness

Drugs	Urinary excretion[a]					Blood acid-base balance[c]	Refractoriness
	Na^+	Cl^-	K^+	HCO_3^-	pH[b]		
Thiazides	↑	↑	↑	→↑[d]	↓	Hypochloremic alkalosis	No
Thiazide-related	↑	↑	↑	→	↓	Hypochloremic alkalosis	No
Loop diuretics	↑	↑	↑	→	↓	Hypochloremic alkalosis	No
K^+-sparing diuretics	↑	↑	↓	↑	↑	Metabolic acidosis	No
Acetazolamide	↑	↓	↑	↑	↑	Metabolic acidosis	Yes

[a] Key: increase (↑); decrease (↓); no change (→).
[b] Urinary pH.
[c] Possible alterations.
[d] Chlorothiazide may produce a slight increase.

BIBLIOGRAPHY

Beermann, B., and M. Groschinsky-Grind: "Clinical Pharmacokinetics of Diuretics," *Clin. Pharmacokinet.* **5**: 221-245 (1980).

Cannon, P.J.: "Diuretics: Their Mechanism of Action and Use in Hypertension," *Cardiovas. Rev. Rep.* **4**: 649-666 (1983).

Hackett, P.H., and D. Rennie: "Incidence, Importance, and Prophylaxis of Acute Mountain Sickness," *Lancet* **2**: 1149-1154 (1976).

Hendry, B.M., and J.C. Ellory: "Molecular Sites for Diuretic Action," *Trends in Pharmacol. Sci.* **9**: 416-420 (1988).

Herbert, S.C., and T.E. Andreoli: "Control of NaCl Transport in Thick Ascending Limb," *Am. J. Physiol.* **246**: F745-F756 (1984).

Koechel, D.A.: "Ethacrynic Acid and Related Diuretics: Relationship of Structure to Beneficial and Detrimental Actions," *Annu. Rev. Pharmacol. Toxicol.* **21**: 265-293 (1981).

Kokko, J.P.: "Site and Mechanism of Action of Diuretics," *Am. J. Med.* **77**: 11-17 (1984).

Lant, A.: "Diuretics: Clinical Pharmacology and Therapeutic Use," *Drugs* **29**: 57-87, 162-188 (1985).

Martinez-Maldonado, M., and H.R. Cordova: "Cellular and Molecular Aspects of the Renal Effects of Diuretic Agents," *Kidney Int.* **38**: 632-641 (1990).

Mujais, S.K., N.A. Nora, and M.L. Levin: "Principles and Clinical Uses of Diuretic Therapy," *Prog. Cardiovasc. Dis.* **35**: 221-245 (1992).

Rybak, L.P.: "Drug Ototoxicity," *Annu. Rev. Pharmacol. Toxicol.* **26**: 79-100 (1986).

Steinmetz, P.R., and B.M. Koeppen: "Cellular Mechanisms of Diuretic Action Along the Nephron," *Hosp. Pract.* **19**: 125-134 (1984).

Stier, C.T., Jr. and H.D. Itskovitz: "Renal Calcium Metabolism and Diuretics," *Annu. Rev. Pharmacol. Toxicol.* **26**: 101-116 (1986).

Velaquez, H., and F.S. Wright: "Control by Drugs of Renal Potassium Handling," *Annu. Rev. Pharmacol. Toxicol.* **26**: 293-310 (1986).

Warren, S.E., and R.C. Blantz: "Mannitol," *Arch. Intern. Med.* **141**: 493 (1981).

Warnock, D.G., and J. Eveloff: "NaCl Entry Mechanism in Luminal Membrane on the Renal Tubule," *Am. J. Physiol.* **242**: F561-F574 (1982).

CHAPTER 32

Antihypertensive Drugs

Cathy A. Bruner

Hypertension is a syndrome characterized by elevated blood pressure. The pathophysiologic basis for 90 to 95 percent of the cases of the disease remains unexplained, and therefore the condition is called *primary*, or *essential, hypertension*. The remaining 5 to 10 percent may be due to a number of known causes, including renal artery stenosis, aortic coarctation, Cushing's syndrome, and pheochromocytoma. Since the hypertension associated with these diseases occur secondarily, the elevated blood pressure is called *secondary hypertension*. Although the cause of primary hypertension is unknown, empirical treatment is generally effective and should be instituted until the etiology of the disease is defined and more specific therapy is employed. This chapter deals with the treatment of primary hypertension.

Sustained elevated blood pressure causes vascular alterations throughout the body. Many studies have concluded that the higher the arterial pressure, whether systolic or diastolic, the higher the morbidity and mortality.

Classification of hypertension on the basis of impact on the risk of other cardiovascular diseases is presented in Table 32-1. All stages of hypertension are associated with increased risk of cardiovascular disease and renal disease. The higher the blood pressure, the greater the risk. Reducing blood pressure with drugs has been clearly demonstrated to decrease the incidence of cardiovascular morbidity and mortality.

PRINCIPLES OF DRUG THERAPY

The goal of drug therapy for hypertension is to maintain blood pressure below 140/90 mm Hg (systolic/diastolic) while controlling other cardiovascular risk factors. The decision to initiate drug treatment is influenced by the severity of hypertension and the presence of other diseases and cardiovascular risk factors. For individuals with Stage 1 or Stage 2 hypertension, drug therapy should be started if blood pressure remains at or above 140/90 mm Hg for 3 to 6 months despite encouragement of lifestyle modifications (e.g., weight reduction, exercise, and reduction of alcohol and sodium intake). Monotherapy is the initial recommended drug therapy for Stage 1 and Stage 2 hypertension. The recommended drug classes for this initial therapy are diuretics or β-adrenergic blockers because these are the only two drug classes that have been shown to reduce cardiovascular morbidity and mortality in controlled, long-term clinical trials. Alternative drug classes are calcium-channel blockers, angiotensin converting enzyme inhibitors, α_1-adrenergic receptor antagonists, and labetalol. These alternate drug classes are efficacious agents for lowering blood pressure, but since they have not been studied in controlled trials to determine their efficacy in reducing morbidity and mortality, they should be reserved for patients in whom diuretics and β-adrenergic receptor blockers cannot be used or are ineffective. Other agents, such as direct-acting vasodilators, α_2-receptor agonists, and adrenergic neuronal blockers are not well suited for initial monotherapy; the side effects of α_2-adrenergic agonists and adrenergic neuronal blockers preclude their use when given alone. Direct-acting vasodilators cause reflex sympathetic stimulation and fluid retention and are best given with a diuretic and a β-adrenergic blocker.

If the response to initial therapy is inadequate, one of the following options should be considered: (1) increase the dose of the first drug toward maximal levels, (2) substitute a drug from another class, or (3) add a second drug from another class. Combination therapy with drugs with different mechanisms of action will often provide effective

TABLE 32-1 Classification of the severity of untreated hypertension in adults based upon both systolic and diastolic blood pressure

Status	Systolic pressure, mm Hg	Diastolic pressure, mm Hg	Estimated risk of morbid events[a]
Normal blood pressure	< 130	< 85	None
Borderline hypertension	130 to 139	85 to 89	Slight
Hypertension			
Stage 1 (Mild)	140 to 159	90 to 99	Long-term risk
Stage 2 (Moderate)	160 to 179	100 to 109	50% in 5 years
Stage 3 (Severe)	180 to 209	110 to 119	40% in 2 years
Stage 4 (Very severe)	> 210	> 120	Medical emergency

[a] Morbid events: stroke, cardiac failure, and renal insufficiency

therapy. If a diuretic was not initially chosen, one may be added, because diuretics usually enhance the effects of other agents.

Modification of the aforementioned principles may be necessary in patients with Stage 3 and Stage 4 hypertension (see Table 32-1). Although some patients may respond adequately to monotherapy, often a second or third agent must be added to achieve blood pressure control.

ANTIHYPERTENSIVE DIURETICS

The mechanism of the antihypertensive effect of diuretics has not been completely elucidated. It appears, however, to be related to a reduction in both total body sodium and extracellular fluid volume. Diuretics reduce elevated blood pressure by enhancing sodium and water excretion via the kidney, with a consequent reduction in extracellular fluid and plasma volume. Although certain diuretics, i.e., the thiazides, relax vascular smooth muscle by a direct action, many antihypertensive diuretics do not. Therefore, it appears that this action is not primarily responsible for the hypotensive response to these drugs.

The various diuretics employed in patients with hypertension and their duration of action are listed in Table 32-2. As a rule, patients are started on an oral diuretic from the thiazide or thiazide-related group. The effects of these drugs are quite similar; milligram dose and duration of action vary. The three main side effects associated with this group are hyperuricemia, hyperglycemia, and electrolyte abnormalities characterized by hypokalemia, metabolic alkalosis, and hypochloremia.

Thiazide diuretics and the thiazide-related drugs can induce increases in the levels of total plasma cholesterol, triglycerides, and low-density lipoprotein (LDL) cholesterol. Some studies have suggested that this effect may wane with long-term use. Dietary modifications may reduce these effects.

Furosemide, although a more efficacious diuretic, has not demonstrated a more potent antihypertensive action than the standard thiazide or thiazide-related group. Oral furosemide is used for those patients who show evidence of hypervolemia and decreased glomerular filtration rates, manifested in elevated serum creatinine or blood urea nitrogen (BUN) concentration. Occasionally a patient with renal insufficiency, on a thiazide diuretic, will exhibit deterioration of renal function and a rising BUN; this has not been noted with furosemide. Torsemide is relatively new and, at present, appears similar to furosemide.

Spironolactone is a competitive inhibitor of aldosterone but does not have side effects such as potassium wasting, hyperuricemia, or deterioration of glucose tolerance. Spironolactone is used as a first-line diuretic for patients with gout or diabetes mellitus or for those who have shown hypokalemic responses to the thiazide group of diuretics. All of the potassium-sparing diuretics are more commonly used in combination with hydrochlorothiazide, but not as first-line therapy for hypertension.

TABLE 32-2 Oral antihypertensive diuretics

Classification and name	Duration of action, h
Thiazide diuretics	
Bendroflumethiazide	6 to 12
Benzthiazide	6 to 18
Chlorothiazide	6 to 12
Hydrochlorothiazide	6 to 12
Hydroflumethiazide	6 to 12
Methyclothiazide	24
Polythiazide	24 to 48
Trichlormethiazide	24
Thiazide-related diuretics	
Chlorthalidone	24 to 72
Metolazone	12 to 24
Indapamide	24 to 36
Loop diuretics	
Furosemide	6 to 8
Torsemide	6 to 8
Potassium-sparing diuretics	
Amiloride	18 to 24
Spironolactone	48 to 72
Triamterene	12 to 16

SYMPATHOLYTIC AGENTS

Centrally-Acting Sympathetic Inhibitors

It has been established that central catecholaminergic neurons are an important factor in the regulation of systemic arterial blood pressure. Stimulation of α-adrenergic receptors in specific areas of the central nervous system (CNS) leads to hypotension and bradycardia. These effects appear to be mediated through the activation of an inhibitory neuronal system in the medullary vasomotor center which decreases sympathetic outflow from this area to the periphery.

A few clinically useful antihypertensive drugs, i.e., clonidine, methyldopa, guanabenz, and guanfacine, appear to act principally by alteration of central sympathetic function. Reserpine and propranolol also have actions on the CNS which may be important to their antihypertensive effects. However, these compounds have significant peripheral actions and are, therefore, discussed in other sections of this chapter.

Clonidine

Clonidine is structurally related to the imidazoline derivative tolazoline, a peripheral vasodilator and α-adrenergic receptor blocker. These actions have not been attributed to clonidine; in fact, the drug is a selective α_2-adrenergic receptor agonist.

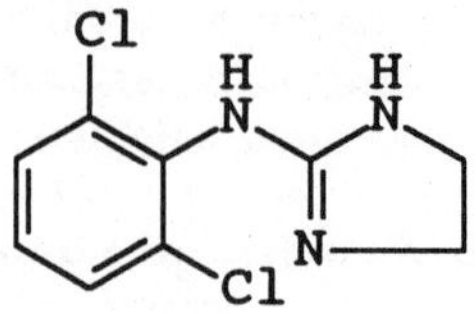

Mechanism of Action The mechanism of action of clonidine is not completely understood. However, it appears that the antihypertensive effects of the drug result mainly from stimulation of α_2-adrenergic receptors in the lower brainstem, probably in the nucleus tractus solitarius. Central α-adrenergic receptor activation causes decreased sympathetic tone from the medullary vasomotor center to the heart, the kidneys, and the blood vessels. In addition, parasympathetic tone from the vagal nucleus is increased which may contribute to the cardiac slowing that is seen with this drug.

Effects on Organ Systems The cardiovascular effects of oral clonidine include decreased arterial blood pressure, heart rate, cardiac output, and peripheral vascular resistance. Orthostatic hypotension is mild and infrequent. There is little effect on renal blood flow and glomerular filtration rate. Renin secretion is suppressed slightly; plasma volume is increased. The serum lipid profile (total cholesterol, triglycerides, LDL, etc.) are unaffected by clonidine.

A transient peripheral α-adrenergic receptor stimulation is evidenced by a transient rise in arterial blood pressure when the drug is given by intravenous injection. However, the central antihypertensive action quickly predominates as clonidine accumulates in the CNS.

In addition to the antihypertensive effects, mediated through the CNS, clonidine may produce drowsiness and sedation. Tolerance to the sedative effect of the drug has been noted during chronic administration. Clonidine reduces salivary flow and causes xerostomia, which appears to be due to a central effect of the drug.

Pharmacokinetics The drug is well absorbed after oral administration and bioavailability is almost 100 percent. Blood pressure falls within 30 to 60 min, with the maximum effect occurring within 2 h. The duration of the antihypertensive effect is at least 6 h, and the elimination half-life ranges between 12 and 16 h. The plasma clearance of clonidine is between 200 and 500 mL/min. The exact biotransformation fate of the compound is not known; 50 percent is eliminated unchanged in the urine.

In addition to the oral route of administration, clonidine is also available in a transdermal delivery system. The drug is released at an approximately constant rate for a week. Three to four days are required to reach steady state levels in plasma. When the patch is removed, plasma concentrations remain stable for about 8 hours then decline over a period of days.

Therapeutic Uses Clonidine is considered a supplemental agent used when the initial therapy fails to achieved the desired result. However, in combination with an oral diuretic such as hydrochlorothiazide, chlorthalidone, or furosemide, clonidine is a drug of choice for the management of various degrees of hypertension. If blood pressure is not adequately controlled with a diuretic-clonidine combination, a peripherally-acting sympathetic inhibitor or a vasodilator may be added to the therapeutic regimen without significant adverse drug-drug interactions. Clonidine can be used in uncomplicated mild to severe hypertensive states or when hypertension is complicated by cerebrovascular insufficiency, ischemic heart disease, or congestive heart failure.

Clonidine has been found to be effective and is still being evaluated in a number of other conditions including reduction of withdrawal symptoms from alcohol, opioids, and nicotine (see Chapter 26); diagnosis of pheochromocytoma; and the treatment of Tourette's Disorder.

Adverse Reactions The most common adverse reactions to clonidine include dry mouth, drowsiness, dizziness, sedation, and constipation. Generally, these side effects diminish as therapy is continued. Serious organ toxicity is rare.

When discontinuing the drug, the dose should be reduced gradually over 2 to 4 days to avoid the potential of a rebound hypertension, observed when clonidine therapy is stopped abruptly. Symptoms include headache, nervousness, abdominal pain, sweating, tachycardia, and a rapid rise in blood pressure. The pathophysiology of this syndrome is unknown but can be reversed by resumption of clonidine therapy or by a combination of phentolamine and propranolol.

The antihypertensive effects of clonidine will be diminished if given concurrently with tricyclic antidepressants. The mechanism responsible for this drug-drug interaction has not been established.

Methyldopa

Methyldopa is the α-methylated derivative of levodopa.

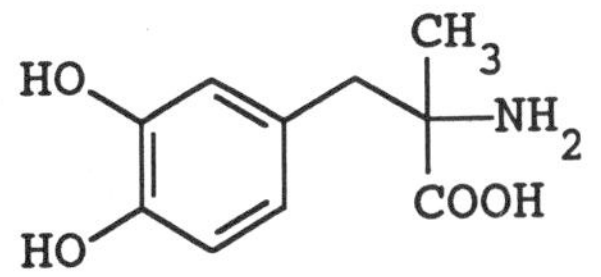

Mechanism of Action It is generally accepted that the major antihypertensive action of methyldopa is on the CNS. The drug enters the CNS, is biotransformed to methylnorepinephrine (the active product), and is stored in adrenergic neurons.

Upon release it activates α_2-adrenergic receptors in the brainstem. This results in decreased sympathetic outflow from the CNS; therefore, it acts in a manner similar to clonidine.

Effects on the Cardiovascular System The cardiovascular effects of this drug are similar to those observed with clonidine. Methyldopa produces less bradycardia and has less effect on plasma renin activity than clonidine; however, it causes somewhat greater orthostatic hypotension than comparable antihypertensive doses of clonidine. Methyldopa has no direct effect on the heart and generally does not alter glomerular filtration rate or renal blood flow and does not affect serum lipid levels.

Pharmacokinetics Methyldopa is incompletely absorbed following oral administration; the average oral bioavailability is 25 percent. The peak antihypertensive effect occurs at about 4 to 6 h, and the duration of action is 12 to 24 h. About 2 days are required to achieve maximal antihypertensive effects. Methyldopa is widely distributed throughout the body; however, this is not reflected in its calculated apparent volume of distribution (0.5 L/kg). Since the drug accumulates in adrenergic nerve endings of the brain and periphery and is not in equilibrium with the circulation, classic pharmacokinetics are of little value.

Plasma protein binding of methyldopa is between 0 and 20 percent. Circulating drug is biotransformed in the liver to the sulfate conjugate, which appears to be inactive. As mentioned previously, methyldopa taken up into adrenergic neurons is biotransformed to the active product, methylnorepinephrine. The parent compound and all biotransformation products are excreted in the urine.

Therapeutic Uses The only indication for methyldopa is hypertension. Like clonidine, it is best given in conjunction with a diuretic. Frequent side effects tend to limit its usefulness.

The ethyl ester of methyldopa, methyldopate, is used by intravenous administration for hypertensive crisis.

Adverse Reactions and Precautions Common adverse reactions include transient drowsiness, headache, and fatigue, which usually diminish as therapy is continued. Paresthesias, parkinsonism-like symptoms, depression, and psychic disturbances including nightmares and mild psychosis may occur.

Cardiovascular reactions may include bradycardia, aggravation of angina pectoris, fluid retention, and orthostatic hypotension.

Drug-related fever, a lupus-like syndrome, and myocarditis have been reported. In addition, gastrointestinal symptoms including nausea, vomiting, abdominal distention, constipation, and diarrhea may occur.

A positive Coombs' test will occur in approximately 20 percent of patients; however, hemolytic anemia is rare (0.2 percent). At the initiation of methyldopa therapy, blood counts should be performed, and periodic blood counts should be done to detect hemolytic anemia.

Methyldopa is contraindicated in active hepatic disease (e.g., hepatitis and cirrhosis) since the drug may cause jaundice and result in abnormal liver function.

Guanabenz and Guanfacine

These are two centrally-acting α_2-adrenergic receptor agonists. Structurally the drugs are similar.

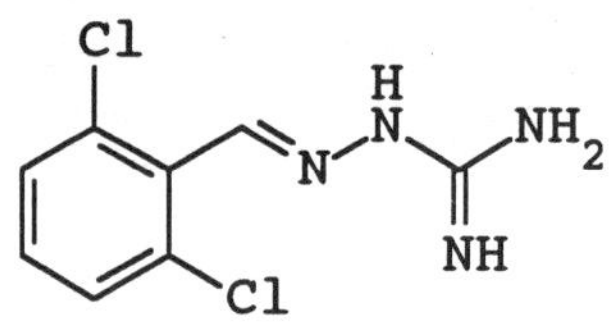

Guanabenz

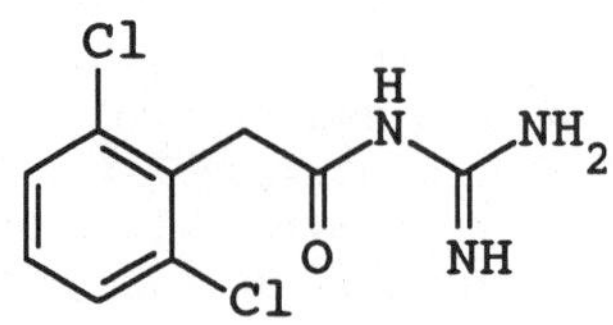

Guanfacine

As with clonidine and methyldopa, stimulation of α_2-adrenergic receptors in the lower brainstem causes inhibition of sympathetic outflow from the vasomotor center in the medulla. Of all of the centrally-acting sympatholytic drugs, guanfacine appears to be the most selective for α_2-adrenergic receptors.

The cardiovascular effects of both guanabenz and guanfacine are similar to clonidine and methyldopa. Reduction of plasma renin activity is somewhat greater with these two compounds. In addition, fluid retention appear to be less problematic with guanabenz and guanfacine. Animal studies suggest that these drug have some diuretic activity; whether this effect is significant in humans is not known at present.

Pharmacokinetics Guanabenz is about 75 percent orally bioavailable. The onset of action is within 1 h and the peak effect occurs in 2 to 4 h. There is extensive biotransformation with less than 1 percent of the unbound drug being present in the urine. The elimination half-life is about 6 h.

The orally bioavailable of guanfacine is 80 percent. The drug is rapidly acting and peak effects occur between 1 and 4 h after a single oral dose. With a large volume of distribution, the drug has a long half-life of 16 to 20 h. About 50 percent of guanfacine is biotransformed, by oxidation of aromatic ring followed by conjugation, and excreted primarily in the urine.

Therapeutic Use Guanabenz and guanfacine are indicated only in the management of primary hypertension. Like the aforementioned centrally-acting drugs, these two compounds may be used alone or in combination with a diuretic.

Adverse Reactions Both drugs have adverse reactions similar to those of clonidine. Sedation and dryness of the mouth are most common. Weakness and orthostatic hypotension are natural consequences of this type of drug. Headache, palpitations, bradycardia, nasal congestion, blurred vision, and gastrointestinal disturbances occasionally occur. Also, as with clonidine, rebound hypertension may occur when the drug is withdrawn abruptly.

Peripherally-Acting Sympathetic Inhibitors

β-Adrenergic Receptor Blockers

The most commonly utilized compounds for the management of hypertension that inhibit the activity of the sympathetic nervous system are the β-adrenergic blockers. The pharmacology of these drugs is discussed in detail in Chapter 9 and only some features relative to their use as antihypertensive agents will be mentioned herein. At the present time, there are twelve of these compounds available for use in the United States as antihypertensive drugs. The drugs are listed in Table 32-3 along with some of their pharmacological properties which may make them preferable for use in certain subgroups of hypertensive patients.

Mechanism of Action Despite years of use, the mechanism of action by which β-adrenergic receptor blockers lower blood pressure is not completely understood. Agreement is certain that they depress myocardial function and decrease cardiac output and heart rate. By competitive blockade of β-adrenergic receptors in the kidney, decreased release of renin from the juxtaglomerular cells occurs, resulting in a reduction in the formation of the vasoconstrictor, angiotensin II; this may be significant in some patients. In addition, sympathetic outflow from the CNS to the heart, kidney, and vasculature may be reduced by those compounds that penetrate through the blood-brain barrier. Theories concerning presynaptic β-adrenergic receptor blockade reducing norepinephrine release and thus reducing vasoconstriction, as well as effects on the prostaglandin and kinase systems are less certain.

In addition to blocking β-adrenergic receptors, labetalol has antagonistic activity at α-adrenergic sites. More specially, labetalol acts as a competitive, selective antagonistic of α_1-adrenergic receptors. In contrast to the other drugs, peripheral vascular resistance will decrease slightly due to the α-adrenergic blocking action. Because of this property, symptoms of postural hypotension can occur with labetalol. Blockade of both receptor types contributes to the antihypertensive effect.

Cardioselectivity Acebutolol, atenolol, betaxolol, bisoprolol, and metoprolol which are primarily β_1-adrenergic receptor antagonists have, at ordinary antihypertensive doses, less activity on β_2 receptors. This would make these drugs more suitable for patients with some degree of sensitivity to bronchospasm. Actually all β-receptor blockers are either contraindicated, or should be used with caution, in persons with bronchial asthma and significant chronic obstructive pulmonary disease because the cardioselectivity is relative rather than absolute.

Intrinsic Sympathomimetic Activity (ISA) Acebutolol, carteolol, penbutolol, and pindolol have the ability to stimulate as well as block β-adrenergic receptors. A number of claims are made for this feature. Theoretically there should be less bradycardia, less risk of congestive heart failure, less increase in peripheral resistance, and more ease of withdrawal of the therapy. Whether these advantages are substantial in clinical practice is still uncertain.

TABLE 32-3 Pharmacologic properties of β-adrenergic blockers which apply to antihypertensive therapy

Drug	Cardioselectivity[a] (selective β_1 blockade)	ISA[b]	MSA[c]	Lipid solubility
Acebutolol	Yes	+	+	Low
Atenolol	Yes	–	–	Very Low
Betaxolol	Yes	–	+	Low
Bisoprolol	Yes	–	–	Moderate
Carteolol	No	+	–	Low
Labetalol	No	–	+	Moderate
Metoprolol	Yes	–	+	Moderate
Nadolol	No	–	–	Low
Penbutolol	No	+	–	High
Pindolol	No	+ +	+	Moderate
Propranolol	No	–	+ +	High
Timolol	No	–	–	Low

[a] At therapeutic dosage
[b] Intrinsic sympathomimetic activity
[c] Membrane stabilizing activity

Membrane Stabilizing Activity (MSA) Acebutolol, betaxolol, labetalol, metoprolol, pindolol, and especially propranolol have MSA. This is believed by some to be important in the control of arrhythmias, mainly premature ventricular contractions PVCs). Actually all β-receptor blockers have the ability to suppress minor arrhythmias by virtue of their sympathetic blocking activity. Whether MSA is a real advantage at therapeutic doses has not been finally determined. Nevertheless, these drugs with MSA might be advantageous in hypertensive patients who also have PVCs.

Lipid Solubility Atenolol has the lowest lipid solubility, enough to allow a claim that it does not significantly cross the blood-brain barrier. All β-adrenergic blocking agents cause varying degrees of dizziness, vertigo, fatigue, mental depression and headache. This has been attributed at least in part to the ability of the drug to cross the blood-brain barrier and have a CNS depressant effect. More likely, the CNS symptoms are due to the lowering of blood pressure and blood supply to the brain. In any event, it sometimes happens that some of the CNS symptoms disappear with the substitution of a less lipophilic agent.

Patient Compliance All of these drugs are equally efficacious as antihypertensives. It is claimed, with some justification, that once daily oral dosing leads to greater compliance by patients. Atenolol, betaxolol, bisoprolol, carteolol, and penbutolol have a pharmacokinetic profile that allows this feature. Acebutolol, metoprolol, and nadolol can sometimes be used once daily, but more commonly need be given twice a day. Pindolol and propranolol are usually given twice daily; however, a sustained-release preparation of propranolol allows once daily dosing.

With respect to parenteral therapy, only labetalol is indicated for the control of blood pressure in severe hypertension. Other β-adrenergic blockers that are available for injection, e.g., propranolol, are indicated for other purposes.

α-Adrenergic Receptor Blockers

Drugs which block α-adrenergic receptors such as phentolamine and phenoxybenzamine (see Chapter 9) have not been successful in treating hypertension. In part, this is because of their side effects but also because of the development of tolerance. There are a few selective α_1-adrenergic receptor antagonists that are very useful in the management of hypertension, i.e., prazosin, terazosin, and doxazosin. In addition, as mentioned above, labetalol has selective α_1-adrenergic receptor blocking activity in addition to β-receptor blockade.

Prazosin was the first of these drugs to be made available for clinical use. It is the prototype compound of a group of piperazinyl quinazoline derivatives (Fig. 32-1).

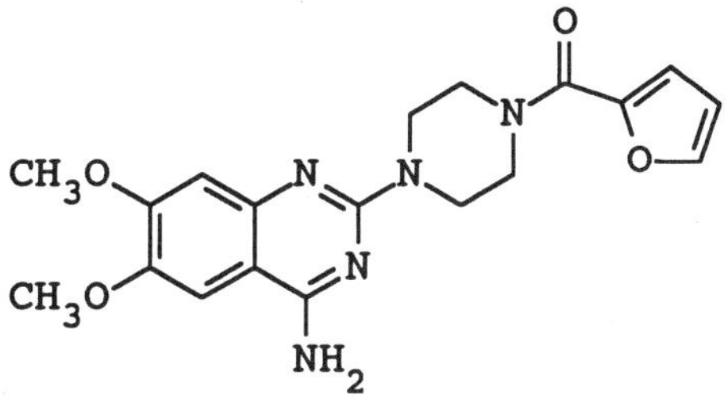

Prazosin

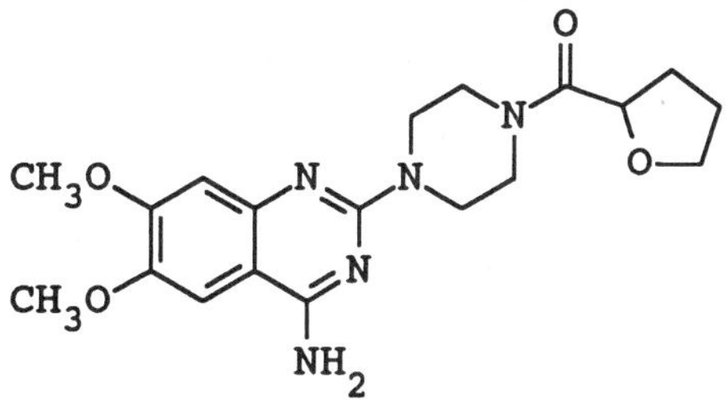

Terazosin

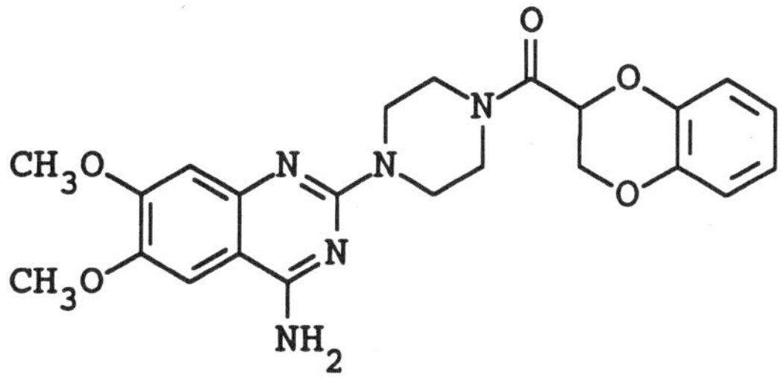

Doxazosin

FIGURE 32-1 *Structures of the selective α_1-adrenergic blocking drugs.*

Mechanism of Action Originally believed to be a direct acting vasodilator, it is now known that prazosin is a selective blocker of peripheral postsynaptic α_1-adrenergic receptors. In contrast to phentolamine and phenoxybenzamine, which block both presynaptic α_2- and postsynaptic α_1-adrenergic receptor sites, at therapeutic doses prazosin leaves the α_2-adrenergic receptor-mediated autoregulatory pathway intact (see Fig. 9-3). In addition to this primary action, prazosin is a relatively potent inhibitor of cyclic nucleotide phosphodiesterase and will directly relax vascular smooth muscle.

Cardiovascular Effects Prazosin causes dilation of arterioles and veins which lead to decreased peripheral resistance and reduced venous return to the heart, respectively. Prazosin elicits less tachycardia than nonselective α-adrenergic blocking drugs and direct-acting vasodilators such as hydralazine. In addition, prazosin tends to reduce total serum cholesterol and triglycerides while increasing high-density lipoproteins (HDLs). These properties are considered to be major advantages of the compound in the management of hypertension. Terazosin and doxazosin are closely related compounds with effects that are qualitatively similar to prazosin; they differ in their pharmacokinetics.

Pharmacokinetics Some of the pharmacokinetics of prazosin, terazosin, and doxazosin are shown in Table 32-4. All of these drugs are well absorbed after oral administration; significant plasma levels are attained within 30 min. Plasma protein binding (mainly to α_1-acid glycoprotein) for all of these drugs is over 90 percent.

Prazosin is extensively biotransformed in the liver by demethylation and conjugation; the demethylated product has some antihypertensive activity. Doxazosin is converted to hydroxylated and O-demethylated metabolites, some of which has some (insignificant) activity. Terazosin undergoes minimal biotransformation. The half-life of prazosin has been estimated at approximately 2.5 h, while that of the other two compounds is longer. All three compounds are primarily excreted via the bile and feces.

Therapeutic Uses These drugs are indicated for the treatment of hypertension. They may be used alone or in combination with other antihypertensive medications such as β-adrenergic blockers or diuretics. Blood pressure (mainly diastolic) is reduced in both the supine and standing positions

TABLE 32-4 Some pharmacokinetics of selective α_1-adrenergic blockers

Parameters	Prazosin	Terazosin	Doxazosin
Oral bioavailability, %	60 to 70	90	65
Plasma protein binding, %	92 to 97	90 to 94	98
Elimination half-life, h	2 to 3	9 to 12	20 to 24
Excretion: feces, %	85 to 90	60	65
Excretion; urine, %	10	40	10

and is unaccompanied by significant changes in cardiac output, heart rate, or renal blood flow. Terazosin and doxazosin have the advantage of once daily dosing.

Adverse Reactions The most common adverse reactions to the selective α_1-adrenergic blockers are dizziness, headache, drowsiness, weakness, cardiac palpitations, and nausea. Postural hypotension, resulting in loss of consciousness, has occurred in some patients within 2 h of the first few doses of the drug. This has been referred to as a "first dose effect". It can be minimized by starting with the lowest dose, taking the first dose at bedtime, and gradually increasing to the maintenance dosage regimen. Tolerance occurs to the first dose effect.

Adrenergic Neuronal Blocking Agents

Reserpine, and related *Rauwolfia* alkaloids, may be employed in the therapy of hypertension (see Chapter 9). Although the antihypertensive effect of reserpine is mild, its use may be advantageous in that it is effective in both the supine and erect postures and adverse reactions are less frequent. The most common side effect of reserpine is psychic depression, occasionally progressing to severe disturbances, including nightmares and severe depressive reactions. Nasal stuffiness, retention of sodium and water with edema, and increased gastric acid secretion also commonly occur.

Guanethidine (see Chapter 9) is a potent long-acting antihypertensive agent; its action is almost exclusively orthostatic, with very little effect on blood pressure when the patient is in a supine position. The most common side effects are related to the orthostatic hypotension, i.e., dizziness, weakness, and syncope. Bradycardia, edema, nasal stuffiness, mild diarrhea, and inhibition of ejaculation may occur. The drug has a notable lack of severe organ toxicity or effects on the CNS. Although guanethidine is occasionally used in monotherapy, most often it is a stage 2 or stage 3 drug in severe hypertension.

Guanadrel, a chemical relative of guanethidine, has similar pharmacologic actions and indications. Both guanethidine and guanadrel should not be used in patients with pheochromocytoma, as they render the patient extremely sensitive to circulating norepinephrine released by the tumor. Both drugs should not be combined with tricyclic antidepressants or phenothiazine derivatives either, which can reverse their effects.

Metyrosine, the drug that competitively inhibits the activity of tyrosine hydroxylase and decreases the endogenous formation of epinephrine and norepinephrine, is indicated for use in patients with pheochromocytoma. The drug is not recommended for the control of essential hypertension (see Chapter 9).

DIRECT-ACTING VASODILATORS

Drugs that elicit vasodilation by a direct action on arterial and/or venous smooth muscle are known as *direct-acting vasodilators*. For the purposes of discussion, these drugs can be classified into two major groups: (1) compounds that relax primarily arterial smooth muscle, with little effect on venous smooth muscle, e.g., hydralazine, minoxidil, and diazoxide, and (2) drugs that affect both arterial and venous tissues, e.g., sodium nitroprusside, nitroglycerin, and the calcium-channel blockers. Diazoxide, sodium nitroprusside, and nitroglycerin are used to treat hypertensive emergencies and will be covered in the last section of this chapter.

Hydralazine

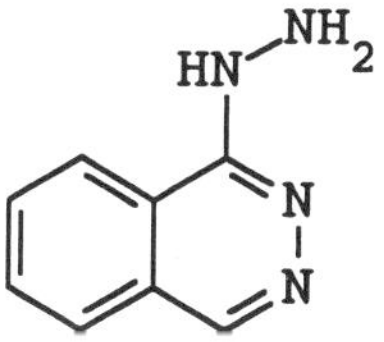

Mechanism of Action The exact mechanism of action of hydralazine on vascular smooth muscle is not completely elucidated. However, it is known that an intact vascular endothelium is necessary for the drug to exert its effect and that hydralazine releases nitric oxide (NO) from blood vessels *in vitro*. Therefore, it is believed that the vasodilation observed with hydralazine is due to the formation of endothelium-derived relaxing factor (EDRF), which is proposed to be either NO or a closely related nitrosothiol intermediate. EDRF stimulates the activity of guanylate cyclase, increases the intracellular concentration of cyclic GMP, which mediates vascular smooth muscle relaxation (see Chapter 29 for a more complete discussion of EDRF and NO).

Cardiovascular Effects Hydralazine exerts an antihypertensive effect by direct relaxation of vascular smooth muscle. Vasodilation is not uniform; the drug primarily affects arteriolar (resistance) vessels with minimal effects on the venous (capacitance) vessels. These actions result in decreased blood pressure (diastolic more than systolic) and decreased peripheral vascular resistance.

Hydralazine no major effects on nonvascular smooth muscle or cardiac tissue. Homeostatic circulatory reflexes remain intact; hydralazine-induced hypotension activates cardiovascular reflexes resulting in increased sympathetic discharge, heart rate, stroke volume, and cardiac output. Therefore, the drug is most effectively employed in combination with a β-adrenergic blocking agent to counteract these cardiac effects.

Pharmacokinetics Hydralazine is well absorbed (80 percent) after oral administration, but bioavailability is low due to a high first pass effect. Peak plasma levels are reached 1 to 2 h after an oral dose. Approximately 85 percent of the circulating drug is bound to plasma proteins. The apparent volume of distribution is low (0.3 to 0.7 L/kg). A major biotransformation pathway involves polymorphic acetylation in the liver; slow acetylators generally attain high blood levels of the drug and require lower maintenance doses. In addition, the compound is hydroxylated and also biotransformed by unidentified processes; therefore, only 12 to 15 percent is excreted unchanged in the urine. The elimination half-life is between 2 and 8 h.

Therapeutic Uses Hydralazine may be employed in a regimen with other drugs in the treatment of primary hypertension. Hydralazine alone is not a drug of choice for chronic therapy even in mild hypertensive states. The drug is tolerated better by patients when combined with a diuretic and a β-adrenergic blocker.

Adverse Reactions Common adverse reactions include headache, palpitations, flushing, anginal pain, anorexia, nausea, vomiting, and diarrhea. Chronic administration of hydralazine can lead to an acute rheumatoid state which can develop into a clinical picture simulating acute systemic lupus erythematosus, e.g., arthralgia, myalgia, fever, dermatoses, and anemia. This syndrome occurs more frequently with high doses (greater than 200 mg daily) and long exposure to the drug and in slow acetylators. The hydralazine lupus-like syndrome is reversible when the drug is stopped.

Minoxidil

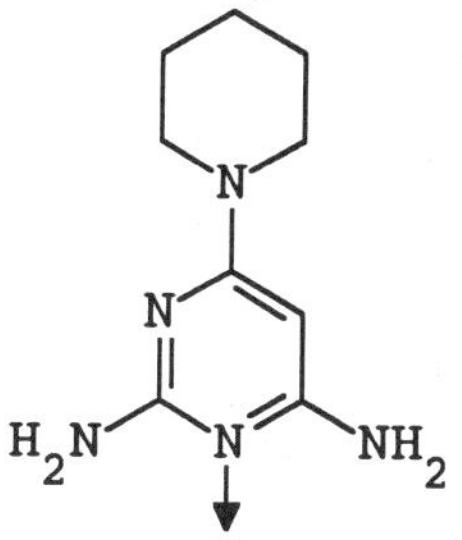

Mechanism of Action Minoxidil is a prodrug that must be biotransformed to the active product, minoxidil N-O sulfate, by hepatic sulfotransferase; this is a minor pathway in the metabolism of the drug. It appears that minoxidil sulfate increases the permeability of membranes of vascular smooth muscle to ionic potassium, resulting in cellular hyperpolarization, and vasodilation.

Cardiovascular Effects Minoxidil is a direct-acting peripheral vasodilator that primarily acts on arteriolar smooth muscle and decreases systolic and diastolic blood pressure. Reflex responses to the hypotension include tachycardia, increased renin secretion, and sodium and water retention. Orthostatic hypotension does not commonly occur.

Pharmacokinetics Minoxidil is almost completely absorbed (90 percent) from the gastrointestinal tract. Blood pressure begins to decline within 60 min; the peak effect occurs in 2 to 3 h. The average plasma half-life is 4.2 h; however, the duration of the antihypertensive effect is approximately 75 h. Therefore, the time course of the effect does not correspond to the drug concentration in the plasma.

Minoxidil does not bind to plasma proteins; it accumulates in arteriolar smooth muscle. Almost 90 percent of the drug is biotransformed predominantly by glucuronide conjugation at the N-oxide position in the pyrimidine ring. Minoxidil and its biotransformation products are excreted in the urine.

Therapeutic Uses Because of potentially serious adverse reactions, this compound is indicated only for severe hypertension that is not controllable by a diuretic plus two other antihypertensive drugs. Minoxidil must usually be used in conjunction with a diuretic and a β-adrenergic blocking agent to reduce sodium and water retention and tachycardia, respectively. Patient acceptance among women is poor due to the development of hypertrichosis.

Since the drug can stimulate the growth of hair, this has led to the local application of a 2% solution of minoxidil to the scalp in patients with male pattern baldness. After 3 to 4 months of daily application, a significant number of patients attain a very modest increase of hair growth. After 8 months, dense growth of hair may occur in about 8 percent of patients. Systemic toxicity may occur from absorption of the drug and patients must be carefully monitored.

Adverse Reactions and Warnings Adverse reactions associated with minoxidil therapy include salt and water retention, tachycardia, pericardial effusion and tamponade, hypertrichosis , ECG abnormalities (negative amplitude of the T wave which usually disappears with continued use), and reduced hematocrit, hemoglobin, and erythrocyte count. In experimental animals, cardiac lesions have been observed after short-term use of minoxidil. Cardiac lesions have been seen at autopsy in patients who have died from various causes and who had received minoxidil for hypertension; however, a causal relationship has never been established. The drug is contraindicated in pheochromocytoma because it may stimulate catecholamine release from the tumor, acute myocardial infarction, and dissecting aortic aneurysm.

Calcium-Channel Blockers

The calcium-channel blockers, also referred to as *calcium antagonists*, inhibit the influx of calcium ions across the cell membrane through voltage-gated calcium channels. As a result, they depress cardiac contractility, automaticity, and conduction velocity, as well as produce relaxation of vascular smooth muscle. The calcium channel blockers are classified by chemical structure and the agents used to treat hypertension are as follows: diphenylalkylamines (verapamil), benzothiazepines (diltiazem), dihydropyridines (amlodipine, felodipine, isradipine, nicardipine, and nifedipine). Although all are effective antihypertensive agents, they differ regarding their selectivity for calcium channels in myocardium, the cardiac conduction system, and vascular smooth muscle (see Chapter 29 for a complete discussion of these drugs). The physiologic effects of each agent depend on the direct effects and the reflex compensations. They are becoming more useful as antihypertensive agents, especially for monotherapy in patients with stage 1 or stage 2 hypertension.

ANGIOTENSIN CONVERTING ENZYME (ACE) INHIBITORS

The Renin-Angiotensin System

Renin, a proteolytic enzyme produced by the juxtaglomerular apparatus of the kidney, acts like a hormone in the sense that it initiates control of physiologic functions of other organs. Increased secretion of renin is stimulated by a fall in renal perfusion pressure as occurs in renal artery stenosis, hemorrhage, dehydration, and sodium depletion. It is also under control of the sympathetic nervous system (via β-adrenergic receptor stimulation and, probably by atrial natriuretic factor, a cardiac peptide hormone discovered several years ago.

Angiotensin I is a decapeptide prehormone which is produced by the proteolytic action of renin on angiotensinogen, an α_2-globulin produced by the liver. Angiotensin I is relatively inactive and is activated to angiotensin II (an octapeptide) by the cleavage of two amino acids by a converting enzyme (known as *dipeptidyl carboxypeptidase*, or *angiotensin converting enzyme (ACE)*) present in the lungs and other tissues. This enzyme not only increases the formation of angiotensin, but also inactivates bradykinin, a potent vasodilator.

Angiotensin receptors are present on the membrane of smooth muscle cells of arterioles and on the adrenal cortex cells of the zona glomerulosa; these are stimulated by angiotensin II. This endogenous peptide has two major effects: (1) constriction of arterioles, and (2) stimulation of the synthesis and secretion of aldosterone. Arteriolar constriction results in increased peripheral resistance; aldosterone acts on the collecting duct in the kidney to cause Na^+ and water retention and the excretion of K^+ and H^+. By a negative feedback loop induced by the rise in blood pressure and renal perfusion, the secretion of renin is reduced.

The role of the renin-angiotensin system in normotensive individuals is probably minor. In hypertensive patients, it is an important mechanism that maintains the elevated arterial pressure by increasing fluid volume and causing arteriolar constriction. Although it might be attractive to surmise that the etiology of essential hypertension is a disturbance of the renin-angiotensin system in every case, the proof of this has never been established. Certainly in renal artery stenosis, reestablishment of flow or removal of the affected kidney cures the hypertension, but a vast majority of hypertensive patients have no demonstrable pathology which might lead to increased production of renin. Nevertheless, ACE inhibitors have proven to be a group of very effective antihypertensive agents and are beginning to replace the β-adrenergic blockers, especially as monotherapy.

Early attempts to block the renin-angiotensin system produced competitive antagonists of angiotensin II. These compounds are variations of angiotensin II, formed by substitution of various amino acids in the peptide structure with other amino acids. The most studied has been *saralasin*, a partial agonist. When given intravenously to normal subjects, saralasin causes a transient rise in blood pressure which is followed by a fall. Saralasin is useful diagnostically because in renin-dependent hypertensive patients there is a sustained fall in blood pressure, whereas in individuals with low-renin hypertension there is a sustained pressor response. Saralasin remains an interesting and important investigative tool; it is not available as a commercial drug.

Captopril and Related Drugs

The inhibitors of the renin-angiotensin system which have proven to be clinically successful are those which inhibit the conversion of angiotensin I to angiotensin II. The drugs included in this class of compounds include benazepril, captopril, enalapril, fosinopril, lisinopril, quinapril, and ramipril.

Chemistry The original inhibitor of ACE was a nonapeptide known as *teprotide*. By analysis of the inhibitory action of teprotide, the amino acid sequence of angiotensin II, and some ingenious deductions on the action of ACE on its substrates, an orally effective, relatively simple chemical (which is essentially a modified and substituted proline derivative) was produced called *captopril*. Later, other compounds followed that were all based upon the original premise of proline derivatives as inhibitors of ACE. The structures of the ACE inhibitors are shown in Fig. 32-2.

Mechanism of Action The ACE inhibitors are very specific in their action. They do not interact with other components of the renin-angiotensin system. In addition to inhibiting the conversion of angiotensin I to angiotensin II, they also inhibit the inactivation of bradykinin. Both of these actions mediate the vasodilator effects of ACE inhibitors; however, the reduction in angiotensin II formation is the principal pharmacologic event. The reduction of angiotensin II synthesis leads to a compensatory adjustment of extra production and blood levels of renin and angiotensin I. This apparently does not contribute to any adverse effects.

Increased prostaglandin (PG) synthesis may play a role in the activity of these drugs. Single doses of captopril have been shown to increase the blood levels and urinary excretion of PGE_2, $PGF_{2\alpha}$, and their metabolites. The antihypertensive effect of ACE inhibitors persist longer than inhibition of the enzyme can be demonstrated.

Cardiovascular Effects A single oral dose of an ACE inhibitor in a normal subject results in only a slight fall in blood pressure. Repeated doses over several days result in a more sustained fall and a slight blunting of postural reflexes. However, if the individual is sodium-depleted, even a single dose of one of these drugs causes a significant fall in blood pressure. After taking an ACE inhibitor, the vascular response to angiotensin II is absent. In addition, the ability of angiotensin II to stimulate the synthesis and secretion of aldosterone is also depressed.

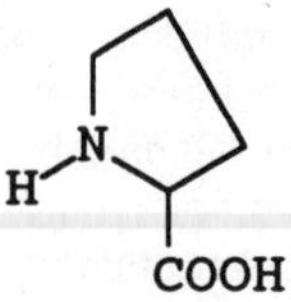

L-Proline

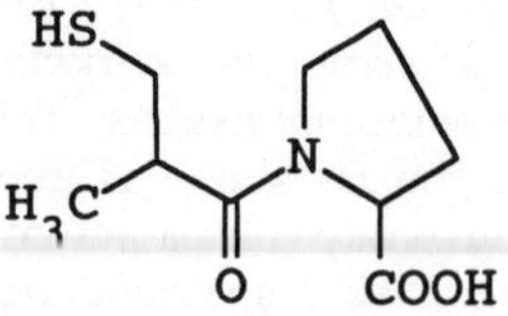

Captopril

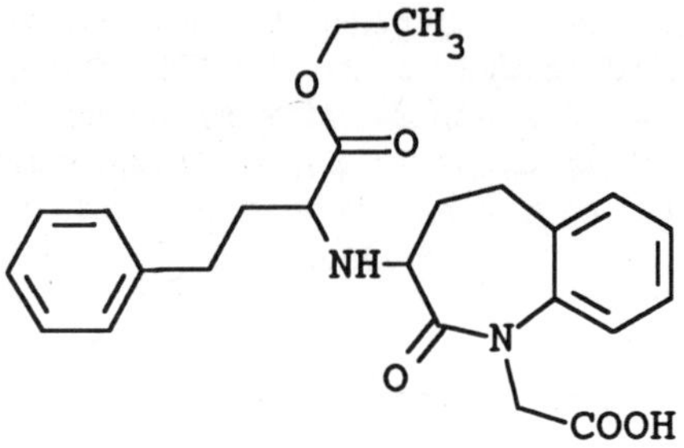

Benazepril

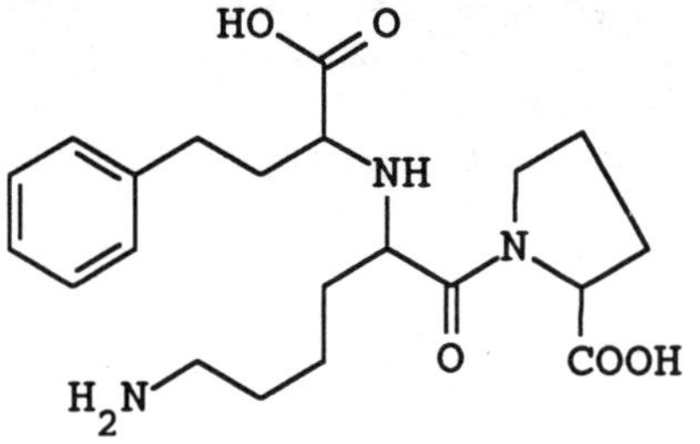

Lisinopril

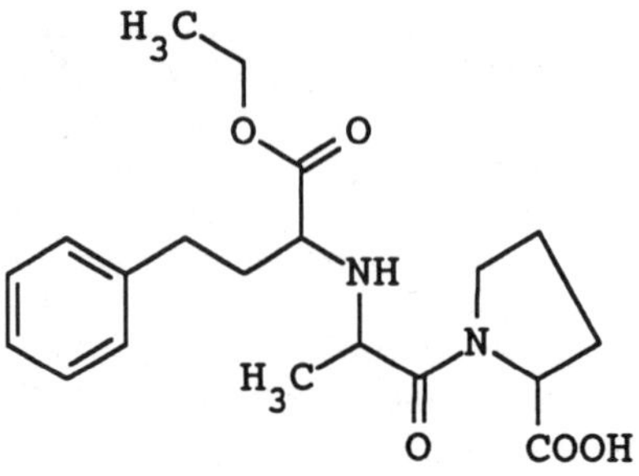

Enalapril

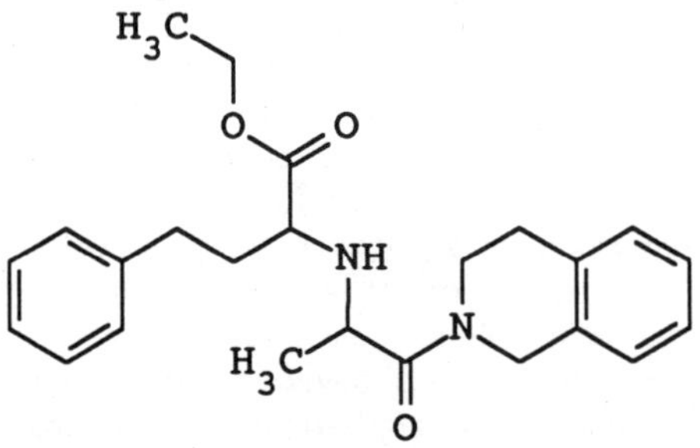

Quinapril

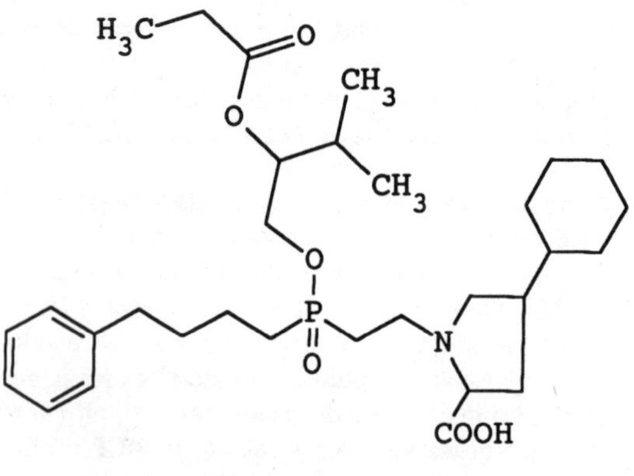

Fosinopril

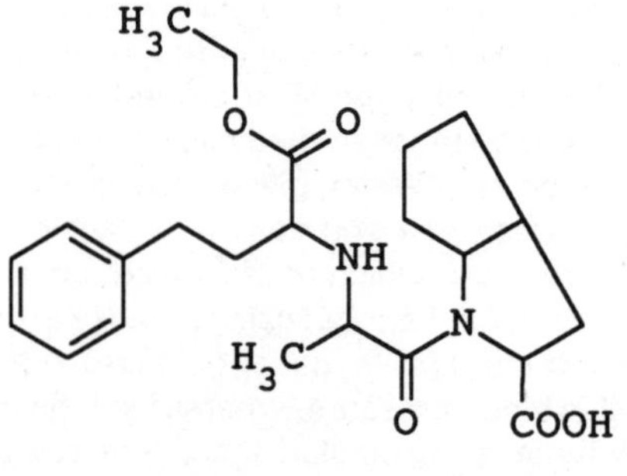

Ramipril

FIGURE 32-2 *Structures of* L*-proline and the angiotensin converting enzyme (ACE) inhibitors.*

In hypertensive patients, whether caused by increased plasma renin levels or not, ACE inhibitors satisfactorily lower both systolic and diastolic blood pressure. Responses to postural changes and exercise are not compromised. Cardiac function is generally not affected; slight increases in stroke volume and cardiac output may occur.

In patients with congestive heart failure, ACE inhibitors reduce cardiac afterload, resulting in an increase in stroke volume and cardiac output. Heart rate is generally reduced. Sodium and water excretion are increased as a result of the improved renal hemodynamics and the reduction in aldosterone secretion.

Pharmacokinetics The ACE inhibitors are rapidly absorbed following oral administration; the oral bioavailability of these drugs is variable (see Table 32-5). The oral absorption of captopril is reduced significantly by food (30 to 40 percent), and therefore an oral dose of this drug should be given 1 h before meals. The absorption of quinapril is reduced by meals with high fat content, and the rate of absorption of ramipril (but not the extent) is delayed by food. The oral absorption of other ACE inhibitors is not affected by meals.

About 50 percent of captopril is metabolized to an inactive product. Lisinopril is not biotransformed. For all of the other compounds the ethyl ester group is hydrolyzed to form products that are more active than the parent drug (see Table 32-5). Enalapril and fosinopril are essentially inactive and are considered prodrugs. The ACE inhibitors and their metabolic products are either conjugated with glucuronic acid prior to excretion or excreted in an unconjugated form mainly into the urine. Although the parent drugs have a short half-life due to rapid metabolism (except for lisinopril), the half-lives of the active metabolites are relatively long and the ACE inhibitors have, therefore, a prolonged duration of action.

The effect of captopril is observed within 15 min of dosing and the duration is up to 6 h. In general for the other drugs, the onset of action is within 1 h and the duration of the antihypertensive effect is about 24 h. Therefore, all of these drugs, except for captopril, are usually given once daily.

Therapeutic Uses The ACE inhibitors are very useful as initial oral monotherapy of essential hypertension. They can be used alone or in combination with other antihypertensive drugs, especially diuretics. The active biotransformation product of enalapril, enalaprilat, is available for intravenous use when oral therapy is not practical.

These drugs also have gained prominence as vasodilator therapy of congestive heart failure (see Chapter 27). Usually, these drugs are used in combination with a diuretic and digoxin, although some physicians have treated patients successfully with an ACE inhibitor alone. Presently only captopril, enalapril, and lisinopril are officially indicated as vasodilators for the treatment of congestive heart failure; the others should be considered as investigational for this purpose.

Since all of these compounds are eliminated through the kidney, and the drugs may cause a reduction in renal function (see below), renal function should be monitored during the first few weeks of therapy. In addition, dosage reduction should be considered in patients with renal impairment.

Adverse Effects All of the ACE inhibitors have the usual side effects associated with the gastrointestinal tract (e.g., diarrhea, nausea, vomiting), the CNS (e.g., headache, dizziness, fatigue), and the cardiovascular system (hypotension) in an incidence of about 0.5 to 2 percent. Most experience has been with captopril, but its toxicities generally apply to the other ACE inhibitors. Transient, reversible elevations of blood urinary nitrogen (BUN) and creatinine may occur, especially in patients with volume depletion or renovascular hypertension. In patients with renal impairment, elevations in serum potassium occur. There is a small incidence of proteinuria and other signs of renal failure. A non-productive cough is a very common side effect of these drugs. In addition, captopril will reduce the sensation of taste (called *dysgeusia*) is up to 5 percent of patients.

Early in the use of captopril, a nephrotic syndrome occurred in about 20 percent of patients; however, a reduction in dosage greatly reduced this complication. Neutropenia and agranulocytoses occur in a small incidence and obviate therapy with ACE inhibitors. The incidence is highest in patients who already have collagen diseases. Cholestatic jaundice is a rare occurrence. Angioedema occurs in an incidence of about 0.1 percent. When life-threatening because of laryngeal edema, epinephrine is to be given.

Excessive hypotension may occur, especially following the first few doses of these drugs, i.e., the *first dose effect*. Although rare, it is more common is patients who are salt/volume depleted or those persons who are being treated vigorously with diuretics. The potential for this may be reduced by reduction of the initial doses.

TABLE 32-5 Some pharmacokinetics of the angiotensin converting enzyme (ACE) inhibitors

Drug	Absorption, %	Time to peak serum levels, h	Plasma protein binding, %[b]	Active metabolite	Half-life, h[b]	Route(s) of elimination[b]
Benazepril	40	0.5 to 1	95 to 97	Benazeprilat	10 to 11	Urine (95%)
Captopril	75[a]	0.5 to 1.5	25 to 30	None	2	Urine (95%)
Enalapril	60	0.5 to 1.5	No data	Enalaprilat	11	Urine (95%)
Fosinopril	40	3	95 to 97	Fosinoprilat	12	Urine (50%) Feces (50%)
Lisinopril	25	7	No data	None	12	Urine (99%)
Quinapril	60[a]	1	95 to 97	Quinaprilat	25	Urine (96%)
Ramipril	55[a]	1	55 to 75	Ramiprilat	13 to 17	Urine (60%) Feces (40%)

[a] Oral absorption reduced by food (see text).
[b] Parent compound and active metabolites, if any.

THERAPEUTIC APPROACHES TO ANTIHYPERTENSIVE THERAPY

Over the past 30 years, the management of hypertension has evolved gradually in a pattern of stepped-care diet and drug therapy which has been eminently satisfactory. Most cases of hypertension are mild to moderate (see Table 32-1) and can be treated on an ambulatory basis. Often the patient may have also minor symptoms so that compliance with drug therapy is difficult especially if the drugs used have many side effects.

The traditional stepped-care therapy of hypertension is as follows:

1. Restrict dietary sodium to 2 g daily. Eliminate risk factors such as obesity, smoking, alcohol. Encourage exercise.

2. Diuretics or β-adrenergic blockers. Alternatively, calcium-channel blockers, ACE inhibitors, selective α_1-adrenergic blockers, or labetalol.

3. Sympatholytic drugs, either centrally or peripherally acting. Most popular are clonidine and prazosin.

4. Add a third drug, usually a direct-acting vasodilator such as hydralazine or minoxidil.

In the past few years there has been a strong movement toward monotherapy with one of four groups of drugs, namely, thiazide diuretics, β-adrenergic blockers, ACE inhibitors, and calcium-channel blockers. Diet therapy and reduction of risk factors is, of course, first advised. However, the drug chosen for monotherapy is titrated to the maximum dose before other therapy is considered. A diuretic is added only after failure to adequately control the blood pressure. Monotherapy will be satisfactory therapy for many mild to moderate hypertensive patients and appears to be simpler, to be less apt to have adverse drug effects and interactions, and to increase compliance.

At the present time there is an intensive effort to determine which is the superior group of drugs for antihypertensive monotherapy. The β-adrenergic blockers have been used for the longest time, and consequently there is more experience with their use. These compounds and thiazide diuretics are the only group of drugs with a proven record of reduction of cardiovascular morbidity and mortality. However, the other two groups, i.e., ACE inhibitors and calcium-channel blockers may be equally effective in this regard.

No therapy thus far developed has succeeded in reducing the incidence of coronary heart disease. This is a paradox in view of the observed reduction in treated hypertensive patients of the incidence of stroke and renal disease. For this reason, attention to the lipid profile of each hypertensive patient must be examined and treated if abnormal.

Finally this chapter does not deal with secondary hypertension such as that caused by pheochromocytoma, aldosteronism, coarctation of the aorta, and renal disease. Therapy used in these diseases is covered under the drugs themselves such as phentolamine, phenoxybenzamine, and metyrosine.

HYPERTENSIVE EMERGENCIES

The patient with hypertensive emergencies requires constant monitoring of blood pressure in an intensive care setting or its equivalent. The availability of diazoxide, sodium nitroprusside, and nitroglycerin has considerably enhanced the ability to deal with hypertensive emergencies. Other drugs, used by the intravenous route, which are valuable for certain hypertensive emergencies include trimethaphan and methyldopate.

Diazoxide

Diazoxide is a non-diuretic thiazide derivative that produces a prompt reduction in blood pressure by directly relaxing smooth muscle of the arterioles. Like hydralazine, this agent has little effect on the venous system or the heart.

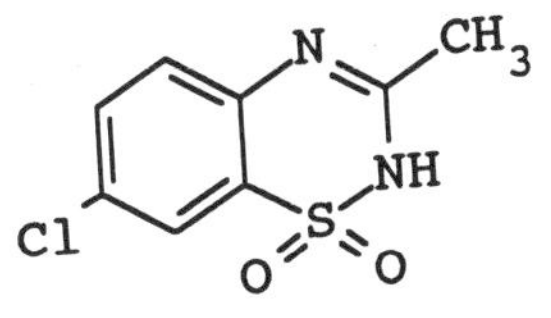

N CH3 NH Cl S O O

Mechanism of Action and Effects Diazoxide stimulates ATP-sensitive K^+ channels in arteriolar smooth muscle, which leads to hyperpolarization of the cells and relaxation. The sympathetic nervous system reflexes are activated, resulting in sodium and water retention (through the renin-angiotensin system) and cardiac stimulation (increased rate, force, and output).

In addition to the hypotensive effects, this drug produces an elevation of blood glucose levels, primarily because of inhibition of insulin release from the pancreas, similar to the thiazide diuretics (see Chapter 31).

Pharmacokinetics Although the oral bioavailability of diazoxide is almost 100 percent, the drug is administered by intravenous injection. Greater than 90 percent is bound to plasma proteins, resulting in a low apparent volume of distribution (0.2 L/kg). The drug is biotransformed to inactive hydroxy and carboxylic acid products, which are subsequently conjugated by sulfate prior to excretion via the kidney. The half-life of the parent compound is 20 to 40 h, largely because of a high degree of renal tubular reabsorption.

Therapeutic Uses Diazoxide has been employed orally in the management of hypoglycemia due to hyperinsulinism associated with islet cell adenoma or carcinoma. However, its major use is in hypertensive emergencies, always administered by the intravenous route (either as a bolus or by infusion) for a prompt, effective, and prolonged response. By intravenous bolus injection, the onset of action is within 30 sec, peak effect occurs between 2 and 5 min, and the duration of action is 3 to 8 h. Diazoxide is not employed for primary hypertension because of its side effects.

Adverse Reactions The major effects of diazoxide on water and electrolyte balance are opposite to those of the thiazide diuretics. Diazoxide causes marked sodium and water retention, expands plasma volume, and can produce edema in patients with inadequate myocardial function. In common with the structurally-related diuretics, diazoxide produces hyperglycemia and hyperuricemia. Other adverse effects include tachycardia, gastrointestinal complaints, flushing, and local pain and inflammation after extravasation. As with minoxidil, long-term administration of diazoxide can cause hypertrichosis.

Sodium Nitroprusside

Sodium nitroprusside, $Na_2Fe(CN)_5NO \cdot 2H_2O$, is a potent, fast-acting intravenous hypotensive agent which is used for reduction of blood pressure in hypertensive crises.

Mechanism of Action and Effects Red blood cells decompose sodium nitroprusside, releasing nitric oxide (NO). NO activates guanylate cyclase in vascular smooth muscle, resulting in vasodilation. The hypotensive effects of the drug are caused by peripheral vasodilatation on both arteriolar and venular blood vessels. Unlike the drugs which primarily affect the arterioles (hydralazine, minoxidil, and diazoxide), tachycardia is only moderate with sodium nitroprusside. The drug also reduces platelet aggregation.

Pharmacokinetics The effects of the drug occur rapidly (within 30 sec) but are of short duration (ending within 3 min after the intravenous infusion is stopped). The effects of the drug are self-limiting because of the short metabolic half-life; sodium nitroprusside reacts with membrane-bound sulfhydryl groups on erythrocytes and blood vessels, dissociates, and releases NO and cyanide. Cyanide is metabolized in the liver by rhodanase to thiocyanate ion, which is eliminated in the urine.

Sodium nitroprusside is also light-sensitive. Ultra-violet light dissociates and inactivates the molecule.

Therapeutic Uses The only indication for sodium nitroprusside is the reduction in blood pressure in patients with hypertensive crisis.

Adverse Reactions Adverse reactions that have been noted by too rapid administration include nausea, apprehension, headache, restlessness, muscle twitching, palpitations, and abdominal pain. Decreased platelet aggregation, tachycardia, and ECG changes may also occur.

If excessive amounts of drug are used, thiocyanate toxicity (tinnitus, flushing, blurred vision, delirium) may result. With gross overdosage or with chronic administration, cyanide intoxication is possible.

Nitroglycerin

Intravenous administration of nitroglycerin is used to control blood pressure in perioperative hypertension associated with surgical procedures and in patients with hypertensive crisis. In the latter case, it is especially useful in those individuals who have angina or myocardial infarction.

Nitroglycerin does not have many of the adverse effects associated with sodium nitroprusside and it is chemically stable. Thus is provides an alternative to sodium nitroprusside.

Nitroglycerin is primarily used for the treatment of angina, by other routes of administration. For a complete discussion of the pharmacology of this compound, see Chapter 29.

BIBLIOGRAPHY

--------: "The Fifth Report of the Joint National Committee on Detection, Evaluation and Treatment of High Blood Pressure, National Institute of Health Publication (JNC V) 1993," *Arch. Int. Med.* **153**: 154-183 (1993).

Amery, A., W. Birkenhager, R. Brixko, C. Bulpitt, D. Clement, et al.: "Efficacy of Antihypertensive Drug Treatment According to Age, Sex, Blood Pressure and Previous Cardiovascular Disease in Patients Over the Age of 60," *Lancet* **2**: 589-592 (1986).

Cruickshank, J.M.: "Antihypertensive Drugs and Cardioprotection," *Blood Press. Suppl.* **1**: 47-55, 56-57 (1992).

Epstein, M., and J.R. Oster: *Hypertension, A Practical Approach*, Saunders, Philadelphia, 1984.

Freis, E.D.: "Veterans Administration Cooperative Study on Nadolol as Monotherapy and in Combination with a Diuretic," *Am. Heart J.* **108**: 1087-1091 (1984).

Gifford, R.W., Jr.: "Role of Diuretics in Treatment of Hypertension," *Am. J. Med.*, 77:102 -106 (1984).

Haber, E., and E.E. Slater: "High Blood Pressure," *Sci. Am. Med.* **1**: 1, **VII**: 1-30 (1988).

Helgeland, A., R. Strommen, C.H. Hagelund, and S. Tretli: "Enalapril, Atenolol and Hydrochlorothiazide in Mild or Moderate Hypertension. A Comparative Multicenter Trial in General Practice in Norway," *Tidsskr. Nor. Laegeforen* **107**: 2937-2940, 2968 (1987).

Lund-Johansen, P.: "Hemodynamic Profiles of Antihypertensive Agents," *Blood Press. Suppl.* **1**: 16-23 (1992).

Kaplan, N.M.: "Non-drug Treatment of Hypertension," *Ann. Intern. Med.* **102**: 359-373 (1985).

McChesney, J.A., and W.J.C. Amend, Jr.: "Minoxidil in the Treatment of Refractory Hypertension Due to a Spectrum of Causes," *J. Cardiavasc. Pharmacol.* **2**: S131--134 (1980).

Sassano, P., G. Chatellier, A.M. Amiot, F. Alhenc-Gelas, P. Corvol, and J. Menard: "A Double-Blind Randomized Evaluation of Converting Enzyme Inhibition as the First-Step Treatment of Mild to Moderate Hypertension," *J. Hypertens. Suppl.* **2**: S75-S81 (1984).

Spivack, C., S. Ocken, and W.H. Frishman: "Calcium Antagonists: Clinical Use in Treatment of Systemic Hypertension," *Drugs* **25**: 154-165 (1983).

CHAPTER 33

Drugs for Chronic Obstructive Pulmonary Diseases

Bruce R. Pitt and William J. Calhoun

Asthma is a clinical syndrome characterized by increased responsiveness, narrowing of the airways, and subsequent episodes of breathlessness, wheezing, and cough. Associated with narrowed airways may be changes in ciliary activity and mucus secretion. Cough may be a major factor during an asthmatic attack. An acute attack can be brought on by external stimuli such as airborne antigen, exercise, cold air, or other unknown triggers. Most studied of these stimuli are exercise and antigen. Clinically, asthma is usually graded as either mild, moderate, or severe. Mild asthma does not usually interfere with normal activities and is controlled by bronchodilators. Moderate asthma may occasionally interfere with normal routine, and it may require steroids for control. Severe asthma limits normal activity considerably and can at times result in life-threatening episodes.

Patients with asthma may quite often demonstrate signs of chronic bronchitis and/or emphysema as well. Chronic bronchitis is characterized by excessive mucus production and is associated with chronic productive cough. Emphysema is defined as a condition of the lung characterized by an abnormal and permanent enlargement of respiratory airspaces accompanied by destruction of their walls without fibrosis. All these disease syndromes lead to episodes of wheezing and coughing. Since the molecular mechanisms of these pathologic changes are largely unknown, therapy for asthma and other chronic obstructive pulmonary diseases (COPDs) is directed toward symptomatic relief of the acute bronchospasm or, in the case of prophylactic drugs like cromolyn sodium, prevention of an attack.

To understand the rationale behind the therapeutic agents of this class, one must have a basic understanding of the pathophysiology involved in an acute or chronic allergy-induced bronchospasm. Our understanding of the mechanism of allergic bronchospasm involves mediation by reaginic antibodies, that is, immunoglobulin E (IgE). IgE is synthesized by plasma cells in response to an initial exposure of allergen in a susceptible individual (Fig. 33-1). These newly synthesized IgE molecules fix themselves to mast cells in the airway mucosa and basophils and mast cells throughout the body.

These fixed IgE molecules are antigen-specific. On subsequent exposure to the same antigen, an antigen-antibody interaction takes place which involves one antigen molecule cross-bridging two IgE molecules, resulting in a perturbation of the cell membrane. Membrane perturbation, or cell activation, is followed by a series of biochemical events including the rapid influx of calcium into the cell and subsequent activation of phospholipase enzymes within the cell (see Fig. 33-1). Phospholipase metabolizes membrane phospholipids to arachidonic acid, which is subsequently metabolized via cyclooxygenase to prostaglandins (PGs) and lipoxygenase to leukotrienes (LTs) and hydroxyeicosatetrenoic acids (HETEs) (Fig. 33-2). Some of the cyclooxygenase products, i.e., $PGF_{2\alpha}$, and thromboxanes, and the sulfidoleukotrienes (LTC_4, LTD_4, and LTE_4), are potent bronchospastic agents. Along with the PGs, LTs, and HETEs, phospholipid metabolism by phospholipase leads to the production of platelet activating factor (PAF), another potent bronchospastic agent which may contribute to the airway narrowing seen in asthma. These newly synthesized mediators are released from the cell along with stored mediators such as histamine and cause smooth muscle contraction, edema, cellular infiltration, and mucus secretion.

Although the immunologic response described above may be responsible for cases of allergic asthma, it is not the only mechanism resulting in

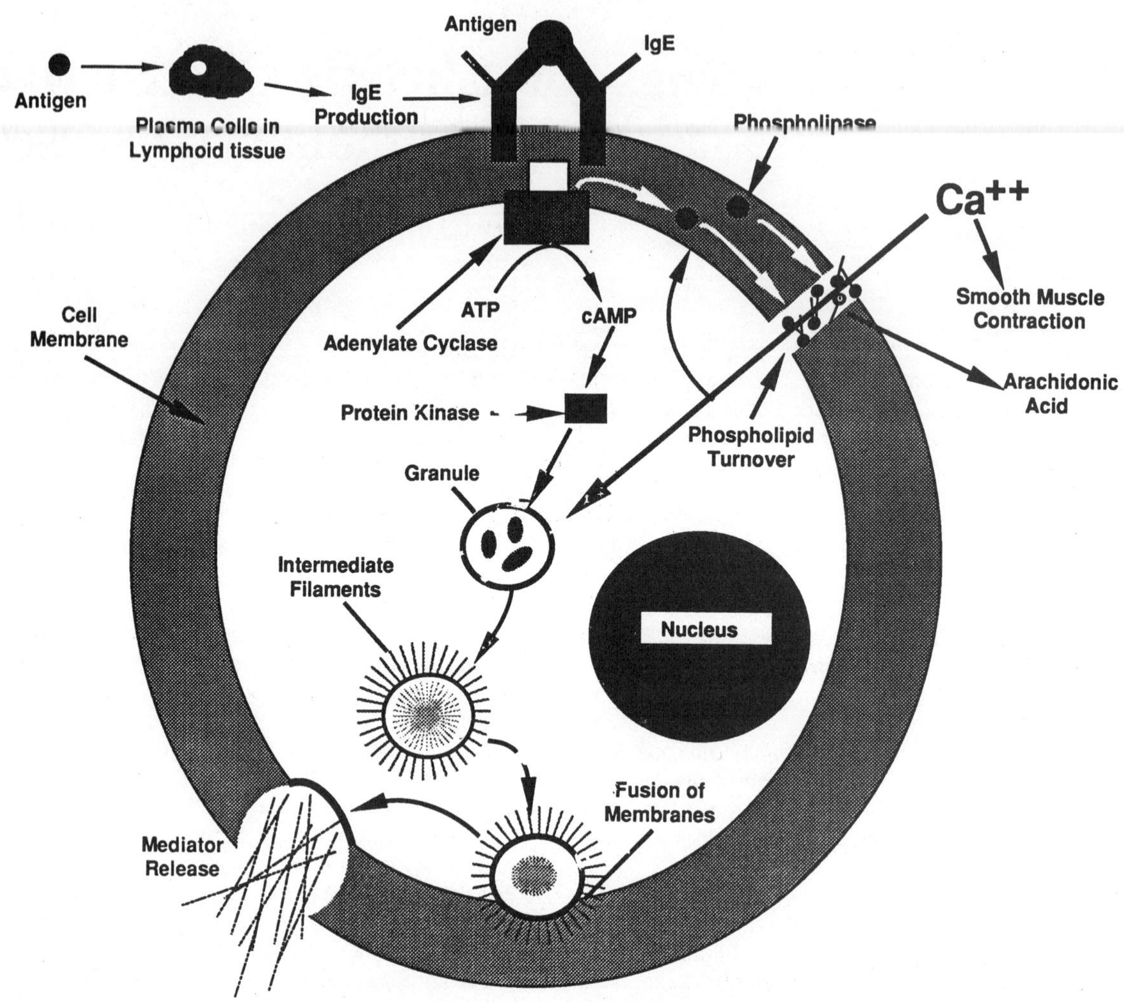

FIGURE 33-1 *Schematic representation of sensitization and exposure to antigen and the resultant mast cell activation.*

bronchospasm. Acute attacks of bronchospasm may be caused by a sensitivity to aspirin, by exercise, or by heat loss from the airways and from other undefined mechanisms. These cases are sometimes referred to as *bronchial hyperreactivity cases* rather than allergic bronchospasm. Airway hyperreactivity appears to be universal in individuals with respiratory disease.

The mechanism behind bronchial hyperreactivity is unknown. However, whatever the mechanism, it appears to be related to released mediators and the interaction of these mediators with neural and humoral pathways involved with homeostatic control of respiratory smooth muscle. With this interaction in mind, it becomes understandable why a variety of types of pharmacologic interventions may have an effect on asthma, albeit not affording a cure. This appears to be the case clinically, since mediator release inhibitors (cromolyn sodium), calcium entry blockers, lipoxygenase-cyclooxygenase inhibitors, specific receptor antagonists (for LTs, histamine, PAF, PGs), as well as physiologic antagonists like theophylline or β-adrenergic receptor agonists may all have some effect in asthma, yet none offers a cure.

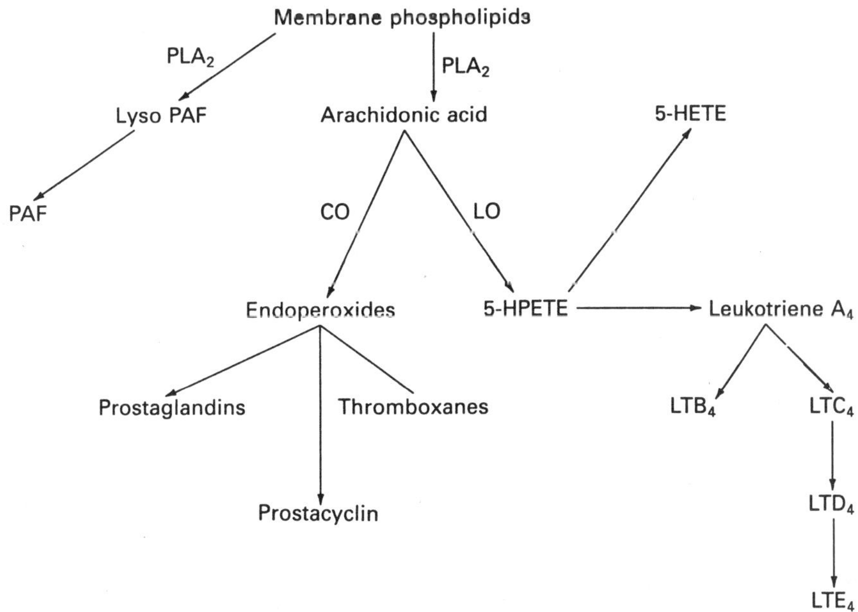

FIGURE 33-2 *Metabolism of membrane phospholipids to products of arachidonic acid metabolism and platelet activating factor (PAF). PLA$_2$ = phospholipase A$_2$; CO = cyclooxygenase; LO = lipoxygenase; 5-HPETE = 5-hydroperoxyeicosatetrenoic acid; 5-HETE = 5-hydroxyeicosatetrenoic acid; LT = leukotriene.*

ANTI-INFLAMMATORY AGENTS

Corticosteroids

Corticosteroids have been used extensively in the treatment of obstructive airways disease. Corticosteroids are not bronchodilators, and it is generally believed that their beneficial effects in chronic airway disease are due to their anti-inflammatory effects. Glucocorticoids readily enter cells and in many tissues, bind to specific receptors in the cytoplasm (or nucleus). The activated steroid-receptor complex binds to DNA and affects the expression of a number of specific messenger RNAs, some of which result in: (1) decreased production of inflammatory mediators; and (2) increased production of anti-inflammatory mediators. Critical cellular targets of transcriptional effects of glucocorticoids include induction of synthesis of lipocortins and β_2-adrenergic receptors. Lipocortins are a group of proteins arising from distinct gene products that are part of the family of calcium- and phospholipid-binding proteins called annexins. All lipocortins are known to inhibit phospholipase A$_2$ thereby decreasing the production of platelet activating factor and arachidonic acid (precursor for prostaglandins, thromboxane and leukotrienes). Enhanced synthesis of β-adrenergic receptors by glucocorticoids presumably contributes to their effectiveness in preventing tachyphylaxis to the bronchodilator response to β_2-adrenergic agonists. Glucocorticoids also directly inhibit the expression of a number of cytokines (Fig. 33-3) in inflammatory cells thereby decreasing activation of macrophages, inhibiting proliferation of T-lymphocytes, reducing mast cell number and down-regulating eosinophil function.

Although glucocorticoids may be administered parenterally or orally, a major advance in the management of chronic obstructive lung disease is the use of aerosol corticosteroids. A group of aerosol corticosteroids are available (see Table 33-1) that have enhanced topical anti-inflammatory potency with lowered systemic effects (secondary to biotransformation in liver to inactive metabolites). These agents are generally administered from a metered-dose inhaler and have been shown to be safe and effective for chronic treatment of asthma, administered in long-term in low doses or

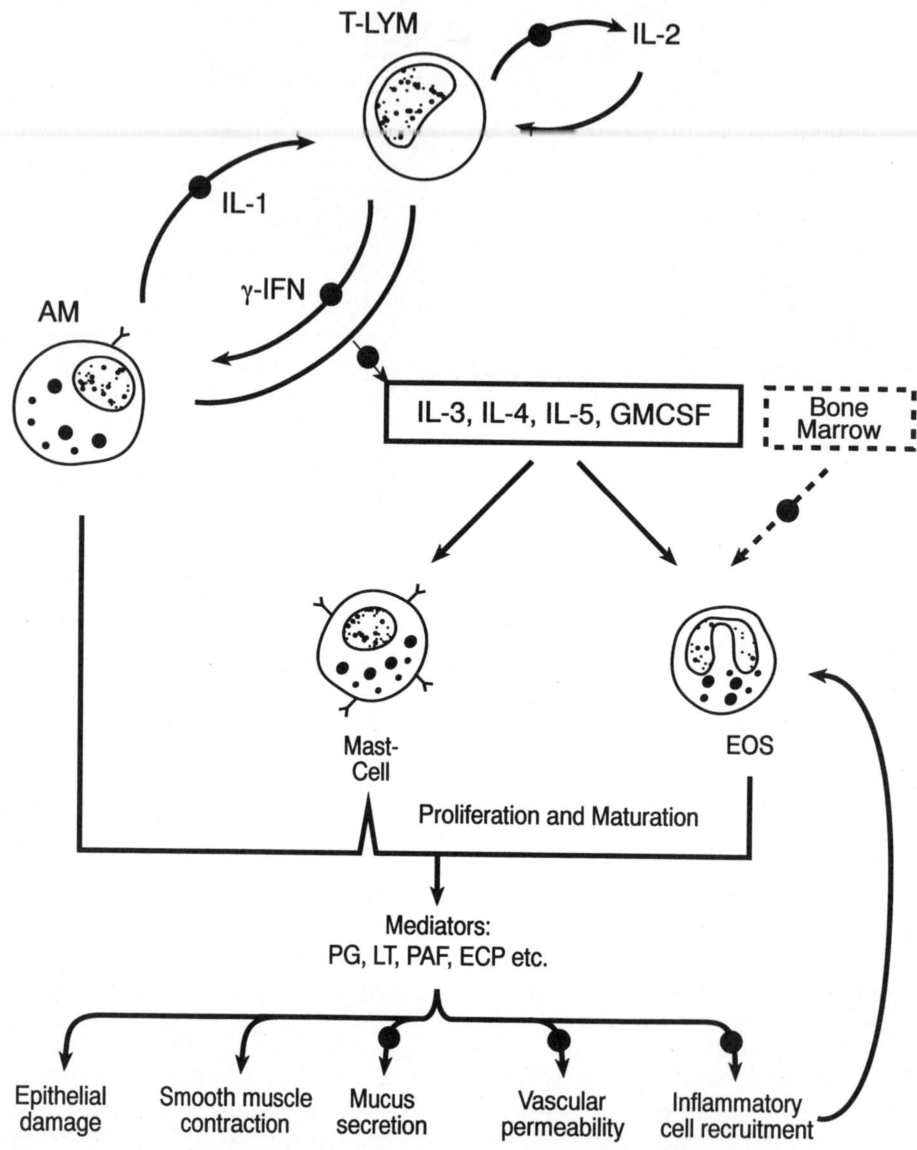

FIGURE 33-3 *Schematic representation of putative interactions between inflammatory cells, cytokines, and inflammatory mediators to cause many of the features characteristic of asthma. The potential inhibitory effects of glucocorticoids are represented by the closed circles placed on several pathways. Glucocorticoids inhibit the release of interleukin-1 (IL-1), IL-2, and interferon gamma (γ-IFN), preventing collaboration between macrophages (AM) and lymphocytes (T-LYM). Release of other interleukins such as IL-3, IL-4, IL-5, and granulocyte-macrophage colony stimulating factor (GMCSF) is also prevented, leading to inhibition of differentiation, proliferation, and activation of mast cells and eosinophils (EOS). In addition, release of inflammatory mediators such as prostaglandins (PG), leukotrienes (LT), platelet-activating factor (PAF), or eosinophil-cationic protein (ECP) may also be prevented by glucocorticoids. Glucocorticoids may therefore be effective at several levels of the inflammatory process in asthmatic airways. [Redrawn from: Chung, K.F., J. Wiggins, and J. Collins: "Corticosteroids," in Weiss, E.B., and M. Stein, (eds.): Bronchial Asthma, Mechanisms and Therapeutics, Third Edition, Little, Brown and Co., Boston, 1993, p. 803.]*

TABLE 33-1 Anti-inflammatory agents available for respiratory disease

CORTICOSTEROIDS
Beclomethasone diproprionate
Dexamethasone sodium phosphate
Flunisolide
Triamcinolone acetonide
NON-STEROIDAL ANTIALLERGIC DRUGS
Cromolyn sodium
Nedocromil sodium

short-term in high doses. Local adverse effects may include oropharyngeal candidiasis and dysphonia and may be minimized by the use of spacer devices in the inhalant apparatus or mouth washing. Systemic effects may occur with lower doses in children, post menopausal women, and patients with Addison's disease. Oral therapy is reserved for patients who are difficult to manage via the topical route. The risk of significant adverse effects secondary to chronic steroid excess via the oral route is substantial and includes reduced hypothalamic-pituitary-adrenal function, potential growth retardation, cataract formation, and osteoporosis.

Non-Steroidal Antiallergic Drugs

The prototype antiallergic drug is cromolyn sodium (disodium cromoglycate), and the history of cromolyn reflects the history of this class of drugs. Many compounds have been synthesized that have similar activity profiles in animal studies, but none has proven as efficacious as cromolyn in the clinic. Cromolyn was first discovered during investigations of khellin (see below), a derivative isolated from Middle Eastern plant *Ammi visnaga*. Many of the derivatives have smooth muscle relaxing properties causing vasodilation and relaxation of airway smooth muscle. Based on the activity of khellin, many analogs, directed toward a more soluble chromone with greater potency, were synthesized in the late 1950s and early 1960s.

Early on, the chromone-2-carboxylic acids were recognized as not having smooth muscle relaxant properties; however, in human volunteers, they inhibited antigen-induced bronchospasm if given prior to antigen as an aqueous aerosol. Animal models showed these compounds to be essentially inactive, so further screening was conducted in humans.

Studies continued with this series, looking for greater potency and longer duration. Significant progress was made when two carboxychromone molecules were attached by an alklyenedioxy chain forming a bis-chromone. One of the early compounds in this series, cromolyn, was found to be active by aerosol as a prophylactic and to have a duration of several hours.

The essential chemical features of cromolyn are the planar chromone rings linked by a 2-hydroxy-trimethylenedioxy group at the 5 position(s) with carboxyl groups in the 2 position(s). Cromolyn is soluble in water up to approximately 5%. It is stable in dilute acids but labile in alkali.

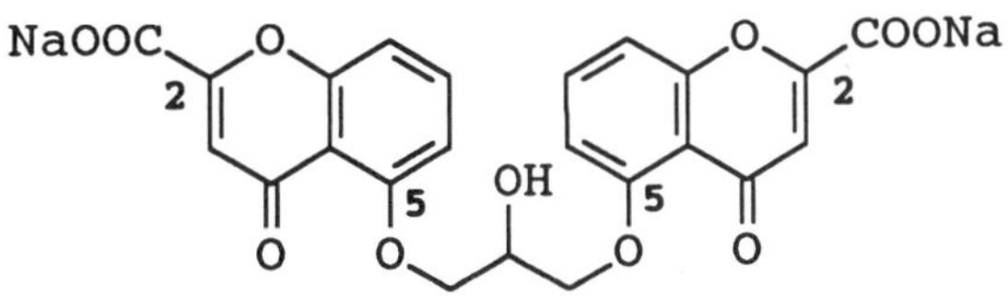

Cromolyn sodium

Although cromolyn is not a bronchodilator, when given prophylactically, it will inhibit the early and later phase of asthma and reduce bronchial hyper-responsiveness. Cromolyn was shown to be effective in antigen-, exercise-, and irritant-induced asthma, and original hypotheses regarding its mechanism of action centered around its purported mast cell stabilizing action. Subsequently it was shown to affect many other inflammatory cells including eosinophils and monocytes. In addition, cromolyn was not a very potent mast cell stabilizer and conversely, other agents that were more potent in this regard possessed considerably less antiasthmatic effects than cromolyn. Subsequent investigations have revealed that cromolyn depresses respiratory neural reflexes, suppresses the response of sensory C fibers and has anti-platelet activating activity.

Cromolyn differs from most medicaments used in obstructive airways disease in that it is useful only as a prophylactic. It inhibits antigen- or exercise-induced bronchospasm if administered prior to exposure but has no bronchodilator properties. Cromolyn lacks oral activity and thus must be administered by inhalation. It is available as a dry powder (Spinhaler), in a metered dose inhaler, or as a solution for use in a nonmetered nebulizer. Cromolyn is also available as a nasal or ophthalmic preparation for use in seasonal rhinitis.

Clinical use of cromolyn in airway disease is restricted to prophylactic use. In asthma, cromolyn is not universally efficacious; however, it is effective in a percentage of patients as measured by a decrease in use of concomitant medications. Patient variability makes it necessary to try cromolyn therapy for at least 4 weeks to determine a therapeutic effect. The consensus that it is particularly effective in children underscores its widespread use as an antiasthmatic in pediatrics. With the exception of local irritant effects in the mouth and airways, and occasionally a powder-induced bronchospasm, adverse reactions to cromolyn are rare.

Cromolyn is best given by aerosol inhalation either as a powder or a solution. When properly administered about 7 to 9 percent is absorbed. The rest is swallowed. Since gastrointestinal absorption is very low (less than 1 percent) most is excreted in the feces.

Nedocromil sodium is a disodium salt of a pyranoquinolone dicarboxylic acid that was developed with the intention of finding a drug possessing an improved pharmacological profile to cromolyn. Although nedocromil is occasionally more potent than cromolyn in affecting asthmogenic activity *in vitro* and *in vivo*, global analysis of current available clinical data reveals they are relatively similar in their effects. Accordingly, nedocromil, like cromolyn, is useful as a prophylactic agent to affect early and late phase aspects of asthma and also reduces hyperreactive bronchomotor function.

TABLE 33-2 Bronchodilators

β-ADRENERGIC RECEPTOR AGONISTS
Selective β_2-receptor agonists
Albuterol
Bitolterol
Isoetharine
Metaproterenol
Pirbuterol
Salmeterol
Terbutaline
Non-selective β-receptor agonists
Ephedrine
Epinephrine
Isoproterenol
XANTHINE DERIVATIVES
Theophylline
Aminophylline
Oxtriphylline
Dyphylline
ANTICHOLINERGIC AGENTS
Ipratropium

BRONCHODILATORS

As shown in Table 33-2, there are three major classes of bronchodilators: β_2-adrenergic receptor agonists, xanthine derivatives, and an anticholinergic drug.

β-Adrenergic Receptor Agonists (Sympathomimetics)

The pharmacology of the β-adrenergic receptor agonists is discussed in Chapter 8. One of their most important uses is in the treatment of obstructive airway disease. These agents relax smooth muscle and inhibit allergic mediator release, presumably by elevation of intracellular cyclic AMP as a result of stimulation of adenylate cyclase activity. Activation of β-adrenergic receptors results in the relaxation of airway smooth muscle, skeletal muscle tremor, and positive inotropic and chronotropic effects in the heart. Non-selective stimulation of β-adrenergic receptors by agents such as epinephrine, ephedrine, and isoproterenol, limit the use of these otherwise effective bronchodilators, owing to cardiac effects. In general, these agents are used in the therapy of acute and severe asthmatic conditions, in combination with other medications for chronic therapy, or as diagnostic agents.

Among the more commonly used agents with longer-lasting, more selective activity on β_2-adrenergic receptors are: albuterol, terbutaline, and pirbuterol (Table 33-2). Most recently, the structures of terbutaline and albuterol have been modified to include a long lipophilic side chain that prolongs the half-life of these β-adrenergic agents. Salmeterol (the long-acting albuterol derivative) has recently become available. At this writing, formoterol (the terbutaline derivative) was not yet marketed in the United States.

With the exception of ephedrine, all of these drugs are available for topical use; albuterol, metaproterenol, terbutaline, and ephedrine may be administered orally, epinephrine can be used by subcutaneous injection, and terbutaline and isoproterenol may be given by the intravenous route.

When given by inhalation, the sympathomimetic drugs listed in Table 33-2 generally act within several minutes. The shorter-acting agents (epinephrine, isoproterenol, and isoetharine) have a duration of action of 1 to 3 h, the others have a duration of 3 to 8 h, and salmeterol and formoterol may have effects for up to 12 to 24 h.

By relaxing bronchial smooth muscle, these drugs are effective in reversing bronchospasm secondary to all stimuli. In addition, this class of bronchodilators has significant antiallergic effects (secondary to stabilization of mast cells) and may also inhibit vagal tone and thus may affect early and late phases of various forms of asthma as well as being useful in improving airway function in other forms of chronic obstructive airway disease. These agents also have a rational use in concurrent therapy and common approaches include administration in combination with theophylline, a corticosteroid, and an anticholinergic agent. The longer-acting agents appear to be effective in nocturnal asthma and may be more effective than the shorter-acting β-adrenergic agonists in preventing late phase aspects of asthma.

As discussed previously, the major side effects associated with β-adrenergic stimulants are cardiac and central nervous system (CNS) effects. Cardiac effects consist of positive inotropic and chronotropic effects, which are easily noticeable to the patient. They also tend to cause cardiac arrhythmias. CNS effects can generally be classified as stimulatory. Although these effects are somewhat minimized with the selective β_2-adrenergic receptor agonists, skeletal muscle tremor is a relatively common, dose-related side effect with these drugs. These compounds also produce a reduction in arterial P_{O2}, perhaps secondary to pulmonary vasodilation and an exacerbation of ventilation perfusion mismatching. β-Receptor agonists may also produce hypokalemia directly via stimulation of Na^+,K^+-ATPase or indirectly via pancreatic β-adrenergic receptor stimulation resulting in insulin secretion.

Epidemiological studies have reported a casual association between the use of β-adrenergic agonists and increases in asthma morbidity and mortality. The potential danger of overuse of pressurized adrenergic aerosols was clearly identified in the late 1960s and led to a keen awareness that therapy with these drugs (for presumptive rescue or breakthrough self-administration) was at least an important marker for severity of chronic obstructive airway disease. In light of the pathophysiological and epidemiologically data, these agents are now viewed in a considerably less cavalier light.

Serious questions still remain regarding issues of tachyphylaxis with β-adrenergic agonists. It is not clear whether actual tolerance develops, i.e., a decrease in β-adrenoceptor responsiveness, or whether the apparent observation of tolerance is due to a worsening of the clinical condition. Chronic therapy has also been associated with bronchial hyperactivity. Both concerns about alterations in airway function during chronic use of these drugs have raised important issues regarding concurrent therapy with inhaled corticosteroids as a rational approach to circumvent these important adverse effects.

Xanthine Derivatives

The three best known naturally occurring methylxanthines are theophylline, theobromine, and caffeine. Major sources of these compounds are tea, cocoa, and coffee, respectively. For example, an average cup of coffee contains approximately 60 to 100 mg of caffeine. Caffeine was first noted over 200 years ago to be an effective remedy for asthma by William Withering and theophylline eventually emerged as the first-line therapy for reversible obstructive airway disease only recently. As contemporary approaches have focused on ant-inflammatory agents (see above) and aerosolized β-adrenergic agonists for rapid bronchodilation, the use of theophylline, which lacks the potent anti-inflammatory effects of steroids and the rapid bronchodilator action of β-adrenergic agonists, has been questioned. Concerns regarding safety of theophylline and its potential for adverse behavioral and cognitive effects in children along with considerable uncertainty regarding its mechanism of action have contributed to the clinical debate regarding the utility of this group of drugs.

The xanthines belong to a family of compounds which contains the purine ring system, one of the most important heterocyclics found in nature. Theophylline is 1,3-dimethylxanthine, and its structure, along with other analogs, is shown in Table 33-3. The three major natural xanthine derivatives, as well as the synthetic drugs (oxtriphylline, dyphylline, and enprofylline) all exert

TABLE 33-3 Commonly used xanthines: structures and pharmacologic comparisons

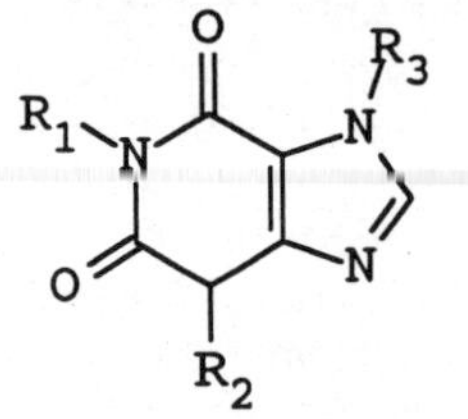

Compound	Chemical groups			Comparison of pharmacologic effects				
	R_1	R_2	R_3	CNS stim.	Broncho-dilation	Diuresis	Cardiac stim.	Skeletal muscle stim.
Caffeine	Methyl	Methyl	Methyl	+ + +	+	+	+	+ + +
Theobromine	H	Methyl	H	+	+	+ +	+ +	+
Theophylline	H	Methyl	Methyl	+ +	+ + +	+ + +	+ + +	+ +
Enprofylline	H	Propyl	H	+	+ + + +	+	+ + + +	—

Increase = + to + + + +

similar biological effects, but differ in their potencies. Theophylline serves as the prototype.

Mechanism of Action The mechanism of action of theophylline as a bronchodilator is unknown. Several theories, however, have been suggested based on the close structural similarity of theophylline with adenosine and cyclic AMP. Theophylline inhibits a cyclic AMP phosphodiesterase, which leads to an increase in cystosolic cyclic AMP and a subsequent relaxation of airway (and other) smooth muscle. Theophylline, however, is not a potent phosphodiesterase inhibitor, and the necessary concentrations may be unobtainable *in vivo*. Theophylline also inhibits reuptake of catecholamines and this can result in an elevation in cyclic AMP with subsequent bronchodilation. An alternative possibility is that theophylline affects cyclic GMP phosphodiesterase. Theophylline has been shown to be a competitive antagonist at adenosine receptors, and this action may be responsible for its bronchodilating properties since it occurs at concentrations within the therapeutic range.

Adenosine is an endogenous mediator which interacts with membrane receptors found in many cells (e.g., A_1 and A_2). Adenosine appears to function both at synapses in the CNS and in the periphery, and has been implicated to be involved in a number of local regulatory mechanisms including maintenance of regional oxygen balance and responses of neurotransmitters at neuroeffector junctions. Adenosine may cause or participate in bronchoconstriction. Theophylline is known to antagonize the binding of adenosine to A_1 and A_2 receptors and thus prevents the bronchospasm produced. Although this mechanism may be important for the action of theophylline, newer xanthine derivatives (e.g., enprofylline) have demonstrated as good or better bronchodilating properties than theophylline while essentially being devoid of adenosine receptor-binding properties.

Effects on Organ Systems Theophylline and the other xanthine derivatives exert pharmacologic effects on a variety of organ systems (Table 33-3). One of their most pronounced effects is the relaxation of respiratory smooth muscle. Additionally, theophylline is a CNS stimulant, relaxes peripheral vascular smooth muscle, increases diuresis, has cardiotonic activity, and stimulates gastric acid secretion. The effects of theophylline on the CNS, cardiovascular, and gastrointestinal systems are the most commonly observed adverse effects of the use of theophylline or congeners as bronchodilators.

The stimulatory effects of theophylline on the CNS is directly related to the dose of compound administered and can include restlessness, anxiety, tremors, and even convulsions at sufficiently high doses. Theophylline also stimulates the medullary respiratory centers, an effect sometimes used therapeutically in cases of respiratory apnea. The nausea and vomiting associated with the use of theophylline are also thought to be centrally-mediated and dose-dependent. Nausea is a particularly common side effect seen with the initial use of the drug. A great deal of concern has been raised by parents regarding theophylline-induced changes in their childrens' mood, behavior, and ability to learn. Clinical laboratory and epidemiological data suggest that this concern over cognitive and behavioral side effects of theophylline is exaggerated.

On the cardiovascular system, the xanthine derivatives exert direct positive inotropic and chronotropic effects on the heart. In the periphery, these drugs cause a decrease in peripheral vascular resistance, except in the cerebral vasculature where theophylline causes vasoconstriction. The inotropic effects of the xanthine derivatives are thought to be mediated via increased calcium influx modulated by cyclic AMP and the effect of the xanthine derivatives on cardiac specific phosphodiesterases.

In the gastrointestinal tract, these drugs stimulate secretion of both gastric acid and digestive enzymes. On the kidney, the xanthine derivatives have diuretic activity, albeit weak. Diuresis may be due to an increased glomerular filtration rate as well as a decreased tubular absorption of sodium. The bronchodilating properties of theophylline are due to direct effects on respiratory smooth muscle. Theophylline also affects skeletal muscle to improve contractile responses. This effect may provide therapeutic effects in cases of diaphragm fatigue.

Pharmacokinetics Theophylline is generally administered orally in sustained-release or controlled-release preparations. Aminophylline (the theophylline-ethylenediamine complex) is available for oral, intravenous, or suppository use. A wide variety of preparations of theophylline are available, and the pharmacokinetics are dependent on which preparation is used.

Generally, theophylline is rapidly and completely absorbed from the gastrointestinal tract. Xanthine derivatives are distributed throughout the body and are able to cross the placenta. Binding to plasma proteins is only about 50 to 60 percent. Metabolism occurs primarily in the liver by oxidation and demethylation with up to 15 percent excreted unchanged in the urine. The half-life of theophylline averages about 3.5 h in children and 8 to 9 h in adults. In smokers, the half-life of theophylline is decreased to approximately half that of nonsmokers. The effectiveness of theophylline as a bronchodilator is usually achieved with attained blood levels of 10 to 20 μg/mL. Nausea, vomiting, and restlessness may be associated with these levels. Blood levels higher than 20 μg/mL may be associated with greater toxicity. Toxic effects associated with elevated serum levels are ventricular arrhythmias, convulsions, and possible death, which may occur without previous warning. It is for this reason (low therapeutic index) that blood levels should be monitored individually to establish a safe and effective dose of theophylline.

Drug Interactions Theophylline interacts with a variety of other therapeutic agents. Most notable are the agents which increase the effects of theophylline, since these agents may lead to severe theophylline toxicity when administered concurrently. Cimetidine (an H_2 receptor antagonist), erythromycin, ciprofloxacin, and troleandomycin (antibiotics), propranolol (a β-adrenergic receptor blocker), and some oral contraceptives may increase theophylline blood levels into the toxic range. It is important to monitor theophylline levels frequently whenever one of these other medications is required. Other interactions with theophylline may occur with lithium, phenytoin, and rifampin leading to decreased effectiveness of one or both drugs. Additionally, concurrent administration of halothane to persons receiving theophylline may result in cardiac dysrhythmias. With such a potential for drug interactions, it is important for the physician to be aware of any other medications being taken by the patient receiving theophylline.

Therapeutic Uses The xanthine derivatives are indicated for use as bronchodilators in cases of acute or chronic obstructive pulmonary disease (COPD). These drugs have been clearly shown to improve spirometry and symptoms (dyspnea) in a wide group of patients with obstructive pulmonary disease. In addition, clinical observation suggest that theophylline may improve mucociliary clearance and increase diaphragmatic strength and delay the onset of fatigue in respiratory muscle in these patients. Additional benefits may also be obtained regarding enhanced central respiratory drive and improved cardiovascular function in patients with COPD. Theophylline also reduces nocturnal asthma and airway hyperresponsiveness suggesting that it may have anti-inflammatory contributions. In light of these and other observations, theophylline continues to be an important part of the chronic management of asthma and may be useful in other forms of obstructive lung disease.

Theophylline is only marginally soluble in water, and thus a few different salts have been prepared. For example, aminophylline (the ethylenediamine salt of theophylline) is very water-soluble and used for intravenous administration by infusion. Oxtriphylline, dyphylline, and enprofylline are all theophylline derivatives. Oxtriphylline is used orally and dyphylline is used by the oral and the intramuscular routes. Enprofylline is not available for use in the United States. All of these theophylline derivatives are less potent (on a mg basis) than theophylline itself. Regardless of which preparation is used or the route of administration, it is important to emphasize that monitoring blood levels of theophylline is required during the initial few days of therapy, during changes in dosage, and every 6 to 12 months during maintenance to prevent toxicity.

Anticholinergics

Anticholinergics (covered in detail in Chapter 11) have been used for centuries in the treatment of obstructive lung disease. Cholinergic blocking drugs affect a variety of tissues and systems and thus have the potential for a wide array of side effects. By inhibiting the action of acetylcholine on respiratory smooth muscle, anticholinergics prevent bronchospasm resulting from vagus nerve discharge. Two important reflexes, spinal and axonal, appear to contribute to airway caliber. Stimuli (irritants, particles, cold air, histamine) may initiate spinal reflexes from upper and lower airways, esophagus, and carotid bodies. Rapidly adapting irritant receptors and unmyelinated C fibers (found in airway epithelium) are the origin of impulses that travel in afferent vagal nerves to the CNS and cause bronchoconstriction via efferent vagal nerves to airway smooth muscle. A second reflex bronchoconstrictor mechanism, axonal reflex, involves local release of substance P, calcitonin gene-related peptide, and other neurokinins by an antidromic mechanism. Among the muscarinic (M) receptor subtypes identified in human airways, inhibition of M_1 and M_3 receptors (peribronchial ganglia and smooth muscle, respectively) results in an inhibitory effect. Inhibition of M_2 receptors may augment cholinergic activity, since it appears to be an autoreceptor. Future efforts are aimed at identifying selective muscarinic receptor antagonists.

Clinically, these agents have been shown to produce bronchodilation in some cases and also to normalize a hyperreactive airway. In many cases of obstructive lung disease, the airways become hyperreactive, i.e., they constrict to an irritant that has no effect on a non-asthmatic patient. This response is apparently due to the airway hyperreactivity or a lower threshold to the stimulus by asthmatics, compared to non-asthmatics. Anticholinergics appear to be especially useful against bronchospastic stimuli including various mediators (histamine, eicosanoids, 5-hydroxytryptamine, bradykinin), psychogenic factors, gases, dusts, irritants, exercise, and exposure to cold air. The drugs are variable in their protection against antigen-induced bronchospasm. Patients with COPD (in addition to asthmatics) have clearly been shown to receive as much benefit with regard to bronchodilation from anticholinergic drugs as they do from β-adrenergic agonists and ipratropium has been suggested as the most efficacious bronchodilator in the long-term management of stable COPD.

Clinically, these agents are generally used by inhalation for the treatment of airway disease. Atropine has been shown to be an effective bronchodilator by aerosol, and its effect can persist for over 4 h. Local side effects by aerosolized atropine can include drying of the mouth and the resultant discomfort. Systemic adverse reactions may include urinary retention, tachycardia, and agitation. Thus the use of aerosolized atropine was abandoned. Systemic side effects of anticholinergic therapy can be minimized by the use of the quaternary ammonium derivative, ipratropium bromide.

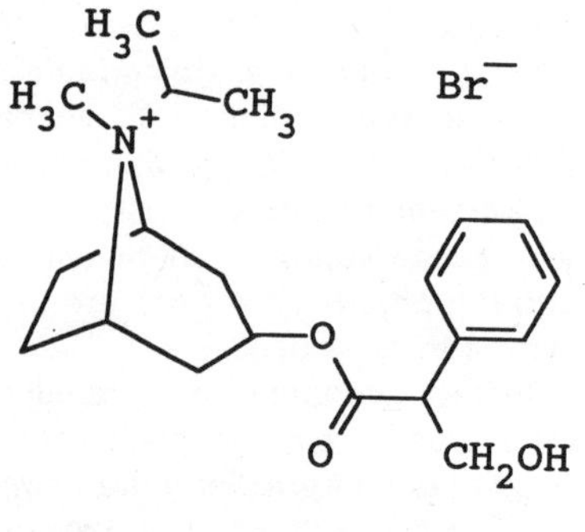

Ipratropium bromide

This compound is poorly absorbed into the systemic circulation and does not cross the blood-brain barrier easily, thus allowing high dose administration to the lung via aerosol. Ipratropium is an effective bronchodilator in some patients, having a duration of action of 3 to 4 h. It can be a valuable agent for use in those individuals who cannot tolerate the β-adrenergic receptor agonists. Adverse effects of ipratropium are largely limited to a brief cough, dry mouth, nausea, and occasionally a paradoxical bronchoconstriction. Approved uses for ipratropium include therapy for emphysema and chronic bronchitis, although work continues for its use in the chronic management of asthma.

MUCOKINETIC AGENTS

Defects in mucociliary clearance are generally considered to be important aspects of the pathogenesis of COPD and, in the case of cystic fibrosis, such dysfunction is paramount to the clinical manifestations of the genetic defect. Although numerous agents have been used to improve mucociliary clearance and sputum elimination, the physiology of this complicated airway function is poorly understood and, just as importantly, is not routinely quantified. Accordingly, a large number of commonly agents are routinely used with little evaluation. These include agents that may stimulate mucus production (bronchomucotropics), increase osmotic transduction of fluid in the airways (bronchorrheics), break down sputum molecules to smaller components (mucolytics), stimulate gastropulmonary vagal reflexes (emetic expectorants), and normalize mucus production (mucoregulators).

Hydration and humidification therapies are generally considered as important elements of the management of the patient with chronic obstructive lung disease although specific directives are often obtuse. Folk remedies have included the use of inhalation aromatic vapor therapies and such flavorful hydration remedies as hot tea, honey, or chicken soup, receive universal clinical support. A brief review of currently available agents that may be useful as mucokinetics is shown in Table 33-4.

Volatile oleoresins including camphenes, pinenes, phenols, and terpenes comprise a group of bronchomucotropics (e.g., terpin hydrate, eucalyptus, menthol, camphor) that have achieved a large following for increasing mucus content and the volume of respiratory tract fluid with little physiological data to support these contentions. These compounds are included in a large number of over-the-counter remedies that are used for a variety of minor respiratory disorders.

Iodide (e.g., saturated solution of potassium iodide, and iodinated glycerol) may work by directly stimulating bronchial glands, but probably shares its bronchomucotropic effect with its expectorant effect (see below) secondary to reflex actions.

Osmotic enhancement of mucus secretion (bronchorrhea) is probably the result of mucosal irritation that can be readily achieved by inhalation of sodium bicarbonate, hypertonic saline, or acetylcysteine. Bronchorrhea presumably accompanies bronchomucotropic and mucolytic effects of various agents and is impossible to currently separate.

Agents that act as mucolytics may break down the fibrillar molecules of mucoproteins into less viscous subunits by breaking down disulfide bridges of the glycoproteins of mucus (e.g., acetylcysteine) or enzymatically digesting compounds of mucus that lead to undesirable enhanced viscosity (recombinant human DNase).

Expectorants comprise an unusually large number of remedies whose effects are to enhance the volume of sputum that can be coughed out more easily. Guaifenesin (glyceryl guaiacolate) is probably the most popular of the expectorants (found in many over-the-counter products) and was originally conceived to have direct effects on bronchial glands. It is becoming clearer that the most common property of expectorants is their emetic potential. Potential for gastropulmonary mucokinetic vagal reflexes suggests that agents that stimulate gastric receptors evoke a reflex via the vagus nerve to lung as well as foregut.

Mucoregulators may directly affect the bronchial gland so as to produce a less viscous output. An interesting agent with this property is S-carboxymethylcysteine. This agent is different than acetylcysteine since it lacks a free thiol and has been shown to be void of mucolytic or expectorant functions. Rather it seems to impair the incorporation of sialic acid residues into the glycoproteins that normally contribute to a highly viscous mucus secretion. Interestingly when garlic is crushed, its major nonodoriferous compound, allicin, is enzymatically converted to diallyl thiosulfinate (diallylallicin) which comprises garlic's unique odor. Allicin may also be converted to S-allyl-cysteine (desoxyallicin) in mammals and this latter compound is remarkably similar to S-carboxymethylcysteine, lending further credence to traditional remedies with garlic.

TABLE 33-4 Actions of major mucokinetic agents

Agent	Mucolytic	Bronchorrheic	Broncho-mucotropic	Emetic expectorants	Mucoregulator
Acetylcysteine	+ + +	+ + +	±	+ +	?
Bromhexine	+	–	–	–	+
Guaifenesin	+	–	–	+ +	+ + +
Iodide	+ +	+	+ + +	+ +	+ +
Saline					
Normal	±	–	–	±	–
Hypertonic	+	+ + +	±	+ + +	–
S-Carboxymethyl-cysteine	–	–	?	–	+ + +
Sodium bicarbonate	+ +	+ +	±	+ +	–

+ + + = marked effect; + + = moderate effect; + = some effect; ± = equivocal effect; – = no effect; ? = not established. [Modified from: Weiss, E.B. and M. Stein, *Bronchial Asthma, Mechanisms and Therapeutics, Third Edition*, Little, Brown & Company, Boston, MA, 1993.]

POTENTIAL THERAPEUTIC CATEGORIES

Antagonists of Mediator Receptor Sites

Leukotrienes (LTs) are a family of compounds which are potent chemotactic factors (primarily LTB_4) and potent bronchospastic agents (LTC_4, LTD_4, and LTE_4). These agents act via membrane receptors on cells of smooth muscle. Therefore, the potential to inhibit their action by specific receptor blockade offers a possible therapeutic approach to inhibiting the bronchospasm and the cellular infiltration associated with their action. Several pharmaceutical companies are currently evaluating specific LTD_4 receptor antagonists for their effects in asthma or acute bronchospasm (Table 33-5). To date, they have proven to be antagonists of leukotriene-induced bronchospasm and have demonstrated mild effects in the bronchospasm associated with some forms of asthma.

Similar to the studies with leukotrienes, various pharmaceutical companies are currently evaluating platelet-activating factor (PAF) antagonists. Many of these compounds are semisynthetic analogs of ginkolides, complex organic molecules of the ginkgo tree. Clinical trials have shown these agents to be effective against exogenous PAF, but to have only modest antiasthmatic activity.

As newer, longer-lasting anti-histamines with higher degrees of specificity and reduced adverse effects are developed, renewed interested in their application for asthma has occurred. In particular, H_1 receptor antagonists such as terfenadine and astemizole block antigen- and histamine-induced bronchospasm. These agents may also affect mast cell release, thereby widening the number of agents with such dual action.

Inhibitors of Allergic Mediator Synthesis

Another approach to prevent the effect of inflammatory mediators is to inhibit their synthesis. A major focus has been the development of orally active 5-lipoxygenase inhibitors. Two first generation agents with this property, piriprost and nafazatrom, did not alter the asthmatic response to inhaled antigen or exercise. Other more effective inhibitors are being currently pursued. Dietary manipulation of eicosanoid levels may also be accomplished by the use of n-3 fatty acids.

TABLE 33-5 Potential therapeutic strategies for chronic obstructive airway disease

Class	Examples	Pharmacologic action
Antagonists of Mediator Receptor Sites	ICI-204,219	LTD_4 receptor antagonist
	WEB-2086	PAF receptor antagonist
	Astemizole, terfenadine	H_1 receptor blockers
Inhibitors of Allergic Mediator Release	Piriprost, nafazatrom	5-Lipoxygenase inhibitors
	Marine fish oils	n-3 fatty acids alter the eicosanoid profile
Potent Anti-inflammatory Agents	Methotrexate, cyclosporine, hydroxychloroquine, gold	Anti-inflammatory activity
Modulators of Ionic Conductance	Nifedipine	Calcium channel blocker
	Lemakalim, cromakalim	Potassium-ATP channel opener
Nitric Oxide	S-nitroso-adenosylar-penicillamine	Nitric oxide donor
	N-monomethyl-L-arsinine	Nitric oxide synthase inhibitor

Marine fish oils rich in eicosapentaenoic acid (EPA) have been shown to reduce levels of leukotrienes and PAF in numerous clinical trials. Although such alternative fatty acid therapy has proven to be beneficial in rheumatoid arthritis and eczema (as well as various chronic cardiovascular disorders), little benefit has been noted in asthmatic patients. Inhibition of cyclooxygenase does not appear to be useful, and a significant subgroup of asthmatic patients have exacerbation of bronchospasm upon exposure to nonsteroidal anti-inflammatory agents.

Potent Anti-Inflammatory Agents

As inflammation becomes increasingly more apparent as a useful target in bronchial asthma, consideration has turned to the use of more potent anti-inflammatory agents than the glucocorticoids discussed above. Agents proven useful in rheumatology and dermatology are currently being investigated for their potential in asthma. Included among these agents is methotrexate and the antirheumatic agents, gold and hydroxychloroquine phosphate. Other agents under consideration for corticosteroid-dependent asthmatics include cyclosporine and colchicine.

Modulators of Ionic Conductances

Critical roles for calcium and potassium homeostasis in smooth muscle contractility is now apparent. Accordingly, agents that modify intracellular calcium or potassium may have applications for bronchial hyperactivity. One approach to block the effect of inflammatory/bronchoconstriction-inducing mediators is to affect ionic calcium flux through voltage-gated calcium channels. Clinical studies on the large group of available calcium channel blockers indicate they are modestly effective against exogenously-induced bronchospasm, but have marginal therapeutic value in antigen- or exercise-induced asthma. In light of this minimal pulmonary effect and the significant cardiovascular liabilities associated with these agents, calcium channel blockers are not exclusively used for respiratory dysfunction in COPD. Nonetheless, the possibility of bronchial specific calcium channel blockers may provide a means of utilizing these agents in bronchial asthma. Drugs that open ATP-dependent potassium channels (lemakalim, cromakalim) will hyperpolarize smooth muscle and physiologically antagonize mediators of bronchoconstriction. Limited clinical data suggest that these agents may be useful against nocturnal asthma and provide an alternative pharmacological approach to the management of asthma. Other potassium channels, including the calcium-sensitive potassium channel, are also presumptive targets and *in vitro* data have shown that charybdotoxin, an inhibitor of such a channel, may be useful in affecting bronchoconstrictor activity of human airway smooth muscle.

Nitric Oxide

Nitric oxide (NO) is a critical signal-transducing and effector molecule discussed in detail elsewhere (see Chapter 29). NO is a bronchodilator and is the neurotransmitter of the non-adrenergic, non-cholinergic innervation of lung. In addition, the potential for generating large amounts of NO via an inducible form of NO synthase is apparently resident within human lung involved in chronic inflammation. These higher concentrations of NO may be cytotoxic and also affect inflammatory cell migration and function. Although there are no clinical data regarding the role of NO in COPD, available NO donors and inhibitors of NO biosynthesis may ultimately be critical components of pharmacotherapy of airway disease.

Gene Therapy

Gene therapy involves the delivery and expression of exogenous DNA to replace and/or restore dysfunctional genes and their products. The two most common inherited lethal disorders of North American caucasians, i.e., α_1-antitrypsin deficiency and cystic fibrosis, have their major manifestations in lung and considerable effort has been devoted towards gene therapy for these disorders. Animal experiments strongly support the possibility that the genes for α_1-antitrypsin and cystic fibrosis (cystic fibrosis transmembrane conductance regulator) can be directly transferred to lung. Current clinical trials using an adenovirus vector or liposomes for DNA delivery are assessing the possibility of such somatic gene transfer in human volunteers. Although genetic targets for such therapy have not been realized in bronchial asthma, topical administration of recombinant DNA for subset of patients with emphysema or cystic fibrosis appears likely in the near future.

MANAGEMENT STRATEGIES FOR SPECIFIC DISORDERS

Asthma

A consensus of expert opinion has been developed by the International Asthma Expert Panel sponsored by the National Institutes of Health. This has substantially changed therapeutic approaches for asthma and COPD. In general, the panel recommends the use of inhaled β-adrenergic agonists as first-line therapy, followed by anti-inflammatory agents. The use of theophylline and other xanthine derivatives is greatly curtailed.

As shown in Table 33-6, asthma can be categorized on the basis of clinical symptoms as mild, moderate, or severe. The first assessment the physician must make in obtaining a history from a new asthmatic patient is the degree to which asthma is interfering with his/her life. Symptoms by which categorization can be made are also shown in Table 33-6.

The management of asthma follows in a stepwise progression based on the strategy outlined in Table 33-7. For asthma which is infrequent in occurrence and mild in intensity, intermittent, as needed (prn) β-adrenergic agonists delivered by a hand-held metered-dose inhaler is often all that is required. However, epidemiologic surveys suggest that asthma is mild only in about

TABLE 33-6 Classification of asthma based on the severity of symptoms

Severity	Frequency of symptoms	Nocturnal symptoms	Exercise tolerance	Interval of symptoms	Emergency room visits
Mild	1 to 2/week	0 to 2/month	Good	None	None
Moderate	Over 2/week	2 to 3/week	Reduced	Some cough, low-grade wheeze: 1 to 3/year	1 to 3/year
Severe	Continuous	Nightly	Very poor	Continuous cough and wheeze	Monthly

TABLE 33-7 Treatment strategies in asthma

Severity	Suggested therapy
Mild	β-Adrenergic agonists as needed
Moderate	β-Adrenergic agonists as needed, plus Anti-inflammatory therapy A. Cromolyn sodium or nedocromil sodium B. Inhaled corticosteroids
Severe	Same as for Moderate, plus A. High-dose inhaled corticosteroids, or B. Systemic corticosteroids

one patient in four. The other three quarters of asthma patients will require more intensive therapy than simply prn β-adrenergic agonists.

Although theophylline has long been the mainstay of bronchodilator therapy in asthma, it is now relegated to second-line therapy. The newer β-adrenergic agonists, administered by metered-dose inhalation, have proven to be superior bronchodilators as compared to theophylline. In addition, theophylline therapy is accompanied by numerous side effects such as nausea; headache; insomnia; tremor; and, on occasion, cardiac arrhythmias and seizures. Theophylline blood levels have to be monitored and there are numerous drug interactions which have to be considered.

In spite of these difficulties, theophylline is very useful when β-adrenergic agonists cannot be tolerated. In selected cases theophylline can be useful in nocturnal asthma. Compliance is usually better with theophylline since the technique of dosing is not a problem and only a few oral doses daily are needed.

The second step in asthma management is the addition of an anti-inflammatory agent. The selection of a particular drug should be left to the clinical judgement and experience of the individual clinician. No infallible guidelines are available to predict which patients will respond well to either cromolyn sodium or nedocromil sodium. A therapeutic trial of 3 to 6 weeks of either, or perhaps both (sequentially) drugs is not unreasonable if the intensity of asthma symptoms and the disturbance of normal activities is not great. For those patients who do not respond to cromolyn sodium or to nedocromil sodium, or whose symptoms are, in the judgement of the clinician, so significant as to preclude a therapeutic trial which may not be helpful, then the administration of inhaled corticosteroids is warranted. Currently, beclomethasone diproprionate, triamcinolone acetonide, and flunisolide are all available by metered-dose inhaler and can be delivered, in most cases, on a twice daily basis. These agents differ considerably in terms of the amount of drug delivered per puff and also in the intrinsic potency of specific steroids. Thus, there is a broad range of anti-inflammatory effect, depending on the compound and dose. However, selecting one of these agents over another must be done based on the clinician's experience and judgement, as comparative clinical trials have not been extensively performed.

Asthma which is severe in degree is a potentially life-threatening condition. These patients should be treated with a short burst and tapering off of oral corticosteroids, and may require either high-dose inhaled corticosteroids or long-term (preferably alternate day) systemic corticosteroids for maintenance.

Chronic Bronchitis and Emphysema

Of the chronic obstructive pulmonary diseases, chronic bronchitis most commonly results from tobacco smoking; a small subset of these patients have the disease due to exposure to a variety of materials in the workplace. Thus, the primary management strategy should be to discontinue exposure to those factors which cause further injury.

Pharmacologically, there are no strategies which reverse the underlying abnormalities. Thus, physicians are left with ameliorating symptoms and preventing further degradation in pulmonary function. Chronic bronchitis and emphysema can visually be differentiated at least in part, on the basis of history and routine clinical tests. Frequent sputum production suggests a component of chronic bronchitis, where as hyperlucency on the chest radiograph, and a diminished diffusing capacity of carbon monoxide when adjusted for alveolar volume, are consistent with a component of emphysema. Regardless of the predominant type of chronic obstructive lung disease, the management of these disorders involves administration of bronchodilator drugs.

Inhaled β-adrenergic agonist bronchodilators, delivered by metered-dose inhaler, remain the most common form of therapy for these disorders. However, in some patients in whom breath holding or coordination of metered-dose inhaler actuation are problems, β-adrenergic agonists can be delivered by a compressor-driven nebulizer. Most authorities avoid delivery of these agents by intermittent positive pressure breathing (IPPB). Some, but not all, obstructive lung disease patients may benefit from the addition of theophylline. The beneficial effect of theophylline in these patients may be rather modest, and the drug should probably not be used if there is a significant contraindication. In addition, many authorities recommend maintaining a therapeutic blood level range of 8 to 12 μg/mL as opposed to the more commonly used range of 10 to 20 μg/mL.

There is less agreement about the use of corticosteroids in COPD. When there is the presence of variable airflow obstruction (episodic wheezing or marked spirometric variation), a therapeutic trial of prednisone, at a dose of about 0.5 mg/kg daily for 2 to 4 weeks, may be considered.

An important diagnostic consideration is distinguishing usual protease excess emphysema (tobacco smoke-induced) from antiprotease deficient emphysema. In the setting of emphysema, it is useful to obtain an α_1-antitrypsin level which will distinguish the common deficient state (the ZZ-phenotype).

In contrast to asthma in which anticholinergic agents have not found a significant role, ipratropium bromide has been shown to produce significant bronchodilation in some patients. The longer duration of action of ipratropium (up to 6 hours) offers additional advantage in the ongoing management of bronchoconstriction of these patients.

BIBLIOGRAPHY

-------- "Inhaled Beta-adrenergic Agonists in Asthma," Position paper of the American Academy of Allergy and Immunology. *J. Allerg. Clin. Immunol.* **91**: 1234-1237 (1993).

-------- "International Consensus Report on Diagnosis and Treatment of Asthma," National Heart, Lung and Blood Institute (Publication No. 92-3091), *Eur. Respir. J.* **5**: 601-641 (1992).

Brogden, R.N., and E.M. Sorkin: "Nedocromil Sodium: An Updated Review of its Pharmacological Properties and Therapeutic Efficacy in Asthma," *Drugs* **45**: 693-715 (1993).

Cott, G.R., and R.M. Cherniack: "Steroids and 'Steroid-Sparing' Agents in Asthma," *N. Engl. J. Med.* **318**: 634-636 (1988).

Gianaris, P.G., and J.A. Golish: "Changing Strategies in the Management of Asthma," *Postgrad. Med.* **95**: 105-110 (1994).

Milgrom, H., and B. Bender: "Current Issues in the Use of Theophylline," *Am. Rev. Resp. Dis.* **147**: S33-S39 (1993).

Weiss, E.B., and M. Stein: *Bronchial Asthma, Mechanisms and Therapeutics, Third Edition*, Little, Brown & Company, Boston, 1993.

Ziment, I.: "Pharmacologic Therapy of Obstructive Openings Disease," *Clin. Chest Med.* **11**: 461-486 (1990).

PART VI

The Hematopoietic System

SECTION EDITOR

Andrew P. Ferko

CHAPTER 34

Antianemia Agents

David L. Topolsky and Sigmund B. Kahn

Anemia is a clinical sign (not a disease per se) indicating a reduction in the red blood cell mass. *Anemia* is defined by a lowered hemoglobin concentration, a reduced red blood cell count, or a reduction in the hematocrit (packed cell volume, PCV). Functionally, anemia may result in tissue hypoxia because of hemoglobin's key role in oxygen transport. Patients with anemia may complain of a variety of nonspecific symptoms, including fatigue, dyspnea, lightheadedness, pallor, or palpitations. The clinical complaints of the patient often do not define the etiology of the anemia. In other words, the cause of anemia is rarely ascertained merely by eliciting signs and symptoms from the patient; however, the ultimate task of the clinician is to define the cause of the anemia before therapy is ordered.

The causes of anemia are quite varied, but several different classification systems are clinically useful. Anemia may be classified pathophysiologically in the following manner: (1) deficiency of building blocks or growth factors needed for normal red blood cell development, (2) deficiency of, or defect in, stem cell proliferation, and (3) excessive loss of red blood cells. The most commonly used and useful first step in defining the etiology of the anemia involves classifying the anemia morphologically. In this schema, the clinician uses the mean corpuscular volume (MCV) and the mean corpuscular hemoglobin concentration (MCHC) to divide the anemias into four categories (Table 34-1). The morphological classification allows the clinician to approach the pathophysiology of the anemia, the next step to determining etiology. These two classifications complement each other since morphology often predicts pathophysiology.

The final necessary step before ordering therapy is determining the etiology of the anemia. Classification schema are complementary to each other. Since many different etiologies can produce anemia via similar pathophysiologic mechanisms, i.e., impaired globin synthesis (thalassemia) and iron deficiency, both cause anemia by interfering with the building blocks of hemoglobin. The classification of anemia by etiology alone might not lead to establishment of the diagnosis rapidly. In practice, therefore, it is best to classify the anemia morphologically, then define its pathophysiology, and finally, it is essential to understand and to determine the etiology before any treatment is suggested.

MICROCYTIC ANEMIA: IRON DEFICIENCY

Iron in the Body

Of the elements found in the body, iron is one of the most multifunctional and essential. Iron is found in hemoglobin, myoglobin, storage compounds (ferritin, hemosiderin), transferrin, and enzymes such as the cytochromes (Fig. 34-1).

Hemoglobin Hemoglobin contains the major portion of body iron. It is a protein that has a molecular mass of 64,658 Da and has approximately 0.35 percent iron by weight. Divalent iron is bound in stable covalent linkage within the porphyrin ring of heme, with additional coordination positions attached to the globin peptide chains. Molecular oxygen is bound reversibly by the iron (ferrous) of hemoglobin. Oxidation of the iron to the ferric state (as in methemoglobin) causes hemoglobin to lose its capacity to carry oxygen. A single molecule of hemoglobin consists of four atoms of iron each inserted into a molecule of protoporphyrin to yield heme. Each of these

TABLE 34-1 Morphologically classified anemias

Class	Number of red blood cells	Size of red blood cells	Amount of Hb/RBC[a]	Usual pathophysiologic mechanism	Some causes
Macrocytic	Decrease	Increase	Slight increase	Megaloblastosis vs. reticulocytosis	Vitamin B_{12} or folate deficiency; hemolytic anemia
Normocytic	Decrease	No change	No change	Marrow failure (usually)	Aplastic anemia; anemia of chronic disease
Simple microcytic	Decrease	Slight decrease	Slight decrease	Marrow failure	Chronic inflammation
Hypochromic microcytic	Slight decrease	Decrease	Marked decrease	Decreased hemoglobin production	Iron deficiency; thalassemias

[a] Hb/RBC = hemoglobin per red blood cell

heme molecules is attached to one of four globin chains, two α and two β (hemoglobin A, the predominant hemoglobin of adult red blood cells). Deficiency of any component (iron, porphyrin, globin) leads to a hypochromic microcytic anemia.

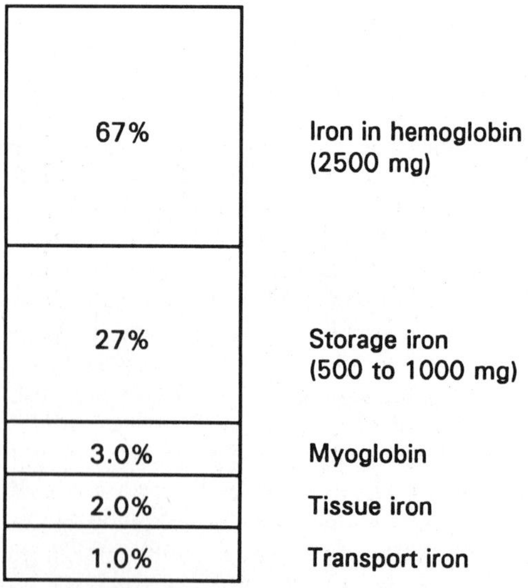

67%	Iron in hemoglobin (2500 mg)
27%	Storage iron (500 to 1000 mg)
3.0%	Myoglobin
2.0%	Tissue iron
1.0%	Transport iron

FIGURE 34-1 *Distribution of iron in the normal adult subject.*

Myoglobin Myoglobin, a protein with a molecular mass of 16,500 Da, is the protein-bound heme of skeletal and cardiac muscle. The concentration of this protein varies greatly in different muscles and is only about 1 percent of the concentration of hemoglobin in blood. The affinity of myoglobin for oxygen is much greater than that of hemoglobin, especially at low oxygen tensions, thus facilitating the transfer of oxygen carried by hemoglobin.

Transferrin Transferrin, which is a beta globulin with a molecular mass of 90,000 Da, has the specific property of binding iron; each transferrin molecule combines with two atoms of ferric iron. The combination is reversible. Transferrin serves to *transport* iron from the gastrointestinal tract to the bone marrow, to other tissue storage sites, and to the cells of the body that require iron. Under physiologic circumstances, about 20 to 35 percent of all available binding sites on the transferrin molecule are occupied by iron atoms. When there is a pathologic increase in body content, the saturation of transferrin increases. Conversely, in iron deficiency the saturation of transferrin falls below 15 percent. The serum iron and serum total iron binding capacity or TIBC (reflecting circulating transferrin levels) can be measured clinically. In practice, these tests serve as rough estimates of the state of iron stores and aid in the establishment of the diagnosis of iron deficiency in the patient.

Ferritin and Hemosiderin Ferritin and hemosiderin are the storage forms of iron in the body. Ferritin, a soluble iron-containing complex, is composed of a protein, apoferritin, within whose matrix iron, in amounts up to about 23 percent by weight, is bound in the form of hydroxide and phosphate complexes. Its major function is as a storage compound, although with its iron in the reduced form it has vasodepressive and antidiuretic properties. A portion of the body stores of ferritin circulates and is clinically measured as the serum ferritin. The serum ferritin has been shown to more accurately reflect iron stores in the body than does the serum iron. This makes the serum ferritin test very important in the diagnosis of disease related to abnormalities of iron metabolism. Hemosiderin, an insoluble iron protein complex, the chief storage form of iron within the mononuclear phagocyte (reticuloendothelial) system, is distinguishable from ferritin by its lack of solubility in water and its increased iron concentration — up to 35 percent iron by weight. Evaluation of bone marrow hemosiderin is a clinically available test which is helpful in the diagnosis of iron deficiency.

Enzymes and Cofactors In cells, iron is an integral part of the heme enzymes (catalases, peroxidases, the cytochromes, and cytochrome oxidase) and of the ferroflavoproteins (succinic dehydrogenase, xanthine oxidase, and NADH cytochrome reductase). Iron also serves as a necessary cofactor for other enzymes. Iron is present in small amounts in a variety of other cell components, including red hair pigment, the muscle proteins (myosin and actin), a protein of human milk, and some compounds found in the brain.

Iron Absorption, Transport, and Storage

Iron is presented to the gastrointestinal tract in a variety of forms. Iron may be ingested in the form of simple inorganic salts derived primarily from cooking and food processing or in the form of heme compounds such as hemoglobin or myoglobin found within meat.

The average American diet contains about 6 mg of elemental iron per 1000 kcal. Thus the average daily intake of iron is 6 to 24 mg daily, provided a balanced diet is being ingested. Only about 5 to 10 percent of the ingested iron, rarely more, is actually absorbed, which closely matches the need, since in the average adult only 0.5 to 1.8 mg of iron is actually lost daily. Factors which tend to increase iron absorption include an acidic pH of the gastric contents, ionization of food iron, solubility of the ingested iron salts, and iron ingested as heme or as other water-soluble chelates. Iron absorption increases in iron deficiency or when the rate of hematopoietic activity in the marrow increases for any cause. It is important to remember that the body has very limited ability to increase the absorption of ingested iron, even in the face of severe iron deficiency.

Absorption of iron can be accomplished at almost any level of the gastrointestinal tract, but it is most efficient in the duodenum and proximal jejunum. Virtually all iron that is absorbed by the intestine enters the body via the bloodstream rather than by lymphatic system. Uptake into the mucosal cell is unidirectional with no excretion of iron into the intestinal lumen except by cell desquamation. Absorption of iron normally balances excretion, with maintenance of fairly constant body composition. Iron absorption depends on a metabolically active two-stage process which is normally at a maximum in the proximal duodenum. Ferrous iron is better absorbed than is the ferric form. The initial rapid stage involves the binding of low molecular weight iron compounds to the cell surface and is virtually complete within an hour. The second, slower stage involves the binding of iron to intracellular proteins, one of which is ferritin. The ferritin actually acts as an intracellular storage depot. By means of signals generated by the body in response to need (the nature of those signals has not been completely defined), the iron absorbed intracellularly is then transferred to the plasma protein, transferrin. The iron, now bound to transferrin, is transferred to tissues for utilization or to mononuclear phagocyte stores for later use. Cells that require iron have transferrin receptors on their surfaces. By a process of endocytosis, the iron-transferrin complex is internalized, the iron removed intracellularly, and the transferrin returned to the circulation.

Iron not transferred to transferrin is maintained within the cell bound to ferritin and, within the 2- to 3-day life span of the gastrointestinal mucosal cell, is lost to the body by desquamation of the cell from the villous tip. This tightly regulated process, in the past called the *mucosal block*, prevents excessive accumulation of iron within the body. Iron stores are located in the mononuclear phagocyte systems and in hepatocytes. About two-thirds of storage iron is in the form of ferritin, and one-third is in the form of hemosiderin. In cases of excessive storage of iron, hemosiderin becomes the chief storage form. Table 34-2 outlines the changes that occur in iron metabolism in various conditions.

Iron Excretion

The capacity of the body to excrete iron is limited. Most excretion is by desquamation of iron-containing cells from the bowel, skin, and genitourinary tract, although some iron is contained in fluids such as bile, urine, and sweat. The total daily iron loss for an adult male or non-menstruating female is about 0.5 to 1.0 mg; an additional daily increment of 0.5 to 0.6 mg is added for normal menstrual loss.

Iron loss as hemosiderin granules in the urinary sediment is found in many patients with massive iron overload and in some patients with brisk intravascular hemolysis. During pregnancy iron is lost from the mother to the fetus and the placental tissues; there is further loss of iron at delivery, and normal iron excretion (minus menstrual losses) continues. The point to remember is that in cases of iron overload, the ability of the body to excrete the excess iron is very limited.

Iron Requirements

Requirements for iron vary during different periods of life and reflect the demands of growth, menstruation, or pregnancy. The effects of these variations superimposed on the baseline excretion are listed in Table 34-3. Men and postmenopausal women ingesting a balanced diet normally maintain an adequate iron balance. Women during their reproductive years and adolescent girls, who must cope with both growth and menstruation, are constantly in precarious iron balance and readily become iron-deficient, since the ability to increase iron absorption is very limited. Similarly, the growth of infants from 6 to 24 months of age, during the period of rapid increase in body size, often outstrips dietary iron supply.

The kinetics of the daily turnover of iron bound to plasma transferrin for a normal subject is schematically summarized in Fig. 34-2. As shown, all iron exchange among the various sites within the body must occur via the plasma, mediated by the binding of the elemental iron to transferrin. In the normal state, the amount of iron entering the plasma is equal to the amount leaving the plasma. The major exchange of iron occurs from the red blood cell (RBC) to the marrow. The erythropoietic labile pool refers to the iron available to RBC marrow precursors for hemoglobin synthesis. Of the 35 mg of iron turned over each day, 21 mg is used to produce hemoglobin for circulating RBC, 11 mg is used to maintain the labile pool, and the remainder is distributed within stores and intracellular fluid. The reader should note that only 1 mg of iron is lost daily and 1 mg is absorbed daily. Should there occur a loss of

TABLE 34-2 Changes in clinically measured parameters of various iron anemias

Condition	Serum iron	Serum transferrin	Serum ferritin
Iron deficiency (i.e., blood loss)	Decreased	Increased	Decreased
Normal pregnancy	Decreased	Increased	Decreased
Hemosiderosis/ Hemochromatosis	Increased	Unchanged	Increased
Anemias not directly caused by changes in iron metabolism:			
Aplastic anemia	Increased	Decreased	Increased
Hemolytic anemia	Unchanged	Unchanged	Unchanged
Megaloblastic anemia	Increased	Unchanged	Unchanged

TABLE 34-3 Estimated dietary iron requirements

	Absorbed iron requirement, mg/day	Daily food iron requirement,[a] mg/day
Normal men and nonmenstruating women	0.5 to 1	5 to 10
Menstruating women	0.7 to 2	7 to 20
Pregnant women	2 to 4.8	20 to 48[b]
Adolescents	1 to 2	10 to 20
Children	0.4 to 1	4 to 10
Infants	0.5 to 1.5	1.5 mg/kg[c]

[a] Assuming 10 percent absorption.
[b] This amount of iron cannot be derived from diet and should be met by iron supplement in the latter half of pregnancy.
[c] To a maximum of 15 mg.

NORMAL IRON KINETICS

Plasma Iron Exchange

Total leaving plasma	**35 mg/day**
Erythropoietic labile pool	*32*
Storage	*1*
Extracellular fluid	*1*
Excretion and loss	*1*
Total entering plasma	**35 mg/day**
Erythrocytes	*21*
Storage	*1*
Extracellular fluid	*1*
Absorption	*1*
Erythropoietic labile pool	*11*

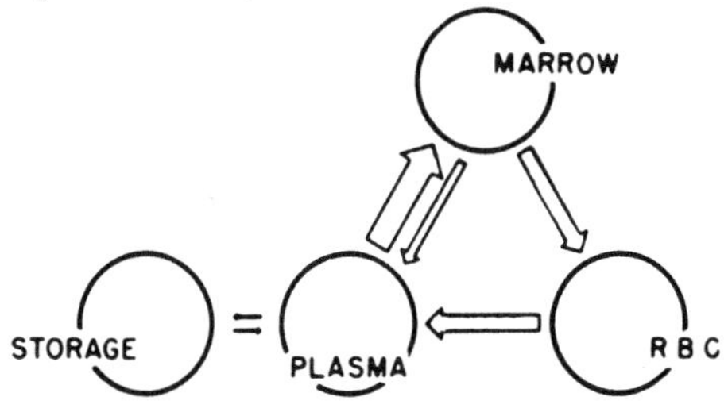

FIGURE 34-2 *Summary of iron kinetics of a normal adult subject.*

RBC from the body through bleeding, the amount of iron lost would be made up by storage iron. Conversely, if absorption of iron is in excess of utilization, the storage pool would increase.

Iron-Deficiency States

In iron-deficiency states, regardless of the etiology, there is an orderly progression of iron depletion, most of which occurs long before clinical signs or symptoms become apparent. The earliest identifiable change is manifest by a loss of storage iron, but with maintenance of normal hemoglobin concentration, iron-dependent enzyme function, and transport iron. This phase is termed *iron store depletion*. Assessment of the patient at this time would be expected to yield low levels of serum ferritin and no stainable iron in the marrow, but normal serum iron concentration, transferrin levels (clinically measured as the total plasma iron-binding capacity, TIBC), hemoglobin concentration, and RBC morphology. As further depletion occurs, there occurs a slow decline in the serum iron concentration, a rise in the TIBC, and a fall in hemoglobin concentration, followed by the development of characteristic microcytic hypochromic red blood cells. It will be at some point along this spiral that the clinical symptoms of anemia would occur.

The diagnosis of iron-deficiency anemia is

based on the finding of small erythrocytes (microcytes) filled poorly with hemoglobin (hypochromia). Only late in the course are cells of bizarre shape (poikilocytosis) and variable size (anisocytosis) sometimes seen. The diagnosis is confirmed by finding a low serum ferritin concentration; alternatively, a low serum iron, coupled with a normal or high TIBC, and the total saturation of the iron-binding protein of less than 15 percent might be noted. Another confirmatory test is the absence of stainable marrow iron. Iron-deficiency anemia constitutes the major cause of hypochromic anemia, the others being the thalassemia syndromes (globin deficiency) and the anemias caused by impaired porphyrin synthesis.

Clinically, iron-deficiency anemia is a sign rather than a disease. In adult males and postmenopausal females, iron deficiency usually signifies the presence of significant blood loss, the cause of which must be diligently sought, most often by careful examination of the gastrointestinal tract. For women of childbearing age, excessive menstrual flow and multiple pregnancies are the most common causes. Infants and children with rapid growth demands on limited dietary iron intake may suffer from iron deficiency. Bleeding related to laboratory testing will add to their iron depletion. Malabsorption of iron as a result of gastrointestinal diseases or surgical alteration of the gastrointestinal tract may be an additional cause of iron-deficiency anemia. Rarely in the United States is pure dietary insufficiency of iron the sole cause of iron-deficiency anemia in adults.

In the treatment of iron-deficiency anemia there are two basic points to consider: (1) recognition and correction of the underlying cause and (2) repletion of body iron. The second of these is usually quite easily achieved, but it is probably the first which is most important in the long run. It is common to find that iron-deficiency anemia is the first sign of a potentially more serious clinical condition (i.e., colon cancer, chronic gastrointestinal bleeding, or genital-urinary bleeding). The task of the clinician is to become aware of etiology of the iron deficiency and correct this problem before prescribing any of the iron compounds listed below.

Iron Compounds for Oral Administration

Ferrous Sulfate Over the years ferrous sulfate has been the standard to which new iron preparations have been compared. Two forms of ferrous sulfate are generally used therapeutically: (1) the hydrated salt ($FeSO_4 \bullet 7H_2O$) contains 20 percent elemental iron by weight and (2) the exsiccated form (80% anhydrous $FeSO_4$) which contains 30 percent elemental iron.

Most ferrous sulfate tablets contain between 40 and 65 mg of elemental iron, and the usual adult with iron deficiency will require between 150 to 200 mg of elemental iron per day. Given an absorption rate of 5 to 20 percent, in order to replete body iron completely, 3 to 6 months of continuous oral therapy are usually required. Liquid forms of ferrous sulfate are also available.

Ferrous Gluconate Ferrous gluconate was introduced in an effort to reduce the side effects of ferrous sulfate. It is supplied as tablets of 320 mg containing 11.5 percent iron, as capsules of 86 mg containing 10 mg of iron, and as an elixir containing 300 mg per 5 mL, equivalent to 36 mg of iron. In order to administer an adequate dose of elemental iron, four to six tablets per day of this preparation would have to be taken.

Ferrous Fumarate Ferrous fumarate is a red-brown iron salt of fumaric acid containing 33 percent elemental iron. It is relatively resistant to oxidation, even in uncoated tables, and is relatively insoluble in aqueous solution except at low pH.

Tolerance and Compliance

The most common reason for failure of oral iron to correct iron deficiency is patient noncompliance, provided the etiology of the blood loss has been corrected. Noncompliance is usually a result of the side effects of the iron preparations. Most troublesome to the patient are the gastrointestinal symptoms of constipation, pyrosis, or loose stool.

Placebo-controlled studies indicate that gastrointestinal intolerance ascribed to medicinal iron ingestion occurs only in 5 to 10 percent of patients given the usual therapeutic doses listed above. Changing the formulation or minor adjustment of dosage coupled with encouragement to continue improves compliance.

Iron Compounds for Parenteral Use

The great majority of patients with iron-deficiency anemia are best treated with orally administered iron. However, the use of a parenteral preparation of iron may be desirable for certain patients: (1) those who are unable to tolerate or unwilling to take iron orally, e.g., those with ulcerative colitis, regional enteritis, colostomies, or extensive bowel resections, as well as those who for various reasons cannot be relied upon to take medications prescribed for them; (2) those who are unable to absorb iron given orally, e.g., patients with idiopathic or post-resection malabsorption syndromes; and (3) those with severe iron deficiency for whom it is impossible to provide iron quickly enough or in sufficient quantity by the oral route.

Iron Dextran This is a complex of ferric hydroxide and low molecular weight dextran (5000 to 20,000 average molecular weight). The compound contains 50 mg of elemental iron per mL. The preparations can be given either by deep intramuscular or intravenous injection. It is recommended that no more than 2 mL be given by either route per day. Total intravenous dose infusion has been used but is not at this time approved in the United States. Intravenous iron therapy has been associated with the infrequent occurrence of anaphylaxis, so it is recommended that a 0.5 mL test dose be given 1 to 2 days prior to the institution of parenteral therapy. A delayed serum sickness-like reaction may also occur. Other toxicities include skin staining at the injection site, local thrombophlebitis, arthralgias, fever, hypotension, bradycardia, myalgias, headaches, abdominal pain, nausea, vomiting, and dizziness. Parenteral iron may also exacerbate arthritis in patients with rheumatoid arthritis or ankylosing spondylitis.

Acute Iron Toxicity

The ingestion of large doses of soluble iron compounds, especially by small children, often results in acute iron intoxication, leading to severe symptoms and death in a high proportion of cases. Lethal doses of ferrous sulfate have varied from 3 to 18 g, although survival has been reported after doses as high as 15 g.

The clinical effects of ingesting toxic doses of iron have been divided into four phases chronologically. The first phase begins with abdominal pain, nausea, and vomiting about 30 to 60 min after the iron tablets are taken. Partially dissolved iron tablets may be vomited together with brown or bloody stomach contents. Irritability, pallor, and drowsiness appear along with frequent black or bloody diarrhea. Signs of acidosis and cardiovascular collapse may become prominent; coma and death ensue within 4 to 6 h in about 20 percent of children taking large doses of iron. The second phase is a period of improvement with subsidence of the initial signs and symptoms spontaneously or in response to treatment. This period, lasting 8 to 16 h, appears to herald the onset of progressive improvement. Often, however, this lull in symptoms is shattered by a third phase of progressive cardiovascular collapse, convulsions, coma, and high mortality about 24 h after iron ingestion. Finally, a fourth phase of gastrointestinal obstruction from scarring of the stomach or small intestine may occur weeks or months after the recovery from the initial episode of iron intoxication.

The most important aspect of management of acute iron toxicity is prevention. Especially in children, in whom accidental ingestion is most common, prevention cannot be overemphasized. In the event of either intentional or accidental ingestion of large amounts of iron, the following is a rational approach to the treatment of the patient: (1) Rid the stomach of its contents by inducing emesis and by lavage with a large-bore tube to remove undissolved iron tablets. With the tube still in place, instill a 1% solution of sodium bicarbonate. Deferoxamine (see below), an iron-chelating compound, may also be instilled to bind residual iron in a poorly absorbable form. Deferoxamine mesylate should also be administered by an intravenous infusion. Follow the gastric lavage with an enema to remove iron from the lower bowel. (2) Institute measures to combat peripheral vascular collapse, including early replacement of body fluids and electrolytes, using isotonic saline solution, Ringer's lactate solution, plasma, dextran, or whole blood. (3) Additional measures of value include treating metabolic acidosis with appropriate solutions of sodium bicarbonate and using oxygen and vasopressor agents to help combat shock. The use of barbiturates or benzodiazepines may be required to control convulsions.

Iron Chelation Therapy: Deferoxamine

Deferoxamine is a powerful iron-chelating agent derived from *Streptomyces pilosus*. The affinity of the compound for iron is high ($K_a = 10^{31}$), whereas its affinity for calcium is much less ($K_a = 10^2$). Deferoxamine will bind iron from transferrin, ferritin, and hemosiderin, but not from hemoglobin or the cytochromes. The major use of this drug and others under development is the removal of excess iron stores in patients with refractory anemia who require lifelong blood transfusion.

Pharmacokinetics Deferoxamine is poorly absorbed from the gastrointestinal tract, making parenteral administration necessary for removal of excess body iron. The drug is metabolized by as yet undefined pathways. It is degraded by plasma enzymes. Metabolites and unchanged drug are excreted in the urine.

Deferoxamine binds ferric iron to form the water-soluble chelate, ferroxamine. Whereas ionized heavy metal ions such as iron salts are highly toxic to tissues, chelates of heavy metals are usually harmless. The newly formed ferroxamine is excreted primarily into the urine (often imparting a reddish color), with lesser amounts eliminated in the bile. The elimination half-life after IV use is approximately 1 hour.

Toxicities and Contraindications Allergic reactions occur commonly and include pruritus, urticaria, skin rashes, and much less commonly, anaphylaxis. Other toxicities include dysuria, abdominal pain, diarrhea, and cataract formation. This drug is contraindicated in pregnancy and renal dysfunction.

Chronic Iron Overload

Excessive amounts of iron may accumulate in the body under a variety of conditions. The following lists the major types of iron-storage diseases:

1. Idiopathic hemochromatosis
2. Transfusion iron overload
3. Medicinal iron overload
   a. Oral
   b. Parenteral
4. Hemolytic iron overload
   a. Refractory anemias
   b. Thalassemia
5. Dietary iron overload
   a. Bantu siderosis
   b. Kaschin-Beck disease

Much confusion results from the nomenclature of clinical disorders of iron overload which reflects an incomplete understanding of the pathogenesis of excessive body-iron storage and associated tissue damage. For the sake of discussion, *hemosiderosis* is defined as an increase in mononuclear phagocyte iron without any associated tissue damage. The term *hemochromatosis* is used to denote increased storage iron with associated tissue damage.

Idiopathic Hemochromatosis and Transfusional Hemosiderosis

Idiopathic hemochromatosis is an uncommon disease that is a result of a regulatory abnormality that involves both the intestinal absorption of iron and the ability of mononuclear phagocyte cells to handle the iron that is absorbed. Excessive absorption over many years leads to accumulation of mononuclear phagocyte iron with eventual "spill-over" into the plasma and the tissues. Particular organs damaged by excessive iron storage are the liver, pancreas, gonads, thyroid, adrenal, heart, and the stomach.

Hemochromatosis is an autosomal recessive inherited disorder. The abnormal gene is present in about 10 percent of the caucasoid population in Europe and the USA. About 3 in 1000 are homozygous. The gene (not yet cloned) is located on chromosome 6, tightly linked to the human HLA locus. Common HLA types of affected individuals include A3, B7, and B14. The gene is distinct from HLA genes since different HLA haplotypes (i.e., other than A3/B7 or A3/B14) may be found in different kindreds. Lifelong increase in daily iron absorption results in iron overload leading to tissue damage. Clinical manifestations of tissue damage are usually first seen in men 40 to 70 years of age. Clinical manifestations are seen less frequently and less often in women because of menstrual loss.

The clinical diagnosis is usually suspected by the demonstration of cirrhosis and excessive iron deposits on biopsy of the liver. Increased iron in skin, gastric mucosa, or urine sediment are confirmatory findings. Elevated plasma iron levels with almost completely saturated iron-binding capacity is generally observed. The serum ferritin level is usually found to be greater than 500 ng/mL and is often even greater than 1000 ng/mL. Bone marrow iron may not show any significant increase, however.

Removal of excess iron by repeated phlebotomy prevents further tissue damage. Patients must be monitored by the serum ferritin level for the remainder of their life.

Transfusion hemosiderosis is a complication of the multiply transfused patient. Each 1 mL of packed red blood cells delivers 1 mg of elemental iron which the body cannot excrete. After 100 or more units of blood, the tissue iron stores become fully saturated and parenchymal organ damage may occur. The picture resembles hemochromatosis. Phlebotomy, as used in idiopathic hemochromatosis, is not feasible, for obvious reasons, in these anemic patients receiving blood transfusions. Alternate means of iron removal involves the use of deferoxamine. A single intravenous dose of 500 to 1000 mg of deferoxamine can mobilize up to 50 mg of iron, which is then excreted in the urine. Deferoxamine is usually given daily intravenously or via continuous intravenous or subcutaneous infusion over a 6 to 9 h period. Treatment is repeated periodically after the initial removal of as much excess iron as possible.

Other iron chelators are under development. Even though deferoxamine is rather nontoxic, it must be given parenterally since it and its chelates are not absorbed orally. Newer agents are active orally but demonstrate toxicity, precluding their use currently.

THE MACROCYTIC MEGALOBLASTIC ANEMIAS: FOLIC ACID (FOLATE) AND VITAMIN B_{12} DEFICIENCY

Deficiency of either vitamin B_{12} or folate will cause macrocytic anemia characterized by a peculiar morphologic appearance of red blood cell precursors in the marrow which is called the *megaloblastic change*. Megaloblastic change was a term coined by Paul Ehrlich in the 1880s. He described bone marrow red blood cell precursors which were larger than normal and which demonstrated nuclear-cytoplasmic maturation dyssynchrony. In such cases, the appearance of the cytoplasm seemed more mature than the nucleus. Actually, it has been shown that nuclear maturation lags behind the maturation of the cytoplasm. After repletion of the missing vitamin, the bone marrow morphology is restored to normal and the anemia is corrected.

Occasionally other deficits in cellular building blocks may give rise to a morphologic picture very similar to vitamin B_{12} or folate deficiency. Examples include blockage of active building block synthesis with antimetabolite therapy (i.e., 6-mercaptopurine, 5-fluorouracil, or methotrexate), hereditary orotic aciduria, and certain refractory anemias. In these instances, vitamin B_{12} and folate replacement will not improve the anemia, nor will administration of these vitamins correct the abnormal morphology. The bone marrow abnormalities noted in the above instances are termed *bone marrow megaloblastoid changes* to distinguish them from true megaloblastosis.

Current evidence suggests that the megaloblast is a cell in a state of "unbalanced growth" due to impaired synthesis of one or more deoxyribonucleotides, the precursors of DNA. Hence the RNA/DNA ratio rises, since the replication of DNA and cell division are blocked, while the synthesis of cytoplasmic components proceeds normally. The roles of vitamin B_{12} and folate in deoxyribonucleotide synthesis are discussed later.

Folic Acid

Chemistry and Nomenclature Folic acid, the common name of pteroylglutamic acid, is a parent compound of a large group of growth factors and coenzymes collectively referred to as *folates*. The folic acid molecule contains three structural units: (1) a pteridine derivative, (2) p-aminobenzoic acid, and (3) glutamic acid (see Fig. 34-3). Pteroylglutamic, or folic acid (F) is metabolically active only after conversion to its coenzyme form, 5,6,7,8-tetrahydrofolic acid (FH_4). Reduction of F to FH_4 occurs in two steps: F is reduced to 7,8-dihydrofolic acid (FH_2), and FH_2 is reduced further to FH_4, both reactions being catalyzed by a single NADPH-linked enzyme, dihydrofolate reductase (DHFR).

Because reduced derivatives of folic acid are extremely sensitive to oxidation in air, they are unstable and difficult to preserve. A notable exception is the stable compound N^5-formyl FH_4, which was isolated from liver and yeast soon after the discovery of folic acid. It was first recognized as a growth factor for *Leuconostoc citrovorum* (since renamed *Pediococcus cerevisiae*) and, thus, it was named *citrovorum factor*. Leucovorin and folinic acid are the currently used names for this compound.

Sources The many different forms of folates are widely distributed in nature. Green leaves, presumed to be sites of active folate synthesis, are especially rich in the vitamin. Though the vitamin is also synthesized by many bacteria, the principal sources in the average diet are leafy vegetables, liver, and fruits. Excessive cooking, particularly with large amounts of water, may remove or destroy a large fraction of the folate in foods. Most food folate exists as polyglutamates with up to six glutamate moieties added to the parent molecule. In nature, folates always exist in a reduced form, but as soon as food folates are exposed to air, oxidation to folic acid occurs.

Absorption and Fate Even though the minimum daily requirement of folate is 50 μg, when 0.2 to 2.0 mg of folic acid is administered orally to a

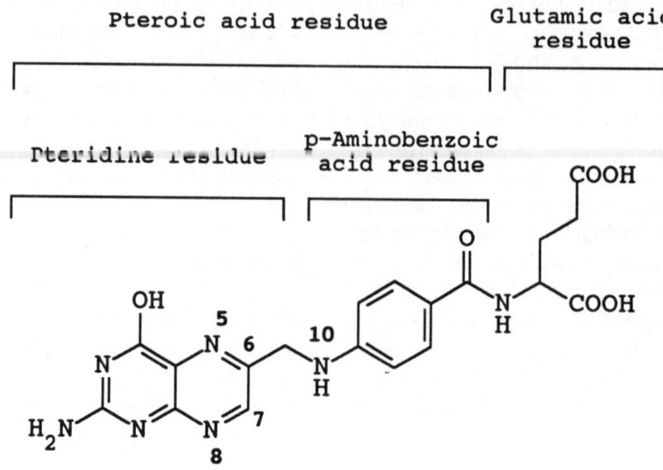

FIGURE 34-3 *Structure of folic acid.*

normal person, more than 65 percent is usually absorbed. About 5 percent of the 0.2 mg dose and 15 percent of the 2.0 mg is excreted in the urine. After a 1 mg oral dose, serum levels can be detected within minutes and reach a peak in about 1 hour.

Gastrointestinal absorption occurs primarily in the upper small bowel and requires DHFR, which is found in high concentrations in the mucosal cells of the duodenum and proximal jejunum. Therefore, any disease process that affects this area of the intestine will have an adverse impact on folate absorption. Although various folates are synthesized by intestinal bacteria, little of the vitamin derived from this source is absorbed, since most of the synthesis of bacterial folate occurs in the colon, which is distal to the major area of folate absorption.

Reduced monoglutamates are absorbed rapidly by simple diffusion, while most polyglutamate folate from food is absorbed by an active process. First, the absorbed polyglutamate must be broken down to monoglutamate forms; after passage into the intestinal cell as polyglutamate, a lysosomal enzyme known as conjugase removes the extra glutamate moieties yielding monoglutamate folate. DHFR then reduces the compound to FH_4, and other enzymes add a single carbon fragment reduced to its methyl form to produce N^5-methyl FH_4. The latter compound then passes to the circulation.

Once the folate is absorbed, it is transported via a nonspecific binding protein to the tissues, where it is either stored or used. Folate uptake by cells involves specific folate binding proteins. Once in the cell, enzymes change monoglutamate folate to polyglutamate folate which facilitates cellular folate enzymatic utilization and retention. As noted, folate is used by all dividing tissues and is stored in the liver. Folate is stored intracellularly in a polyglutamate form. While most folate coenzymes are monoglutamates, some of their coenzymatic activity involves polyglutamate forms also. Body stores are maintained by food intake and an active enterohepatic circulation of the vitamin. The liver secretes folate into the bile, which is then reabsorbed by the intestinal cells. Most of the folate lost from the body is through the urine, but some is lost through the feces.

Metabolic Functions In metabolism, FH_4 is a catalytic self-regenerating acceptor-donor of one-carbon units in reactions involving one-carbon transfers from a carbon-containing donor compound, X-C, to an acceptor, Y:

$$\text{X-C} + FH_4 \longrightarrow \text{X} + \text{C-}FH_4$$
$$\text{C-}FH_4 + \text{Y} \longrightarrow \text{Y-C} + FH_4$$

$$\text{Sum: X-C} + \text{Y} \longrightarrow \text{Y-C} + \text{X}$$

The varieties of C-FH_4 differ only in the identity to the one-carbon unit and the site of its attachment to FH_4: one-carbon units can attach to either N^5, N^{10}, or to both nitrogens (Fig. 34-3).

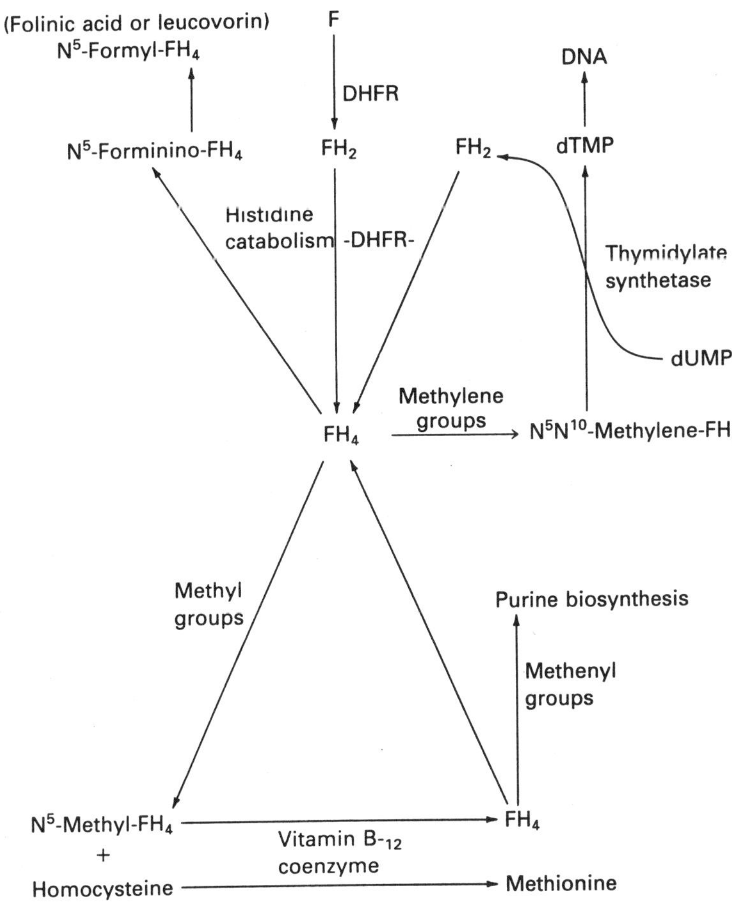

FIGURE 34-4 *The metabolic reactions of folate and their relationship to vitamin B_{12} (see text for details).*

Figure 34-4 shows the metabolic action of FH_4. Methylene, methenyl, and methyl groups are found among the one-carbon units carried by FH_4. Specific enzymes are known which interconvert many of these compounds. In human folate deficiency, the reaction, whose impairment produces the major clinical manifestations, is that which catalyzes thymidylate synthesis. The methylation of deoxyuridylate (dUMP) to thymidylate (dTMP), catalyzed by the thymidylate synthetase, is an essential preliminary step in the synthesis of DNA. The coenzyme of reaction, N^5,N^{10}-methylene FH_4, transfers a one-carbon group and also acts as a hydrogen donor in converting (reducing) the transferred group to a methyl group. This reaction generates FH_2, which dihydrofolate reductase must reduce to FH_4 before it can again be utilized as a folate coenzyme. Limitation of thymidylate synthesis in folate deficiency results in the defective DNA synthesis manifested by megaloblast formation.

Impairment of folate metabolism occurs in vitamin B_{12} deficiency. In Fig. 34-4 the only reaction in which N^5-methyl FH_4 may be utilized is by the donation of its methyl group to homocysteine to form methionine. Since this reaction depends on the vitamin B_{12} coenzyme, when there is vitamin B_{12} deficiency (see section on vitamin B_{12}), the N^5-methyl FH_4 remains "trapped". Since only N^5,N^{10}-methylene FH_4 can be used for DNA synthesis, the FH_4 trapped as N^5-methyl FH_4 is unavailable for synthesis of N^5,N^{10}-methylene FH_4 and for other FH_4 reactions. This creates relative "folate deficiency." This mechanism may account for the megaloblastosis seen in vitamin B_{12} deficiency. Evidence supporting this mechanism includes the fact that intracellular folates are low in vitamin B_{12} deficiency, while serum folate, whose major form is N^5-methyl FH_4, is raised in vitamin B_{12} deficiency.

Requirements and Distribution The minimum daily requirement for folic acid in the normal adult is approximately 50 μg. Although the average diet contains several times this amount in the form of various food folate compounds, body reserves of folic acid are relatively smaller than are those of vitamin B_{12}. Reducing folate acid intake from a normal to a low daily intake of 5 μg/day results in the development of megaloblastic anemia in about 4 months. The majority of folate is stored within the liver.

Folate Deficiency The principal causes of folate deficiency are inadequate dietary intake, defective intestinal absorption, abnormally increased requirements, and impaired utilization in the tissues. In contrast to the vitamin B_{12}-deficiency syndromes, malnutrition is an important cause of folate deficiency. This is often associated with chronic alcoholism.

Various forms of malabsorption, tropical sprue, and nontropical sprue (adult and infantile celiac disease) are also causes of folate deficiency. In tropical sprue, treatment with folate alone may reverse all abnormalities, including the defective absorption of the vitamin itself. In nontropical sprue, as in most other forms of malabsorption, folate treatment corrects only the folate deficiency, without affecting the absorptive defect. Low serum folate levels in patients receiving phenytoin and other anticonvulsants have been attributed to a reversible drug-induced malabsorption of folate.

Increased requirements for folate occur in chronic hemolytic anemias, leukemia, other malignant diseases, and pregnancy, which increases requirements three- to six-fold.

A major mechanism of folate "deficiency" is the inhibition of folate reduction caused by administration of various pharmacologic agents. The 4-aminofolic acid analogs, such as methotrexate, are powerful inhibitors of DHFR. Other, weaker inhibitors of DHFR in widespread use are trimethoprim and pyrimethamine. Oral contraceptives have been reported to impair folate metabolism and produce folate depletion; the effect is mild and anemia or megaloblastic changes rarely occur.

Diagnosis of Folate Deficiency If there is a clinical suspicion of folate deficiency (e.g., chronic alcoholism, or malabsorption), or a macrocytic anemia, or findings on peripheral smear suggestive of deficiency (e.g., hypersegmented polymorphonuclear leukocytes), the diagnosis should be confirmed with a serum folate. This should always be done before any replacement therapy is given, as even a small amount of oral folate may increase serum values appreciably.

It is essential to distinguish between folic acid and vitamin B_{12} deficiencies so that the pathogenetic mechanism may be understood and appropriate therapy given. (Gastrointestinal features of folate deficiency may also be similar to those of pernicious anemia.) Neurologic abnormalities are said to occur only in vitamin B_{12} deficiency, although scattered recent reports have suggested that neurologic changes may occur in pure folate deficiency. It should be remembered that neuropathies may result from deficiencies of other vitamins that may accompany a deficiency of folate (i.e., alcoholic polyneuropathy often accompanies folate deficiency).

Therapy of Folate Deficiency The sole indication for folic acid therapy is folate deficiency or, as in pregnancy, anticipated folic acid deficiency. It has also been recommended that folate be given to all pregnant women to prevent neural tube defects in the fetus. All therapeutic effects are attributable to reversal or prevention of the deficiency state.

The vitamin is available as tablets and the sodium salt of folic acid (folate sodium) is available as a parenteral solution which may be given by intramuscular, intravenous, or subcutaneous injection. Although the parenteral administration of folic acid has no advantage over oral administration, this route may be preferred when the folate deficiency is caused by malabsorption rather than by ingestion of inadequate amounts.

Calcium leucovorin, tablets or injection, the clinically available preparation of N^5-formyl FH_4, is used in the presence of severe intoxication by folic acid antagonists (such as methotrexate), which act by blocking the reduction of FH_2 to FH_4. No purpose is accomplished in ordinary folate deficiency by giving this compound in place of folic acid. Suggestions that impaired reduction of folate in liver disease may respond to leucovorin have not been clinically proved.

Adverse reactions caused by folic acid have not been observed even with doses 100 times higher than the usual minimum daily requirement (MDR). In patients on phenytoin or primidone, folate administration may cause seizures, probably because of concomitant changes in serum levels of anticonvulsant.

Vitamin B_{12}

Chemistry and Nomenclature Chemically, the structure of vitamin B_{12} relates it to the corrinoid compounds; the *cobalamin* (introduced before the structure was known) is frequently used to refer to the vitamin B_{12} molecule minus the cyano group (Fig. 34-5). Vitamin B_{12} itself then becomes cyanocobalamin. The cyano moiety of cyanocobalamin may be replaced by a hydroxyl group to yield hydroxocobalamin. Cobalamin, in either the cyano or hydroxy form, is readily converted to deoxyadenosylcobalamin in tissues by a coenzyme synthetase system. This compound is known as vitamin B_{12} coenzyme. In this reaction, the deoxyadenosyl moiety of ATP is transferred intact to the vitamin to form the coenzyme. Most natural sources of vitamin B_{12} contain the coenzyme or hydroxocobalamin.

Sources Only bacteria can synthesize vitamin B_{12}. Vitamin B_{12} is required by all living cells. Plants obtain their supply from soil bacteria, while animals obtain their supply by diet. Foods especially rich in vitamin B_{12} include liver, seafood, meat, eggs, and milk. The average daily dietary intake of vitamin B_{12} is between 5 and 30 μg. The MDR is 1 to 3 μg. The vitamin is widely distributed throughout body tissues. In the human being, the total body content is 4 to 5 mg, about 1 mg being in the liver.

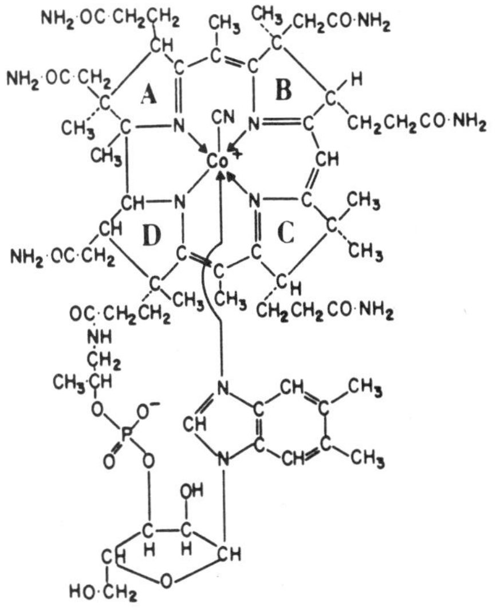

FIGURE 34-5 *Chemical structure of vitamin B_{12}.*

Absorption and Fate Human gastric intrinsic factor (IF) binds dietary vitamin B_{12} and small oral doses of pure cyanocobalamin. Intrinsic factor is a glycoprotein with a monomeric molecular mass of 50 to 60 kDa. When it binds vitamin B_{12}, it forms a dimer of molecular mass of 114 to 119 kDa. The dimeric molecule binds two molecules of vitamin B_{12}. Vitamin B_{12} in fact must be released from various food proteins by pancreatic digestive enzymes.

The intrinsic factor-vitamin B_{12} complex is carried through the intestine to the terminal ileum, where the complex attaches to specific receptors on the microvilli of the terminal ileum. The vitamin B_{12} is then internalized by an active metabolic process, while the IF is released to be lost with the fecal contents. This accounts for the delay of several hours in the appearance of the ingested vitamin in the bloodstream. Small physiologic doses of vitamin B_{12} are absorbed very efficiently in this fashion, while larger oral doses are absorbed by simple diffusion, both in normal and pernicious anemia subjects. In these instances, the vitamin appears almost immediately in the blood. The range of blood levels of vitamin B_{12} is 200 to 1000 pg/mL.

Normal plasma contains at least two vitamin B_{12}-binding proteins, termed *transcobalamin I* and *transcobalamin II* (TC I and TC II). The former, an α_1-globulin, binds most of the circulating endogenous vitamin B_{12}. TC I is derived from the white blood cells and their precursors. TC II, a β-globulin, normally one-third to two-thirds saturated, is derived from the mononuclear phagocyte system and mediates the transfer of vitamin B_{12} to other cells in the body. Thus, TC II binds most of the ingested or injected vitamin B_{12}. Small injected doses of vitamin B_{12} are almost completely retained, while the major portion of doses of more than 50 μg are lost in the urine, since this dose exceeds the binding capacity of the TC II. Free vitamin B_{12} is filtered by the glomerulus and is lost in the urine, since there is no tubular reabsorption.

Vitamin B_{12} is excreted in the bile. There is an active enterohepatic circulation of vitamin B_{12}. The total amount of vitamin B_{12} in feces exceeds the sum of that excreted in the urine plus the unabsorbed vitamin because there is new synthesis by colon bacteria. Vitamin from the latter source is not available to the human host. As yet, there is little information concerning the degradation of vitamin B_{12} in human tissues.

Metabolic Functions As currently understood, the biochemical systems impaired in human vitamin B_{12} deficiency are (1) the metabolism of methylmalonyl CoA and, thus, propionate catabolism, and (2) methionine synthesis and, thus, N^5-methyl-FH_4 demethylation (see section on folate). While the exact role for vitamin B_{12} in the maintenance of neurologic function is unknown, it has been suggested that impairment of methylmalonyl CoA conversion accounts for the neurologic damage of human vitamin B_{12} deficiency. The cobalamin-dependent isomerization of methylmalonyl CoA is a step in the catabolism of propionic acid. Propionic acid metabolism resulting from fatty acid oxidation in animal tissue involves the biotin-dependent carboxylation of propionyl CoA to methylmalonyl CoA. After a racemization step, methylmalonyl CoA mutase catalyzes the reversible conversion of methylmalonyl CoA to succinyl CoA (Fig. 34-6), which can then enter the tricarboxylic acid cycle after conversion to succinate. Nondividing nerve cells are not engaged in DNA synthesis, but they do synthesize myelin and other lipids. Vitamin B_{12} deficient humans excrete abnormal quantities of methylmalonate and acetate. Data suggest that the presence and severity of neurologic symptoms correlate with the degree of acetic aciduria, but not of methylmalonic aciduria. These results, as well as evidence from isotopic studies of propionate metabolism in human vitamin B_{12} deficiency, are compatible with the view that distorted lipid metabolism may be responsible for neurologic damage.

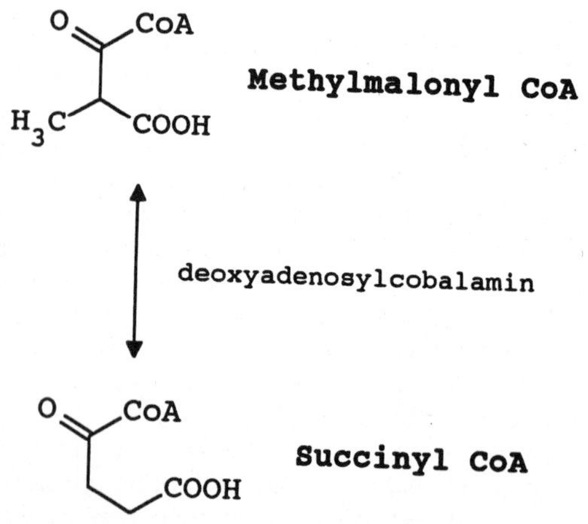

O CoA
H_3C COOH
Methylmalonyl CoA

deoxyadenosylcobalamin

O CoA
COOH
Succinyl CoA

FIGURE 34-6 *The conversion of methylmalonyl CoA to succinyl CoA. The source of methylmalonyl CoA is propionate.*

The interrelationship between folate and vitamin B_{12} metabolism has been discussed previously. The trapping of folate caused by vitamin B_{12} deficiency has been presented as an explanation for the megaloblastic anemia seen in vitamin B_{12} deficient patients (Fig. 34-4).

Vitamin B_{12} Deficiency States Deficiency of vitamin B_{12} may be caused by the following mechanisms: (1) decreased ingestion, (2) decreased absorption, (3) increased requirement, and (4) impaired utilization and increased loss. Vitamin B_{12} deficiency secondary to decreased ingestion occurs in persons who are strict ovo-lacto-vegetarians and is quite rare because all organisms require vitamin B_{12} and, therefore, most food supplies contain vitamin B_{12}. The most common cause of vitamin B_{12} deficiency is decreased absorption secondary to the loss of the intrinsic factor. Increased requirement for vitamin B_{12} is more a theoretical than a real clinical problem. Impaired utilization of vitamin B_{12} involves a number of hereditary conditions involving intrinsic factor, transcobalamine, lysosomal and cytologic metabolizing enzymes, and enzymes involved in succinate and methionine synthesis. Chronic inhalation of nitrous oxide also impairs the metabolic function of the vitamin.

Clinically, the major effect of vitamin B_{12} deficiency is macrocytic anemia. The deficiency may also result in degenerative changes of the dorsal and lateral columns of the spinal cord and peripheral nerves yielding disturbances of vibratory sense, proprioception, and pyramidal-tract function. Mental aberrations, ranging from mood changes to frank psychosis, may occur. Optic atrophy and toxic amblyopia (usually associated with tobacco use) may be associated with vitamin B_{12} deficiency. Rarely, neurologic symptoms in the absence of anemia may dominate the clinical picture.

Clinical Presentation and Diagnosis of Vitamin B_{12} Deficiency The major clinical manifestations of vitamin B_{12} deficiency are (1) macro-ovalocytic anemia and its many sequelae, (2) gastrointestinal symptoms, including glossitis and the dyspepsia caused by gastric mucosal atrophy, and (3) diverse neurologic abnormalities with degenerative changes of the dorsal and lateral columns of the spinal cord and peripheral nerves.

In the proper clinical setting and with the characteristic peripheral blood findings, in all regards similar to that seen in folate deficiency, a serum vitamin B_{12} level should be obtained. A low value supports the diagnosis of vitamin B_{12} deficiency. Then, an assessment of the cause of the vitamin B_{12} deficiency must be undertaken. If the history suggests no obvious etiology (e.g., malabsorption syndrome), the usual first step is the Schilling test, which involves measuring the amount of absorption of an orally administered tracer dose of radioactive vitamin B_{12} (^{60}Co-labeled). There is reduced absorption of the radioactive vitamin B_{12} in instances where vitamin B_{12} absorption is impaired. If the results of the first Schilling test show low absorption of the vitamin, the test is repeated with orally administered IF given with the tracer vitamin B_{12}. If the second test is normal, then the cause of the deficiency is an absence of IF.

It is important to note that anyone suspected of having vitamin B_{12} deficiency should also be evaluated for concomitant folate deficiency, since the two may coexist. It should again be stressed that the hematologic picture of vitamin B_{12} deficiency is the same as that of folate deficiency.

Therapy of Vitamin B_{12} Deficiency Vitamin B_{12} is usually administered intramuscularly or subcutaneously as cyanocobalamin (vitamin B_{12}) injection. These routes of administration are used, since in most cases vitamin B_{12} deficiency is due to intestinal malabsorption due to IF lack.

The most common cause of lack of IF is the disease, pernicious anemia, in which gastric atrophy and parietal cell loss occur. IF deficiency may also be caused by surgical gastrectomy, destruction of the gastric lining secondary to ingestion of corrosives, and rarely anti-IF antibodies in the gastric secretions. Many different intestinal diseases as well as the ingestion of para-aminosalicylic acid, colchicine, neomycin, ethanol, and potassium chloride impair the absorption of the vitamin. Other causes of decreased absorption of vitamin B_{12}, not involving IF, include infestation with the vitamin B_{12} devouring fish tapeworm *Diphyllobothrium latum*, intestinal bacterial overgrowth syndromes, blind loop syndromes, and chronic pancreatitis. Theoretically, increased requirements for the vitamin include multiple pregnancies, malignancies, and chronic hyperthyroidism. Impaired utilization is the least frequent cause and may be seen in certain rare enzyme deficiencies or chronic nitrous oxide administration. Increased loss is quite rare and occurs in congenital absence of transcobalamin II.

About 90 percent of the total body stores of vitamin B_{12} must be depleted before hematologic evidence of a deficiency state develops. Since the daily requirement of vitamin B_{12} is 1 to 3 μg, an interval of many years must elapse before deficiency symptoms develop after abrupt loss of vitamin B_{12} absorption from any cause.

Many different dosing schemes exist of vitamin B_{12} to replete a deficient patient, and are equally effective, as long as stores of vitamin B_{12} are repleted and all reversible signs and symptoms are corrected. Actually, more than half of the pharmacologic dosages are lost in the urine.

There are oral vitamin B_{12} preparations available. Except for the rarely seen dietary deficiency of vitamin B_{12}, oral preparations have no use in the management of vitamin B_{12} deficiency (e.g., pernicious anemia, or malabsorption), since absorption of these materials is not predictable. It also is axiomatic that use of vitamin B_{12} in the management of anemia not caused by vitamin B_{12} deficiency is contraindicated.

Adverse reactions to vitamin B_{12} are rare. Patients with intrinsic heart disease who become anemic due to deficiency of vitamin B_{12} may develop heart failure following vitamin B_{12} therapy if their blood volume expands rapidly. Rarely, a patient with vitamin B_{12} deficiency may develop polycythemia vera, which had been masked by the lack of vitamin B_{12}.

THE HYPOPROLIFERATIVE NORMOCYTIC ANEMIAS

Aplastic anemia, pure red blood cell aplasia, and anemia of chronic disease are caused by impaired production of mature erythrocytes by the red blood cell (RBC) stem cells of the bone marrow (i.e., marrow failure). Many of these anemias are caused by impaired production of or response to erythropoietin. Others are due to primary loss of the stem cell. Thus, in aplastic anemia, the earliest pluripotent or multi-potent stem cells are affected, and thus, all three mature hematopoietic cell lines are diminished or absent. In pure red blood cell aplasia, the immediate precursor erythroid stem cells are affected thus resulting in anemia alone. The anemia of chronic disease or inflammation occurs in patients with inflammatory or metabolic disease. It, too, is almost always associated with marrow failure, normochromic and normocytic, and is associated with relative or absolute reticulocytopenia. It is these anemias which are associated with inadequate production of or impaired response to erythropoietin.

The most common causes of marrow failure are exposure to environmental toxins, drugs and other chemicals, infectious states usually involving viruses (i.e., hepatitis B virus, human immunodeficiency virus (HIV)), chronic renal failure, and chronic inflammatory states.

The first step in managing a patient with either primary or secondary marrow hypo-proliferation is an investigation of etiology. If the etiology can be reversed or an offending toxin discontinued, then resolution of the anemia may occur. Unfortunately, the etiology of the disorder is often impossible to find, or if found, the damage done to marrow stem cells may be permanent. In either of these two situations, pharmacologic stimulation of the marrow might be attempted. Until recently, only indirect or nonspecific stimulation of the erythroid marrow was possible, but with the cloning and testing of erythropoietin, a more specific therapy is now available.

Erythropoietin

Chemistry and Physiology In 1906, Caznot and Deflandre first suggested that arterial hypoxia generated a humoral factor that was capable of stimulating RBC production. However, it was not until 1977 that this humoral agent was isolated and purified. In 1985, its gene was located on chromosome 7 which allowed sequencing and cloning. The production of recombinant human erythropoietin by molecular genetic technology has allowed its testing in those conditions associated with failure of RBC production. Currently, there are two recombinant human erythropoietin products that are commercially available (under the generic name *epoetin alfa*).

Erythropoietin is a glycosylated α-globulin with a molecular mass of about 30 kDa. In human beings, its primary site of synthesis is in the kidney. This appears to occur within the peritubular cells of the proximal tubule, cortical interstitial cells, or even glomerular cells. Extra-renal sources, primarily the liver, have also been identified but their physiologic importance is unknown.

Physiologic control of erythropoietin production appears to be related primarily to the degree of hypoxemia in the renal circulation. The mechanism by which hypoxemia leads to changes in erythropoietin synthesis and secretion is poorly understood, but it may be mediated through prostaglandin E, cyclic AMP, or changes in intracellular calcium concentration. Direct loss of erythropoietin-producing cells, as seen in progressive renal failure, can lead directly to erythropoietin deficiency with a resultant hypoproliferative anemia. Conversely, erythroid marrow insensitivity to circulating erythropoietin may also result in a hypoproliferative anemia that may be overcome with pharmacologic dosing of the glycoprotein. In inflammatory states, erythropoietin insensitivity may be the result of increased levels of inflammatory cytokines such as interferon gamma.

Mechanism of Action Erythropoietin promotes differentiation of committed erythroid precursors (i.e., burst forming units - erythroid, BFU-E; colony forming units - erythroid, CFU-E) within the marrow microenvironment. Its role during the earlier stages of erythropoiesis is unclear. Erythroid committed stem cells up to the BFU-E possess small numbers of erythropoietin receptors, suggesting a limited role for erythropoietin in the growth of these early forms. The most receptor rich cells are those of the CFU-E and the earliest identified RBC precursor, the pronormoblast. These cells are considered to be the pharmacologic target of erythropoietin therapy. The effect of erythropoietin is to greatly increase the proliferation and maturation of the CFU-E to pronormoblasts. Maturation of these early forms results in reticulocytosis in several days. In 2 to 6 weeks, an increase in circulating RBC mass will result.

Indications In general, the most specific indication for the use of epoetin alfa is in the treatment of a hypoproliferative anemia caused by absolute deficiency of erythropoietin. In addition, epoetin alfa may be used as a drug in hypoproliferative anemias where there is erythropoietin insensitivity that can be overcome by pharmacologic dosing of the hormone. Currently, recombinant human erythropoietin has been approved for only three clinical types of anemias.

1. *Anemia of chronic renal failure* — This disorder is characterized by a loss in the number of erythropoietin-producing cells in the kidney. It produces anemia directly from deficiency or complete lack of erythropoietin.
2. *Zidovudine-treated HIV-infected patients* — This drug-induced anemia has been shown to be due in part to an inappropriately low level of circulating erythropoietin in relation to the anemia. Specifically, in patients with circulating levels of erythropoietin less than 500 mU/mL a significant improvement in the transfusion requirements occurs when these patients are treated with pharmacologic doses of erythropoietin.

3. *Cancer patients on chemotherapy* — Although the anemia of cancer has been shown to be multifactorial, a number of trials have shown a dose-dependent improvement in transfusion requirement if treated with pharmacological doses of erythropoietin. Response also appears to be related to the baseline level of plasma erythropoietin.

Adverse Effects Overall, epoetin alfa is extremely well-tolerated, but significant side effects have been reported in small numbers of patients. These include exacerbation of pre-existing hypertension, seizures, thrombotic events, headaches, arthalgias, and nausea. Some, if not all of these complaints may be related to a rise in the hematocrit. In addition, some patients have reported tachycardia, shortness of breath, hyperkalemia, and flu-like syndrome. Serious allergic reactions with anaphylaxis have not been reported. Occasional reports of skin rashes and urticaria have been noted. There is no evidence of erythropoietin antibody production impairing response to the recombinant products.

Pre-Therapy Iron Evaluation and Folate Supplementation Relative or absolute iron deficiency may occur in patients on chronic hemodialysis. When epoetin alfa is administered, iron stores, if present, may not be mobilized rapidly enough to maximize the erythropoietic response to the drug. In addition, these patients may be folate deficient (because of inadequate diet or excessive plasma folate binding). Thus, it is imperative that all patients who are to undergo therapy with erythropoietin be evaluated for iron deficiency. It is customary to administer supplemental iron and folate to these patients (and to others) who are being treated with erythropoietin.

BIBLIOGRAPHY

Bergeron, R.J., R.R. Streibb, E.A. Creary, R.D. Daniels, Jr., W. King, G. Luchetta, J. Weigand, T. Moerker, and H.H. Peter: "A Comparative Study of the Iron-Clearing Properties of Desferrithiocin Analogues with Desferrioxamine B in a Cebus Monkey Model," *Blood* **81**: 2166-2173 (1993).

Bilgrami, S., A. Bartolomeo, V. Synnott, and F.R. Rickles: "Management of Hemosiderosis Complicated by Coexistent Anemia with Recombinant Human Erythropoietin and Phlebotomy," *Acta Haematol.* **89**: 141-143 (1993).

Carmel, R., and B.S. Skikne: "Serum Transferrin Receptor in the Megaloblastic Anemia of Cobalamin Deficiency," *Eur. J. Haematol.* **49**: 246-250 (1992).

Crosby, W.H.: "Hemochromatosis: Current Concepts and Management," *Hosp. Pract.* **22**: 173-192 (1987).

Dallman, P.R.: "Manifestation of Iron Deficiency," *Semin. Hematol.* **19**: 19-20 (1982).

Dallman, P.R.: "Iron Deficiency and the Immune Response," *Am. J. Clin. Nutr.* **46**: 329-334 (1987).

Das, K.C., and V. Herbert: "Vitamin B-12 and Folate Interrelations," *Clin. Haematol.* **5**: 697-725 (1976).

English, E.C.: "Anemia," *J. Fam. Pract.* **24**: 521-527 (1987).

Erslev, A.J.: "The Discovery of Erythropoietin," *ASAIO J.* **39**: 89-92 (1993).

Eschback, J.W., J.C. Egrie, J.C. Downing, J.K. Browne, and J.W. Adamson: "Correction of the Anemia of End Stage Renal Disease with Recombinant Human Erythropoietin," *N. Engl. J. Med.* **316**: 73-78 (1987).

Finch, C.A., and H. Huebers: "Perspectives in Iron Metabolism," *N. Engl. J. Med.* **306**: 1520-1528 (1982).

Hallberg, L.: "Bioavailability of Dietary Iron in Man," *Annu. Rev. Nutr.* **1**: 123-147 (1981).

Kellermeyer, R.W.: "General Principles of Evaluation and Therapy of Anemias," *Med. Clin. North Am.* **68**: 533-543 (1984).

Mohler, Jr., E.R.: "Iron Deficiency and Anemia of Chronic Disease. Clues to Differentiating these Conditions," *Postgrad. Med.* **15**: 123-128 (1992).

Scott, J.M., J.J. Dinn, P. Wilson, and D.G. Weir: "Pathogenesis of Subacute Combined Degeneration: A Result of Methyl Group Deficiency," *Lancet* **2**: 334-337 (1981).

CHAPTER 35

Anticoagulant and Procoagulant Drugs

Carl Barsigian and José Martinez

The proper maintainance of the fluid nature of blood is critical for adequate perfusion of vital organs and tissues which constitute the living organism. If damage to a blood vessel should occur, however, the ability of blood to clot becomes important in order to prevent the loss of blood or the leakage of blood into the parenchymal tissue of organs. Thus the homeostatic state is a balance between anticoagulant and procoagulant mechanisms which operate to keep the vascular system intact. Perturbation of the endogenous controls of the anticoagulant and procoagulant pathways may have serious consequences. On the one hand, initiation of coagulation in areas of vascular pathology, such as overlying an atherosclerotic plaque, may lead to thrombosis with subsequent ischemia, myocardial infarction, and death. On the other hand, failure of coagulation to occur normally may result in hemorrhage.

Treatment of thrombotic or hemorrhagic disorders frequently involves drug therapy. The rational use of drugs that influence clot formation or dissolution is based on an understanding of the fundamental concepts of the coagulation and fibrinolytic pathways. Our understanding of the basic biochemistry of these processes is rapidly expanding. The following discussion outlines current concepts of these biochemical mechanisms as a foundation for understanding the pharmacology of the anticoagulant and procoagulant drugs.

THE COAGULATION PATHWAY

Hemostasis (i.e., the arrest of bleeding) involves a complex interplay between formed elements such as platelets and endothelial cells, soluble plasma proteins known as clotting factors, and components of the subendothelial extracellular matrix. Within seconds after injury to the vascular endothelium, platelets adhere to the damaged area via interactions between specific platelet-membrane receptors and proteins of the exposed subendothelium. One well-characterized mechanism is mediated by the von Willebrand factor (vWF), a glycoprotein that functions as a molecular bridge between subendothelial matrix components (e.g., collagen fibrils) and a specific vWF receptor, glycoprotein Ib, present on platelet plasma membranes. Adhesion is rapidly followed by platelet aggregation, resulting in formation of the primary hemostatic plug. Aggregation is mediated by the binding of fibrinogen to a receptor, glycoprotein IIb/IIIa, which is exposed on the platelet plasma membrane following platelet activation by agonists such as collagen, thrombin, and adenosine diphosphate (ADP). The latter agonist, which is released from platelets that have been activated by contact with subendothelial collagen, subsequently binds to its platelet receptor, resulting in the synthesis of thromboxane A_2 (Chapter 14), a potent platelet-activating agent that initiates a secondary wave of aggregation with subsequent enlargement of the primary hemostatic plug.

The primary hemostatic plug is fragile and can be disrupted by the shear stress imposed by the flowing of blood. With time, however, the platelet plug undergoes stabilization due to biochemical platelet-platelet interactions and to the localized initiation of the coagulation pathway involving the blood-clotting factors. The consequence of these events is the formation of the secondary hemostatic plug consisting of a network of covalently cross-linked fibrin overlying and intermingled with aggregated platelets and other entrapped vascular cells.

The formation of cross-linked fibrin is the end result of the intricate and tightly regulated series of enzymatic and nonenzymatic reactions and interactions depicted in Fig. 35-1. The clotting

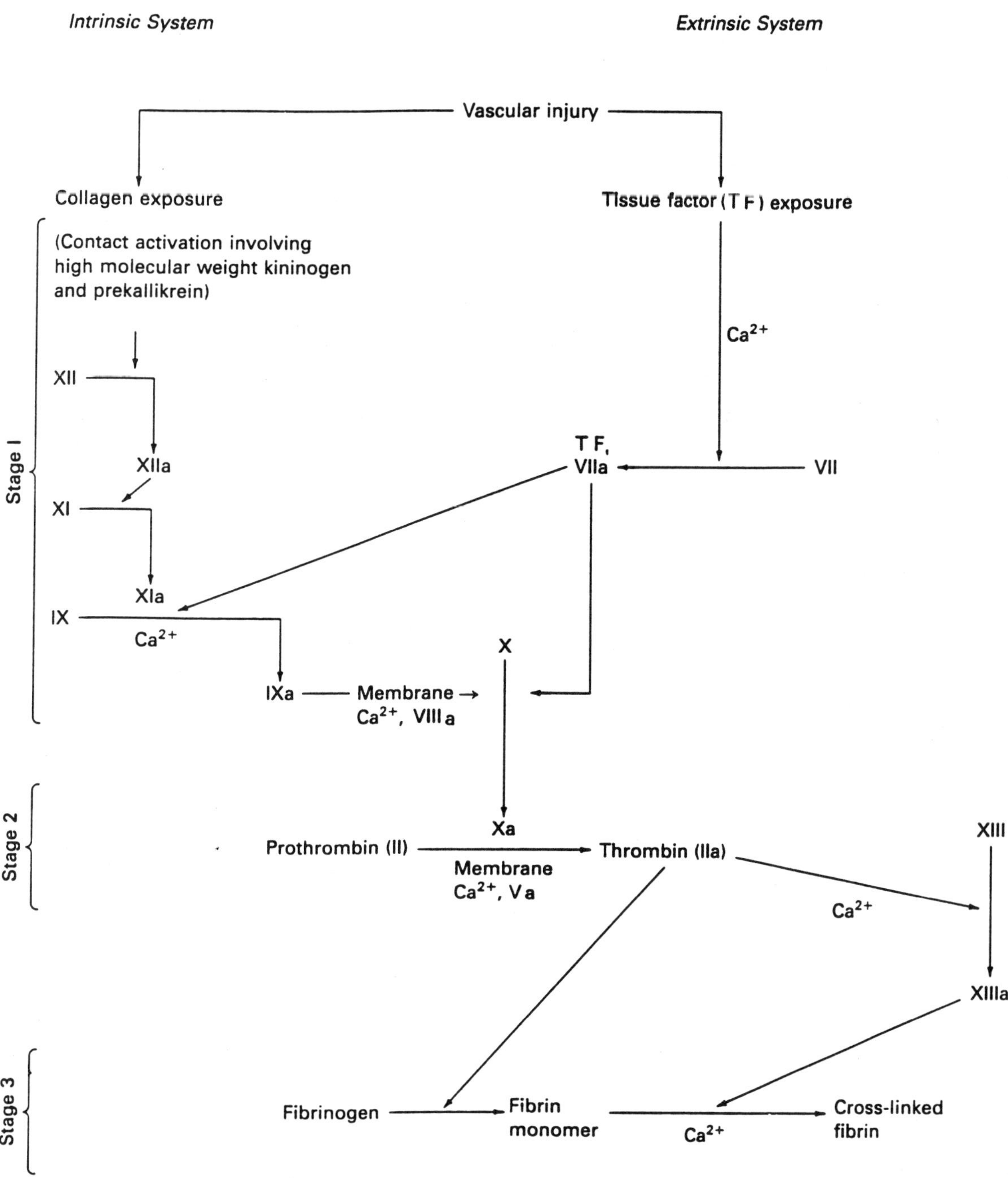

FIGURE 35-1 *The coagulation pathway. Blood coagulation can be viewed as proceeding through three stages: (1) the activation of factor X to factor Xa (which can be initiated via either the intrinsic or extrinsic systems), (2) the conversion of prothrombin to thrombin, and (3) the transformation of fibrinogen into fibrin. Fibrin monomers then spontaneously polymerize and undergo factor XIIIa-mediated cross-linking to form a stabilized fibrin clot.*

factors (Table 35-1) involved in coagulation can be classified either as enzymes or as enzyme cofactors. With the exception of factor XIII, which is a transglutaminase, the other enzymes involved in coagulation are serine proteases which circulate as inactive proenzymes or zymogens. When coagulation is initiated, the zymogens are converted to the active serine proteases by limited proteolysis involving cleavage of a specific bonds in the zymogen molecules. For didactic purposes, the coagulation pathway may be represented as occurring in three stages (Fig. 35-1): (1) the activation of factor X to factor Xa, (2) the conversion of prothrombin (factor II) to thrombin (factor IIa), and (3) the thrombin-mediated transformation of fibrinogen to fibrin. The biochemistry of each of these stages will now be discussed in greater detail.

The first stage of coagulation involves components of both the extrinsic and intrinsic pathways (Fig. 35-1). The extrinsic pathway is thought to initiate coagulation *in vivo*, with the intrinsic pathway contributing to the amplification of coagulation once initiated via the extrinsic system. Both pathways interact to culminate in the activation of factor X to factor Xa. The extrinsic pathway is so named because it requires components not normally present in blood. When a blood vessel is injured in such a way as to result in damage to the endothelial cell lining, blood is exposed to subendothelial fibroblasts and smooth muscle cells which constitutively express a transmembrane glycoprotein known as tissue factor (TF) or thromboplastin. Factor VII (or factor VIIa which may be present in plasma in trace amounts) then binds to TF to form factor VIIa/TF complexes. Once formed, the factor VIIa/TF complex can directly activate factor X, without the involvement of the factor IXa-VIIIa-platelet complex (described below), or it can activate factor IX to IXa, thereby mediating factor Xa generation through an arm of the intrinsic pathway. The activity of the factor VIIa/TF complex is tightly regulated by an inhibitor, known as the tissue factor pathway inhibitor (TFPI), which is associated with the endothelial cell surface and with plasma lipoproteins. The TFPI inhibits the continued activation of factor X to Xa by binding and inactivating the initial factor Xa which is generated. A quaternary complex is formed consisting of TFPI/Xa/VIIa/TF which inhibits further conversion of factor X to Xa and of factor IX to IXa by the factor VIIa/TF complex. However, the inhibitory function of TFPI can be bypassed through the activation of factor IX to IXa mediated by factor XIa which is formed from factor XI, possibly by the action of the initial small amount of thrombin that is generated when coagulation is initiated via the extrinsic system.

As explained above, the intrinsic system is thought to amplify *in vivo* coagulation which is initiated via the extrinsic system. However, it is also possible that blood coagulation *in vivo* may involve surface activation of the intrinsic pathway when blood comes into contact with negatively charged molecules found in the subendothelium. This would be similar to *in vitro* conditions, where the initiation of coagulation via the intrinsic system involves surface or contact activation mediated by four major plasma proteins: high molecular mass kininogen, prekallikrein, factor XII, and factor XI. A major feature of contact activation is the initiating effect of negatively charged artificial surfaces such as kaolin, dextran, or glass. These early events involve the binding of the contact-activation factors to the negatively charged surfaces, resulting in activation and amplification of the procoagulant biochemical reactions. None of these reactions are calcium-dependent, in contrast to the majority of those that follow. In the first calcium-dependent step of the intrinsic pathway,

TABLE 35-1 Clotting factors

International nomenclature	Common name
I	Fibrinogen
II	Prothrombin
III	Tissue factor (thromboplastin)
IV	Calcium
V	Proaccelerin
VII	Proconvertin
VIII	Antihemophilic factor
IX	Christmas factor
X	Stuart-Prower factor
XI	Plasma thromboplastin antecedent
XII	Hageman factor
XIII	Fibrin-stabilizing factor

factor XIa activates factor IX to factor IXa. Factor IXa then activates factor X to factor Xa by a unique mechanism in which a cofactor (factor VIIIa) binds to the platelet surface and serves as a receptor site for the assembly of the calcium-dependent factors IXa and factor X on the platelet surface and dramatically increases the rate at which factor IXa converts factor X to factor Xa.

When factor Xa is generated, the second stage of coagulation is initiated, and prothrombin (factor II) is converted to the active serine protease thrombin (factor IIa). At this step, factor Va (a nonenzyme) serves as a cofactor much in the same manner as does factor VIIIa in the formation of factor Xa. By binding to the surface of activated platelets, factor Va acts as a binding site for factor Xa and prothrombin, thereby greatly accelerating factor Xa-mediated conversion of prothrombin to thrombin. The thrombin formed is released from the platelet surface and activates additional factor V and factor VIII, resulting in a marked increase in further thrombin generation.

When thrombin becomes available in the blood, the third stage in clot formation can proceed. This reaction is the transformation of fibrinogen to fibrin, a unique proteolytic modification that is not calcium-dependent. The action of thrombin as a catalyst promotes the conversion of fibrinogen to fibrin monomers that spontaneously polymerize, resulting in the formation of insoluble fibrils and fibers of fibrin. Simultaneously, thrombin activates factor XIII to factor XIIIa (a transglutaminase, as opposed to a serine protease), which in the presence of Ca^{2+} covalently cross-links the polymerized fibrin, resulting in the formation of a stable fibrin clot. In addition, thrombin may activate factor XI to factor XIa, which can then activate factor IX (Fig. 35-1).

Thrombin plays a central role in the coagulative pathway in that it manifests both procoagulant and anticoagulant properties. As a procoagulant, thrombin functions by promoting platelet aggregation, by activating factors VIII, V, and XI, by transforming fibrinogen to fibrin, and by converting factor XIII to factor XIIIa, which promotes covalent cross-linking of fibrin polymers. In addition to these coagulative properties, thrombin also displays significant anticoagulant activity, which is initiated when it binds to a receptor (thrombomodulin) present on endothelial surfaces (Fig. 35-2). Once bound to thrombomodulin, thrombin is rendered inactive as a procoagulant, but is transformed into a potent anticoagulant by virtue of its ability to activate protein C to protein Ca, which, together with its cofactor protein S, inactivates the two major clotting cofactors (factors VIIIa and Va) thus depressing the coagulation mechanism.

THE FIBRINOLYTIC PATHWAY

Fibrinolysis (i.e., clot resolution) is mediated principally by plasmin, a plasma serine protease derived from the inactive zymogen known as *plasminogen*. Conversion of plasminogen to plasmin involves cleavage of a single peptide bond (Arg_{560}—Val_{561}), resulting in generation of a two-chain disulfide-linked molecule (Fig. 35-3). The heavy chain (N terminus) contains five disulfide-bonded loops, or "kringles," which act as lysine-binding sites and are responsible for the binding of plasminogen and plasmin to specific lysine residues in polymerized fibrin. The light chain (C terminus) contains the active catalytic site of the molecule. Plasminogen activation to plasmin can be mediated via endogenous or exogenous activators. Endogenous activation of the fibrinolytic mechanism can be initiated by the extrinsic or intrinsic fibrinolytic pathways. As in extrinsic activation of coagulation, extrinsic activation of fibrinolysis requires the exposure of blood to factors produced by the blood vessel, while initiation by the intrinsic system involves factors normally present in blood. Activation of the fibrinolytic mechanism initiated by the extrinsic system involves tissue-type plasminogen activator (t-PA), which is synthesized by vascular endothelial cells and released at the local site of thrombosis. The extrinsic system is thought to be the principal plasminogen activator pathway for initiation of fibrinolysis *in vivo*. The t-PA binds to binding sites on fibrin which are in close proximity to plasminogen bind sites. Once the t-PA binds to fibrin, it activates the fibrin-bound plasminogen to fibrin-bound plasmin which initiates fibrinolysis and also converts prourokinase to urokinase (see below) which itself enhances fibrin-bound plasminogen activation thus amplifying the fibrinolytic response to t-PA.

The intrinsic system involves contact activation of factor XII to factor XIIa with subsequent factor XIIa-mediated conversion of prekallikrein to kallikrein, which may result in kallikrein-mediated activation of plasminogen. Kallikrein may also convert plasma prourokinase (also called single-chain urokinase-type plasminogen activator, scu-PA), an endogenous plasminogen activator normally present in plasma but synthesized by extravascular cells such as fibroblasts, to urokinase (also

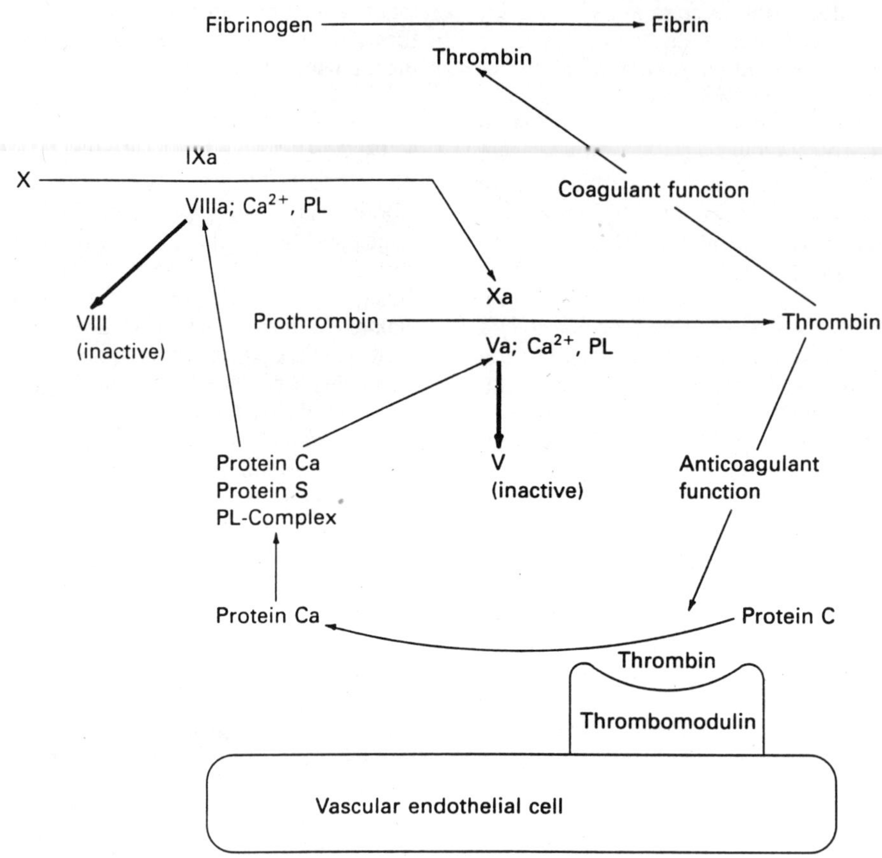

FIGURE 35-2 *The protein C—thrombomodulin anticoagulant pathway. Upon binding to thrombomodulin, a vascular endothelial cell receptor, thrombin is rendered inactive as a procoagulant and transformed into a potent anticoagulant by virtue of its ability to activate protein C to protein Ca, which, in complex with protein S and membrane phospholipids (PL), inactivates factors VIIIa and Va, thereby retarding procoagulant mechanisms.*

called two-chain urokinase-type plasminogen activator, tcu-PA), which is approximately 20,000 times more active than kallikrein in activating plasminogen.

The primary exogenous plasminogen activator, streptokinase, does not occur endogenously in humans, hence the term *exogenous*. Each of these plasminogen activators, with the exception of streptokinase, is a serine protease that activates plasminogen by selective cleavage of the Arg_{560}—Val_{561} peptide bond. Plasmin itself can also cleave this bond and act, in positive feedback fashion, as a plasminogen activator. Once formed, plasmin degrades the insoluble fibrin clot into a series of soluble proteolytic fragments, resulting in the dissolution of the clot (Fig. 35-3). The ability of plasminogen and plasmin to bind to fibrin is important in limiting the proteolytic degradation of circulating fibrinogen and other plasma proteins.

Localized fibrinolysis is a finely tuned homeostatic mechanism much in the same sense as the coagulative mechanism. As mentioned earlier, plasminogen binding to fibrin serves to confine the proteolytic action of plasmin in areas of thrombosis. However, should plasmin become free in plasma, it is normally rapidly inactivated by a specific inhibitor, α_2-antiplasmin, so that circulating fibrinogen (and factors VIII and V) is protected. However, should plasmin generation exceed the capacity of the α_2-antiplasmin neutralizing system, a systemic "lytic state" may result, leading to consumption of fibrinogen, factor VIII, factor V, and other plasma proteins. Localization of fibrinolysis is also mediated by endothelial cells, which

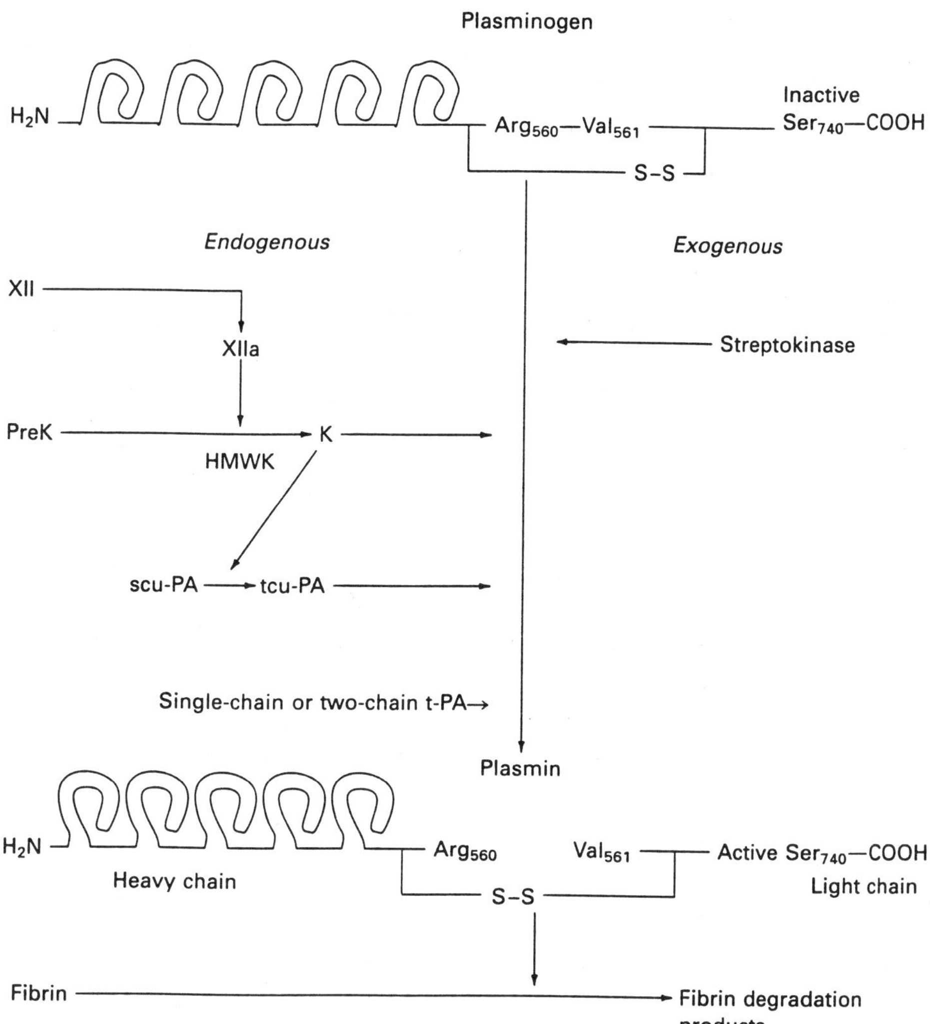

FIGURE 35-3 *The fibrinolytic pathway. Fibrinolysis is mediated by the serine protease plasmin, which is derived from inactive precursor plasminogen. Endogenous plasminogen activators include the enzyme kallikrein (K), single-chain and two-chain urokinase-type plasminogen activators (scu-PA and tcu-PA, respectively), and single-chain or two-chain tissue-type plasminogen activators (t-PA). Streptokinase is a nonhuman protein, and is therefore classified as an exogenous plasminogen activator. Each of these plasminogen activators (with the exception of streptokinase) functions by cleaving the* Arg_{560}*—*Val_{561} *bond of plasminogen, thus generating the two-chain disulfide-linked plasmin molecule.*

synthesize and secrete t-PA, which binds to fibrin and selectively activates the fibrin-bound plasminogen. However, significant amounts of t-PA do not appear to be released at the early stages of clot formation. During this phase, plasminogen activator inhibitors (PAI-1 and PAI-2) are released from platelets and endothelial cells, thereby allowing the assembly of a functional hemostatic clot. Subsequently, inhibitor production decreases and t-PA production increases, with the end result being the breakdown of the fibrin clot and recanalization of the damaged vessel. Several of the plasmin-derived degradation products of cross-linked fibrin (the fibrin-split products) can be assayed in plasma as evidence of active coagulation and fibrinolytic mechanisms.

ANTICOAGULANT DRUGS

Heparin

Heparin is a naturally occurring sulfated polysaccharide found principally in the mast cell granule. During synthesis within the mast cell, polysaccharide chains of molecular masses up to 100,000 Da are covalently linked to polypeptide core proteins forming proteoglycan structures. The polysaccharide chains undergo extensive postsynthetic modifications, and the resulting highly sulfated proteoglycans are stored within basophilic granules. The lysosomes of the mast cell contain proteases and glycosidases which, presumably upon release of granular contents, degrade the heparin-proteoglycan, resulting in the generation of a diverse heterogeneous population of sulfated oligosaccharides (molecular masses from 5000 to 30,000 Da), which constitute the heparin present in extracellular tissue spaces and in the purified preparations that are used clinically. Commercial sources of heparin include porcine intestinal mucosa and bovine lung. The final extracts must be standardized by biologic assay, and the potency of each preparation must be expressed in terms of USP units of heparin activity. Currently, all heparin preparations contain at least 120 USP units per milligram.

Chemistry The heparin molecule is composed of three monosaccharides that occur as repeating disaccharide units of D-glucosamine linked with either D-glucuronic acid or L-iduronic acid (Fig. 35-4). Individual heparin molecules vary considerably in length, and therefore commercial heparin is a molecularly heterogeneous preparation. A majority of the monosaccharides are modified by being either N-acetylated, N-sulfated, or O-sulfated, thereby accounting for the strong negative charge of heparin molecules. Sulfation at critical positions is essential for functional activity (Fig. 35-4), as discussed later.

Mechanism of Action The anticoagulant action of heparin requires the presence of the plasma serine protease inhibitor, antithrombin III (AT-III). The ability of this natural inhibitor to inactivate thrombin is increased markedly in the presence of heparin. A specific pentasaccharide sequence (Fig. 35-4) within the heparin molecule mediates the high-affinity binding of AT-III by heparin. Only about one-third of the molecules present in unfractionated heparin preparations contain this pentasaccharide structure. These molecules are primarily responsible for the antithrombin activity of commercially available heparin.

Binding of AT-III to the pentasaccharide sequence is essential but not sufficient for thrombin neutralization by heparin, as evidenced by the finding that the synthetic pentasaccharide, though still exhibiting high-affinity AT-III binding, fails to inhibit thrombin activity. Because larger oligosaccharides (of greater than 14 monosaccharide units) containing the pentasaccharide structure exhibit both thrombin binding and neutralizing activity, it has been proposed that heparin acts as an anticoagulant by serving as a template to bring in close proximity AT-III and thrombin. Once bound to heparin, a stable bond is rapidly formed between the active center serine of thrombin and a specific arginine residue of AT-III. The thrombin—AT-III complex dissociates from the heparin molecule, freeing the latter to interact with other AT-III molecules and to inactivate additional thrombin.

Experimentally, the heparin—AT-III complex can also neutralize the activity of factors IXa, Xa, XIa, and XIIa. In fact, certain low molecular weight heparins may act as anticoagulants primarily through neutralization of factor Xa rather than thrombin. Theoretically, therefore, heparin can be considered to retard all three stages of blood coagulation: (1) the formation of factor Xa, (2) the factor Xa-mediated conversion of prothrombin to thrombin, and (3) the thrombin-mediated transformation of fibrinogen to fibrin.

Pharmacokinetics Because heparin is a largely negatively charged molecule, it is not absorbed via the oral, sublingual, or rectal routes and is therefore administered parenterally. Intravenous or subcutaneous administration is preferred, since intramuscular injection commonly results in hematomas at the injection site. Heparin is highly bound to plasma proteins (approximately 95 percent), and its apparent volume of distribution is 0.05 to 0.2 L/kg. Depending on the dose, the half-life of heparin varies considerably among patients. The half-life after commonly employed doses of the drug can vary between 1 and 5 h. Because of its extensive binding to plasma proteins, heparin is only minimally available for passive excretion by the kidney. Heparin is biotransformed, by liver heparinase, to inactive products which are excreted in the urine. Heparin itself appears in the urine only after the intravenous administration of large doses. Low urinary excretion, however, fails to account for the rapid loss of heparin from the peripheral blood. The

BACKBONE MONOSACCHARIDES

Glucosamine Glucuronic acid Glucosamine Iduronic acid Glucosamine

(a) $H_2COSO_3^-$ COO^- H_2COR'' (b) OSO_3 COO^- $H_2COSO_3^-$

OH OH OH OH

NH OH $HNSO_3^-$ (a) OSO_3^- $HNSO_3^-$ (a)

R'

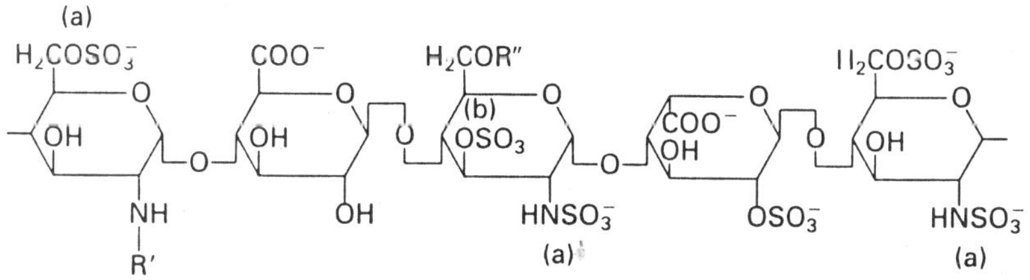

R' = $-SO_3^-$ or $-COCH_3$

R'' = $-H$ or SO_3^-

a = essential for AT-III binding

b = unique to AT-III binding region

FIGURE 35-4 *The antithrombin III binding sequence of heparin. A pentasaccharide sequence consisting of substituted moieties of glucosamine, glucuronic acid, glucosamine, iduronic acid, and glucosamine functions as the antithrombin III (AT-III) binding structure within the heparin molecule. The critical substitutions to these monosaccharides that are involved in the binding of AT-III are depicted in the figure.*

latter observation may be due to extensive binding of heparin to the surface of endothelial cells throughout the vascular tree. Also, it is hypothesized that mast cells may act as a storage depot for exogenously administered heparin. Heparin does not cross the placenta or pass into maternal milk, and is therefore the recommended anticoagulant for use during the first trimester of pregnancy, since warfarin crosses the placenta and can cause fetal malformations.

Adverse Reactions The major toxicity of heparin is bleeding, which may frequently occur from mucous membranes or open wounds. Intracranial hemorrhage can also occur and represents one of the most serious toxicities of heparin therapy. Because of the short duration of action of aqueous heparin, treatment of such hemorrhagic phenomena usually involves decreasing the dose or frequency of injections. Alternatively, the anticoagulant action of heparin can be directly antagonized by the intravenous administration of protamine sulfate, a strongly basic, low molecular weight protein that reacts directly with acidic heparin thus forming an inactive complex. When protamine is used, it is essential to determine the amount of heparin remaining in the patient and to administer equimolar amounts of protamine, because excess protamine can itself induce bleeding, by virtue of its ability to bind to platelets, fibrinogen, and other plasma proteins. To minimize hypotension, bradycardia, or dyspnea, which may result from histamine release from mast cells, protamine should be administered intravenously at a very slow rate of not more than 50 mg in a 10 min period.

Long-term use of heparin (3 months or more of therapy) may cause osteoporosis with spontaneous fractures. Mild to severe thrombocytopenia can occur, which appears to be due to heparin-induced platelet aggregation (mild thrombocytopenia) or to the production of heparin-dependent antiplatelet antibodies (severe thrombocytopenia). The severe form of thrombocytopenia occurs only after several days of therapy and is not dose-related. Platelet aggregation resulting from this mechanism may result in venous or arterial thrombosis, such as stroke or gangrene. Heparin therapy in these patients should therefore be discontinued. Hemorrhage may also result due to the development of thrombocytopenia. Transient and reversible alopecia represents an undesirable but less serious adverse reaction to heparin therapy.

Therapeutic Uses Heparin is indicated as an anticoagulant in the prevention and treatment of deep venous thrombosis (DVT), pulmonary embolism, and arterial thrombosis. For the prophylactic prevention of DVT, the ability of the heparin—AT-III complex to neutralize factor Xa appears to be more important than its inhibitor effect on thrombin. Low-dose heparin (5000 units given subcutaneously two to three times a day) is used prophylactically to prevent thromboembolic complications following surgery, in certain cases of trauma such as fractures, and in patients with acute coronary thrombosis. Whether prophylactic treatment is instituted depends on many factors, such as the age of the patient, the degree of bed rest, the presence of a history of previous thromboembolic disease, and the absence of specific contraindications.

Heparin therapy is monitored by using the activated partial thromboplastin time (aPTT), which normally varies between 20 and 35 sec. Low-dose prophylactic therapy does not require that the aPTT be prolonged. For the therapeutic treatment of established acute thrombotic episodes, larger doses of heparin are used, and the marked inhibitory action of the heparin—AT-III complex on preformed thrombin is central. In the aggressive treatment of DVT or pulmonary embolism, the daily administration of 16,000 to 30,000 units of heparin by continuous intravenous infusion is required so that the aPTT is prolonged 1.5 to 2 times that of baseline. After the initial thrombotic episode is resolved, long-term therapy with adjusted-dose heparin (i.e., subcutaneous injections of increasing doses of heparin every 12 h until the midinterval aPTT is prolonged 1.5 times over baseline) is very effective in preventing the recurrence of venous thrombosis and is associated with a low incidence of bleeding.

Heparin may also be useful as an adjunct in the treatment of coronary occlusion with acute myocardial infarction, especially after fibrinolytic therapy or angioplasty. Anticoagulant therapy reduces the frequency of arterial embolism in patients with arterial fibrillation, mitral stenosis, or prosthetic heart valves. As mentioned above, heparin is the recommended anticoagulant for use during the first trimester of pregnancy, since warfarin crosses the placenta and can cause embryopathy. After the first trimester, however, warfarin may be used because bone and brain development are adequately advanced. Unfortunately, experience has shown that approximately one-third of all pregnancies will terminate in premature delivery or stillbirth. Heparin therapy also carries significant risk of hemorrhage for the mother, and the rational use of anticoagulants during pregnancy remains a controversial area.

Since heparin exerts its anticoagulant effect by combining with preformed factors present in plasma, it is effective not only *in vivo* but also *in vitro*. In this context, it is utilized to prevent coagulation during extracorporeal oxygenation of blood, during hemodialysis, and in blood samples drawn for laboratory analysis. Moreover, it is used routinely in maintaining the patency of indwelling vascular catheters.

Enoxaparin Sodium

One of the disadvantages of heparin is its short duration of action, necessitating 2 or 3 subcutaneous injections daily to maintain prophylactic anticoagulation. Only 15 to 20 percent of subcutaneously injected heparin is absorbed, and it is the low molecular weight fraction which accounts for absorption from the unfractionated product. Knowledge of this fact has lead to the development of a low molecular weight heparin product, enoxaparin sodium, with a mean molecular weight of 2000 to 8000 Da. Enoxaparin is prepared from heparin by chemical depolymerization followed by ion exchange chromatography. It is 90 percent absorbed from subcutaneous sites and can be given twice daily for prophylaxis. The indication for enoxaparin is in hip replacement surgery to prevent deep venous thrombosis. The drug is injected subcutaneously within 24 hours postoperatively and is continued for up to 14 days.

The mechanism of action of the low molecular weight heparin agent is not clear, since antithrombotic properties can be evident in the absence of any alterations in laboratory coagulation studies. However, the neutralization of factor Xa is greater than that of thrombin, since the compound is too small to serve as a template for the AT-III-dependent neutralization of thrombin. Moreover, enoxaparin also has powerful effects on cell-mediated aspects of thrombosis involving endothelial cells and blood cells, and it is likely that its mechanism of action is quite complex, involving several of the biochemical processes which play important roles in the pathogenesis of thrombosis.

Oral Anticoagulants

Warfarin

In contrast to heparin and enoxaparin sodium, warfarin (and all other currently employed oral anticoagulants) is effective only *in vivo*, since it acts by altering the hepatic synthesis of several essential blood-clotting factors.

Chemistry Warfarin, the most commonly employed oral anticoagulant, and dicumarol, the first oral anticoagulant used clinically, are both structural analogs of 4-hydroxycoumarin (Fig. 35-5.) Dicumarol (bishydroxycoumarin) is a dimeric derivative of 4-hydroxycoumarin, which was isolated from spoiled sweet clover and shown to be the causative agent of "sweet clover disease," a fatal hemorrhagic diathesis of cattle prevalent in the 1920s. Dicumarol has been largely replaced by warfarin, which is prepared as the sodium salt of the racemic mixture. Interestingly, the levorotatory isomer of warfarin is several times more potent than the dextrorotatory form.

O O
OH
4-Hydroxycoumarin
(nucleus required for activity)

O O
CH
OH
CH_3
C=O
CH_3
Warfarin

O O O O
CH_2
OH OH
Dicumarol
(Bishydroxycoumarin)

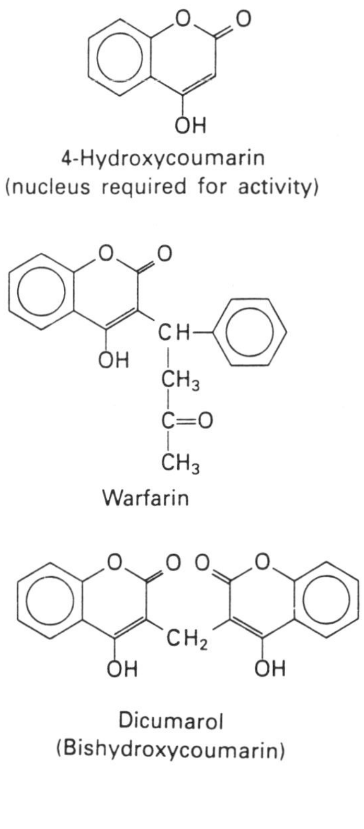

FIGURE 35-5 *Structure of oral anticoagulants. The intact 4-hydroxycoumarin nucleus is essential to the anticoagulant activity of warfarin and dicumarol. Commercial warfarin is supplied as the racemic mixture; however, the levorotatory isomer is severalfold more potent than the dextrorotatory form.*

Mechanism of Action The therapeutic action of warfarin depends on its ability to suppress the formation of biologically functional factors II, VII, IX, and X by the liver. These factors (along with protein C and protein S) are referred to as the *vitamin K-dependent clotting factors*, since their biosynthesis by the hepatocyte is partially linked to hepatic vitamin K metabolism. Vitamin K can be supplied to the liver either from dietary plant sources (vitamin K_1, phylloquinone) or as a metabolite of intestinal flora (vitamin K_2, menaquinone). Though the relative contribution of either form *in vivo* is unknown, it is clear that the quinone form of the vitamin must be reduced to the hydroquinone, which functions as a cofactor in the synthesis of active vitamin K-dependent proteins. Conversion of the hydroquinone to the epoxide form of vitamin K is catalyzed by vitamin K epoxidase and is coupled to vitamin K-dependent carboxylase-mediated γ-carboxylation of glutamic acid residues present in the N-terminal regions of the polypeptide backbones of each of the vitamin K-dependent factors (Fig. 35-6). The exact nature of the coupling between epoxidation and γ-carboxylation remains elusive, but it is well established that γ-carboxylation contributes Ca^{2+}-binding properties to these proteins, conferring on them the capacity to bind to phospholipid surfaces such as platelet membranes and endothelial cell membranes. It appears that a single Ca^{2+} serves as an ionic bridge between 2 (or possibly 3) intramolecular γ-carboxyglutamic acid residues present in the proteins, thereby exposing membrane-binding domains. Whether Ca^{2+} actually serves to link the vitamin K-dependent proteins to the cell membranes remains unknown. However, in the absence of adequate γ-carboxylation, the vitamin K-dependent factors cannot bind to membranes and therefore are nonfunctional in coagulation, even though present at near normal concentrations in plasma.

Warfarin acts as a vitamin K antagonist primarily by blocking the reduction of the epoxide to the quinone form of vitamin K. This reaction is mediated by a poorly characterized vitamin K epoxide reductase that utilizes an unknown endogenous dithiol, *in vivo*, or dithiothreitol, *in vitro*, as cofactor. Conversion of the quinone form to the active hydroquinone appears to be mediated by two enzymes: (a) a warfarin-sensitive enzyme that may be identical or very similar to the dithiol-dependent vitamin K epoxide reductase and (b) a warfarin-insensitive vitamin K reductase that utilizes NAD(P)H, rather than a dithiol, as cofactor (Fig. 35-6). Though the pathway mediated by the

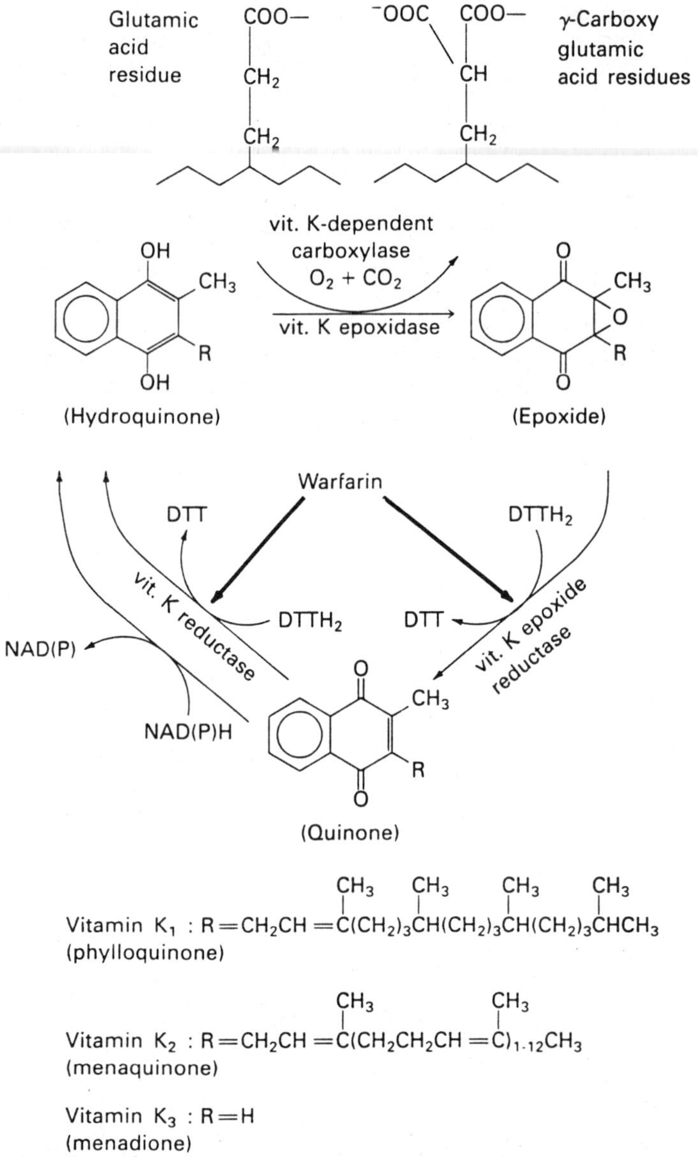

Glutamic acid residue COO^- / CH_2 / CH_2 → ^-OOC COO^- / CH / CH_2 γ-Carboxy glutamic acid residues

vit. K-dependent carboxylase
$O_2 + CO_2$
vit. K epoxidase

(Hydroquinone) (Epoxide)

Warfarin
DTT
$DTTH_2$
vit. K reductase
$DTTH_2$
DTT
vit. K epoxide reductase
NAD(P)
NAD(P)H

(Quinone)

Vitamin K_1 : $R{=}CH_2CH{=}C(CH_3)(CH_2)_3CH(CH_3)(CH_2)_3CH(CH_3)(CH_2)_3CH(CH_3)CH_3$
(phylloquinone)

Vitamin K_2 : $R{=}CH_2CH{=}C(CH_3)(CH_2CH_2CH{=}C(CH_3))_{1\text{-}12}CH_3$
(menaquinone)

Vitamin K_3 : R=H
(menadione)

FIGURE 35-6 *The vitamin K cycle and the mechanism of action of warfarin. Conversion of the hydroquinone form of vitamin K to the epoxide is catalyzed by vitamin K epoxidase and is coupled to γ-carboxylation of glutamic acid residues present in vitamin K-dependent proteins. The γ-carboxylation reaction is catalyzed by vitamin K-dependent carboxylase. Neither epoxidation nor carboxylation is affected by warfarin. Rather, warfarin inhibits the dithiol ($DTTH_2$)-dependent conversion of the quinone to the hydroquinone. See text for further details.*

latter enzyme is only minimally active *in vivo*, the inhibitory effects of warfarin on synthesis of the vitamin K-dependent factors can be overcome by the administration of large doses of the vitamin, which increase vitamin K shunting through this pathway.

Pharmacokinetics Warfarin is absorbed rapidly and completely from the gastrointestinal tract, whereas dicumarol is absorbed more slowly and erratically. Under certain circumstances, sodium warfarin may be administered parenterally. The coumarin anticoagulants are largely confined to the circulation. Binding of warfarin to serum albumin, for example, is approximately 99 percent, resulting in a low apparent volume of distribution (0.1 L/kg). Warfarin is completely biotransformed by the liver drug-metabolizing microsomal system to hydroxylated derivatives that have weak anticoagulant activity. The metabolic half-life of warfarin is approximately 2 days, but the hydroxylated biotransformation products may be excreted in the urine for up to 4 weeks after a single dose.

Adverse Reactions The principal toxicity of warfarin is the direct effect of overdosage, resulting in marked hypoprothrombinemia manifest as ecchymoses and, if not recognized and corrected, fatal hemorrhage. The hypoprothrombinemia can be treated with fresh plasma, which supplies functional vitamin K-dependent blood coagulation factors. In extreme emergency, vitamin K-dependent factor concentrates may be used. Large doses of vitamin K_1 (phytonadione) may also help by increasing shunting through the warfarin-insensitive NAD(P)H-dependent reductive pathway (Fig. 35-6). Vitamin K_3 (menadione) is less effective in this regard. The action of vitamin K begins within 30 minutes following intravenous administration; however, there is a latent period of several hours before its effect on the prothrombin time is obtained. Therefore, when hemorrhage occurs (and depending on its severity), the dose of the anticoagulant should be reduced or discontinued, and vitamin K_1 or fresh plasma may be administered.

Adverse reactions of warfarin, other than hemorrhage, are uncommon and may include alopecia, urticaria, dermatitis, nausea, diarrhea, abdominal cramps, and, on rare occasions, skin necrosis. Warfarin is also contraindicated in the first 10 weeks of pregnancy due to potential embryopathy, which most commonly involves the development of nasal hypoplasia and stippled epiphyses. This type of classic warfarin embryopathy may be due to the biosynthesis of a nonfunctional acarboxy form of the vitamin K-dependent protein osteocalcin, which plays a role in bone ossification. Independent of embryopathy, central nervous system abnormalities have been described when warfarin is used between 10 and 40 weeks of gestation.

Perhaps no other group of drugs is more subject to drug interactions than are the oral anticoagulants. The reason is that the hypoprothrombinemic effect is directly related to the free plasma level of the drug, which is determined not only by the dose but also by the extent of plasma protein binding and by the rate of biotransformation. Table 35-2 lists drugs that may alter the activity of the anticoagulants. In general, the mechanisms responsible for enhanced anticoagulant effects include (1) decreased absorption of vitamin K from the gastrointestinal tract, (2) displacement of the anticoagulant from binding sites on plasma proteins, (3) inhibition of hepatic biotransformation of the anticoagulant, (4) inhibition of platelet aggregation, and (5) reduction in the production of clotting factors. On the other hand, decreased anticoagulant effects may result from (1) induction of the drug-metabolizing microsomal system, or (2) enhancement of the production of clotting factors. These interactions become especially problematic after a patient has become stabilized on an anticoagulant dosage regimen. For example, all the drugs that induce increased activity of the liver microsomal enzyme system cause an increased inactivation of the oral anticoagulants. This decreases their effect for a given dose, so the clinician observing this effect may tend to increase the dose. If at this point the inducing drug is discontinued, the anticoagulant will have a much greater effect and hemorrhage may result. Conversely, the coumarin derivatives are known to increase the blood level of phenytoin and to increase the effect of oral hypoglycemic drugs.

Therapeutic Uses Warfarin and other oral anticoagulants are routinely used for the prophylaxis and treatment of deep venous thrombosis (DVT) and pulmonary embolism. As a result of the mechanism of action of the oral anticoagulants, the therapeutic effect of these agents only occurs *in vivo* and requires several days to become manifest. The anticoagulant action of warfarin is monitored by measuring the prothrombin time (PT), which has a normal range of 11 to 13 sec. Although synthesis of the vitamin K-dependent factors by the liver is decreased almost immediately following absorption of the drug, some time is required before blood levels of the preformed factors fall as a result of normal utilization. Factor VII activity falls rapidly (within 1 day) due to its short biologic half-life (5 to 6 h). This affects the PT but may not prevent thrombosis. Factor IX activity is depressed within about 2 days and also affects the PT. Most importantly though, patients are not adequately anticoagulated until 4 or 5 days, at which time the activities of all factors are sufficiently depressed to provide clinically apparent therapeutic anticoagulation (PT of 1.4 to 2 times control, depending on the nature of the clinical disorder). For this reason, when rapid reduction in

TABLE 35-2 Drug interactions with oral anticoagulants

Mechanism	Drugs
ENHANCED ORAL ANTICOAGULANT ACTIVITY	
Decreased vitamin K absorption	Antibiotics Mineral oil
Displacement from plasma proteins	Salicylates Phenylbutazone Chloral hydrate Clofibrate
Inhibition of biotransformation	Allopurinol Disulfiram Metronidazole Chloramphenicol
Inhibition of platelet aggregation	Aspirin Indomethacin Sulfinpyrazone Dipyridamole
Decreased production of clotting factors	Quinidine
DEPRESSED ORAL ANTICOAGULANT ACTIVITY	
Enzyme induction	Barbiturates Glutethimide Griseofulvin
Increased production of clotting factors	Vitamin K Oral contraceptives

coagulation is required, as in cases involving active thrombosis, heparin is preferred, since it inhibits coagulation almost instantaneously. The time required for the PT to return to normal when oral anticoagulant therapy is discontinued varies more than the time required to produce an effect, and, depending on the drug, may be from 1 to 8 days.

Current therapeutic regimens to treat thrombosis usually start with the administration of heparin to establish immediate anticoagulation during the 4 to 5 days required for the anticoagulant effects of warfarin to reach therapeutic levels. Warfarin therapy is usually continued, under close medical supervision, for 4 to 6 months following an episode of DVT or pulmonary embolism. In patients with DVT, the PT should be maintained at about 1.4 times baseline. In the treatment of arterial embolization in patients with mitral valve disease, warfarin therapy is usually continued for the life of the patient. Warfarin is also indicated for most patients with mechanical prosthetic heart valves.

ANTIPLATELET DRUGS

Platelets play a major role in the pathogenesis of thrombosis by adhering and aggregating at the site of blood vessel damage and by releasing potent vasoconstrictor and pro-aggregative agents, such as thromboxane A_2. The effect of aspirin in reducing platelet aggregation by blocking the synthesis of thromboxane A_2 is discussed elsewhere in this book. A novel approach to pharmacologic blockade of platelet aggregation involves the use of fibrinogen receptor antagonists which prevent fibrinogen from binding to its platelet receptor, glycoprotein IIb/IIIa. Two basic types of fibrinogen receptor antagonists are currently being tested in clinical trials. These include synthetic mimicking-peptides containing the Arg-Gly-Asp tripeptide sequence, which is the motif in the fibrinogen molecule that is recognized by glycoprotein IIb/IIIa, and monoclonal antibodies directed against various regions of the glycoprotein IIb/IIIa molecule. The fibrinogen receptor antagonists are being tested as adjunctive therapy to prevent occlusion of coronary arteries following thrombolytic therapy with fibrinolytic drugs.

Antithrombin III

Deficiencies of antithrombin III (AT-III) can either be hereditary or acquired. Acquired deficiency of AT-III can arise as a result of (1) impaired synthesis such as in acute liver failure, (2) increased loss such as occurs with nephrotic syndrome or during therapeutic plasmapheresis, or (3) increased consumption with conditions such as disseminated intravascular coagulation or acute infections. As a result of AT-III deficiency, patients are predisposed to a variety of thrombotic conditions. The use of AT-III for the prophylaxis or therapy of these thromboembolic episodes is an efficacious treatment which gives greater increases in circulating levels of AT-III, with less volume expansion, than does the infusion of fresh-frozen plasma.

AT-III (human) is a preparation produced from pooled human serum that is available for therapeutic use. It is assayed biologically and dosage is expressed in international units (IUnits)/kg. The drug is used by intravenous infusion for patients with hereditary deficiency to control acute thrombotic episodes or to prevent thrombosis following surgical procedures.

FIBRINOLYTIC DRUGS

Heparin and oral anticoagulants are ineffective in reducing the size of preformed fibrin clots. For this purpose, activation of the endogenous fibrinolytic mechanism via the administration of plasminogen activators such as streptokinase and urokinase is most frequently employed. However, since these first-generation fibrinolytic agents activate plasminogen that is free in plasma, their use is associated with a significant risk of bleeding due to plasma degradation of fibrinogen and other coagulation factors. The discovery of endothelial cell tissue-type plasminogen activator (t-PA), a potent activator of fibrin-bound plasminogen (but not of soluble plasminogen), has generated tremendous interest in the potential development of this agent as a clot-specific fibrinolytic drug.

Streptokinase

Streptokinase (SK), a protein secreted by group C hemolytic streptococci, was the first clinically useful fibrinolytic agent. Unlike other plasminogen activators, SK is not an enzyme and does not itself cleave any bonds within the plasminogen molecule. Rather, it forms an equimolar complex with plasminogen, resulting in SK-plasminogen. Formation of this complex induces a conformational change within the plasminogen that results in exposure of the active site within the molecule forming the SK-plasminogen activator complex which can convert other SK-plasminogen complexes to SK-plasmin complexes or can activate free plasminogen to plasmin, the net result being the lysis of fibrin clots. However, since the drug activates plasminogen which is free in plasma and not bound to fibrin, considerable degradation of plasma fibrinogen can occur resulting in a systemic lytic state. The drug, which has a plasma half-life of 15 to 30 min, is used intravenously to treat patients with acute massive pulmonary embolism and extensive thrombi of deep veins. It is also employed via the intra-coronary or intravenous routes in the treatment of acute myocardial infarction. In this regard, it is crucial to begin fibrinolytic therapy very early (if possible, within 1 h following the onset of symptoms) in order to achieve maximum therapeutic benefit (i.e., increased survival). It is quite clear that fibrinolytic therapy begun later than 6 h following the onset of symptoms is associated with a lower success rate.

The major complication associated with streptokinase therapy is bleeding due to the dissolution of hemostatic plugs and to the consumption of fibrinogen and other coagulation factors. When used via the intra-coronary route in the treatment of acute myocardial infarction, however, the incidence and severity of bleeding are lower, due to the smaller doses used compared with the therapeutically equivalent intravenous dose. On the other hand, intravenous streptokinase therapy is easier to initiate within the crucial first few hours following the onset of symptoms of acute myocardial infarction. Because streptokinase is a foreign protein, it is pyrogenic and antigenic and therefore allergic reactions, including anaphylaxis, may occur.

Anistreplase

Various streptokinase derivatives have been introduced for their use as fibrinolytic agents. The best characterized of these is anistreplase, the anisoylated plasminogen streptokinase activator complex (or APSAC). In this product, the conformationally altered plasminogen molecule of the SK-plasminogen activator complex is acylated at its active center serine and is therefore inactive as such. This prevents the *in vivo* inactivation by α_2-antiplasmin and the activation of free plasminogen, but not the binding of the anistreplase to fibrin. The fibrin-bound anistreplase undergoes spontaneous deacylation with concurrent local generation of active SK-plasminogen activator complex and a more fibrin-selective lytic activity. The half-life of anistreplase is also much longer than that of streptokinase, allowing administration by intravenous bolus injection with sustained fibrinolytic activity and greater protection against re-thrombosis.

Urokinase

Urokinase (UK) is a two-chain disulfide-linked enzyme extracted either from human urine or human kidney cells, which directly cleaves the Arg_{560}—Val_{561} peptide bond in the plasminogen molecule, thus activating plasminogen to plasmin. As with streptokinase, urokinase can produce systemic plasminogen activation with development of the lytic state. Prourokinase (i.e., scu-PA) is relatively more clot-specific than urokinase and therefore produces less systemic plasminogen activation with a lower incidence of bleeding.

The indications for these intravenous products are similar to those for streptokinase. Urokinase is used in the treatment of peripheral arterial thrombosis and for flushing indwelling catheters. Since urokinase and prourokinase are endogenous proteins, they are not antigenic. Nevertheless, allergic reactions such as skin rash, bronchospasm, and febrile reactions do occur.

Alteplase

Tissue-type plasminogen activator (t-PA) is a glycoprotein of 70 kDa which is synthesized by vascular endothelial cells. In contrast to most other serine proteases, t-PA does not appear to occur in zymogen form. The enzymatic activity of t-PA can be increased by treatment with plasmin, which cleaves a single peptide bond converting the single-chain t-PA to a disulfide-linked two-chain form. In the presence of fibrin, however, both forms exhibit similar activity. Alteplase is a t-PA produced by recombinant DNA technology, biologically equivalent to natural t-PA.

Serving as the major endogenous promoter of fibrinolysis, alteplase binds avidly to fibrin, where it proteolytically cleaves the Arg_{560}—Val_{561} bond of fibrin-bound plasminogen, converting the latter to the active disulfide-linked, two-chain plasmin molecule, which mediates the degradation of the cross-linked fibrin clot (Fig. 35-3). Alteplase is extremely inefficient at activating plasminogen which is not bound to fibrin. Consequently its action is preferentially localized to areas of thrombosis, and the tendency of alteplase to produce systemic fibrinogenolysis is much lower than that of either streptokinase or urokinase.

Experimentation has revealed a significant dose-related fibrinolytic effect of alteplase. Furthermore, clinical trials using the drug have demonstrated recanalization of occluded coronary arteries within 30 to 60 min with re-perfusion rates that range from 70 to 85 percent of normal. However, clinically significant bleeding occurs in some patients, presumably due to lysis of good clots in areas of vascular injury, manifest principally as cerebral hemorrhage. The incidence of other adverse reactions associated with alteplase are very low, and it does not produce the allergic reactions and hypotension seen with streptokinase. It is, however, much more expensive than streptokinase.

Both natural t-PA and alteplase have very short biologic half-lives (approximately 3 min) and are removed from the circulation mainly by the liver. For this reason, alteplase is administered by continuous intravenous infusion. In the treatment of acute infarction, the intravenous route of administration is as efficacious as the intra-coronary route. This is due to the clot-specific nature of the substance.

PROCOAGULANT DRUGS

Systemic Procoagulants

The systemic procoagulant drugs currently employed act either by replacement of deficient clotting factors (antihemophilic factor and factor IX complex), by increasing the plasma concentrations of endogenous clotting factors (desmopressin), or by inhibition of the natural fibrinolytic mechanism (aminocaproic acid and tranexamic acid).

Antihemophilic Factor Hemophilia A is an X-linked genetic disorder characterized by a deficiency of factor VIII (antihemophilic factor). As a consequence, these patients experience episodic bleeding disorders such as hemarthroses, intramuscular hematomas, hematuria, and intracranial hemorrhage.

Factor VIII manifests a half-life of 8 to 12 h and can be supplied as fresh (or fresh-frozen) plasma, cryoprecipitate, or lyophilized concentrates (the latter two are prepared from fresh or fresh-frozen human plasma). Antihemophilic factor is also produced by recombinant DNA technology; this product is a purified glycoprotein with the same biological activity as factor VIII found in human plasma. Fresh or fresh-frozen plasma contains, by definition, 1.0 IUnit of factor VIII coagulant activity per mL, and is therefore frequently unsuitable for replacement therapy due to potential volume overload, which may result if administration of high levels of factor VIII activity is required. The other preparations offer an advantage in this regard since they are more concentrated; for example, when reconstituted, cryoprecipitate contains 50 to 150 times as much factor VIII as an equal volume of fresh plasma. In addition, the various concentrates are convenient for self-administration by the patient and can be stored at ambient temperatures. The foregoing preparations are effective in reducing spontaneous hemarthroses, deep hematomas, and bleeding after trauma or surgery.

A major problem with the administration of factor VIII-containing products derived from human plasma is the risk of iatrogenic non-A, non-B hepatitis and acquired immune deficiency syndrome (AIDS). Various purification modalities (e.g., monoclonal antibody immunoaffinity chromatography) have been employed to eradicate the AIDS virus from factor VIII preparations; however, the risk of non-A, non-B hepatitis still poses a potential (but rare) clinical problem. Factor VIII prepared in this manner is 99.9 percent pure and is virtually free of infectious hepatitis or AIDS viruses. The development of factor VIII by recombinant DNA technology will even further reduce the chances of viral infection and will no doubt result in diminished use of factor VIII concentrates which have been the mainstay of therapy in the past.

Factor IX Complex A highly purified human factor IX complex is used to replace factor IX in patients with hemophilia B, who suffer from an X-linked genetic deficiency of factor IX. Patients treated with the complex manifest a dose-dependent increase in plasma factors IX, X, XI, and XII. Since all of the available preparations are heat-treated fractions of human plasma, all pose the small risk of viral infections.

Desmopressin Desmopressin functions by increasing the titers of endogenous clotting factors. This agent, which is a structural analog of the pituitary hormone vasopressin, functions by stimulating the release of endogenous pools of factor VIII into the circulation. As a result of this action, it is used to promote hemostasis in mild classic hemophiliac patients or patients with von Willebrand's disease who undergo minor surgery such as tooth extraction or tonsillectomy. It is ineffective in patients with severe classic hemophilia, since these patients do not have sufficient endogenous pools of factor VIII. Only patients with baseline titers of factor VIII over 5 percent of normal usually respond. The antidiuretic action of desmopressin may lead to electrolyte imbalance and fluid overload, though this is rare. For this purpose, desmopressin is administered intravenously.

Aminocaproic Acid Aminocaproic acid, though not a procoagulant per se, is effective in decreasing hemorrhage with surgical procedures. Aminocaproic acid is a structural analog of lysine, differing only by the absence of the α-amino group. Because binding of plasminogen or plasmin to fibrinogen or fibrin is mediated by lysine groups present within the fibrin or fibrinogen structure, aminocaproic acid functions as a competitive inhibitor of plasmin(ogen) binding to fibrin, thus reducing the activity of the fibrinolytic mechanism and shifting the homeostatic balance in favor of coagulation. Aminocaproic acid can be administered orally or intravenously. It is rapidly absorbed from the gastrointestinal tract, has a serum half-life of 1 to 2 h, and is excreted unchanged in the urine (greater than 90 percent within 24 h). Its concentration in urine can be up to 100-fold greater than in plasma, and it is therefore very useful for treating bleeding from the urinary tract.

Tranexamic Acid Like aminocaproic acid, tranexamic acid is a lysine analog that functions as a competitive inhibitor of plasmin(ogen) binding to fibrin(ogen). Tranexamic acid lacks the α-amino group of lysine, but contains two additional carbon atoms that form a six-membered ring structure. As a result of these molecular differences, it is 6 to 10 times more potent than aminocaproic acid, but overall the two drugs manifest very similar pharmacokinetic profiles.

Topical Procoagulants

Thrombin Thrombin is prepared from bovine plasma and is used topically to arrest minor bleeding and oozing of blood from abraded or otherwise open vessels when it is impractical to use ligation or pressure techniques or when these techniques are unsuccessful.

Absorbable Gelatin Absorbable gelatin is a specially prepared form of gelatin (denatured collagen) that has been processed so that it is porous, nonantigenic, and completely absorbed after application. The material is available as a sterile film and sterile sponge for topical use in many fields of surgery and as a sterile powder for decubitus ulcers and chronic leg ulcers.

Oxidized Cellulose Oxidized cellulose is surgical gauze that has been treated with nitrogen dioxide. When it comes in contact with tissue fluid, it forms a sticky and gummy artificial clot that provides mechanical hemostasis.

BIBLIOGRAPHY

Benedict, C.R., S. Mueller, H.V. Anderson, and J.T. Willerson: "Thrombolytic Therapy: A State of the Art Review," *Hosp. Prac.*, **June 15**: 61-72 (1992).

Broze, G.J.: "The Role of Tissue Factor Pathway Inhibitor in a Revised Coagulation Cascade," *Semin. Hematol.* **29**: 159-169 (1992).

Collen, D.: "Human Tissue-type Plasminogen Activators: From the Laboratory to the Bedside," *Circulation* **72**: 18-20 (1985).

Collen, D., and H.R. Lijnen: "Fibrinolysis and the Control of Hemostasis," in *The Molecular Basis of Blood Diseases*, Stamatoyannopoulos, G., A.W. Nienhuis, P. Leder, and P.W. Majerus (eds.), Saunders, Philadelphia, 1987, pp. 662-668.

Collen, D., D.C. Strump, and H.K. Gold: "Thrombolytic Therapy," *Ann. Rev. Med.* **39**: 405-423 (1988).

Fareed, J., D.A. Hoppensteadt, and J.M. Walenga: "Current Perspectives of Low Molecular Weight Heparins," *Semin. Thrombos. Hemost.* **19**: 1-11 (1993).

Furie, B., and B.C. Furie: "The Molecular Basis of Blood Coagulation," *Cell* **53**: 505-518 (1988).

Hirsh, J., and M.N. Levine: "Low Molecular Weight Heparin," *Blood* **79**: 1-17 (1992).

Hull, R., and J. Hirsh: "Long-term Anticoagulant Therapy in Patients with Venous Thrombosis," *Arch. Int. Med.* **143**: 2061-2063 (1983).

Jorgensen, M.J., B.C. Furie, and B. Furie: "Vitamin K-Dependent Blood Coagulation Proteins," Arias, I.M., W.W. Jakoby, H. Popper, D. Schachter, and D.A. Shafritz, (eds.), in *The Liver: Biology and Pathobiology, 2nd ed.*, Raven Press, New York, 1988, pp. 495-503.

Lindahl, U., and L. Kjellen: "Biosynthesis of Heparin and Heparin Sulfate," in *Biology of Proteoglycans*, Wight, T.N., and R.P. Mecham (eds.), Academic Press, Orlando, 1987, pp. 59-104.

Marder, V.J., and S. Sherry: "Thrombolytic Therapy: Current Status: 1," *N. Eng. J. Med.* **318**: 1512-1520 (1988).

Marder, V.J., and S. Sherry: "Thrombolytic Therapy: Current Status: 2," *N. Eng. J. Med.* **318**: 1585-1595 (1988).

Miescher, P.A., and E.R. Jaffe (eds.): "Human Factor VIII:C Purified Using Monoclonal Antibody to von Willebrand Factor," *Semin. Hematol.* **25 (Suppl. 1)**: 1-45 (1988).

Nemerson, Y.: "Tissue Factor and Hemostatis," *Blood* **71**: 1-8 (1988).

Rappaport, S.I., and Rao, L.V.M.: "Initiation and Regulation of Tissue Factor-Dependent Blood Coagulation," *Arteriosclerosis and Thrombosis* **12**: 1111-1121 (1992).

Rosenberg, R.D.: "The Heparin-Antithrombin System: A Natural Anticoagulant System," Colman, R.W., J. Hirsh, V.J. Marder, and E. W. Salzman (eds.), in *Hemostasis and Thrombosis: Basic Principles and Clinical Practice, 2nd ed.*, J.B. Lippincott, Philadelphia, (1987), pp. 1373-1392.

Schafer, A.I.: "Focusing on the Clot: Normal and Pathologic Mechanisms," *Ann. Rev. Med.* **38**: 211-220 (1987).

Verstraete, M., and D. Collen: "Thrombolytic Therapy in the Eighties," *Blood* **67**: 1529-1541 (1986).

PART VII

The Gastrointestinal System

SECTION EDITOR

Joseph R. DiPalma

CHAPTER 36

Vitamins

David R. Schneider

Vital substances found in fruits, green vegetables, and certain other foods, that prevent or eliminate particular diseases or suffering complications in humans have been known since ancient times. The actions of these essential substances, which have been classified as vitamins, have always been taught intuitively from one generation to another. Now these substances are among some of the new therapies for cancer, endocrine diseases, blood disorders, and mental health as a result of our increasing knowledge of how they act in altering the function of cells.

Vitamins are classified into two major categories according to their solubility in lipids or water. Eleven agents are commonly organized and understood to be vitamins. Four of these are fat-soluble substances, and include vitamins A, D, E and K. The remaining seven are water-soluble, and include thiamine (vitamin B_1), riboflavin (Vitamin B_2), pyridoxine (vitamin B_6), niacin (nicotinic acid), ascorbic acid (vitamin C), folic acid, and cyanocobalamin (vitamin B_{12}). The latter two agents are discussed under the subject of antianemia agents (Chapter 34). Information concerning Vitamin K is discussed in the chapter on anticoagulants (see Chapter 35).

From a pharmacologic point of view, there is little difference between food and drugs. Both are handled by the body as chemicals which have to be absorbed, metabolized, and excreted. If the substance happens to be a carbohydrate, protein, or fat, it can be utilized to produce energy and provide building blocks for body structures (amino acids for example). The vitamins and certain minerals are essential as cofactors in specific metabolic reactions. Ordinarily vitamins cannot be synthesized and must be obtained from outside sources (exceptions: vitamin D and niacin). Minerals also cannot be manufactured by the body and must be supplied from external sources. The concept then is that nutritionally there is a daily requirement of caloric-producing substances (carbohydrates, fats, and proteins) plus essential vitamins and minerals.

FEDERAL REGULATION

In the United States the Food and Drug Administration (FDA) regulates the labeling of vitamin and minerals sold as food or drugs. The FDA has adopted as official the U.S. RDA (Recommended Daily Allowances) which is produced by the Food and Nutrition Board of the National Research Council. It is revised every 5 years and recommends daily doses of vitamins and minerals which are certain to prevent deficiencies and also are not so large as to cause toxicity. The RDAs are most useful in the preparation of diets by hotels and hospitals and to provide, as mentioned, the labeling basis of all prepared food items. The public has learned to read these labels and thus insure themselves of an adequate intake of vitamins. Actually vitamins are so well promoted that additional vitamins are taken by most Americans. Most nutritionists advise that supplemental doses of vitamins be taken only under conditions of an inadequate diet, pregnancy, and unusual physical stress.

Supplemental doses are usually only 1.5 to 3 times the RDA. There is fad of calling certain vitamin preparations *megadoses*. These are seldom more than 3 to 5 times the RDA. Vitamin C has been recommended in doses of 2 to 8 g a day (33 to 133 times the RDA) which is obviously excessive. Fortunately vitamin C is relatively nontoxic. However, doses of vitamins in excess of 10 times the RDA must be considered as pharmacologic and presumed to have effects beyond the ordinary metabolic function of the vitamin. For example, niacin is used as a drug to lower blood lipids in doses of 2 to 8 g a day. It has entirely different pharmacologic actions than when it is used in the RDA dose to cure pellagra. Vitamins A and D cannot be administered in daily doses exceeding 2 times the RDA because they are extremely toxic. Fat-soluble vitamins are stored in the body and thus accumulate contributing to toxicity.

THE FAT-SOLUBLE VITAMINS: A, D, E, and K

Vitamin A

Research into carotenoids and retinoids has attracted the attention of many scientists since the discovery of vitamin A. Recent developments into the possible roles of these substances, apart from their classical purpose in vision, have focused on their properties in human nutrition. In particular, their actions in cancer development and prevention are of great interest.

Vitamin A is found in a number of foods, but especially in eggs, milk, vegetables, and in fish liver oils. The precursors to vitamin A, known as the carotinoid pigments, are present in colored vegetables and fruits. The RDAs for vitamin A range from 1,400 International Units (IU) for infants, to 5,000 IU for adult males and 6,000 IU for pregnant females.

Biochemistry, Pharmacology, & Molecular Biology
Because the effects of vitamin A vary with tissue type and often with the form of vitamin A itself, a complete understanding of the mechanism(s) of action still has not been attained. For example, the action of vitamin A may be at the level of genomic expression, at the membrane level, or both. Intercellular and intracellular transport of vitamin A are facilitated by specific binding proteins but probably not in the cellular uptake of vitamin A. Subcellularly, vitamin A may exert a direct effect on transit through the Golgi apparatus, as observed from both biochemical and morphological studies. Recent work using cell-free systems has shown that retinol stimulates transition vesicle formation from endoplasmic reticulum in a GTP-requiring step.

Two pathways have been suggested for the conversion of carotenoids to vitamin A in mammals: central cleavage and eccentric cleavage. An enzyme, β-carotenoid-15,15'-dioxygenase, has been partly purified from the intestines of several species and has been identified in several other organs and species. The enzyme converts β-carotene into two molecules of retinol, requires molecular oxygen, and is inhibited by sulfhydryl-binding and iron-binding reagents. Most provitamin A carotenoids, including the β-apo-carotenols, are cleaved to retinol by these enzymes.

Retinoids, including retinol and retinoic acid (RA), achieve their effects by binding to intracellular proteins, the retinoic acid receptors (RAR), which include: RAR-α, RAR-β, and RAR-γ. These proteins bind retinol, retinaldehyde, and retinoic acid for purposes of protection against decomposition, solubilizing them in aqueous medium, rendering them nontoxic, and for transporting them within cells to their site of action. Binding proteins also function by presenting the retinoids to appropriate enzymes for metabolism.

Finally, RA-binding proteins function in the nucleus by attaching to promoter regions of a number of specific genes to stimulate their transcription and thus affect growth, development, and differentiation. These receptors function as transcription factors by binding to RA-responsive elements of multiple genes. Once bound to the gene through this mechanism, retinoids play a role in vision; embryogenesis; immune modulation; growth and differentiation of normal, premalignant, and malignant tissues; the suppression of carcinogenesis; and the inhibition of tumor growth in experimental systems and humans.

Vitamin A (retinol) and its metabolite, retinoic acid, are major factors involved in differentiation and in maturation of the lungs. Lack of this dietary micronutrient causes a reversible keratinizing squamous metaplasia of the bronchopulmonary tree. Vitamin A is also involved in pulmonary gene expression. Both adult and fetal lungs accumulate retinyl esters, the storage form of vitamin A, and both contain specific retinol- and RA-binding proteins. Lung tissue expresses several isoforms of nuclear RAR, and it is these proteins which are involved in the activation and repression of specific genes regulated by retinoic acid. Finally, prematurely born human neonates who are given vitamin A, show significant improvement and reduced morbidity as a result of an acceleration in lung maturation.

Many cell types require a continuous supply of retinol, and in mammals, liver perisinusoidal stellate cells play an important role as a main store of body retinol. Extrahepatic vitamin A-storing stellate cells are found in higher vertebrates when excessive doses of vitamin A are administered.

However, at this time it is not clear whether these cells also play a role in retinol metabolism under normal conditions.

Role in Metabolism (Nutrition) Vitamin A function depends not only on adequate tissue stores of the vitamin, but also on the ability of cells to generate functionally active forms of the vitamin. Among endogenous and exogenous factors that adversely affect vitamin A homeostasis are the polyhalogenated aromatic hydrocarbons. These substances, universally present as environmental pollutants, will cause disturbances in vitamin A metabolism, often evident by the accelerated metabolism of vitamin A and its metabolites and an overall depletion of vitamin A from the body, a sequence of events which accounts for vitamin A deficiency-like symptoms with polyhalogenated aromatic hydrocarbon intoxication.

Vitamin A as a Teratogen It is well-known that toxic levels of vitamin A have the possibility of acting as a teratogen. In several reports, experimental evidence points to the teratogenicity of natural and synthetic retinoids in animals. Data confirming an effect in humans are not as good; nevertheless, case series, case reports, and some epidemiological data regarding isotretinoin suggest that synthetic retinoids are teratogenic in humans. High dosages of vitamin A and retinoids are teratogenic and the use of isotretinoin in pregnancy is associated with a high risk of congenital malformations. Some retinoid metabolites (e.g., 4-oxo-transretinoic acid and retinyl palmitate) have also been related to teratogenicity. Studies in premature infants support the concept that supplements of vitamin A (to achieve normal serum retinol concentrations) reduces the pulmonary damage caused by hyperoxia. Thus, on the side of potential therapeutic applications, injudicious use of vitamin A is associated with previously unsuspected toxicity in the fetus and newborns. Until more is known about the mechanisms of placental transfer and control as well as about the dose-related teratogenicity of vitamin A at different stages of gestation, there are few justifications for routine ingestion by fertile women of supplemental vitamin A in excess of 8,000 to 10,000 IU. Exceptions may be made when clinical signs are evident and normal diets are unusually deficient. Even then, however, high dosages should be restricted to single administrations followed by frequent or daily dosages not exceeding 10,000 IU. Available evidence indicates that high-dosage supplements of β-carotene can be taken safely.

Deficiency Syndrome The initial indication of vitamin A deficiency in humans is an inability to see in dim light. This effect is due to a deficit in the amount of rhodopsin or visual purple present in the retina. The second clinical sign is the appearance of white spots that are observable in the retina with an ophthalmoscope. After the appearance of these two clinical signs, vitamin A deficiency will proceed through a series of corneal changes beginning with xerosis and progressing through keratomalacia. If such conditions are reached, there is a high probability of permanent deformity of the cornea, iris or lens.

During clinical conditions of vitamin A deficiency, a general failure of mucus and tear secretion by the lacrimal glands, which lubricate and moisten the eyes, lead to infections and ulceration. Partial or complete blindness may result. Prolonged and severe vitamin A deficiency will also become manifest in clinical signs affecting other epithelial tissues, including the skin, the gastrointestinal tract, the urinary tract, the lung, and the respiratory tract.

Vitamin A deficiency is a serious problem throughout the developing world. An estimated 25 to 50 million children may well suffer the physiologic consequences of vitamin A deficiency; about 5 million develop xerophthalmia, of whom 250,000 to 500,000 go blind every year; and untold numbers are at increased risk of diarrhea, respiratory disease, and death. Even mild vitamin A deficiency has been associated with up to a tenfold increase in mortality, and controlled field trials have demonstrated vitamin A supplements can reduce childhood death rates by 30 to 70 percent.

Three general intervention strategies exist for improving vitamin A status of high-risk, rural, economically deprived populations. These include: nutrition education leading to increased dietary intake, vitamin A fortification of centrally-processed, widely consumed dietary items, and periodic administration of large doses of vitamin A. At present, the latter is far and away the most widely employed intervention activity, because of its immediate impact, and because it can be implemented through the existing (and specialized) health care infrastructure.

Pharmacological Use High levels of vitamin A have been advocated as a preventative measure in order to maintain a healthy epithelium in persons exposed to respiratory pollutants (e.g., cigarette smoke). Some animal studies have indicated that vitamin A can lessen carcinogenesis in animals exposed to respiratory carcinogens.

General Toxicity Indiscriminate use of vitamin A can cause serious toxicity. Toxic manifestations in children consist of hyperostosis, giving rise to painful swellings. In adults, dry, itching skin; hyperkeratosis; and altered liver function, with coarse, dry and sparse hair are seen. Acute toxicity causes hypertension, an increase in cerebral spinal fluid pressure, headache, nausea and vomiting.

Toxicity has been associated with abuse of vitamin A supplements and with diets extremely high in preformed vitamin A. Consumption of 25,000 to 50,000 IU/day for periods of several months or more can produce multiple adverse effects. The lowest reported intakes causing toxicity have occurred in persons with liver function compromised by drugs, viral hepatitis, or protein-energy malnutrition. Certain drugs or other chemicals may markedly potentiate vitamin A toxicity in animals. Especially vulnerable groups include children, with adverse effects occurring with intakes as low as 1,500 IU/kg/day, and pregnant women, with birth defects being associated with maternal intakes as low as approximately 25,000 IU/day. The maternal dose threshold for birth defects cannot be identified from present data. An identifiable fraction of the population surveyed consumes vitamin A supplements at 25,000 IU/day and a few individuals consume much more. β-Carotene is much less toxic than vitamin A.

Any assessment of the toxic effects of vitamin A derivatives must distinguish between vitamin A (i.e., retinol and retinoic acid) and its synthetic derivatives. And, just as no single description is universally applicable to the mode of action of vitamin A derivatives, so too do their toxic effects defy generalization. Recommendations from 1982 may be chemically logical, but unusable for the description of effects or side effects of vitamin A derivatives. Retinol, frequently used as synonym for vitamin A, can eliminate all symptoms of vitamin A deficiency if it is taken in sufficient quantity with the diet. Retinoic acid and its derivatives (including the synthetic ones) might be referred to as retinoids, since they do not cover the whole spectrum of effects exerted by retinol and because they also vary markedly in their side effects. Retinoic acid cannot be reduced to retinol in the organism.

Neurotoxicity Vitamins contain reactive functional groups necessary to carry out their established roles as coenzymes and reducing agents. These active site are thought to be responsible for the production of cellular injury if vitamin concentrations, their distribution, or their metabolism are altered. However, identification of vitamin toxicity has been difficult. The only well-established human vitamin neurotoxic effects are those due to hypervitaminosis A (pseudotumor cerebri) and pyridoxine (sensory neuropathy). In each case, the neurological effects of vitamin deficiency and vitamin excess are similar.

Closely related to the neurological symptoms of hypervitaminosis A are symptoms including headache, pseudotumor cerebri, and embryotoxic effects reported in patients given a vitamin A analog or a retinoid. Most tissues contain retinoic acid and vitamin A receptors, members of a steroid receptor superfamily known to regulate development and gene expression.

Vitamin A toxicity is also a good general model of vitamin neurotoxicity, because it shows the importance of the ratio of vitamin and vitamin-binding proteins in producing vitamin toxicity and of permeability barriers of the central nervous system (CNS). Because vitamin A and analogs enter the CNS better than most vitamins, and because retinoids have many effects on enzyme activity and gene expression, vitamin A neurotoxicity is more likely than that of most, perhaps all, other vitamins.

Megadose vitamin therapy may cause injury that is confused with disease symptoms. High vitamin intake is more hazardous to peripheral organs than to the nervous system, because the entry of vitamins into the CNS is restricted. Vitamin administration into the brain or cerebrospinal fluid, recommended in certain disease states, is hazardous and best avoided. The lack of controlled trials prevents defining the lowest human neurotoxic dose of any vitamin. Large differences in individual susceptibility to vitamin neurotoxicity probably exist, and ordinary vitamin doses may harm occasional patients with genetic disorders.

The Link Between Cancer and Vitamin A There are now a significant number of epidemiologic studies establishing that vitamin A is associated with a reduced risk for some forms of human cancers. These types of studies have also attempted to distinguish effects of retinol from those of β-carotene. Major findings consistently show that β-carotene is associated with reduced risk for a number of human cancers, particularly epithelial cancers. By contrast, retinol is generally found to be either not associated with, or positively associated with, an increased risk for many cancers, including those associated with the esophagus, oral cavity, pharynx, larynx, stomach, colon, and rectum.

When dietary studies alone are considered, the findings have been notably consistent, showing an approximate 50 percent reduction in risk associated with high vs. low consumption of carotene-containing fruits and vegetables. Most studies in which serum β-carotene was assayed have found lower levels of β-carotene in people who subsequently developed lung cancer. Unlike carotene, blood retinol levels do not reflect dietary intake under normal conditions and, as might be expected, have failed to show a consistent relation with risk of lung cancer. Although epidemiological studies have not strongly supported the role of preformed retinol as a protective agent, animal studies have provided convincing evidence that retinol and synthetic retinoids are protective against epithelial tumors including those of the lung.

In contrast to retinol or β-carotene however, a strong connection for cancer prevention and vitamin A exists in the field of lung cancer. The incidence of lung cancer in the United States has stabilized in recent years, but it remains a major cause of death. Secondary prevention, aside from removing tobacco from the environment, suggests there might be a reduction in such cancers with chemoprophylactic treatment of smokers and ex-smokers. Results of clinical trials in head and neck cancer have demonstrated effective inhibition of the development of second primary tumors with the synthetic retinoid 13-*cis*-retinoic acid, encouraging investigators that similar results can be repeated in patients with lung cancer.

Therapeutic Uses of Other Retinoids In addition to the therapeutic uses of vitamin A and β-carotene, there are a number of retinoid derivatives useful in severe and refractive dermatological diseases.

Tretinoin (*trans*-retinoic acid, vitamin A acid) is used topically and indicated for the therapy of acne vulgaris. Unlabeled uses include certain forms of skin cancer, lamellar ichthyosis, and Darier's Disease. A popular and widespread use is to cure wrinkles in aging skin. The evidence that it is actually of benefit in this condition is doubtful. The compound has all of the toxicities of vitamin A, but is much safer when used as a topical preparation. Toxicity is usually restricted to the skin and consists of an inflammatory response which may proceed to blistering and crusting. Exposure to ultraviolet light is to be avoided when tretinoin is being used.

Isotretinoin (13-*cis*-retinoic acid) is a drug used systemically for the therapy of a severe form of nodulocystic acne vulgaris. It should not be used for less severe forms of acne since it is extremely toxic. It has been used in the therapy of keratosis follicularis and other forms of skin diseases characterized by keratosis and ichthyosis. Isotretinoin has also found use in various forms of skin and mucous membrane cancers such as mycosis fungoides and leukoplakia. Since it is actually high dose vitamin A therapy, all of the toxicities of this vitamin are possible. Extreme care must be exercised to avoid teratogenic effects. Females of child-bearing age must have a pregnancy test before therapy and must use strictly controlled contraceptive measures.

Etretinate, another retinoid used systemically, is an aromatic compound for the therapy of severe refractory psoriasis. It is of little use in acne and should only be used in psoriasis when other treatments have failed. Etretinate is often combined with psoralen/ultraviolet light photochemotherapy. Like isotretinoin, etretinate has all the toxicities of vitamin A. Precautions must be exercised against teratogenicity. The pharmacokinetic properties of the drug makes it even more potentially dangerous than vitamin A or isotretinoin. Etretinate and its active metabolities accumulate in fat and plasma after continuous administration. The half-life for elimination is at least 100 days and it has been detected in plasma as long as 3 years after termination of therapy. Consequently, it is not known how many years must elapse before safe pregnancy can be allowed.

Vitamin D

Vitamin D is a general term for the description of steroids that increase the absorption of calcium and phosphorus from the intestine. Under ultraviolet irradiation, various steroid procurers will produce different vitamin Ds. At present there are three major forms of vitamin D, identified as vitamins D_1, D_2 and D_3. Vitamin D_3 is present in fish liver oils, and is produced in the skin by the action of sunlight on 7-dehydrocholesterol. Ergocalciferol, vitamin D_2, is obtained by the irradiation of ergosterol.

Besides its classical actions in calcium metabolism (see Chapter 38), it is clear that the hormonal form of vitamin D has many functions, which have only been discovered following the elucidation of its receptor. In addition, because of the vitamin D-based endocrine system, the use of vitamin D compounds in treating a variety of diseases has been expanded. For example, it is now known that in addition to stimulating the intestine to absorb calcium and phosphorus, the bones to mobilize calcium and phosphorus, and the kidney to cause increased renal reabsorption of calcium, 1,25-dihydroxy vitamin D_3 (1,25-$(OH)_2$ D_3, calcitriol) can also stimulate and suppress parathyroid hormone actions. Moreover, vitamin D is a developmental hormone necessary for the recruitment of cells for osteoclast formation, for female reproduction, for development of skin, and for the treatment of certain malignant conditions.

Vitamin D_3 is hydroxylated by mixed-function monooxygenase NADPH-cytochrome P-450 ferredoxin/ferredoxin reductase systems in liver parenchyma and renal proximal tubular cells, to 25-hydroxy vitamin D_3, and finally to 1,25-$(OH)_2$ D_3, the active hormone. Advanced methods for measuring components of the vitamin D endocrine system have been developed and involve column extractions, liquid chromatographic purifications (also HPLC) and protein- and receptor-binding assays as well as mass spectrometry. These have facilitated elucidation of vitamin D physiology (also in pregnancy and lactation) and of metabolic defects in classical, vitamin D resistant and renal rickets and osteomalacia, in sarcoidosis and in the possible involvement of the vitamin in cell differentiation (e.g., in myeloid leukemia), and breast cancer.

Role in Metabolism (Nutrition) The hormonally active form of vitamin D, 1,25-$(OH)_2$ D_3, is a secosteroid and the principle mediator of vitamin D, producing biological effects in over 28 target tissues. Within target tissues, biological responses can be generated either by a signal transduction mechanism, which involves a nuclear receptor for 1,25-$(OH)_2$ D_3 that modulates gene transcription, or a signal transduction pathway which involves rapid opening of calcium channels which are located externally on the plasma membranes.

It is well established that 1,25-$(OH)_2$ D_3 can up-regulate or down-regulate the expression of genes involved in cell proliferation, differentiation, and mineral homeostasis. Genomic effects are brought about through interactions of the hormone with its receptor, a member of the superfamily of hormone-activated nuclear receptors that regulate eukaryotic gene expression. Ligand-bound receptor acts as a transcription factor that binds to specific DNA sequences (HREs) in target gene promoters. DNA-binding domains of the steroid hormone receptors are highly conserved, and contain two zinc-finger motifs that recognize HREs. Both the spacing and orientation of the HRE half-sites, as well as the HRE sequence, are critical for proper discrimination by the various receptors.

Deficiency Syndrome A deficiency of vitamin D results in the clinical condition of rickets, a disorder characterized by a disturbance of calcification of bones and teeth in children. In this insufficiency, bones become soft, have swollen epiphyses, and lack a normal calcification. This clinical situation sets up further conditions in which bones bend and distort under muscular movements. In adults, osteomalacia can occur.

Pharmacological Uses Vitamin D therapy involves one of two available sources. The more important source is cholecalciferol (vitamin D_3), which is produced photochemically in the skin from the provitamin; the other source, 7-dehydrocholesterol or the vitamin D ingested with food, is of secondary importance, but assumes a critical role when an individual is deprived of solar exposure. Both rickets and/or osteomalacia are easily reversed by the provision of sunlight or small oral doses of the vitamin. Alternatively, ergocalciferol (vitamin D_2) can be used.

There are other conditions in which small doses of the vitamin are ineffective, whereas larger doses of vitamin D can achieve healing of the bone disease. Collectively, these conditions are called vitamin D-resistant diseases and include: hypoparathyroidism, genetic and acquired hypophosphatemic osteomalacias, renal osteodystrophy, vitamin D-dependent rickets, and the osteomalacia associated with liver disease and intestinal malabsorption. Unfortunately, large doses of vitamin D continue to be prescribed for a wide variety of diseases in which there is little scientific evidence of their efficacy.

Vitamin D and Cancer It was proposed in 1980 that vitamin D and calcium could reduce the risk of colon cancer, based on studies showing a decreasing gradient of mortality rates from north to south, and suggesting a mechanism related to the influence of ultraviolet light-induced vitamin D metabolites on calcium metabolism. More recently, a study of 1,954 Chicago men found a 50 percent reduction in colorectal cancer with a dietary intake of greater than 3.75 μg of vitamin D; if the accompanying intake of calcium was at least 1,200 mg daily, there was a 75 percent reduction in colorectal cancers.

Psoriasis Calcitriol, the physiologically active metabolite of vitamin D_3, as previously noted, has the ability to regulate growth and differentiation in many cell types. Among the more responsive cells are epidermal keratinocytes. As a result of this interaction, calcitriol has been used in trials involving hyper-proliferative and immune-mediated diseases. In double-blind, placebo-controlled multicenter studies, topical calcitriol has been shown to be both efficacious and safe for the short-term and long-term treatment of plaque-type psoriasis. Additional studies are ongoing involving the use of this compound in the treatment of itchy noses, cancer, and autoimmune diseases. Results from such investigations illustrate that it is possible to separate the vitamin D effects on the cellular level from those on calcium metabolism not only *in vitro*, but also in a clinical setting.

Bone Loss Osteoporosis Osteoporosis, a disease that results in approximately 1.2 million fractures each year in the U.S., has a substantial morbidity and mortality as well as financial impact each year. Considerable progress in our understanding of this disorder is underway, even though most clinical studies include only early postmenopausal individuals. It is clear that major epidemiologic, physiologic, and clinical differences exist between early postmenopausal and older individuals.

The role of vitamin D (hormonally active) seems indispensable in the dual processes of bone formation (mediated by osteoblasts) and bone resorption (mediated by osteoclasts). A substantial amount of evidence now supports the claim that vitamin D_3 tightly regulates differentiation of osteoclast progenitors into osteoclasts. Osteoclast progenitors, believed to be derived from the monocyte-macrophage lineage, are modulated by osteoblastic stromal cells, one of the target cells for the nuclear actions of vitamin D_3.

Toxicity Vitamin D is pharmacologically inactive except for its influence on calcium and phosphorus metabolism. As discussed above, large doses of vitamin D can mobilize bone calcium. The movement of large amounts of calcium will produce rarefaction of bone and metastatic calcification in the kidney, as well as in the eye, where the effects are particularly prominent in the cornea and conjunctiva.

Vitamin D can be associated with significant morbidity when prescribed in large doses. Clinically, vitamin D intoxication can be manifest as periarticular calcinosis, and nephrocalcinosis with hypertension and chronic renal failure and hearing loss. Prolonged therapy with prednisone, a phosphate-binding antacid, phenytoin, and etidronate disodium provides an improvement of calcinosis but no improvement in renal function or hearing loss.

Vitamin E

Vitamin E is commonly recognized to be a group of eight naturally occurring fat-soluble nutrients called *tocopherols*. Dietary intake of vitamin E is essential in many species including humans. In humans, of all the tocopherols, α-tocopherol has the highest biological activity and the highest molar concentration of lipid-soluble antioxidants. α-Tocopherol is absorbed through the lymphatic pathway and is transported in association with chylomicrons. In plasma, α-tocopherol is found in all lipoprotein fractions, but is most often associated with apo B-containing lipoproteins in man. After intestinal absorption and transport with chylomicrons, α-tocopherol is generally transferred to liver parenchymal cells where most of this vitamin is stored. α-Tocopherol is secreted in association with very-low-density lipoproteins (VLDLs) from the liver. Most α-tocopherol is located in mitochondrial fractions and in the endoplasmic reticulum of tissues; little is found in cytosol and peroxisomes.

It is the high-affinity receptor for low-density lipoproteins (LDLs) which has been demonstrated to function as a mechanism for delivery of vitamin E to cells. LDL, as a carrier, is specific for D-α-tocopherol, the most active biological form of vitamin E in humans.

Vitamin E is well accepted as one of the most effective lipid-soluble, chain-breaking antioxidant agents. In humans, it can protect cell membranes from peroxidative damage resulting from free radical-mediated pathology. In addition to immediate damage to cells in stroke, or ischemia, free radical damage has been implicated in the development, over time, of degenerative diseases and conditions, including cancer, aging, circulatory conditions, arthritis, cataracts, pollution, and strenuous exercise.

Biochemistry α-Tocopherol performs an antioxidant role in biological membranes by acting as a one-electron reductant. Singlet molecular oxygen, $^1O_2$, has been shown to be generated in biological systems and is capable of damaging proteins, lipids, and DNA. Tocopherols and thiols, compounds with low quenching rate constants, occur at higher levels in biological tissues and contribute almost equally to the protection of tissues against the deleterious effects of $^1O_2$. Vitamin E is also effective in preventing the nitrosation of amino substrates under physiological conditions, and if used together with vitamin C provide an even stronger inhibiting effect on the formation of N-nitrosamine. Such a mechanism is suggested as a means to reduce human exposure to carcinogenic N-nitrosamine.

Role in Metabolism (Nutrition) Vitamin E is found in many vegetable oils, and is especially high in wheat germ oil. It is so widely distributed that a dietary deficiency is all but impossible to achieve, except for a transient problem in premature infants. In most adults, it is an absorption defect that is responsible for deficiency. Adults also have a larger tocopherol requirement when the intake of large amounts of unsaturated fats occurs.

Individuals with an assortment of enteropathies, hemolytic anemias, acute respiratory distress syndrome, hepatitis, or Gaucher's disease, as well as those on total parenteral nutrition and/or hemodialysis, often have low ("deficient") blood levels of vitamin E.

In persons with glucose-6-phosphate dehydrogenase deficiency, sickle-cell anemia, or P-thalassemia, the administration of 800 IU/day of vitamin E results in an improvement of clinical hematological parameters. A supplement of 300 IU/day over a 3 to 6 month period can improve walking distances and blood flow in patients with intermittent claudication. In a series of limited controlled studies, 300 to 600 IU/day has resulted in improvement in premenstrual syndrome, tardive dyskinesia, and arthritis. And finally, epidemiological studies suggest that high plasma levels of vitamin E are associated with lower risk of certain cancers, cardiovascular disease, and infections.

In some instances, high tissue and/or plasma levels of vitamin E are difficult to obtain by diet alone. High levels of vitamin E are contraindicated in subjects who are receiving vitamin K antagonists as anticoagulant therapy. However, except for this interaction with vitamin K, there are no specific side effects associated with high doses of vitamin E. Consequently, there may be reasons for supplements with vitamin E and, with the exception of an interaction with vitamin K, the risks associated appear to be quite low.

Deficiency Syndrome A deficiency of vitamin E is often apparent by an observation of accelerated red blood cell destruction and neuromuscular deficit. Neurological dysfunction has been observed in adults with prolonged vitamin E deficiency resulting from lipid malabsorption.

The most common clinical signs of a vitamin E deficiency are associated with neurological dysfunction, myopathies and, as noted above, a diminished erythrocyte life span. There is a well-known detrimental effect of vitamin E deficiency on the nervous system of humans and several experimental animal models. However, only in the past 10 years has vitamin E become recognized as essential for the maintenance of the structure and function of nerves in humans. The discovery of a neurologic role for vitamin E is primarily a result of the identification of a degenerative neurologic syndrome in children and adults with chronic vitamin E deficiency, a problem brought about by gastrointestinal diseases impairing fat and vitamin E absorption.

In various animal species, a deficiency of vitamin E is known to result in specific clinical problems. Among these are infertility and muscle and brain impairments. Some of these conditions have counterparts in human situations. Yet, vitamin E treatment of any of these conditions does not show a significant therapeutic effect. A vitamin E deficiency syndrome has been described in premature infants however, that is characterized by edema, anemia, thrombocytosis, and erythematous papular eruption of the skin, followed by a desquamation. This condition is treatable with vitamin E. A second example is shown in children with severe chromic steratorrhea, and low blood levels of α-tocopherol, who have a high creatinuria; this condition can also be reversed by the administration of α-tocopherol.

As suggested above, in the absence of absorption defects, clinically manifest vitamin E deficiency is extremely rare in the adult. Besides a general diet with a supply exceeding the average RDAs, vitamin E is widely advertised in health magazines for the treatment of multiple conditions, including dermatoses and idiopathic leg cramps to cardiovascular disease and for the improvement of athletic ability and sexual performance.

Treatment of Vitamin E Deficiency Megadoses of vitamin E, ranging to 1 g/day, are generally well-tolerated by adults. Data from animal studies however indicate that there are possible inhibitory effects of such treatments, with major problems involving collagen synthesis, wound repair, and importantly, in the utilization of vitamin A.

Cancer There are numerous *in vivo* and *in vitro* experiments that illustrate that supplementing of diet with vitamin E, within a certain dose range, will reduce the risk of chemical- and radiation-induced cancers. *In vitro* studies have shown that α-tocopheryl succinate could induce differentiation and growth inhibition in certain animal and human tumor cells in culture. By contrast, neither α-tocopherol by itself, α-tocopheryl acetate, nor α-tocopheryl nicotinate were effective. The succinate form of α-tocopherol has other actions as well: reducing basal and ligand-stimulated adenylate cyclase activity, and the expression of c-*myc* and H-*ras* oncogenes in tumor cells in culture.

The relative efficacy of various forms of vitamin E in cancer prevention for either animal or human models has not been evaluated; however, some human trials utilizing vitamin E alone or in combination with other nutrients are in progress. In one series of experiments, serum α-tocopherol concentration was studied for its prediction of cancer in a cohort of 36,265 adults in Finland. During a follow-up over 8 years, cancer was diagnosed in 766 persons. Levels of serum α-tocopherol determined from stored serum samples from these cancer patients and from matched control subjects indicated that individuals with low levels of α-tocopherol had about a 1.5-fold risk of cancer compared with those with a higher level. The strength of the association between the serum α-tocopherol level and cancer risk varied for different cancer sites, but was strongest for some gastrointestinal cancers and for the combined group of cancers unrelated to smoking. The association was also strong for men who did not smoke and among women with low levels of serum selenium. In other studies however, the results of such studies on whether vitamin E intake reduces the risk of cancer do not generally support the hypothesis of its protective effect.

Cardiovascular Myocardial ischemia is a disease process characterized by reduced coronary blood flow, such that the supply of nutritive blood to heart muscle (myocardium) is insufficient for normal myocardial aerobic metabolism. Reestablishment of coronary flow, either by invasive or noninvasive clinical procedures, is the most direct and effective means of limiting myocardial damage in ischemic heart disease patients. It is also known that re-perfusion carries with it an injury component that reflects, in some degree, toxic effects of partially reduced oxygen species and their participation in degenerative cellular processes, e.g., membrane lipid peroxidation.

Vitamin E, as a lipophilic, chain-breaking antioxidant, is a prominent membrane constituent in heart muscle. In that tissue it modulates and regulates various aspects of heart muscle cellular metabolism and function. The beneficial effects of vitamin E against experimentally-induced oxidative damage to the heart, together with inverse epidemiological correlations between plasma vitamin E levels and either anginal pain or mortality due to ischemic heart disease, suggests that vitamin E might have protective and therapeutic roles against myocardial ischemic re-perfusion injury.

Laboratory investigations have demonstrated that vitamin E supplements protects isolated hearts against ischemic re-perfusion injury. Other more limited data document the cardioprotective effects of vitamin E in some animal models of myocardial ischemic re-perfusion. These effects are most prominent when the vitamin is administered prior to the ischemic period.

Clinical attempts to establish whether vitamin E has therapeutic benefit in ischemic heart disease patients remain inconclusive at this time, because they have generally relied on non-uniformly controlled protocols and only a single, rather subjective endpoint (anginal pain). Compelling clinical evidence regarding the therapeutic potential of vitamin E in the ischemic heart disease patient is lacking at this time.

Other animal experiments suggest that a deficiency in vitamin E may be related to arterial lesions. Pharmacological studies in animal models of spontaneous atherosclerosis and some retrospective epidemiological studies in man suggest that vitamin E, as the principal (if not sole) lipid-soluble chain-breaking tissue antioxidant, might have therapeutic benefit as an antiatherosclerotic agent. Such a suggestion has gained support from *in vitro* evidence illustrating the influence of vitamin E on cells and lipoproteins most likely involved in the pathogenesis of spontaneous atherosclerosis.

Immune Function In addition to its role in relieving certain neurologic syndromes, there is evidence that vitamin E supplements improve both *in vivo* and *in vitro* parameters of immune function. Presently, certain investigators believe that vitamin E may be crucial for maintenance of high levels of immune response. It is thought that supplemental vitamin levels, and especially both vitamins A and E, activate alveolar macrophages. Alveolar macrophages are primary immune targets and are believed to be especially important in preventing pulmonary infection and cancer.

Abnormalities of immune components present in the acquired immunodeficiency syndrome (AIDS) are similar to those stimulated or restored by intake of high doses of vitamin E. Dietary supplements of vitamin E with an adequate nutrition support or concomitant use of this vitamin with current drug therapies (e.g., zidovudine) is suggested to improve the therapeutic efficiency of such agents and to enhance any immune resistance to opportunistic infections associated with AIDS. A moderately high dose of vitamin E may be used to target and stimulate some specific immune cells destroyed by human immunodeficiency virus (HIV) infection.

Toxicity Commonly available publications on the "prophylactic" and "therapeutic" use of vitamin E allow the conclusion that toxicity of vitamin E in adults is extremely low. And, in animal experiments it is concluded that vitamin E has neither mutagenic, teratogenic, nor carcinogenic properties. As a result, based on studies in humans, a daily dosage of 100 to 300 mg vitamin E can be considered harmless from a toxicological point of view.

From double-blind studies involving a large number of subjects, it has been demonstrated that large oral doses of up to 3,200 USP Units/day led to no consistent adverse effects. It should be noted however that an oral intake of high levels of vitamin E could exacerbate the blood coagulation defect of vitamin K deficiency caused by malabsorption or anticoagulant therapy.

Reports of toxicity to orally administered vitamin E are rare in infants; however, reports suggest an increased risk of sepsis and necrotizing enterocolitis when plasma (or serum) vitamin E levels exceed 3.5 mg/dL. Levels this high are seldom seen when intake is 25 mg of α-tocopherol equivalent/(kg/day) or less.

THE WATER-SOLUBLE VITAMINS: THIAMINE, RIBOFLAVIN, NIACIN, PYRIDOXINE, and ASCORBIC ACID

Many of the water-soluble vitamins are essential parts of coenzymes and have major functions in the enzymatic machinery of the cell. Because these substances are water-soluble, absorption from the gastrointestinal tract is usually not a problem; however, their water solubility makes them easy to be excreted by the kidney. Through kidney excretion, significant amounts of any of these factors can be removed. None of these vitamins are stored in the body, and if not replenished, are rapidly depleted.

Thiamine (Vitamin B_1)

Biochemistry Thiamine, in the form of thiamine pyrophosphate or co-carboxylase, is essential in the decarboxylation of α-ketoacids, e.g., pyruvic acid and α-ketoglutarate. This substance also functions as a connecting link between the glycolytic cycle, the high-energy producing (Krebs) citric acid cycle, and the hexose monophosphate shunt. Thiamine is unique among the B vitamins in that it activates the guanylate cyclase/cyclic GMP system and not the adenylate cyclase/cyclic AMP system. Thiamine pyrophosphate, the active coenzyme of thiamine, is an antiberiberi substance.

Thiamine itself is a pharmacologic antagonist of acetylcholine, and this has been used as an explanation for nerve lesions seen in thiamine deficiency. There are multiple sources of thiamine, including liver, pork, yeast, and rice-polishings. Certain common foods, e.g., tea leaves and the viscera of fresh water fish, are known to contain antithiamine factors.

A recent study has shown a significant variability in the excretion of the water-soluble vitamins, and especially vitamin B_1 (range 11 to 25 percent) by normal individuals over a 24 hour period. This uncertainty did not improve even when laboratory values were expressed on the basis of creatinine. If accurate determinations are necessary, more than twice weekly sampling of blood levels are suggested, and daily monitoring of urine excretion may be required.

Role in Metabolism (Nutrition) Thiamine is found in many foods, whole grain cereals, milk, meats, fish, and eggs. The RDA ranges from 0.3 mg/day for infants to 2.0 mg/day for physically active men, women, and children.

Deficiency Syndrome The original disease in which thiamine was deficient was known as *beriberi*, and was due to the consumption of polished rice. Now, with fortified cereals and breads, this disease is never seen the United States. However, deficiencies are seen in the United States in alcoholics, and in Korsakoff's psychosis. Beriberi may be classified into three types:

Dry beriberi: a chronic form in which neurologic involvement is prominent,

Wet beriberi: an acute form with congestive heart failure and in a less acute state, in which edema is the most characteristic manifestation, and,

Infantile beriberi: still found in the Far East; it has manifestations of cardiology problems, labored breathing, cyanosis, and finally cardiac arrest.

A thiamine deficiency neuropathy, with typical complaints of weakness and burning feet, are often regarded as trivial by attending physicians. Unfortunately, this disorder is increasing in incidence in our society. Sensitive electrophysiologic studies often provide supportive evidence to aid a diagnosis, especially when chronic pain therapy is ineffective.

Pharmacological Uses The treatment of thiamine deficiency is usually with oral administration of thiamine. In medical emergencies, thiamine can be administered by intramuscular injection. Because thiamine is a quaternary ammonium compound, intravenous administration may manifest a curare-like action; even more of a problem would be the introduction of a fatal anaphylactic shock due to vasodilatation and rapid fall in blood pressure.

Since patients with beriberi often exhibit multiple deficiencies, they should also receive the other water-soluble vitamins in therapeutic quantities.

Specific Therapies with Thiamine The long-term use of furosemide in patients with congestive heart failure is associated with clinically significant thiamine deficiency via urinary loss. This deficit may be prevented or corrected by appropriate thiamine supplements.

Several neuropathological reports in the last 5 years have described brain lesions characteristic of Wernicke's encephalopathy in patients with AIDS. Thiamine deficiency in these patients most likely results from the cachexia and catabolic state characteristic of AIDS. A recent study now recommends that dietary thiamine supplements be initiated in all newly diagnosed cases of AIDS or AIDS-related complex. Conventional wisdom suggests that Korsakoff's psychosis, an amnesiac disorder associated with prolonged alcohol consumption, is the chronic outcome of a thiamine deficiency first exhibited as Wernicke's encephalopathy. Studies in alcoholics with Wernicke's encephalopathy suggest that during the acute stage, there is bilateral damage to the blood-brain barrier that is completely relieved after a one week course of treatment with thiamine.

Toxicity Oral thiamine has a very low toxicity. As suggested above, thiamine deficiency is not uncommon in certain populations and clinical disease states such as Wernicke's encephalopathy or beriberi. For such conditions, rapid parenteral repletion may be required. Questions about the safety of intravenous thiamine have been raised because of reports of anaphylaxis. However, a prospective evaluation of the safety of thiamine hydrochloride, given as a 100 mg intravenous bolus, when tested in 989 consecutive patients (1,070 doses) found only 12 adverse reactions (1.1 percent).

Riboflavin (Vitamin B_2)

Riboflavin is present in the body as flavin mononucleotide and as flavin adenine dinucleotide, a coenzyme of the flavoprotein enzymes. Riboflavin influences epithelial integrity, tissue flavin concentrations, the rates of prostaglandin biosynthesis, and the rate of glutathione metabolism. In addition to their importance in sustaining life, each of these interactions have important implications for carcinogenesis.

Sources Riboflavin occurs in milk, green leafy vegetables, egg yoke, and in liver, kidney, and other meats. The RDA ranges from 0.4 mg for infants to 1.5 mg for active adult males.

Role in Metabolism (Nutrition) NADPH-dependent methemoglobin reductase, first detected in erythrocytes sixty years ago, has the ability to catalyze the intracellular reduction of administered riboflavin to dihydroriboflavin. A reinvestigation of this capability suggested that this system might be exploited to protect tissues from oxidative damage. When tested, the hypothesis was supported by findings that dihydroriboflavin reacts rapidly with Fe(IV)O and Fe(V)O oxidation states of heme proteins. It is these oxidative states that have been implicated in tissue damage associated with ischemia and re-perfusion. The preliminary studies confirmed that the administration of low concentrations of riboflavin protects both isolated rabbit heart from re-oxygenation injury, rat lung from injury following a systemic activation of complement, and rat brain from damage caused by four hours of ischemia, and that flavin therapy could protect tissues from the oxidative injuries of myocardial infarction, acute lung injury, and stroke.

Deficiency Syndrome Riboflavin deficiency almost always occurs in association with deficiencies of other B vitamins. For most individuals, the symptoms include angular stomatitis, dermatitis, photophobia and corneal vascularization. In extreme cases of riboflavin deficiency, neuropathies and anemia can occur.

Riboflavin deficiency diminishes the rate of growth of spontaneous tumors in experimental animals but enhances the carcinogenicity of specific drugs such as azo dyes, which are degraded by a microsomal hydroxylase system requiring riboflavin. Human esophageal cancer has been epidemiologically associated with riboflavin deficiency, but the precise role of riboflavin in this tumor remains to be defined.

In a study evaluating the nutritive status of 24 healthy elderly females, where, by history, riboflavin intake was greater than or equal to the RDA in 21 of the group. By contrast, in these same 24 women, calcium intake was shown to adequate in only four women. A sufficient calcium intake was found to be gained from the total dietary intake of riboflavin, which was being derived from milk and dairy products. It was determined that individuals who took a daily multivitamin supplement showed a corresponding increase in their urinary excretion of riboflavin. These data indicate that, in the elderly, even if an individual consumes additional riboflavin, they will not retain any extra capacity, but will lose any extra vitamin about as fast as they consume it.

Pharmacological Uses There is little pharmacology related to riboflavin outside of its vitamin properties. A possible exception suggests that the administration of riboflavin (with vitamin B_1 and vitamin B_6) could improve the therapeutic actions of some antipsychotic agents (see below). Large doses can be administered without untoward effects. There are, however, a significant number of drug interactions that influence the availability of riboflavin. Moreover, there could be a substantial problem maintaining therapeutic or normal levels of the vitamin because of its significant excretion by the kidney in elderly persons.

In a recent clinical study, fourteen geriatric inpatients with depression were paired with identical depressed controls, and were administered low concentrations of vitamins B_1, B_2, and B_6. Those participants receiving supplements of both vitamins B_2 and B_6 showed improvement in ratings of depression and cognitive function. It was suggested that B-complex vitamin supplementation could augment the treatment of depression in a geriatric population.

Drug Interactions Alterations in various aspects of flavin metabolism have been observed following administration of antimalarial, antimicrobial, anticancer, as well as tricyclic antidepressants and antipsychotic agents. Aside from drugs, other factors known to influence urinary excretion of vitamins include the level of the vitamin in the diet, the degree of tissue saturation of the vitamin, and the extent of protein binding of the vitamin. Drugs can induce vitamin deficiencies by altering their intestinal absorption, transport, storage, and/or metabolic conversions.

Of more than 35 agents evaluated in interaction with riboflavin, only boric acid and its derivatives and the antipsychotic agent, chlorpromazine, have been shown to promote riboflavinuria in man. Boric acid complexes with the polyhydroxyl ribitol side chain of riboflavin and greatly increases its water solubility. Individuals who have accidentally consumed boric acid or one of its derivatives excrete high levels of riboflavin within the first 24 to 48 hours following ingestion. A molecular complex between the phenothiazine ring of chlorpromazine (and related derivatives), and the isoalloxazine ring of riboflavin will form *in vitro*. Studies have extended these findings to humans. Finally, the co-administration of agents that alter the urinary riboflavin excretion are of special concern for high-risk patients who are already nutritionally compromised as a result of illness or disease. Enhanced urinary excretion of vitamins induced by drugs is a major factor in development of vitamin deficiencies.

Cancer Chemotherapy Doxorubicin has been shown to form a 1:1 stoichiometric complex with riboflavin, as well as to compete for binding to tissue proteins. Several studies have now shown that doxorubicin can inhibit the metabolism of riboflavin. Findings in animal models now raise the possibility that defects of riboflavin nutriture, either dietary or drug-induced, may be a determinant of doxorubicin toxicity.

Toxicity The toxicity of riboflavin at the present time is limited to the possible acceleration of carcinogenesis, which is caused by certain agents in drug and carcinogen metabolism. Vitamin B_2 interacts in such biochemical sequences through a flavin cofactor interaction.

Niacin

Nicotinic acid, in its amide form, is an integral part of two important coenzymes: NAD (nicotinamide adenine dinucleotide) and NADP (nicotinamide adenine dinucleotide phosphate). These two substances act as acceptors or donors of hydrogen and reduction equivalents in enzymatic reactions, including the metabolism of many drugs through the cytochrome P-450 microsomal enzyme systems.

Role in Metabolism (Nutrition) Niacin is found in lean meats, in liver, dried yeast, and eggs. For many years both in the United States and in other developed countries, niacin has been added to all flour used to produce enriched breads. The RDA ranges from 5 mg for an infant to 20 mg for active, adult males.

Niacin can be synthesized in the body from tryptophan with the aid of pyridoxine. Corn, a vegetable deficient in both niacin and tryptophan, is grown in the southern United States, and as a result of diets high in corn in that region of the country, epidemic pellagra often occurred.

Deficiency Syndrome A deficiency state of niacin is associated with the illness known as *pellagra*. Pellagra is a disease characterized by skin lesions, gastrointestinal mucosal changes with accompanying diarrhea, and neurological symptoms, including mental disorders. Dietary deficiencies, generally more common until about 1950, have been resolved by the production of breads and other foodstuffs which provide the minimum RDA for all water-soluble vitamins.

Pellagra-like disorders have been observed in alcoholics. A hereditary affliction known as Hartnup Disease, where tryptophan is abnormally metabolized, also provides pellagra-like skin lesions. All pellagra-like syndromes are responsive to either oral or intravenous niacinamide.

Pharmacological Uses Together with the form of nicotinic acid administered, the individual kinetics have been proposed as the reason for differences in efficacy and toxicity of nicotinic acid. Nicotinic acid has two metabolic fates: the formation of nicotinamide adenine dinucleotide (NAD) and the formation of nicotinuric acid, the glycine conjugate of nicotinic acid. Catabolism of NAD releases nicotinamide, which is subsequently methylated and/or oxidized to form a number of metabolites; for most individuals, 2-pyridone is found to be the major metabolite.

There appears to be a marked difference in the metabolism of unmodified and timed-release nicotinic acid in humans. When humans are given unmodified nicotinic acid, their excretion of nicotinuric acid increases up to four times over that when timed-release nicotinic acid is administered. At the same time, excretion of the major metabolite of nicotinic acid, 2-pyridone, varies only minimally when these two forms of nicotinic acid are given.

Lipid Metabolism Niacin is used in hyperlipidemia to reduce plasma lipid levels in an attempt to reduce or revert the arteriosclerotic processes believed due to elevated blood lipid levels. At present however, niacin is a second or third choice for isolated hypercholesterolemia because of a high incidence of side effects, especially those involving glucose tolerance. However, it has a therapeutic advantage as a monotherapy when reduction of both low-density lipoprotein (LDL) cholesterol and triglycerides are needed in patients with severe combined hyperlipidemia. Moreover, niacin can be used in combination with other cholesterol-lowering agents to maximize lipid-lowering activity. From several research studies however, niacin appears to lower the production of very-low-density lipoproteins (VLDLs) in the liver while activating lipoprotein lipase. It may also influence the metabolism of high-density lipoprotein (HDL) cholesterol. The exact mechanism of action is not known (See Chapter 30).

Pharmacological intervention for altering plasma levels of lipoproteins is usually aimed at reducing atherogenesis and preventing coronary heart disease. In high doses, nicotinic acid, lowers total plasma cholesterol, LDL cholesterol, and VLDL triglycerides, while raising HDL cholesterol in otherwise normal (non-diabetic) patients with Type II, III, IV, and V hyperlipoproteinemias.

Patients receiving isoniazid therapy for tuberculosis may become pyridoxine deficient (see Chapter 48) and thus also may have a lowered conversion of tryptophan to niacin. Malignant carcinoid tumors may divert large amounts of tryptophan to 5-hydroxytryptophan (serotonin) causing a niacin deficiency.

Niacin has also been used in the treatment of schizophrenia. As pellagra symptoms may mimic schizophrenia, this treatment was probably the rationale for such trials. More recent protocols and rationale include ideas that niacin participates in transmethylation processes. Most authorities agree that niacin has no role in the therapy of schizophrenia.

Toxicity Niacin and niacinamide have a very low order of toxicity, however, these compounds do have intrinsic pharmacological actions. Niacin, but not the amide, is a vasodilator, and will cause a noticeable flushing of the skin when administered. Previous claims of cerebral vasodilation have been discounted. Aspirin antagonizes the flushing, suggesting a mechanism involving prostaglandins.

As niacin causes harmless side effects such as the hot skin flushes, it is an excellent agent to be used as a "reinforcement placebo". However, because it may give an abnormal glucose tolerance test, these types of treatments should be used with caution in diabetics. Rare duodenal ulcers and abnormalities in hepatic function have also been reported.

Pyridoxine (Vitamin B_6)

Over the past 50 years there has been an increased awareness of the importance of pyridoxine in human nutrition. In its active form, pyridoxine, as pyridoxal or pyridoxamine, is an essential coenzyme in the decarboxylation, transamination, and racemization of amino acids. In each of these ways this vitamin assists in the conversion of tryptophan to niacin. It may also assist in the transport of amino acids across membranes and in the synthesis of unsaturated fatty acids. Normal red blood cell formation is highly dependent upon its presence.

Indices for vitamin B_6 status can be separated into direct and indirect measures. Among the direct measures, plasma levels of pyridoxal 5'-phosphate (PLP) is considered the most relevant. Monitoring the urinary excretion of xanthurenic acid following a tryptophan load provides an indirect measure of determining a valid functional index for otherwise healthy persons. Evaluation of erythrocyte transaminase activity and stimulation with PLP provide an estimate of vitamin B_6 taken over an extended period of time. Levels of plasma pyridoxal and erythrocyte PLP are newer measures of status and, with further refinement of methodology, may provide additional insight into vitamin B_6 status.

There are several conditions in clinical neurology that might be responsive to pyridoxine as a therapeutic agent, including headache, chronic pain, and depression. Observations that a serotonin deficiency is a common thread between these symptoms, and that pyridoxine can raise serotonin levels, has opened a wide range of therapeutic options. It has been suggested that several of these problems may result from exposure to "toxic" concentrations of pyridoxine antagonists. Such a hypothesis suggests that supplements with pyridoxine could minimize or reduce indices of hyperactivity and aggressive behavior.

In addition, it has been demonstrated that vitamin B_6 can play an important role in the immune response. Data from a vitamin B_6 depletion-repletion study suggest that a pyridoxine deficiency impairs both the production of interleukin-2 as well as subsequent lymphocyte proliferation.

Role in Metabolism (Nutrition) Pyridoxine is present in significant amounts in yeast, liver, and whole grain cereals. The principal metabolic function of vitamin B_6 is in amino acid metabolism, although the greater part of the body's vitamin B_6 is in muscle, associated with glycogen phosphorylase. The vitamin also has an important role in the actions of steroid hormones.

Most often vitamin B_6 requirements are calculated with respect to protein intake. An adequate intake to meet the requirements of most populations is 15 μg/g of dietary protein, a number which has become the basis of RDAs in most countries. Current RDAs range between 1.5 and 2.2 mg/day. A minimum safe intake, below which an individual would have a high probability of deficiency, is 11 μg/g of dietary protein. Of course, higher intakes are required in pregnancy and lactation (although there are problems in determining the requirement of the infant), and possibly also in the elderly.

Average intakes of vitamin B_6 in developed countries meet the target of 15 μg/g of dietary protein, although there is biochemical evidence of inadequate vitamin B_6 nutritional status in 10 to 25 percent of the population. There is little evidence that pharmacological doses of vitamin B_6 have any beneficial effect, and neurological damage has been reported at extremely high intakes (in excess of 500 mg/day). As a result of these findings, more modest doses (50 to 100 mg/day) cannot be regarded as being entirely without hazard.

There have been a number of reported cases of a genetic pyridoxine dependency, in which chronic administration of high dosages of pyridoxine may be required. Permanent requirements may reach levels of 10- to 100-fold the minimum RDA of unaffected persons. In individuals exhibiting these syndromes, there is a conformational change in the enzyme so that abnormally high levels of coenzyme are required to maintain normal levels of function.

Deficiency Syndrome Pyridoxine deficiency, due to a dietary insufficiency, does not ordinarily occur. In the 1960s there was a brief epidemic concerning hundreds of infants that had been put on a proprietary substitute milk formula which had been mishandled so that pyridoxine was destroyed. Hyperirritability and convulsions occurred, which were relieved with the administration of pyridoxine. A significant symptom of deficiency is the appearance of a hypochromic anemia.

Pharmacological Uses There are a number of drugs that interfere with vitamin B_6 utilization. By way of illustration, both isoniazid and hydralazine form inactive derivatives and increase vitamin B_6 requirements; penicillamine and cycloserine act as antimetabolites of vitamin B_6. Iatrogenic polyneuritis may appear as a complication of therapy with these agents. All or most of these symptoms can be relieved by large doses of pyridoxine.

A newer pharmacologic use for vitamin B_6 supplements has been for the treatment of young women on contraceptive steroids that have an abnormal tryptophan metabolism. Such persons can easily be adjusted to a normal level of tryptophan by the administration of supplemental pyridoxine, e.g., 25 mg/day.

Toxicity The pharmacodynamic effects of pyridoxine are few. In animals, convulsions have been reported when extremely large dosages are administered intravenously. Orally, there are no effects noted. Megatherapy dosages are known which extend from 100 mg up to several grams, with a duration lasting from weeks to years. After a long-term intake of megatherapy dosages, toxic effects often occur in the form of a peripheral sensory neuropathy. The threshold above which toxic effects occur appears to be between 300 and 500 mg/day, although systematic investigations in this dose range have never occurred. Among megatherapy cases, there appears to be an inverse relationship between the dose and the time of occurrence of toxic symptoms.

The real danger with pyridoxine megatherapy is considerably less when controlled applications are undertaken by a physician. It is the self-medication by laymen on the basis of promises in obscure health magazines which constitutes the larger problem.

Ascorbic Acid (Vitamin C)

Ascorbic acid is a strong reducing agent, and probably helps to maintain the oxidation-reduction conditions appropriate for many enzymatic activities. It is thought to function in the metabolism of tyrosine, and is important in the formation of collagen.

Biochemistry Well-known active oxygen species have been implicated in the demonstration of several pathological conditions, including aging, arthritis, carcinogenesis, atherosclerosis, and muscular dystrophy. And, although it is known that ascorbate plays a key role in protecting cells against oxidative damage, in the presence of ferric ion (Fe^{3+}) or cupric ion (Cu^{2+}), ascorbate can promote the generation of the same reactive oxygen species ($\cdot OH$, O_2, H_2O_2, and ferryl ion) it is known to destroy. This pro-oxidant activity derives from the ability of ascorbate to reduce Fe^{3+} or Cu^{2+} to Fe^{2+} or Cu^{+}, respectively, and to reduce O_2 to O_2^{-} and H_2O_2. Damage to nucleic acid and proteins results from the binding of either Fe^{2+} or Cu^{+} to metal binding sites on these macromolecules, followed by reaction of the metal complexes with H_2O_2. It is these reactions that lead to the production of active oxygen species that attack functional groups at or near the metal binding sites.

In humans, there are two well-known actions of ascorbate in serum: its interaction with urate, and its role in copper transport. Urate serves as a potent antioxidant by means of its radical ion scavenging and reducing activities. Such an antioxidant action is partly manifested by its interaction with ascorbic acid, and is particularly evident in species that lack the ability to synthesize ascorbic acid. Urate not only behaves as a radical scavenger but also stabilizes ascorbate in biological fluids, an effect particularly evident in human serum and largely due to iron chelation by urate. Unlike radical-scavenging reactions, the urate protective effect is not associated with the depletion of serum urate, because a stable, non-catalytic urate iron complex is formed. However, serum urate depletion quickly results in the oxidation of ascorbate, which is largely iron-dependent.

Because scurvy-like symptoms have been seen in experimental copper deficiency, a role for vitamin C in copper metabolism has been sought and finally determined. Ascorbate is known to antagonize intestinal copper absorption, and most recent studies have characterized a post-absorption role for ascorbate in the transfer of copper ions into cells. Vitamin C reacts with ceruloplasmin, the serum copper protein, to specifically mobilize bound copper atoms and ease their transport across membranes. The mechanism is unclear but nonetheless suggests both positive and negative regulatory functions for ascorbate in copper metabolism.

Reactions understood at the molecular level make it apparent that ascorbic acid does not directly participate in enzyme-catalyzed conversion of substrates to products. Instead, the vitamin regenerates prosthetic metal ions, in these enzymes, in their required reduced forms. Such a mechanism is in agreement with other antioxidant functions of vitamin C, e.g., scavenging of free radicals. However, it remains unclear how the deficiency of ascorbate leads to the pathological symptoms found in scurvy.

Role in Metabolism (Nutrition) Dietary sources of vitamin C include citrus fruits, berries, tomatoes, potatoes, and green leafy vegetables. The RDA ranges from 35 mg for infants to 80 mg or more for lactating women. When included in the diet, ascorbic acid has a complex multi-function, acting as a hydrogen donor, as a metal inactivator, and as a peroxide destroyer.

Deficiency Syndrome The classic picture of ascorbic acid deficiency is *scurvy*, described as involving red and swollen gums, which bleed upon slight pressure. Scurvy is mostly attributed to the decreased synthesis of collagen. This nutritional deficit includes other obvious examples of collagen-bone interactions, e.g., loosening of the teeth, resorption of alveolar bone in the jaws, and anemia. Bleeding may also occur into tissue or body cavities, and subcutaneous hemorrhages are quite common. Joint swelling, edema, and anemia are commonly found, and a delayed healing of wounds is conspicuous.

During early stages of vitamin C deficiency, the concentration of ascorbic acid first decreases in plasma to the vanishing point. After plasma levels are depleted, the amounts in circulating leukocytes and in fixed tissues are markedly decreased. At this second level of deficiency, lassitude, weakness, fatigue, and shortness of breath are noticed. Clinically, pains in the joints and bones are a common complaint. The individual in vitamin C deficiency will show a skin condition that is dry, rough, and increasingly pigmented. This individual will also display respiratory difficulty, and precordial oppression. Convulsions and shock will just precede death if treatment is not instituted.

Infant scurvy is similar in most respects to the adult form. Children show notable subperitoneal hemorrhages in the shafts of long bones and swellings involving the growing epiphyses of the long bones.

Pharmacological Uses Although the RDA for ascorbic acid is, at most, 45 mg/day, doses of 50-fold that amount are quite commonly used by persons who stress improved health through the ingestion of megadoses of vitamins and minerals. In particular, daily high doses of vitamin C have been advocated for both the prevention and cure of the common cold.

A number of studies have indicated the frequency and severity of the cold may be reduced by such large supplements. In one study, for example, 26 percent, or 106 of 407 subjects, taking supplemental ascorbic acid remained free of cold symptoms, while only 19 percent, or 78 of 411 individuals, taking a placebo remained symptom free. However, the benefits observed in different studies show a large variation and, therefore, the clinical significance may not be clearly inferred from them.

In addition to preventing cold symptoms, the claims for high dosages of ascorbic acid do not include enhancement of wound healing, prevention of deep vein thrombosis, or the reduction of elevated blood cholesterol levels. Ascorbic acid appears to function in ameliorating cold symptoms through a mechanism involving the reduction of disulfide bridges in bronchial mucus, with subsequent thinning of the material and easier expectoration.

The biochemical explanation for the benefits may be based on the antioxidant property of vitamin C. In an infection, phagocytic leukocytes become activated and produce oxidizing compounds which are released from the cell. By reacting with these oxidants, vitamin C may decrease their inflammatory effects. However, vitamin C also participates in several other reactions, such as the destruction of a multitude of oxidizing substances.

The common cold studies indicate that the amounts of vitamin C which safely protect from scurvy may still be too low to provide an efficient rate for other reactions, possibly antioxidant in nature, in infected people.

There are three additional areas in therapeutics where vitamin C is under active investigation and clinical trials: (1) in the treatment of cardiovascular disease, (2) as an adjunct in cancer treatment, and (3) in the prevention of cataracts.

Cardiovascular Disease The concept that ascorbic acid supplements protects against coronary heart disease was developed in the late 1970s when the daily vitamin C intakes of persons in industrialized nations were lower than at present. Supplementation with vitamin C in these persons showed that this agent had an ability to lower plasma total cholesterol and, among some elderly men, to raise HDL cholesterol. However, among people in initially good vitamin C nutriture, these effects are usually not seen. In five populations of essentially healthy people, blood pressure has been found to correlate negatively with vitamin C status. However, recently, in a placebo-controlled, double-blinded study, extra ascorbic acid for 6 weeks was found to lower both systolic and pulse pressure in a small group of borderline hypertensive subject.

Cancer Therapy Epidemiologic evidence of a protective effect of vitamin C for non-hormone-dependent cancers is strong. Of 46 studies in which a dietary vitamin C index was calculated, 33 were found to have a statistically significant protection, with high intake conferring approximately a two-fold protective effect compared with low intake. Of 29 additional studies that assessed fruit and vitamin C intake, 21 found significant protection. Evidence is strong for a protective effect in cancers of the esophagus, oral cavity, stomach, and pancreas. There is also substantial evidence of a protective effect in cancers of the cervix, rectum, and breast. Even in lung cancer, for which carotenoids show a consistent protective effect, there is recent evidence of a role for vitamin C.

Cataracts The ocular lens, which is continually exposed to light and ambient oxygen, is at high risk of photo-oxidative damage resulting in cataracts. Oxygen free radicals appear to impair not only lens crystallins, which appear to aggregate and precipitate and form opacities, but there is also impairment of lens proteolytic enzymes, whose function it is presumed is to eliminate damaged proteins. Apart from an enzymatic defense system consisting of superoxide dismutase, catalase, and glutathione peroxidase against excited oxygen species, the lens contains the antioxidant vitamins C and E as well as β-carotene as yet another line of defense. *In vitro* and *in vivo* studies in different animal species have demonstrated a significant protective effect of vitamins C and E against light-induced cataracts. In such trials, sugar and steroid cataracts were prevented as well.

Epidemiological evidence in humans suggests that persons with comparatively higher intakes or blood concentrations of antioxidant vitamins are at a reduced risk of cataract development. These positive findings, established by several research groups, justify extensive intervention trials with antioxidant vitamins in humans using presenile cataract development as a model.

Toxicity Vitamins contain reactive functional groups necessary to their established roles as coenzymes and reducing agents. Their reactive potential may produce injury if vitamin concentration, distribution, or metabolism is altered. The lack of controlled trials prevents us from defining the lowest human neurotoxic dose of any vitamin. Large differences in individual susceptibility to vitamin neurotoxicity probably exist, and ordinary vitamin doses may harm occasional patients with genetic disorders.

Ascorbic acid influences CNS function after peripheral administration and influences brain cell differentiation and 2-deoxyglucose accumulation by cultured glial cells. Megadose vitamin therapy may cause injury that is confused with disease symptoms. High vitamin intake is more hazardous to peripheral organs than to the nervous system, because vitamin entry into the CNS is restricted. Vitamin administration into the brain or CSF, recommended in certain disease states, is hazardous and best avoided.

As described above, there are a number of investigators who have raised objections to the general use of high doses of ascorbic acid. Several studies have failed to demonstrate clearly the effectiveness of such treatment in preventing or reducing cold symptoms. Furthermore, in individuals without frank ascorbic acid deficiency, most supplemental vitamin is excreted rather rapidly in the urine. However, the main problem is the lack of knowledge of possible side effects associated with a long-term use of high doses of ascorbic acid. For example, excessive blood levels of ascorbic acid may be associated with renal excretion of large amounts of oxalic acid and subsequent renal stone formation. In addition, results of some animal studies indicate that supplementary ascorbic acid may lead to mobilization of calcium and phosphate from the skeleton and, in the absence of adequate protein intake, may have toxic effects in bones, cartilage, and in other cellular functions. Concern has also been expressed about the possibility that the mucolytic activity of large doses of this vitamin may affect fertility by changing the viscosity of the cervical mucus. And finally, it has been suggested that consistent long-term use of large doses of ascorbic acid may facilitate the development of deficiency symptoms if there were a sudden reduction or cessation of vitamin intake.

It can be concluded from these examples, that large doses of ascorbic acid may alleviate the symptoms of viral colds in some people, although the mechanism of this action is not known. Taking such moderately large amounts of ascorbic acid is probably not harmful, but there is enough evidence to warrant monitoring for possible side effects, especially in patients taking more than 1 to 2 g of the vitamin daily.

There are extreme contradictions in the question of an optimum intake of vitamin C. Reports suggesting that gram doses of ascorbic acid are beneficial for the prevention and treatment of several disorders have led to widespread ingestion of vitamin C supplements. The RDA in the United States, Great Britain, and many other countries range from 30 to 60 mg for an adult man or woman, whereas the proponents of megadoses recommend as much as 18,000 mg per day. On the basis of correlations of the hepatic vitamin C levels in guinea pigs with the rate of cholesterol degradation and the activity of microsomal detoxification systems, it is suggested that an optimum intake to form a body pool and steady state levels of vitamin C in the tissues would require a dose of 100 to 200 mg; in conditions of stress, the requirement could exceed 200 mg per day. However, despite contradictory reports, the consensus from an extensive literature is that these adverse health effects are not induced in healthy persons by ingesting large doses of ascorbic acid.

BIBLIOGRAPHY

General

Food and Nutrition Board: *Recommended Dietary Allowances, 10th Ed.*, National Academy of Sciences, Washington, D.C., 1989.

Shils, M.E., and J.R. Young: *Modern Nutrition in Health and Disease, 7th Ed.*, Lea & Febiger, Philadelphia, 1988.

Vitamin A

Biesalski, H.K.: "Comparative Assessment of the Toxicology of Vitamin A and Retinoids in Man," *Toxicol.* **57**: 117-161 (1989).

Blomhoff, R. K. and Wake: "Perisinusoidal Stellate Cells of the Liver: Important Roles in Retinol Metabolism and Fibrosis," *FASEB J.* **5**: 271-277 (1991).

Chytil F.: "The Lungs and Vitamin A," *Am. J. Physiol.* **202**: 517-527 (1992).

Gorodischer, R.: "Micronutrients and Drug Response: Vitamin A and Vitamin E in the Fetus and in the Newborn," *Develop. Pharmacol. Therap.* **15**: 166-172 (1990).

Goss, G.D., and M.W. McBurney: "Physiological and Clinical Aspects of Vitamin A and Its Metabolites," *Crit. Rev. Clin. Lab. Sci.* **29**: 185-215 (1992).

Hathcock, J.N., D.G. Hattan, M.Y. Jenkins, J.T. McDonald, P.R. Sunderasan, and V.L. Wilkening: "Evaluation of Vitamin A Toxicity," *Am. J. Clin. Nutrit.* **52**: 183-202 (1990).

Lippman, S.M., S.E. Benner, and W.K. Hong: "Chemoprevention Strategies in Lung Carcinogenesis," *Chest* **103**: 15S-19S (1993).

Mayne, S.T., S. Graham, and T.Z. Zheng: "Dietary Retinol: Prevention or Promotion of Carcinogenesis in Humans?," *Cancer Causes and Control* **2**: 443-450 (1991).

Morre D.M.: "Intracellular Actions of Vitamin A," *Int. Rev. Cytol.* **135**: 108 (1992).

Olson, J.A.: "Provitamin A Function of Carotenoids: The Conversion of Beta-carotene into Vitamin A," *J. Nutrit.* **119**: 105-108 (1989).

Pinnock, C.B., and C.P. Alderman: "The Potential for Teratogenicity of Vitamin A and its Congeners," *Med. J. Australia* **157**: 804-809 (1992).

Snodgrass, S.R.: "Vitamin Neurotoxicity," *Molec. Neurobiol.* **6**: 41-73 (1992).

Tee, E.S.: "Carotenoids and Retinoids in Human Nutrition," *Crit. Rev. Food Sci. Nutrit.* **31**: 103-163 (1962).

Underwood, B.A.: "Teratogenicity of Vitamin A," *Int. J. Vitamin Nutrit. Res.* **30**: 42-55 (1989).

Zile, M.H.: "Vitamin A Homeostatis Endangered by Environmental Pollutants," *Proc. Soc. Exper. Biol. Med.* **201**: 141-153 (1992).

Vitamin D

Allen, S.H., and J.H. Shah: "Calcinosis and Metastatic Calcification Due to Vitamin D Intoxication. A Case Report and Review," *Hormone Res.* **37**: 68-77 (1992).

Boyan, B.D., Z. Schwartz, and L.D. Swain: "In Vitro Studies on the Regulation of Endochondral Ossification by Vitamin D," *Crit. Rev.*

Oral Biol. Med. **3**: 15-30 (1992).
Dabek, J.: "An Emerging View of Vitamin D" *Scand. J. Clin. Lab. Invest.* **201**: 127-133 (1990).
Davies, M.: "High-dose Vitamin D Therapy: Indications, Benefits and Hazards," *Int. J. Vitamin Nutrit. Res.* **30**: 81-86 (1989).
DeLuca, H.F.: "New Concepts of Vitamin D Functions," *Ann. N.Y. Acad. Sci.* **669**: 59-68 (1992).
Garland, C.F., F.C. Garland, and E.D. Gorham: "Can Colon Cancer Incidence and Death Rates Be Reduced with Calcium and Vitamin D," *Am. J. Clin. Nutrit.* **54**: 193S-201S (1991).
Kragballe, K.: "Treatment of Psoriasis with Calcitriol and Other Vitamin D Analogues," *J. Am. Acad. Dermatol.* **27**: 1001-1008 (1992).
Kragballe, K.: "Vitamin D_3 and Skin Diseases," *Arch. Dermatol. Res.* **284**: S30-S36 (1992).
Lowe, K.E., A.C. Maiyar, and A.W. Norman: "Vitamin D-Mediated Gene Expression," *Crit. Rev. Eukaryotic Gene Express.* **2**: 65-109 (1992).
Menne, T. and K. Larsen: "Psoriasis Treatment with Vitamin D Derivatives," *Semin. Dermatol.* **11**: 278-283 (1992).
Norman, A.W.: "Bone Biochemistry and Physiology From the Perspectives of the Vitamin D Endocrine System," *Curr. Opin. Rheumatol.* **4**: 375-382 (1992).
Norman, A.W., I. Nemere, L.X. Zhou, J.E. Bishop, K.E. Lowe, A.C. Maiyar, E.D. Collins, T. Taoka, I.L. Sergeev, and M.C. Farach-Carson: "1,25(OH)2-Vitamin D3, A Steroid Hormone That Produces Biologic Effects via Both Genomic and Nongenomic Pathways," *J. Steroid Biochem. Molec. Biol.* **41**: 231-240 (1992).
Rubin, C.D.: "Age-Related Osteoporosis," *Am. J. Med. Sci.* **301**: 281-298 (1991).

Vitamin E

Bell, E.F.: "Upper Limit of Vitamin E in Infant Formulas," *J. Nutrit.* **119 (Suppl. 12)**, 1829-1831 (1989).
Bisby, R.H.: "Interactions of Vitamin E with Free Radicals and Membranes," *J. Free Radical Res. Commun.* **8**: 299-306 (1990).
DiMascio, P., T.P. Devasagayam, S. Kaiser, and H. Sies: "Carotenoids, Tocopherols and Thiols as Biological Singlet Molecular Oxygen Quenchers," *Biochem. Soc. Transact.* **18**: 1054-1056 (1990).
Dorgan, J.F., and A. Schatzkin: "Antioxidant Micronutrients in Cancer Prevention," *Hematol.-Oncol. Clin. North Am.* **5**: 43-68 (1991).
Drevon, C.A.: "Absorption, Transport and Metabolism of Vitamin E," *J. Free Radical Res. Commun.* **14**: 229-246 (1991).
Gonzalez, M.J.: "Serum Concentrations and Cellular Uptake of Vitamin E," *Med. Hypotheses* **32**: 107-110 (1990).
Janero, D.R.: "Therapeutic Potential of Vitamin E Against Myocardial Ischemic-Reperfusion Injury," *Free Radical Biol. Med.* **10**: 315-324 (1991).
Janero, D.R.: "Therapeutic Potential of Vitamin E in the Pathogenesis of Spontaneous Atherosclerosis," *Free Radical Biol. Med.* **11**: 129-144 (1991).
Kappus, H., and A.T. Diplock: "Tolerance and Safety of Vitamin E: A Toxicological Position Report," *Free Radical Biol. Med.* **13**: 55-74 (1992).
Kishino, Y., and S. Moriguchi: "Nutritional Factors and Cellular Immune Responses," *Nutrition and Health* **8**: 133-141 (1992).
Knekt, P.: "Role of Vitamin E in the Prophylaxis of Cancer," *Ann. Med.* **23**: 3-12 (1991).
Knekt, P., A. Aromaa, J. Maatela, R.K. Aaran, T. Nikkai, M. Hakama, T. Hakulinen, R. Peto, and L. Teppo: "Vitamin E and Cancer Prevention," *Am. J. Clin. Nutrit.* **53**: 283S-286S (1991).
Lathia, D., and A. Blum: "Role of Vitamin E as Nitrite Scavenger and N-Nitrosamine Inhibitor: A Review," *Int. J. Vitamin Nutrit. Res.* **59**: 430-438 (1989).
Machlin, L.J.: "Use and Safety of Elevated Dosages of Vitamin E in Adults," *Int. J. Vitamin Nutrit. Res.* **30**: 56-68 (1989).
Odeleye, O.E. and R.R. Watson: "The Potential Role of Vitamin E in the Treatment of Immunologic Abnormalities During Acquired Immune Deficiency Syndrome," *Prog. Food Nutrit. Sci.* **15**: 1-19 (1991).
Packer, L.: "Protective Role of Vitamin E in Biological Systems," *Am. J. Clin. Nutrit.* **53**: 1050S-1055S (1991)
Prasad, K.N., and J. Edwards-Prasad: "Vitamin E and Cancer Prevention: Recent Advances and Future Potentials," *J. Am. Coll. Nutrit.* **11**: 487-500 (1992).
Sokol, R.J.: "Vitamin E and Neurologic Function in Man," *Free Radical Biol. Med.* **6**: 189-207 (1989).

Vitamin B_1 (Thiamine)

Butterworth, R.F., C. Gaudreau, J. Vincellete, A.M. Bourgault, F. Lamothe, and A.M. Nutini: "Thiamine Deficiency and Wernicke's Encephalopathy in AIDS," *Metabol. Brain Dis.* **6**: 207-212 (1991).

Schroth, G., W. Wichmann, and A. Valavanis: "Blood-Brain-Barrier Disruption in Acute Wernicke Encephalopathy: MR Findings," *J. Comput. Assist. Tomography* **15**: 1059-1061 (1991).

Seligmann, H., H. Halkin, S. Rauchfleisch, N. Kaufmann, M. Motro, Z. Vered, and D. Ezra: "Thiamine Deficiency in Patients with Congestive Heart Failure Receiving Long-Term Furosemide Therapy: A Pilot Study," *Am. J. Med.* **91**: 151-155 (1991).

Skelton, W.P., 3rd, and N.K. Skelton: "Thiamine Deficiency Neuropathy. It's Still Common Today," *Postgrad. Med.* **85(8)**: 301-306 (1989).

van Dokkum, W., J. Schrijver, and J.A. Wesstra: "Variability in Man of the Levels of Some Indices of Nutritional Status Over a 60-Day Period on a Constant Diet," *Eur. J. Clin. Nutrit.* **44(9)**: 665-674 (1990).

Wrenn, K.D., F. Murphy, and C.M. Slovis: "A Toxicity Study of Parenteral Thiamine Hydrochloride," *Ann. Emerg. Med.* **18**: 867-870 (1989).

Vitamin B_2 (Riboflavin)

Alexander, M., G. Emanuel, T. Gotlin, J.T. Pinto, and R.S. Rilin: "Relation of Riboflavin Nutriture in Healthy Elderly to Intake of Calcium and Vitamin Supplements: Evidence Against Riboflavin Supplementation," *Am. J. Clin. Nutrit.* **39**: 540-546 (1984).

Bell, I.R., J.S. Edman, F.D. Morrow, D.W. Marby, G. Perrone, H.L. Kayne, M. Greenwald, and J.O. Cole: "Vitamin B_1, B_2, and B_6 Augmentation of Tricyclic Antidepressant Treatment in Geriatric Depression with Cognitive Dysfunction," *J. Am. Coll. Nutrit.* **11**: 159-163 (1992).

Hultquist, D.E., F. Xu, K.S. Quandt, M. Shlafer, C.P. Mack, G.O. Till, A. Seekamp, A.L. Betz, and S.R. Ennis: "Evidence That NADPH-Dependent Methemoglobin Reductase and Administered Riboflavin Protect Tissues from Oxidative Injury," *Am. J. Hematol.* **42**: 13-18 (1993).

Pinto, J., G.B. Raiczyk, Y.P. Huang, and R.S. Rivlin: "New Approaches to the Possible Prevention of Side Effects of Chemotherapy," *Cancer* **58**: 1911-1914 (1986).

Pinto, J.T. and R.S. Rivlin: "Drugs That Promote Renal Excretion of Riboflavin," *Drug-Nutrient Interact.* **5**: 143-151 (1987).

Rivlin, R.S.: "Riboflavin," *Adv. Exper. Med. Biol.* **206**: 349-355 (1986).

Vitamin B_3 (Niacin)

DiPalma, J.R., and W.S. Thayer: "Use of Niacin as a Drug," *Am. Rev. Nutrit.* **11**: 169-187 (1991).

Drood, J.M., P.J. Zimetbaum, and W.H. Frishman: "Nicotinic Acid for the Treatment of Hyperlipoproteinemia," *J. Clin. Pharmacol.* **31**: 641-650 (1991).

Miller, N.E.: "Pharmacological Intervention for Altering Lipid Metabolism," *Drugs* **40**: 26-31, (1990).

Stern, R.H., D. Freeman, and J.D. Spence: "Differences in Metabolism of Time-Release and Unmodified Nicotinic Acid: Explanation of the Differences in Hypolipidemic Action?," *Metab. Clin. & Exper.* **41**: 879-881 (1992).

Vitamin B_6 (Pyridoxine)

Bassler, K.H.: "Use and Abuse of High Dosages of Vitamin B_6," *Int. J. Vitamin Nutrit. Res.* **30**: 120-126 (1989).

Bender, D.A.: "Vitamin B_6 Requirements and Recommendations," *Eur. J. Clin. Nutrit.* **43**: 289-309 (1989).

Bernstein, A.L.: "Vitamin B_6 Clinical Neurology," *Ann. N.Y. Acad. Sci.* **585**: 250-260 (1990).

Leklem, J.E.: "Vitamin B-6: A Status Report," *J. Nutrit.* **120**: 1503-1507 (1990).

Vitamin C (Ascorbic Acid)

Block, G.: "Epidemiologic Evidence Regarding Vitamin C and Cancer," *Am. J. Clin. Nutrit.* **54**: 1310S-1314S (1991).

Gerster, H.: "Antioxidant Vitamins in Cataract Prevention," *J. Nutrit. Sci.* **28**: 66-75 (1989).

Ginter, E.: "Ascorbic Acid in Cholesterol Metabolism and in Detoxification of Xenobiotic Substances: Problem of Optimum Vitamin C Intake," *Nutrition* **5**: 369-374 (1989).

Harris, E.D., and S.S. Percival: "A Role for Ascorbic Acid in Copper Transport," *Am. J. Clin. Nutrit.* **54**: 1193S-1197S (1991).

Hemila, H.: "Vitamin C and the Common Cold," *Br. J. Nutrit.* **67**: 3-16 (1992).

Padh, H.: "Cellular Functions of Ascorbic Acid," *Biochem. Cell Biol.* **68**: 1166-1173 (1990).

Padh, H.: "Vitamin C: Newer Insights into its Biochemical Functions," *Nutrit. Rev.* **49**: 65-70 (1991).

Sevanian, A., K.J. Davies, and P. Hochstein: "Serum Urate as an Antioxidant for Ascorbic Acid," *Am. J. Clin. Nutrit.* **54**: 1129S-1134S (1991).

Snodgrass, S.R.: "Vitamin Neurotoxicity," *Molec. Neurobiol.* **6**: 41-73 (1992).

Stadtman, E.R.: "Ascorbic Acid and Oxidative Inactivation of Proteins," *Am. J. Clin. Nutrit.* **54**: 1125S-1128S (1991).

CHAPTER 37

Gastrointestinal Drugs

Joan S. DiPalma

Of all the vital organs that comprise the human body, the gastrointestinal tract gives rise to the greatest amount of disease symptomatology. Disorders such as peptic ulcer, constipation, diarrhea, nausea and vomiting, and inflammatory bowel disease are the most common. Over-the-counter medications abound for most of these disorders as well as for simple dyspepsia, bloating, and epigastric burning. Yet, until 1977 when the first H_2 receptor antagonist was introduced there was a relative paucity of effective gastrointestinal drugs. Today the H_2 receptor blockers enjoy a yearly market share of 2 billion dollars alone, while antacids and the newly developed gastrointestinal drugs have very widespread applications.

This chapter discusses the gastrointestinal drugs from the viewpoint of their mechanism of action, based as much as possible on the pathophysiology of disease states. Clinical uses (including treatment of peptic ulcers, diarrhea, constipation, emesis, and inflammatory bowel disease) will be interpreted from this viewpoint.

PEPTIC ULCER DISEASE

Peptic ulcers are sores on the mucosal surface of the alimentary tract. They are common, occurring in one out of every ten people. The stomach and duodenum are most commonly affected. Presenting symptoms, which vary in magnitude of expression, are abdominal pain, vomiting, and gastrointestinal bleeding. Research during the past thirty years has resulted in a great deal of information on the etiology of ulcers and medications to treat ulcers are among the largest selling prescription drugs.

Gastric acid is secreted by parietal cells in the oxyntic glands, located in the gastric body and fundus. The baseline acid milieu of the stomach ($pH < 3.0$) is required for activation of the proteolytic enzyme pepsin and for digestion and absorption of carbohydrates, proteins, and lipids. In light of the constant exposure of gastric mucosa to extremely low pH, it is remarkable that ulceration does not occur more frequently.

Figure 37-1 illustrates the formation of gastric acid (hydrochloric acid, HCl) by the parietal cell. The three major stimuli of gastric acid secretion are acetylcholine (ACH), gastrin, and histamine, which activate the cell's ATPase-dependent H^+,K^+ pump through stimulation of a protein kinase. ACH and gastrin theoretically do this by increasing the intracellular concentration of free calcium ions; histamine activates adenylate cyclase, which increases the concentration of intracellular cyclic AMP. There is a proposed interaction between the calcium and the cyclic AMP pathways *in vivo*. Receptors on the parietal cell are specific for ACH (muscarinic), gastrin, or histamine (H_2). The stimuli are derived via paracrine (histamine), neurocrine (ACH), and endocrine (gastrin) transmission. Ulcer formation occurs when there is an imbalance between the actions of "ulcerogenic" mechanisms and "protective" mechanisms, as listed in Table 37-1.

Pharmacotherapy of peptic ulcer disease includes an attempt to tailor a particular medical regimen to an individual patient. Factors such as location of the ulcer, severity of symptoms, and proposed etiology are taken into consideration. Examples of drugs used as antiulcer agents are listed in Table 37-2.

Antisecretory agents, compounds that neutralize stomach acidity, and cytoprotective drugs are discussed in this chapter. Anti-infective agents are not covered; the reader should refer to the chapters on Antimicrobials (Chapters 45 to 48) which discuss the therapy against organisms such as *Helicobacter pylori*.

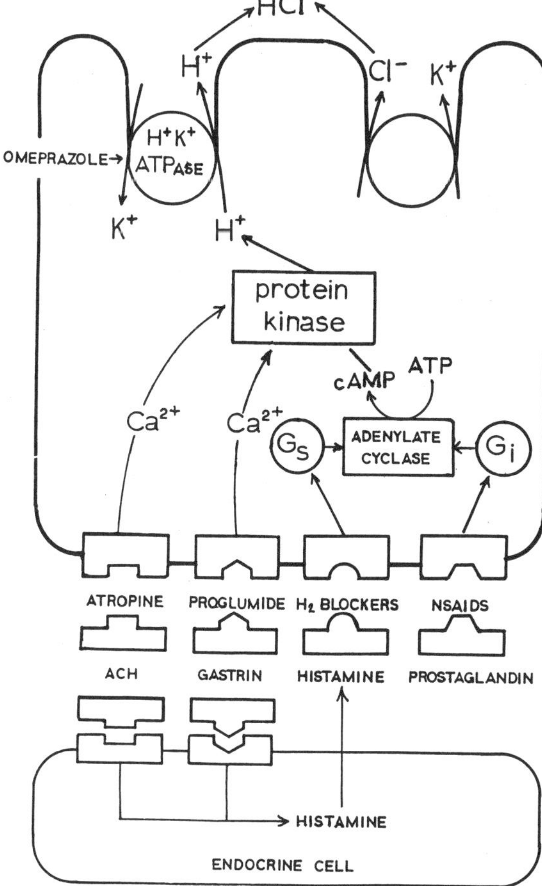

FIGURE 37-1 *Diagram of the parietal cell (top) showing the proposed mechanisms of acid secretion from the luminal membrane. Receptors for acetylcholine (ACH), gastrin, histamine, and prostaglandin are located on the basolateral membrane. The drugs which block the actions of these agonists i.e., atropine, proglumide, H_2 receptor blockers, and nonsteroidal anti-inflammatory drugs (NSAIDs), are also shown. (Proglumide is an experimental drug and not available clinically.) Note that histamine and prostaglandin affect message transduction through the G-protein stimulatory (G_s) and inhibitory (G_i) systems involving adenylate cyclase, cyclic AMP, and protein kinase. ACH and gastrin affect protein kinase through a Ca^{2+} transduction system. Omeprazole affects the H^+,K^+-ATPase proton pump directly. ACH and gastrin also have activity on endocrine cells, producing histamine. This partially explains why H_2 blockers are more effective in reducing acid secretion than cholinergic blocking drugs.*

TABLE 37-1 Proposed "ulcerogenic" and "protective" mechanisms which play a role in peptic ulcer formation

ULCEROGENIC
Acid hypersecretion
Idiopathic
Gastrin Hypersecretion
(e.g., Zollinger-Ellison Syndrome)
Pepsin
Bile Acid Reflux
Infection
Helicobacter pylori
Medications / Irritants
Nonsteroidal anti-inflammatory drugs
Corticosteroids
Ethanol
Cigarette smoking
Stress
Head trauma
Cushings ulcer
Shock / Sepsis
Emotional (?)
Genetic predisposition
PROTECTIVE
Mucosal integrity
Prostaglandins
Tight junctions between cells
Mucus secretion (mucous neck cells)
Cellular regeneration
Bicarbonate secretion
Blood flow

ANTISECRETORY AGENTS

H_2 Receptor Antagonists

The four H_2 receptor antagonists (cimetidine, ranitidine, famotidine, and nizatidine) are discussed comprehensively in Chapter 13. The discussion in this chapter is restricted to their therapeutic applications.

All four H_2 receptor antagonists are equally

TABLE 37-2 Antiulcer medications

- Antisecretory Drugs
  - H_2 receptor antagonists
  - Omeprazole
  - Anticholinergics
- Cytoprotective Drugs
  - Prostaglandins
  - Sucralfate
  - Bismuth
- Anti-Infective Agents
  - Bismuth
  - Antibiotics
    - Erythromycin
    - Amoxicillin
    - Metronidazole
- Acid-neutralizing Compounds
  - Antacids

effective antisecretory agents, with famotidine being the most potent on a mg dose basis. All of the H_2 receptor blockers are relatively free of severe adverse reactions. This contributes to their popularity, the propensity for use just for simple dyspepsia, and a tendency for long-term usage. Cimetidine appears to inhibit the hepatic cytochrome P-450 system more than do the other drugs and thus has a greater incidence of drug interactions. The choice between the four drugs depends more on cost than efficacy or toxicity. Cimetidine, having been on the market for the longest period of time, is the least expensive.

The Food and Drug Administration (FDA) has approved the use of the H_2 receptor antagonists for: acute therapy of and maintenance therapy of duodenal ulcers, gastric ulcers, pathological hypersecretory conditions (e.g., Zollinger-Ellison syndrome), and gastroesophageal reflux disease (GERD). However, treatment of gastrointestinal hemorrhage due to known peptic ulcer disease, prophylaxis against ulcers induced by nonsteroidal anti-inflammatory drugs (NSAIDs), and protection against aspiration of gastric acid during anesthesia are FDA-unapproved uses currently being explored. Therapy with these drugs for nonspecific gastrointestinal symptoms (e.g., nausea, diarrhea, and non-ulcer dyspepsia) is not recommended or FDA-approved.

H_2 receptor blockers are now the first line agents for the cure of duodenal ulcers, achieving an 80 to 90 percent cure rate in 8 to 12 weeks. This is as good or better than antacid therapy with a greater incidence of compliance and less adverse effects. Nearly as good results are achieved in the therapy of gastric ulcers and GERD.

Omeprazole

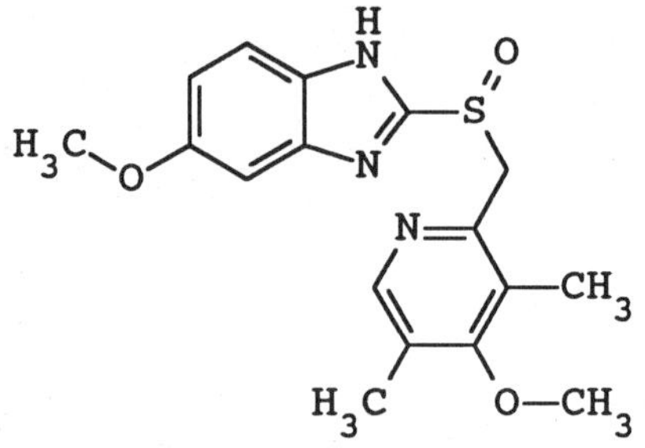

Mechanism of Action Omeprazole greatly decreases gastric acid secretion by inhibiting the ATPase-dependent H^+,K^+ pump in the parietal cell (Fig. 37-1). Omeprazole, a weak uncharged base (pH 4.0), reaches the parietal cell through the systemic circulation following intestinal absorption. Its lipophilic nature causes it to pass through the parietal membrane. Once inside the parietal cell secretory canaliculus (pH 2), the drug converts to a pronated (charged) form and is unable to exit the cell. It is then further converted to the cationic sulfenamide, which reacts with cysteines to irreversibly inhibit the H^+,K^+-ATPase pump. Because the conversion of omeprazole only takes place in an acid environment, its inhibition of the H^+,K^+-ATPase is specific to parietal cells.

Effects The main effect of omeprazole is inhibition of gastric acid secretion. Individuals treated regularly with omeprazole show a 75 to 90 percent reduction in gastric acid secretion. Studies suggest that standard doses of omeprazole are 10 to 100 times more potent at inhibiting gastric acid secretion than standard doses of H_2 receptor antagonists. Increased doses of omeprazole lead to increased inhibition of gastric acid secretion. Discontinuing omeprazole does not cause rebound gastric hypersecretion. Omeprazole has no known effect on gastric emptying time or lower esophageal sphincter pressure. Parietal cells also secrete intrinsic factor, but this process (as well as vitamin B_{12} absorption) is not inhibited by omeprazole. Pepsinogen is secreted by chief cells in the gastric glands, and it is converted to its active form, the proteolytic enzyme pepsin. Omeprazole does not directly inhibit pepsinogen secretion, however, it reduces gastric pepsin activity by 40 percent by reducing gastric acidity.

Pharmacokinetics Oral doses of omeprazole alone are denatured by gastric acid. Therefore, omeprazole is incorporated into pH-sensitive granules, and is released when the pH exceeds 6. Absorption takes place in the small intestine. Peak plasma concentration is achieved 2 to 4 hours after ingestion.

The oral bioavailability of omeprazole is about 50 percent. After a few days of use, oral bioavailability and plasma concentrations increase slightly. This is presumably due to decreased gastric acid secretion, leading to decreased omeprazole inactivation in the stomach. Although the plasma half-life of omeprazole is about 1 h, its duration of action is about 24 hours. This is due to its irreversible binding to the H^+,K^+-ATPase. The half-life of the enzyme is about 18 hours. The extent of inhibition of gastric acid secretion is best related to the area under the plasma concentration-time curve.

Plasma protein binding of the drug is approximately 95 percent. Omeprazole is biotransformed by the hepatic cytochrome P-450 system to at least six metabolic products. The three major metabolites, hydroxyomeprazole and the sulfide and sulfone derivatives of omeprazole, have insignificant antisecretory activity. These are excreted in urine (80 percent), and feces (20 percent) via the biliary tract. The metabolism of omeprazole is decreased and bioavailability is increased in elderly patients and in those with liver dysfunction. However, dosage adjustment is not required in these patients.

Adverse Effects and Drug Interactions Adverse reactions associated with this drug are generally mild. Headache, diarrhea, nausea and vomiting, and rash are the more common untoward effects. A post marketing survey of other adverse effects is in progress. Long-term use of the drug has not resulted in alterations in laboratory test values, including thyroid and liver function tests.

Omeprazole interacts with the hepatic cytochrome P-450 system. Therefore, blood levels of drugs such as warfarin, phenytoin, and diazepam may increase and must be monitored during omeprazole use. Drug interactions with propranolol and theophylline are probably not as significant.

Therapeutic Uses The ability of omeprazole to markedly decrease gastric acid secretion makes it an attractive option when considering the management of acid-peptic disease. Many studies have been performed testing the efficacy of omeprazole in treating these disorders.

Omeprazole is effective in healing duodenal ulcers, and in relieving ulcer symptoms. In the initial phases of duodenal ulcer treatment (usually 2 to 4 weeks), it is significantly more effective than H_2 receptor antagonists. However, as the treatment period progresses (8 to 12 weeks), this difference becomes much less dramatic. Omeprazole is excellent at healing duodenal ulcers resistant to H_2 blockers. However, once discontinued, the ulcer relapse rate is similar to that of H_2 receptor antagonists.

Omeprazole is 92 to 100 percent effective in healing ulcers both in the gastric body and antrum after 8 weeks of therapy. This effect is only slightly better than that of the H_2 blockers, and the gastric ulcer relapse rate is comparable to that of the latter compounds. The major benefit of omeprazole in gastric ulcer therapy is in the treatment of "resistant" ulcers.

Omeprazole is effective in healing moderate to severe reflux esophagitis in 8 weeks. Reflux esophagitis symptoms, such as heartburn, are relieved dramatically. The greatest role of the drug is in the treatment of "resistant" esophagitis. Unfortunately, the relapse rate after 8 to 12 weeks of therapy is high and many patients require maintenance therapy with H_2 receptor antagonists.

Zollinger-Ellison syndrome results from increased gastrin secretion due to gastrinomas, which are usually located within the gastrointestinal tract. This results in duodenal and jejunal ulcerations, secretory diarrhea, and malabsorption. Omeprazole is currently the drug of choice in the treatment of Zollinger-Ellison syndrome. Effective gastric acid suppression can be achieved with twice a day dosing (albeit at higher doses than recommended for treatment of duodenal or gastric ulcer alone). A five year experience treating several Zollinger-Ellison syndrome patients with omeprazole has been promising.

Anticholinergics

Prior to the mid 1970s, when the more recent antisecretory medications were developed, anticholinergics were used to treat peptic ulcer disease. The pharmacologic actions, effects, and uses of the anticholinergics are described extensively in Chapter 11. Basically, they are competitive antagonists of acetylcholine at the muscarinic receptors.

The general, or "classical", anticholinergics (e.g., atropine and propantheline) are nonselective blockers of acetylcholine at muscarinic (M) receptors, i.e., they inhibit the activity of acetylcholine at all muscarinic receptor sites. Therefore, they act on multiple organs and tissues and have numerous side effects. General anticholinergics decrease gastric acid secretion by 40 to 50 percent. Although intestinal motility is only minimally affected, gastro-duodenal motility is decreased, leading to a relief of ulcer pain.

Despite adequate absorption, the response to general anticholinergics varies from patient to patient. This results in difficulties in determining dosage. There have been no recent studies comparing general anticholinergics to placebo or to currently utilized therapies for the treatment of peptic ulcer disease. This lack of demonstrated benefit, coupled with multiple side effects, put the general anticholinergics low on the priority list for treatment of acid-peptic disease.

Two selective anticholinergics, *pirenzepine* and *telenzepine* are complex tricyclic compounds. Both inhibit acetylcholine primarily via M_1 receptors. Because of their selective action, they decrease both basal and stimulated gastric acid and pepsin secretion, but have less effect than general anticholinergics on gastric emptying and heart rate. Both drugs are hydrophilic and, therefore, do not cross the blood-brain barrier, minimizing central nervous system effects.

In general, these selective anticholinergics are less effective inhibitors of gastric acid secretion than H_2 receptor antagonists. Pirenzepine has been shown to be more effective at healing duodenal ulcers than placebo, but it is equally as effective as H_2 receptor antagonists at healing duodenal ulcers and relieving symptoms. Ulcer recurrence rates are similar between pirenzepine and H_2 blockers. The efficacy of telenzepine seems to be similar to that of pirenzepine, although it is more effective at inhibiting gastric acid secretion.

Side effects of these drugs include dry mouth, blurred vision, and constipation; however the incidence of adverse reactions appears to be less than with the general anticholinergics. Their use is not contraindicated in patients with glaucoma, or prostatic hypertrophy, unlike the general anticholinergics. Selective anticholinergics are presently used in Europe to treat peptic ulcers, but are not available in the United States.

CYTOPROTECTIVE AGENTS

Misoprostol

Although prostaglandin E_1 analogs have been used in Europe to treat duodenal and gastric ulcers whether caused by NSAIDs or not, misoprostol is the first one to be available in the United States. Misoprostol is comprised of four stereoisomers in approximately equal proportions. As can be seen, its structure resembles other eicosanoid derivatives (see Chapter 14).

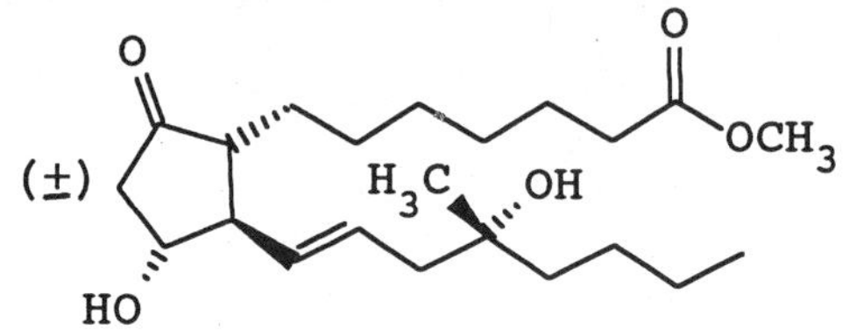

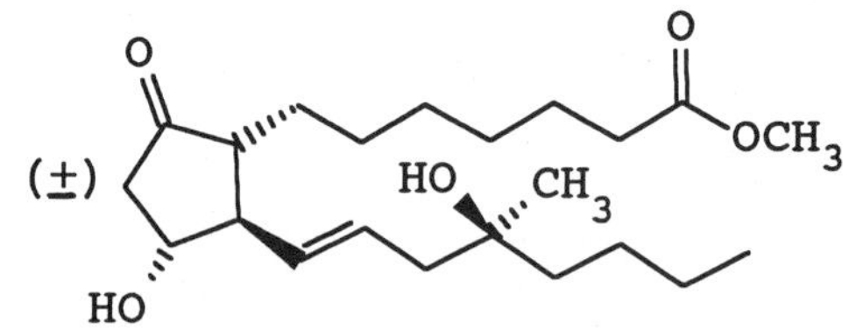

(±) O, HO, H_3C, OH, O, OCH_3

(±) O, HO, HO, CH_3, O, OCH_3

Effects As a prostaglandin analog, the major effect of misoprostol on the gastrointestinal mucosa is cytoprotection. The gastro-duodenal mucosa is protected from injury from hydrochloric acid, bile reflux, toxins, etc., via cytoprotective mechanisms. These mechanisms are dose-dependent and independent of gastrin levels or gastric acid secretion. They include: (1) enhanced secretion of mucus and bicarbonate ion, (2) stimulation of cell proliferation, (3) preservation of the microcirculation, (4) maintenance of mucosal sulfhydryl groups, and (5) stabilization of tissue lysosomes.

In addition to cytoprotection, misoprostol also inhibits gastric acid secretion. This effect is expressed only at higher doses of the drug. Misoprostol binds to and stimulates E-type prostaglandin receptors on the parietal cell, and through the activation of G_i nucleotide protein, leads to inhibition of adenylate cyclase, and a reduction in acid secretion (see Fig. 37-1).

Pharmacokinetics Rapidly and completely absorbed in the gastrointestinal tract, misoprostol undergoes de-esterification to the free acid which is the active form. After oral administration, peak plasma concentrations of the acid metabolite occur in 12 to 15 minutes. The elimination half-life is only 20 to 40 minutes. Approximately 80 percent of an oral dose of misoprostol appears in the urine.

Adverse Effects The major adverse effects of misoprostol come from the stimulatory activity of prostaglandins on smooth muscle. Abdominal cramps, nausea and vomiting, flatulence, dyspepsia, and diarrhea are seen with misoprostol use. The incidence of diarrhea is high (15 to 40 percent), it is dose-dependent, but usually self-limiting. Increased uterine contractions are another important adverse effect of misoprostol, resulting in bleeding or spontaneous abortions. Therefore, the use of misoprostol is contraindicated in pregnancy and the drug is to be used with caution in women capable of child-bearing. Other gynecological disorders, such as menstrual irregularities and cramps, have been reported.

Misoprostol has no effect on the hepatic cytochrome P-450 system and there are few drug interactions. Its use has been reported to increase propranolol levels via unknown mechanisms.

Therapeutic Uses Although duodenal and gastric ulcer healing rates with misoprostol are superior than placebo, they are comparable to those of H_2 receptor antagonists. Misoprostol is not effective at relieving ulcer symptoms. Therefore, the drug has no benefit over H_2 receptor blockers as a first line drug for peptic ulcer therapy.

NSAIDs are commonly used to treat arthritis. Unfortunately, by inhibiting cyclooxygenase systemically, they decrease prostaglandin production, which leads to damage to the gastro-duodenal mucosa. This damage can be expressed as gastritis, or as gastric or duodenal ulceration. Symptomatically, NSAID-induced gastropathy can range from minimal symptomatology to abdominal pain, gastrointestinal hemorrhage, and even perforation. In short-term trials, (4 to 12 weeks), misoprostol has been shown to be effective at preventing gastritis and gastric ulcer caused by NSAIDs. Minimal protection from duodenal ulcer or abdominal pain was demonstrated. Currently, misoprostol is recommended and approved for the prevention of NSAID-induced gastric ulcers in susceptible patients. Usually, these are patients who are elderly, have had ulcers or ulcer complications in the past, or who are on steroid therapy.

Sucralfate

Sucralfate is an aluminum salt of sucrose octasulfate. The general structure of sucralfate is:

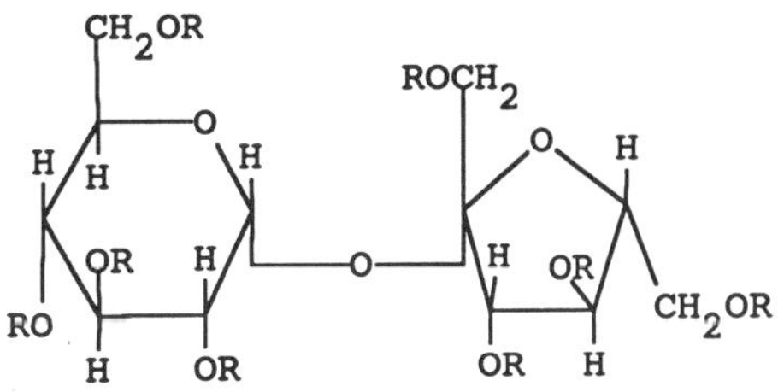

$$R = SO_3[Al_2(OH_2)_5\text{-}(H_2O)_2]$$

Effects Sucralfate has no ability to neutralize gastric acid or to inhibit gastric acid secretion; its major effect is one of cytoprotection. Sucralfate is insoluble in aqueous solutions. In the gastric milieu, it interacts with hydrochloric acid to form a viscous, negatively charged substance, which reacts with positively charged proteins at the base of ulcers. It therefore binds preferentially to inflamed or abnormal mucosa. The viscous protective "barrier" that forms prevents injury by blocking the mucosal-damaging effects of hydrochloric acid, pepsin, and bile. Sucralfate is believed to have a trophic effect on gastric mucosa by its ability to bind salivary epidermal growth factor, stimulate re-epithelization, and preserve vascular integrity and mucosal blood flow. Other proposed mechanisms of action of sucralfate are enhancement of mucosal bicarbonate ion secretion and mucus secretion, and stimulation of local prostaglandin release.

Pharmacokinetics Because of its high polarity and poor solubility, sucralfate is poorly absorbed, and 95 to 97 percent is excreted unchanged in the feces. Sucralfate is 3 to 5 percent absorbed as an aluminum base and sucrose octasulfate, which is excreted unchanged in the urine. Aluminum excretion occurs via the kidneys. There have been no reported changes in aluminum bone levels, but aluminum serum levels must be monitored in patients with renal failure.

Adverse Effects Sucralfate has few adverse effects, due to its poor absorption. Constipation, diarrhea, nausea, vomiting, indigestion, and flatulence have been reported. Bezoar formation is seen rarely in patients who are tube fed or have gastrointestinal motility disorders. As mentioned above, serum levels of aluminum and phosphate may be altered, especially in patients with renal failure. Sucralfate may alter the absorption of several drugs, some of which are listed in Table

TABLE 37-3 Examples of drugs whose absorption is affected by sucralfate

Digoxin	Warfarin
Phenytoin	Amitriptyline
Cimetidine	Ciprofloxacin
Ranitidine	Norfloxacin
Tetracycline	Ofloxacin

37-3. It is suggested that sucralfate be given 2 hours from the administration of these drugs.

Therapeutic Uses Sucralfate is recommended and approved for acute treatment of duodenal ulcers, and for maintenance therapy in the prevention of duodenal ulcer recurrence. It has proven to be superior to placebo and equivalent to H_2 receptor antagonists for this purpose. No synergistic effect was seen when sucralfate was used together with H_2 receptor antagonists for the treatment of duodenal ulcer.

Sucralfate is effective in the treatment of reflux esophagitis, and its efficacy is equivalent to that of cimetidine. When used concomitantly with cimetidine, it has a better efficacy at healing reflux esophagitis than cimetidine alone.

Although sucralfate does promote healing in NSAID-induced gastropathy, complete remissions have not been achieved. Prostaglandin analogs, such as misoprostol, are superior for this purpose.

Sucralfate has been used to treat recalcitrant inflammatory conditions, such as radiation enteritis or esophagitis, chemotherapy induced mucositis, portal gastropathy and "pouchitis" following ileorectal anastomosis post-proctocolectomy. Although sucralfate use shows some promise in these clinical situations, further investigation is in order before it is officially recommended and approved.

Bismuth

Preparations containing bismuth have been used to treat a variety of gastrointestinal ailments for two centuries. The most commonly used preparations are bismuth subsalicylate, bismuth subcitrate, and bismuth subnitrate. Only bismuth subsalicylate is approved for use and commercially available in the United States.

Bismuth is the heaviest nonradioactive element. The action of nitric acid on free bismuth results in the formation of bismuth nitrate, which is hydrolyzed to bismuth subnitrate. Bismuth subnitrate together with soluble basic salts in solution results in the formation of bismuth subcarbonate, subgallate, subsalicylate, or subcitrate.

Effects The major actions of bismuth are its bacteriocidal and its cytoprotective properties. For years, the antispirochital activity of bismuth has been known and it was originally used as a treatment for syphilis. Bismuth has also been shown to have *in vitro* bacteriocidal activity against enterotoxigenic *Escherichia coli*, *Clostridium difficile*, *Bacteroides fragilis*, and *Helicobacter pylori*. There is also evidence of the ability of bismuth to bind cholera toxin *in vitro*. The salicylate present in bismuth subsalicylate may also have antibacterial properties, by antagonizing the effects of *E. coli*, *Shigella*, and *Salmonella* toxins on intestinal secretion.

Preliminary studies, primarily with bismuth subcitrate, have demonstrated cytoprotection of the gastro-duodenal mucosa via binding to abnormal mucosa, pepsin, and bile acids. There is also evidence that bismuth preparations may enhance prostaglandin production and bicarbonate ion secretion in the stomach. Bismuth preparations do not alter gastric acid secretions, nor do they neutralize acid.

Pharmacokinetics Bismuth salts are generally insoluble in water (with the exception bismuth subcitrate), and gastric acid only increases this solubility slightly. In the stomach, insoluble precipitates of bismuth are formed (e.g., Bi_2O_3, $Bi(OH)_3$, and BiOCl). Trace amounts of bismuth are absorbed from the intestine by phagocytosis into enterocytes. Serum levels of bismuth, using therapeutic doses of bismuth subsalicylate, are far below toxic levels. The half-life of serum bismuth is 5 days, and excretion occurs via urine and bile. In the oral cavity and colon, hydrogen sulfide produced by bacteria converts bismuth salts to bismuth sulfide, which has a black color. When bismuth subsalicylate is ingested, bismuth dissociates from salicylate in the stomach. The salicylate is well absorbed in stomach and duodenum. However, chronic (13 week) use of bismuth subsalicylate results in salicylate levels well below the toxic range.

Adverse Effects Due to poor absorption of bismuth preparations, adverse effects are minimal, except for black-colored stools and reversible dark staining of teeth and oral mucosa. Large doses of bismuth preparations used chronically have lead to encephalopathy, due to bismuth toxicity. These reports came out of France and Australia, and were reported after use of bismuth subcarbonate and bismuth subgallate, which are rarely used today.

Because of its salicylate content, bismuth subsalicylate should be used with caution in patients with salicylate sensitivity or who are already on therapeutic doses of salicylate. It must also be used with caution in patients with renal disease. Fecal impaction may occur in infants and in elderly, debilitated patients. The compound may interfere with radiological examinations of the gastrointestinal tract.

Therapeutic Uses Bismuth subsalicylate is approved for use in treating abdominal symptoms, such as indigestion, heartburn, nausea, abdominal cramps, and diarrhea. It is found in a number of over-the-counter preparations in both tablet and liquid forms.

As mentioned above, bismuth has cytoprotective properties. In addition, it has been shown to be bacteriocidal to *H. pylori*, an S-shaped, gram negative bacteria which lives under the mucus layer coating the gastric epithelium and in areas of the duodenum with gastric metaplasia. The organism does not invade mucosal cells, but lies above and between them in tight junctions. *H. pylori* has been associated with upper gastrointestinal symptoms, gastritis, and peptic ulcer disease. It has been implicated as one of the main reasons for ulcer recurrence. About 80 percent of gastritis and 90 to 95 percent of duodenal ulcers are associated with *H. pylori*, identified histologically or via urea production (breath test).

Bismuth preparations (bismuth subsalicylate and bismuth subcitrate) have been found effective at eradicating *H. pylori*. When used to treat duodenal ulcers, healing rates are similar to those of H_2 receptor antagonists. Bismuth subcitrate, used in conjunction with H_2 receptor antagonists, leads to lower relapse rates of duodenal ulcer. Because of the importance of eliminating, *H. pylori*, trials have been instituted using bismuth subsalicylate or bismuth subcitrate together with antibiotics in the treatment of duodenal ulcers. The antibiotics being tried are ampicillin, erythromycin, tetracycline, and metronidazole. Many of these trials have been quite successful, but further study is required before the proper place of bismuth preparations in ulcer therapy is defined.

ACID-NEUTRALIZING COMPOUNDS: ANTACIDS

Antacids are weak bases, whose main function is that of gastric acid neutralization. They also have a considerable placebo effect and have been used for hundreds of years to treat a variety of gastrointestinal symptoms. The most frequently used antacids are: aluminum hydroxide ($Al(OH)_3$), magnesium hydroxide ($Mg(OH)_2$), calcium carbonate ($Ca(CO)_3$), and magnesium aluminum trisilicate. These can be used alone, but are frequently combined in proprietary preparations.

Effects The most widely used antacids for clinical situations are *nonsystemic* antacids (aluminum, calcium, and magnesium salts), those which form insoluble complexes in the stomach and intestine. Therefore, most of their effects are local, they are poorly absorbed, and they do not elicit systemic effects. In contrast, a *systemic* antacid (e.g., sodium bicarbonate) is readily absorbed and produces transient systemic changes in electrolytes and alkalosis. The following are the chemical reactions of commonly used antacids:

$$Al(OH)_3 + 3\ HCl \longrightarrow AlCl_3 + 3\ H_2O$$

$$Mg(OH)_2 + 2\ HCl \longrightarrow MgCl_2 + 2\ H_2O$$

$$Ca(CO)_3 + 2\ HCl \longrightarrow CaCl_2 + H_2O + CO_2$$

The potency of an antacid is described as its *acid-neutralizing capacity* (ANC). The ANC is defined as the mEq of hydrochloric acid (HCl) required to keep an antacid suspension (1 mL of antacid plus 100 mL of distilled water) at pH 3.0 for 2 h. The ANC of aluminum hydroxide, magnesium hydroxide, and calcium carbonate are 30 mEq/g, 30 mEq/g, and 13 to 17 mEq/g, respectively. Suspensions have greater ANC than tablets or capsules.

The rate of gastric emptying can effect the neutralization abilities of an antacid. Administering an antacid on an empty stomach results in rapid evacuation of the antacid and poor acid neutralization. An ingested meal usually delays gastric emptying and increases gastric pH to 5. This will prolong an antacid's acid neutralizing effect. Antacids do not decrease gastric acid secretion. By increasing gastric pH, gastrin secretion is stimulated which may even enhance gastric acid secretion.

Adverse Effects The availability and frequent use of antacids would suggest considerable safety. However, antacids have the potential for significant adverse effects and need to be used with caution in some patients and in certain clinical situations. In addition, many nonsystemic antacids have an unpleasant "chalky" taste, which is tolerable for occasional use, but which contributes to poor compliance in cases where regular chronic use is recommended. Attempts have been made to enhance the palatability of antacids by the addition of various flavorings to the preparations. Many antacids contain considerable amounts of sodium. The sodium content needs to be taken into consideration when treating patients on sodium restricted diets.

Aluminum-containing antacids can cause constipation, due to the ability of aluminum to bind bile acids. Aluminum is absorbed, especially in patients with renal failure, and can rarely precipitate an encephalopathy. In the intestine, aluminum binds with phosphate ion and is excreted in the feces. This action is beneficial in some patients with renal failure, preventing secondary hyperparathyroidism. However, excessive antacid use can lead to the "phosphate depletion syndrome." This consists of hypophosphatemia, hypercalciuria, osteomalacia, bone pain, malaise, muscle weakness, convulsions, and anorexia.

Antacid preparations containing magnesium frequently cause loose stools or diarrhea, via the ability of magnesium to increase intestinal motility. This side effect is dose-related and magnesium hydroxide is used as a laxative (see below). Magnesium can be absorbed systemically, and magnesium levels must be watched carefully in patients with renal failure.

Carbonate-containing antacids may cause abdominal distention, flatulence, and belching, due to the release of carbon dioxide. The effect of these compounds on intestinal motility are variable; however, constipation occurs more frequently than a laxative effect. Sodium bicarbonate generally only causes belching.

The milk alkali syndrome was first described in the 1940s in patients ingesting large quantities of antacids (usually sodium bicarbonate or calcium carbonate) and milk. The pathogenesis of milk alkali syndrome, which consists of hypercalcemia without hypercalciuria or hypophosphatemia, alkalosis, calcinosis, and renal failure, is unknown. The clinical presentation is headache, nausea, vomiting, and irritability. Treatment of the milk alkali syndrome is via hydration and dietary restriction.

Critically ill patients on respirators have an increased incidence of pneumonia following antacid use. It is thought that antacids may contribute to this problem via two mechanisms. First, raising gastric pH may increase bacterial colonization of the stomach, increasing the infectious nature of aspirated gastric contents. Second, antacids increase gastric volume which may further enhance the incidence of gastroesophageal reflux and aspiration in these patients.

Drug Interactions Antacids can alter the plasma levels of several drugs and when these are administered in combination with other drugs, potential drug interactions must be kept in mind. For example, by increasing the gastric pH, the absorption of weak acids (e.g., digoxin, phenytoin, isoniazid) is reduced, possibly decreasing their effects; the absorption of weak bases (e.g., pseudoephedrine and levodopa) may be enhanced. Drugs such as the tetracyclines form complexes with divalent (Mg^{2+} and Ca^{2+}) and trivalent (Al^{3+}) cations and absorption is reduced.

Increased urinary pH (especially with sodium bicarbonate), may inhibit the excretion of weak bases (e.g., quinidine, amphetamines) and may enhance the elimination of weak acids (e.g., salicylates). Administering a drug 2 hours from the ingestion of an antacid minimizes the effects on drug plasma levels.

Therapeutic Uses Antacids have anecdotal efficacy in treating a great number of gastrointestinal disorders. Unfortunately, there are few carefully controlled studies as to their true efficacy in treating dyspepsia, peptic ulcer disease, and stress-associated gastritis and hemorrhage. The increase in therapeutic modalities available for the treatment of acid-peptic disease makes interpretation of existing studies difficult. This leaves the clinician and patient unclear as to which is the most effective and safest modality to utilize in a particular clinical situation. A summary of the available literature on the efficacy of antacids for various gastrointestinal conditions is presented in Table 37-4.

ANTIDIARRHEAL AGENTS

The bowel is presented with 9 to 12 liters of fluid per day (ingested fluid in addition to gastrointestinal secretions). Normal stool volume does not exceed 100 to 200 g/day. Therefore, the intestine is extremely efficient at water absorption. Water

TABLE 37-4 Summary of therapeutic uses of antacids

GASTROESOPHAGEAL REFLUX

No controlled studies with placebo
Improvement of esophagitis over baseline
No benefit shown over H_2 receptor antagonists

GASTRIC ULCER

Efficacy in healing ulcer comparable to H_2 receptor antagonists
Relief of symptoms superior with ranitidine

DUODENAL ULCER

Superior to placebo at healing ulcer (not relieving symptoms)
Equal to H_2 receptor antagonists at healing ulcer
As effective as H_2 receptor antagonists in treating ulcer symptoms
Equal to H_2 receptor antagonists at preventing ulcer recurrence and relieving symptoms
No benefit in using antacids together with H_2 receptor antagonists in healing ulcer

STRESS RELATED GASTRITIS/HEMORRHAGE

Superior to placebo and cimetidine at maintaining pH > 3.5
Superior to placebo and cimetidine at controlling gastrointestinal hemorrhage
Most effective when administered as continuous drip

is not actively transported out of the bowel lumen, but moves passively as an osmotic response to the transport of electrolytes (Na^+, K^+, Cl^-) and organic solutes (glucose and amino acids) into the enterocyte and intracellular and subcellular spaces.

Diarrhea is usually defined as an excessive loss of water and electrolytes in the stools, due to an inability of the intestine to absorb the volume of fluid presented to it. Clinical symptoms are frequent watery stools, lassitude, and weight loss, which can progress to dehydration.

The movement of sodium and chloride into the enterocyte takes place in the villus tips of the enterocytes. Low intracellular Na^+, maintained by Na^+,K^+-ATPase on the basolateral junction, is the main driving force for Na^+ and fluid absorption. The three major mechanisms for sodium absorption are:

1. Diffusion of Na^+ coupled with Cl^- down its "electrical" gradient via a pericellular pathway.

2. Neutral sodium chloride (NaCl) co-transport. This transport is responsible for most of the sodium and chloride presented to the intestine. This process is inhibited by cholera toxin, enterotoxins, and rotavirus.

3. Absorption of water soluble organic solutes (glucose and amino acids) coupled to Na^+ absorption.

Sodium and fluid absorption in the colon is also stimulated by short-chain fatty acids, produced by the action of colonic bacteria on undigested carbohydrate. Short-chain fatty acids facilitate coupled Na^+ and Cl^- via their own absorption.

Electrolyte and fluid secretion take place primarily in the villus crypts. Again, the low intracellular Na^+ created by Na^+,K^+-ATPase promotes the accumulation of chloride in the enterocyte. Chloride channels in the apical membrane of the crypt cells open to permit Cl^- to proceed from enterocyte to intestinal lumen, forming a negatively charged potential difference. This stimulates Na^+ and, in turn, fluid secretion. The Cl^- channels are controlled by proteins, which stimulate their opening after phosphorylation. Increased intracellular cyclic AMP, cyclic GMP, calcium, and (possibly) calmodulin, initiate this process.

The complex mechanisms of controlling water and electrolyte flux in the bowel are subject to further systemic control. Four systems regulate water and sodium balance within the bowel: (1) the enteric nervous system, (2) the endocrine system, (3) the immune system, and (4) bacterial endotoxins. These systems play a role in the rate of absorption of fluid secretion by affecting transport mechanisms directly and/or by altering motility and transit time.

There are two major goals in the treatment of diarrhea. The first is to reestablish adequate hydration and electrolyte balance. This can be done via oral or intravenous rehydration. Oral rehydration solutions containing glucose take advantage of the fact that sodium absorption (and therefore fluid absorption) is enhanced by coupling to glucose. Most oral rehydration solutions also contain sodium and chloride as well. In severe dehydration, intravenous rehydration is necessary. Continued assessment of the patient's fluid and electrolyte status during therapy is imperative.

The second goal in the treatment of diarrhea, is to identify and treat, if indicated, the underlying cause of the diarrhea. Potential etiologies for diarrhea are listed in Table 37-5.

Once a particular etiology for the diarrhea is cited, it is then determined how or whether to treat the diarrhea. This is an important consideration in many clinical situations. For example, treating a *Salmonella*-induced gastroenteritis with antibiotics may actually prolong the diarrheal symptoms. Management of the patient with diarrhea must be a careful balance between relieving symptoms, maintaining hydration, and avoiding long term sequelae.

TABLE 37-5 Differential diagnosis of diarrhea

Infection: Bacterial, Viral, Parasitic
Inflammation
Drugs, including abuse of laxatives
Endocrine disorders
Tumors
Malabsorption: Fats, Carbohydrates, or Proteins
Functional: Irritable bowel syndrome

Adsorbents

Currently, there are many over-the-counter preparations marketed as antidiarrheal agents that contain natural or synthetic substances which act to adsorb water into themselves. This theoretically leads to thicker stools and decreased frequency and volume of stools. Intestinal fluid secretion is not affected. Most of these preparations contain attapulgite, psyllium husk, methylcellulose, or calcium polycarbophil and are indicated for the treatment of diarrhea; attapulgite is also used for abdominal cramping. Side effects such as abdominal bloating and pain can occur after use of these drugs.

Opioids

Opium and its derivatives have been used for thousands of years as antidiarrheal agents. The complete pharmacology of the opioids are described in detail in Chapter 23.

Opioids affect the bowel by their inhibitory effect on motility. Intestinal transit time is decreased, resulting in more contact time for absorption. Opium, codeine, and morphine are rarely used for their gastrointestinal effects alone, because of their central nervous system effects and abuse potential. There are three synthetic opioids commonly used in antidiarrheal preparations, diphenoxylate, difenoxin, and loperamide.

Diphenoxylate has ten times the antidiarrheal effect of morphine with little central nervous system or analgesic effects. Difenoxin is an active biotransformation product of diphenoxylate. Both compounds are marketed combined with an anticholinergic (atropine sulfate) so as to discourage opioid abuse. Adverse effects on the gastrointestinal tract include constipation, toxic megacolon (if used in an exacerbation of ulcerative colitis) and nausea. Diphenoxylate and difenoxin will have morphine-like central nervous system adverse effects if taken in large doses.

Loperamide is a potent antidiarrheal agent, having 45 to 50 times the effect of morphine. Due to poor oral absorption, its action is largely confined to the intestine, and the small amount that is absorbed does not cross the blood-brain barrier. Therefore, there are few central nervous system effects and little chance for abuse. Proposed actions of loperamide are decreased intestinal secretion (via inhibition of calmodulin) and decreased intestinal motility. The major gastrointestinal side effect is constipation.

Octreotide

Octreotide is a long-acting, synthetic analog of somatostatin that contains 8 amino acids, and has pharmacologic actions that are similar to the natural peptide. Somatostatin is a peptide containing 14 amino acids, that is located in many sites throughout the body including the central nervous system and the gastrointestinal tract. Somatostatin is generally an inhibitory peptide. In the gastrointestinal tract, somatostatin inhibits both endocrine and exocrine secretion, as well as smooth muscle contraction. The half-life of somatostatin is 1 to 3 min, requiring continuous intravenous infusion for administration; this makes somatostatin impractical for clinical trials, clinical research, and therapeutic use.

Like somatostatin, octreotide is an inhibitory peptide. It decreases the secretion of the gastrointestinal hormones, vasoactive intestinal peptide (VIP) and motilin. It also decreases the secretion of intestinal fluid and electrolytes and decreases intestinal motility.

Absorption is poor when octreotide is taken enterally. Therefore, administration is by subcutaneous injection. Peak blood levels are achieved in 30 min and maximum effects occur in about 2 h. Approximately 65 percent is bound in the plasma, mainly to lipoprotein and, to a lesser extent, albumin. The plasma half-life is 90 minutes. Elimination occurs via hepatic and renal mechanisms, and 10 to 30 percent is excreted in the urine. Therefore, octreotide must be used with caution in renal failure patients.

Because of its efficacy as an antidiarrheal agent, octreotide has been studied in patients with a number of gastrointestinal diseases. It is indicated for use as an antidiarrheal drug in patients with metastatic carcinoid tumors or VIPomas.

Octreotide has a number of adverse effects, but those that occur are usually mild and transient. Nausea, vomiting, abdominal pain, and pain at the injection site are seen in 3 to 10 percent of patients. Other less frequently seen adverse effects include headache, dizziness, fatigue, flushing, and hypoglycemia.

Bismuth

Bismuth compounds are described in detail earlier in this chapter. Bismuth subsalicylate has been found to have antisecretory, antimotility, and antibacterial properties and is effective in patients with travelers diarrhea (especially that related to toxicogenic *E. coli*). Bismuth subsalicylate has also been shown to be effective at treating nonspecific diarrhea of childhood.

LAXATIVES

Constipation is one of the most common digestive complaints presented to the physician. In the United States alone, $400 million a year are spent on laxative preparations.

The definition of constipation varies widely, mostly according to personal opinion and cultural belief. In certain populations, "regular" bowel movements are imperative to general well-being. Therefore, it is important for the physician to develop his or her own parameters as to the necessity of intervention. In most medical circles, constipation suggests not infrequent bowel movements (1 to 2 per week), but difficulty in passing bowel contents. This difficulty consists of obstipation (abdominal obstruction associated with constipation), severe pain on defecation, abdominal cramps, rectal bleeding, hemorrhoids, and/or recurrent anal fissures. Straining with bowel movements may prove to be physically stressful for some cardiac or post-operative patients. Transient use of laxatives is helpful in these situations. Patients with spinal cord abnormalities or neuromuscular disease may benefit from the medical management of constipation.

Alterations in life-style are the most effective and safest means of managing constipation. Regular exercise has been shown to decrease intestinal transit time, thus allowing for more frequent bowel movements. Increasing the amount of total dietary fiber per day to 25 to 30 g is important. Dietary fiber is plant cell material which is not digested by intestinal enzymes; examples are wheat bran and fibers obtained from fresh fruits and vegetables. Fiber will add bulk or mass to the stool, but also draws water into itself, decreasing water absorption from the colon. Thus, the stools are more moist. Fiber also decreases intestinal transit time and decreases intracolonic pressure, thereby, reducing abdominal cramps.

Laxatives are divided into several major types based upon their action. These include bulk laxatives, stimulant laxatives, saline laxatives, and hyperosmotic laxatives. In addition, stool softeners and a lubricant are available for patients who should not strain during defecation.

Bulk Laxatives

There are many brands and preparations of non-dietary fiber that are used as bulk-producing laxatives. The most common naturally-derived fiber is psyllium hydrophilic mucilloid, derived from the husk of the psyllium seed (*Plantago ovata*). Another natural fiber product is barley malt extract. Methylcellulose and polycarbophil are synthetically derived fibers. In addition to absorbing water and decreasing intestinal transit, fibers are also fermented by bacterial flora, resulting in the formation of short-chain fatty acids. These increase the osmolarity of the luminal contents and enhance intestinal secretion. Some fibers are also believed to sequester bile acids in the small intestine, which enhances water secretion by the colon. The laxative effect of these drugs is generally seen within 12 to 24 h.

Fiber preparations are available in powder, wafer, granules, or tablet form. It is critical that the patient be on adequate oral fluid during fiber therapy (at least 32 fl. oz. per day). A fiber program deficient in fluid supplementation may lead to severe constipation. Fiber preparations are generally considered safe. They are rarely associated with abdominal cramps or bloating. Because of their effect of increasing stool bulk, they are contraindicated in cases of intestinal narrowing or obstruction.

Some fiber preparations contain sugar, which needs to be monitored in diabetics. Fiber can also bind to drugs, altering their absorption. Plasma levels of salicylates and cardiac glycosides need to be monitored in patients on fiber therapy.

Stimulant Laxatives

Stimulant laxatives are thought to work via enhancement of colonic motility. These compounds stimulate sensory nerve ending in the mucosa or submucosal plexi of the large intestine, initiating parasympathetic reflexes and increased peristaltic contractions of the colon. Although this mechanism may still be a valid, stimulant laxatives are also believed to alter the colonic water and electrolyte transport mechanism, promoting fluid accumulation in the colon. The three major stimulant laxatives are: anthraquinones (cascara sagrada, senna, casanthranol), polyphenolic laxatives (phenolphthalein, bisacodyl), and castor oil.

Anthraquinones These compounds are either synthetic, i.e., casanthranol, or glycosides derived from plant sources: cascara sagrada (the dried bark of *Rhamnus purshiana*), senna (the dried pod of *Cassia acutifolia* or *C. augustifolia*). Once ingested, the plant products reach the colon unabsorbed, where the inactive precursor glycosides are hydrolyzed by the bacterial flora into the active form. Casanthranol is a free, active anthraquinone rather than a glycoside.

In addition to stimulation of intestinal peristalsis (decreasing transit time), the active anthraquinones are also thought to enhance intestinal fluid secretion. By inhibiting intestinal Na^+,K^+-ATPase, the major pump for sodium absorption, anthraquinones also inhibit water absorption. All of the substances are efficient laxatives; their onset of action is delayed (6 to 10 h) and they have short durations of action (2 to 6 h). Prolonged use of these drugs can cause irritation to the intestinal mucosa and melanosis coli, a benign increase of melanotic pigment in enterocytes.

Polyphenolic Laxatives The two polyphenolic laxatives are phenolphthalein and bisacodyl. Both act to increase colonic peristalsis and to enhance fluid and electrolyte secretion into the bowel. Phenolphthalein is present in prunes and contained in many oral laxative preparations. Up to 15 percent is absorbed following oral administration, metabolized by conjugation with glucuronic acid, and excreted in urine and bile. The urine and stool will become red or pink if sufficiently alkaline. Bisacodyl is available in oral and rectal forms; it is very poorly absorbed orally (up to 5 percent). Following oral administration, phenolphthalein and bisacodyl act within 6 to 12 h; bisacodyl rectal suppositories initiate an effect in 15 to 60 min. Both drugs are relatively non-toxic since little reaches the systemic circulation.

Castor Oil Castor oil, which is one of the oldest known laxatives, is derived from the seed of *Ricinus communis* and is composed of the triglyceride of ricinoleic acid. Unlike other stimulant laxatives, castor oil acts in the small intestine. At this site, castor oil is hydrolyzed into glycerol and ricinoleic acid by pancreatic lipase. Ricinoleic acid is irritating to the intestinal mucosa, and can result in disruption of villi. It also decreases sodium and fluid absorption by inhibiting intestinal Na^+,K^+-ATPase and increases intestinal secretion by increasing intracellular cyclic AMP. Ricinoleic acid also enhances intestinal and uterine contractibility, making its use in pregnancy undesirable. Any absorbed ricinoleic acid is metabolized like other fatty acids.

Saline Laxatives

The saline laxatives include magnesium citrate, magnesium sulfate, magnesium hydroxide, sodium phosphate, and sodium biphosphate. These salts are slowly and incompletely absorbed from the intestinal tract; thus, they increase luminal osmolarity and peristalsis is stimulated indirectly. It has been suggested that magnesium salts increase the secretion of cholecystokinin, which increases intestinal motility.

Saline laxatives are available for oral and rectal administration. The oral preparations have an onset of action of 3 to 6 h and a duration of action of 6 to 8 h; rectal administration acts within minutes and has a short duration. These compounds are generally well-tolerated, but must be used with caution in patients with renal failure, cardiac disease, ileostomies or colostomies, or in patients on diuretics. Oral magnesium hydroxide is also used as an antacid (see above).

Hyperosmotic Laxatives

The two hyperosmotic laxatives are glycerin and lactulose. Glycerin is a trihydroxy alcohol which absorbs water and irritates the bowel, both actions induce peristalsis when administered rectally (via suppository or enema). It is effective in 2 to 6 h and causes occasional rectal discomfort as its only major adverse effect.

Lactulose, a disaccharide (containing galactose and fructose), is administered orally. It is not absorbed and not metabolized by human intestinal enzymes; therefore, it acts as an osmotic agent enhancing the secretion of water into the intestinal lumen. Once it reaches the colon, lactulose is processed by intestinal flora into low molecular weight acids (lactic acid, formic acid, acetic acid) and carbon dioxide which increase the osmotic load and enhance intestinal motility. Since the intestinal contents become more acidic than the blood, ammonia (NH_3) diffuses from the blood to the colon. Ammonia reacts with the acidic bowel contents, forming ammonium ion (NH_4^+), which become trapped (ion trapping mechanism), is not reabsorbed, and is expelled by the laxative effect of the drug. This effect of lactulose on ammonia metabolism makes it useful in the management of hepatic encephalopathy.

Small amounts of lactose are in lactulose, therefore, it is to be avoided in patients with lactose intolerance. Although lactulose is well-tolerated, there are occasional complaints of abdominal cramps, diarrhea, bloating, flatulence, and nausea and vomiting.

Stool Softeners

Stool softeners include calcium, potassium, or sodium salts of docusate (dioctyl sodium sulfosuccinate). They were originally believed to act as surfactants, allowing water and lipids to penetrate into the stool. They are also thought to decrease colonic water absorption and to enhance intestinal secretion. Stool softeners are effective as mild laxatives, but are not recommended for prolonged use.

Only a small amount of docusate is absorbed following oral administration. Even large doses have not produced significant adverse effects.

Lubricant Laxatives

The basis of all lubricant preparations is mineral oil, a hydrocarbon derived from petroleum. Mineral oil has minimal absorption from the bowel and primarily acts to lubricate stool and ease passage of the stool. It is especially effective in some post-operative patients or in those with anal fissures and pain. In general, mineral oil is safe and easily tolerated. There is some suggestion that prolonged use may lead to malabsorption of fat soluble vitamins. In large doses, mineral oil can "leak" out of the anus, this can lead to embarrassment, staining, and anal irritation. Oral aspiration of mineral oil can lead to a severe lipoid pneumonia. Therefore, mineral oil is contraindicated in patients with vomiting or significant respiratory symptoms. Lipoid granulomas in the reticuloendothelial system have been found in patients after prolonged use of mineral oil.

Miscellaneous Laxatives

There is a preparation called polyethylene glycol-electrolyte solution (PEG-ES) which consists of an isotonic solution of sodium sulfate, sodium bicarbonate, sodium chloride, potassium chloride, and polyethylene glycol which causes a marked catharsis without resulting in dehydration. It is usually taken orally in large quantities (the adult dose is 4 liters). The usefulness of PEG-ES is limited to bowel cleansing prior to gastrointestinal procedures such as barium enemas or endoscopy. However, its use has been suggested in severe chronic constipation or in the meconium ileus equivalent syndrome of cystic fibrosis. PEG-ES is generally well-tolerated, but can produce nausea, abdominal fullness, and bloating in up to 50 percent of patients.

It must be stressed that laxative use needs to be recommended judiciously. The over-the-counter nature of these preparations may lead the patient and physician into a false sense of security concerning their safety. In most situations, the only laxatives that are tolerated well with chronic use are the dietary and non-dietary fiber preparations accompanied by adequate fluid intake. The *cathartic colon syndrome* can result after chronic laxative use and it is possibly related to laxative dependency. On barium enema, the colon is dilated, hypomotile, and demonstrates decreased haustral markings. The syndrome can progress to hypokalemia and malabsorption of carbohydrates, fat, fat soluble vitamins, and calcium.

TABLE 37-6 Clinical situations treated by prokinetic and antiemetic drugs

Vomiting
Chemotherapy-induced
Gastroesophageal reflux
Gastroparesis (bloating, early satiety)
Diabetes
Collagen vascular disease
Post-operative
Intestinal pseudo-obstruction
Collagen vascular disease
idiopathic
Chronic, severe "resistant" constipation
Placement of feeding tubes

PROKINETIC AND ANTIEMETIC DRUGS

The physiology of gastrointestinal motility is not completely understood. Factors that play a major role in motility are the neuropeptides, originating from the central nervous system or the enteric nervous system. Amount of bowel motility, contractile strength, and coordination of contractions all contribute to uncomplicated and efficient transit through the gastrointestinal tract. Disorders of gastrointestinal motility can lead to a variety of symptoms, such as vomiting, bloating, constipation, dysphagia, and abdominal distension. Prokinetic and antiemetic drugs are used to manage several motility disorders (Table 37-6). A prokinetic drug is one that stimulates motility of the gastrointestinal tract; antiemetic drugs reduce or abolish vomiting. Metoclopramide, bethanechol, and cisapride are all prokinetic drugs and will be discussed in this section; metoclopramide also has antiemetic effects. Other antiemetics, such as anticholinergics, antihistamines, and phenothiazines are discussed in depth in Chapters 11, 13, and 20, respectively.

Metoclopramide

Effects Metoclopramide stimulates motility of the upper gastrointestinal tract. It increases the tone of the esophageal sphincter (increasing lower esophageal sphincter pressure), increases contractions of the stomach, relaxes the pyloric sphincter, and increases peristaltic activity of the duodenum and jejunum. The result is an increase in gastric emptying and intestinal transit. The colon is unaffected and the drug does not stimulate gastric, pancreatic, or biliary secretions.

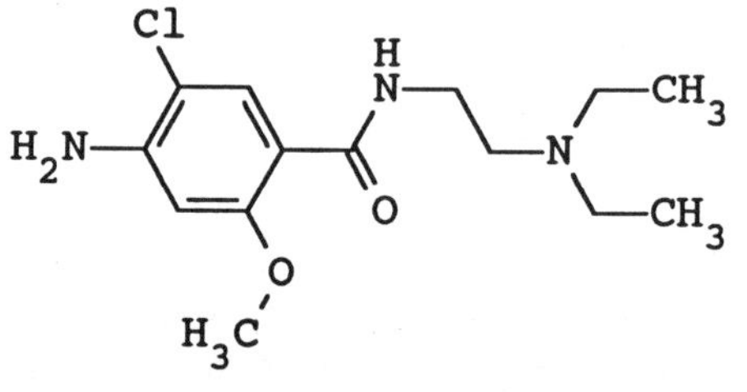

Although the mechanism of action of its prokinetic effect is unknown, metoclopramide has cholinomimetic properties and is a potent dopamine receptor antagonist. The drug does not act directly at cholinergic receptors, but is believed to sensitize intestinal tissues to the action of acetylcholine. Some evidence suggests that it increases acetylcholine release from enteric neurons. By inhibiting peripheral and central dopaminergic receptors, metoclopramide allows cholinergic effects to gain prominence.

Centrally, metoclopramide has a direct antiemetic effect by blockade of dopamine receptors in the chemoreceptor trigger zone. This is demonstrated by inhibition of nausea and vomiting induced by dopamine and apomorphine, a dopamine receptor agonist, at the chemoreceptor trigger zone.

Pharmacokinetics After oral ingestion, metoclopramide is rapidly and well absorbed (oral bioavailability over 85 percent). The elimination half-life of metoclopramide is 5 to 6 h. The drug is conjugated with glucuronic acid in the liver and the parent compound and conjugated metabolites are excreted in the urine. The elimination of the drug is prolonged up to 24 h in patients with renal failure.

Adverse Effects Because metoclopramide crosses the blood-brain barrier, it will induce central nervous system adverse effects in up to 20 percent of patients. These include restlessness, drowsiness, fatigue, confusion, mental depression, and (rarely) hallucinations. Since the compound blocks central dopaminergic receptors, parkinson-like symptoms (extrapyramidal reactions, tardive dyskinesia) and increased prolactin secretion and gynecomastia can occur. The extrapyramidal reactions are usually reversible and can be managed with centrally-acting anticholinergic such as benztropine; tardive dyskinesia is not always reversible. The central nervous system effects of metoclopramide must be monitored, especially in patients on chronic therapy or higher (antiemetic) doses. Metoclopramide can also lead to cholinergic side effects, diarrhea and abdominal cramps.

Drug Interactions Due to its prokinetic effect on the stomach and bowel, metoclopramide may alter the absorption of drugs given concomitantly. The absorption of acetaminophen, tetracycline, ethanol, and levodopa is enhanced by metoclopramide. The absorption of cimetidine and digoxin are decreased when used with metoclopramide.

When used with anticholinergic drugs or opioid analgesics, the effects of metoclopramide are decreased. Extrapyramidal effects of metoclopramide are enhanced when used with phenothiazines or butyrophenones.

Therapeutic Uses Metoclopramide is approved for use in the treatment of diabetic gastroparesis. It has been shown to improve symptoms and to enhance gastric emptying in these patients. If oral administration is tolerated poorly, intramuscular or intravenous injections may be used.

Metoclopramide is used for the prevention and post-operative nausea and vomiting. It is also approved for use as an antiemetic in patients undergoing chemotherapy. The drug has also been approved for use in facilitating the passage of naso-jejunal tubes for therapeutic or diagnostic purposes.

Bethanechol

Bethanechol is a derivative of acetylcholine and a cholinergic agonist. The pharmacology of the drug is described in detail in Chapter 10. In the gastrointestinal tract, bethanechol increases contractility, mostly of the upper tract. It increases the amplitude and velocity of esophageal contractions and increases lower esophageal sphincter pressure. Bethanechol has no effect on gastric emptying or small bowel transit time. However, due to its cholinergic effects, it will increase saliva and gastric acid secretion.

Adverse effects of bethanechol are mainly due to its cholinergic actions, and include abdominal cramping, fatigue, blurred vision, and increased micturition. These effects can occur in 10 to 15% of patients treated with bethanechol.

Bethanechol has been used to treat gastroesophageal reflux in children and adults. Treatment resulted both in improvement of symptoms and in esophageal histology.

Cisapride

This compound is the newest of the approved prokinetic drugs.

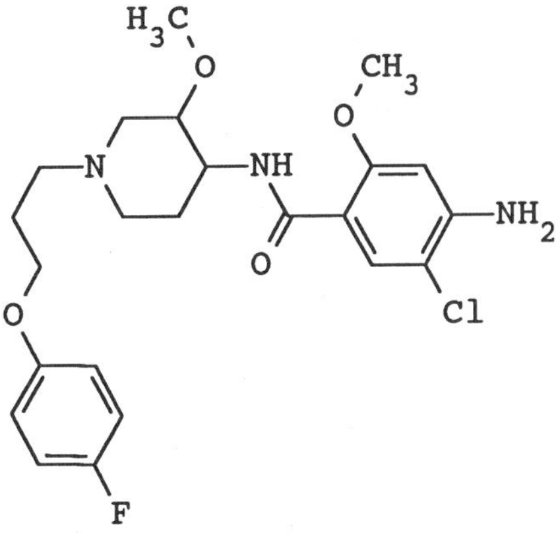

Effects Unlike metoclopramide, cisapride has no effect on dopamine receptors and no direct antiemetic effect. Its prokinetic actions are due to its ability to facilitate acetylcholine release from the myenteric plexus, and possibly, its ability to affect various neuropeptides. Cisapride is known to increase levels of pancreatic polypeptides, cholecystokinin, gastrin, and insulin. *In vitro* the compound acts as an agonist at type 4 5-hydroxytryptamine (5-HT_4) receptors; this may be involved in the increased gastrointestinal motility induced by the drug.

Cisapride exerts its effects on the entire gastrointestinal tract. It increases the amplitude of distal esophageal contractions and increases lower esophageal sphincter pressure. Gastric tone and emptying are enhanced by cisapride, as are central duodenal and ileal contractions. Cisapride decreases colonic transit time.

Pharmacokinetics When administered orally, cisapride is rapidly and adequately absorbed; the oral bioavailability is 35 to 40 percent. The onset of action is about 30 to 60 min. Peak plasma levels are reached in 1 to 1.5 h and the plasma half-life is 7 to 10 hours. Cisapride is 98 percent bound to plasma proteins, mainly to albumin. However, the volume of distribution is large, indicating extensive distribution to tissues. The drug is extensively biotransformed by N-dealkylation and hydroxylation in the liver. Its major metabolite is norcisapride, which is excreted in the urine and feces. The drug and its metabolites will accumulate in individuals with hepatic and renal disease and in the elderly.

Adverse Effects The more common adverse effects of this drug include abdominal cramps, diarrhea, constipation, dyspepsia, flatulence, rhinitis, fatigue, and headache. Cardiovascular and hematologic adverse effects are rare. There is a suggestion that cisapride may lower the seizure threshold.

Like metoclopramide, the ability of cisapride to increase the rate of gastric and intestinal transit may alter the absorption of other drugs. Cisapride enhances the anticoagulant effects of warfarin by competition for plasma protein binding sites. The oral absorption of cimetidine and ranitidine is increased by cisapride.

Therapeutic Uses Cisapride has been approved for oral use in the treatment of idiopathic gastroesophageal reflux disease (GERD) and GERD associated with diabetes, cystic fibrosis, and scleroderma. It has proven superior to placebo and metoclopramide and equal to H_2 receptor antagonists in reversing histological reflux esophagitis. Cisapride has been used to treat a number of other gastrointestinal diseases including gastroparesis associated with diabetes and anorexia nervosa, progressive systemic sclerosis, severe chronic constipation, non-ulcer dyspepsia, and intestinal pseudo-obstruction. Although it has shown promise for many conditions, studies are ongoing and no definitive recommendations of approval have been made.

INFLAMMATORY BOWEL DISEASE

There are two major diseases under the general heading of inflammatory bowel disease (IBD): Crohn's disease and ulcerative colitis. These are chronic idiopathic inflammatory disorders of the bowel which result in a great deal of morbidity. A lengthy discussion of IBD is beyond the scope of this book. Basically, Crohn's disease is a transmural inflammation of the entire gastrointestinal tract, mouth to anus. The most common sites of involvement are the terminal ileum and colon. Because of the potential for small bowel involvement, malabsorption, vitamin deficiencies, growth failure, and a functional short bowel syndrome can ensue. The transmural inflammation can result in the formation of inflammatory masses, fistulas, and perianal disease. Crohn's disease can reoccur once a diseased portion of the bowel has been removed.

Ulcerative colitis involves the colon alone and the inflammation exists only in the mucosa. Therefore, the primary symptoms are diarrhea, abdominal cramps, and rectal bleeding. Colectomy is a "cure" for ulcerative colitis. Patients who suffer from chronic ulcerative colitis have a higher incidence of colon cancer than the general population.

Although the symptoms of IBD are primarily gastrointestinal, there are some systemic or extraintestinal manifestations. These include skin rashes, fever, iritis, arthritis, and liver disease (sclerosing cholangitis).

Investigations are underway to uncover the etiology and pathogenesis of the inflammation in IBD. It is currently thought that an excess amount of tissue damaging proteases, free radicals, and peroxidases are released from granulocytes (polymorphonuclear leukocytes and monocytes) located in the bowel. Leukotriene B_4 (LTB_4), interleukin 2, platelet activating factor (PAF), and tumor necrosis factor all lead to enhanced attraction and activation of more granulocytes, which sets up a cascade of progressive inflammation. The initial event in stimulating this cycle is unknown, but may be a foreign antigen or bacterial endotoxin that "leaks" from the bowel epithelium to the lamina propria.

Before drug therapy for IBD is discussed, it must be mentioned that one of the cornerstones of effective therapy for IBD is nutrition. Excellent nutrition is paramount in the successful management of IBD, and can be achieved enterally or parenterally. Drug therapy for IBD is based on management of bowel inflammation and its mediators.

Sulfasalazine

Sulfasalazine consists of sulfapyridine linked to 5-aminosalicylic acid by an azo bond.

5-aminosalicylic acid

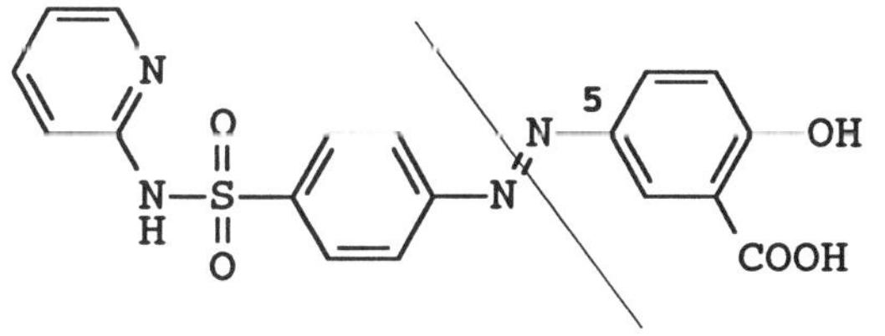

sulfapyridine

Effects Although sulfasalazine has been used successfully to treat IBD for over sixty years, its exact mechanism of action in reducing inflammation is not know. Theories include inhibition of the synthesis of prostaglandins and leukotrienes (which enhance inflammation) by 5-aminosalicylic acid and the ability to scavenge oxygen free radicals (cytotoxic products of granulocytes).

Pharmacokinetics After oral ingestion, most sulfasalazine (over 70 percent) is not absorbed. It arrives intact in the terminal ileum and colon, where its biotransformation begins. Sulfasalazine is split by bacteria into sulfapyridine and 5-aminosalicylic acid (5-ASA) by reduction of the azo bond. Sulfapyridine is absorbed by the colon, metabolized by the liver, and excreted in the urine. A small amount of the 5-ASA is absorbed and excreted in the urine as an N-acetylated derivative; however, most of the 5-ASA is not absorbed and is excreted unchanged in the feces.

Adverse Effects Adverse effects occur in up to 20 percent of patients on sulfasalazine and include gastrointestinal intolerance (nausea, vomiting, anorexia, dyspepsia), headache, and hematologic effects (hemolysis, leucopenia, impaired folate absorption). Hypersensitivity reactions (pneumonitis, hepatitis, pancreatitis, neuropathy) have been attributed to the sulfapyridine portion of the compound. Sulfasalazine has no known teratogenic effects and is not contraindicated in pregnant woman or nursing mothers.

Therapeutic Uses Sulfasalazine has been a cornerstone in the treatment of IBD since its introduction in the early 1940s. It is used for the management of acute, mild to moderate ulcerative colitis. Sulfasalazine is also used prophylactically in ulcerative colitis, in order to prevent relapses. Crohn's disease, ileitis with colitis, but not ileitis alone, can be managed with sulfasalazine. The ability to prevent recurrence of exacerbations in Crohn's disease with sulfasalazine has not been clearly demonstrated.

Mesalamine and Olsalazine

These two aminosalicylates have been developed as alternatives to sulfasalazine for the treatment of IBD. Mesalamine is 5-ASA. Olsalazine is a dimer of 5-ASA connected through the azo bond; cleavage of the azo bond occurs in the colon by azo reductase produced by bacteria.

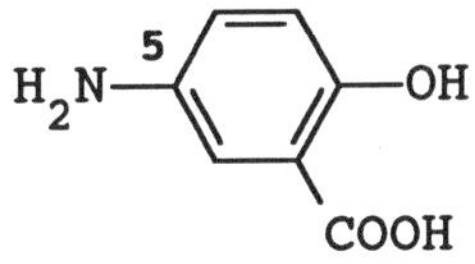

Mesalamine

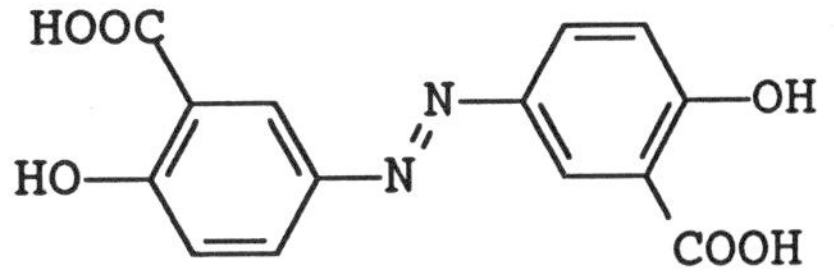

Olsalazine

Effects The exact anti-inflammatory mechanism of the aminosalicylate preparations has not been defined, but appears to be topical rather than systemic. It is thought that 5-ASA may block the cyclooxygenase and 5-lipoxygenese pathways of arachidonic acid metabolism in the colon, interfering with the formation of mediators of inflammation. 5-ASA may also inhibit platelet activating factor (PAF) or interleukins.

Pharmacokinetics After oral administration, about 30 percent of 5-ASA (mesalamine) is absorbed from the proximal bowel and will be biotransformed via N-acetylation in the liver. N-acetyl-5-ASA is excreted by the kidneys. Unabsorbed 5-ASA will also be biotransformed to N-acetyl-5-ASA by the colonic epithelium.

Since oral mesalamine preparations are intended for local action on the ileum and colon, tablets are made to delay absorption. This is accomplished by using tablets coated with an acrylic-based resin that delays the drug release. Release of the drug from these tablets is pH-dependent (occurring at pH > 6), allowing the coating to dissolve when delivered to the terminal ileum and colon.

Mesalamine is also available as rectal suppositories and a rectal suspension. These have poor absorption from the rectal mucosa and thus exert a local effect. Depending on the retention time in the colon, only 10 to 30 percent of the drug is absorbed systemically by this route.

Olsalazine is very poorly absorbed orally; over 98 percent of an oral dose will reach the colon where it is split into two molecules of 5-ASA. At this point, the fate of the compound is the same as described above for mesalamine.

Adverse Effects Both mesalamine and olsalazine are well tolerated, and demonstrate the same, but less frequent, adverse effects than sulfasalazine. Patients having excessive adverse reactions to sulfasalazine will be able to use either of these drugs chronically 85 percent of the time. However, 10 to 20 percent of sulfasalazine-sensitive patients will continue to have reactions to mesalamine and olsalazine. Anal irritation has been reported after topical use of mesalamine. Diarrhea has been reported in up to 13 percent of patients on olsalazine. Other adverse effects include hair loss and, rarely, hypersensitivity reactions (pancreatitis, pericarditis, myocarditis, and a Kawasaki-like syndrome).

Therapeutic Uses Mesalamine and olsalazine have been found to be of equal or greater benefit than sulfasalazine in treating mild to moderate active ulcerative colitis. They are also equally effective at maintaining remission in ulcerative colitis. There is some evidence that the delayed-release oral mesalamine preparation may be effective in treating ileal involvement in Crohn's disease. Rectal mesalamine is very effective in treating distal colitis (enemas) and proctitis (suppositories), especially in ulcerative colitis. These preparations are showing promise in the management of colitis refractory to other therapies, and in maintaining remission in IBD.

Currently, the exact place of these drugs in the treatment of IBD is unclear. Olsalazine is indicated only for those patients with a known sensitivity to sulfasalazine. In general, the oral preparations are useful in the management of active ulcerative or Crohn's colitis and for maintenance of remission. Rectal mesalamine preparations are helpful in the treatment of active distal ulcerative colitis, and in preventing relapses.

Corticosteroids

Corticosteroids are discussed in depth in Chapter 42. They have been used successfully in the treatment of IBD for many years. Intravenous, topical, and oral preparations are used. The precise anti-inflammatory mechanism of the corticosteroids in relation to IBD is unknown. Proposed mechanisms include (1) inhibition of arachidonic acid metabolism leading to decreased prostaglandin and leukotriene synthesis, (2) modification of the immune response, (3) decreased release of interleukin 2, and (4) decreased production of helper T cells.

Corticosteroids are superior to sulfasalazine in achieving remission in moderate to severe colitis. Oral and topical preparations suffice in mild to moderate colitis, but intravenous preparations are often recommended for severe colitis. None of the corticosteroid preparations are effective in maintaining remissions in colitis, and long-term chronic use is discouraged.

Again, corticosteroids are more effective at treating active Crohn's disease (regardless of location) than sulfasalazine. Studies have not shown that corticosteroids can maintain remission; therefore, long-term corticosteroid use in Crohn's disease is not recommended. There is some suggestion that high dose corticosteroids may actually worsen progression of perianal disease.

Immunosuppressives

Although not officially indicated for this purpose, azathioprine and 6-mercaptopurine have been used to treat IBD for several years. The pharmacology of these drugs are thoroughly discussed in Chapter 44 and 43, respectively. In the management of inflammation in IBD, azathioprine and mercaptopurine are thought to exert their effects by their ability to decrease killer T lymphocytes. Because of their potential for toxicity and slow onset of clinical effect (2 to 3 months), these compounds are not first-line drugs in the management of IBD. They are generally effective in treating refractory IBD and in patients who are unable to be weaned off corticosteroids, due to recurrent exacerbations. Azathioprine and mercaptopurine have been shown to be particularly effective in the management of fistulae and perianal disease in Crohn's disease.

Antibiotics

Metronidazole has been used in the management of Crohn's disease for several years. It is as effective as sulfasalazine in treating ileitis and colitis, and in the management of perianal disease. Metronidazole has shown no significant effectiveness in the treatment of ulcerative colitis. Its mechanism of action is unknown, but it is thought to decrease bowel inflammation by altering colonic and anaerobic flora and by suppressing cell mediated immunity. The pharmacology of metronidazole is discussed in Chapter 47.

BIBLIOGRAPHY

Adler, D.J., and B.I. Korelitz: "The Therapeutic Efficacy of 6-Mercaptopurine in Refractory Ulcerative Colitis," *Am. J. Gastroenterol.* **85**: 727-722 (1990).

Baker, D.: "Misoprostol," *Prac. Gastroenterol.* **13**: 8-14 (1989).

Buhl, K., and H.R. Clearfield: "Omeprazole: A New Approach to Gastric Acid Suppression," *Am. Fam. Physician* **41**: 1225-1227 (1990).

D'Arienzo, A., A. Panarese, F.P. D'Armiento, C. Lancia, P. Quattrone, F. Giannattasio, A. Boscaino, and G. Mazzacca: "5-Aminosalicylic Acid Suppositories in the Maintenance of Remission in Idiopathic Proctitis or Proctosigmoiditis: A Double-Blind Placebo-Controlled Clinical Trial," *Am. J. Gastroenterol.* **85**: 1079-1082 (1990).

DiPalma, J.R.: "Metoclopramide: A Dopamine Receptor Antagonist," *Am. Fam. Physician* **41**: 919-924 (1990).

DiPalma, J.R.: "Misoprostol: A Prostaglandin for Peptic Ulcer," *Am. Fam. Physician* **40**: 217-219 (1989).

Feldman, M., and M.E. Burton: "Histamine2-Receptor Antagonists. Standard Therapy for Acid-Peptic Diseases," *N. Engl. J. Med.* **323**: 1672-1680 (1990).

Figueroa-Quintanilla, D., E. Salazar-Lindo, R.B. Sack, R. Leon-Barua, S. Sarabia-Arce, M. Campos-Sanchez, and E. Eyzagurre-Maccan: "A Controlled Trial of Bismuth Subsalicylate in Infants with Acute Watery Diarrheal Disease," *N. Engl. J. Med.* **328**: 1653-1658 (1993).

Hanauer, S.B., and M.B. Smith: "Rapid Closure of Crohn's Disease Fistulas with Continuous Intravenous Cyclosporin A," *Am. J. Gastroenterol.* **88**: 646-649 (1993).

Harig, J.M., K.H. Soergel, R.A. Komorowski, and C.M. Wood: "Treatment of Diversion Colitis with Short-Chain-Fatty Acid Irrigation", *N. Engl. J. Med.* **320**: 23-28 (1989).

Hyams, J.S., and W.R. Treem: "Cyclosporine Treatment of Fulminent Colitis," *J. Pediatr. Gastroenterol. Nutr.* **9**: 383-387 (1989).

Jaros, W., J. Biller, S. Greer, T. O'Dorisio, and R. Grand: "Successful Treatment of Idiopathic Secretory Diarrhea of Infancy with the Somatostatin Analogue SMS 201-995, *Gastroenterology* **94**: 189-193 (1988).

Knodel, L.C., and A.A. Allerman: "Formulary Update: Treatment of Peptic Ulcer Disease: Focus on Sucralfate," *Prac. Gastroenterol.* **15**: 46-50 (1991).

Lanza, F.L., and C.M. Sibley: "Role of Antacids in the Management of Disorders of the Upper Gastrointestinal Tract. Review of Clinical Experience 1975-1985, "*Am. J. Gastroenterol.* **82**: 1223-1241 (1987).

Linn, F.V., and M.A. Peppercorn: "Drug Therapy for Inflammatory Bowel Disease Part I," *Am. J. Surg.* **164**: 85-92 (1992).

Livingston, E.H., and P.H. Gutn: "Peptic Ulcer Disease," *Am. Scientist* **80**: 592-598 (1992).

Lochs, H., H.J. Steinhardt, B. Klaus-Wentz, M. Zeitz, H. Vogelsang, H. Sommer, W.E. Fleig, P. Bauer, J. Schirrmeister, and J. Melchow: "Comparison of Enteral Nutrition and Drug Treatment in Active Crohn's Disease. Results of the European Cooperative Crohn's Disease Study. IV," *Gastroenterology* **101**: 881-888 (1991).

Mahalanabis, D.: "Fluid Therapy of Diarrhea," In W.A. Walker, P.R. Durie, J.R. Hamilton, J.A. Walker-Smith and J.B. Watkins, (eds.), *Pediatric Gastrointestinal Disease*, B.C. Decker, Inc. Philadelphia, 1991, pp. 1561-1567.

Marshall, B.J.: "The Use of Bismuth in Gastroenterology. The ACG Committee on FDA-Related Matters. American College of Gastroenterology," *Am. J. Gastroenterol.* **86**: 16-25 (1991).

Maton, P.N.: "Omeprazole," *N. Engl. J. Med.* **324**: 965-975 (1991).

McCallum, R.W.: "Cisapride: A New Class of Prokinetic Agent. The ACG Committee on FDA-Related Matters. American College of Gastroenterology," *Am. J. Gastroenterol.* **86**: 135-149 (1991).

Riley, S.A., et al.: "Comparison of Delayed-Release 5-Aminosalicylic Acid (Mesalazine) and Sulfasalazine as Maintenance Treatment for Patients with Ulcerative Colitis," *Gastroenterology* **94**: 1383-1389 (1988).

Singleton, J.W., S.B. Hanauer, G.L. Gitnick, M.A. Peppercorn, M.G. Robinson, L.D. Wruble, and E.L. Krawitt: "Mesalamine Capsules for the Treatment of Active Crohn's Disease: Results of a 16-Week Trial," *Gastroenterology* **104**: 1293-1301 (1993).

Soll, A.H.: "Pathogenesis of Peptic Ulcer and Implications for Therapy," *N. Engl. J. Med.* **322**: 909-916 (1990).

Van Outryve, M., R. Milo, J. Toussaint, and P. Van Eeghem: "'Prokinetic' Treatment of Constipation-Predominant Irritable Bowel Syndrome: A Placebo-Controlled Study of Cisapride," *J. Clin. Gastroenterol.* **13**: 49-57 (1991).

Walt, R.P.: "Misoprostal for the Treatment of Peptic Ulcer and Antiinflammatory-Drug-Induced Gastroduodenal Ulceration," *N. Engl. J. Med.* **327**: 1575-1580 (1992).

Wolfe, M.M. (ed): *Gastrointestinal Pharmacotherapy*, W.B. Saunders, Philadelphia, 1993.

Yazdi, A.J., and E.B. Chang: "The Pharmacologic Basis of Treatment of Diarrhea," *Pract. Gastroenterol.* **17**: 29-35 (1992).

PART VIII

Endocrines

SECTION EDITOR

Andrew P. Ferko

CHAPTER 38

Thyroid and Parathyroid Drugs

Jeffrey L. Miller and Leslie I. Rose

THYROID HORMONES AND ANTITHYROID DRUGS

The thyroid gland exerts a profound metabolic control over the body through two iodine-containing amino acid hormones, triiodothyronine (T_3) and thyroxine (tetraiodothyronine, T_4). These hormones regulate general body metabolism by controlling the rate of the cellular oxidative processes. The activity of the thyroid gland is directly regulated by the thyroid-stimulating hormone (TSH, thyrotropin) produced and secreted by the pituitary gland.

Anatomically, the thyroid is a bilateral organ in the neck. It consists of vesicles lined by cuboidal epithelium surrounding a follicular cavity containing the colloidal iodinated protein thyroglobulin. In addition to follicular cells which secrete thyroid hormones, the thyroid gland has other cells which secrete a third hormone, calcitonin, which is involved in calcium homeostasis and is discussed later.

Normal Thyroid Function

The absorption of iodide, as well as biosynthesis, secretion, and degradation of active thyroid hormones, occurs by means of complex metabolic pathways. The major steps are described here and summarized in Table 38-1.

Dietary Intake Molecular inorganic iodine is reduced in the gastrointestinal tract to iodide which is absorbed. Dietary inorganic iodide (I^-) is absorbed as such. Organic iodine compounds are absorbed and then biotransformed by reductive dehalogenation in the liver, yielding inorganic iodide to the iodide pool.

Human dietary intake varies considerably, according to the local iodine content of the soil and water and the variations among culturally determined eating habits. The euthyroid individual may ingest 150 to 250 μg of iodine daily (up to 700 μg daily in the United States) and eliminate the same amount in the urine and feces. About 80 to 90 percent of the iodine is excreted in the urine, while 10 to 20 percent is eliminated in the feces. The metabolic products of the thyroid hormones are excreted in the feces.

Iodide Uptake by Thyroid Usually about half of the daily intake of iodine is "trapped" by the thyroid gland, while most of the remainder is excreted by the kidney. In the normal thyroid, this active transport system is capable of sustaining an intracellular iodide concentration 25 to 40 times higher than that of the extracellular fluid; TSH stimulates this uptake. The iodide "trapping mechanism" of the thyroid requires energy, which is supplied by actively respiring thyroid cells and has been linked to potassium transport. Since there is little free iodine in the thyroid gland (less than 0.2 percent of the total thyroidal iodine), this trapping process can be regarded as the rate-limiting step in thyroid hormone formation.

Iodide Oxidation and Organification The sequential reactions involved in iodide oxidation and organification are (1) oxidation of iodide ion to a form that serves as an iodinating reagent, (2) iodination of tyrosyl groups in preformed thyroprotein to form iodotyrosines, and (3) coupling of two iodotyrosines to form iodothyronines.

The oxidation of iodide is catalyzed by a thyroid peroxidase in the microsomal fraction. The reaction requires molecular oxygen and a source of hydrogen peroxide. The product of this peroxidation has not been identified because of its extreme reactivity, which results in instantaneous iodin-

TABLE 38-1 Steps in iodide oxidation, organification, and secretion

Step	Stimulated by	Inhibited by
1 Uptake of circulating iodide ion by thyroid	TSH	Thiocyanate, nitrite, perchlorate ions
2 Enzymatic oxidation of iodide ion to active iodine		Propylthiouracil, methimazole
3 Reaction of active iodine with tyrosyl residues on thyroglobulin to form MIT and DIT		
4 Combination of MIT and DIT on thyroglobulin to form T_4 and T_3		
5 Storage of iodinated thyroglobulin in the colloid of the thyroid gland		
6 Proteolysis of iodinated thyroglobulin and secretion of T_4 and T_3	TSH	Iodide ion (high concentrations)
7 Conversion of T_4 to T_3 by liver and kidney		propylthiouracil, glucocorticoids, amiodarone, propranolol
8 Circulating T_4 and T_3 on α-globulin and prealbumin inhibits TSH secretion by the anterior pituitary		

ation of the tyrosyl groups. Hypoiodite (IO^-) or iodinium ion (I^+) has been postulated as the intermediate. Tyrosine groups of thyroglobulin readily react with the highly active iodine, forming monoiodotyrosine (MIT) and diiodotyrosine (DIT) (see Fig. 38-1). Two DIT molecules or one DIT molecule and one MIT molecule aerobically condense to form T_4 and T_3 (Fig. 38-1), respectively, in the approximate ratio of 4:1. Two MIT molecules do not condense because the nature of the biosynthetic reaction is such that DIT must remain in peptide linkage during the coupling reaction; consequently, DIT must be at least one of the two reaction partners. T_3 and T_4 are stored in the colloid of the follicular cavity as a moiety of the thyroglobulin molecule.

Thyroglobulin is a large protein (670 kDa) containing 5900 amino acid residues, of which 110 to 120 are tyrosyl residues. As the thyroglobulin molecule is folded, only about 10 percent of the tyrosines are iodinated, and of these only a few are coupled to form thyronine. Thus there are only about three thyronines per molecule of thyroglobulin. The iodine in thyroglobulin is distributed approximately as follows: 30 percent in T_4, 3 percent in T_3, 20 percent in MIT, and 40 percent in DIT.

Circulating Thyroglobulin It has been customary to believe that thyroglobulin, which is a prohormone and a very large molecule, remains in the thyroid gland. The development of radioimmunoassay, and particularly a double-antibody technique, enabled the detection of the minute amounts present in the bloodstream of euthyroid subjects (5.1 ng/mL average, range 1.6 to 20.7 ng/mL). Patients with Graves' disease show elevated thyroglobulin blood levels. This is consistent with the finding that a thyroid-stimulating immunoglobulin is the etiological cause of hyperthyroidism in these patients. What role, if any, thyroglobulin plays as a thyroid hormone in the peripheral tissues is not clearly defined.

Secretion of T_3 and T_4 Thyroglobulin is stored as colloid droplets within the thyroid gland. Upon stimulation for hormone synthesis, the thyroglobulin is first hydrolyzed, separating out iodotyrosines (MIT and DIT) and T_3 and T_4. The iodotyrosines are deiodinated within the thyroid gland, and their

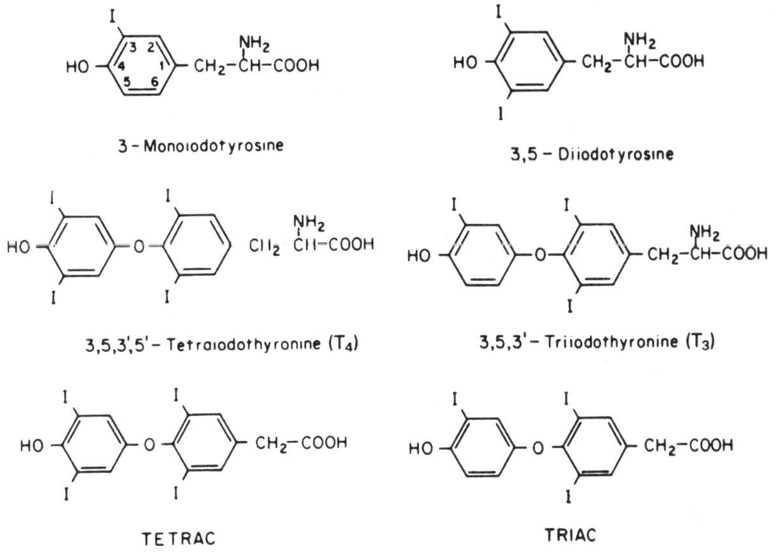

3-Monoiodotyrosine

3,5-Diiodotyrosine

3,5,3',5'-Tetraiodothyronine (T_4)

3,5,3'-Triiodothyronine (T_3)

TETRAC

TRIAC

FIGURE 38-1 *Thyroid iodoamino acids and the metabolites.*

iodide rejoins the general iodide pool where it can be reused to synthesize new hormone. The iodothyronines, T_3 and T_4, are released into the circulation. Normally, 80 μg of T4 is secreted daily. Approximately 33 μg of T_3 is produced daily, of which 20 percent is the result of direct secretion by the thyroid gland; the remaining 80 percent is produced by peripheral conversion of T_4 to T_3 (mainly by the liver and kidney).

Plasma Binding and Transport of Thyroid Hormones T_4 and T_3 are transported into the blood stream bound firmly, but reversibly, to plasma proteins. Most of the thyroid hormones are bound to an α_2-globulin, thyroxine-binding globulin (TBG) or to a prealbumin, thyroxine-binding prealbumin (TBPA). Only 0.02 percent of T_4 and 0.3 percent of T_3 circulate unbound. The binding protects the thyroid hormones from loss in the urine and also serves as a reservoir which regulates the peripheral supply of hormone in the active free form. Tissue utilization of thyroid hormones results in a reduction in the peripheral level of T_3 and T_4, shifting the balance to favor dissociation of the protein-bound complex. By this mechanism, it is possible for the free hormone to be delivered to the peripheral tissues at rates proportional to the metabolic requirement of each tissue.

Degradation of Thyroid Hormone The liver is the major site of biotransformation of T_3 and T_4; however, kidney and muscle are other sites where conjugation to glucuronides and sulfates occurs. In the liver, T_4 is conjugated mainly as the glucuronide, while T_3 is conjugated mainly as the sulfate. After excretion via the bile duct, the conjugates are hydrolyzed in the intestine, and most of the T_4 and T_3 reenter the blood stream via the hepatic portal circulation. Approximately 10 to 20 percent of thyroid hormone conjugates are excreted in the feces.

Tetraiodothyroacetic acid (TETRAC) and triiodothyroacetic acid (TRIAC) are two other metabolites produced by the liver and kidney by oxidative deamination of the alanine side chains of T_4 and T_3 (see Fig. 38-1). These products are subject to conjugation and deiodination as are the parent compounds.

Regulation of Synthesis and Release of Thyroid Hormones The hypothalamus secretes thyrotropin-releasing hormone (TRH), which stimulates the pituitary to produce and secrete TSH. Studies in humans indicate that TSH induces the synthesis and release of thyroglobulin. Thyroid hormones inhibit the release of both thyroglobulin from the thyroid gland and TSH from the pituitary.

Hormonal Actions of T_3 and T_4 Consistent with present theories of hormone action, receptors in the cell nucleus are postulated for thyroid hormones. Measurements of hormone-receptor binding both *in vivo* and *in vitro* suggested that T_3 rather than T_4 is the physiologically active ligand. Other metabolites do bind, but their contribution appears to be minor. Solubilized T_3-receptor complex also binds to DNA, and this may explain the nuclear localization. Histones also participate in the localization of T_3 receptors in chromatin material. In contrast to steroid hormones, where the hormone-receptor complex has to translocate to the nucleus, thyroid hormone receptors are already allied to chromatin material and translocation is unnecessary (Fig. 38-2).

Extranuclear modes of action for thyroid hormone are still a valid concept, and some of the actions of this hormone may be apart from the regulation of macromolecular synthesis. Thus the transport of amino acids is enhanced in the presence of thyroid hormone when protein synthesis is blocked.

The actions of thyroid hormone may now be described. At very low concentrations, the thyroid hormones initiate normal growth and development. The mechanism of this growth-promoting quality is thought to be initiation of the incorporation of amino acids into specific proteins. At higher concentrations, the thyroid hormones have been shown to induce many oxidative enzymes and to uncouple oxidative phosphorylation. This results in increased heat production and oxygen consumption. Although liver, muscle, kidney, and heart, among others, are involved, some tissues, such as the brain, lymph nodes, spleen, and testes, are apparently not stimulated in this manner by the thyroid hormones.

Many aspects of carbohydrate and lipid metabolism are affected by thyroid hormones, either alone or in combination with other hormones. These affect many biologic events and include:

1. Increased intestinal absorption of glucose and galactose
2. Potentiation of the glycogenolytic-hyperglycemic and lipolytic actions of epinephrine
3. Potentiation of insulin-induced glycogen synthesis and glucose utilization
4. Reduced serum cholesterol level
5. Increased uptake of glucose by adipose tissue
6. Increased mobilization of free fatty acids from adipose tissue (in part through potentiation of epinephrine)
7. Maturation of the central nervous system (CNS)

Thyroid hormones decrease the level of serum cholesterol by stimulating cholesterol degradation in excess of biosynthesis. These hormones also increase coenzyme and vitamin requirements probably indirectly through increased metabolic demand.

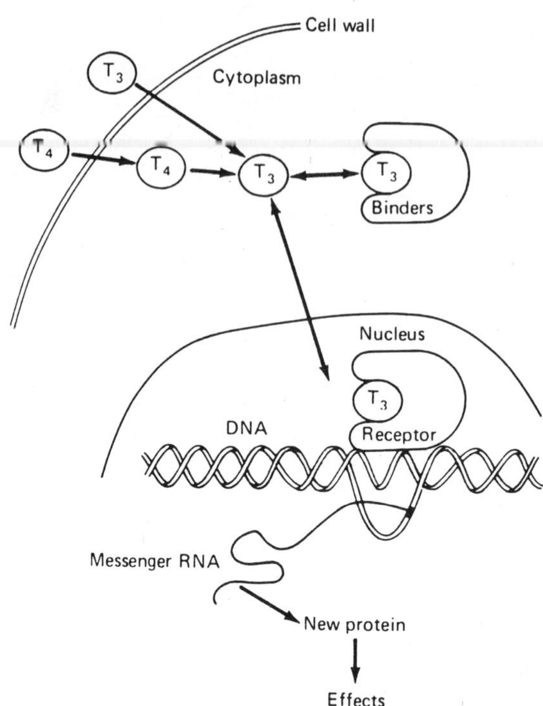

FIGURE 38-2 *Schematic diagram of a tissue cell response to thyroid hormone. Circulating T_4, the predominant form of thyroid hormone, enters the cell where, in the cytoplasm, it is converted to T_3. Binders for T_3 are present in the cytoplasm. Receptors bind the T_3 which enters the nucleus. This hormone-receptor complex is in close conjunction with DNA. This brings about changes in specific mRNAs, which are involved in the synthesis of new proteins and reflect the thyroid hormone response. [Modified from Baxter, J.D., and J.W. Funder: N. Engl. J. Med.* ***301:*** *1149-1161 (1979).]*

Disorders of Thyroid Function

Thyroid hormone disease states may be the result of overproduction of thyroid hormones, *hyperthyroidism*, or underproduction of thyroid hormones, *hypothyroidism*. In either case, goiter may be present.

Hypothyroidism Hypothyroidism may be due to failure of the thyroid gland to develop or to synthesize thyroid hormones appropriately, damage to the thyroid gland (e.g., surgery, scarring from irradiation or autoimmune disease), or failure of the pituitary and/or hypothalamus to secrete the stimulatory hormones necessary for thyroid hormone secretion, TSH and TRH. At birth, cretins (babies with congenital hypothyroidism) may be recognized by a puffy expressionless face, decreased muscle tone, coarse features, and a large tongue. Irreversible mental retardation will occur unless thyroid hormone replacement therapy is instituted promptly. Hypothyroidism (myxedema) in adults can be recognized by coarse, dry skin, bradycardia, anemia, and delayed relaxation of the deep tendon reflexes, especially prominent in the Achilles tendon. While findings may be subtle in early hypothyroidism, in later stages of disease, if untreated, coma may ensue. Juvenile hypothyroidism (postinfancy) presents similarly to adult hypothyroidism, with concurrent growth retardation.

Drugs Used in Hypothyroidism Therapy consists of thyroid hormone replacement. Levothyroxine (L-T_4) is the preferred form of therapy. It is converted *in vivo* to T_3, which is the active form of the hormone. Levothyroxine therapy provides constant serum levels of both T_4 and T_3 and is therefore the treatment of choice for hypothyroidism. Liothyronine (T_3) and preparations containing a combination of T_4 and T_3 (liotrix) have no advantage over levothyroxine. Administration of these produce rapid peaks and troughs of serum T_3 concentrations, as contrasted to the stable hormone concentrations achieved with levothyroxine therapy. These preparations are less accurately titrated and stabilized in individual patients than is levothyroxine.

Levothyroxine Sodium (L-T_4) is pure synthetic T_4. The oral absorption of L-T_4 is approximately 80 percent. A single dose will be eliminated in 6 to 7 days. L-T_4 is also available in a parenteral form for treatment of myxedema coma. Daily therapy may then be instituted with 50 μg of L-T_4 daily parenterally until enteral intake is possible. Some improvement in condition may be seen 6 h after the initial dose; the full therapeutic benefit may not be evident for over 24 h. Serum T_4 concentrations usually return to normal within 24 h.

Liothyronine Sodium (L-T_3) is a pure synthetic hormone. The oral absorption is approximately 90 percent. It has a more rapid onset of action and elimination than does L-T_4, peaking within several hours of administration. Its major indication is in patients who must be withdrawn from L-T_4 therapy for weeks (e.g., for thyroid scans) to provide temporary hormonal therapy that may be rapidly withdrawn while avoiding the adverse effects of hypothyroidism. Liothyronine is also available in a parenteral form for emergency treatment of myxedema coma.

Desiccated Thyroid (made mainly of bovine, ovine, and porcine thyroid glands) is standardized by its organic iodine content. Both T_3 and T_4 are present.

Liotrix is a 4:1 mixture of synthetic L-T_4 and L-T_3. It has no advantage over pure L-T_4.

In addition to these thyroid hormone preparations that are commonly used, dextrothyroxine (D-T_4), the dextrorotatory isomer of L-T_4, deserves comment. It was introduced as a cholesterol-lowering agent. However, it is usually contaminated with up to 1 percent L-T_4. It should not be used for therapy of hypothyroidism. In addition, it is not a drug that is widely used to reduce serum cholesterol.

Iodine deficiency is a cause of goiter and hypothyroidism in some countries, but is virtually nonexistent in the United States due to the addition of iodide to table salt and bread. Therefore, iodine has no role in treating hypothyroidism in this country, and it may cause hyperthyroidism if given to patients with goiters (Jod-Basedow syndrome).

Adverse Reactions Untoward effects of thyroid hormone therapy may result from overdosage. These effects take the form of symptoms of hyperthyroidism variably accompanied by psychotic behavior, angina pectoris, cardiac decompensation, myalgia, and severe diarrhea. It is now well recognized that subclinical hyperthyroidism (suppressed TSH with normal T_4 level in an individual who is clinically euthyroid) results in significant decrease in bone mineral density with resultant possible premature osteoporosis. To avoid this problem of overdosage with levothyroxine used for replacement therapy, the dose should be titrated to have TSH within the normal reference range. In addition, acute Addison's crisis may occur in patients with undiagnosed and/or untreated concomitant adrenal insufficiency.

Sucralfate and compounds containing iron such as ferrous sulfate should not be administered at the same time the levothyroxine is taken. They can markedly decrease absorption of the thyroid medication. It is safe to administer them 3 hours after taking levothyroxine.

Hyperthyroidism Excessive production of thyroid hormones may be due to the presence of autoantibodies which bind to the TSH receptor and stimulate it. Rarely, it may be due to a TSH-secreting pituitary neoplasm. Symptoms include weight loss, increased appetite, perspiration, fever, tachycardia, diarrhea, muscle weakness, anxiety, tremors, and eyelid retraction, causing a typical stare. Signs and symptoms may be subtle, especially in elderly patients.

Treatment of hyperthyroidism consists of drugs to inhibit excessive thyroid hormone synthesis, radioactive iodine to destroy the overactive gland, or surgery to remove the overactive thyroid gland. Because surgery is very dangerous and may result in a potentially lethal episode of acute hyperthyroidism (thyroid storm), it is usually reserved for pregnant women in whom other therapeutic modalities are contraindicated or in patients first rendered euthyroid when all other modalities of therapy have failed.

Drugs Used in Hyperthyroidism

Thioamide (Thiocarbamide) Drugs

Thioamides are the primary agents useful in the long-term therapy of hyperthyroidism. Presently only two compounds are available: propylthiouracil and methimazole.

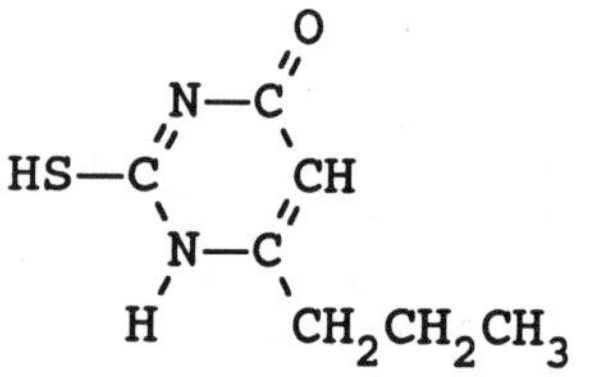

```
            O
           //
       N—C
      //    \
HS—C        CH
      \     //
       N—C
      /     \
     H      CH2CH2CH3
```

Propylthiouracil

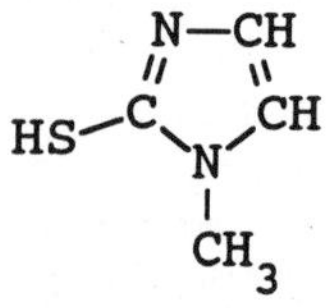

```
      N—CH
      //  \\
HS—C       CH
      \   /
        N
        |
        CH3
```

Methimazole

Mechanism of Action Thioamides are reducing agents. They inhibit the synthesis of thyroid hormones by inhibiting organification of iodine and the coupling of iodotyrosines. In addition, propylthiouracil, but not methimazole, also inhibits the peripheral conversion of T_4 to T_3. Once stores of preformed thyroid hormones are depleted, concentrations of circulating thyroid hormones fall.

Pharmacokinetics These drugs are about 80 to 90 percent absorbed after oral administration. Propylthiouracil has its onset of action 20 to 30 min after administration. Serum levels peak approximately 1 h after administration. Its half-life is 1 to 2 h. Methimazole has a longer duration of action than does propylthiouracil, with a half-life of 6 to 13 h and serum concentrations peaking 2 h after administration.

Therapeutic Use Thioamides may be employed as the sole therapeutic agent in the treatment of hyperthyroidism. There is a delay in the patient's therapeutic response to the drugs until circulating levels of thyroid hormones are reduced. The drugs may be taken for years; studies indicate that less than 25 percent of people with hyperthyroidism will have spontaneous remission within 2 years, and many of these will relapse. These drugs may also be used in conjunction with iodide to prepare patients for surgery, and they may be used following radioactive iodide administration until the latter takes effect. Overly aggressive treatment with these drugs may result in hypothyroidism.

Adverse Reactions Adverse reactions consist of fever, skin rash, urticaria, myalgia, jaundice, edema, gastrointestinal upset, hepatitis, nephritis, lymphadenopathy, and arthralgia. In addition, potentially fatal agranulocytosis may occur in less than 1 percent of patients. This occurs without warning, and may occur immediately, within months of starting therapy or even after more than a year of treatment. Patients should be warned of this complication and should have emergent white blood cell counts checked if fever or sore throat develops. These drugs cross the placenta, and maternal overdose may result in the birth of a goitrous cretin. In this regard, transplacental passage of methimazole is high, that of propylthiouracil is low. Both drugs are secreted into breast milk (methimazole greater than propylthiouracil) and therefore should not be given to nursing mothers.

Other Drugs

Iodide in large doses inhibits the release of thyroid hormones as well as their synthesis by blocking the organification of iodine. These effects are short-lived, however, and hyperthyroidism may be exacerbated by outpouring of preformed thyroid hormones as well as new synthesis of thyroid hormones. Thyroid storm may result. Iodide is usually used in conjunction with thioamide drugs to prepare patients for surgery. Usually, one of two preparations are used: Lugol's solution (5 g iodine and 10 g potassium iodide per 100 mL solution, yielding 6 mg of iodine per drop; 5 drops daily), or saturated solution of potassium iodide (100 g potassium iodide per 100 mL solution, yielding 50 mg iodide per drop; 1 drop three times daily). Sodium iodide (0.5 to 1.0 g daily) may be administered intravenously. Side effects include acute hypersensitivity reactions with angioedema, hemorrhagic skin lesions, and serum sickness. *Iodism* is a chronic toxicity characterized by unpleasant taste, burning in the mouth, swelling of parotid and submaxillary glands, increased salivation, rhinitis, headache, productive cough, gastric irritation, bloody diarrhea, depression, and skin lesions; these symptoms usually resolve several days after discontinuation of iodine.

Radioactive sodium iodide (^{131}I) has been used to partially or totally destroy the thyroid gland for treatment of hyperthyroidism. It has a half-life of 8 days, and it emits both beta particles and gamma rays. The beta particles have ionizing properties and thus destroy cells, but they have poor penetration through tissues (1 to 2 mm) and are undetectable outside the body. Gamma rays penetrate further and can be used for diagnostic purposes. Radioactive iodide is also used as an adjuvant to surgery for treatment of many types of thyroid cancer. The major adverse effect is permanent hypothyroidism (which is treated with replacement thyroid hormone therapy). Radiation-induced thyroiditis may occur in some patients but is of limited duration. Resultant hypoparathyroidism is exceedingly rare.

The *β-adrenergic blocking agent* propranolol is often useful in temporarily blocking the peripheral manifestations of hyperthyroidism while the patient undergoes definitive therapy. It does not inhibit thyroid gland function, but it masks the adrenergic manifestations of tremor, stare, and tachycardia. The use of propranolol for thyrotoxicosis symptoms is discussed in Chapter 9.

Drug Use to Assess Thyroid Gland Function

Protirelin is a synthetic tripeptide, identical to natural TRH. The sole indication for protirelin is the assessment of thyroid gland function as an adjuvant to other diagnostic procedures. Patients

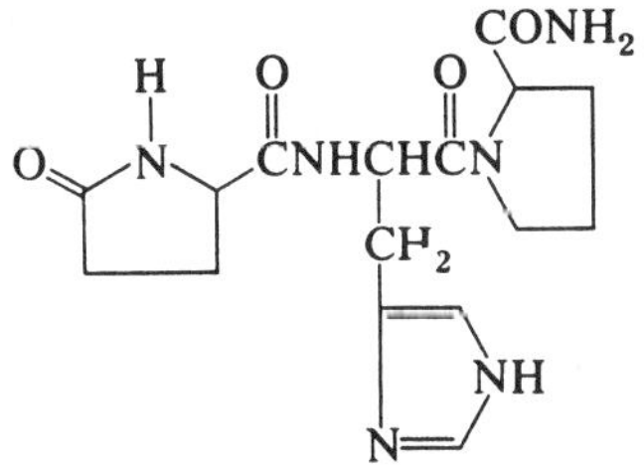

H O O CONH$_2$
O N CNHCHCN
CH$_2$
NH
N

with hyperthyroidism will not respond to administration with elevated TSH levels. Patients with hypothyroidism due to hypothalamic disease or to intrinsic thyroid disease (primary hypothyroidism) show a greater response than do those with pituitary dysfunction. The supersensitive TSH assay, which is able to distinguish low from normal TSH levels, often makes this test unnecessary.

Protirelin is given intravenously; its half-life is 5 min. TSH levels peak in 20 to 30 min following administration in normal individuals and fall to baseline over the next several hours. Side effects include marked changes in blood pressure (both hypotension and hypertension), headache, flushing, nausea, the urge to urinate, a bad taste in the mouth, and chest pressure. Rarely, pituitary apoplexy has occurred when protirelin was given to a patient with a pituitary adenoma.

CALCIUM, PARATHYROID HORMONE, CALCITONIN, AND VITAMIN D

Calcium

An adult human contains approximately 1200 g of calcium, about 10 g is found in the extracellular fluid and soft tissues, while the remainder (approximately 99 percent) is deposited in bone. The normal concentration of total plasma calcium, which is divided about equally between free ionic calcium and calcium loosely bound to plasma proteins, is 8.8 to 10.3 mg per 100 mL of plasma. This range of concentrations of calcium in plasma also is apparently ideal for normal growth and development of the skeleton and for the maintenance of healthy bone.

One of the principal functions of calcium is at the cellular membrane: a decrease causes less stability, an increase causes greater stability. For instance, nerve fiber membranes in the presence of low calcium become partially depolarized and therefore transmit repetitive and uncontrolled impulses. Spasm or tetany of skeletal muscles may result. Very high concentrations of calcium ions depress neurons in the CNS presumably because membranes will not depolarize.

Calcium Homeostasis Despite the many functions of calcium described above, its main role is the preservation of the integrity of bone. Certainly the main signs and symptoms of disorders of calcium metabolism relate to bony defects and calcification of soft tissues. For these reasons, the homeostasis of calcium is of critical importance to the bodily economy. Unfortunately calcium homeostasis involves many interrelating factors which are difficult to compose into a conceptual model. At the least, calcium metabolism is controlled by three main hormones: parathyroid hormone (PTH), vitamin D, and calcitonin (CT). If the intake is adequate (15 mg/kg body weight in the young adult), the concentration of blood calcium will depend on the rate of intestinal absorption, deposition or resorption in bone, and renal excretion. Thus it is the control of these latter factors by vitamin D, PTH, and CT which determines calcium metabolism at any given moment.

A model, called the "butterfly" model, has been devised which aids the comprehension of the interaction of the main factors and elements in calcium metabolism (Fig. 38-3). The critical factor in the butterfly model is the serum calcium level (SCa^{2+}). If for any reason it falls (lower central point of loops), there will be induced an increased secretion of PTH and a decrease in the secretion of CT. This brings about increased bone resorption (1A); 1,25-$(OH)_2D_3$, the active form of vitamin D, causes increased intestinal absorption of calcium and also, by a minor feedback loop, increases the resorption of bone (2A). Meanwhile the renal excretion of calcium is decreased (3A) while the serum phosphate (SP) declines as a result of increased renal excretion of urinary phosphate (UP). This results in an increase in serum calcium. Should the serum calcium attain a level above the normal, the opposite events will occur (loops 1B, 2B, and 3B).

Obviously, such a model oversimplifies a very complicated series of events. Unfortunately, neither the time constants of the various events nor the magnitude of the response are known. Both PTH and CT respond relatively rapidly compared with vitamin D. However, the potential contribution of vitamin D (reserve capacity) is much greater than that of PTH or CT. That is, over a period of time vitamin D can have a dominant effect simply because, although slower, its capacity to achieve a determinate action is greater. The components of the model can now be examined in detail.

Parathyroid Hormone

Source and Chemistry Parathyroid hormone is a polypeptide hormone secreted by the parathyroid glands. There are usually four parathyroid glands, but supernumerary glands are common. Each gland normally weighs 25 to 75 mg. They are generally situated near the thyroid gland. Histologically, normal parathyroid glands consist of sheets of chief cells, measuring 4 to 8 μm in diameter. These cells contain secretory granules and secrete PTH. Oxyphil cells, larger (6 to 10 μm in diameter) with eosinophilic cytoplasm, are also present. These cells are believed to be a degenerative form of chief cells and generally do not secrete PTH.

PTH is a polypeptide composed of 84 amino acids. It is biosynthesized in the form of a larger precursor, pre-pro-PTH (115 amino acids), which is then converted to pro-PTH (90 amino acids). Pro-PTH is then cleaved to PTH in the parathyroid glands. Pre-pro-PTH and pro-PTH have little biologic activity. The first (N-terminal) 34 amino acids of PTH confer its biologic activity and a synthetic polypeptide hormone, teriparatide, consisting of these 34 amino acids, is available for use as a diagnostic agent.

Physiological Effects The major physiologic function of PTH is to raise the plasma calcium ion concentration to the optimum level for efficient neuromuscular activity. After total parathyroidectomy, plasma calcium concentrations may fall below 6 mg/dL; without therapy seizures, tetany, and death may ensue. In hyperparathyroidism, excess circulating PTH causes hypercalcemia. The sites of action of PTH are bone, kidney, and intestine.

Bone PTH increases the resorption of bone, the chief reservoir of calcium within the body. It increases osteoclast activity while inhibiting osteoblastic function. In normal adults, osteoclastic and osteoblastic functions are balanced. In states of excess PTH secretion, the rate of bone resorption increases without an increase in bone formation, and serum calcium levels rise. In states

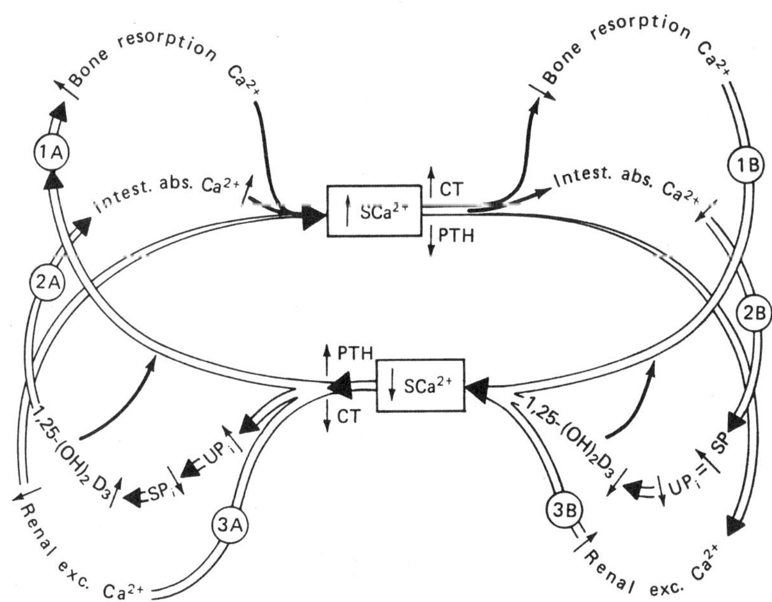

FIGURE 38-3 *The "butterfly" model of calcium homeostasis depicted by three overlapping loops operating by negative feedback. The loops relate to one another through the blood concentration of ionic calcium (Ca^{2+}), parathyroid hormone (PTH), and calcitonin (CT). Loop 1 represents bone resorption; on the left, limb 1A indicates increased bone resorption and limb 1B decreased bone resorption. Loops 2 and 3 deal in a similar manner with intestinal absorption and renal excretion of calcium, respectively. Also shown are the relationships of 1,25-$(OH)_2D_3$ (the active form of vitamin D) and the role of the concentration of serum phosphate (SP) and urinary phosphate (UP). The influence of 1,25-$(OH)_2D_3$ in stimulating bone resorption is shown by a minor feedback loop (2A to 1A and 2B to 1B). (See text for further details.) [Modified from Arnaud, C.D.: Fed. Proc.* ***37****: 2557-2560 (1978).]*

of PTH deficiency, bone resorption decreases without a decrease in bone formation, and serum calcium levels fall.

Kidney PTH enhances the fractional reabsorption of calcium from the glomerular filtrate. It inhibits phosphate reabsorption by the renal tubules (i.e., enhances phosphate excretion), and stimulates the release of cyclic AMP in the urine.

Intestine PTH stimulates intestinal absorption of calcium indirectly by stimulating renal 1-hydroxylation of 25-hydroxycholecalciferol (25-OH-D) to 1,25-dihydroxycholecalciferol (1,25-$(OH)_2$-D). Vitamin D is the principal factor responsible for promoting the absorption of calcium from the intestine.

Teriparatide This drug elicits all of the effects of natural PTH. It is indicated for use as a diagnostic agent in patients presenting with hypocalcemia and is used to discriminate between hypoparathyroidism or pseudohypoparathyroidism. The drug is used by intravenous infusion. Patients with hypoparathyroidism generally respond to this compound with increased urinary cyclic AMP and phosphate excretion; patients with pseudohypoparathyroidism (target-organ resistance to PTH) show a blunted response.

Adverse reactions to teriparatide administration include nausea, abdominal cramps, the urge to defecate, flushing, tachycardia, tingling of the fingers, dizziness, and lightheadedness. Patients may experience pain at the injection site. Allergic and hypersensitivity reactions have been observed.

Calcitonin

When hypercalcemic blood is perfused through the thyroid gland, a hypocalcemic hormone, calcitonin (thyrocalcitonin), is secreted by the parafollicular, or C, cells of the thyroid gland. Calcitonin has been isolated from humans and other mammals, as well as birds and fish. In all species, it is a 32 amino acid polypeptide with an N-terminal seven-membered disulfide ring and a C-terminal proline-amide. The individual amino acids differ from species to species. Salmon calcitonin and human calcitonin are both available for use.

Mechanism of Action Calcitonin's action is hypocalcemic and hypophosphatemic. However, the normal output of calcitonin by the thyroid gland is not sufficient to produce hypocalcemia. Removal of the thyroid gland does not result in hypercalcemia in usual circumstances.

The major site of action of calcitonin is bone, where it inhibits osteoclastic function. It also inhibits PTH-stimulated bone resorption. In pharmacologic doses, it has a direct calciuric effect. These effects are mediated by cyclic AMP, which is formed through activation of adenylate cyclase by calcitonin.

Regulation of Secretion The rate of secretion of calcitonin is regulated by the ionic calcium concentration of blood flowing through the thyroid gland. As the plasma calcium concentration rises, the secretion of calcitonin increases; as the calcium concentration falls, calcitonin secretion decreases.

Drug Administration Calcitonin is ineffective if given orally. It is active when administered parenterally. Synthetic human and salmon preparations are available and are used to treat hypercalcemia of various causes. While the hypocalcemic effect is rapid (within 24 to 48 h), it is short-lived, because tachyphylaxis may develop within several days. Glucocorticoids may prevent this.

Calcitonin is also used in the treatment of Paget's disease. Paget's disease is a bone disorder characterized by a rapid uncontrolled increase in bone resorption and formation, with the new bone formed being structurally abnormal. Symptoms may include bone pain, thickening of the skull, compression of spinal and cranial nerves, and hearing loss. Serum alkaline phosphatase and urinary hydroxyproline are usually elevated.

Adverse Reactions Nausea and vomiting are the most frequent side effects and may occur in 50 percent of patients. These symptoms are usually mild and do not necessitate discontinuation of therapy. Facial flushing is also common. Local inflammatory reactions at the site of injection may develop. Less commonly, abdominal cramps, diarrhea, itching, urinary frequency, and urticaria may develop.

Vitamin D

Precursors of vitamin D are present in many foods of vegetable and animal origin. The liver of fish is especially rich in vitamin D, and cod liver oil has been a traditional source. In the past, confusion existed as to the most desirable preparation, since the active form of vitamin D was not known; nor was it realized that vitamin D acted as a hormone in the body rather than as a vitamin. It does so because it is capable of being synthesized in the body, in contrast to classic vitamins, and also because it actually functions as a messenger substance with control action rather than entering into a critical metabolic step of synthesis or as a cofactor for an enzyme.

Present understanding of the pathway of biotransformation of vitamin D includes the following. 7-Dehydrocholesterol is converted to cholecalciferol (vitamin D_3) by the action of ultraviolet light on the skin. With the aid of a plasma-binding protein (vitamin D-binding globulin), vitamin D_3 is transported to the liver. Here a 25-hydroxylase catalyzes the hydroxylation of carbon-25 of vitamin D_3 to produce the major circulating form of vitamin D, 25-hydroxy vitamin D_3 (25-OH D_3), which is inactive at physiologic concentrations. Again with the aid of a plasma-binding protein, 25-OH D_3 is transported to the kidney. In this organ, it is converted to 1,25-dihydroxy vitamin D_3 (1,25-$(OH)_2$ D_3), when hypocalcemia and hypophosphatemia are present. This is the most active form of vitamin D, and it is highly effective in causing increased intestinal absorption of calcium and also resorption of calcium from bone. PTH is also a tropin for the renal synthesis of 1,25-$(OH)_2$ D_3. In the absence of stimulation by PTH and with normal serum calcium and phosphate, the kidney converts 25-OH D_3 to 24,25-$(OH)_2$ D_3 (which is only weakly active) and then to 1,24,25-$(OH)_3$ D_3 (which is inactive). Table 38-2 summarizes these events.

The substances designated as vitamin D, were shown to be a mixture of antirachitic substances. A commonly used form of vitamin D in commercial preparations is ergosterol, which is also present in irradiated bread and milk. Ergosterol is the provitamin for vitamin D_2 (ergocalciferol). Ergocalciferol and cholecalciferol are metabolized by the same pathway and have similar biologic activities.

The major storage form of vitamin D in the body is vitamin D_3. Ordinarily, with average daily intake of milk, meat, and fish and with some exposure to sunlight, supplemental amounts of

TABLE 38-2 Metabolism of vitamin D

Organ	Metabolic effect		
Skin (UV light)	7-Dehydrocholesterol →		Cholecalciferol (Vitamin D_3) ↓
Liver			25-OH D_3 ↓
Kidney	Influence of PTH, low serum calcium, low serum phosphate		$1,25\text{-}(OH)_2\ D_3$ ↓
	Influence of normal serum calcium, normal serum phosphate	$24,25\text{-}(OH)_2\ D_3$ (weakly active) ↓ $1,24,25\text{-}(OH)_3\ D_3$ (inactive)	
Intestine	Increases absorption of calcium		$1,25\text{-}(OH)_2\ D_3$ (active) ↓
Bone	Causes resorption of calcium		$1,25\text{-}(OH)_2\ D_3$ (active)

Abbreviations — PTH: parathyroid hormone; 25-OH D_3: 25-hydroxy vitamin D_3; $1,25\text{-}(OH)_2\ D_3$: 1,25-dihydroxy vitamin D_3; $24,25\text{-}(OH)_2\ D_3$: 24,25-dihydroxy vitamin D_3; $1,24,25\text{-}(OH)_3\ D_3$: 1,24,25-trihydroxy vitamin D_3

vitamin D are not needed. Poor diet, malnutrition, infancy, pregnancy and lactation, and lack of exposure to sunlight are generally considered indications for supplementation. Even under these circumstances, the recommended daily allowance (RDA) of 400 IU of vitamin D should not be exceeded.

Hypervitaminosis D This is perhaps the most common of the vitamin toxicity syndromes. It is easily caused by overenthusiastic medication, either professionally or self-prescribed. The syndrome in mild form consists of hypercalcemia with nausea, weakness, weight loss, vague aches and stiffness, constipation or diarrhea, anemia, and mild acidosis. Eventually impaired renal function results with polyuria, nocturia, polydipsia, hypercalcinuria, and azotemia. If allowed to progress, eventual nephrocalcinosis takes place along with calcification of other soft tissues. Marked CNS symptoms such as mental retardation and convulsive states occur. Osteoporosis may cause fractures in adults; in children there is a decreased rate of linear growth.

Treatment of hypervitaminosis D consists of withdrawal of vitamin therapy, a low calcium diet, increased fluid intake, and acidification of the urine along with symptomatic and supportive treatment. A loop diuretic (e.g., furosemide) may aid in the elimination of calcium. In desperate cases, dialysis may have to be used. Recovery is the rule if irreversible damage has not occurred.

Therapeutic Uses of Vitamin D and Vitamin D Analogs Cholecalciferol (vitamin D_3) is used as a dietary supplement and in the treatment of, or in the prophylaxis of, vitamin D deficiency; usually 400 to 1000 IU daily satisfies the individual's needs in this regard. Alternatively, ergocalciferol (vitamin D_2) can be used.

In severe hypocalcemic states, larger doses of vitamin D preparations are indicated. For example, in the treatment of refractory rickets (also known as vitamin D-resistant rickets), oral doses of 12,000 to 500,000 IU daily of ergocalciferol has been used. Hypoparathyroidism requires oral doses of ergocalciferol of 50,000 to 200,000 IU daily. Intramuscular therapy with this drug is required in patients with gastrointestinal, liver, or biliary diseases that are associated with the malabsorption of vitamin D.

For patients with hypocalcemia due to chronic renal dialysis, calcitriol (1,25-$(OH)_2$ D_3) and calcifediol (25-(OH) D_3) are available. Calcitriol is indicated in patients with impaired ability to convert 25-(OH) D_3 to 1,25-$(OH)_2$ D_3. Because it is the most active hormone, it has the most rapid onset of action of all the vitamin D preparations. The usual oral dosage is 0.25 μg daily. Oral doses of calcifediol range from 300 to 350 μg per week, given daily or on alternate days. In most instances, therapy with either drug requires that additional calcium be given in the diet (at least 1 g daily) and serum calcium levels should be monitored. Hypoparathyroidism and pseudohypoparathyroidism also respond to treatment with calcitriol.

Dihydrotachysterol is a synthetic compound and a close isomer of vitamin D. Unlike cholecalciferol and ergocalciferol, dihydrotachysterol is active in nephrectomized patients and does not require hydroxylation in the kidney. It is used to treat severe hypocalcemia and hypoparathyroidism.

HYPERCALCEMIA

Hypercalcemia may be caused by malignancy, granulomatous diseases, endocrinologic diseases, genetic disorders, prolonged immobilization, and drugs. Hyperparathyroidism is usually treated surgically; in other cases, removal of the cause should be attempted. Frequently, other therapeutic interventions are necessary to control the hypercalcemia in the acute setting.

Saline hydration is important, and all patients with hypercalcemia should be kept well hydrated. Saline hydration promotes renal excretion of calcium. Furosemide, a loop diuretic, may be added to saline hydration to increase renal calcium excretion. This agent is discussed in Chapter 31.

Phosphates may be administered as neutral phosphate or potassium phosphate. Phosphate forms complexes with calcium, resulting in a fall of serum calcium. These are generally given orally, because rapid intravenous administration may result in extraskeletal precipitation of calcium salts; if these precipitate in the kidneys, renal failure may result. Gastrointestinal side effects include diarrhea and nausea.

Plicamycin is a cytotoxic antibiotic often used as a cancer chemotherapeutic agent. It blocks calcium resorption from bone. Serum calcium concentrations usually fall within a few days; however, they may fall within hours of plicamycin administration. The duration of the response is variable. Plicamycin may be administered again should hypercalcemia recur. Adverse effects include hepatic and renal toxicity, nausea, vomiting, and thrombocytopenia.

Gallium nitrate exerts a hypocalcemic effect by inhibiting calcium resorption from bone. It is used by the intravenous route in hospitalized patients with cancer-related hypercalcemia. Adverse effects are numerous and involve the renal, cardiovascular, hematologic, and respiratory systems.

Pamidronate disodium is a biphosphonate, chemically related to etidronate disodium (see below). Both this compound and its congener are available for intravenous use the treatment of hypercalcemia associated with malignancies.

ETIDRONATE DISODIUM

This drug is a biphosphonate that acts primarily on bone. The major pharmacologic action is inhibition of normal and abnormal bone resorption; the drug also inhibits bone formation. Although the mechanism of action is not completely understood, etidronate disodium inhibits hydroxyapatite crystal formation, growth, and dissolution. The activity of both osteoclasts and osteoblasts appear to be reduced. A significant reduction in serum calcium is usually seen by the third day after intravenous administration of etidronate disodium. Oral etidronate disodium has been shown to maintain normal serum calcium concentrations.

Although oral absorption is poor (1 to 6 percent), etidronate disodium is used by this route, as well by intravenous injection. Approximately half of the dose that reaches the systemic circulation is taken up by bone. While the plasma half-life is approximately 6 h, the half-life of the drug in bone is over 90 days. Etidronate is not biotransformed and is excreted unchanged in the urine.

Adverse reactions to etidronate disodium are generally mild. Patients may experience a metallic, altered, or loss of taste during and shortly after both oral or intravenous administration. Diarrhea and nausea may occur. Hyperphosphatemia may be observed; this generally resolves after therapy is discontinued and has not been of clinical significance. In addition, hypersensitivity reactions have been reported.

Oral etidronate disodium is indicated for the treatment of symptomatic Paget's disease. The parenteral form is used in patients with hypercalcemia associated with a variety of malignancies, with or without metastases.

BIBLIOGRAPHY

Aaron, J.E., M.C. deVernejoul, and J.A. Kanis: "Bone Hypertrophy and Trabecular Generation in Paget's disease and in Fluoride-treated Osteoporosis," *Bone and Mineral* **17**: 399-413 (1992).

Arnaud, C.D.: "Calcium Homeostasis: Regulatory Elements and Their Integration," *Fed. Proc.* **37**: 2557-2560 (1978).

Baxter, J.D., and J.W. Funder: "Hormone Receptors," *N. Engl. J. Med.* **301**: 1149-1161 (1979).

Bilezikian J.P.: "Management of Acute Hypercalcemia," *N. Engl. J. Med.* **326**: 1196-1203 (1992).

Cooper, D.S., and E.C. Ridgway: "Clinical Management of Patients with Hyperthyroidism," *Med. Clin. North Amer.* **69**: 953-971 (1985).

Habener, J.F., and H.M. Kronenberg: "Parathyroid Hormone Biosynthesis: Structure and Function of Biosynthetic Precursors," *Fed. Proc.* **37**: 2561-2566 (1978).

Hay, I.D., and G.G. Klee: "Thyroid Dysfunction," *Endocrinol. Metab. Clin. North Amer.* **17**: 473-509 (1988).

Kanis, J.A., G.H. Urwin, R.E.S. Gray, M.N.C. Beneton, E.V. McCloskey, N.A.T. Hamdy, and S.A. Murray: "Effects of Intravenous Etidronate Disodium on Skeletal and Calcium Metabolism," *Amer. J. Med.* **82 (Suppl. 2A)**: 55-70 (1987).

Kumar, R., and B.L. Riggs: "Vitamin D in the Therapy of Disorders of Calcium and Phosphorus Metabolism," *Mayo. Clin. Proc.* **56**: 327-333 (1981).

Paul, T.L., J. Kerrigan, A.M. Kelly, L.E. Braveman, and D.T. Baran: "Long-term L-Thyroxine Therapy is Associated with Decreased Hip Bone Density in Premenopausal Women," *J. Amer. Med. Assoc.* **259**: 3137-3141 (1988).

Ross D.S.: "Monitoring L-Thyroxine Therapy: Lessons from the Effects of L-Thyroxine on Bone Density," *Amer. J. Med.* **91**: 1-4 (1991).

Shapiro, L.E., M.I. and Surks: "Managing Hypothyroidism," *The Endocrinologist* **1**: 343-347 (1991).

Van Herle, A.J., G. Vassart, and J.E. Dumont: "Control of Thyroglobulin Synthesis and Secretion," *N. Engl. J. Med.* **301**: 239-248, 307-314 (1979).

CHAPTER 39

Insulins and Oral Hypoglycemic Agents

Norman Altszuler

Insulin and oral hypoglycemic agents are useful in the treatment of diabetes mellitus. This disease is now considered to be a heterogeneous syndrome, consisting of several different diseases, each with its own etiology and appropriate treatment. While the primary manifestation of diabetes mellitus is hyperglycemia, it is also associated with abnormalities in lipid and protein metabolism. The chronic state is associated with neurologic damage, macrovascular and microvascular pathology in the extremities, eyes, kidneys, and heart. The clinical manifestations of the vascular abnormalities include impaired wound healing, gangrene of the foot, blindness, uremia, and coronary artery disease.

CLASSIFICATION OF DIABETES MELLITUS

The two major types of diabetes mellitus (DM) are Insulin Dependent Diabetes Mellitus (IDDM or Type I) and Non-Insulin Dependent Diabetes Mellitus (NIDDM or Type II). Of the 14 million Americans believed to have diabetes, about 80 to 85 percent have NIDDM. IDDM is caused by an absolute deficiency of insulin due to autoimmune destruction of the pancreatic beta cells. A predisposition for this is carried in genes of the major histocompatibility complex (the human leukocyte antigen system). However, environmental factors must also be involved since there is only a 50 percent incidence of IDDM in homozygous twins. The destruction is believed to be initiated by a virus which causes the beta cell of the pancreas to produce a membrane antigen that, in susceptible individuals, is attacked by the T killer cells of the immune system. The destructive process is believed to occur gradually, but the clinical manifestations occur abruptly when over 80 percent of the islets are lost. When specific markers become available to identify, early on, the genetically predisposed individuals, it may be feasible to prevent the islet destruction.

Insulin replacement is essential for maintenance of life in IDDM. Severe deficiency of insulin leads to life-threatening ketoacidosis, which may progress to coma and death if not treated promptly. The acidosis is due to impaired ketone utilization, which increases blood levels of the organic acid, dihydroxybutyrate, and of acetone, which gives the breath the characteristic odor.

NIDDM may appear to be less insidious a disease than IDDM, but nonetheless, it can result in all the long-term complications cited above and its incidence worldwide is increasing. It usually occurs after age 35 to 40, although in one subset, Maturity Onset Diabetes of the Young (MODY), it occurs earlier. A number of the individuals are obese. The disease tends to run in families, suggesting a genetic influence, but it does not involve the immune system. Unlike in IDDM, these individuals secrete insulin but there is a lesser tissue response to the insulin. Such resistance to insulin occurs either at the initial signal transduction or, more likely, at sites beyond the insulin receptor. There may also be a deficient "early phase" insulin response; the nonobese individuals have low levels of circulating insulin. Because ketone body formation can be suppressed by very small amounts of insulin, the incidence of ketosis and diabetic coma in NIDDM is quite low. However, they can develop a hyperglycemic-hyperosmotic, nonketotic coma. This is more likely to occur in the elderly at times when the insulin secretion is inadequate to prevent glucosuria and dehydration. As the latter becomes severe, urine output decreases and the glucose level in the blood rises, increasing the osmolarity which can result in coma.

Treatment of NIDDM always begins with diet regulation and weight reduction. If these measures are inadequate to maintain acceptable glucose regulation, oral hypoglycemic agents are used. Insulin may be added as warranted.

INSULIN

In 1921, Banting, a Canadian surgeon, and Best, who was a second-year medical student, succeeded in obtaining a pancreatic extract which lowered blood glucose levels when injected into a depancreatized dog. This activity was due to the insulin in the extract and heralded the beginning of life saving therapy in patients with severe deficiency of insulin.

Chemistry and Biosynthesis

Insulin is a polypeptide consisting of 51 amino acids (molecular mass of 6 kDa), arranged in two chains (A = acidic and B = basic; see Fig. 39-1). It is formed in the rough endoplasmic reticulum from a single-chain polypeptide, preproinsulin, which loses 16 amino acids to form proinsulin, the immediate precursor of insulin. The proinsulin is transported to the Golgi apparatus where it is encapsuled. Within the capsule, two amino acids at each of two sites are excised from the proinsulin, giving rise to the double-chained insulin and the connecting peptide (C peptide). Three pairs of insulin dimers then bind to one zinc atom, forming the histologically recognized granules. The encapsuled granules migrate along microtubules toward

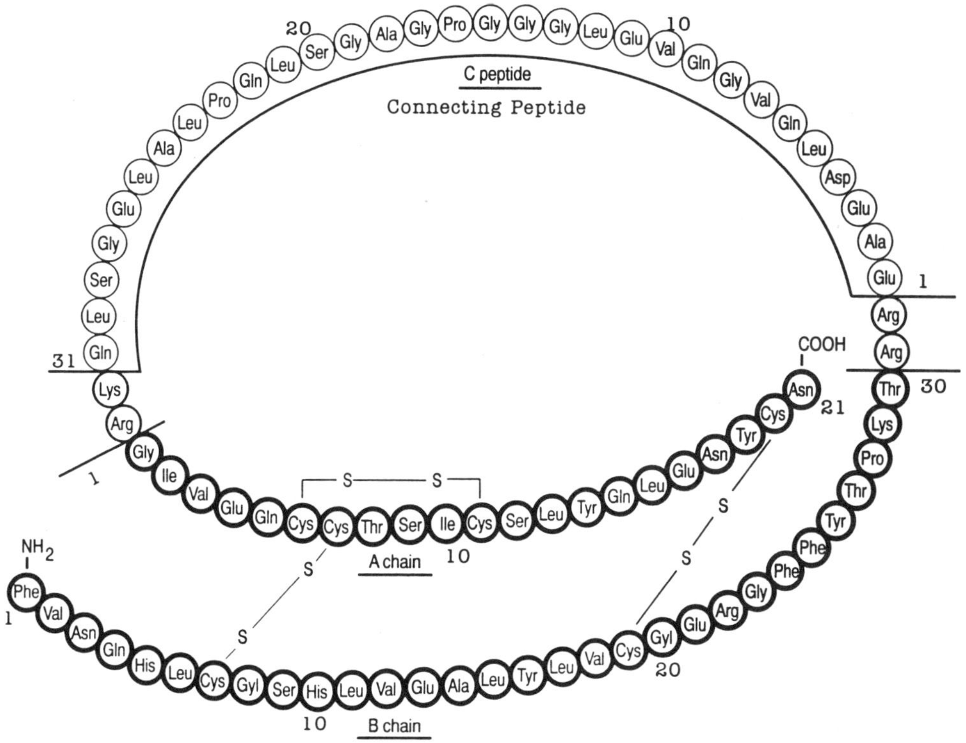

FIGURE 39-1 *Amino acid sequence of human proinsulin. Two basic amino acids (Arg—Lys and Arg—Arg) at each end of the C peptide are excised to form insulin (amino acid chains with the darker circles show the human insulin molecule). In pig insulin, threonine at B_{30} is replaced by alanine. In bovine insulin, threonine at B_{30} is replaced by alanine, threonine at A_8 by alanine, and isoleucine at A_{10} by valine.*

the plasma membrane and, following fusion of the two membranes, the capsule content is secreted by exocytosis. The entire process from synthesis to readiness for secretion takes about 1 h.

The C peptide and insulin are secreted in a 1.1 ratio, along with intact proinsulin, which normally represents about 5 to 10 percent of the total secretion. Proinsulin has one-sixth to one-tenth of the biological activity of insulin. Whether this is of physiologic relevance is unclear, but it has been suggested that increased secretion of proinsulin, as occurs from pancreatic tumors, could bind to insulin receptors and thereby diminish the effectiveness of insulin. The radioimmunoassay (RIA) commonly used to measure insulin also measures proinsulin, but such interference is commonly ignored. The amino acid composition of the A and B chains differ slightly in different species (see legend of Fig. 39-1) which explains the antigenicity and serum binding of insulin derived from human, porcine, or bovine pancreas.

The C peptide is believed to have no biologic effects, although a recent report claims that infusion of C peptide into IDDM patients, increased to normal the blood flow and capillary diffusion capacity in muscle during exercise. The human C peptide can be measured by a specific RIA and has been used to assess endogenous insulin secretion in individuals receiving insulin, and to differentiate between illicit insulin injection or increased endogenous insulin secretion in suspicious cases of hypoglycemic coma. Injected insulin would decrease endogenous insulin and C peptide release from the pancreas, whereas increased secretion of insulin would increase C peptide release.

Secretion and Degradation

The secretion of insulin can be stimulated by ingestion of proteins as well as carbohydrates and it can be affected by a variety of agents. The main stimulus for insulin secretion is the level of circulating glucose. The islets of the pancreas are freely permeable to D-glucose (but not to L), which has to be phosphorylated by a specific beta cell glucokinase to initiate the signal for insulin secretion; this enzyme has been called the "glucose sensor". The probable mechanism whereby glucose stimulates insulin secretion is shown in Fig. 39-2. The metabolism of glucose increases the ATP/ADP ratio, which closes the ATP sensitive K^+ channels; the decrease in cation efflux from the cell makes the electrical potential across the membrane less negative and depolarizes the cell to a threshold which activates the voltage-dependent Ca^{2+} channel and increases Ca^{2+} influx. The increased Ca^{2+} content stimulates insulin secretion. Other stimuli, e.g., oral hypoglycemic drugs, may have similar effects on K^+ channels but act through different receptors; some insulin secretagogues may not use all the steps outlined above, but probably require Ca^{2+} to induce exocytosis.

Conversely, agents which decrease insulin secretion, such as diazoxide, epinephrine, and various diuretics, open the K^+ channels, increasing cation efflux and making the cells more negative; this causes hyperpolarization of the cell, decreasing Ca^{2+} influx and thus decreasing insulin secretion.

Secretion of insulin in response to glucose has a biphasic pattern. Within a few minutes there is a prompt but brief increase in insulin secretion, the "first phase" or "early peak", which is followed by a more gradual increase in insulin release. A diminished first phase insulin secretion (the sum of the plasma insulin level at 1 and 3 min during a standard intravenous glucose tolerance test) has been suggested as a possible marker to identify susceptible individuals likely to develop NIDDM diabetes.

The plasma half-life of insulin is about 5 min. It circulates in the plasma largely in the free form, with a small amount bound to albumin. Its concentration is usually measured by RIA, using ^{125}I-labelled insulin, and normal fasting plasma values range from 5 to 20 μU/mL in conventional units (30 to 120 pmol/L in Systeme International units; to convert multiply conventional units by 6) and may rise to 100 μU/mL in response to a meal or glucose load. The insulin content of the human pancreas is about 200 U, and the total daily secretion is about 30 to 40 U.

The major sites of degradation of endogenous and exogenous insulin are the liver and, to a lesser degree, the kidneys. Endogenous insulin is carried to the liver by the portal vein and about 50 percent of the insulin is removed prior to its release into the general circulation. It is degraded in stepwise fashion by an insulin-specific protease, which cleaves the B chain, thus unhinging the molecule and allowing further cleavage by non-specific endopeptidases and reduction of the disulfide bridges by a glutathione-insulin-transhydrogenase (insulinase). The degradation products are excreted by the kidneys. In addition, insulin is filtered by the glomeruli, then is largely reabsorbed and metabolized within the proximal tubules, with small amounts of free insulin also excreted in the urine.

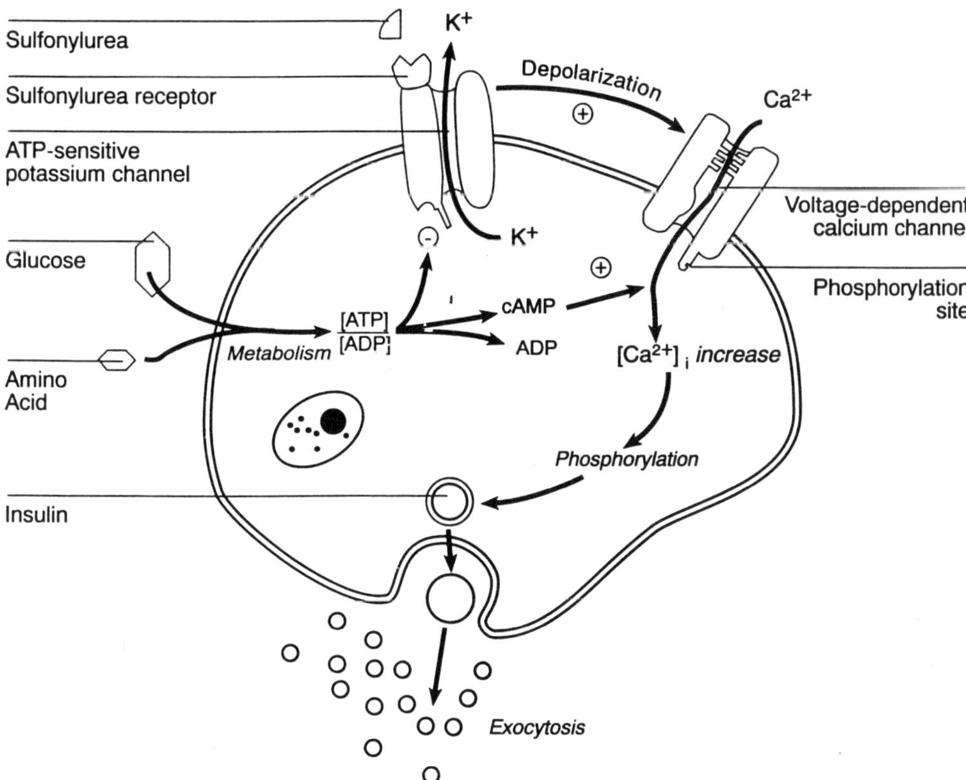

FIGURE 39-2 *Proposed mechanism for stimulation of insulin release by various agents. Sulfonylureas bind to ATP-sensitive potassium channels or closely associated protein and inhibit potassium efflux through the channel. Metabolism of glucose or amino acids by an increasing ATP/ADP ratio inhibits the same channel at the inner surface of the plasma membrane. The inhibition leads to depolarization, opening voltage-dependent calcium channels to allow the entry of extracellular calcium and thereby to trigger exocytosis. An increase in the cyclic AMP concentration also can gate the voltage-dependent calcium channel to increase calcium influx. [From A.E. Boyd, 3rd: "Intracellular Signalling Mechanisms and the Pathophysiology of Disease," Current Concepts, The Upjohn Co., Kalamazoo, 1991.]*

Mechanism of Action

The biologic effects of insulin are initiated by its binding to specific receptors located on the surface of various cells (see Chapter 3, Fig. 3-3 and Table 3-4). The insulin receptor is a tetrameric protein complex, composed of two α subunits and two β subunits; the α subunits form the extracellular domain and the β subunits form the membrane-spanning and cytoplasmic domains. Insulin binds only to the extracellular domain, causing dimerization of these receptors and initiation of a signal that is transmitted to the β subunit. The latter contains intrinsic protein tyrosine kinase activity as well as distinct phosphorylation regulatory sites at tyrosine, serine, and threonine residues; these are part of a complex signal transduction system which ultimately results in the observed biological responses.

One important response to insulin is the mobilization of glucose transporters from intracellular compartments to the cell membrane where they facilitate inward glucose transport. To date, at least five specific glucose transporter proteins (GLUT 1 to 5) have been identified. Since insulin elicits a variety of responses, it is likely that each response is regulated by a specific internal signalling circuit and this is a subject of intense investigation.

Following activation of the receptor, the insulin-receptor complex migrates to special invaginated areas in the membrane which are coated with the protein *clathrin*, and these "coated pits" are then internalized by endocytosis. The coated pits break up into vesicles and are ingested by special organelles that have an internal pH of 4.5 to 5, which causes dissociation of the hormone-receptor complex. The receptor is then recycled to the membrane while the insulin is taken up by lysosomes and degraded.

Biologic Effects

Insulin initiates its biologic effects through activation of insulin receptors. Most tissues, including brain, erythrocytes, lymphocytes, and heart, have insulin receptors, but the role of insulin in many of the tissues is not clear. Insulin has been shown to have effects on development, growth, and sodium excretion, but our focus has been largely on carbohydrate, lipid, and protein metabolism and the major tissues involved: liver, skeletal muscle, and adipose tissues. Since insulin is required to facilitate glucose uptake by these tissues, they are commonly referred to as "insulin sensitive". By contrast, glucose uptake by brain or erythrocytes is not dependent on insulin.

Effect on Carbohydrate Metabolism Endogenous insulin or insulin administered exogenously lowers plasma glucose levels by decreasing glucose release from the liver into the circulation and by increasing glucose uptake, mainly by muscle and to a lesser extent by fat tissue. The liver is quite sensitive to insulin, which when infused can decrease glucose release at doses that have little effect on glucose uptake by muscle. Even in the fasting state, the circulating insulin exerts a restraining effect on glucose release; this can be shown by injecting an antibody to neutralize circulating insulin, which results in a prompt increase in hepatic glucose release and a marked hyperglycemia. Insulin decreases glucose release by the liver by two mechanisms: it stimulates glycogen synthetase thereby shunting glucose into glycogen, and it inhibits gluconeogenesis by inhibiting several key enzymes: phosphoenolpyruvatecarboxykinase, fructose-1,6-bisphosphatase, glucose-6-phosphatase, and glycogen phosphorylase. The converse is seen in insulin deficiency, with increased release of glucose from the liver and decreased uptake of glucose by muscle and fat.

The insulin-induced increase in glucose uptake occurs largely in muscle, resulting in increased glycogen deposition due to stimulation of glucokinase and glycogen synthetase; glucose uptake by fat tissue is also increased and this provides the alpha glycerophosphate moiety to esterify the free fatty acids and be deposited as triglycerides. Although the glucose uptake by fat tissue accounts for only about 5 percent of the total glucose uptake following a meal (postprandial state), the triglycerides represent the most abundant and most efficient means of storing energy. In addition to increasing glucose uptake, insulin also increases glycolysis and oxidation of the glucose by stimulating several key enzymes: phosphofructokinase and pyruvate kinase. In insulin deficiency the converse is seen: glucose release from the liver is increased and glucose uptake by muscle and fat is decreased.

Effect on Lipid Metabolism Insulin increases lipogenesis and decreases lipolysis and ketogenesis. Fat is stored in cells as triglycerides which are hydrolyzed and released into the circulation by a hormone-sensitive lipase. This enzyme, which is stimulated by epinephrine and norepinephrine, is inhibited by insulin, thereby decreasing the release of free fatty acids and consequently decreasing ketone body formation. Insulin increases lipogenesis by stimulating synthesis of a lipoprotein lipase in adipose tissues; the enzyme is secreted, becomes associated with the endothelial cells of capillaries, and is responsible for hydrolysis of chylomicrons to yield free fatty acids, which are then taken up by cells. The concurrent increase in glucose uptake provides the α-glycerol phosphate needed to form the triglyceride. Insulin deficiency results in the opposite effects, namely increased lipolysis and decreased lipogenesis.

Effect on Protein Metabolism Insulin stimulates the active transport of various amino acids into cells, increasing protein synthesis and growth of tissues. Indeed, insulin is an anabolic hormone and can also interact with receptors for insulin-like growth factor (IGF-1, somatomedin) which is responsible for the growth-promoting actions of growth hormone. The effects of insulin on amino acid uptake are independent of its effect on glucose uptake. In insulin deficiency, plasma amino acid levels are elevated, making more amino acids available for gluconeogenesis and the production of glucose. In addition, the absence of insulin removes its normal suppressive effect on the enzymes associated with gluconeogenesis.

Insulin Preparations

The commercially available preparations consist of porcine, bovine, or human (obtained by recombinant DNA techniques) insulins; they differ mainly in times of onset and maximal activity and in duration of action. These differences are achieved by conjugating regular insulin, which is soluble in solution, with protamine and/or zinc, to form a precipitate which retards absorption and prolongs the duration of action.

The various insulin preparations can be divided into three major groups: (A) *rapid-acting* preparations with a fast onset of action and a relatively short duration of action, (B) *intermediate-acting* preparations with a rapid onset and an intermediate duration of action, and (C) *long-acting* preparations with a delayed onset and a long duration of action (Table 39-1). Insulins are available in 10 mL vials, in concentrations of 100 U/mL, and also at 500 U/mL for emergency treatment requiring large doses of insulin, such as insulin resistance or ketoacidosis. There are at least 25 different insulin preparations on the market, but with changing patterns of treatment, manufacturers are discontinuing a number of preparations. Insulin is also packaged in special cartridges for use in pen injectors, making it more convenient for frequent dosing regimens. New formulations are also being tested for intranasal and transdermal administration. Human insulin preparation carry designation of R, L, U, and N for regular, lente, ultralente and NPH, respectively.

Rapid-acting Insulins Insulin Injection is also known as Regular Insulin and Crystalline Zinc Insulin Injection. This type of insulin comes as a clear solution which contain regular, unmodified, completely dissolved crystalline zinc insulin in a phosphate buffer. This insulin, which is in aggregates of three pairs of insulin dimers bound to one atom of zinc, is disassembled in the body to monomer insulin, the active form. The time of onset of action is a function of dose, site of injection, and blood circulation. Intravenous injection begins to produce effects within 5 min. Injection into abdominal subcutaneous tissue can produce effects within 15 min, with a duration of 4 to 6 h. This site is a preferred one because absorption is fast and is less affected by factors which alter rate of absorption, such as exercise and increased blood flow. Muscle has more extensive blood circulation than subcutaneous tissue, which shortens the duration of action of injected insulin. Human insulin is absorbed somewhat more rapidly than the animal types. Currently several human insulin preparations are being explored in which replacement of some amino acids results in a faster rate of absorption. The advantage of such preparations would be that insulin could be injected at the time of the meal rather than 15 to 30 min before as is the case with the current insulins. Premixed preparations containing regular insulin and isophane insulin (an intermediate-acting insulin) are described below.

Intermediate-acting Insulins These insulins are produced by the addition of protamine or zinc to regular bovine, porcine, or human insulin, in a phosphate buffer, forming an insulin precipitate which slightly retards absorption and prolongs the duration of effect. Protamine, a basic peptide obtained from fish sperm, is the agent used in NPH insulin (neutral protamine Hagedorn), which also contains a small amount of zinc. Since the protamine and insulin are mixed in a stoichiometric ratio, there is no excess of either and hence it is also called "isophane" insulin.

The NPH suspensions of beef, pork, and human insulin vary somewhat in their kinetics. Human NPH begins acting in about 1 to 2 h following subcutaneous injection, reaches a peak by 6 to 10 h and its effects wane by 18 h. Pork or beef NPH have a slightly longer onset, peak and duration, but activity is usually dissipated by 24 h.

In the "Lente" preparations (insulin zinc suspensions) only zinc is added in the presence of an acetate buffer which results in the formation of a precipitate. The degree of insolubility, and hence absorption, can be altered by varying the size of crystals formed. Small crystals dissolve rapidly leading to a rapid onset of effect and a short duration, while large crystals dissolve slowly and resulting in a delayed onset and a prolonged duration. Compared to NPH, lente insulin has only slightly longer onset and a similar duration of effect; and ultralente (extended insulin zinc suspension) is longer-acting (Table 39-1). Semilente (prompt insulin zinc suspension) was a shorter-acting insulin preparation, but it is no longer available since it was rarely used.

An important advance has been the introduction of premixed preparations containing both short- and intermediate-acting insulins. The combination provides insulin for prompt absorption at meal time as well as slow and prolonged release to cover the periods between meals. Previously, the patient would draw insulin from two different bottles, either into one syringe or inject each separately. The new preparations decrease dosing

TABLE 39-1 Comparison of various insulin preparations[a]

Type of insulin	Onset of effect, h	Maximum effect, h	Duration of effect, h
RAPID-ACTING			
Insulin Injection (Regular)	0.5 to 1	2.5 to 5	6 to 8
INTERMEDIATE-ACTING			
Isophane Insulin Suspension (NPH)	1 to 2	8 to 10	18 to 26
Insulin Zinc Suspension (Lente)	2	8 to 10	18 to 26
70% Isophane Insulin Suspension + 30% Insulin Injection	0.5	2 to 12	up to 24
50% Isophane Insulin Suspension + 50% Insulin Injection	0.5	2.5	up to 24
LONG-ACTING			
Extended Insulin Zinc Suspension (Ultralente)	4 to 6	16 to 18	30 to 36

[a] The times of onset, maximum, and duration of effect are estimates and vary from one patient to another.

errors as well as the number of injections. In the United States, the two preparations available consist of mixtures of 70% isophane insulin and 30% regular insulin (70/30) and 50% isophane insulin and 50% regular insulin (50/50). Since both types of insulins are in the same buffer (i.e., phosphate), these insulins may be mixed in any proportion. However, since the buffers are different in isophane (NPH) insulin (phosphate buffer) and lente insulin (acetate buffer), these cannot be mixed because a physical incompatibility will result in an inactive precipitate.

The usefulness of the premixed insulins is demonstrated in the following example: a patient is prescribed a morning dose of 20 U of isophane insulin and 10 U of regular insulin. The patient draws 30 U (0.3 mL) of the 70/30 mixture, which provides 21 U (70%) of the isophane insulin and 9 U (30%) of the regular insulin. Preparations with additional ratios are available in Europe.

Long-acting Insulins Protamine zinc insulin was introduced in 1936 as the first long acting preparation. Its onset of action occurs in 4 to 6 h and it acts for 24 to 48 hours and possibly longer. Since the preparation contains an excess of protamine, it cannot be mixed with regular insulin because the protamine will bind it and retard its absorption. Concern about the immunogenic potential of protamine has diminished the use of protamine zinc insulin and the product is now no longer available.

Ultralente insulin (as described above) contains only zinc as the precipitant and is used more widely. The human ultralente insulin has a similar onset of action (4 to 6 h) but a shorter duration of action (about 24 h) compared to the animal ones (about 36 h). It is noteworthy that the absorption of the long-acting insulin is sufficiently slow, which provides a prolonged plateau plasma level without an abrupt peak. Superimposing injections of short-acting insulins at meal time, on such constant levels of insulin, mimics the physiologic pattern of insulin secretion.

Insulin Therapy

A number of factors may increase insulin requirements. These include: (1) increased metabolic needs of the body, e.g., thyrotoxicosis and fever; (2) stress from situations such as surgery, injury, infection, myocardial infarction, or psychic trauma; (3) reduced muscular exercise; (4) increased caloric intake and weight gain; (5) development of resistance to insulin through immune mechanisms or various endocrinopathies such as acromegaly, Cushing's syndrome, thyrotoxicosis, and increased estrogen secretion in pregnancy; (6) reduction in insulin receptor number, signal transduction, or post-receptor defects; and (7) administered drugs which reduce the effectiveness of insulin by as yet unknown mechanisms. Conversely, increased sensitivity to insulin occurs in adrenal glucocorticoid deficiency, adrenalectomy, and hypophysectomy, but replacement therapy adequately ameliorates the insulin hypersensitivity.

Complications of Insulin Therapy

Hypoglycemia is undoubtedly the most significant complication of insulin therapy. Mild degrees of hypoglycemia result in fatigue, drowsiness, and headaches. More severe and abrupt decreases in blood glucose, to below 50 to 60 mg/dL, may lead to autonomic symptoms (e.g., sweating, tremors, palpitations, cold hands, hunger, and anxiety), and to neurogenic symptoms (e.g., blurred vision, confusion, aggressiveness, lack of concentration, and loss of consciousness (insulin shock)). Awareness of hypoglycemic symptoms may differ among individuals. Also some reports claim that there is less awareness of hypoglycemia when using human insulin, but this has been disputed and the issue remains unresolved. The incidence of hypoglycemia may be reduced by adherence to a prescribed regimen of diet, exercise, and insulin dosage. Guidelines for medical care of patients with diabetes mellitus have been prepared by the American Diabetes Association.

The various symptoms of hypoglycemia can be relieved by the administration of glucose. The conscious individual, experiencing mild hypoglycemia, can obtain relief by ingestion of any sugar-containing liquid. In the unconscious individual, intravenous injection or infusion of a 50% glucose solution provides effective relief. Glucagon, which stimulates glycogenolysis and raises plasma glucose, is also available.

Coma can also be due to insulin deficiency. It may be of the hyperglycemic-hyperosmotic, nonketotic type or as a consequence of diabetic ketoacidosis. Both are life-threatening emergencies and need to be quickly differentiated from hypoglycemic insulin shock. The latter results in symptoms of sympathetic activation, while those seen in hyperglycemic diabetic coma include dry and flushed skin, weak pulse and low blood pressure, dehydration, abdominal pain, exaggerated (Kussmaul) respiration, and acetone odor of the breath in the case of ketoacidosis. The specific treatments consist of insulin infusion along with correction of the electrolyte and water losses. Improvement is gradual, usually becoming evident by 6 to 12 hours of treatment.

Other adverse effects of insulin therapy consist of allergic reactions and these may be either local or systemic. Local allergic reactions include the formation of an erythematous area at the site of injection. This reaction appears within an hour and may persist for several days. It usually occurs within a few days after initiation or reinstitution of insulin therapy, suggesting prior sensitization to some proteins in the insulin injection. Such reactions may be avoided by switching from the usual mixed beef and pork insulin preparation to the less allergenic pork only or human insulin products. Local irritation may also be due to factors not directly related to insulin such as the injection procedure and irritation from disinfectant and cleansing solutions.

Systemic allergic reactions may occur with or without local reactions, and may consist of nausea, vomiting, diarrhea, dyspnea, and bronchial asthma. Rarely angioedema, hypotension, shock, and death may occur. Systemic manifestations from therapeutic doses of insulin usually occur in patients with a history of allergic reactions to other drugs or patients treated with insulin intermittently. This type of allergy may be treated by desensitization, using repeated injections of small amounts of insulin.

Insulin may also affect lipid stores at sites of injection, causing atrophy or hypertrophy of subcutaneous fat tissue. The atrophy may have an immunologic basis and is ameliorated by using highly purified insulin preparations; local hypertrophy perhaps due to the lipogenic action of insulin, may be avoided by rotating sites of injection.

Local infections at sites of injection are now quite uncommon. This is due in part to inclusion of bacteriostatic agents in the insulin preparations and greater use of disposable needles; cleaning injection sites with water rather than alcohol does not appear to increase the incidence of infection.

GLUCAGON

Glucagon is a single-chain polypeptide, consisting of 29 amino acids. It is produced by pancreatic alpha cells and is secreted in greater amounts in response to hypoglycemia. It raises plasma glucose levels acutely by stimulating cyclic AMP-mediated hepatic glycogenolysis. Chronically, or in large doses, it also stimulates gluconeogenesis and ketogenesis. The plasma glucose levels in the basal state are fine-tuned by the plasma glucagon-insulin ratio; therefore, decreasing insulin levels, without changing the glucagon levels will increase glucose output by the liver, whereas suppression of both insulin and glucagon, e.g., by somatostatin, will lower the plasma glucose acutely, albeit transiently.

In addition to its action on plasma glucose levels, glucagon increases myocardial contractility, relaxes smooth muscles of the gastrointestinal tract, and decreases gastric and pancreatic secretions.

Glucagon, used parenterally, has three main uses: (1) in the emergency treatment of hypoglycemia in the unconscious individual, (2) to reverse the hypoglycemia in psychiatric patients undergoing insulin shock therapy, and (3) in radiology, to relax the smooth muscles of the gastrointestinal tract to allow better X-ray visualization of the stomach and intestines.

ORAL HYPOGLYCEMIC AGENTS

At present the only orally effective drugs for regulating blood glucose in NIDDM are the sulfonylureas and biguanides and only the former are used therapeutically in the United States.

Sulfonylurea Derivatives

The hypoglycemic effect of the sulfonylurea drugs was discovered in France in 1942, as a side effect of a sulfur-containing bacteriostatic which was used to treat typhoid fever. Their plasma glucose lowering effect is due to the sulfonylurea moiety, but they will not act in individuals who have less than 30 percent of their islet beta cells in the pancreas, thus they are ineffective in IDDM. The first generation compounds introduced into clinical use include: tolbutamide, acetohexamide, tolazamide, and chlorpropamide (Table 39-2). The use of these compounds declined markedly with the 1976 report of a long-term study (University Group Diabetes Program, UGDP) which questioned their efficacy and suggested an increased risk of cardiovascular complications. These results were vigorously challenged, and by 1984 the introduction of glyburide and glipizide, as the second generation of such drugs (Table 39-2), contributed to greater acceptance of their use again. Indeed, it is estimated that about 40 percent of those with NIDDM in the United States are treated with these drugs.

Mechanism of Action The first and second generation drugs contain the sulfonylurea moiety but differ in the various substitutions which affects their pharmacologic profile. They all appear to act by the same, although incompletely understood, mechanism. Since they are ineffective in the de-pancreatized or severely insulin-deficient individuals, it is evident that their action requires the presence of insulin. The beta cells of the pancreas have high affinity binding sites ("receptors") for sulfonylurea derivatives. These sites appear to be structural components of the ATP-sensitive potassium channels; these channels are closed by the sulfonylurea derivatives, which leads to depolarization of the membrane and an influx of ionic calcium due to activation of the voltage-dependent calcium channel, resulting in insulin secretion (Fig. 39-2). Acutely, the sulfonylurea derivatives stimulate insulin secretion, elevate plasma insulin levels and enhance the second phase insulin response to glucose and other nutrients. However, when NIDDM patients are treated with these drugs for several months, the fasting plasma insulin levels are no longer elevated, but plasma glucose levels are still reduced, suggesting an extra-pancreatic action. The latter has not been convincingly demonstrated, but NIDDM patients treated with the sulfonylureas show a decrease in their elevated hepatic glucose production as well as a diminished insulin resistance in peripheral tissues. Sulfonylurea receptors have been shown in nerve cells, cardiac muscle, skeletal muscle, and smooth muscle, and low affinity binding sites in myocytes and adipocytes, but all of them are believed to contribute little to the therapeutic effects of the drugs.

Pharmacokinetics The sulfonylurea derivatives are weak acids and are distributed in the extracellular space (apparent volume of distribution of 10 to 15 L). All are rapidly and completely absorbed from the small intestines and are extensively bound to plasma proteins (> 95 percent). The first generation compounds, because of their ionic

TABLE 39-2 Sulfonylurea derivatives

Generic name	Chemical structure[a]
Tolbutamide	H_3C—⟨benzene⟩—[SO_2—NH—C(=O)—NH]—$(CH_2)_3CH_3$
Chlorpropamide	Cl—⟨benzene⟩—SO_2—NH—C(=O)—NH—$(CH_2)_2CH_3$
Acetohexamide	H_3C—CO—⟨benzene⟩—SO_2—NH—C(=O)—NH—⟨cyclohexyl⟩
Tolazamide	H_3C—⟨benzene⟩—SO_2—NH—C(=O)—NH—N⟨CH_2—CH_2—CH_2 / CH_2—CH_2—CH_2⟩
Glyburide	(Cl, OCH_3)⟨benzene⟩—$CONHCH_2CH_2$—⟨benzene⟩—$SO_2NHCONH$—⟨cyclohexyl⟩
Glipizide	H_3C—⟨pyrazine (N, N)⟩—$CONHCH_2CH_2$—⟨benzene⟩—$SO_2NHCONH$—⟨cyclohexyl⟩

[a] The sulfonylurea group is indicated by the boxed area on tolbutamide

binding, are more readily displaced by other drugs from these binding sites, and thus are more prone to cause side effects due to drug interactions, than the nonionic-bound second generation drugs. The drugs also have important differences in onset and duration of action, nature of metabolites, route of elimination, and intrinsic potency (Table 39-3). The drugs also differ in their plasma half-lives, but these do not correlate with duration of their plasma glucose-lowering effect.

Tolbutamide is the least potent and shortest acting of the drugs and may not prevent hyperglycemia in NIDDM as effectively as the other drugs. It is also least likely to cause serious side effects. It is metabolized in the liver to inactive compounds that are excreted in the urine. Its duration of action is 6 to 12 hours, so it is commonly taken several times a day.

Acetohexamide is the only one of the drugs that is metabolized to a hydroxylated product that is more potent than the parent drug and both compounds contribute to the glucose-lowering effects. The kidneys are the route of elimination for both. The drug has not been used widely and even less so since the introduction of newer drugs.

Tolazamide is metabolized in the liver to products with weak hypoglycemic activity, which are excreted in the urine.

Chlorpropamide has the longest duration of action, up to 70 hours, and is administered once daily. It is metabolized to relatively weak compounds which are eliminated by the kidneys. However, about 20 percent of a dose is excreted

TABLE 39-3 Doses and pharmacokinetic properties of the sulfonylurea derivatives

	Tolbutamide	Acetohexamide	Tolazamide	Chlorpropamide	Glyburide	Glipizide
Usual dose, mg/day	1500	500	250	250	10	10
Dose range, mg/day	500 to 3000	250 to 1250	100 to 500	100 to 500	1.25 to 20	2.5 to 20
Hepatic metabolism	Inactive products	Active product	Weakly active product	Inactive products	Weakly active product	Inactive products
Excretion	Renal	Renal	Renal	Renal	Renal and biliary	Renal
Biologic half-life, h	4 to 5	6 to 8	7	36	10	2 to 4
Onset of action, h	1 to 4	1 to 2	4 to 6	1 to 3	2 to 4	1 to 1.5
Peak activity, h	4 to 6	3	4 to 8	4 to 6		
Duration of action, h	6 to 12	12 to 24	12 to 24	24 to 60	16 to 24	12 to 24

unchanged and impaired renal function may result in drug accumulation to levels which produce severe hypoglycemia. It is the most common drug involved in hypoglycemic episodes.

Glyburide and glipizide are the second generation sulfonylurea derivatives. Their mechanism of action is the same as for the older drugs, but they have greater intrinsic potency (100 to 150 times more potent than tolbutamide on a molar basis) and thus are used in much smaller doses; their side effects are similar to those produced by the first generation compounds. The two drugs differ in their kinetics and metabolism. Peak plasma levels are attained earlier by glipizide (1 h) than by glyburide (3 h), but its duration of action is somewhat shorter (16 vs. 24 h). The longer duration of action of glyburide has been cited as explaining the better normalization of the fasting plasma glucose levels than that seen with glipizide, while the greater release of insulin in response to a meal seen with glipizide treatment has been attributed to its faster onset of action. These differences are still a matter of debate. Glipizide is metabolized in the liver to inactive products which are excreted in the urine. Glyburide is also metabolized in the liver and about 50 percent of a dose is excreted in the bile and the rest in the urine. One of the products, 4-hydroxyglyburide, retains about 15 percent of the hypoglycemic activity of the parent drug and is eliminated in the urine.

Adverse Effects Hypoglycemia is the most common adverse effect of the sulfonylureas. It occurs most frequently with chlorpropamide, as might be anticipated from its long duration of action. It is more likely to be associated with large doses of the drugs, failure to maintain adequate diet, presence of hepatic or renal disease, and concomitant use of other medication. Large doses will prolong the duration of action of these drugs. Skipping meals or an insufficient diet will likewise extend and exacerbate a hypoglycemic state. Since most of the sulfonylurea derivatives are oxidized in the liver to inactive metabolites, impaired liver function can prolong their effects. Likewise, active metabolites of sulfonylureas that are excreted by the kidneys may produce hypoglycemia in patients with renal dysfunction.

Some adverse effects of these drugs are independent of their antidiabetic actions. For example, chlorpropamide may cause an inappropriate secretion of anti-diuretic hormone, causing water retention and hyponatremia. The drug also can cause a flushing of the face and neck in response to alcohol ingestion. These adverse effects are not seen with the second generation drugs.

Less common side effects for sulfonylurea drugs consist of gastrointestinal, dermatological, and hematologic reactions. These include nausea, vomiting, dyspepsia, rashes, pruritus, exfoliative dermatitis, hemolytic anemia, and bone marrow aplasia.

Drug Interactions The concomitant use of other drugs can either enhance or diminish the effectiveness of the sulfonylurea drugs to lower plasma glucose levels. The hypoglycemic effects may be enhanced by drugs which: (1) can displace the sulfonylureas from binding to plasma proteins, e.g., aspirin, the antihyperlipidemic fibric acids, sulfonamides, and trimethoprin, or (2) inhibit metabolism of the sulfonylurea compound by inhibiting the cytochrome P-450 drug-metabolizing system, e.g., acute alcohol ingestion, H_2 receptor antagonists, oral anticoagulants, and monoamine oxidase inhibitors. Probenecid, allopurinol, sulfonamides, and salicylates may also inhibit the urinary excretion of the sulfonylurea metabolites. Also, some drugs have an additive effect because of their intrinsic hypoglycemic activity, e.g., alcohol, salicylates, guanethidine, and insulin.

Diminishing the effectiveness of the sulfonylurea derivatives can be brought about by drugs which: (1) induce their metabolism e.g., barbiturates and rifampin, or (2) inhibit insulin secretion, e.g., thiazide and loop diuretics, phenytoin, β-adrenergic receptor blockers, and diazoxide. The latter compound can actually be used to reduce insulin secretion in emergency treatment of acute hypoglycemia due to the sulfonylureas.

Biguanides

Instead of the sulfonylurea moiety, these compounds contain two adjoining molecules of guanidine with one amino group removed. The two main biguanides: phenformin and metformin became available in 1957, but only phenformin was used in the United States. Phenformin was withdrawn after a number of reports that it caused an often fatal lactic acidosis. The drug is available only through the Food and Drug Administration (FDA) and can be used only in patients with nonketotic NIDDM who have severe symptoms, are not controlled through diet and sulfonylureas, and cannot take insulin because of disability and have no means to receive medical assistance.

Metformin has a safer record, and has been used for over 20 years in Canada and Europe and more recently in Japan. It is expected to be approved for use in the United States. Its structure is:

$$(H_3C)_2N{-}C(=NH){-}NH{-}C(=NH){-}NH_2$$

Metformin is antihyperglycemic rather than hypoglycemic since it lowers the elevated plasma glucose levels in NIDDM, but does not cause clinical hypoglycemia and does not cause hypoglycemia in nondiabetic patients. Its mechanism of action is unclear; it does not increase insulin secretion acutely, but still requires the presence of insulin for its action. In NIDDM, metformin decreases the elevated basal hepatic glucose output, increases insulin-mediated glucose uptake and non-oxidative metabolism (glycogen formation) by muscle. It diminishes intestinal absorption of carbohydrates. It also increases the anaerobic glycolysis in the intestines and the resulting lactate is used by the liver to increase gluconeogenesis; this detracts from the drug's inhibitory effect on glucose output, but prevents hypoglycemia. Noteworthy, it does not increase weight gain as insulin does, and reduces the insulin resistance seen in the obese NIDDM patient. Metformin lowers plasma triglyceride levels, mainly by decreasing very low density lipoproteins (VLDL) in nondiabetic patients and in NIDDM.

Metformin is not bound to plasma proteins, is not metabolized, and is excreted by the kidneys. It has a plasma half-life of 2 to 4 h, thus is given three times a day with meals. The onset of action is 1 to 1.5 hours. The drug achieves a peak effect in 2 hours and has a duration of action between 10 and 12 hours. Side effects of the drug are seen in up to 20 percent of the patients and consist mainly of gastrointestinal disturbances including nausea, diarrhea, anorexia, and metallic taste, but these are usually transient and can be minimized by slowly increasing the dose to the therapeutic level and taking it with meals. Curiously, less than 10 percent of patients fail to respond to the drug. Because of its different mode of action, metformin has been used in combination with sulfonylurea derivatives with reasonable success.

THERAPY OF DIABETES MELLITUS

Management of IDDM usually depends on the therapeutic goals of the physician and the cooperation of the patient. Goals may vary from a minimum of eliminating diabetic symptoms to a maximum of attaining normoglycemia. Until recently it was not clear whether the long-term complications of diabetes, such as neuropathy, nephropathy, and retinopathy, were genetically predetermined and therefore progressed independently of insulin treatment or if they were due to the disease process and the attending hyperglycemia and therefore might be controlled by prevention of the hyperglycemia. To this end, a multicenter study, the Diabetes Control and Complications Trial (DCCT), was begun in 1983 to compare the incidence of complications between: (1) the conventional treatment consisting of one or two doses of insulin per day and single daily self-testing of blood glucose, and (2) intensive therapy for tighter control of blood glucose, involving 3 to 5 daily insulin injections and 4 to 7 daily self-testing of blood glucose. The results of the 10 year study revealed that intensive therapy reduced significantly (by 50 to 70 percent) the progression of diabetic retinopathy, nephropathy, and neuropathy. Although this study was quite demanding on the patients and required extensive professional staff support, it was recommended that the majority of IDDM patients should be treated with intense therapy. Various protocols for insulin treatment have appeared in the literature and more should be forthcoming as a result of the DCCT findings.

Therapy of NIDDM usually begins with weight reduction and exercise. If these measures are inadequate, an oral hypoglycemic agent is added. If maximal doses do not attain the desired plasma glucose levels, insulin may be added. Various schedules for the combined treatment have been reported. One approach is to inject an intermediate-acting insulin (e.g., NPH) at bedtime to provide a near normal glycemia in the morning and adding the oral agents during the day. The initial lowering of the plasma glucose makes the oral hypoglycemic drugs more effective. Also, since persistent hyperglycemia produces pancreatic islet toxicity, lowering of plasma glucose by insulin serves to protect the islets and likely extends the duration of effectiveness of the oral agents.

About 20 percent of patients do not respond to the sulfonylureas (primary failure), and of those who do respond, 5 to 10 percent lose their response each year (secondary failure). The basis for these failures in not known. Best candidates for successful therapy are those who developed NIDDM after the age of 30 and have had it for less than 5 years. No beneficial effects are likely to occur in individuals who are on diet therapy and still have fasting plasma glucose levels over 250 mg/dL. Also in patients with newly diagnosed NIDDM, who have such high plasma glucose levels, oral therapy should not be started until the fasting glucose levels are significantly reduced by insulin treatment. Patients who exhibit primary or secondary failure with tolbutamide, acetohexamide or tolazamide may respond to chlorpropamide, glyburide, or glipizide; however, those who fail to respond to the latter group are unlikely to respond to the former group.

Monitoring of Diabetes Control

The development of pen- or pocket-size, inexpensive glucometers has drastically changed the management of diabetes. It allows frequent daily measurement of blood glucose, which is essential for multiple-dose insulin therapy. Assessment of glucose control over more extended periods of time is made by measuring the degree to which glucose interacts with several circulating proteins, i.e., hemoglobin and albumin. These are non-enzymatic reactions and the percent of glycation of the protein is a function of the glucose concentration and the duration of exposure of the protein; the latter is dependent on the half-life of the protein being measured. If the average age of the red blood cells is 60 days (their approximate life span is 120 days) then the percentage of hemoglobin glycated reflects glycemic control over a 60 day period. The values are given as percentage of hemoglobin A_{1c} (Hb A_{1c}) or total hemoglobin (multiply A_{1c} value by 1.2). Such measurements are now routinely carried out as part of patient care. Measurement of "fructosamine", which determines the extent of glycation of plasma albumin, provides monitoring of glycemic control over a 14 day period (the approximate half-life of albumin). Desirable levels of control of various parameters in patients with diabetes are given in Table 39-4.

New Approaches for Therapy of NIDDM

Hyperglycemia and insulin resistance are the major abnormalities in NIDDM and a number of new drugs are directed at these problems. These drugs are in various stages of clinical use at this time and include the following:

TABLE 39-4 Biochemical indexes of metabolic control in patients with diabetes mellitus[a]

Index	Range			
	Good	Acceptable	Fair	Poor
Fasting plasma glucose level, mg/dL	80 to 120	120 to 140	140 to 180	> 180
Postprandial plasma glucose level[b], mg/dL	80 to 140	140 to 180	180 to 235	> 235
Hemoglobin A_{1c} level, percent[c]	< 6.0	6.0 to 7.5	7.5 to 9.0	> 9.0
Total plasma cholesterol level, mg/dL	< 200	200 to 220	200 to 240	> 240
Plasma HDL[d] cholesterol level, mg/dL	> 40	35 to 40	30 to 35	< 30
Plasma triglyceride level, mg/dL	< 150	< 150 to 200	< 200 to 240	> 240

a Based on recommendations of the American Diabetes Association and the European NIDDM Policy Group.
b Measured two hours after eating.
c For total glycosylated hemoglobin, multiply values by 1.2.
d HDL denotes high density lipoprotein.

[Modified from Gerich, J.E.: "Oral Hypoglycemic Agents," New Engl. J. Med. 321: 1231-1245 (1989).]

Acarbose — it is taken orally to inhibit the intestinal α-glucosidase, which digests complex carbohydrates to allow their absorption,

Thiazolidinedione derivatives (e.g., pioglitazone) — these agents appear to amplify some post-insulin receptor step which increases glucose uptake by muscle,

2-Oxiranecarboxylates (e.g., methylpalmoxirate and clomoxir) — they inhibit oxidation of long-chain fatty acids which provides the energy source for gluconeogenesis (acetyl CoA for activation of pyruvate carboxylate; and reducing equivalents (NADH) and thereby reduce hepatic glucose production,

Insulin-like growth factor 1 (IGF-1) — its high degree of homology with insulin allows it to react with insulin and IGF receptors, although it is only 6% as potent as insulin in lowering plasma glucose in nondiabetic patients; in a small trial in patients with extreme insulin resistance (acanthosis nigricans), the recombinant IGF-1 decreased plasma glucose as effectively as in nondiabetic patients, opening the possibility for such use in the future, and

Glucagon-like peptide-1 (7-36) amide, "insulinotropin" — this peptide, which lacks the first 6 amino acids, occurs naturally in humans, is released in response to a meal or oral glucose load and potentiates glucose-induced insulin release. In IDDM patients, it decreased significantly their insulin requirements and lowered their plasma glucagon levels.

BIBLIOGRAPHY

---------- "Clinical Practice Recommendations," American Diabetes Association, 1992-1993, *Diabetes Care* **16 (Suppl. 2)**: May, 1993.

Bailey, C.J.: "Biguanides and NIDDM," *Diabetes Care* **15**: 755-772 (1992).

Boyd, A.E., 3rd: "Intracellular Signalling Mechanisms and the Pathophysiology of Disease," *Current Concepts*, The Upjohn Co., Kalamazoo, 1991.

Bressler, R., and D. Johnson: "New Pharmacological Approaches to Therapy of NIDDM", *Diabetes Care* **15**: 792-805 (1992).

Davidson, M.B.: "How to Get the Most Out of Insulin Therapy," *Clinical Diabetes* **8**: 65 Sept/Oct (1990).

Fajans, S.S.: "Scope and Heterogeneous Nature of MODY", *Diabetes Care* **13**: 49-64 (1990).

Gerich, J.E.: "Oral Hypoglycemic Agents," *N. Engl. J. Med.* **321**: 1231-1245 (1989).

Groop, L.C.: "Sulfonylureas in NIDDM," *Diabetes Care* **15**: 737-754 (1992).

Gutniak, M., C. Orskov, J.J. Holst, B. Ahren, and S. Efendic: "Antidiabetogenic Effect of Glucagon-like Peptide-1 (7-36) Amide in Normal Subjects and Patients With Diabetes Mellitus," *N. Engl. J. Med.* **326**: 1316-1322 (1992).

Johansson, B.L., B. Linde, and J. Wahren: "Effects of C-peptide on Blood Flow, Capillary Diffusion Capacity and Glucose Utilization in the Exercising Forearm of Type 1 (Insulin-Dependent) Diabetic Patients," *Diabetologia* **35**: 1151-1158 (1992).

Lebovitz, H.E.: "A Look at Sulfonylurea Drugs," *Diabetes Spectrum* **4**: 314-319 (1991).

Nathan, D.M.: "Long-term Complications of Diabetes Mellitus," *N. Engl. J. Med.* **328**: 1676-1685 (1993).

Panten, U., M. Schwanstecher, and C. Schwanstecher: "Pancreatic and Extrapancreatic Sulfonylurea Receptors," *Horm. Metab. Res.* **24**: 549-554 (1992).

Rosenbloom, A.L.: "Intracerebral Crises During Treatment of Diabetic of Ketoacidosis," *Diabetes Care* **13**: 22-33 (1990).

Skyler, J.S., and M.D. Fili: "Intensive Therapy of Type 1 Diabetes," In: Sakamoto, N., K.G.M. M. Alberti, and N. Hotta, (eds): *Current Status of Prevention and Treatment of Diabetic Complications*, Amsterdam, The Netherlands: Excerpts Medica; 235-242 (1990).

Widen, E.I., J.G. Eriksson, A.V. Ekstrand, and L.C. Groop: "Metformin Normalizes Nonoxidative Glucose Metabolism in Insulin-Resistant Normoglycemic First-Degree Relatives of Patients with NIDDM," *Diabetes* **41**: 354-358 (1992).

Wu, M.S., P. Johnston, W.H. Sheu, C.B. Hollenbeck, C.Y., Jeng, I.D. Goldfine, Y.D. Chen and G.M. Reaven: "Effect of Metformin on Carbohydrate and Lipoprotein Metabolism in NIDDM Patients," *Diabetes Care* **13**: 1-8 (1990).

CHAPTER 40

Female Sex Hormones, Oral Contraceptives, and Fertility Agents

Ira Weinstein

In the female, the ovaries have two main functions, the production of ova and the synthesis and secretion of the steroidal hormones, estrogen and progesterone. These hormones serve to regulate the development and maintenance of the female sexual characteristics and the processes essential for fertilization of the ova, pregnancy, and parturition. The inter-relationship that exists between the ovarian steroids and the peptide hormones of the hypothalamus and anterior pituitary are essential for the reproduction of the species. The feedback controls exerted by the gonadal steroids on these higher centers in the brain are utilized in pharmacologic interventions that control fertility in the female.

The gonadal steroids modify behavior by actions in the brain. Although quite evident in lower animals, however, in primates behavior modification is complex. Virilization of the female fetus does occur when androgen excess is present. Mood swings accompanying the menstrual cycle, postpartum, and the menopause may have an origin, in part in steroid hormone imbalance, mediated by their effects on higher centers.

Clearly pharmacologic intervention to correct a hormone deficiency, to interfere or promote the fertilization process, and to modify selected metabolic processes observed with gonadal hormonal imbalance are indications for therapy either with gonadal steroids, hypothalamic peptides, gonadotropins, antiestrogens, antiprogestins or inhibitors of lactation. In this chapter the pharmacology of estrogens, progestins, oral contraceptives, and fertility agents will be reviewed. A discussion on the intramuscular use of medroxyprogesterone acetate and the subdermal implantation of levonorgestrel for long-term contraceptive effects is also presented. In addition, the pharmacology of mifepristone (RU 486) is discussed. In order to understand more fully the pharmacology of the female sex hormones and related compounds, a brief review of the physiology of menses is presented.

MENSTRUAL CYCLE

The menstrual cycle is a repetitive ovulatory sequence with a mean duration of 28 days. The cycle consists of two phases, a follicular (proliferative) phase commencing on the first day of menstruation and a luteal (secretory) phase beginning just prior to ovulation. The pituitary hormones involved with ovarian stimulation and function are the follicle-stimulating hormone (FSH) and luteinizing hormone (LH). Figure 40-1 illustrates the variation in hormonal levels and their effects on the uterus during a typical cycle.

Pituitary gonadotropin secretion is regulated by the episodic pulsatile release of hypothalamic LH-releasing hormone (LHRH) into the hypophyseal portal veins. There are LHRH receptors on pituitary cells specialized to secrete the glycoprotein hormones, FSH and LH. These gonadotrophic hormones, in turn, promote both steroid hormone production and the requisite growth and delivery of gametes to achieve reproduction. Follicular growth, ovulation, maintenance of the corpus luteum, and maintenance of early pregnancy are regulated by the pituitary. Overall control mechanisms are homologous in males and females. The discussion here will be confined to the female.

The first events in the ovarian cycle are initiated by FSH. Early in the cycle FSH brings about stimulation of follicle growth and enlargement of the ovum itself, along with increased proliferation of granulosa and theca interna cells. The theca interna cells produce 17β-estradiol (90 to 1500 μg/day) under the influence of LH. In

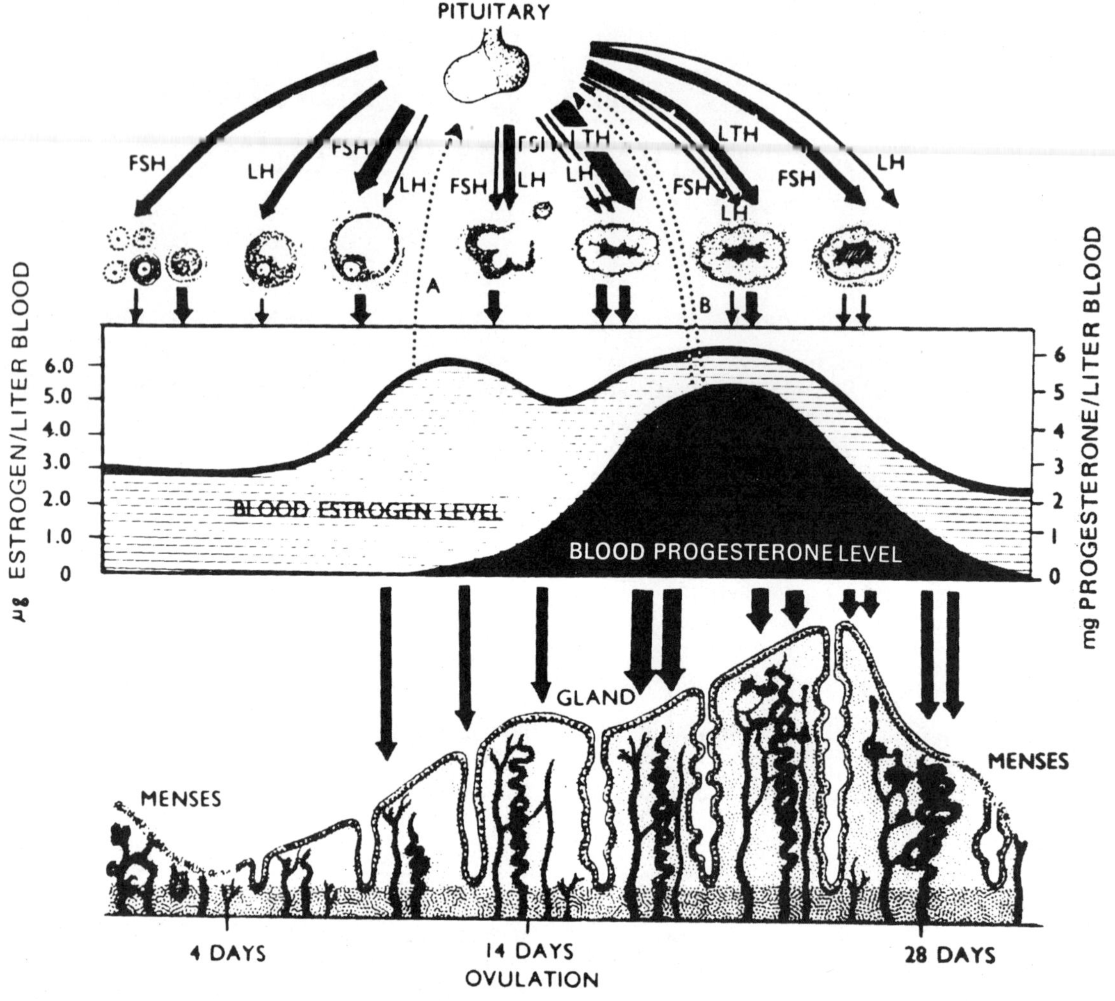

FIGURE 40-1 *Variations in pituitary and ovarian hormone secretion, and endometrial morphology during the menstrual cycle. The top graph demonstrates the alterations in follicle-stimulating hormone (FSH) and luteinizing hormone (LH) concentrations during the cycle in relation to effects on the follicle. The bottom graph shows the level of blood estrogen and progesterone as related to glandular secretions.*

addition, FSH increases the amount of fluid in the Graafian follicle to form the mature follicle.

As the follicle matures, it secretes increasing amounts of estrogen; when the appropriate level of estrogen is achieved, a brief excessive release of LH occurs (LH surge). Ovulation takes place on day 14, approximately 36 hours after the onset of the LH surge. The combined action of FSH and LH (and perhaps prostaglandins), is needed for the rupture and liberation of the mature ovum from the follicle. The liberated follicle then undergoes certain changes to form the corpus luteum; this is followed by the elaboration of progesterone by the granulosa cells (20 to 30 mg/day). The compound, 17β-estradiol, (200 to 250 μg/day) continues to be released from the theca interna cells.

LH maintains the functioning of the corpus luteum for approximately 10 days postovulation. If fertilization does not take place, the corpus luteum will begin to regress, hormone production is reduced and eventually ceases functioning altogether. The onset of menses will then follow at about the twenty-eighth day of the cycle.

Simultaneously with ovulation, the endometrium manifests cyclic alterations. These changes result from the influence of 17β-estradiol and progesterone on this tissue. In the first part of the cycle, as estrogen is being secreted, the endometrium enters its proliferative phase (approximately 11 days). During this phase the tissue increases in thickness, with progressive growth of glandular and vascular elements. Under the combined influence of 17β-estradiol and progesterone on the endometrium following ovulation, the secretory phase (approximately 13 days) is established. During this period there is further development of blood vessels and glandular structures, and an elaboration of the contents of the glandular epithelial cells. If implantation of a fertilized ovum does not occur, the levels of progesterone and estrogen gradually decrease. The myometrium contracts and the endometrium then begins to undergo desquamation, and menses ensues.

If the egg is fertilized, the syncytiotrophoblast is the source of production of a new series of protein substances, among which is human chorionic gonadotropin (HCG). One of the many effects of HCG is to prolong the secretory life span of the corpus luteum for the duration of pregnancy. However, beyond the first trimester of pregnancy, the progesterone production by the placenta is many times that produced by the corpus luteum, the latter being unnecessary for the maintenance of normal pregnancy in humans.

The entire ovary is capable of synthesizing three classes of steroid hormones: progesterone (one of the C-21 steroids, i.e., compounds that contain 21 carbons), androstenedione (a C-19 steroid), and 17β-estradiol (a C-18 steroid). Plasma low-density lipoprotein (LDL) cholesterol ester is the major source of steroidogenic cholesterol from which the steroids are derived. The overall steroidogenic pathways are presented in Fig. 40-2.

Cholesterol liberated from LDL apoproteins is transported to the mitochondria, where side chain cleavage takes place, releasing pregnenolone. This occurs in all steroidogenic tissue and is, in general, regulated by LH in the gonads and adrenocorticotropic hormone (ACTH) in the adrenal cortex through the mediation of cyclic AMP.

Progesterone is derived from pregnenolone by the action of Δ^5-3β-ol-dehydrogenase-Δ^4-5-isomerase (3β-HSD). The enzymes which subsequently metabolize progesterone are found in interstitial cells and theca cells. There is a dual enzyme complex with produces 17β-hydroxyprogesterone and Δ^4-androstenedione. The Δ^4-androstenedione can be metabolized further to either testosterone or to estrone. Aromatase catalyzes the conversion of androstenedione to estrone and testosterone to 17β-estradiol.

ESTROGENS

Chemistry and Synthesis

Estrogen is a general term used to describe chemical compounds which have estrogenic activity. Estrogen can be divided into two chemical categories: those with a steroid nucleus (endogenous) and those without one (synthetic). Endogenous estrogens, some synthetic estrogens, (the nonsteroidal estrogens), and antiestrogens of major interest are illustrated in Fig. 40-3.

The compound, 17β-estradiol, is an 18-carbon, cyclopentanophenanthrene molecule with an aromatic ring and a hydroxyl group in the C-17 position. It is the major estrogen synthesized and secreted by the normal human ovary. There is little storage of ovarian steroidal hormones, so that synthesis and release of either estrogens or progesterone are closely associated. The oxidized derivative, estrone, is also secreted by the premenopausal ovary, but in much smaller quantities. Biosynthesis of 17β-estradiol from cholesterol takes place in both granulosa and theca interna cells of the follicular ovary and in the human corpus luteum. The complete enzymatic pathway for estrogen biosynthesis (cholesterol to estrogen) is not present in the placenta. Nevertheless, it can transform C-19 steroids of fetal and maternal origin to estrogen.

Gonadotrophic regulation of ovarian estrogen production involves the "steroidogenic" hormone LH, which enhances the rate of cholesterol conversion to pregnenolone via cyclic AMP-mediated reactions. Within the follicular apparatus, the theca interna cells produce the C-19 precursors which are aromatized to estradiol. The granulosa cell aromatase enzyme system is induced by FSH. The capacity to aromatize C-19 androgens efficiently determines which follicle will become the dominant follicle and, therefore, ovulate.

A variety of tissues such as fat, muscle, liver, skin, endometrium, and even hypothalamus also have the aromatase enzyme system necessary to transform C-19 steroids to estrogen. Fat is an important nonovarian tissue locus of total estrogen production in obese postmenopausal patients. Androgens secreted by the adrenal cortex are aromatized to estrone by fat cells.

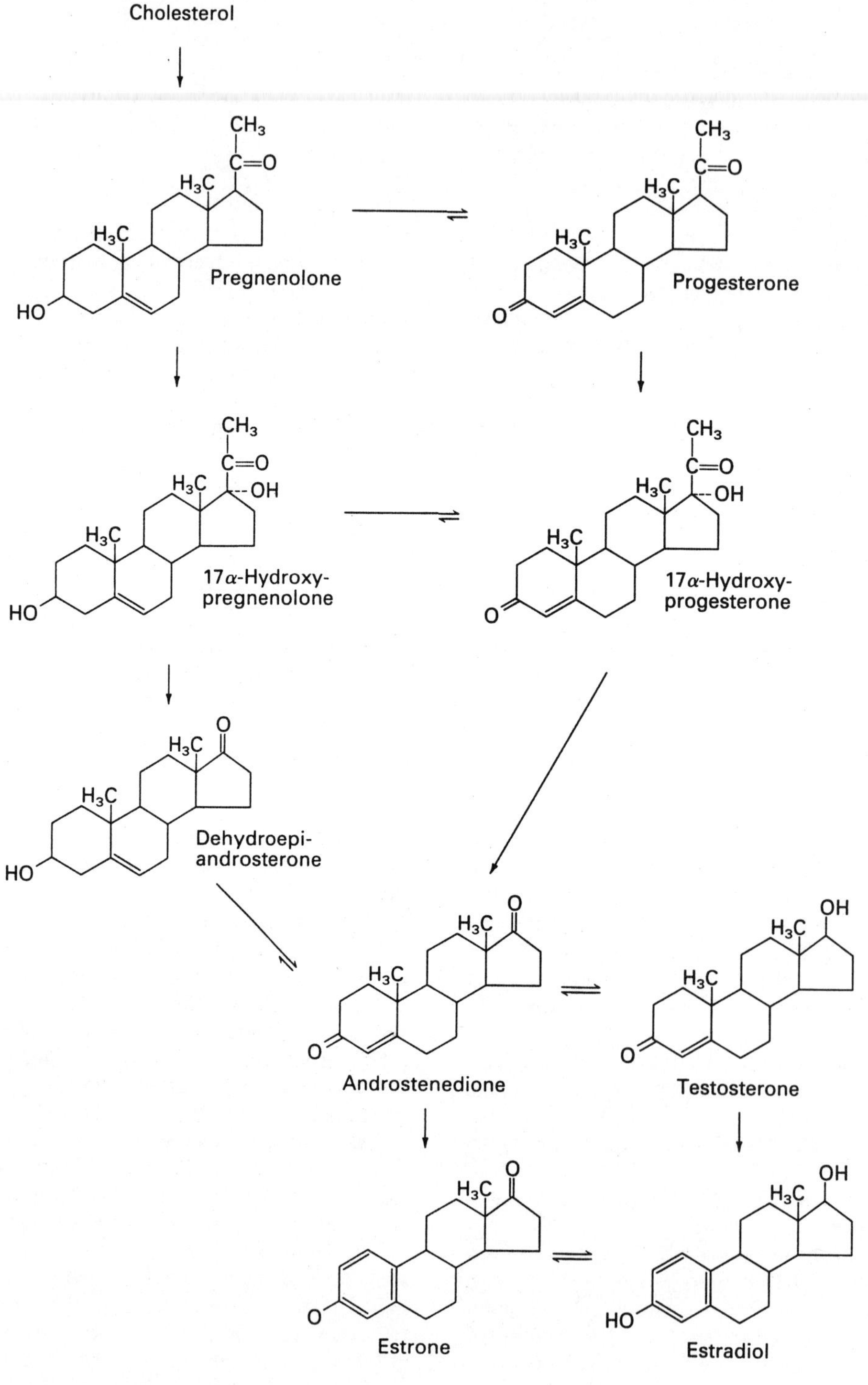

FIGURE 40-2 *Synthetic pathways of sex steroids.*

ENDOGENOUS ESTROGENS

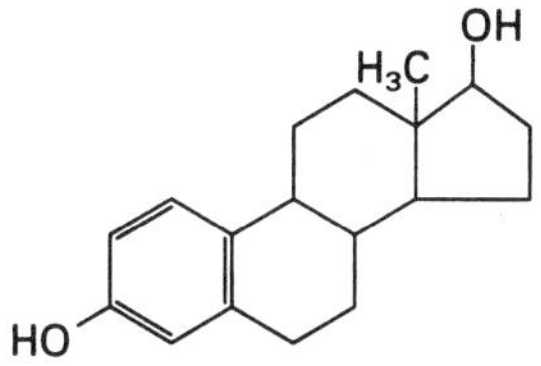

Estradiol

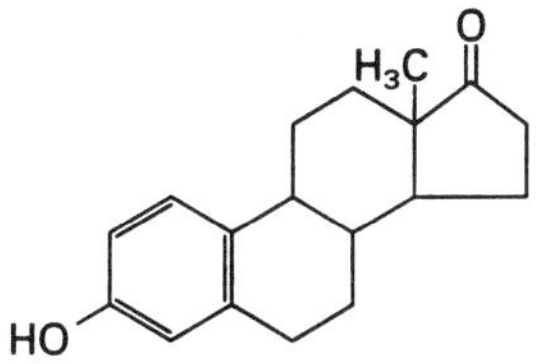

Estrone

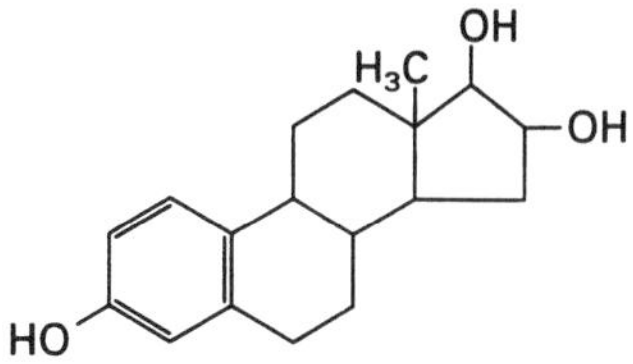

Estriol

SYNTHETIC, STEROIDAL

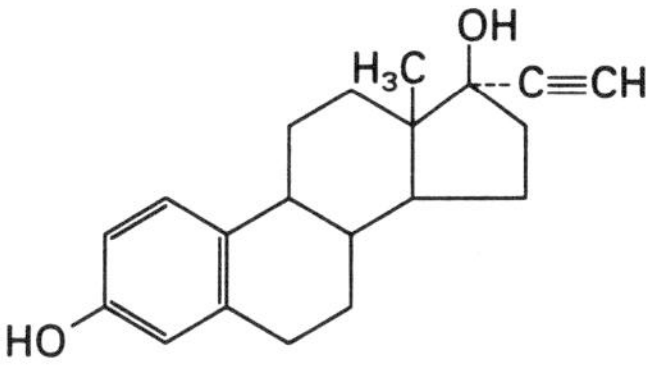

Ethinyl estradiol

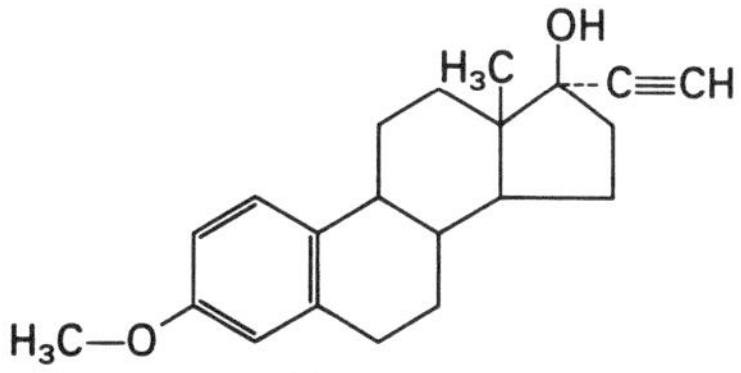

Mestranol

SYNTHETIC, NONSTEROIDAL

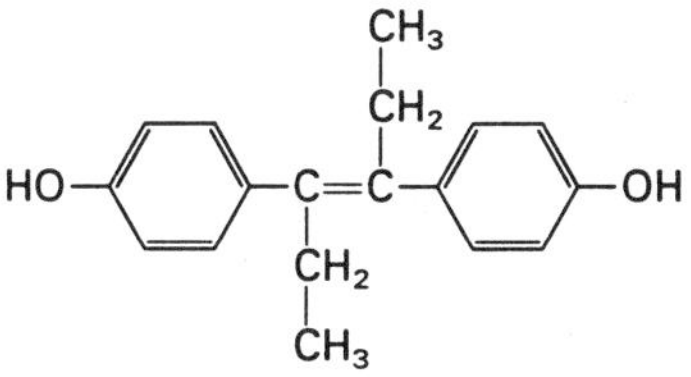

Diethylstilbestrol

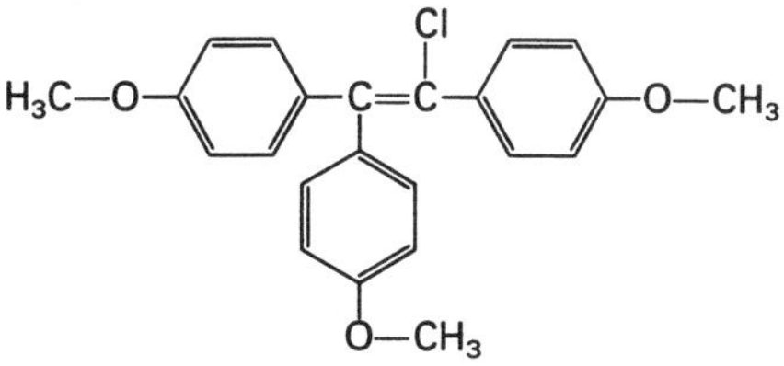

Chlorotrianisene

ANTIESTROGENS

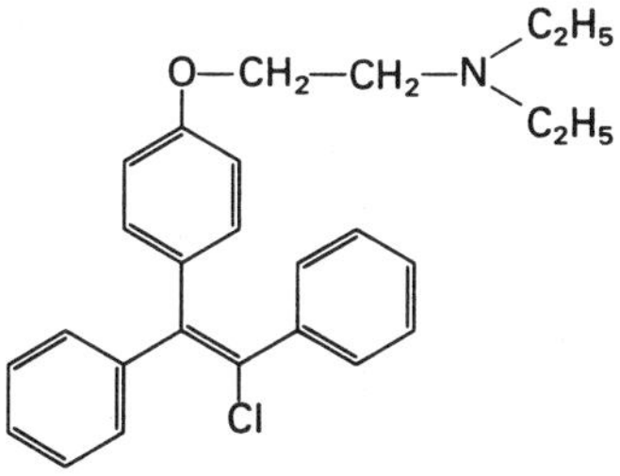

Clomiphene

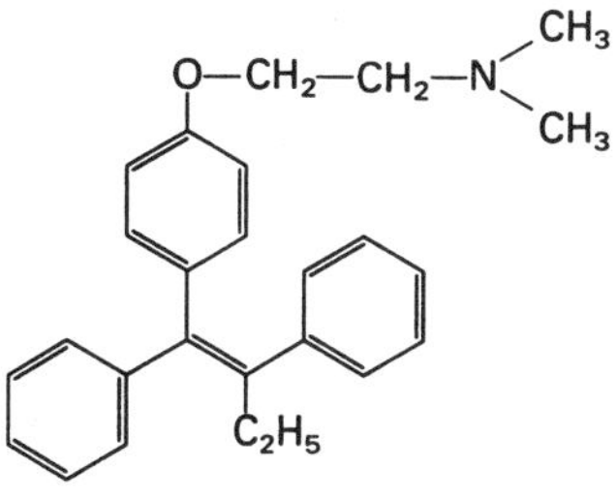

Tamoxifen

FIGURE 40-3 *Chemical structures of endogenous and clinically important estrogens and antiestrogens.*

Estriol is a major metabolite of 17β-estradiol in which an additional hydroxyl group is added in the 16 position of the steroid nucleus. This takes place in the liver. In the fetoplacental unit, 17β-estradiol is produced through a series of steps in which dehydroepiandrosterone, produced by the fetal adrenal gland, is hydroxylated in the fetal liver and aromatized to 17β-estradiol in the placenta.

Conjugating 17β-estradiol with straight-chain fatty acids results in a marked prolongation of the serum half-life of these estrogens and, therefore, in the marked enhancement of their biologic activity. Parenteral administration of short-chain fatty acid conjugates of 17β-estradiol or orally effective estrone (when conjugated with sulfate) have been used for many years for long-term estrogen replacement therapy.

Mechanism of Action

The gonadal steroids (as well as the adrenal steroids) enter most cells by simple diffusion as a result of their lipophilic nature. In target cells, the gonadal steroids bind to specific macromolecules (receptors). The receptor is a 4S protein (75,000 Da). These receptors for estrogenic steroids and their congeners have a finite binding capacity, high affinity, estrogen specificity and tissue or cellular specificity. The principal target tissues are in the reproductive tract (vagina, cervix, uterus, and in the mammary glands), the anterior pituitary, and hypothalamus. These tissues contain 15,000 to 20,000 high affinity estrogen binding sites per cell ($K_d \approx 0.6$ nmol/L) whereas nonreproductive structures which respond to estrogens contain smaller number of sites, e.g., liver, kidney, and adrenal. The specific receptors are very large molecules that are found in both the cytoplasmic and nuclear compartments. Once the gonadal steroid binds to its receptor, a poorly defined allosteric change occurs. The transformed receptor is a 5S protein (140,000 Da). The conformational change in the receptor results in its activation. The activated receptor (steroid-receptor complex) has a very high affinity for various nuclear binding sites. These sites have been shown to be regulatory DNA sequences as well as nonhistone sites. The conformational change may occur in either the cytoplasm or nuclear compartments. Once the binding of the activated steroid hormone receptor complex to the regulatory DNA sequence occurs, transcription ensues. The RNA polymerase is derepressed and messenger RNA (mRNA) is produced. The mRNA is translated to the ribosomes in the cytoplasm and the specific protein is synthesized. These proteins manifest the actions observed by gonadal steroids, i.e., cell function, growth, and differentiation. The specific gene receptor interaction may also result in a reduction in gene activity. The expression of estrogen receptors is affected by progesterone and prolactin. Progesterone decreases receptor expression in the reproductive tract, and perhaps the liver, whereas prolactin increases the number of estrogen receptors in the mammary gland and liver, but has no effect on those found in the uterus.

The cellular action of the steroid hormones is terminated by the re-establishment of the unoccupied receptor by a series of reactions that are not well defined. The receptor may dissociate from the steroid and be converted to a form that binds more hormone. Alteratively the gonadal steroid may undergo metabolism to intermediates that do not bind to the receptor and these metabolites diffuse out of the cell.

Effects on Organ Systems

In the female, 17β-estradiol and other estrogenic steroids have separate and distinct effects on sexual and nonsexual organ systems. These steroids have a general tonic effect on most tissues of the body. They are specifically involved in the development and maintenance of primary and secondary sexual characteristics. In general, the estrogens are of a stimulatory nature. They have an anabolic action on the reproduction system. In the genital system, they are associated with hypertrophy, hyperplasia, increased blood supply, accumulation of amino acids, synthesis of proteins, and retention of water and electrolytes. In the genital system, the cervix, vagina, uterus, fallopian tubes, and mammary glands, the estrogens act in conjunction with progesterone. 17β-estradiol induces the synthesis of progesterone receptors in primary target tissues. Thus cyclical changes that occur with the menstrual cycle, the cervical secretions conducive to sperm transport, movement of the sperm through the fallopian tubes, implantation of the blastocyst, proliferation and enhanced secretory function of the alveoli of the mammary gland, pregnancy, and parturition are some examples of this interaction.

The role of steroid sex hormones in the pubertal growth of bones is poorly understood. Estrogen is believed to stimulate pubertal growth by increasing production of an insulin-like growth factor. Estrogen deprivation, either because of ovariectomy or menopause, results in accelerated osteoporosis.

The synthesis of many proteins is not restricted to those involved in the genital system. The synthesis of lipoproteins, hormone binding globulins, clotting factors, renin substrate (angiotensinogen), and renin are also increased by estrogens.

Lipid metabolism and fat deposition are affected by estrogens. Estrogens elevate the concentrations of very low-density lipoproteins (VLDLs) and high-density lipoproteins (HDLs), especially HDL-2 and its apolipoproteins A1 and A2, in plasma. Estrogens decrease total cholesterol and LDLs. The fact that HDL levels are higher and LDL levels are lower in premenopausal females, as compared to similarly aged males, is believed to contribute to the protected state of younger women from coronary heart disease.

In the male, estrogens decrease libido, the activity of sebaceous glands, and the growth of the prostate gland. Gynecomastia can occur when estrogen excess is present.

Pharmacokinetics

Estrogens are absorbed via the skin and mucous membranes as well as from subcutaneous and intramuscular sites. Esterification of estrogen can be used to delay the rate of absorption from parenteral sites. Systemic effects may occur from direct absorption through the skin.

Oral administration of estrogens results in rapid absorption from the gastrointestinal tract. However, the hormone is carried directly to the liver via the portal vein, where it is readily inactivated. Estriol undergoes little biotransformation and has the shortest serum half-life. Minor structural changes, such as the presence of an ethinyl group at position 17 (e.g., as in ethinyl estradiol) results in a decreased rate of liver inactivation which increases its efficacy when administered orally. When 17β-estradiol is administered (as the micronized preparation), it is almost completely converted to estrone prior to absorption. The transdermal route is being used in estrogen replacement therapy and appears to be a safe and effective method.

The physiologically active and major estrogen in the body is 17β-estradiol. Estrogens circulate in the blood in both conjugated and unconjugated forms. Estrogenic steroids are generally conjugated through the hydroxyl group at C-3 with inorganic sulfate or glucuronic acid. Conjugation takes place in the liver. The estrogens are highly bound to specific plasma globulins (50 to 80 percent). Only the unbound or "free" estrogens are biologically active. Conjugated steroids are more water soluble, and thus their excretion into the urine is facilitated.

With the exception of estriol, large amounts of estrogen in the free form of endogenous, as well as exogenous origin, are excreted by the liver into the bile. An enterohepatic circulation of estrogens (except estriol) exists in which estrogens conjugated in the liver are excreted into the bile, hydrolyzed within the gastrointestinal tract, and reabsorbed.

There are many other transformations of 17β-estradiol which take place in the liver, such as hydroxylation in the 2 position of estrogen, resulting in dramatic decreases in the activity of the estrogen. With hydroxylation in the 16 position of 17β-estradiol, the biological activity is maintained. These congeners have been shown to be of considerable biologic and clinical significance.

Conjugating estrogens with straight-chain fatty acids results in a marked prolongation of the biologic activity of these estrogens. The "conjugated estrogens," because of their extremely long half-lives and increased bioactivity, may be involved in the development of endometrial and/or breast cancer. The concomitant administration of a progestin is important to consider if the estrogen is administered for a prolonged period.

Diethylstilbestrol (DES), a nonsteroidal compound, is orally active and has a relatively long duration of action. Following oral administration, it is slowly biotransformed in the liver, with its metabolites excreted by the kidney.

Adverse Reactions

The adverse effects of estrogens are related directly to either the dosage or length of time the drug is given. The adverse effects can be relatively minor and may disappear with continued therapy; these include nausea (without loss in weight), chloasma, acne, vaginal infections and vaginal bleeding, mucoid leukorrhea, and edema. Higher doses of estrogen may induce anorexia, vomiting, and diarrhea. The anabolic action of estrogen can result in endometrial hyperplasia and an exacerbation in estrogen receptor-positive mammary tumors. The estrogens may also produce adverse effects on the cardiovascular system that are potentially severe. These effects include an enhancement of thromboembolic disease by promoting the synthesis of clotting factors II, VIII, IX, and X; hypertension, stroke, and myocardial infarction. Some conflicting reports exist that show estrogen replacement therapy may reduce the risk of cardiovascular disease. Clear cell adenocarcinoma of the cervix and vagina is a rare disease particularly in young women 15 to 22 years of age. Daughters of mothers given DES during the first trimester of pregnancy to prevent abortion, have an increased incidence of this pathological condition.

It is unknown if steroidal estrogen preparations induce carcinoma of the vagina or cervix. An increase in the incidence of genital abnormalities in both male and female progeny has been reported. Estrogens should not be given during the first few months of pregnancy when development of the reproductive organs occurs.

There are several strong contraindications of estrogen replacement therapy; these include estrogen-dependent malignancy, undiagnosed abnormal vaginal bleeding, thrombophlebitis, thromboembolic phenomena, cerebral vascular disease or coronary occlusive disease, estrogen-induced hypertension, markedly impaired liver function, history of obstructive jaundice of pregnancy, and congenital hyperlipidemias. These conditions are discussed in more detail in the section on oral contraceptives.

TABLE 40-1 Estrogens of clinical importance for hormone replacement therapy

ORALLY ACTIVE PREPARATIONS
Conjugated estrogens
Estrone sulfate[a]
Ethinyl estradiol
Esterified estrogens
Mestranol[b]
Micronized estradiol
PARENTERAL PREPARATIONS
Conjugated estrogens
Estradiol cypionate
Estradiol valerate
Estrone aqueous suspension
VAGINAL ESTROGEN PREPARATIONS
Estradiol vaginal cream
Dienestrol vaginal cream
Estropipate vaginal cream
NONSTEROIDAL ESTROGENS
Diethylstilbestrol
Quinestrol
TRANSDERMAL PREPARATIONS
Estradiol

[a] This preparation is available as the piperazine salt known as estropipate.

[b] Available in the United States only in oral contraceptives.

Therapeutic Uses

Estrogen replacement therapy is used in agonadal, menopausal, and hypothalamic amenorrheic states (i.e., in primary hypogonadism and hormonal therapy in postmenopausal women). Estrogens commonly used for hormone replacement therapy are presented in Table 40-1.

As in other clinical endocrine disorders, once the diagnosis of hypoestrogenism is established, replacement therapy is recommended. There are several special considerations for estrogen replacement therapy. First, in the normal younger woman, estrogen is secreted on a daily basis. Therefore, administration of estrogens for only 21 to 25 days can frequently result in estrogen deprivation symptoms, such as hot flashes, irritability, and insomnia. With time, the affected patient will report a decrease in these symptoms. Nevertheless about 25 percent of menopausal women will seek medical advice. Optimal physiologic estrogen replacement therapy should utilize daily estrogen administration, in conjunction with monthly 14-day courses of progestins. Any abnormal vaginal bleeding is investigated by physical examination, pap smear, and endometrial biopsy.

A special indication exists for the administration of very large doses of intravenous estrogens; it is the occasional patient with dysfunctional uterine bleeding which may have life-threatening hemorrhage. The problem may be controlled by intravenous administration of conjugated estrogen.

In patients being treated for acute painful osteoporosis, large doses of estrogen are started. There will be a clinical response in terms of decreased back pain within days and/or weeks. Once this effect is accomplished, the dose can be decreased. Estrogen will prevent bone loss for as long as it is administered, but will not reverse osteoporosis that is established. It should be noted that exercise and increased intake of calcium salts along with fluoride can effect an improvement either in combination with or without estrogen. Therefore prophylactic use of exogenous therapy with estrogen alone is hard to justify. Recently, the biphosphonate, etidronate, has been shown to be efficacious in the treatment of postmenopausal osteoarthritis.

Estrogen has seen some therapeutic usefulness in the treatment of hirsutism, acne, and suppression of postpartum lactation. Dysmenorrhea can be relieved by inhibition of ovulation by estrogen since this disorder results from production of prostaglandins, the treatment of choice would be nonsteroidal anti-inflammatory drugs.

To prevent conception, postcoital use of extremely large doses of 17β-estradiol for 5 days or two tablets of an estrogen-progestin combination taken immediately after unprotected coitus followed by two more tablets 12 hours later, have proven to be effective. Nausea and vomiting may occur resulting in the loss of pills. The benefits of estrogen-progestin therapy results from the lower dose of estrogen used, treatment is completed in one day, and frequency and severity of adverse effects is reduced. The estrogen-progestin combination has replaced the use of DES as the "morning after" pill. DES is not as widely used because of increased incidence of vaginal and cervical adenocarcinoma. DES is used in the treatment of inoperable carcinoma of the prostate. Estrogens along with progestins have a major use as oral contraceptives. This therapeutic use will be discussed later in this chapter.

ANTIESTROGENS

The weakly estrogenic triphenylethylene derivative, chlorotrianisene, was observed to block the 17β-estradiol induced enlargement of the rat pituitary. Three orally active congeners were synthesized with more potent antiestrogenic activity and are used clinically. These compounds are tamoxifen, clomiphene (see Fig. 40-3) and danazol and they have mixed agonist/antagonist actions depending upon the tissue.

Tamoxifen

Tamoxifen is a competitive inhibitor of 17β-estradiol. It is used in the palliative treatment of estrogen receptor-positive breast cancer. It should be used in conjunction with chemotherapeutic agents more effective in killing rather than suppressing the cancer cells.

Tamoxifen is absorbed from the gastrointestinal tract following oral administration. Peak plasma levels are reached in 4 to 7 hours. It has a nuclear retention time of 24 to 48 hours. The initial serum half-life ranges from 7 to 14 hours. Most of the drug is conjugated in the liver, then excreted by the kidney. Less than 30 percent is excreted unchanged or hydroxylated. The drug undergoes enterohepatic recirculation.

The most common adverse reactions include nausea or vomiting and hot flashes. Other estrogen deficiency type side effects occur, but are much less common.

Clomiphene

Clomiphene acts by enhancing new follicular growth with resultant ovulation. The drug attaches to cytosolic estrogen receptors, but the clomiphene-receptor complex does not bind to nuclear receptors for estrogen. This is interpreted by the hypothalamus as a hypoestrogenic state. The hypothalamic response is the increased secretion of LHRH, which enhances gonadotropin secretion. The increased FSH and LH secretion initiates sequential follicular growth and eventual ovulation.

Clomiphene is administered orally. It has a long half-life; only about one-half of an ingested dose is excreted in 5 days. The drug is eliminated primarily in the feces, with small amounts in the urine. Some of its antiestrogenic effects may persist for several weeks.

The major indication for clomiphene is to induce ovulation in anovulatory women who have some basal estrogen production. It works much less effectively in hypoestrogenic anovulatory disorders such as hypothalamic amenorrhea. Clomiphene is used to enhance the fertility of women who are oligo-ovulators; that is, if a woman has three or four ovulatory cycles per year, her fertility will be enhanced by ovulating on a monthly basis. Clomiphene is also used to gain predictability of ovulations in women undergoing artificial insemination. Ovulation induction is most commonly accomplished by administering tablets once a day from the fifth through the ninth day of the menstrual cycle.

Since an expected effect of clomiphene is to induce follicular growth, higher doses may induce the growth of multicystic ovaries. There is also a reported 8 to 10 percent incidence of twins with this drug, but multiple births of more than two babies are considered rare. Ovarian cysts may occur in 5 to 15 percent of patients. Massive cystic enlargement of the ovaries is a rare but a serious side effect. When clomiphene induces ovulation, it has been shown to reduce the length of the luteal phase in some patients. This luteal phase deficiency can be treated by administration of human chronic gonadotropin or progesterone. Other adverse reactions include menopausal-type hot flashes, headaches, occasional reversible hair loss, and less commonly gastrointestinal distress and breast engorgement. Symptoms are reversible when therapy is discontinued.

Clomiphene has also been used with or without testosterone to stimulate spermatogenesis in patients with oligospermia who had been exposed to large doses of estrogen *in utero*.

Danazol

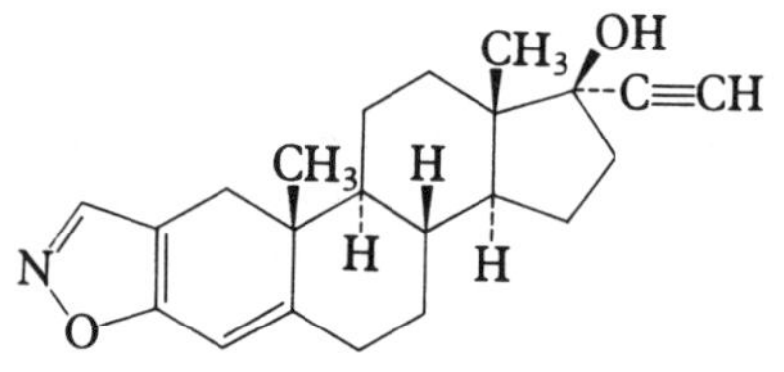

CH₃ OH —C≡CH CH₃ H H H N O

The progestin, ethisterone, was modified to produce danazol. It is effective in altering the hypothalamic pituitary axis. The mid-cycle surge of gonadotropins is inhibited in a dose-dependent manner. Hypoestrogenism is produced with higher dosage regimes. Danazol has both antiestrogenic and androgenic actions. The antiestrogenic action of danazol produces regression of normal and ectopic endometrial tissue in patients with endometriosis and produces a decrease in the rate of growth and modularity of abnormal breast tissue in patients with fibrocystic breast disease. Its androgenic action results in increased levels of the 4 component of complement, which reduces the frequency and severity of attacks in patients affected with hereditary angioedema. In some patients, danazol improves systemic lupus erythematosus and premenstrual syndrome. Danazol is bound to receptors for androgens, progesterone, and glucocorticoids but only the danazol-androgen receptor complex is translocated to the nucleus where it binds with DNA. Danazol does not bind to the intracellular estrogenic receptor and acts directly on the ovary to inhibit ovarian steroidogenesis.

Danazol is absorbed orally, but the amount absorbed is not proportional to the dose administered. The compound undergoes hepatic biotransformation, but little is known of its distribution in the body and route(s) of excretion.

The drug is contraindicated in patients with renal or cardiac disease because it causes electrolyte and water retention. In patients with hepatic disease the drug may accumulate. It should be avoided in patients with undiagnosed abdominal bleeding and patients with uncharacterized breast nodules or masses. Danazol may produce headache, dizziness, sleep disorders, and behavioral changes. Its androgenic action may induce hirsutism, acne, deepening of the voice, clitoral enlargement, and change in libido.

Isoflavone Phytoestrogens

Vegetarian diets (mainly plant foods and low in animal products, as well as low in fat and high in fiber content), have been associated with a lower incidence of cancers of the breast, endometrium, and prostate. The antiestrogenic effects of these diets is associated with their content of isoflavone phytoestrogens. The antiestrogenic effects of phytoestrogens may be attributed either to decreasing the enterohepatic circulation of estrogen, decreasing the availability of estrogen by increasing sex hormone binding globulin (SHBG), decreasing the sulfation of estrogen by the liver, or any combination of these actions. However, the antiestrogenic effects of isoflavone phytoestrogens may exacerbate cardiovascular disease and osteoporosis in high risk women.

PROGESTINS

The term progestin (or progestogen) includes progesterone and other compounds which share its physiologic actions. Progesterone is the active hormone secreted by the corpus luteum and placenta. It is ineffective when given orally because of extensive metabolism before reaching the peripheral circulation. It must therefore be administered parenterally or transvaginally, usually in the form of suppositories. The major orally active progestins were developed for use in oral contraceptives.

Progestins induce secretory changes in the uterine glandular epithelium and decidual changes in the stroma. Normal menstruation ensues when the corpus luteum stops producing progesterone approximately 14 days after ovulation. Progestational agents given about 6 to 7 days after ovulation and continued for 3 or more weeks will result in a delay of menstruation until 2 to 3 days after the hormone is stopped.

Chemistry

The structures of several progestins are presented in Fig. 40-4. Progesterone loses much of its biologic activity with the addition of a hydroxyl group at the C-17 position. Esterifying this hydroxyl group with a long-chain fatty acid, such as caproic acid, results in a long-acting progestin for parenteral administration (hydroxyprogesterone caproate).

Progestins derived from nortestosterone may have higher androgenic properties than those derived from the C-21 steroid nucleus. Norethindrone, the C-17 ethinyl derivative, is a very potent oral progestin and is the progestational component of several oral contraceptives.

Mechanism of Action

Progesterone acts as discussed above for estrogens, on specific steroid receptors found in the cytoplasmic and nuclear compartments. The progesterone-receptor complex translocates to the nucleus, where it stimulates production of specific mRNA which results in the synthesis of specific proteins. Unlike the estrogen receptor which requires a phenolic A ring, the Δ^4-3-one substituent is required for the progesterone to bind with its receptor. This accounts for the glucocorticoid, mineralocorticoid, and androgenic actions of progesterone and other progestins. The specific progesterone receptor is confined to the female reproductive tract. Estrogen appears to induce an increase in the number of progesterone receptors. Conversely, progesterone decreases the content and/or the biologic efficacy of estrogen receptors in the target tissues as discussed above.

Pharmacokinetics

Progesterone undergoes first-pass metabolism. Therefore, although readily absorbed, little unmetabolized progesterone reaches the general circulation. Its metabolic clearance rate is approximately 2100 L/day, while the hepatic blood flow is about 1500 L/day, suggesting an extrahepatic clearance. Progesterone binds to corticosteroid-binding globulin; the physiologic significance of this is unclear. It is also bound weakly to plasma albumin.

One of the major metabolites of progesterone is pregnanediol. It is excreted in the urine as the monoglucosiduronate, and its measurement has been used to assess corpus luteum function. During the luteal phase, 2 to 4 mg/day are excreted in the urine, whereas with pregnancy, the excretion increases to 50 to 70 mg/day prior to parturition.

The clinical situations in which progesterone itself must be given, instead of other progestins, are those in which an embryo or fetus could be affected or harmed by the other drugs. In these situations, progesterone must be given either as an intramuscular injection or as a vaginal suppository.

Effects on Organ Systems

The physiologically important effects of progesterone occur on estrogen primed tissues. These effects include the induction of a secretory endometrium and decreased myometrial contractility. Progesterone is essential for early implantation of the embryo and maintenance of pregnancy to term. Progesterone withdrawal is an important part of the mechanism necessary for the initiation of labor.

Progesterone induces an elevation of basal body temperature, a thermogenic action which is clinically useful in detecting ovulation. In the breast, progesterone stimulates growth of alveolar epithelium and is necessary for the prolactin-mediated postpartum induction of lactation. Progesterone stimulates respiration and reduces the arterial P_{CO2}. It appears to stimulate urinary sodium excretion by antagonizing the effects of aldosterone on the collecting duct of the kidney. In contrast, some other progestins induce fluid retention. The effects of individual progestins are best considered in conjunction with the simultaneous administration of estrogens in certain oral contraceptive medications.

Therapeutic Uses

Progestins of clinical importance are listed in Table 40-2. These drugs are used in the therapy of various abnormal gynecological conditions, such as menstrual abnormalities, endometriosis, and

A. Progestins derived from (C-21) progesterone

Progesterone

17α-Acetoxy-progesterone

6-Methyl-17α-acetoxy-progesterone (medroxyprogesterone acetate)

6α-methyl-6-dehydro-17α-acetoxyprogesterone (megestrol acetate)

B. Progestins derived from (C-18) 19-nortestosterone

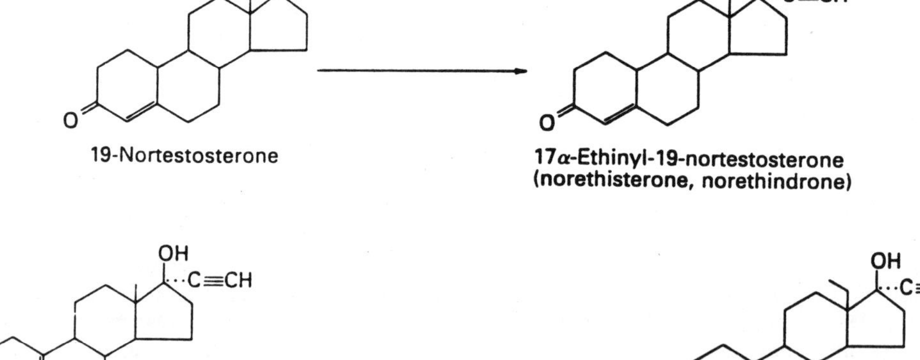

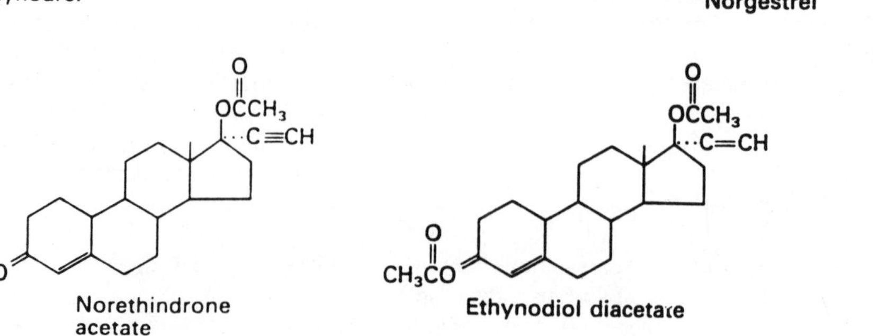

FIGURE 40-4 *Chemical structures of some progestins.*

Table 40-2 Progestins of clinical importance

PROGESTERONE AND DERIVATIVES
Progesterone
Hydroxyprogesterone caproate
Medroxyprogesterone acetate
Megestrol acetate
19-NORTESTOSTERONE DERIVATIVES
Norethindrone
Norethindrone acetate
Norethynodrel
Desogestrel[a]
Ethynodiol diacetate[a]
Norgestrel[a]
Norgestimate[a]
Levonorgestrel[b]

[a] Available in the United States only in oral contraceptives.
[b] Available in the United States in oral contraceptives and in a contraceptive implant.

dysmenorrhea. They are also of some use in the treatment of endometrial carcinoma. They are also used in conjunction with estrogen in hormone replacement therapy. Their greatest use is as components of contraceptives alone or in combination with estrogen.

Progestins are used in the differential diagnosis of amenorrhea as a result of a dysfunctional endometrium, anovulatory dysfunctional uterine bleeding as a result of patients who do not have an LH surge, and in premenopausal dysfunctional uterine bleeding as a result inadequate follicular growth resulting from insufficient number of FSH receptors on ovarian follicles.

Even though nonsteroidal anti-inflammatory drugs are the preferred method of therapy in dysmenorrhea, relief of dysmenorrhea can also be accomplished with combined progestin and estrogen therapy for 5 to 15 days or estrogen for 20 days combined with the progestin for 5 days. In either case menstruation is prompt. However, in severe cases, combined with estrogen, ovulation is inhibited and relief is achieved. Severe dysmenorrhea accompanies endometriosis. In contrast to cyclical therapy for the treatment of gynecologic problems discussed above, continuous progestin therapy has been used successfully to cause regression of the ectopic uterine masses and restoration of fertility. The prolonged amenorrhea produced, results in the resorption of the ectopic endometrium presumably by peritoneal macrophages. Norethindrone acetate is particularly effective in this regard; in 80 percent of the cases symptomatic relief is realized and in 50 percent of the patients fertility is restored. Changes in hormone levels and serum electrolytes appear to contribute to the episodic irritability premenstrual syndrome. There is no convincing evidence that therapy with progestins is efficacious.

Progestins have been used with and without estrogens in the suppression of postpartum lactation. Progestins have been used in the palliative treatment of endometrial carcinoma and in renal and breast carcinoma as well. With respect to endometrial carcinoma, only the highly differentiated and hormonally dependent forms can be controlled by continuous long term therapy with progestins.

Medroxyprogesterone acetate Medroxyprogesterone acetate is a progestin that, when given intramuscularly, will inhibit ovulation. It is given every 3 months and is as effective as combination oral contraceptives. It acts like other progestins to inhibit the mid-cycle surge of LH secretion. Fertility is delayed following cessation of therapy. The variable rates of absorption and metabolism among patients could account for the prolonged effects. This drug is of use in patients who are noncompliant, when estrogens are contraindicated, and in intellectually or psychological impaired patients. The most common adverse effect that necessitates discontinuation of therapy, is irregular menstrual cycles. Other common side effects include headache, depression, weight gain, and abdominal bloating.

Levonorgestrel Levonorgestrel is a progestin that is implanted subdermally in 6 Silastic capsules which results in its long-term contraceptive actions. Initially for the first 6 to 18 months 80 μg/day is released and subsequently the release gradually declines to 25 to 30 μg/day for the remainder of 5 years. The contraceptive protection is evident for 5 years, after which its efficacy diminishes. After removal of the implants, fertility returns in 20 ± 13 days to rates like those in the general population. The released levonorgestrel is 95 percent bound to SHBG, albumin, and α_1-acid glycoprotein. After metabolism by the liver, the drug is secreted in the urine, primarily conjugated with glucuronide and sulfate. The serum half-life is approximately 28 hours.

Levonorgestrel implants would be used either in patients who desire long-term reversible contraception (such as patients 35 years or older), to improve compliance, or in patients in which estrogens are contraindicated. Headache, weight gain, depression, and disruption of the menstrual cycle are common adverse effects.

PROGESTIN ANTAGONIST

Mifepristone (RU 486)

Mifepristone (a congener of norethindrone) is a progesterone receptor antagonist with weak agonistic activity. It has been used in Europe since 1988 as an abortifacient in women during early pregnancy.

Mifepristone can prevent ovulation if given in the follicular phase of the menstrual cycle by preventing the action of progesterone at the level of the pituitary and/or hypothalamus. Its abortifacient effect results from its induction of contraction of the myometrium and subsequent detachment of the embryo. In addition to its antagonism of progesterone, it is also a potent glucocorticoid receptor antagonist; it has been used successfully to treat patients with Cushing's syndrome.

Mifepristone is rapidly absorbed after oral dosing. Peak plasma levels occur between 1 and 3 h after a single dose. The compound is 94 percent bound to albumin and α_1-acid glycoprotein. It is biotransformed in the liver and three active products have been identified. Most of the compound and its metabolites are eliminated in the feces with a half-life of between 20 and 50 hours; renal excretion is minimal.

This drug is given in a single dose or multiple doses for 5 to 7 days, followed by a dose of a prostaglandin to induce abortion. The single dose regimen has a success rate of 72 to 94 percent, especially if followed by a prostaglandin. This dose of mifepristone is sufficient to saturate all of the myometrial progesterone receptors. The effect of the multiple dose regimen is more variable, with a 10 to 85 percent success rate. Common adverse effects include nausea and excessive heavy bleeding during mifepristone-induced menses.

ORAL CONTRACEPTIVES

Historically since the knowledge of the relationship between coitus and pregnancy became known, mankind has sought ways to limit the number of children as well as to abort unwanted pregnancy. The contemporaries of Aristotle were the first to provide written accounts of attempts at contraception. The world population continues to increase particularly in Third World nations and as such, puts tremendous strain on the ability of the world to feed itself. Additionally, the advances in medicine and public health have decreased mortality and increased life expectancy. This in turn has led to the desire to regulate conception therapeutically. Drugs in the form of natural hormones and their congeners have been synthesized and are effective in the control of fertility. There are two main types of preparations taken orally on a regular basis to prevent conception: (1) an estrogen and a progestin taken as fixed combination (i.e., monophasic preparations) or in variable combinations (biphasic and triphasic preparations), and (2) a progestin alone (the "minipill"). Representative formulations are shown in Table 40-3.

The primary pharmacologic effect of oral contraceptives is to inhibit ovulation. Either estrogen (by inhibiting the secretion of FSH) prevents follicular development or progestin (by inhibiting the secretion of LH) does not allow the corpus luteum to develop. Thus the combination is particularly effective in the prevention of conception. These actions of the estrogen and progestin components of the oral contraceptive, mimic actions of endogenous hormones on gonadotropin secretion and the menstrual cycle which were discussed earlier in this chapter. The estrogenic component is responsible for the inhibition of ovulation, whereas cessation of progestin intake on the 21st day induces withdrawal menstrual bleeding that approximates normal physiological function.

The efficacy of the combination preparations results from their actions on other reproduction organs. The progestin causes the cervical mucus to thicken which impedes the passage of sperm and which could also interfere with capacitation. Together the compounds alter the histology of the endometrium and impede implantation. Fertilization occurs in the upper third of the fallopian tubes. By affecting muscle contractility in the fallopian tube, sperm movement is impaired and the sperm's capacity to fertilize the ova may be prevented.

In an attempt to more closely approximate events that occur in a normal menstrual cycle, preparations have been formulated with varying amounts of estrogen and progestin, i.e., the biphasic and triphasic oral contraceptives (see

TABLE 40-3 Representative formulations of oral contraceptives

Trade name	Estrogen	Progestin
FIXED DOSE-COMBINATIONS OF ESTROGEN AND PROGESTIN		
MONOPHASIC PREPARATIONS		
Brevicon, Modicon, Nelova 0.5/35E	Ethinyl estradiol, 35 μg	Norethindrone, 0.5 mg
Demulen 1/35	Ethinyl estradiol, 35 μg	Ethynodiol diacetate, 1.0 mg
Demulen 1/50	Ethinyl estradiol, 50 μg	Ethynodiol diacetate, 1.0 mg
Desogen, Ortho-Cept	Ethinyl estradiol, 30 μg	Desogestrel, 0.15 mg
Levlen, Nordette	Ethinyl estradiol, 30 μg	Levonorgestrel, 0.15 mg
Loestrin 21 1/20	Ethinyl estradiol, 20 μg	Norethindrone acetate, 1.0 mg
Loestrin 21 1.5/30	Ethinyl estradiol, 30 μg	Norethindrone acetate, 1.5 mg
Lo/Ovral	Ethinyl estradiol, 30 μg	Norgestrel, 0.3 mg
Nelova 1/35E, Norethin 1/35E, Norinyl 1 + 35, Ortho-Novum 1/35	Ethinyl estradiol, 35 μg	Norethindrone, 1.0 mg
Nelova 1/50M, Norethin 1/50M, Norinyl 1 + 50, Ortho-Novum 1/50	Mestranol, 50 μg	Norethindrone, 1.0 mg
Ortho-Cyclen	Ethinyl estradiol, 35 μg	Norgestimate, 0.25 mg
Ovcon-35	Ethinyl estradiol, 35 μg	Norethindrone, 0.4 mg
Ovcon-50	Ethinyl estradiol, 50 μg	Norethindrone, 1.0 mg
Ovral	Ethinyl estradiol, 50 μg	Norgestrel, 0.5 mg
BIPHASIC PREPARATIONS		
Nelova 10/11, Ortho-Novum 10/11	Ethinyl estradiol, 35 μg (21 tabs)	Norethindrone, 0.5 mg (10 tabs); 1.0 mg (11 tabs)
TRIPHASIC PREPARATIONS		
Ortho-Novum 7/7/7	Ethinyl estradiol, 35 μg (21 tabs)	Norethindrone, 0.5 mg (7 tabs); 0.75 mg (7 tabs); 1.0 mg (7 tabs)
Ortho Tri-Cyclen	Ethinyl estradiol, 35 μg (21 tabs)	Norgestimate, 0.18 mg (7 tabs); 0.215 mg (7 tabs); 0.25 mg (7 tabs)
Tri-Levlen, Triphasil	Ethinyl estradiol, 30 μg (6 tabs); 40 μg (5 tabs); 30 μg (10 tabs)	Levonorgestrel, 0.05 mg (6 tabs), 0.075 mg (5 tabs); 0.125 mg (10 tabs)
Tri-Norinyl	Ethinyl estradiol, 35 μg (21 tabs)	Norethindrone, 0.5 mg (7 tabs); 1.0 mg (9 tabs); 0.5 mg (5 tabs)
PROGESTIN ONLY ("MINIPILLS")		
Micronor, Nor-Q.D.		Norethindrone, 0.35 mg
Ovrette		Norgestrel, 0.075 mg

Table 40-3). Some physicians believe that these preparations are not as effective as the monophasic combination preparations and are more complicated for the patients. For these reasons, these drugs are not as popular as the monophasic combination preparations.

The contraceptives composed of a progestin alone (the "minipills") have some limitations to their use. Inhibition of ovulation is variable and inconsistent. The minipill is less reliable than the combination preparations and missing a dose may result in conception. Finally, with continued daily dosing menstruation occurs, but the duration of the cycle is variable and a greater likelihood of breakthrough bleeding during the cycle exists. However, they can be given after parturition because they do not inhibit lactation as do the estrogen-containing tablets.

Therapeutic use of oral contraceptives is rare among drug regimens, in that these very potent drugs are given to relatively healthy women for prolonged periods. These drugs have been surveyed for their acute and chronic effects on the normal physiology of the women. These effects are attributed to the estrogen or progestin alone, or their combination. Some of the adverse effects are minor whereas other effects have major consequences for the patient.

Adverse Effects

Minor Adverse Effects These are not infrequent and often times disappear with continued use. The adverse response may necessitate changing the preparation or cessation of therapy. The preparations with lower concentrations of estrogen and progestin have a lower incidence of side effects associated with their use. These minor effects due to the presence of the estrogenic component include chloasma, nausea, weight gain, headaches (even migraine), breakthrough bleeding, and amenorrhea. Minor adverse effects attributed to the progestin component include fullness in the breasts, depression, and delayed onset of menses. Effects that are attributed to progestins with androgenic potential include acne, hirsutism, increased appetite with weight gain, and increase in libido. Effects that are attributed to both components include vasomotor symptoms, irritability, breakthrough bleeding, and spotting.

Major Adverse Effects These are less frequently encountered but are of considerable concern. Epidemiological studies have confirmed the existence of several problems and, although rare, they may have serious consequences for the patient. There is an increased incidence of thrombophlebitis, venous thrombosis, and embolism. Under the influence of estrogen, the synthesis of clotting factors is increased. In turn, the incidence of thromboembolism is increased in cerebral and pulmonary veins and deep vein thrombosis. These studies prompted the recommendation that the estrogen content of the preparation should not exceed 50 μg. The incidence or attack rate of thromboembolism is estimated to be 1 in 1500 to 1 in 2000 per year.

Oral contraceptives have been associated with an increased risk of hypertension, stroke, and myocardial infarction. The risk factor is three times that of the general population and is more likely to be increased if the patient is over the age of 30, smokes cigarettes, drinks excessively, does not exercise, or is a diabetic.

Estrogen stimulates the synthesis and release of VLDL from the liver and decreases hepatic lipase activity. The incidence of gallbladder disease, an acute attack of hepatitis, and a decrease in glucose tolerance are increased in the oral contraceptive user. The combination preparations should be avoided in patients with estrogen receptor-positive tumors.

Contraindications to the use of oral contraceptives include preexisting cardiovascular disease, liver disease, cerebrovascular disease, diabetes, hormonally dependent tumors, hyperlipidemia, and development of serious headaches or migraine.

Table 40-4 compares some of common methods of contraception, and it also summarizes their mechanisms of action, failure rates, and most prominent adverse effects.

Drug Interactions

Antibiotics alter the gastrointestinal flora and can result in a decreased potency of oral contraceptives. The mechanism is believed to be via an altered enterohepatic circulation of the hormones, resulting in decreased hormone efficacy. Anticoagulant therapy for any indication requires discontinuation of oral contraceptives because oral contraceptives can cause a hypercoagulable state.

Drugs which induce liver microsomal enzymes will cause a more rapid metabolism of the hormones and therefore decrease their efficacy. Such drugs include barbiturates, primidone, carbamazepine, phenytoin, rifampin, griseofulvin, and benzodiazepines such as chlordiazepoxide and diazepam.

TABLE 40-4 Methods of contraception

Method	Mechanism of action	Failure rate[a]		Some adverse effects
		Low	High	
No method		85.0%	85.0%	
Sperimicide alone	Inactivation of sperm	21.6%	25.6%	Irritation can occur
Sponge with spermicide	Mechanical barrier to sperm; inactivation of sperm	16.0%	51.9%	Increased risk of vaginal infection
Withdrawal		14.7%	27.8%	
Periodic abstinance	Avoidance of coitus during presumed fertile days	13.8%	19.2%	
Diaphragm or cervical cap with spermicide	Mechanical barrier to sperm; inactivation of sperm	12.0%	38.9%	Increased risk of urinary tract or vaginal infection
Condom	Mechanical barrier to sperm	9.8%	18.5%	Allergic reactions
Oral contraceptive, fixed-combination	Suppression of ovulation, changes in cervical mucus and endometrium	3.8%	8.7%	Estrogen-related risk of thromboembolism, stroke; myocardial infarction in older smokers; hypertension
Oral contraceptive, progestin only	Changes in cervical mucus & endometrium, possibly suppression of ovulation	——[b]	3.0%	Irregular, unpredictable bleeding in some
Medroxyprogesterone acetate	Changes in cervical mucus & endometrium, suppression of ovulation	<1.0%	<1.0%	Menstrual irregularities; headache; weight gain
Levonorgestrel subdermal implants	Changes in cervical mucus & endometrium, suppression of ovulation	<1.0%	<1.0%	Menstrual irregularities; headache; weight gain

[a] Percent accidental pregnancy during first year of use. "Low" and "high" refer to rates among women in the United States more and less likely than average to use the method correctly and consistently.

[b] No data found.

*[Modified from The Medical Letter **34**: 111-114 (1992).]*

FERTILITY AGENTS

Gonadotropins

Human chorionic gonadotropin (HCG) is a purified extract of human placental tissue. It has predominantly LH-like activity in that it binds to all LH receptors. It is more widely available and less expensive than human pituitary LH. HCG differs from LH in that it has a different B chain, has higher a sugar content, and has a longer serum half-life. Its use is limited to induction of ovulation, for which it is administered intramuscularly as a bolus to replace the LH surge. In smaller daily doses, it is used to support corpus luteum function in those patients with luteal-phase defects.

Human menopausal gonadotropin (HMG) is a purified extract of human menopausal urine. The final product has 75 IUnits each of FSH and LH. The biological activity is determined by bioassay. Successive doses of HMG are given by intramuscular injection to stimulate the development of the follicles. However, if ovulation does not occur, it may be induced by an appropriately timed dose of HCG. The success rate is 30 to 50 percent, providing the ovary is functional and steroids are secreted in response to the injected gonadotropin. Multiple ovulations may occur and multiple births are common (about 20 percent). Indication for the use of HMG therapy include hypopituitarism, hypothalamic amenorrhea that is unresponsive to clomiphene, and patients with polycystic ovarian disease who are resistant to induction of ovulation.

Adverse effects resulting from excessive stimulation of the ovary are quite serious. Excessive levels of estrogens are produced by the ovary which necessitates careful monitoring of plasma steroid concentrations. In the overly-stimulated ovary, cysts may develop which, if they burst, can result in intra-abdominal hemorrhage and death. Detection of enlarged, overly-stimulated ovaries mandates cessation of therapy.

Inhibitors of Prolactin Secretion

Prolactin is secreted by the mammotrophin cells of the anterior pituitary. Prolactin participates along with progesterone, thyroid hormone, glucocorticoids, somatotropin, and insulin in the initiation and maintenance of postpartum lactation. Dopamine is secreted by the hypothalamus and prevents prolactin from being secreted. Prolactin in turn regulates the dopaminergic neurons of the hypothalamus to regulate its own secretion. Hypoprolactinemia from a variety of pathological conditions will result in anovulatory hypoestrogenic amenorrhea and attendant premature osteoporosis. Hyperprolactinemia is believed to be responsible for 30 percent of cases of infertility in women. Gynecomastia results in patients receiving antidopaminergic neuroleptic drugs (e.g., phenothiazines and butyrophenones) or oral contraceptives.

Bromocriptine

Bromocriptine is a dopaminergic agonist, which binds to the dopamine receptors on pituitary lactotropes. The net effect is to decrease pituitary prolactin secretion in a dose-dependent manner.

Side effects include nausea, anorexia, hypotension, headaches, nasal stuffiness, and depression. Peripheral prolactin levels are followed and the dose of bromocriptine is increased until normal prolactin levels are obtained. The drug is as effective in pituitary prolactin-secreting tumors as it is in pituitary hyperplasia. The drug can be stopped as soon as pregnancy is established. In very large pituitary tumors, therapy is continued throughout pregnancy.

Bromocriptine is also used to suppress postpartum lactation. The older treatment for this condition, i.e., huge doses of estrogen, is contraindicated.

This drug also is useful for treating most pituitary tumors, whether they are actively secreting hormones or simply causing symptoms because of the effects of the tumor mass. This antitumor effect frequently results in a reduction of tumor size and/or symptoms within weeks of beginning therapy.

LHRH Agonists and Antagonists

Luteinizing hormone-releasing hormone (LHRH) is a linear decapeptide found in highest concentrations in nerve ending of the median eminence of the hypothalamus. The secretion of LHRH is influenced by catecholaminergic, serotonergic, cholinergic, and peptidergic (e.g., opioid peptides) neurohumors as well as by various hormones. The final common pathway of these stimuli can be conceptually visualized as a "pulse generator" with which LHRH induces the pulsatile secretion of the gonadotropins FSH and LH.

The most important physiologic concept of the role of LHRH on pituitary FSH and LH secretion is that pulsatile LHRH is necessary for normal ovulatory function. Conversely, constant infusion of LHRH induces "down-regulation" of the LHRH receptors, resulting in a cessation of gonadotropin secretion and a profound hypogonadal state.

LHRH has a very short half-life. It is used clinically in two situations. It is used in a "stimulation or provocative test" to help distinguish pituitary from hypothalamic hypogonadism. Following basal LH and FSH determination, an intravenous bolus of LHRH is given with concomitant assay of FSH and LH in the blood. It is also commonly used to induce ovulation. LHRH is administered in a pulsatile manner, intravenously. Several pumps are commercially available, which are worn by the patient during the several weeks required to induce ovulation.

Leuprolide acetate is an LHRH agonist, approved for inducing a profound hypogonadal state in males with metastatic prostate carcinoma. Leuprolide and other LHRH agonists are being extensively investigated in a variety of clinical conditions such as treatment for endometriosis, treatment of sex hormone-dependent malignancies, suppression of precocious puberty, shrinkage of leiomyomata uteri, and suppression of endogenous gonadotropin secretion prior to HMG/HCG induction of ovulation in anovulatory patients with high endogenous LH secretion (such as patients with polycystic ovarian disease). These hormones must be given as daily subcutaneous injections.

The side effects of treatment with leuprolide include profound nausea, which resolves after several months, hypogonadal osteoporosis, which will worsen as a function of the duration of treatment, and profound "menopausal" hot flashes in both men and women.

BIBLIOGRAPHY

Baulieu, E.E.: "Contraception and Other Clinical Applications of RU 486, an Antiprogesterone at the Receptor," *Science* **245**: 1351-1357 (1989).

Beller F.K. and C. Ebort: "Effect of Oral Contraceptives on Blood Coagulation: A Review," *Obstet. Gynecol. Surv.* **40**: 425-436 (1985).

Bush, T. and I. Barret-Conner: "Noncontraceptive Estrogen Use and Cardiovascular Disease," *Epidemol. Rev.* **7**: 80-104 (1985).

Carson, S.L.: "Contraceptive Efficacy of a Monophasic Oral Contraceptive Containing Desogestrel," *Am. J. Obstet. Gynecol.* **168**: 1017-1020 (1993).

Clark, J.H., W.T. Schrader, and B.W. O'Malley: "Mechanisms of Action of Steroid Hormones," In Wilson, J.D., and D.W. Foster (eds.), *Williams Textbook of Endocrinology*, Saunders, Philadelphia, 1992, pp. 35-90.

Henzl, M.R.: "Contraceptive Hormones and Their Clinical Use," In Yen, S.S., and R.B. Jaffe (eds.), *Reproductive Endocrinology, Physiology, Pathophysiology and Clinical Management, 2nd ed.*, Saunders, Philadelphia, 1986, pp. 643-682.

Heuson, J.C., and A. Coune: "Hormone-Responsive Tumors," In Felig, P., J.D. Baxter, A.E. Broadus, and L.A. Frohman (eds.), *Endocrinology and Metabolism, 2nd ed.*, McGraw-Hill, New York, 1987, pp. 1736-1767.

Hommani, Z.T., H. Yavetz, L. Yogev, R. Rotem, and G.F. Pas: "Clomiphene Citrate Treatment in Oligozoospermia: Comparison Between Two Regimens of Low Dose Treatment," *Fertil. Steril.*, **50**: 801-804 (1988).

Jordan, V.C.: "Biochemical Pharmacology of Antiestrogen Action," *Pharmacol. Rev.* **36**: 245-276 (1984).

Kaplan, N.M.: "Cardiovascular Complications of Oral Contraceptives," *Annu. Rev. Med.* **29**: 31-40 (1987).

Maguire, P.J.: "Estrogen Replacement Therapy and Breast Cancer," *J. Reproduct. Med.* **38**: 183-185 (1993).

Shoupe, D., and D.R. Mishell: "Norplant: Subdermal Implant System for Long Term Contraception," *Am. J. Obstet. Gynecol.* **160**: 1286-1292 (1989).

Sullivan, J.M., R. Vander Zwaag, G.F. Lemp, J.P. Hughes, V. Maddock, F.W. Kroetz, K.B. Ramanathan, and D.M. Mirvis: "Postmenopausal Estrogen Use and Coronary Atherosclerosis," *Ann. Intern. Med.* **108**: 358-363 (1988).

Tayob, Y.: "Oral Contraceptives: An Epidemiological Perspective," *Internat. J. Fertil.* **37 (Suppl. 4)**: 199-203 (1992).

Yen, S., C.C. Hsieh, and B. MacMahon: "Extrahepatic Bile Duct Cancer and Smoking, Beverage Consumption, Past Medical History and Oral Contraceptive Use," *Cancer* **59**: 2112-2116 (1987).

Zumoff, B.: "Biological and Endocrinological Insights into the Possible Breast Cancer Risk from Menopausal Estrogens Replacement," *Steroids* **58**: 196-204 (1993).

CHAPTER 41

Androgens, Anabolic Steroids, and Inhibitors

Gerald H. Sterling

Androgens, designated as the male sex hormones, are steroid hormones; testosterone being the principal androgen secreted by the testes. The adrenal gland and the ovaries also secrete androgenic hormones, but to a much lesser degree than do the testes. Androgens have both masculinizing and growth-stimulating, or anabolic, effects. Those synthetic analogs possessing greater growth-promoting than androgenic effects are termed anabolic steroids and have been abused by many aspiring and professional athletes. Thus, androgens and anabolic steroids have been declared Schedule III controlled substances. More recently, compounds which inhibit the synthesis or actions of androgens have been made available, primarily for treatment of prostatic cancer and androgen hypersecretory states.

CHEMISTRY

All androgens possess the cyclopentanophenanthrene nucleus (three benzene rings and a five-carbon ring), typical of steroid hormones. Testosterone is the major naturally occurring androgen. The structures of testosterone and selected clinically available compounds are shown in Fig. 41-1. Structural analogs of testosterone have been synthesized for clinical use to maximize bioavailability from various routes of administration and prolong the androgenic effects.

PHYSIOLOGIC REGULATION

Testosterone is synthesized and secreted by the Leydig cells in the testes. An adult male produces between 2.5 and 10 mg of testosterone daily, in a circadian pattern with highest amounts in the early morning hours. Androgens are also secreted by the adrenal glands, but are generally less potent.

Synthesis of testosterone is under control of the hypothalamopituitary system. Steroidogenesis in the Leydig cell is stimulated by the anterior pituitary hormone, luteinizing hormone (LH), previously called interstitial cell-stimulating hormone (ICSH). Luteinizing hormone acts through increased synthesis of cyclic AMP and calmodulin. Testosterone, in conjunction with follicle-stimulating hormone (FSH) stimulate spermatogenesis in the seminiferous tubules. The hypothalamus secretes gonadotropin releasing hormone (GnRH) which regulates the pituitary secretion of LH and FSH. Testosterone, in a classic negative feedback system, suppresses pituitary secretion of LH and FSH. Estradiol, secreted by the testes or synthesized by peripheral conversion of testosterone, also inhibits secretion of gonadotropins. Inhibin, a glycoprotein secreted by the Sertoli cells, works in conjunction with dihydrotestosterone to reduce secretion of FSH.

MECHANISM OF ACTION

All steroids, including testosterone, being highly lipid soluble, exert their effects primarily by binding to intracellular receptors in target tissues. The androgenic effects of testosterone in many tissues (e.g., prostate seminal vesicles) depend on conversion of testosterone to its more active metabolite, 5α-dihydrotestosterone (DHT) by the enzyme, 5α-reductase in these target tissues. Dihydrotestosterone binds 10 times more tightly to the androgen receptor than does testosterone. The androgen receptor has been demonstrated to belong to a group of steroid-receptor proteins which act in the cell nucleus. The androgen receptor gene has been localized on the X chromosome, and cloning

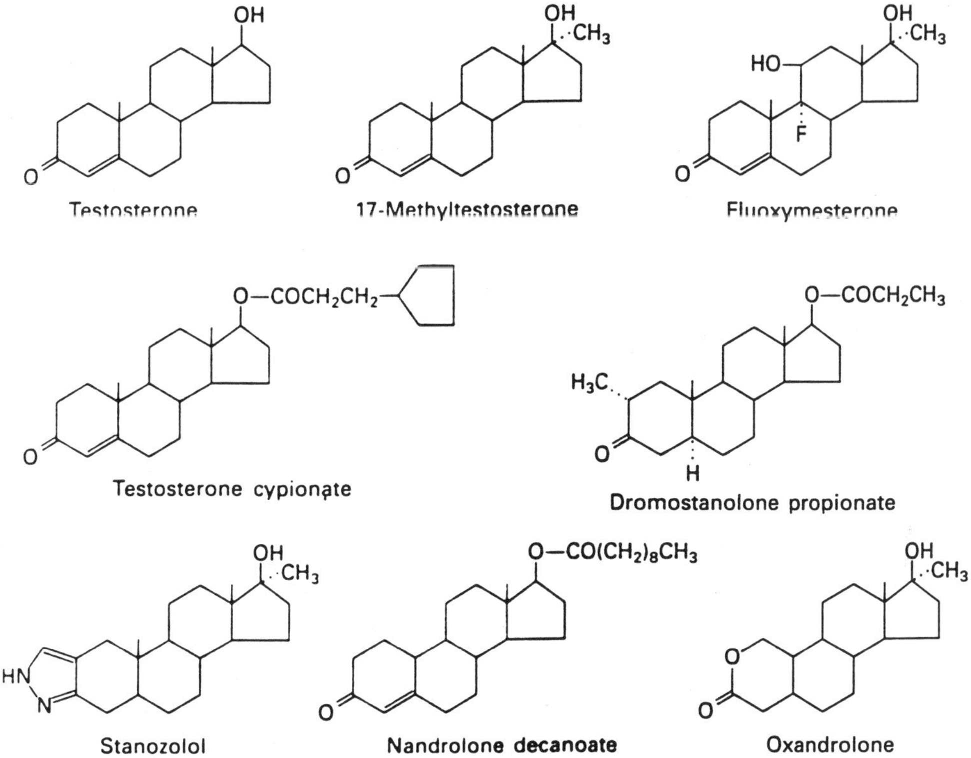

FIGURE 41-1 *Structures of selected clinically used androgenic and anabolic steroids.*

of androgen receptor complementary DNA has been accomplished. The receptor protein contains several regions which have different functions, namely, an area involved with binding to the nonhistone portion of DNA, one responsible for binding to the androgen, and another that activates transcription of messenger RNA (mRNA). Thus, binding of androgen to the receptor induces a series of events causing its target tissue effect by activating the transcription of specific mRNAs, which in turn direct the synthesis of specific proteins involved in regulation of growth and cell division. The receptor has been widely thought to be cytosolic with binding causing translocation of the androgen-receptor complex to the nucleus. Recent evidence suggests that steroids can enter the nucleus and thus bind directly to receptors in the nucleus.

PHARMACOKINETICS

As indicated, endogenous androgens are primarily produced in the testes. Androgens may also be produced by the theca cells in the ovarian cortex. Most of these androgens are aromatized to estrogens by the granulosa cells of the ovary; some are secreted into the peripheral circulation as androgens. Androgens and androgenic precursors (17 ketosteroids) secreted by the ovary can be converted to testosterone in peripheral tissues. The adrenal cortex also is responsible for the production of androgens and androgenic precursors. When an enzyme defect exists in the adrenal cortex, such as in congenital adrenal hyperplasia, large quantities of androgens and androgen precursors may be secreted with masculinizing effects. Although little testosterone is actually secreted by the adrenal, peripheral conversion of other androgens to testosterone is again important. Once testosterone is released to the peripheral circulation, 98 to 99 percent of testosterone is bound to sex hormone binding globulin (SHBG) and albumin, while 1 to 2 percent is in the free form. Testosterone reduces hepatic synthesis of SHBG, while estrogen increases production. It is the free form of testosterone which exerts an effect on target tissues. The half-life of endogenous testosterone is 10 to 20 min. Metabolism of endogenous testosterone results in production of an active metabolite, DHT, as well as estrogenic compounds (e.g., estradiol). See Fig. 40-2 in the previous chapter for details of the interrelationship of testosterone to other steroid hormones.

Biotransformation of androgens occurs primarily in the liver. Testosterone is converted to androstenedione, which can then be reduced to the 17-ketosteroids, androsterone, and etiocholanolone. These products have significantly less androgenic potency. The 17-ketosteroids are then excreted in the urine. Small amounts of testosterone glucuronide and sulfate are also excreted. About 6 percent is excreted unchanged in the feces. Since adrenal and gonadal androgens share a common metabolite in the 17-ketosteroids, urinary ketosteroid determinations may not accurately reflect plasma levels of gonadal or exogenous androgens.

When testosterone is administered orally or parenterally, it is rapidly absorbed and inactivated by the liver. Biochemical modifications of testosterone are necessary for its clinical pharmacologic use, to reduce its biotransformation and prolong its duration of action. Modifications to protect the compound from biotransformation include esterification of the 17β-hydroxy group (e.g., testosterone cypionate), methylation of the 17α-position (e.g., methyltestosterone), halogenation of the ring (e.g., fluoxymesterone) and alterations of the ring structure. In addition to side chain modifications, aqueous solutions for parenteral injection can be prepared to delay absorption. Esterification of androgens followed by suspension in oil for intramuscular injection can also delay absorption and allow for continued availability of the steroid over a period of several days. Thus, drugs such as methyltestosterone and fluoxymesterone are effective orally and drugs such as testosterone cypionate can be given in intervals of 2 to 4 weeks. The prolonged bioavailability of the modified injectable androgens makes them particularly attractive for replacement therapy in the hypogonadal male. The various testosterone esters available for intramuscular injection have different absorption properties but prolonged action. The oral preparations are primarily analogs alkylated in the 17α-position. A microparticulate testosterone for oral use is available in other countries. Preparations being examined include subcutaneous implants of testosterone-containing siloxane capsules and a testosterone-impregnated adhesive film for transdermal administration. See Table 41-1 for a list of available drugs.

EFFECTS OF ANDROGENS ON ORGAN SYSTEMS

Male

Physiologic effects of testosterone and other androgens are seen throughout development, beginning in early fetal life and varying as growth and development of the organism proceed in the male. Androgens produced by the testes cause masculinization of the genital tract of the male fetus early in gestation. In puberty, androgens are responsible for development of the secondary male sexual characteristics. Androgens produce an increase in the size of the penis and testes, growth of the beard, and growth of the pubic and axillary hair. Androgens are also necessary for spermatogenesis and sperm maturation. They cause proliferation of sebaceous glands and increase secretion from these glands. Other effects at puberty in the male include growth of the larynx, which results in deepening of the voice, and increase in skeletal muscle mass, especially of the shoulder girdle. This increase in skeletal muscle mass is a manifestation of the anabolic effects of androgens. Testosterone also has a growth-promoting effect on bone, which is mediated by growth hormone. In studies of boys with constitutional delay of growth, testosterone has been shown to increase endogenous growth hormone levels as well as increase rates of linear growth. Androgens also stimulate epiphyseal maturation and closure, which ultimately limit the phase of accelerated linear growth that occurs in puberty. The stimulatory effect on epiphyseal growth by androgens is much less than that seen with estrogens.

Female

Androgens produced by the ovary and adrenal glands are important in the pubertal development of the female, also. Growth of pubic and axillary hair is attributed to androgenic stimulation. In the normal female, the total rate of production of the weaker androgens, androstenedione and dihydroepiandrosterone, far exceeds the rate of production of testosterone.

In both males and females, androgens have a negative feedback effect on the secretion of gonadotropins from the pituitary. This is an important aspect of the function of the hypothalamic-pituitary-gonadal axis in pubertal develop-

TABLE 41-1 Selected androgenic compounds in clinical use

Drug preparation	Relative activity	
	Androgenic	Anabolic
FOR INTRAMUSCULAR INJECTION		
Testosterone (aqueous suspension)	1	1
Testosterone esters (in oil suspension)		
Testosterone propionate	1	1
Testosterone cypionate	1	1
Testosterone enanthate	1	1
Nandrolone phenpropionate (oil suspension)	1	3 to 5
Nandrolone decanoate (oil suspension)	1	3 to 4
FOR ORAL OR BUCCAL ADMINISTRATION (AS TABLETS)		
Methyltestosterone	1	1
Fluoxymesterone	1	1 to 2
Oxymetholone	1	3
Stanozolol	1	3 to 5
Oxandrolone	1	3 to 13

ment as well as in adult life. Pharmacologic doses of androgens certainly suppress pituitary gonadotropin secretion, which may have adverse effects on normal gonadal function.

Hematopoietic Effects

Androgens have a stimulatory effect on normal hematopoietic cells, which is mediated by erythropoietin. Steroids may enhance the effects of erythropoietin as well as increase its production. Steroids may also have a direct growth-promoting effect on erythroid stem cells. The higher levels of circulating androgens in males are responsible for the normally higher hemoglobin, hematocrit, and red blood cell mass in males than females.

THERAPEUTIC USES

Male Hypogonadism

The use of androgenic steroids is clearly indicated as replacement therapy for the male with gonadal failure. Testicular deficiency can be congenital or an acquired condition. In either case, the treatment is the same, with goals of induction of puberty, maintenance after puberty or treatment of infertility. In congenital hypogonadism in the male, puberty will not occur unless androgens are administered. Masculinizing features as well as the pubertal growth spurt are lacking without replacement therapy. In cases of constitutional growth delay, normal development will usually occur by 18 years of age without drug therapy, but androgens may be used for brief periods after the age of 14 years to induce puberty. Androgens have also been useful in treatment of cryptorchidism and micropenis.

Testosterone esters (e.g., testosterone enanthate, testosterone propionate and testosterone cypionate) are usually administered parenterally in cases of replacement therapy, with careful monitoring of the response of penile and testicular growth. The intramuscular preparations have greater potency and are less hepatotoxic than the oral preparations. Although patients with hypogonadotropic hypogonadism (hypothalamic-pituitary dysfunction) can be treated with exogenous gonadotropins to stimulate the gonads, frequently the administration of synthetic androgens is a simpler and less expensive means of achieving the same results.

Growth Deficiency

Androgens have been used alone, or in conjunction with growth hormone to enhance growth in boys prior to puberty. The doses of androgens used must be carefully monitored to avoid premature closure of the epiphyseal plate which would reduce expected adult height rather than enhance it.

Anemia

Androgens have been reported to enhance red blood cell production by increasing the production of erythropoietic-stimulating factor. Androgens have thus been used for treatment of various forms of refractory anemias. For example, patients with anemia based on lack of bone marrow proliferation of red blood cell precursors or due to chronic renal failure may respond to large dose androgen therapy. Unfortunately, the response of these patients is unpredictable and may not be sustained. Also, patients often do not tolerate the side effects of the steroids; studies have been undertaken in anemic patients to identify factors which may predict response to androgen therapy. Testosterone esters administered by injection have better results than orally administered agents.

Breast Cancer

Androgens have been used secondarily in the treatment of breast carcinomas, particularly in women who are 1 to 5 years postmenopausal. Their effect seems to be primarily palliative and may be a result of the antiestrogenic properties of androgens. This type of therapy only benefits women with a hormone-sensitive tumor. Use of specific antiestrogens such as tamoxifen may be more effective and better tolerated by the patient with an estrogen-responsive breast tumor.

Endometriosis

Danazol is the isoxazole derivative of the synthetic steroid 17α-ethinyltestosterone. It has weak androgenic potential and multiple endocrine effects, which combine to make it an effective medical therapy for endometriosis in women. Danazol binds to androgen, progesterone, and glucocorticoid receptors, but not estrogen receptors. It inhibits the midcycle surge of LH and FSH, thus suppressing ovarian function.

In addition to treatment of endometriosis, danazol is also used for the treatment of angioneurotic edema, an autosomal dominant immune disorder that results in random activation of the complement cascade and release of local factors responsible for angioedema. Its effect is mediated through synthesis of inhibitory proteins by the liver that prevent activation of the complement system. Danazol has been used in treatment of fibrocystic disease of the breast and hematologic disorders including idiopathic thrombocytopenic purpura. A complete discussion of danazol is found in Chapter 40.

ADVERSE REACTIONS AND PRECAUTIONS

The most frequent side effect of androgenic steroids is virilism. Signs of virilism in the prepubertal male include growth of pubic hair, increase in penile size and increase frequency of erections and priapism. Androgens may also cause premature closure of the epiphyseal plate and reduce attainable adult height. Prolonged use in males can lead to feminization, such as gynecomastia, due to reduced release of endogenous gonadotropins and peripheral conversion of testosterone to estrogen. Androgen-induced prostatic hypertrophy has been reported. In females, untoward effects of androgen therapy include hirsutism, clitoral enlargement, acne, deepening of the voice, and menstrual irregularities. Other undesirable effects associated with these agents are liver dysfunction, hypercalcemia, and retention of sodium and water, which may lead to edema and hypertension. Liver dysfunction is especially noted with the 17α-alkyl derivatives (e.g., methyltestosterone, fluoxymesterone and other orally effective agents). They have rarely been reported to cause hepatocellular and endothelial carcinomas and hepatic adenomas. These compounds should be avoided in patients with liver disease. Large doses taken by athletes may cause atherogenic changes in blood lipids. Androgenic compounds are contraindicated in pregnant women and in patients with prostatic or estrogen-insensitive breast carcinoma.

USE OF ANABOLIC STEROIDS BY ATHLETES

Anabolic steroids are closely related structurally to testosterone and though they possess both androgenic and anabolic activities, they produce greater anabolic than androgenic effects. These compounds were originally designed to induce weight gain and improve nitrogen balance in individuals with recent or chronic debilitating illness, serious infections, trauma or use of cytotoxic drugs. However, the widespread use of androgens and anabolic steroids by athletes, is a major concern of both the athletic and medical communities. Androgens and anabolic steroids were therefore, declared Schedule III controlled substances in the Anabolic Steroids Control Act of 1990. Because of their known growth promoting properties, many male and female athletes, in early adolescence through adulthood, use androgens and anabolic steroids in alarmingly high doses to improve performance and enhance muscle strength. A comparison of androgenic and anabolic activity of these compounds is shown in Table 41-1.

There is conflicting evidence of any benefits to athletes. Although some studies document small improvements in muscle strength associated with steroid use, particularly in trained athletes, these findings are not consistently reproduced. Most investigators agree that significant weight gain results from administration of oral and injectable androgens by athletes. However, the weight gain may be the result of fluid retention and not increased tissue growth. Steroids also improve appetite, and weight gain may partially result from the combined effects of athletic training and increased intake of nutrients.

Changes in athletic performance may be related to the psychologic effects of steroids. Androgens have long been linked to the behavioral changes that take place in puberty. Athletes report increased aggression and mood changes during steroid usage which may be looked upon as beneficial in competitive performance.

Many athletes obtain anabolic steroids from black-market sources, but a surprising number may get the drugs from legitimate sources such as pharmacists, physicians, and trainers. Drug use regimens may combine oral and parenteral agents over a period of weeks to months and usually have a 4 to 6 week drug holiday prior to competitions when drug testing is carried out.

Regardless of the benefits perceived by athletes who use these compounds, the adverse effects can be quite significant. Females can become virilized, as evidenced by hirsutism, voice changes, clitoral enlargement, and menstrual irregularities. Conversely, males may exhibit feminization because high levels of circulating androgens inhibit release of gonadotropins from the hypothalamopituitary system, thus reducing endogenous testosterone secretion by the testes and increasing conversion to estrogen. The most common effect of steroid use in males is gynecomastia. Decrease in testicular size and reduction in spermatogenesis may also result. Although this is a reversible side effect, resumption of baseline testicular function may not be seen until 4 to 6 months after the drugs are discontinued. When androgens and anabolic steroids are administered to young males who have not completed puberty, premature epiphyseal closure can occur, causing reduction in adult height.

Liver damage may result from use of anabolic steroids, especially with orally active preparations with 17α-methyl substitutions. The damage may be mild, resulting in jaundice, or severe enough to result in hepatocellular carcinoma.

Reports of psychiatric effects, ranging from depression to psychosis, are becoming more frequent with use of anabolic steroids by athletes. Increased aggression, increased energy, increased libido, delusions, and manic episodes are associated with steroid use. Depression and suicidal ideation have been reported upon discontinuance of the drugs. Psychiatrists clearly recognize that these steroids can commonly cause mental disturbances.

Anabolic steroids also have effects on the cardiovascular system. These drugs decrease high-density lipoproteins (HDLs) while increasing low-density lipoproteins (LDLs) and total cholesterol; this may increase the risk of coronary heart disease. It is unclear whether short term alterations in lipid metabolism secondary to steroid use actually have long term effects. In addition, retention of fluid and electrolytes associated with usage may cause hypertension.

In summary, androgens and anabolic steroids have significant adverse effects. The risks of serious complications of drug therapy are generally more acceptable when use is in treatment of a disease state. Use of these compounds by athletes, in attempts to enhance performance, is unacceptable and dangerous.

TREATMENT OF MALE INFERTILITY

There are several drugs which have proven useful

in the treatment of male infertility. These drugs include: bromocriptine mesylate, clomiphene citrate, human chorionic gonadotropin (HCG), and menotropins. Bromocriptine is used in the treatment of infertility in males associated with elevated prolactin; it acts by stimulating dopamine receptors in the pituitary, thus inhibiting prolactin secretion. Clomiphene, a nonsteroidal compound with partial estrogenic activity, stimulates spermatogenesis by blocking negative feedback to the hypothalamopituitary axis, thus leading to an increased secretion of LH and FSH. HCG is a placental hormone obtained from the urine of pregnant women; it is used in the diagnosis of males with delayed puberty to evaluate their ability to secrete androgens. Menotropins, human menopausal gonadotropin obtained from the urine of postmenopausal women, contains FSH and LH and is used in combination with HCG in hypogonadal male infertility. These agents are discussed in more detail in the preceding chapter (Chapter 40).

ANTIANDROGENS AND ANTAGONISTS

A search for effective therapy for prostate carcinoma and hypersecretion of testosterone has led to the development of compounds which reduce either the synthesis or actions of endogenous androgens. These compounds include analogs of gonadotropin releasing hormone (GnRH), androgen receptor blockers, and a drug which inhibits the formation of dihydrotestosterone (DHT).

Gonadotropin Releasing Hormone Analogs

It is recognized that the pulsatile release of GnRH from the hypothalamus stimulates the synthesis and secretion of FSH and LH (therefore, GnRH is also known as luteinizing hormone-releasing hormone (LHRH)). However, sustained levels of GnRH reduce the secretion of the pituitary gonadotropins. Synthetic analogs of GnRH include nafarelin acetate, leuprolide acetate, goserelin acetate, and histrelin acetate.

Nafarelin

Nafarelin is a derivative of GnRH. Similar to natural GnRH, initially the drug stimulates the release of FSH and LH and then, with continued administration, decreases the release of FSH and LH and reduces gonadal steroids. Nafarelin is given by a nasal spray and is used in the treatment of endometriosis in women and in the therapy of central (gonadotropin-dependent) precocious puberty in children of both sexes.

Leuprolide, Histrelin, and Goserelin

Leuprolide and histrelin are nonapeptide derivatives of GnRH and goserelin is a decapeptide analog of this releasing hormone. Initially these compounds stimulate the secretion of FSH and LH and cause an increase in serum levels of testosterone and DHT in males and an elevation of serum estradiol levels in females. Chronic administration however, produces suppression of gonadotropins with a subsequent reduction in serum testosterone levels, similar to those present in castrated males. In females, serum estradiol concentrations are reduced by chronic treatment to values seen in postmenopausal females. Both leuprolide and goserelin are indicated for the treatment of prostatic cancer (by subcutaneous injection) and in the management of endometriosis (intramuscular depot administration). Histrelin, as well as leuprolide, is used in children of both sexes with central precocious puberty.

Androgen Receptor Antagonists

Flutamide

Flutamide is a nonsteroidal competitive androgen receptor antagonist that blocks the effects of endogenous androgens. Following oral administration, the drug is completely absorbed from the gastrointestinal tract. Flutamide is quickly biotransformed in the body with the formation of an active alpha-hydroxylated metabolite and a number of inactive products. The alpha-hydroxylated derivative has a half-life of approximately 6 hours in younger patients; in geriatric patients the half-life of the active product is about 8 to 9 hours. The protein binding of flutamide and its active metabolite is greater than 90 percent.

Flutamide, in conjunction with a GnRH analog such as leuprolide, is indicated for the treatment of metastatic prostatic carcinoma. The combination essentially causes a chemical castration and may alleviate the need for orchiectomy. Adverse reactions include hot flashes, loss of libido, impotence, gynecomastia, gastrointestinal disturbances and reversible hepatic dysfunction.

Spironolactone

An aldosterone antagonist, spironolactone, has also been shown to competitively inhibit binding to androgen receptors. It has been used in treatment of hirsutism in women.

Androgen Synthesis Inhibitors

Finasteride

Finasteride is a 4-azasteroid useful orally in the treatment of benign prostatic hyperplasia. The size and integrity of the prostate gland depends on DHT which is formed from testosterone via the enzyme 5α-reductase. Finasteride is a competitive inhibitor of 5α-reductase and causes decreased formation of DHT. With the decrease in DHT levels a reduction in the size of the prostate glands occurs. Prolonged administration increases urine flow and relieves symptoms of urinary obstruction due to prostate hypertrophy. The drug is not effective in all patient who have benign prostatic hypertrophy; although the prostate gland may be reduced in size, some patients still experience difficulty in urination or have symptoms associated with prostatic hypertrophy. The oral bioavailability of finasteride is approximately 65 percent. Food does not interfere with its absorption. Its binding to plasma proteins is about 90 percent. The drug undergoes extensive biotransformation and its metabolites are found in urine and feces. The elimination half-life of finasteride is about 6 hours. It appears that dosage reduction is not required for patients with kidney dysfunction or in elderly patients. Adverse reactions include impotence, decreased libido, and decreased volume of ejaculate.

Ketoconazole

Ketoconazole, an effective antifungal agent, inhibits synthesis of glucocorticoids and androgens in the adrenal. Experimental use in the treatment of prostatic cancer has been discouraging.

BIBLIOGRAPHY

Barbieri, R.L., and K.J. Ryan: "Danazol: Endocrine Pharmacology and Therapeutic Applications," *Am. J. Obstet. Gynecol.* **141**: 454-463 (1981).

Cicardi, M., L. Bergamashini, M. Cugno, E. Hack, G. Agnostoni, and A. Agnostoni: "Long-term Treatment of Hereditary Angioedema with Attenuated Androgens: A Survey of a 13-Year Experience," *J. Allergy Clin. Immunol.* **87**: 768-773 (1991).

Fotherby, K., and F. James: "Metabolism of Synthetic Steroids," *Adv. Steroid Biochem. Pharmacol.* **3**: 67-165 (1972).

Gormley, G.J., E. Stoner, R.S. Rittmaster, H. Gregg, D.L. Thompson, K.C. Lassiter, P.H. Vlasses, and E.A. Stoner: "Effects of Finasteride (MK-906), a 5-α-Reductase Inhibitor, on Circulating Androgens in Male Volunteers," *J. Clin. Endocrinol. Metab.* **70**: 1136-1140 (1990).

Lukas S.E.: "Current Perspectives on Anabolic-Androgenic Steroid Abuse", *Trends in Pharmacol. Sci.* **14**: 61-68 (1993).

Malarky, W.B., R.H., Strauss, D.J. Leizman, M. Liggett, and L.M. Demers: "Endocrine Effects in Female Weight Lifters who Self-administer Testosterone and Anabolic Steroids," *Am. J. Obstet. Gynecol.* **165**: 1385-1390 (1991).

Miller, W.L.: "Molecular Biology of Steroid Hormone Synthesis," *Endrocrin. Rev.* **9**: 295-318 (1988).

Perlmutter, G., and D.T. Lowenthal: "Use of Anabolic Steroids by Athletes," *Am. J. Fam. Pract.* **32**: 208-210 (1985).

Pope, H.G., Jr., and D.L. Katz: "Psychiatric Effects of Anabolic Steroids," *Psychiatric Ann.* **22**: 24-29 (1992).

Whitcomb, R.W., and W.F. Crowley, Jr.: "Diagnosis and Treatment of Isolated Gonadotropin-releasing Hormone Deficiency in Men," *J. Clin. Endocrinol. Metab.* **70**: 3-7 (1990).

Yesalis, C.E., N.J. Kennedy, A.N. Kopstein, and M.S. Bahrke: "Anabolic-Androgenic Steroid Use in the United States," *J. Am. Med. Assoc.* **270**: 1217-1221 (1993).

CHAPTER 42

Corticotropin and Corticosteroids

Jeffrey L. Miller and Leslie I. Rose

The term *corticosteroids* designates those steroid hormones normally secreted by the adrenal cortex: glucocorticoids, mineralocorticoids, and sex steroids. Production of these hormones is under direct control of adrenocorticotropic hormone (ACTH, corticotropin) originating from the anterior pituitary. The first section deals with the pharmacology and clinical applications of ACTH. Glucocorticoids and mineralocorticoids are addressed in the second section. Sex steroids were discussed in the preceding chapters.

CORTICOTROPIN

Source and Chemistry

ACTH is a polypeptide hormone secreted by the corticotropic cells of the anterior pituitary gland. It is derived by proteolytic cleavage from a precursor glycoprotein, pro-opiomelanocortin.

Human ACTH is composed of 39 amino acids with a molecular mass of 4500 Da. Its structure is shown in Fig. 42-1. It differs from the ACTH of various animal species in the sequence between amino acids 29 and 33. However, ACTH (1-24) is 100 percent conserved in mammalian species and retains its biologic activity. Its synthetic form, *cosyntropin*, is used clinically to assess adrenocortical function. Other sources of ACTH include extraction from animal pituitary glands of chromatographic or electrophoretic, techniques and synthesis of the entire human ACTH polypeptide, but there are few clinical indications for their use.

Regulation of Secretion and Effects of ACTH

Regulation of Secretion Secretion of ACTH is regulated by corticotropin-releasing factor (CRF), a 41 amino acid peptide formed in the median eminence of the hypothalamus. CRF reaches the pituitary corticotropic cells through the hypothalamic portal venous system.

Plasma cortisol (hydrocortisone) modulates ACTH secretion by a negative-feedback mechanism both at the hypothalamic and pituitary level. This simple negative feedback can be overridden in periods of stress such as exercise, surgery, hypovolemia, hyperthermia, and hypothermia as well as psychologic stress. ACTH secretion also occurs in bursts 7 to 13 times a day, independent of plasma cortisol levels and in a pattern reproducible for any given person. This diurnal rhythm is under hypothalamic control and does not submit to negative feedback.

Action on the Adrenal Cortex Some of the actions of ACTH on the adrenal cortex occur within minutes, whereas others become apparent only after several hours or days of exposure. Within 1 min of administration of a bolus of ACTH, the concentration of adenosine-3′,5′-monophosphate (cyclic AMP) rises within the adrenal. This in turn stimulates the formation of the labile protein which activates the conversion of cholesterol to pregnenolone. Pregnenolone will then be converted by various enzyme systems to other steroid hormones. This entire process requires about 3 min. More prolonged exposure to ACTH promotes adrenal growth, stimulates protein and cholesterol synthesis, increases the functional capacity of the enzyme systems, and leads to depletion of adrenal ascorbic acid.

Extra Adrenal Effects Corticotropin can affect lipid and carbohydrate metabolism. These effects have been demonstrated mostly *in vitro* and with pharmacologic doses of ACTH. It stimulates lipolysis by activation of a "hormone-sensitive

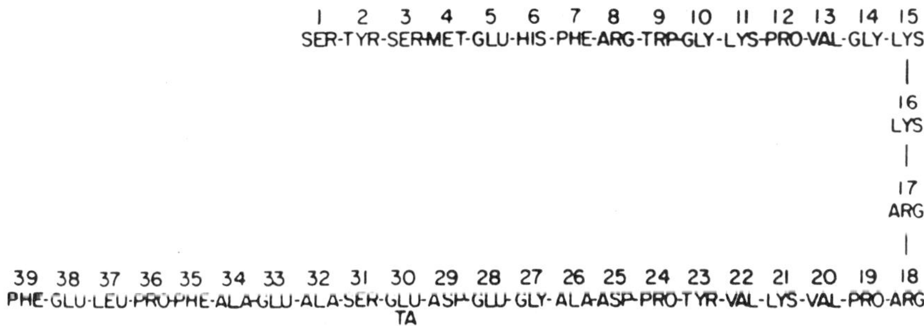

FIGURE 42-1 *Amino acid sequence of human adrenocorticotropic hormone (ACTH, corticotropin).*

lipase" in adipose tissue, mediated by cyclic AMP. This leads to a rise in plasma free fatty acids, an increase in hepatic fat, and accelerated ketogenesis. ACTH improves glucose tolerance and increases muscle glycogen by stimulating insulin secretion. Prolonged exposure to ACTH, on the other hand, can induce insulin resistance as well as cutaneous hyperpigmentation.

Pharmacokinetics

ACTH is destroyed by proteolytic enzymes and thus cannot be given orally. Similarly, when administered subcutaneously or intramuscularly, much of it is inactivated before reaching the circulation. When given intravenously, its half-life is about 15 min. The amount of ACTH in the urine is negligible, indicating inactivation in the tissues. Maximal stimulation of the adrenal cortex can be obtained with more prolonged exposure, and corticosteroid secretion shows a linear increase with the duration of ACTH infusion.

Therapeutic and Diagnostic Applications

At present corticotropin has no therapeutic usefulness, with the possible exception of multiple sclerosis. Adrenal insufficiency, its main potential indication, is better treated with oral synthetic corticosteroids. Its important use is in the diagnosis of adrenal insufficiency. The rapid ACTH stimulation test measures the rise of plasma cortisol 30 to 50 min after intramuscular or intravenous injection of ACTH or cosyntropin. In the event of a subnormal response, a more prolonged simulation can be done by infusing cosyntropin over 6 to 24 h. Primary adrenal insufficiency (Addison's disease) is characterized by the absence of a cortisol response to ACTH or cosyntropin. A mild increase in cortisol is seen in secondary adrenal insufficiency (hypopituitarism).

Adverse Reactions

Adverse reactions are mostly a result of the increased rate of secretion of corticosteroids and include fluid retention, hypokalemic alkalosis, and glucose intolerance. Hypersensitivity reactions are rare. They range from fever to life-threatening anaphylactic reactions. Synthetic ACTH, though less antigenic than the natural peptide, also rarely induces hypersensitivity.

CORTICOSTEROIDS

This section deals with two groups of corticosteroids: (1) glucocorticoids, which influence carbohydrate, lipid, and protein metabolism and possess anti-inflammatory properties; and (2) mineralocorticoids, which affect fluid and electrolyte balance. However, the biologic properties of the various corticosteroids are within a spectrum that ranges from strict glucocorticoid to strict mineralocorticoid activity.

Source and Chemistry

The naturally occurring steroid hormones originate from cholesterol. The rate-limiting step is the side-chain cleavage of cholesterol to form pregnenolone and isocaproic aldehyde. This reaction occurs in the mitochondria and requires molecular oxygen and NADPH. All corticosteroids are pregnane derivatives (Fig. 42-2) with ketone groups on C-3 and C-20, an unsaturated bond between C-4 and

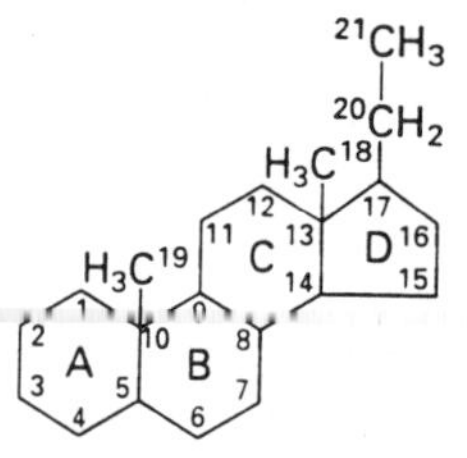

FIGURE 42-2 *Pregnane: the backbone structure of the corticosteroids.*

C-5 (denoted as Δ^4); and a 17β-CO-CH_2OH side chain. They vary in the presence or absence of an 11-keto, 11β-hydroxyl, 17α-hydroxyl group, and/or 18-oxygen function. These differences determine the main physiologic and pharmacologic actions of the end products and of some of their precursors. The main endogenous glucocorticoid is cortisol (hydrocortisone), and the main endogenous mineralocorticoid is aldosterone. Figure 42-3 shows the structural formulas of the major endogenous steroids. Figure 42-4 shows the structural formulas of commonly used synthetic corticosteroids.

Relation of Structure to Function

The relationship of chemical structure to function for corticosteroids is extremely complex, but a number of basic generalizations can be made. Generally, structural modifications alter receptor affinity, the rate of biotransformation of the compounds, and the degree of glucocorticoid or mineralocorticoid action. For glucocorticoid activity, the 11β-hydroxyl and 17α-hydroxyl groups are important. For adequate mineralocorticoid activity, the presence of oxygen at C-11 and C-18, or absence of oxygen at both C-11 and C-17, is required. In general, glucocorticoid binding occurs on the surface of the receptor, especially involving the 11β-hydroxyl and 17β-CO-CH_2OH groups, which project above the plane of the ring. Since the 11β-hydroxyl group is generally essential for glucocorticoid activity, it seems likely that this group is involved in the primary steroid-receptor combination with a secondary combination with the 17β-CO-CH_2OH side chain. Thus bulky beta substitutes would interfere with binding and decrease activity, while equatorial or alpha substitutes would not.

Since 11-desoxycorticosterone has no glucocorticoid activity but is a potent mineralocorticoid and has only two potentially reactive substitutes, receptor combination must involve the 3-keto and/or the 17β-CO-CH_2OH groups. Some association with the alpha surface of the molecule of rings A, C, and D may also be involved. The fact that the modifications affecting the D ring markedly affect mineralocorticoid activity suggests that the 17β-CO-CH_2OH side chain may be more important. 9α-Fluorination increases the mineralocorticoid potency of both 11-hydroxy (cortisol) and 11-desoxy (desoxycorticosterone) compounds. Furthermore, the influence of the 18-aldehyde group as in aldosterone is unknown. Conceivably it influences the reactivity of the 11-oxygen function, but it could also change the D ring or influence the 17β side chain.

Pharmacokinetics

Corticosteroids are well absorbed following oral administration. These compounds are also injected intramuscularly, intravenously, and intra-articularly. Glucocorticoid preparations can be applied locally to the skin, nasal mucosa, and eyes. Although topical application of these drugs limits systemic absorption, it is possible to produce systemic adverse reactions with glucocorticoids when they are used on large areas of skin or applied excessively to the eye.

Corticosteroids are reversibly bound in plasma to two proteins: corticosteroid-binding globulin (transcortin), a specific high-affinity α_2-globulin; and albumin, which has nonspecific, low-affinity binding properties. These compounds are biotransformed in the liver and to some extent in the kidney. They can undergo reduction, hydroxylation, and conjugation reactions and are then excreted in the urine.

Mechanism of Action

Steroids enter target cells by simple diffusion due to their high lipid solubility. Upon entering the cell the steroid molecule binds to a cytoplasmic receptor, which is a polypeptide. This steroid-receptor complex then undergoes a conformational change with the dissociation of a heat shock protein (hsp90). This activated steroid-receptor complex is then translocated into the nucleus where it binds to a specific site in chromosomal DNA. The attached transformed steroid-receptor complex on DNA initiates gene activation to cause transcription to produce specific mRNA which eventually

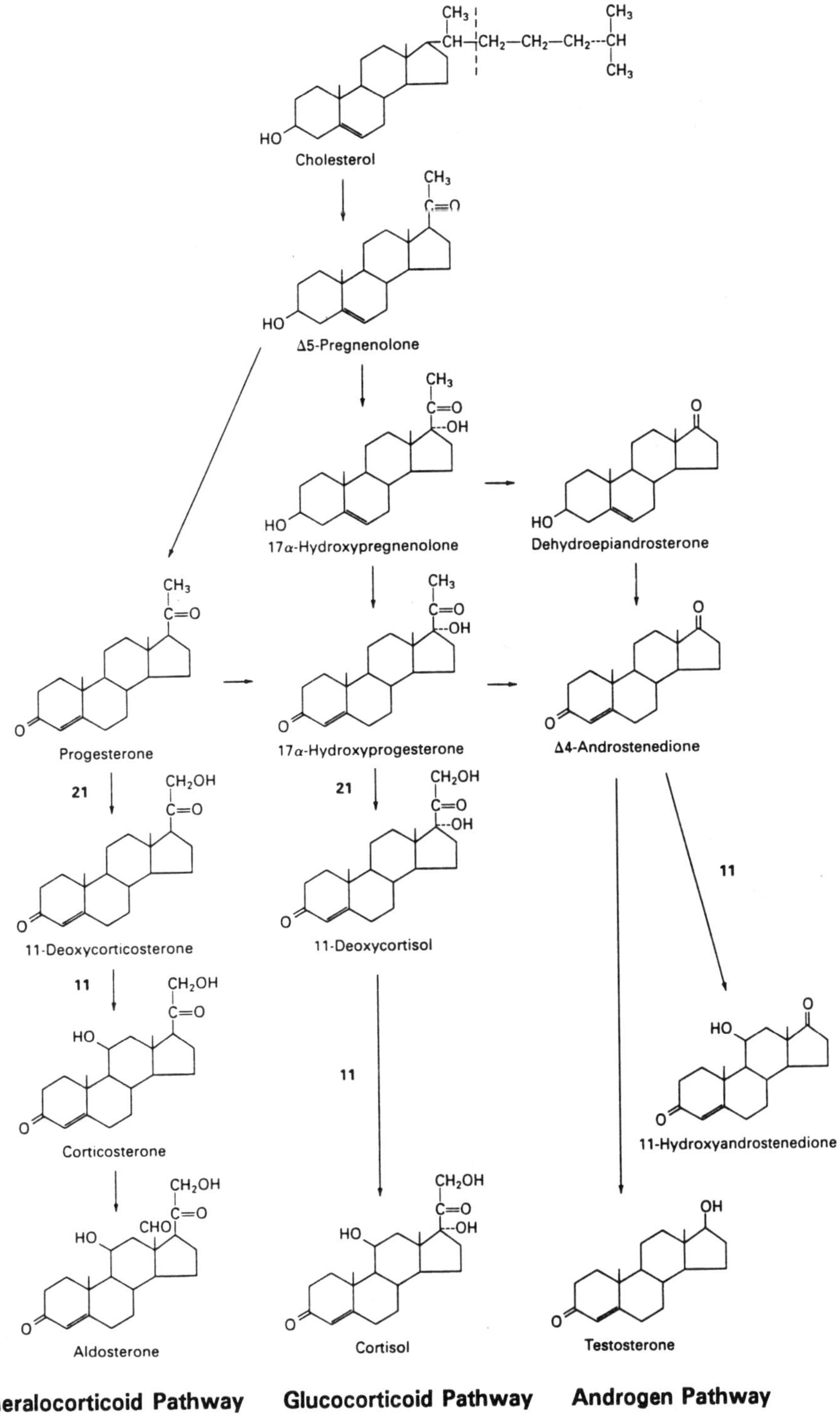

Cholesterol

Δ5-Pregnenolone

17α-Hydroxypregnenolone

Dehydroepiandrosterone

Progesterone

17α-Hydroxyprogesterone

Δ4-Androstenedione

11-Deoxycorticosterone

11-Deoxycortisol

Corticosterone

11-Hydroxyandrostenedione

Aldosterone

Cortisol

Testosterone

Mineralocorticoid Pathway **Glucocorticoid Pathway** **Androgen Pathway**

FIGURE 42-3 *Biosynthetic pathways of adrenal corticosteroids.* ***21*** *= C-21 hydroxylase;* ***11*** *= C-11 hydroxylase.*

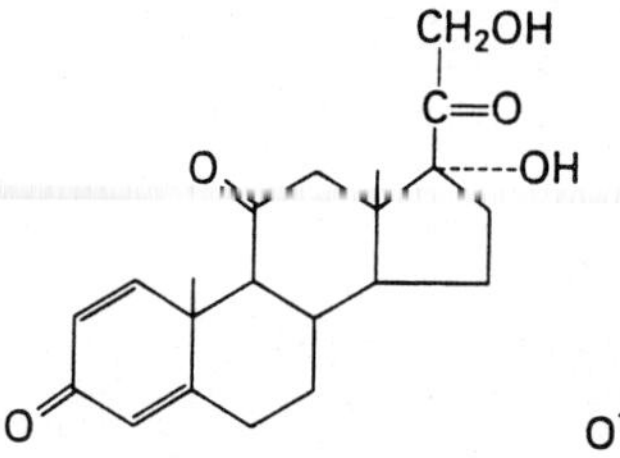

FIGURE 42-4 *Structural formulas of commonly used synthetic corticosteroids.*

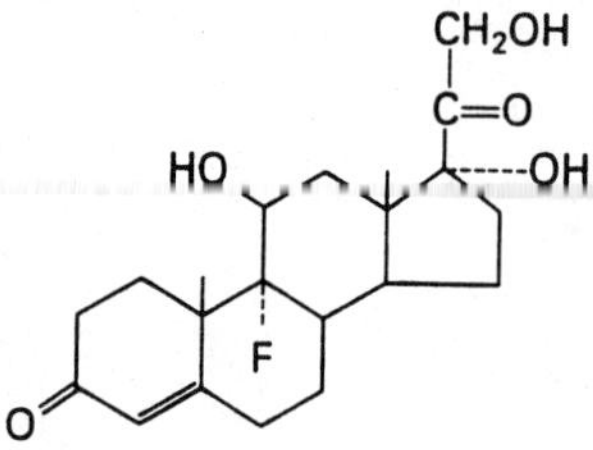

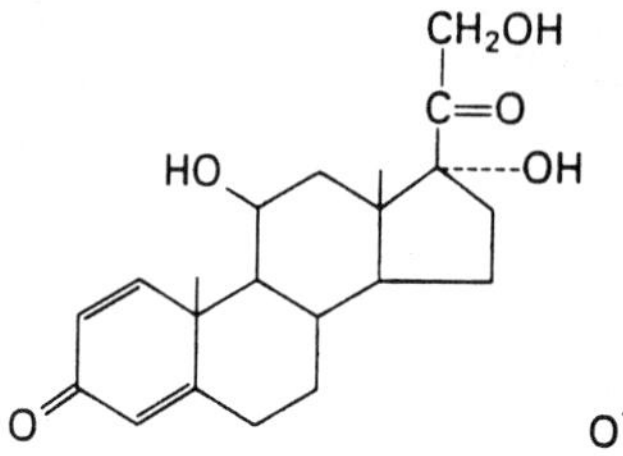

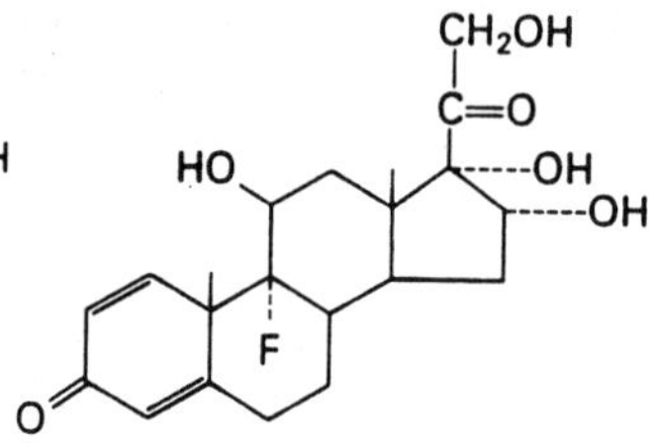

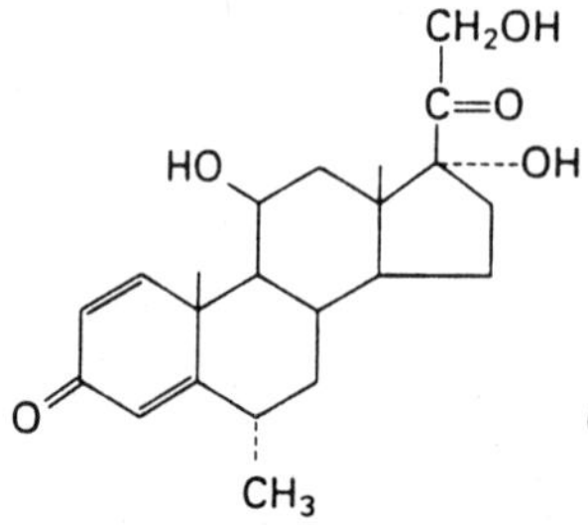

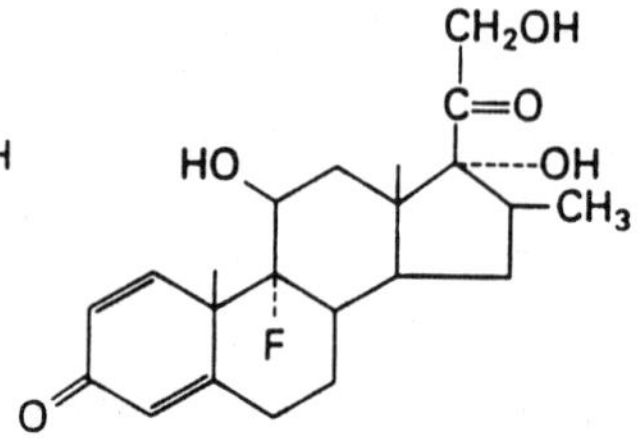

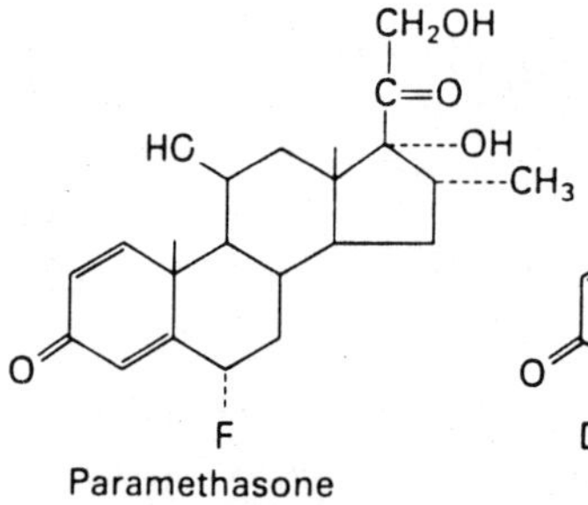

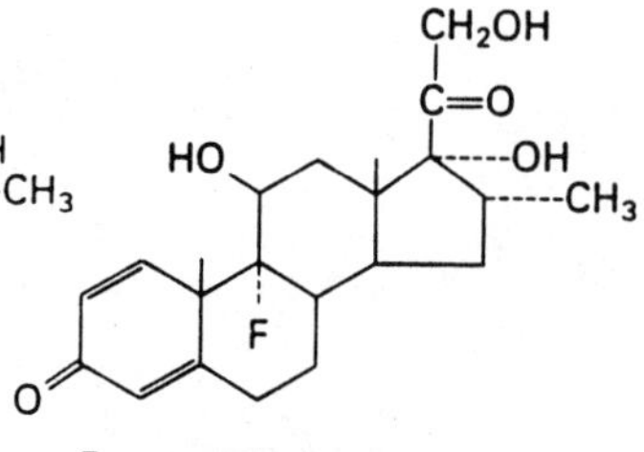

leads to protein formation and modification of cellular activity.

Anti-inflammatory and Immunosuppressive Actions

Glucocorticoids display both anti-inflammatory and immunosuppressive characteristics through complex and, at times, shared mechanisms. They act on the different components of the inflammatory process, which includes various cell types, enzymes, and vascular responses. They increase the polymorphonuclear count by accelerating the transfer of mature neutrophils from the bone marrow but inhibit their passage from blood to the site of inflammation. Glucocorticoids also cause lymphocytopenia, monocytopenia, and eosinopenia by several mechanisms, which probably include redistribution of these cells into other compartments, including the bone marrow, lymphoid tissue, and spleen. In addition, there is a delayed release of monocyte precursors from the bone marrow. The end result is decreased influx of leukocytes to the inflammatory site.

Prostaglandins and leukotrienes are involved in the inflammatory process. Glucocorticoids cause the formation of lipocortin which inhibits the catalytic activity phospholipase A_2 to release arachidonic acid from cellular membranes which results in prevention or decrease in the synthesis of prostaglandins and leukotrienes. Glucocorticoids also inhibit the inflammatory effects of interleukin-1 (IL-1), tumor necrosis factor (TNF), and macrophage migration-inhibitory factor (MIF). The actions of these substances are described below in the discussion on the immune response and glucocorticoids. In addition, glucocorticoids suppresses the vasodilation which is responsible for increased capillary permeability and edema in inflammation.

Most immunologic processes display an inflammatory component upon which glucocorticoids can act. Although all subpopulations of lymphocytes are decreased, the depression of cell-mediated immunity is probably not the sole result of direct action of corticosteroids on T lymphocytes; rather, steroids seem to act preferentially, by direct or indirect means, on the macrophages. Thus, decreased recruitment of the latter leads to blunted cutaneous delayed hypersensitivity. The effect of MIF and macrophage aggregating factor (MAF) is suppressed, resulting in decreased access of these cells to the sites of inflammatory and immunologic processes. Other components of the immune response that are inhibited by glucocorticoids include TNF, IL-1, interleukin-2 (IL-2), and interferon gamma. TNF enhances the inflammatory process, and IL-1 activates resting T cells. Activated T cells elaborate interleukins 2, 3, 4, 5, and 6 and interferon gamma. IL-1 also increases proliferation and maturation of B cells to plasma cells which produce antibodies. IL-1 can stimulate the formation prostaglandin E_2. IL-2 may activate cytotoxic lymphocytes and promotes division of activated T cells and interferon gamma enhances the ability of macrophages and B cells to handle antigens. TNF and IL-1 are released from macrophages following macrophage interaction with an antigen (cell-mediated immunity). Corticosteroids inhibit the passage of immune complexes across basement membranes and decrease the levels of complement. There is some evidence that glucocorticoids do not suppress antibody production (a hormonal immune response); however, they do inhibit the effects of interleukins and interferon gamma on B cells.

Effects on Organ Systems

Glucocorticoids influence virtually every tissue and organ in the body. The end result of their action is the induction (anabolism) or suppression (catabolism) of protein synthesis. For example, following glucocorticoid administration, there is a marked increase in the concentration and activity of liver enzymes such as glucose-6-phosphatase, fructose-6-diphosphatase, and phosphoenolpyruvate carboxykinase. But glucocorticoids can also suppress DNA synthesis; induce protein breakdown in muscle; suppress inflammatory responses; and inhibit cell proliferation in epithelial, lymphoid, connective, and bone tissue. In lymphatic cells, glucocorticoids stimulate the synthesis of an "inhibiting protein" responsible for the catabolic action.

Mineralocorticoids (e.g., aldosterone) facilitate the transport of sodium across the distal renal tubule epithelium and collecting duct. They increase the activity of enzymes involved in the generation of adenosine triphosphate (ATP), which will act as an energy source for the sodium pump. They also increase phospholipase activity, fatty acid synthesis, and acyltransferase activity. These actions play a role in the regulation of the sodium transport.

Table 42-1 shows the relative anti-inflammatory and sodium-retaining potencies of some natural and synthetic corticosteroids.

TABLE 42-1 Relative potencies of some natural and synthetic corticosteroids

Drug	Relative anti-inflammatory effect[a]	Relative sodium-retaining effect[a]	Equivalent dose for systemic anti-inflammatory activity, mg
Glucocorticoids			
Short-acting drugs (biologic half-life: 8 to 12 h)			
Hydrocortisone (cortisol)	1.0	1.0	20
Cortisone	0.8	0.8	25
Prednisone	4.0	4.0	5
Prednisolone	4.0	4.0	5
Methylprednisolone	5.0	5.0	4
Intermediate-acting drugs (biologic half-life: 12 to 36 h)			
Triamcinolone	5.0	0	4
Paramethasone	10.0	0	2
Long-acting drugs (biologic half-life: over 36 h)			
Dexamethasone	30.0	0	0.75
Betamethasone	30.0	0	0.6
Mineralocorticoids			
Aldosterone	0	300 to 900	
Fludrocortisone	10.0	250	

[a] Based on hydrocortisone as 1.0

Carbohydrate and Protein Metabolism When glucocorticoids are administered acutely to normal fasting humans, their catabolic action mobilizes amino acids from protein in muscle and plasma, increasing their flow to the liver, where they serve as substrates for gluconeogenesis. Glucose utilization by peripheral tissues is inhibited. Fatty acids are mobilized from adipose tissue and replace glucose as an energy source for muscle. This results in a rise in plasma glucose, stimulating insulin release to prevent ketogenesis. More prolonged exposure to glucocorticoids can cause a diabetogenic effect. The glucocorticoids stimulate the release of glucagon, which promotes gluconeogenesis and decreases sensitivity to insulin, and can cause hyperglycemia. The overall effect of glucocorticoids on energy metabolism is the conservation of carbohydrate (in the form of glycogen) and the use of proteins and lipids as alternative sources of fuel.

Lipid Metabolism Lipogenesis is normally initiated when glucose, under the action of insulin, enters the adipocytes. It is then metabolized to acetyl CoA, which will be used for fatty acid synthesis. Fatty acids, in turn, are esterified with glycerol phosphate to form triglycerides. This anabolic cascade is inhibited by glucocorticoids; this blockade can be overcome by large doses of insulin. Glucocorticoids can promote lipolysis. Lipolysis occurs with stimulation of an adipocyte "hormone-sensitive lipase" by catecholamines and various hormones such as ACTH, glucagon, and thyroid-stimulating hormone (TSH). However, the presence of glucocorticoids is usually necessary for this activation. Insulin blocks this effect. Thus the antagonistic actions of glucocorticoids and insulin participate in the regulation of lipid metabolism. Clinically, patients with glucocorticoid excess exhibit a characteristic redistribution of fat, which accumulates in the face ("moon face"), interscapular area ("buffalo hump"), supraclavicular fossae, and omentum (truncal obesity).

Electrolyte and Water Metabolism Aldosterone is the most potent endogenous mineralocorticoid. It acts on the distal renal tubules and collecting ducts, where it promotes sodium reabsorption and increases urinary excretion of potassium and hydrogen ions. Adrenal insufficiency is characterized by hyponatremia, hyperkalemia, acidosis, contraction of extracellular volume, cell hydration, and increased urinary excretion of sodium. In the absence of exogenous mineralocorticoid, most patients can be maintained alive with sodium chloride solution.

Hypercorticism results in a positive sodium balance, normal or increased plasma sodium concentration, hypokalemic hypochloremic alkalosis, and increased extracellular volume. If this state persists, sodium excretion eventually increases until it equals sodium intake, thus averting gross edema. However, despite this poorly understood "escape phenomenon," the excessive urinary excretion of potassium and hydrogen ions continues.

Glucocorticoids also can possess mineralocorticoid activity and can cause salt and water retention, but they are 1000 times less potent than aldosterone, thus limiting the amount of free cortisol available to compete for mineralocorticoid-binding sites. Newer synthetic compounds are essentially devoid of mineralocorticoid effects.

Central Nervous System In states of hypercorticism (Cushing's syndrome), there are profound effects on the CNS. Up to 20 percent of patients are psychotic. Other psychologic manifestations include irritability, insomnia, difficulty in concentrating, and hallucinations. When Cushing's syndrome is drug-induced, the most common manifestation is euphoria.

Patients with Addison's disease commonly exhibit apathy, depression, and fatigue. There is a lowered threshold for the senses of taste, smell, and hearing. An EEG shows diffuse high-amplitude slowing of activity.

The exact mechanism of glucocorticoid action on the central nervous system is not well understood. Glucocorticoids regulate cerebral blood flow and the movement of sodium and potassium across cell membranes. They also modulate neural conduction by their stimulatory effect on neurotransmitter release; in high doses they increase neuronal excitability and lower the seizure threshold.

Cardiovascular System The effect of mineralocorticoids on sodium and water retention, hence on plasma volume, has already been discussed. However, the cardiovascular actions of corticosteroids are complex and still poorly understood. Adrenal insufficiency is characterized by hypotension and decreased cardiac output. Heart size is reduced and myocardial contractility is depressed. Arteriolar tone is diminished, partly through decreased inhibition of prostacyclin (PGI_2) synthesis. Capillary permeability is increased. These phenomena do not respond to volume expansion or administration of catecholamines, but they respond dramatically to intravenous cortisol.

Cushing's syndrome is also accompanied by depressed cardiac output. This effect, however, is a result of prolonged arterial hypertension and is not totally reversible after treatment of the hyperadrenocortical state.

Gastrointestinal System High-dose glucocorticoids are associated with an increased incidence of gastric and duodenal ulcers. However, the incidence of such ulcers in patients with natural Cushing's syndrome is the same as in the normal population. High-dose steroids increase gastric secretion of acid and pepsin, but this effect is probably not a major contributing factor, since patients with achlorhydria can also develop steroid-induced ulcers. More importantly, glucocorticoids decrease the rate of gastric mucous secretion and reduce the rate of renewal of gastric surface epithelial cells, thus weakening the physical barrier and delaying the healing of mucosal lesions.

Musculoskeletal System Excess glucocorticoids cause muscle weakness and can, with chronic use, lead to muscle atrophy. This steroid-induced myopathy is a result of increased protein breakdown. Adrenal insufficiency is associated with weakness and fatigability, but this may be due to the compromised cardiovascular state rather than to a primary effect on muscle. In primary aldosteronism, the observed weakness is secondary to hypokalemia.

Children treated with supraphysiologic doses of glucocorticoids exhibit a delay in linear growth and skeletal maturation. Osteopenia is a frequent complication of chronic steroid therapy and is the end result of two distinct mechanisms: (1) direct inhibition of osteoblasts, and (2) inhibition of intestinal calcium absorption, leading to secondary hyperparathyroidism and consequently to stimulation of osteoclastic activity. Cartilage breakdown may occur, leading to joint degeneration. The analgesic properties of glucocorticoids might facilitate the prolonged, painless traumatization of the joint and development of a severe arthropathy. Avascular necrosis of bone is another complication of glucocorticoid excess. Its mechanism remains poorly understood.

Skin and Connective Tissue The main cutaneous finding in adrenal insufficiency is the slow development of a diffuse hyperpigmentation, more pronounced over exposed areas of skin, areas subject to pressure and friction such as the knees and axillae, and, more characteristically, in the creases of palms and soles. Normally pigmented areas such as the nipples and genital skin appear darker. This phenomenon is a result of increased plasma levels of melanocyte-stimulating hormone (MSH, melanocortin) which, along with ACTH, is derived by proteolytic cleavage from a common precursor glycoprotein, pro-opiomelanocortin. Vitiligo may appear, interspersed with hypermelanosis, indicating the presence of "idiopathic" adrenal insufficiency, an acquired autoimmune disorder. Body hair is diminished and at times absent.

Excessive glucocorticoids inhibit fibroblast activity, resulting in decreased collagen formation. Patients with Cushing's syndrome exhibit thinning of skin and the development of purplish striae, predominantly on the lower abdomen and hips. The loss of collagen support around subcutaneous blood vessels lead to easy bruising and purpura. Skin ulcers may develop as a result of minor trauma and wound healing is delayed. The changes in fat distribution have been described earlier. Women may display mild hirsutism and acne secondary to increased production of androgens by the adrenals. Hyperpigmentation, such as in Addison's disease, can be seen in Cushing's disease, in which a pituitary adenoma secretes large amounts of ACTH.

Endocrine Effects The hypothalamic-hypophyseal-adrenal axis, like many other endocrine systems, is regulated by a negative-feedback mechanism. Glucocorticoids inhibit release of ACTH. Administration of exogenous corticosteroids for more than 3 weeks causes decreased stimulation of the adrenals by ACTH, resulting in atrophy of the adrenal cortex. The degree of atrophy is dose-dependent. Even a low-dose regimen, such as prednisone, 5 mg/day, or its equivalent, can induce detectable adrenal suppression. The fascicular and reticular zones are most affected. The zona glomerulosa, which secretes aldosterone, is minimally dependent on ACTH and thus is least sensitive to pituitary suppression. The clinical implication of adrenal atrophy is the development of primary adrenal insufficiency. The exogenous corticosteroids are sufficient to replace output by the deficient gland under basal conditions. However, in stressful situations such as surgery, major illness, or trauma, when a normal adrenal would increase in production by up to tenfold, larger doses of steroids should be administered to avoid development of a state identical to adrenal crisis. When chronic steroid therapy is discontinued, increased production of ACTH stimulates the adrenal once again. However, during the first 9 to 12 months following interruption of therapy, the gland, which has not fully recovered from its prolonged suppression, remains in a state of relative insufficiency and is unable to meet the increased demands in conditions of stress. Such patients are at risk of developing acute adrenal insufficiency, and should be covered with large doses of exogenous steroids throughout the duration of their illness.

Functional Tests

Dexamethasone Suppression Tests Hypercortisolism (Cushing's syndrome) can be the result of abnormal adrenal hyperactivity secondary to adrenal adenoma or carcinoma, an ACTH-secreting pituitary adenoma, or ectopic production of ACTH or CRF. However, hypercortisolism can also be a normal physiologic response to stress.

Dexamethasone is a potent synthetic glucocorticoid which can suppress the pituitary-adrenal axis at a dose which will not affect plasma or urinary concentrations of endogenous steroids. Its structure is shown in Fig. 42-4.

Overnight Dexamethasone Suppression Test Dexamethasone (1.0 mg) is given orally at 11:00 PM. The plasma cortisol level at 8:00 AM the next day should be less than 5 μg/dL, indicating normal negative feedback. Higher cortisol levels are suggestive, but not diagnostic, of hyperadrenocorticism. In Cushing's syndrome, levels are usually greater than 20 μg/dL. This is a rapid test, frequently used for screening purposes, with the knowledge that false positive results are not infrequent.

Low-Dose and High-Dose Dexamethasone Suppression Tests These tests are done consecutively over a 6-day period. During the first 2 days,

24-h urine samples are collected for free cortisol and creatinine. On days 3 and 4, dexamethasone (0.5 mg) is given orally every 6 h, starting at 8:00 AM, as urine collection continues. On days 5 and 6, dexamethasone (2.0 mg) is given orally every 6 h, while urine collection proceeds. Plasma cortisol is measured at 4:00 PM on days 4 and 6. A normal suppression on low-dose dexamethasone is indicated by a greater than 50 percent drop in urine cortisol or a plasma cortisol level less than 5 μg/dL. On high-dose dexamethasone, a greater than 50 percent fall in urine cortisol or a plasma cortisol less than 10 μg/dL indicates partial suppression and is suggestive of an ACTH-producing pituitary adenoma (Cushing's disease). Failure to suppress suggests adrenal tumor or ectopic production of ACTH or CRF.

False positive results can be seen in some patients with endogenous depression. Patients on phenytoin or phenobarbital also fail to suppress, secondary to the accelerated rate of metabolism of dexamethasone. Other drugs such as sympathomimetics, nasal decongestants, and oral contraceptive agents can also inhibit dexamethasone suppression. Finally, as mentioned earlier, stress is a frequent cause of false positive results, especially among hospitalized patients.

ACTH Stimulation Test The secretory reserve of the adrenal cortex can be determined by its response to exogenous ACTH. A 24-h infusion of cosyntropin is initiated with a concomitant 24-h urine collection for 17-hydroxycorticosteroids. A partial rise in 17-hydroxycorticosteroids is suggestive of secondary adrenal insufficiency (hypopituitarism); failure to respond is characteristic of primary adrenal failure (Addison's disease). Sometimes, a more prolonged, 48-h, infusion is necessary to separate those two entities. A quicker alternative is the rapid cosyntropin test; 0.25 mg (about 25 units) of cosyntropin is injected intravenously or intramuscularly. Plasma cortisol and aldosterone are measured before and 30 or 60 min after injection. Normally, cortisol should rise by more than 7 μg/dL from baseline with a peak level greater than 20 μg/dL. Primary adrenal insufficiency is characterized by a subnormal response of cortisol and aldosterone. A normal rise in aldosterone with a subnormal cortisol response is indicative of secondary adrenal insufficiency.

Metyrapone Test Metyrapone is one of several drugs designed to block steroidogenesis. Specifically, it inhibits 11β-hydroxylase, the enzyme which catalyzes the addition of a hydroxyl group on position 11 of 11-deoxycortisol and 11-deoxycorticosterone to form cortisol and corticosterone, respectively (see Fig. 42-3).

Metyrapone has been used as a diagnostic test for hypothalamic-pituitary-ACTH function. The use of metyrapone as a diagnostic test has decreased because of nonspecific results and that ACTH plasma levels can be directly determined. The drug, however, has been used in investigational studies to treat Cushing's syndrome, since metyrapone can block the synthesis of cortisol as does aminoglutethimide.

Clinical Uses of Corticosteroids

Corticosteroids do not cure any disease, but they are nevertheless used in a variety of conditions where their anti-inflammatory, immunosuppressive, and mineralocorticoid properties are applied. They also serve as replacement therapy in patients with adrenal insufficiency. Corticosteroids can be life-saving in status asthmaticus, severe allergic reactions, and transplantation rejection. They are available as nasal sprays for allergic rhinitis. They are effective in noninfectious granulomatous diseases, such as sarcoid, and in man, collagen vascular diseases, particularly rheumatoid arthritis and systemic lupus erythematosus. Intra-articular injection is indicated in some rheumatoid disorders. They have been used in treatment of leukemia. They can also be applied topically as ointments, creams, lotions, and sprays for treatment of dermatologic and ophthalmologic diseases.

A wide variety of corticosteroid preparations are available as to potency, concentration, and formulation. Topical corticosteroid preparations are generally formulated as creams, lotions, ointments, gels, and solutions. Selected corticosteroid dermatologic preparations are list in Table 42-2. For example, low to moderate potency preparations may be used to treat most cases of atopic dermatitis, facial psoriasis, and seborrheic dermatitis, while the more potent anti-inflammatory preparations are used in such conditions as discoid lupus erythematosus, lichen simplex chronicus, and allergen-induced contact dermatitis. In cases

TABLE 42-2 Selected Corticosteroid Dermatological Preparations

Low Potency
- Alclometasone dipropionate, 0.05%
- Desonide, 0.05%
- Dexamethasone, 0.01 - 0.04%
- Fluocinolone acetonide, 0.01%
- Hydrocortisone, 0.25 - 2.5%

Moderate Potency
- Betamethasone benzoate, 0.025%
- Fluocinolone acetonide, 0.025%
- Flurandrenolide, 0.025 - 0.5%
- Hydrocortisone valerate, 0.2%
- Triamcinolone acetonide, 0.025 - 0.1%

High Potency
- Amcinonide, 0.1%
- Desoximetasone, 0.25%
- Halcinonide, 0.1%
- Triamcinolone acetonide, 0.5%

Highest Potency
- Betamethasone dipropionate, 0.05%
- Clobetasol propionate, 0.05%
- Diflorasone diacetate, 0.05%
- Halobetasol propionate, 0.05%

of acute, severe allergic contact dermatitis injectable or oral corticosteroids may be needed.

Although steroids are applied topically to the cutaneous inflammation, these preparations can cause adverse reactions of a systemic nature. Adverse reactions such as thinning of skin, purpura, hypopigmentation, increased intraocular pressure, iatrogenic Cushing's syndrome, and growth suppression in children have been reported.

Adverse Reactions

Corticosteroids are very potent drugs, and it is virtually impossible to achieve clinical improvement on pharmacologic doses of steroids without inducing side effects. Consequently, they should be used at the smallest effective dose and over the briefest period (in short-lived illnesses). There are no absolute contraindications for their use, especially in life-threatening situations. However, continued use of large doses can result in iatrogenic Cushing's syndrome. Corticosteroid therapy can also lead to peptic ulceration with or without hemorrhage, cataracts, and increased susceptibility to infection. Osteoporosis may be induced by chronic use in the elderly. Myopathy is an uncommon but serious complication. Psychosis can also occur. Therefore, caution should be exercised when administering corticosteroids to patients with peptic ulcer disease, osteoporosis, tuberculosis, and other chronic infections and psychological disorders.

In intensive corticosteroid therapy, sudden cessation results in withdrawal symptoms consisting mainly of signs of adrenal insufficiency, but they may also include fever, myalgia, arthralgia, and malaise. It is advisable to reduce corticosteroid doses gradually rather than terminate therapy abruptly.

Dosage

By far the most serious complication of chronic steroid therapy (more than 3 weeks duration) is suppression of the hypothalamic-pituitary-adrenal axis (HPA axis). Dosage should thus be frequently adjusted according to disease activity to avoid overtreatment. Moreover, the choice of steroids is important, since preparations with long half-lives, such as dexamethasone, cause more suppression than those preparations with shorter half-lives such as hydrocortisone or prednisone. Similarly, the more potent drugs have more potential for suppression (Table 42-1). During full-blown disease activity, patients are placed on a several-times daily, relatively large dose corticosteroid regimen. If clinical improvement occurs but the primary stimulus for the disease process is still present, steroid administration is reduced to one daily morning dose. As remission is maintained, an alternate-day regimen is substituted, whereby double the daily dose is given as a single dose every, other day. This method is thought to minimize inhibition of the HPA axis while keeping disease activity in a stable subclinical state. If relapse occurs, a temporary return to divided-dose daily corticosteroids will be necessary.

Glucocorticoid Inhibitors

There are certain patients with endogenous Cushing's syndrome in whom surgery can not be performed. In these patients it may be necessary to pharmacologically decrease glucocorticoid levels. Aminoglutethimide and ketoconazole can inhibit steroidogenesis. These modalities offer palliation only. Their main side effect is adrenocortical insufficiency. Aminoglutethimide inhibits the conversion of cholesterol to pregnenolone. The drug is given orally and the dosage is titrated to the desired plasma cortisol level. Ketoconazole inhibits the cytochrome P-450 system in many organs including the adrenal glands. Thus it can be effective in decreasing steroid levels when administered orally. Ketoconazole is used in the adjunctive medical management of Cushing's syndrome where surgery fails or is not possible. When it is used, adverse effects need to be closely monitored, particularly hepatic toxicity.

Spironolactone

Mineralocorticoids such as aldosterone increase renal tubular reabsorption of sodium and chloride and augment potassium excretion. Spironolactone is a synthetic compound which belongs to the group of 17-spirolactone steroids.

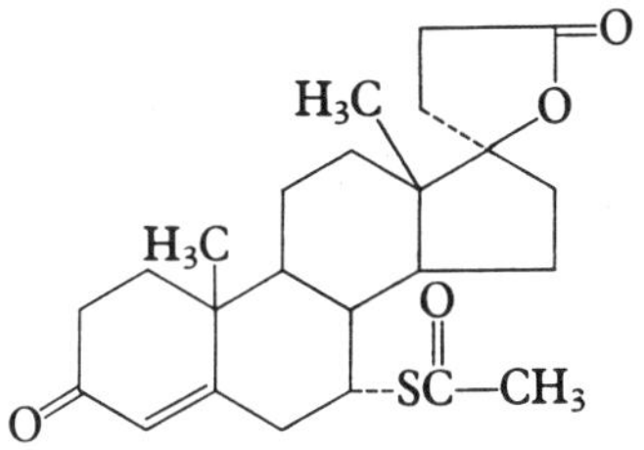

Spironolactone has no positive intrinsic activity. It is a competitive aldosterone antagonist, binding to the same receptor sites as the natural hormone. Spironolactone thus is only effective in the presence of aldosterone and is indicated in the treatment of primary and secondary hyperaldosteronism. Its pharmacology is discussed in Chapter 31 ("Diuretics") since spironolactone is used as a potassium-sparing diuretic.

BIBLIOGRAPHY

Baxter, J.D.: "The Effects of Glucocorticoid Therapy," *Hosp. Pract.* **15**: 111-114 (1992).

Ellis, E.F.: "Steroid Myopathy," *J. Allergy Clin. Immunol.* **76**: 431-432 (1985).

Hers, H.G.: "Effects of Glucocorticoids on Carbohydrate Metabolism," *Agents Actions,* **17**: 248-254 (1985).

Milgrom, H., and B.G. Bender: "Psychologic Side Effects of Therapy with Corticosteroids", *Amer. Rev. Resp. Dis.* **147**: 471-473 (1993).

Pratt, W.B.: "Transformation of Glucocorticoid and Progesterone Receptors to the DNA-Binding State," *J. Cell. Biochem.* **35**: 51-68 (1987).

Reisine, T.: "Neurohormonal Aspects of ACTH Release," *Hosp. Pract.* **77**: 96 (1988).

Rose, L.I., G.H. Williams, P.I. Jagger, and D.P. Lawler: "The 48-Hour Adrenocotrophin Infusion Test for Adrenocortical Insufficiency," *Ann. Intern. Med.* **73**: 49-54 (1970).

Sheeler, L.R.: "Cushing's Syndrome-1988," *Cleve. Clin. J. Med.* **55**: 329-337 (1988).

Snow, K., N.S. Jiang, P.C. Kao, and B.W. Scheithauer: "Biochemical Evaluation of Adrenal Dysfunction: The Laboratory Perspective," *Mayo Clin. Proc.* **67**: 1055-1065 (1992).

Sonino, N.: "The Use of Ketoconazole as an Inhibitor of Steroid Production," *N. Engl. J.Med.* **317**: 811-818 (1988).

Szefter, S.J.: "Anti-inflammatory Drugs in the Treatment of Allergic Disease," *Med. Clin North Amer.* **74**: 953-975 (1992).

Taylor, A.L., and L.M. Fishman: "Corticotropin-Releasing Hormone," *N.Engl. J. Med.*, **319**: 213-222 (1988).

PART IX

Antineoplastic Agents

SECTION EDITOR

Joseph R. DiPalma

CHAPTER 43

Cancer Chemotherapy

Pamela A. Crilley and Michael J. Styler

The cure of a patient with cancer depends on the success of removal or destruction of every cancer cell within the body. Currently, even with the best and most efficiently applied detection procedures, only 50 percent of all newly diagnosed cancer patients will be cured of their disease. The reason for failure to cure is not delay in diagnosis; it is because cancer has spread beyond the confines of its primary location, making any local form of therapy inadequate. In essence, these patients need some form of systemic treatment.

Surgery, chemotherapy, and radiation constitute the three forms of treatment for cancer, but only chemotherapy can effectively treat systemic disease.

Cancer chemotherapy is totally nonspecific. By that it is meant that the drugs kill not only cancer cells but also normal cells that happen to be dividing. Because of the nonspecificity of killing, strategies have been developed to increase the relative cancer-killing potential of these agents by lessening the toxic impact on normal tissues. These strategies require a knowledge of the pharmacology of the drugs as well as a knowledge of tumor cell kinetics.

It has been recognized for decades that cancers grow at different rates than the tissues from which they are derived. Paradoxically, and contrary to what is expected, normal tissues often grow faster than the cancerous ones. Thus normal tissues may recover from the cytoinhibitory effects of cancer chemotherapy faster than the cancer being treated. By "cycling" the drug therapy being given, differential cytotoxicity favoring cancer cytoreduction may occur. Then it is incumbent upon the clinician to recognize these patients for optimum therapy to be given.

Much has been written about the side effects and toxicities of cancer therapy. One should distinguish the difference between a noncytotoxic toxicity (e.g., nausea and vomiting) and a cytotoxic effect on normal tissue (e.g., bone marrow suppression). Similarly, the clinician should recognize why chemotherapy may fail. Cytokinetic failure and lethal adverse effects created in normal tissues are obvious reasons. Repair of cellular damage, impaired cellular drug penetrance, increased cellular drug excretion, and drug detoxification are other mechanisms for failure of therapy. A molecular biological approach in which specific drug receptors are identified and where cellular metabolism is defined has made possible a more efficient selective toxicity for the malignant cell, as compared to the normal cell.

THE CELL CYCLE

Cell division by both normal and neoplastic cells progresses through an orderly sequence of events collectively called the *cell cycle*. The biochemical changes that occur within growing cells during the cell cycle have been divided into four major phases (Fig. 43-1). The M phase is the period of mitosis (cell division); the S phase is the time during which DNA is synthesized. The G_1 phase is usually the longest phase and is the interval during which RNA synthesis, protein synthesis, and cellular growth occur. The G_2 phase is the interval during which formation of specialized proteins, in preparation for mitosis, occurs. Cells that are dormant or in a resting state, but which retain the potential to divide, are in phase G_0.

Most cancer chemotherapy drugs cause cell death by affecting the ability of cells to divide. This means the drugs inhibit one or more of the phases of the cell cycle or prevent a cell in G_0 from entering into the cycle. Drugs that inhibit cell replication during a phase of the cycle are termed *cell cycle-specific cytotoxic agents*. Methotrexate

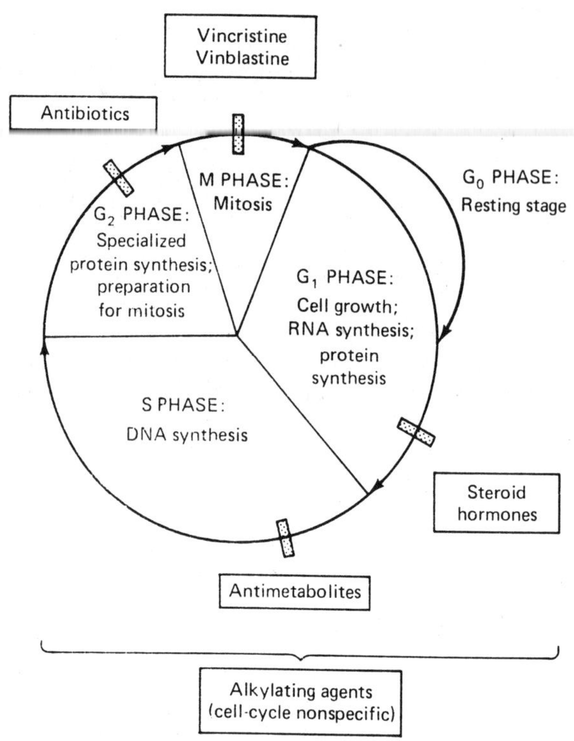

FIGURE 43-1 *The cell cycle. This diagram indicates where some cancer chemotherapeutic agents act during the cell growth cycle. Antibiotics, for example, are cell cycle-specific for the G_2 phase; alkylating agents are cell cycle-nonspecific and affect cell growth during all phases.*

for example, is a cell cycle-specific antimetabolite that inhibits DNA synthesis during the S phase. Because its cytotoxic action is restricted to one phase of the cell cycle, methotrexate is termed a *phase-specific cytotoxic agent*. Agents that are active while the cancer cells are dividing but whose action spans more than one phase of the cycle are termed *cycle-specific agents*. *Cell cycle-nonspecific drugs* (e.g., mechlorethamine, an alkylating agent) affect cellular division at all phases of the cell cycle as well as cells within G_0. Figure 43-1 shows an outline of the site of action of various cancer chemotherapeutic agents in the cell cycle. Cells that are in the G_0 phase are relatively resistant to most chemotherapy drugs and require increased dosages to attain any response. The toxicity of cycle-specific drugs is proportional to the length of exposure, whereas the toxicity of the cycle-nonspecific drugs is purely dose-related. Therefore cycle-specific drugs given by continuous infusion become much more toxic than the same total dose given as an intravenous bolus. This is because during increased exposure time, an increased proportion of cells will pass through the specific phase affected by the drug.

Malignant neoplasms are composed of *dividing cells, nondividing cells* (G_0), and *end-stage cells*, which have permanently lost the capacity to divide and will eventually die. The *growth fraction* relates the fraction of cells in cell cycle to the portion of nonproliferating cells (G_0 and end-stage cells). Chemotherapy is most effective against dividing cells. As cancers enlarge, the growth fraction usually decreases, and consequently the number of cells sensitive to chemotherapy decreases. Chemotherapy also tends to be more cytotoxic against cells with a short cycle length (e.g., lymphoma and leukemia) than those with a long cycle length (e.g., colon cancer and lung cancer).

Mathematical models have been developed to describe the complex growth of neoplasms. At low tumor burden (< 10,000 cells), growth of cancers is exponential. This rapid growth phase reflects a short cycle length, minimal cell loss, and a high growth fraction. These facts mean that the time it takes for the total number of cells within a given neoplasm to double (doubling time) is short. With time, however, the doubling time increases, the growth fraction decreases, and a graph of tumor size versus time demonstrates a plateau. The equation for this type of growth pattern was originally described by the eighteenth-century mathematician Gompertz and is known as *Gompertzian growth*. For these reasons, advanced cancers are generally less responsive to chemotherapy than those treated earlier.

In order for chemotherapy to be effective for neoplasms with a low growth fraction, the noncycling (G_0) cells need to be forced back into cycle where they will be more vulnerable. A combination of drugs, usually including cycle-nonspecific agents, are given initially. The cycle-nonspecific drugs usually reduce tumor bulk and recruit resting cells into cycle. After a rest period of several weeks to allow recovery of normal tissues, a different combination of drugs (i.e., phase- or cycle-specific) is administered. This strategy enhances tumoricidal effectiveness, reduces clinical side effects, and decreases the emergence of multiple drug-resistant clones.

Chemotherapy is often administered in cycles every 3 or 4 weeks to allow recovery of normal tissues. Each cycle kills malignant cells by first-order kinetics; that is, a constant fraction of cells is killed each month, not a constant number of cells. Therefore the ability to reduce the tumor cell number to zero (and cure the patient) is related to the *fraction* of cells killed per cycle, the number of cells initially present (which may also predict the number of inherently resistant cells), the length of time between cycles (which allows for regrowth of tumor cells), and the number of cycles given.

GENERAL TOXICITIES TO NORMAL TISSUES

Chemotherapeutic agents are not selectively toxic to neoplastic cells. Therefore, inhibition of cell division of normal cells also occurs. Toxicity to normal tissues often is proportional to dose and/or duration of therapy. In general, the most common dose-limiting toxicities of chemotherapy drugs relate to their inhibition of rapidly proliferating tissues such as bone marrow and gastrointestinal tract epithelium.

Nausea and vomiting are common and are caused by both a central nervous system (CNS) effect at the chemoreceptor trigger zone and through gastrointestinal irritation. Many chemotherapeutic drugs cause temporary arrest of the cellular proliferation of the gastrointestinal mucosa necessary to maintain the integrity of the lining of the gastrointestinal tract. This can cause severe oral and esophageal pain (i.e., mucositis). If mucosal damage is severe, abdominal pain, diarrhea, gastrointestinal bleeding, gram negative sepsis, and bowel perforation can result.

Most chemotherapy drugs cause dose-related reversible bone marrow suppression, resulting in leukopenia and thrombocytopenia, which is most pronounced 10 to 14 days after administration. Bone marrow recovery is complete by 3 to 4 weeks. This places some patients at a temporary risk of severe infection and bleeding.

Hematopoiesis is a carefully regulated process which is mediated by humoral factors called hematopoietins. Although the physiologic roles of these proteins have not yet been fully elucidated, several hematopoietic growth factors are now available for clinical use. Granulocyte-colony stimulating factor (G-CSF) and granulocyte macrophage colony stimulating factor (GM-CSF) appear to regulate myeloid cell proliferation. Several clinical trials have suggested that they can reduce the severity and duration of chemotherapy-induced neutropenia.

Filgrastim is a non-glycosylated G-CSF product produced in *E. coli* through recombinant DNA technology. It is administered as a subcutaneous injection once daily and has a mean plasma half-life of 3.5 hours. The mode of clearance is not known. When therapy is started 24 hours following myelosuppressive chemotherapy, studies have shown a significant decrease in the number of neutropenic days and episodes of febrile neutropenia. The most common side effect is bone pain, seen in approximately one quarter of the patients treated. Other toxicities include transient elevations of liver transaminases and uric acid (see Chapter 44 for additional information).

GM-CSF is available as **sargramostim**, a yeast-derived recombinant glycosylated form of GM-CSF (an *E. coli*-derived product is also being studied which appears to have similar efficacy). When given by intravenous infusion, the distribution (α) half-life of sargramostim is 12 to 17 min and the elimination (β) half-life is 2 h. Extensive clinical trials in bone marrow transplant patients have demonstrated that engraftment is accelerated with consequent decreases in the number of infectious episodes, the duration of infections, and the length of hospitalization. Major side effects include fluid retention, serositis, bone pain, myalgia, fevers, and headaches.

Certain chemotherapeutic drugs may be used in extremely high doses in conjunction with bone marrow or peripheral stem cell rescue. Theoretically, dosage escalation may overcome the resistance of cancer cells to conventional doses and possibly cure more patients. Limitations to dosage escalation include extramedullary toxicities. Bone marrow or peripheral stem cells removed before high dose or "supra-lethal" chemotherapy subsequently rescue the patient from marrow failure. Not all chemotherapeutic agents can be thus dose escalated. Drugs such as busulfan, cyclophosphamide, thiotepa, melphalan, and ifosfamide, lend themselves to dosage escalation. Such transplants may be curative, particularly for leukemias and the lymphomas. Other tumor types are currently under investigation.

DRUG CLASSIFICATION

Drugs discussed in this chapter are divided into six major groups, as shown in Table 43-1. This arbitrary division provides a convenient basis both for describing the action of the drugs and for helping choose drugs for particular clinical circumstances. The pharmacokinetic characteristics of the drugs are discussed, as well as common adverse reactions and more severe toxicities associated with their use. In addition, their indications for treatment of various neoplasms is also listed in the text.

ANTIMETABOLITES

Antimetabolites are structural analogs of naturally occurring substances. They interfere with various metabolic processes and disrupt cell function and proliferation. These drugs may act in two ways: (1) by incorporation into a metabolic pathway and formation of a "false" metabolite which is nonfunctional, or (2) by inhibition of the catalytic function of an enzyme or enzyme system. Included in the antimetabolite group are the folic acid antagonists (methotrexate), purine derivatives (mercaptopurine, thioguanine, fludarabine, cladribine, and pentostatin), and pyrimidine derivatives (fluorouracil, floxuridine, and cytarabine). Figure 43-2 shows some useful antimetabolites, which are discussed below, compared structurally with their corresponding metabolite.

Folate Antagonists

Methotrexate

Mechanism of Action The principal action of methotrexate is to compete with folic acid for the active binding sites on the enzyme dihydrofolate reductase. This enzyme's function is to keep folic acid in its reduced state, 5,6,7,8-tetrahydrofolic acid (FH_4) (Fig. 43-3). This reduction occurs in two steps: the first is an NADPH-dependent reduction of folic acid to 7,8-dihydrofolic acid (FH_2), and the second is an NADH- or NADPH-dependent reduction of FH_2 to FH_4. The reduced folates are the active forms, and they function as carriers of one-carbon groups which are required during the synthesis of purines and the pyrimidine thymidylate. Specifically, FH_4 is required for methylation of deoxyuridine monophosphate to deoxythymidine monophosphate and for the addition of formate to the purine precursor inosinic acid. The FH_4 is oxidized to inactive FH_2 during this reaction. Therefore during the S phase a constant supply of dihydrofolate reductase is needed to maintain a pool of reduced folates within the cell. After methotrexate exposure, oxidized folates build up and DNA synthesis is inhibited. The affinity of dihydrofolate reductase for the antimetabolite is far greater than its affinity for the normal substrates, folic acid, and FH_2. Because of the marked affinity of the enzyme for methotrexate, even very large doses of folic acid given simultaneously fail to reverse the effects of methotrexate. If folic acid is given 1 h prior to methotrexate, the drug effects can be prevented, since this allows time for the reduction of folic acid to the active derivatives. Leucovorin (folinic acid, citrovorum factor), if given with or shortly after methotrexate, also prevents its effects, since leucovorin (N^5-formyl FH_4) is a derivative of the product (FH_4) of the blocked reaction (Fig. 43-3) and can directly supply a source of reduced folate. There is, however, no selective block of toxic effects, and except in special circumstances (see Therapeutic Uses, below), the use of leucovorin can prevent both the therapeutic and toxic effects of methotrexate.

Pharmacokinetics Methotrexate is well absorbed from the gastrointestinal tract in doses less than 25 mg. Erratic absorption is seen with larger doses. Peak blood concentration occurs after 1 h. After intravenous or intramuscular injection, the drug rapidly distributes in the extracellular fluid.

TABLE 43-1 Some examples of cancer chemotherapeutic agents

Antimetabolites

Folate antagonists: methotrexate
Purine derivatives: mercaptopurine, thioguanine, fludarabine, cladribine, pentostatin
Pyrimidine derivatives: fluorouracil, floxuridine, cytarabine

Alkylating Agents

Nitrogen mustards: mechlorethamine, chlorambucil, cyclophosphamide, melphalan, thiotepa, ifosfamide
Nitrosoureas: lomustine, carmustine, streptozocin
Triazenes: dacarbazine
Alkyl sulfonates: busulfan
Platinum derivatives: cisplatin, carboplatin
Methylhydrazines: procarbazine

Antibiotics

Dactinomycin (actinomycin D)
Plicamycin (mithramycin)
Bleomycin
Anthracyclines: doxorubicin, daunorubicin, idarubicin,
Mitoxantrone
Mitomycin (mitomycin C)

Plant Derivatives

Vinca Alkaloids: vincristine, vinblastine
Podophyllotoxins: etoposide (VP-16), teniposide (VM-26)
Taxanes: paclitaxel
Topotecan

Miscellaneous

Asparaginase
Hydroxyurea

Hormones

Estrogens: estradiol, diethylstilbesterol, estramustine
Progestins: hydroxyprogesterone, megestrol
Adrenocorticoids: prednisone, prednisolone
Androgens: testosterone, fluoxymesterone
Antiestrogens: tamoxifen
Gonadotropin analogs: leuprolide
Antiandrogens: flutamide

Methotrexate enters cells by carrier-mediated active transport, although passive diffusion may occur with very large doses. After a short distribution phase, its elimination is biphasic. The primary elimination half-life is 2 to 3 h and is followed by a terminal half-life of 8 to 10 h. Increased toxicity due to prolongation of either half-life occurs with renal disease. Accumulation of drug in pleural or peritoneal fluid can increase toxicity by prolongation of the terminal half-life. The highest tissue levels are found in the kidney and liver. The drug is approximately 50 percent

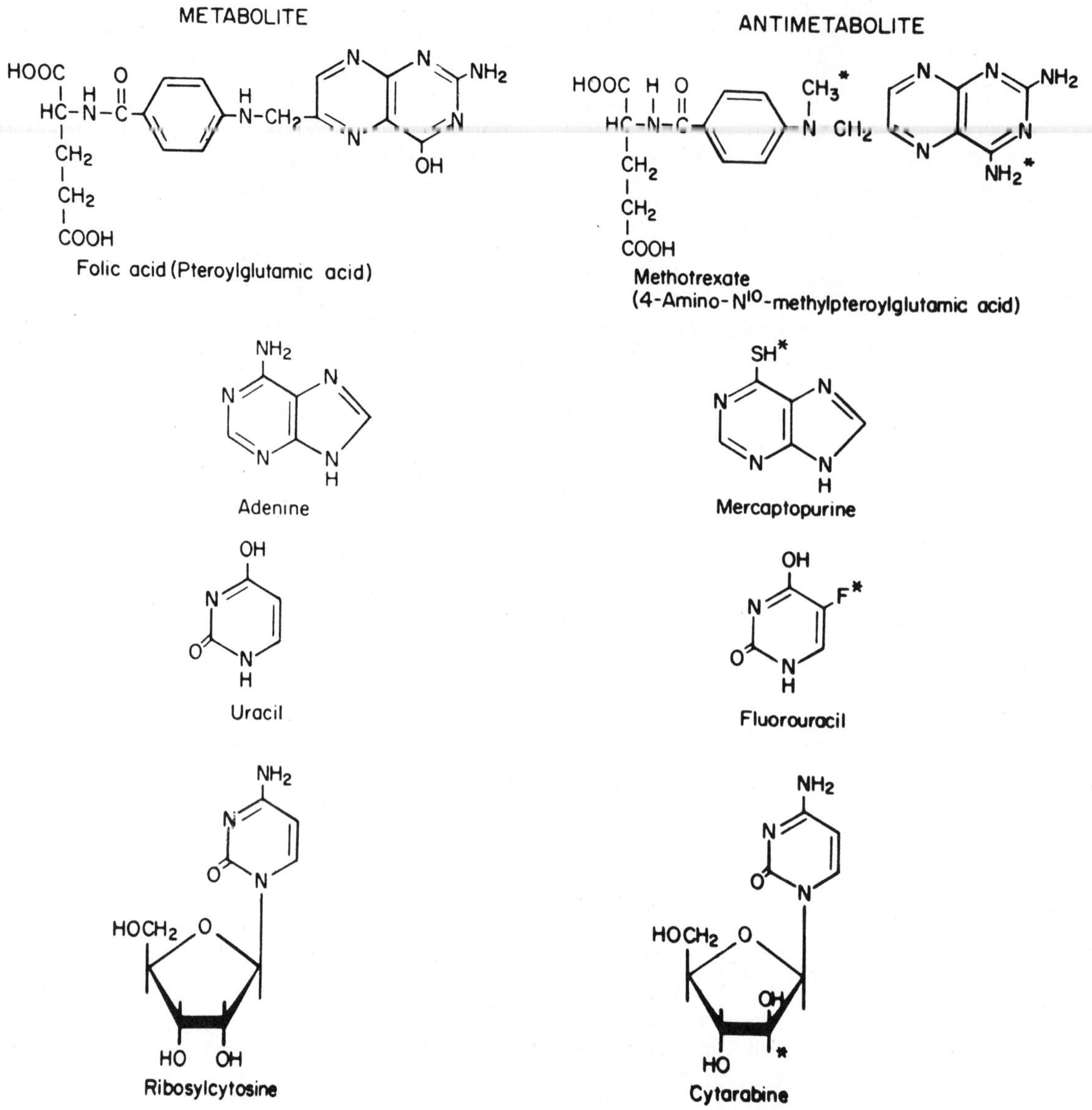

METABOLITE

Folic acid (Pteroylglutamic acid)

ANTIMETABOLITE

Methotrexate (4-Amino-N^{10}-methylpteroylglutamic acid)

Adenine

Mercaptopurine

Uracil

Fluorouracil

Ribosylcytosine

Cytarabine

FIGURE 43-2 *Examples of antimetabolites with the corresponding metabolites. (The asterisk indicates the structural change.)*

bound to plasma proteins.

Methotrexate penetrates the blood-brain barrier poorly, and when used in conventional doses its concentration in the cerebrospinal fluid (CSF) is less than 10 percent of that in the blood. When given intrathecally, the concentration of the drug can be maintained in the CSF for long periods of time. Transport of the drug from the CSF to the systemic circulation does occur. Although methotrexate can be biotransformed in the liver to much less active metabolites, its major route of elimination is the kidney. Methotrexate should be used cautiously in the presence of renal insufficiency.

Therapeutic Uses Methotrexate is indicated for the treatment of acute lymphatic leukemia (ALL), choriocarcinoma, non-Hodgkin's lymphoma (NHL),

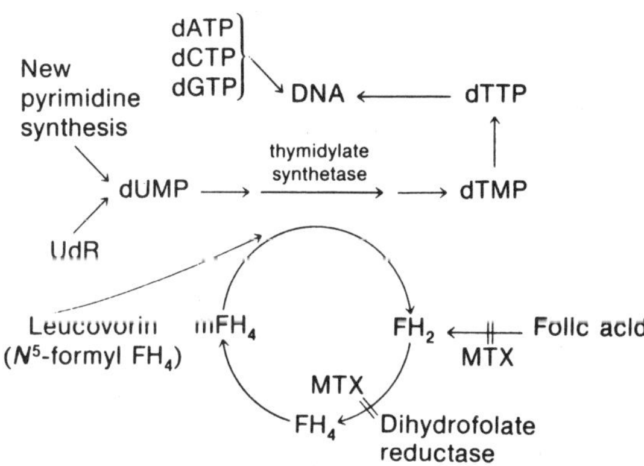

FIGURE 43-3 *A schematic representation of the formation of DNA from precursors. The relationship of the generation of thymidylate synthetase cofactor is shown. FH_2 = dihydrofolate; FH_4 = tetrahydrofolate; mFH_4 = N^5,N^{10}-methylenetetrahydrofolate; MTX = methotrexate; UdR = uridine; dUMP = deoxyuridylate; dTMP = thymidylate; dATP, dCTP, dGTP, dTTP = deoxyribonucleotide triphosphates of adenine, cytosine, guanine, and thymine, respectively.*

mycosis fungoides, sarcoma of the bone, and cancers of the head and neck, breast, and lung. It is also used intrathecally for the treatment of meningeal involvement by carcinoma, lymphoma, or leukemia.

In an attempt to overcome resistant cells, very high dosage regimens have been used with "rescue" by leucovorin 18 to 36 h after the start of the methotrexate infusion. These regimens have achieved cytotoxic CNS levels. They require rigorous hydration to avoid acute renal failure and careful monitoring of methotrexate blood levels to avoid life-threatening toxicity.

Adverse Reactions The most common adverse reactions are myelosuppression, nausea, vomiting, abdominal pain, ulceration, and severe mucositis. Hepatic fibrosis can occur with chronic maintenance therapy for ALL or psoriasis. Acute liver atrophy and allergic pneumonitis may be seen rarely. With high dosage regimens, acute renal failure can occur due to precipitation of methotrexate and its metabolites in the renal tubules.

Purine Derivatives

Analogs of the purine nucleotides were first developed in the early 1950s. The guanine derivatives mercaptopurine and thioguanine were soon found to be highly active in the treatment of acute leukemia. Another guanine analog, allopurinol, was found to be a potent inhibitor of xanthine oxidase, useful for prevention of gout. Recently, three adenosine derivatives, fludarabine, cladribine (2-chlorodeoxyadenosine), and pentostatin, have shown great promise for treating lymphoid malignancies.

Mercaptopurine and Thioguanine

Mechanism of Action Mercaptopurine and its amino analog, thioguanine, differ from guanine by the substitution of a sulfhydryl group for the 6-hydroxyl group in the purine ring (Fig. 43-4). Both compounds readily enter cells, where they are converted to their active nucleotide forms by hypoxanthine-guanine phosphoribosyl transferase. The monophosphate forms block *de novo* purine synthesis through inhibition of inosine monophosphate synthesis. They also inhibit the conversion of inosine monophosphate to adenine and guanine nucleotides. In addition, the triphosphate forms of mercaptopurine and thioguanine are incorporated into DNA as fraudulent bases, resulting in DNA strand breaks.

Pharmacokinetics Both mercaptopurine and thioguanine are administered orally. Their absorption, however, is incomplete and erratic, with only

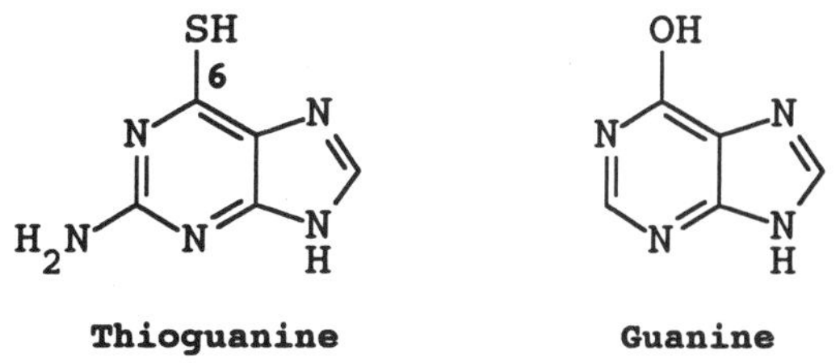

Mercaptopurine **Allopurinol**

Thioguanine **Guanine**

FIGURE 43-4 *Structures of guanine and three of its drug analogs: mercaptopurine, thioguanine, and allopurinol.*

30 to 50 percent reaching the systemic circulation. The half-lives of mercaptopurine and thioguanine are 20 to 60 min and 90 min, respectively. Both drugs are metabolized in the liver. Mercaptopurine is converted to the inactive metabolite 6-thiouric acid via a pathway mediated by xanthine oxidase. Thioguanine is methylated to 6-methyl thioguanine and excreted by the kidney.

Therapeutic Uses Mercaptopurine is primarily used for remission maintenance in acute lymphatic leukemia, while thioguanine is used in induction regimens for acute nonlymphatic leukemia.

Adverse Reactions The major toxicities of these agents are myelosuppression, nausea, vomiting, diarrhea, and mucositis. Cholestatic jaundice is seen frequently with mercaptopurine but it is usually reversible with discontinuation of the drug.

Drug Interaction Allopurinol is a potent inhibitor of xanthine oxidase (Fig. 43-4), which is responsible for the conversion of hypoxanthine and xanthine to uric acid. Consequently, allopurinol is used to treat the excessive production of uric acid seen in gout, leukemia, and lymphoma, particularly where treatment results in the rapid dissolution of neoplastic cells with liberation of their nucleic acid purines and subsequent oxidation of these purines to uric acid. Since mercaptopurine is also a substrate for xanthine oxidase, the concurrent administration of allopurinol delays the oxidative degradation of mercaptopurine and markedly increases its toxicity. The dose of mercaptopurine should therefore be reduced to one-third to one-fourth of the usual dose if allopurinol is to be given concurrently. Since thioguanine is degraded by other pathways not dependent on xanthine oxidase, its toxicity is not enhanced by allopurinol and, therefore, it may be used more safely than mercaptopurine in clinical situations where allopurinol is needed. Allopurinol produces few adverse reactions, although about 5 percent of patients develop an allergic rash, which is promptly responsive to withdrawal of the medication.

Fludarabine Phosphate

Mechanism of Action Fludarabine phosphate was the first of the new adenosine analogs to enter clinical trials. It was specifically designed to overcome the shortcomings of 9-β-arabinofuranosyladenine (ara-A, vidarabine), a potent antitumor agent that had poor aqueous solubility and was rapidly deaminated by the enzyme adenosine deaminase. The 2-fluoro derivative of ara-A is resistant to deamination, while the addition of a 5′-monophosphate confers improved solubility.

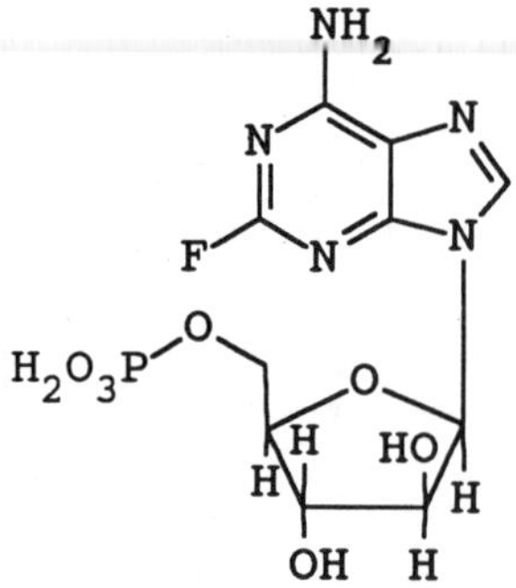

Fludarabine phosphate is rapidly dephosphorylated in plasma. It then enters cells by a carrier-mediated process where it undergoes phosphorylation to 2-fluoroadenine arabinoside triphosphate (2-fluoro-ara-ATP). The triphosphate is incorporated into DNA with resultant inhibition of DNA polymerase. Fludarabine phosphate is also active in non-dividing cells where its cytotoxicity may be due to inhibition of DNA ligase I.

Pharmacokinetics Fludarabine phosphate is administered by intravenous infusion. It undergoes rapid dephosphorylation in the liver to the active product 2-fluoro-ara-A, with a mean half-life of the phosphate form of about 5 min. 2-Fluoro-ara-A is then widely distributed to the tissues. Its terminal half-life is 8 to 10 h. It is eliminated through renal excretion and the dose should be reduced in patients with renal insufficiency.

Therapeutic Uses Fludarabine phosphate is effective in the treatment of chlorambucil-resistant chronic lymphocytic leukemia. It also has activity against myeloid leukemias and indolent non-Hodgkin's lymphoma (NHL).

Adverse Reactions The primary toxicity of fludarabine phosphate is reversible myelosuppression. In particular, a profound decrease in lymphocytes is seen with an increased risk of opportunistic infections. Peripheral sensorimotor neuropathy is also common. At high doses, delayed neurotoxicity occurring 3 to 6 weeks following therapy has been described. Neurologic symptoms included cortical blindness, optic neuritis, seizures, and altered mental status. These phenomena have not been reported when conventional doses of fludarabine phosphate are used.

Cladribine (2-Chlorodeoxyadenosine, 2-CdA)

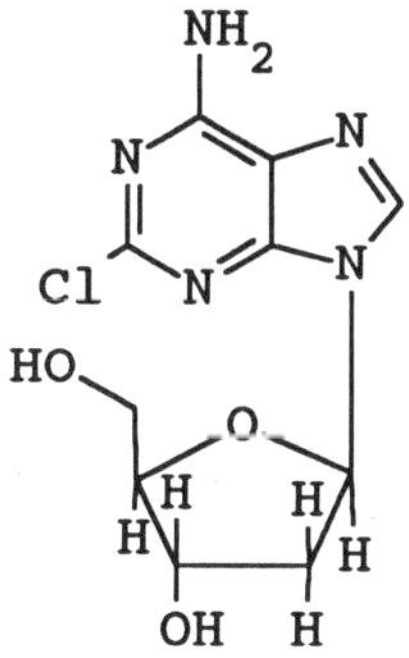

Mechanism of Action Cladribine is a purine analog which differs from deoxyadenosine by the substitution of a chlorine for a hydrogen atom in the 2 position of the purine ring. This modification confers resistance to degradation by adenosine deaminase. Cladribine enters cells by passive diffusion and is converted to 2-chlorodeoxyadenosine monophosphate (2-CdAMP) by deoxycytidine kinase. Since adenosine deaminase is inhibited, 2-CdAMP accumulates intracellularly and is ultimately converted to the triphosphate, 2-CdATP. This compound is then incorporated into the DNA of dividing cells and, subsequently, impairs DNA synthesis.

Cladribine is also active in non-dividing cells. The mechanism appears to be due to inhibition of repair of DNA strand breaks by the high concentrations of intracellular 2-CdATP. The effects of cladribine are especially pronounced in lymphoid cells since they are deficient in the alternate degradation enzyme deoxynucleotide deaminase.

Pharmacokinetics Cladribine is given by continuous intravenous infusion. It has a biphasic half-life with the initial (α) half-life of approximately 36 min, followed by a terminal (β) half-life of 7 h. Little is known about the metabolism or excretion of the drug. The effect of impairment of renal or hepatic function on cladribine clearance has not been established.

Therapeutic Uses Cladribine has shown dramatic activity in the treatment of hairy cell leukemia, with an overall 88 percent response rate from a single 7 day course of treatment, demonstrated in two clinical trials. Cladribine is also effective against chronic lymphocytic leukemia, NHL, and myeloid leukemias.

Adverse Reactions Myelosuppression has been observed in 20 percent of patients, mainly when bone marrow function was already impaired by previous therapy. Lymphopenia and monocytopenia are seen routinely. Fevers are seen in up to 70 percent of patients. When given in high doses, renal failure and neurologic toxicity were observed.

Pentostatin (Deoxycoformycin)

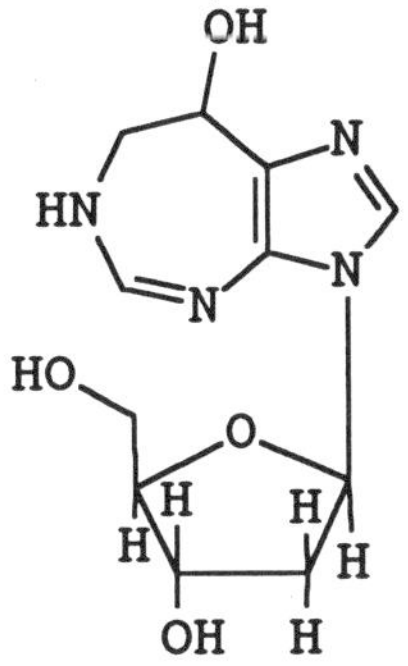

Mechanism of Action Pentostatin is another inhibitor of adenosine deaminase. This inhibition results in the accumulation of intracellular deoxy-ATP. Through feedback inhibition, the activity of the enzyme ribonucleotide reductase is reduced, leading to a decrease in the other deoxynucleotides. Consequently, DNA synthesis and repair are inhibited. Additionally, pentostatin appears to inhibit 5-adenosyl methionine-dependent methylation reactions in RNA transcription. Thus, it is active in both dividing and non-dividing cells. Like other adenosine deaminase inhibitors, pentostatin is most active against lymphoid cells due to their deficiency of deoxynucleotide deaminase.

Pharmacokinetics Pentostatin is administered intravenously and exhibits biphasic clearance from the plasma. The terminal half-life is 6 h. Thirty to 50 percent of administered doses are excreted unchanged in the urine. Therefore, dose adjustments should be made when renal function is impaired.

Therapeutic Uses Pentostatin is effective against hairy cell leukemia, indolent non-Hodgkin's lymphomas, and chronic lymphocytic leukemia.

Adverse Reactions Pentostatin is generally well-tolerated with fever, mild nausea, and rashes being the most frequent side effects seen with conventional doses. At higher doses, renal failure, elevation of hepatic enzymes, confusion, and coma have been described. Pentostatin is also highly immunosuppressive.

Pyrimidine Derivatives

Numerous pyrimidine analogs have been synthesized as potential anti-cancer drugs; they are either nucleosides or bases that have some structural difference from the endogenous compounds. The most intensively studied of these have been two fluorinated derivatives, fluorouracil and floxuridine, and a cytosine derivative, cytarabine.

Fluorouracil (5-FU) and Floxuridine (5-FUdR)

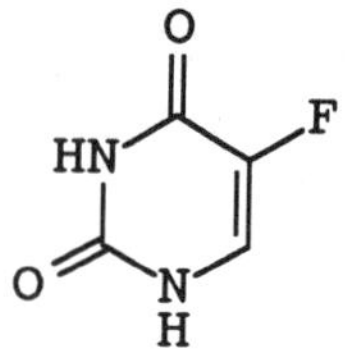

Fluorouracil

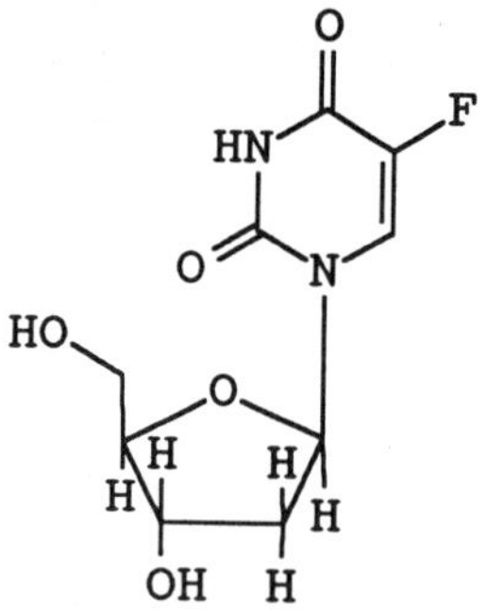

Floxuridine

Mechanism of Action Probably the most important mechanism of action of the fluorinated pyrimidines is the inhibition of thymidylate synthetase and thus interference with DNA production (Fig. 43-3). This action is accomplished by formation of an active metabolite, 5-fluorodeoxyuridine monophosphate (FdUMP), from both fluorouracil and floxuridine. FdUMP forms a complex with the reduced folate N^5,N^{10}-methylene tetrahydrofolate. This complex inhibits thymidylate synthetase and decreases the methylation of 2-deoxyuridylic acid to form thymidylic acid. The thymidine deficiency which results interferes with cell division and causes cellular injury and death. Also, the triphosphate form of fluorouracil can be incorporated into RNA and interferes with protein synthesis.

Pharmacokinetics Floxuridine is rapidly biotransformed to fluorouracil in the liver. Its oral absorption is poor and the drug is only used by continuous intra-arterial infusion.

Fluorouracil is absorbed irregularly from the gastrointestinal tract and is degraded by the liver when ingested. Its bioavailability is less than 15 percent when taken orally. For these reasons it is only used intravenously. After an intravenous bolus injection, fluorouracil rapidly distributes throughout the body and enters cells by passive diffusion; it has a half-life of only 10 min. Eighty percent is metabolized by the liver to inactive products (carbon dioxide, urea, and α-fluoro-β-alanine), and these products appear in the urine; 90 percent of the carbon dioxide is expired through the respiratory tract. Although fluorouracil has a short half-life, the active metabolite, FdUMP, may persist intracellularly for an extended period.

Therapeutic Uses Fluorouracil administered intravenously is indicated in the management of carcinomas of the head and neck, colon, rectum, breast, stomach, and pancreas. Topical application of the drug is effective for multiple actinic or solar keratoses. This method of administration is also useful in the treatment of superficial basal cell carcinomas.

The combination of high-dose leucovorin followed by fluorouracil has been effective in the treatment of metastatic colon and stomach cancer. Leucovorin supplies a source of reduced folates which may occur in insufficient quantities within neoplastic cells. Leucovorin enhances the formation of the FdUMP-N^5,N^{10}-methylene tetrahydrofolate.

Floxuridine is used for hepatic artery infusion of patients with colon cancer metastatic to liver. Its rapid first pass metabolism allows greater dosage with lessened systemic toxicity.

Adverse Reactions The effects of fluorouracil and floxuridine are most prominent on the rapidly proliferating tissues of the bone marrow and gastrointestinal tract. Toxicity includes bone marrow suppression, mucositis, diarrhea, gastrointestinal ulceration, and bleeding. The use of leucovorin in conjunction with fluorouracil increases toxicity to the gastrointestinal tract, particularly diarrhea. Toxicities of fluorouracil are related to the dose and schedule of administration. After prolonged intravenous infusion, the major adverse effects are mucositis and diarrhea, whereas after bolus administration the major toxicity is bone marrow suppression.

Cytarabine (Cytosine Arabinoside, Ara-C)

Mechanism of Action Cytarabine is an antimetabolite effective in the treatment of leukemias. Similar to the other pyrimidine antimetabolites, cytarabine must be "activated" by biotransformation to the corresponding nucleotide. Ara-cytosine triphosphate (ara-CTP) is the active form of the drug. Cytarabine inhibits DNA polymerase and Ara-CTP is incorporated into DNA, which inhibits DNA synthesis.

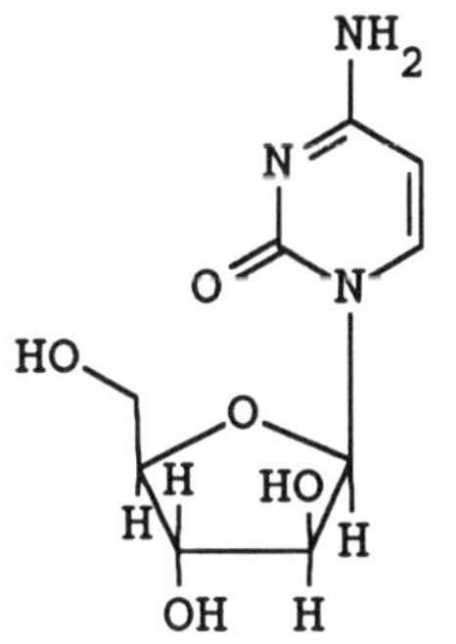

Pharmacokinetics Less than 20 percent of cytarabine is absorbed after oral administration; therefore it is administered by the parenteral route. Within several hours of intravenous infusion of cytarabine, there are concentrations of the drug in the cerebrospinal fluid which are approximately 50 percent of plasma levels. The drug has a biphasic half-life. The initial distributive half-life is approximately 10 to 20 min; the terminal elimination half-life about 1 h. The drug is primarily deaminated in the liver. About 75 to 90 percent of the drug is excreted in the urine as an inactive metabolite, ara-uracil.

Therapeutic Uses Cytarabine is primarily used in the treatment of the acute leukemias. When administered by continuous intravenous infusion in combination with an anthracycline derivative (e.g., doxorubicin or daunorubicin), complete remission rates of 70 to 80 percent are achieved in acute myelogenous leukemia (AML). High dosage schedules of cytarabine have been used both in induction regimens for AML and at relapse with success. These doses yield cytotoxic cerebrospinal fluid levels.

Cytarabine can also be given by the intrathecal route which achieves high cerebrospinal fluid levels. Thus the drug is useful for meningeal leukemia.

Adverse Reactions Cytarabine produces profound bone marrow suppression and gastrointestinal toxicity. High dosage regimens of cytarabine can cause elevated liver enzymes and cerebellar toxicity with ataxia. A cytarabine-induced syndrome characterized by fever, myalgia, bone pain, rash, conjunctivitis, and malaise has been described.

ALKYLATING AGENTS

Bis(β-chloroethyl)sulfide (mustard gas) was the most effective war gas used during World War I. In 1935, a nitrogen-containing analog of sulfur mustard, tris(β-chloroethyl)amine, was synthesized. This drug and the related series of compounds subsequently prepared have been called *nitrogen mustards*. Many analogs of nitrogen mustard and related agents (e.g., the nitrosoureas) have been synthesized and tested in various biologic systems.

Mechanism of Action The alkylating agents are highly reactive compounds with the ability to form covalent bonds with nucleophilic (electron-rich) sites on molecules such as nucleic acids, phosphates, amino acids, and proteins. Alkylation refers to the formation of a new covalent bond between the above molecules and one of the carbon atoms of an alkylator. This is usually accomplished through the formation of a positively charged carbonium ion ($—CH_2^+$). This unstable intermediate may attack any electron-rich site, but it has a predilection for the N-7 position of guanine. For the platinum derivatives, i.e., cisplatin and carboplatin, the formation of a doubly charged platinum (Pt^{2+}) becomes the active moiety. Representative chemical reactions are shown in Fig. 43-5.

The cytotoxic effects of the alkylating agents most likely reflect their ability to bind to the nucleotides of DNA. This results in DNA misreading, single- and double-strand breaks, and DNA interstrand cross-linking. Cell death occurs through interference with DNA replication and mitosis. The bifunctional alkylators have the capacity to form DNA interstrand cross-linkages, which makes them more cytotoxic than the monofunctional alkylators. The alkylators have an effect during any part of the cell cycle (cell-cycle nonspecific), but cells in the late G_1 or S phases (especially if rapidly dividing) are most susceptible.

General Properties

Chemistry The structures of the alkylating agents used most commonly in cancer chemotherapy are shown in Fig. 43-6. Note that all but lomustine (CCNU) contain two or three alkylating groups and are thus known as *bifunctional* or *polyfunctional* alkylating agents. Although the alkylating agents share a common mechanism of

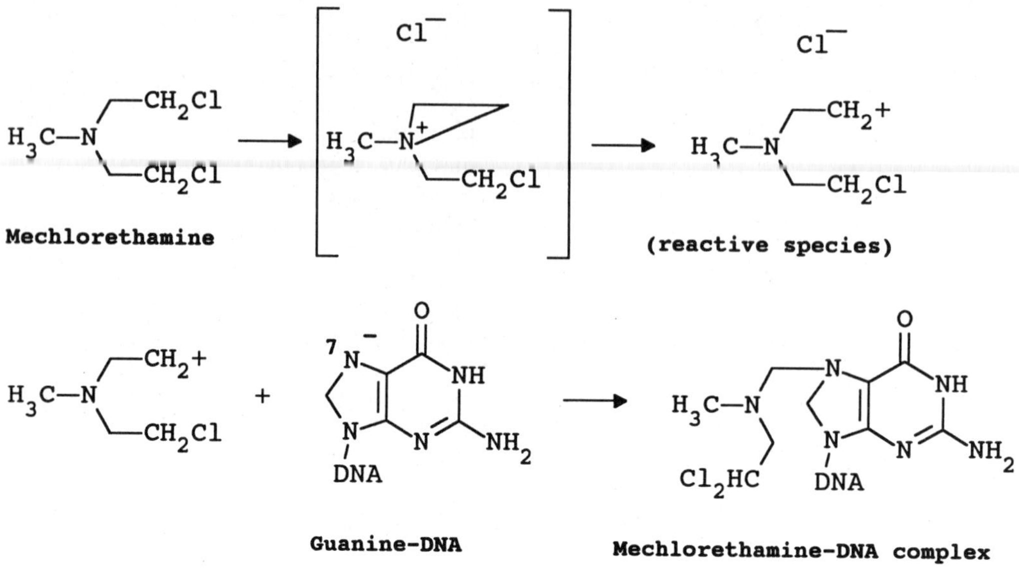

FIGURE 43-5 *Reactions of an alkylating agent (mechlorethamine) with guanine of DNA. At physiologic pH, mechlorethamine converts to an unstable intermediate and then to the active, carbonium ion-containing species. The active species reacts with guanine of DNA to form a stable drug-DNA complex. The other functional group of mechlorethamine can react at a site on the complementary DNA strand to form an interstrand cross-linkage or at another site on the same DNA strand to form an intrastrand cross-linkage.*

action, their clinical utility varies because of differences in pharmacokinetics, metabolism, lipid solubility, ability to cross cell membranes, and toxicities. They can be classified into six groups: (1) nitrogen mustard derivatives, (2) nitrosoureas, (3) triazene derivatives, (4) alkyl sulfonates, (5) platinum derivatives, and (6) methylhydrazines.

Pharmacokinetics Generally, the alkylating agents are eliminated by metabolic pathways with partial excretion of those metabolites through the kidney. Cisplatin, however, is excreted in the urine predominantly unchanged. Additional pharmacokinetics are included below in the monographs for each drug.

Adverse Reactions The adverse reactions of the alkylating agents as a group include:

1 *Myelosuppression*, manifested by a dose-related leukopenia and thrombocytopenia.

2 *Gastrointestinal toxicity* including nausea, vomiting, mucositis, diarrhea, and possible intestinal mucosal ulceration.

3 *Alopecia*.

4 *Reproductive toxicity* with impairment of spermatogenesis, menstrual irregularities, and possible irreversible sterility.

5 *Pulmonary fibrosis* has been a rare complication of almost all alkylating agents.

6 *Teratogenic effects*. An increased incidence of fetal birth defects has been associated with the use of alkylating agents during the first trimester of pregnancy.

7 *Carcinogenic effects*. The use of alkylating agents has been shown to increase the incidence of AML, non-Hodgkin's lymphoma, and other secondary tumors. Although this was first recognized with the use of cyclophosphamide, melphalan, and chlorambucil, most alkylating agents have been implicated. A marked increase in AML has been demonstrated, for example, in patients with polycythemia vera treated with chlorambucil and with the use of nitrogen mustards for Hodgkin's disease. In Hodgkin's disease, the incidence of AML at 10 years varies between 2 and 10 percent in different reports. The use of combined modality therapy (i.e.,

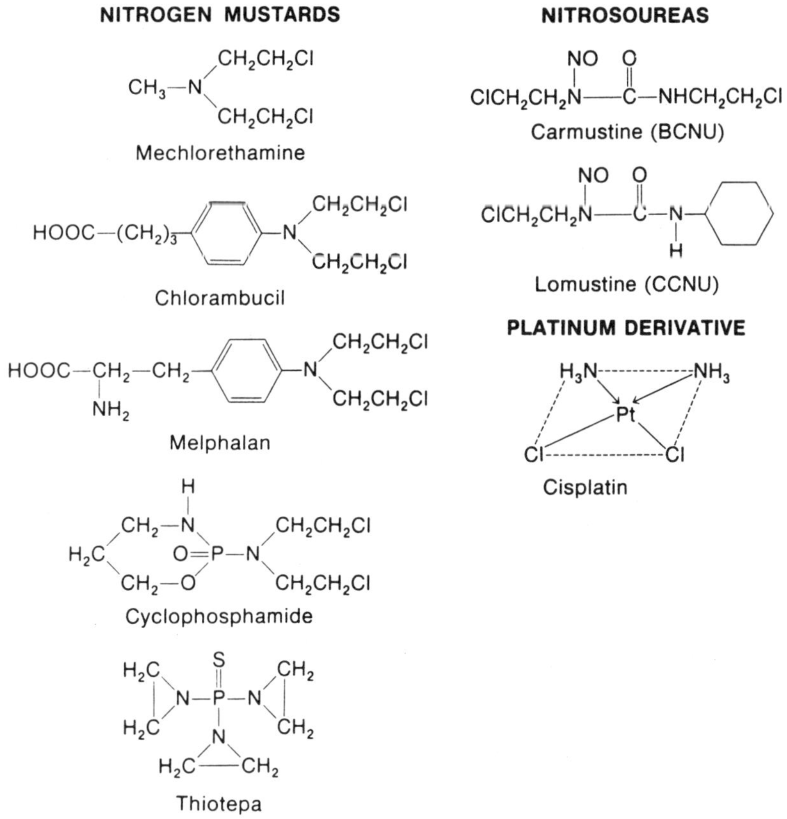

NITROGEN MUSTARDS

Mechlorethamine

Chlorambucil

Melphalan

Cyclophosphamide

Thiotepa

NITROSOUREAS

Carmustine (BCNU)

Lomustine (CCNU)

PLATINUM DERIVATIVE

Cisplatin

FIGURE 43-6 *Chemical structures of some alkylating agents.*

chemotherapy and radiation) appears to be most leukemogenic. A vast majority of cases occur 2 to 9 years after treatment.

Toxicities that are specific to each drug are mentioned in the drug monographs below.

Individual Agents

Nitrogen Mustards *Mechlorethamine (Nitrogen Mustard)* Mechlorethamine is a highly reactive drug which was the first clinically-tested alkylating agent. It causes the formation of DNA interstrand cross-linkages and DNA-protein cross-linkages. Generally, nitrogen mustard is administered by the intravenous route, but it is a potent vesicant which can cause tissue necrosis with extravasation. Its cytotoxic and vesicant properties make it useful for intrapleural administration for malignant pleural effusions. Nitrogen mustard has most commonly been used as a component of the MOPP (nitrogen mustard, vincristine, procarbazine, and prednisone) regimen for Hodgkin's disease. Topical nitrogen mustard has proven effective in the therapy of mycosis fungoides.

Chlorambucil Chlorambucil is available only for oral use and is well absorbed. It is rapidly metabolized in the liver to 2-[4-bis(2-chloroethyl)aminophenyl] acetic acid (phenylacetic acid mustard), which has antineoplastic activity, and then is excreted in the urine. The plasma half-life is approximately 90 min. The primary use of chlorambucil has been in lymphoid malignancies such as chronic lymphocytic leukemia, indolent lymphomas, and Hodgkin's disease.

Cyclophosphamide Cyclophosphamide is available for intravenous or oral use. It is a prodrug that requires biotransformation by the liver to phosphoramide mustard, the active form of the drug. Cyclophosphamide is well absorbed after oral administration and is approximately 55 percent bound to plasma protein. The half-life averages 6 h. Ten to 20 percent of a dose is excreted unchanged in the urine. Cyclophosphamide is one of the most commonly used chemotherapeutic agents. It is not a vesicant, but can cause severe hemorrhagic cystitis especially with high intravenous doses or with prolonged administration. Patients should be well hydrated before administration. Metabolites such as acrolein have been suggested as the cause of hemorrhagic cystitis. Mesna disulfide may detoxify these metabolites and alleviate hemorrhagic cystitis. With high doses, a syndrome of inappropriate antidiuretic hormone can occur and myocardial necrosis has rarely been reported. Cyclophosphamide is used for the treatment of non-Hodgkin's lymphoma, acute lymphatic leukemia, chronic lymphocytic leukemia, myeloma, breast and ovarian cancers, neuroblastoma, and in high dose preparative regimens for marrow transplantation. It has also been used as an immunosuppressant in non-malignant disorders such as connective tissue diseases.

Melphalan Melphalan or L-phenylalanine mustard (L-PAM), is administered either orally or by the intravenous route. Oral absorption is variable, with 20 to 50 percent excreted in the stool. Food and alkaline pH decrease the absorption by about 30 percent. The drug is transported into cells by the L-amino acid transport system which also mediates the cellular uptake of leucine and glutamine. The plasma half-life is approximately 90 min. About 15 percent is excreted intact in the urine. Therefore, melphalan should be used cautiously in patients with decreased renal function. It is used in the treatment of multiple myeloma, lymphomas, breast and ovarian cancers. High dosage regimens with bone marrow transplant have been investigated for multiple myeloma, AML, and neuroblastoma.

Thiotepa (N,N′,N″-Triethylenethiophosphoramide) Thiotepa is a complex alkylating agent which causes DNA adducts and strand breaks. Thiotepa can be administered by the intravenous, intrapleural, intravesicular, or intrathecal routes. About 15 percent of the drug is metabolized to triethylene phosphoramide (TEPA); approximately 85 percent is excreted in the urine unchanged. The dose-limiting side effect of thiotepa is myelosuppression. The primary indications for the drug are breast and ovarian cancers and, more recently, as high-dose therapy with autologous bone marrow transplant. Thiotepa has also proven useful in the intravesicular treatment of superficial bladder carcinoma. With high dose therapies, additional toxicities may be seen such as mucositis, CNS toxicities, and darkening of the skin.

Ifosfamide Ifosfamide is a closely related structural analog of cyclophosphamide. Like cyclophosphamide, it is activated by the hepatic P-450 mixed function oxidase system, though significantly more slowly than its analog. It can be administered either orally or intravenously and has a plasma half-life of 5 to 6 h. Oral bioavailability is close to 100 percent. A number of stable metabolites have been identified, most of which are eliminated in the urine. The clinical spectrum of this drug is similar to that of cyclophosphamide but a different pattern of toxicity is seen. Myelosuppression is less, but the risk of hemorrhagic cystitis is much greater, requiring the prophylactic administration of mesna disulfide. Significant neurologic toxicity including cerebellar dysfunction, seizures, and altered mental status have been reported, particularly in patients with impaired hepatic function.

Nitrosoureas *Lomustine (CCNU)* Lomustine is available for oral use only. It is very lipid-soluble and is rapidly and completely absorbed after oral administration. Peak levels occur in 3 h. Cerebrospinal fluid levels may approach 50 percent of the plasma levels. Lomustine is biotransformed in the liver to several cytotoxic products. The plasma half-life of the drug is variable, with a range of 16 to 72 h. Sixty percent of a dose is excreted through the kidneys as metabolites. Lomustine can cause delayed cumulative bone marrow toxicity, with a white blood cell nadir occurring 4 to 6 weeks following therapy. Therefore, 6-week intervals or more are recommended between doses to allow for adequate recovery of the bone marrow. Kidney damage can occur with prolonged administration, particularly with a large cumulative dose. Lomustine is active against NHL, brain tumors, small-cell lung cancer, and gastrointestinal cancers.

Carmustine (BCNU) Carmustine is available for intravenous use only. It is highly lipid-soluble and freely crosses into the cerebrospinal fluid where levels are at least 50 percent of those found in plasma. The drug is rapidly metabolized with 60 to 70 percent of a dose excreted in the urine; about 10 percent is eliminated as respiratory carbon dioxide. The plasma half-life of the drug is 15 to 30 min. Pulmonary fibrosis has been associated with the use of carmustine and is usually dose-related. Renal toxicity can occur as with lomustine. Delayed bone marrow toxicity is also seen. Carmustine is useful for NHL, multiple myeloma, and brain tumors.

Streptozocin This drug is available for intravenous use. Its plasma half-life is 35 min. Sixty to 70 percent is excreted by the kidney, of which 20 percent is the unchanged drug. Streptozocin has a predilection for the beta cells of the pancreatic islets. It is active against pancreatic islet cell tumors and carcinoid. It may cause mild glucose intolerance. It commonly causes severe dose-related kidney damage. Myelosuppression is mild.

Triazene Derivatives *Dacarbazine (DTIC)* Dacarbazine is available for intravenous use. It requires hepatic microsomal demethylation for activation. This generates an active methyl cation for alkylating activity. In addition to its function as an alkylating agent, a metabolic side product, methyltriazinoimidazole carboxamide inhibits purine incorporation into DNA. Although considered to be cell-cycle nonspecific, dacarbazine appears to be most active in the G_2 phase. The drug is only 5 percent bound to plasma proteins. The plasma elimination is biphasic, with an initial half-life of 19 min and a terminal half-life of 5 h. Up to 50 percent of an administered dose is excreted unchanged in the urine. Toxicity includes severe nausea, vomiting, moderate myelosuppression, a flu-like syndrome, and fulminant hepatic veno-occlusive disease. The latter is characterized by fever, eosinophilia, and acute hepatic necrosis; it is often fatal. Dacarbazine is active against Hodgkin's disease, soft tissue sarcomas, and melanoma.

Alkyl Sulfonates *Busulfan* Although busulfan is classified as a bifunctional alkylating agent, it binds poorly to DNA and has not been shown to cause interstrand cross-linking. Unlike other alkylating agents, it has little effect on lymphocytes and is much less immunosuppressive. It has potent cytotoxic properties and the ability to kill stem cells and cells in the G_0 phase of the cell cycle. Busulfan is available for oral use and is well absorbed. It is used in the myeloproliferative disorders, especially chronic myelogenous leukemia and polycythemia vera. Busulfan has a significant effect on stem cells and, thus, has been increasingly used as part of a preparative regimen for bone marrow transplantation, particularly for the leukemias. It has not been shown to increase the incidence of secondary leukemia, in contrast to other alkylating agents. It produces little mucositis or gastrointestinal disturbance in conventional doses. Blood counts must be carefully followed during prolonged use as irreversible marrow suppression can occur. A clinical syndrome that resembles adrenal insufficiency has been rarely reported.

Platinum Derivatives *Cisplatin (cis-Diaminedichloroplatinum, cis-DDP)* Cisplatin is an inorganic platinum-containing compound which functions like an alkylating agent. It produces interstrand and intrastrand cross-linking of DNA. The mechanism by which intrastrand DNA adducts cause cell death is not fully understood. Other effects on the cells, including suppression of mitochondrial respiration and inhibition of microtubule assembly, have been reported. Cisplatin has a triphasic half-life and its excretion is dependent on adequate renal function. Toxicities of cisplatin include renal dysfunction, nausea and vomiting, peripheral neuropathy, high-frequency hearing loss, and myelosuppression. Rarely, seizures and ischemic vascular effects are seen. Nephrotoxicity is common, however, but can be lessened by the administration of hydration with hypertonic saline. Cisplatin is an extremely important drug which can be curative for testicular and ovarian cancers. It is also highly effective in head and neck and bladder cancers, as well as lymphoma.

Carboplatin Carboplatin is a platinum analog with a mechanism of action similar to cisplatin. A larger concentration of carboplatin is required to achieve DNA cytotoxicity equivalent to cisplatin. Carboplatin is also excreted by the kidneys and the dose should be reduced for impaired renal function. The dose-limiting toxicity is myelosuppression. Carboplatin has a clinical spectrum similar to that of cisplatin.

Methylhydrazines *Procarbazine* Procarbazine was initially synthesized as a monoamine oxidase (MAO) inhibitor. The mechanism of action as an antineoplastic drug is not clearly understood but it is believed to function as an alkylating agent. Procarbazine is completely absorbed after oral administration and crosses well into the cerebrospinal fluid. It has a half-life of only 7 min after intravenous use. Procarbazine is metabolized in the liver to cytotoxic products and is excreted by the kidneys as N-isopropylterephthalamic acid. Procarbazine can be used intravenously or orally and is active in Hodgkin's disease and brain tumors. Adverse reactions include nausea, skin rash, myelosuppression, and neurotoxicity. Since it is a weak MAO inhibitor, foods with a high tyramine content should be avoided. In addition, procarbazine has a disulfiram-like reaction manifested by flushing and headache after alcohol ingestion.

ANTIBIOTICS

Antitumor antibiotics are a diverse class of chemotherapeutic agents all of which are natural products of microbial metabolism. The majority were isolated from various species of *Streptomyces*. Despite their varied structural features, antitumor antibiotics primarily affect DNA. Therefore, they typically are most effective against metabolically active, dividing cells.

Dactinomycin (Actinomycin D)

Mechanism of Action The actinomycins were the first antibiotics to be isolated from *Streptomyces parvullus*. Dactinomycin is a chromopeptide with a phenoxazone ring and two cyclic polypeptides. Dactinomycin forms a complex with DNA involving selective binding to and intercalation between the guanine-cytosine segments, with a specific block in DNA-dependent RNA synthesis. The greatest effect of the drug occurs in early S phase. Another cytotoxic effect of dactinomycin is to cause single-stranded breaks in DNA.

Pharmacokinetics Dactinomycin is available for intravenous use. It is rapidly concentrated in nucleated cells and minimally metabolized. It does not penetrate into the cerebrospinal fluid. The plasma half-life is approximately 36 h. Most of the drug is excreted unchanged in the urine and bile.

Therapeutic Uses Dactinomycin is effective against Wilms' tumor, Ewing's sarcoma, rhabdomyosarcoma, testicular carcinoma, gestational choriocarcinomas, lymphoma, and Kaposi's sarcoma.

Adverse Reactions The most frequent toxicity is myelosuppression. Gastrointestinal toxicities can include stomatitis, nausea, vomiting, and diarrhea. Abnormalities of liver and kidney functions have been reported. Dactinomycin can enhance radiation injury. Extravasation can produce significant tissue necrosis.

Plicamycin (Mithramycin)

Mechanism of Action Plicamycin is a cytotoxic antibiotic from *Streptomyces plicatus*. Its mechanism of action is similar to dactinomycin in that it inhibits the synthesis of DNA-dependent RNA synthesis.

Pharmacokinetics Plicamycin is available for intravenous use only. Its metabolism and excretion are poorly understood; however, it clears the blood quickly (within 2 h) and will cross the blood-brain barrier. Most of the drug is eliminated in the urine. Caution should be used in the presence of liver or kidney disorders.

Therapeutic Uses Plicamycin is useful in the treatment of malignant hypercalcemia and testicular germ cell neoplasms. It blocks calcium reabsorption from bone and reduces serum calcium concentration within hours of administration.

Adverse Reactions The major adverse effects of plicamycin include nausea and vomiting, hepatic and renal toxicities, and a hemorrhagic diathesis associated with severe thrombocytopenia and decreased synthesis of certain clotting factors.

Bleomycin Sulfate

Mechanism of Action Bleomycin is a mixture of glycopeptide antibiotics derived from a strain of *Streptomyces verticillus*. Bleomycin has antitumor, antiviral, and antibacterial activity. The drug binds with DNA to produce single- and double-strand breaks. DNA is cleaved at the guanine-cytosine and guanine-thymine sequences. RNA and protein synthesis is also inhibited. Bleomycin is cell-cycle specific; major effects are observed during the G_2 and M phases of the cell cycle.

Pharmacokinetics Bleomycin is administered via the parenteral route. After intravenous use, its initial plasma distribution half-life is 10 to 20 min. After intramuscular use, peak levels occur in 30 to 60 min and are approximately one-third of those achieved with intravenous administration. Bleomycin is metabolized in the tissues by bleomycin hydrolase and then excreted by the kidney. Approximately 30 to 40 percent is excreted in the urine as unchanged drug. The terminal elimination half-life is approximately 2 h. It is advisable to decrease the dose of bleomycin by at least 50 percent in the presence of renal insufficiency.

Therapeutic Uses Bleomycin is active in testicular cancer, Hodgkin's and non-Hodgkin's lymphomas, and squamous cell carcinomas of the head and neck, cervix, esophagus, and lung. Bleomycin can also be given into the pleural space to treat malignant pleural infusions.

Adverse Reactions An important toxicity of bleomycin is interstitial pneumonitis, which may progress to pulmonary fibrosis. This pulmonary toxicity is dose-related. Abnormalities in the diffusion capacity of the lungs are most commonly seen with total doses above 250 mg. Mucocutaneous reactions are common and include skin ulceration, hyperpigmentation, erythema, and stomatitis. Myelosuppression is rare. Pyrexia, which is particularly common in lymphoma patients, may occur either alone or in combination with wheezing, hypotension, and vomiting.

The Anthracyclines

The structure of the anthracycline antibiotics includes the amino sugar daunosamine with a planar naphthacenequinone nucleus. There are three compounds in this group that are presently being used: doxorubicin, daunorubicin, and idarubicin. Doxorubicin is a hydroxylated derivative of daunorubicin; idarubicin lacks the 4-methoxy group of daunorubicin.

Doxorubicin

Mechanism of Action Doxorubicin is an antibiotics derived from *Streptomyces peucetius*. The drug primarily acts by DNA intercalation. It also participates in oxidation-reduction reactions, impairs DNA repair, chelates divalent cations, interferes with cell membranes to alter their function, and triggers topoisomerase II-dependent DNA fragmentation.

Pharmacokinetics Doxorubicin is given by intravenous injection. It binds extensively to plasma proteins and does not cross the blood-brain barrier. It is cleared from the plasma with triphasic half-lives of 12 min, 3 h, and 30 h. Doxorubicin is metabolized by carbonyl reduction to the active alcohol, doxorubicinol, and to inactive products. Although a minor amount is excreted by the kidneys, most of the inactive metabolites are recovered in the bile. Doses need to be decreased in the presence of liver disease.

Therapeutic Uses Doxorubicin is extremely active in acute leukemia, lymphoma, breast and ovarian cancers, sarcoma, and several other solid tumors.

Adverse Reactions Bone marrow suppression and mucositis are the major adverse effects of doxorubicin. Nausea, vomiting, and alopecia will occur in the majority of patients. Drug extravasation of doxorubicin can cause severe tissue injury. A dose-limiting adverse effect of doxorubicin is cardiac toxicity. One form of cardiotoxicity is acute with either arrhythmias or pump failure, which is not dose-dependent. The second form is a cumulative dose-dependent cardiomyopathy, which typically occurs at doses greater than 550 mg/m^2 of body surface area. Prolonged intravenous infusions or repeated weekly small doses appear to produce less cardiac toxicity. Endocardial biopsy can identify characteristic pathologic features.

Daunorubicin

Mechanism of Action Daunorubicin is derived from a *Streptomyces coeruleorubidus*. Although the precise mechanism of action is unknown, daunorubicin, like doxorubicin is believed to intercalate into DNA. Other actions associated with doxorubicin appear to occur with daunorubicin.

Pharmacokinetics Daunorubicin is used only by the intravenous route. The drug is highly bound to plasma protein, and about 25 percent concentrates in liver. It does not enter the cerebrospinal fluid to any significant extent. Similar to its congener, daunorubicin is metabolized by carbonyl reduction to the active alcohol, daunorubicinol. It is eliminated from the plasma with triphasic half-lives of 10 to 30 min, 3 h, and 26 h. About 25 percent is eliminated as the active drug by urinary excretion, and 40 percent through the bile. Doses need to be decreased in the presence of liver disease.

Therapeutic Uses Daunorubicin is highly effective in acute nonlymphocytic leukemia (myelogenous, erythroid, and monocytic) and acute lymphocytic leukemia.

Adverse Reactions Adverse reactions are similar in most respects to doxorubicin. Nausea, vomiting, alopecia, bone marrow suppression, and mucositis are the most common untoward effects.

Idarubicin

Mechanism of Action Idarubicin is a synthetic analog of daunorubicin which is given by the intravenous route. The absence of the 4-methoxy group confers increased lipid solubility to the compound which results in increased cellular uptake and may decrease the incidence of cardiac toxicity. Its mechanism of action is similar to the other anthracyclines, with inhibition of DNA synthesis through DNA intercalation and interaction with topoisomerase II.

Pharmacokinetics The pharmacokinetics of idarubicin are similar to those for daunorubicin with a terminal elimination half-life of 22 h. Similar to the parent compound, the primary metabolite, idarubicinol, retains significant activity and has a terminal half-life exceeding 45 h. Dose reduction is not recommended in the presence of hepatic dysfunction. Most of the compound and its metabolic products are eliminated by biliary excretion.

Therapeutic Uses Idarubicin has a profound effect on acute nonlymphocytic leukemia and also some activity in acute lymphocytic leukemia, myelodysplasia, and breast cancer.

Adverse Reactions The toxicities of idarubicin are similar to the other anthracyclines with the suggestion of less cardiac toxicity.

Mitoxantrone

Mitoxantrone is a synthetic anthracenedione antibiotic; the drug is chemically related to the anthracyclines but was designed to have reduced side effects. It lacks the amino sugar moiety of the anthracyclines which is believed to be largely responsible for the cardiac toxicity.

Mechanism of Action Mitoxantrone retains the planar polycyclic aromatic ring structure of the anthracyclines and, therefore, has DNA intercalating activity. In addition, it appears to stabilize topoisomerase-DNA cleavable complexes, preventing rejoining of strand breaks. Mitoxantrone also generates free radicals which induce DNA and RNA strand breaks. It is a cell-cycle nonspecific agent.

Pharmacokinetics Mitoxantrone is used intravenously. It has a large volume of distribution. Disappearance from plasma follows triphasic kinetics, with half-lives of 3 to 10 min, 0.3 to 3 h, and up to 12 days. The drug is partially biotransformed to inactive products; these and the active drug are excreted mainly in the bile.

Therapeutic Uses Mitoxantrone has shown activity in the treatment of breast cancer, non-Hodgkin's lymphoma, and acute nonlymphatic leukemia. Dosage should be reduced in patients with hepatic dysfunction and in those with pleural effusions or ascites.

Adverse Reactions Adverse reactions include myelosuppression, nausea, vomiting, and mucositis. Cardiotoxicity has been reported, but appears to be less frequent than with the anthracyclines.

Mitomycin (Mitomycin C)

Mechanism of Action Mitomycin is an antibiotic isolated from *Streptomyces caespitosus*. This compound acts like an alkylating agent and inhibits DNA synthesis by cross-linking at guanine-cytosine sites on DNA. Mitomycin is most active in the cell cycle in late G and early S phases.

Pharmacokinetics Mitomycin is administered by the intravenous route, is minimally bound to plasma proteins, and has a half-life between 10 and 30 min. The liver is the major site of biotransformation, but metabolism occurs at other tissue sites. Approximately 10 percent is excreted in the urine unchanged.

Therapeutic Uses Mitomycin has primarily been used in combination with other chemotherapeutic drugs in the treatment of adenocarcinoma of the stomach, or pancreas.

Adverse Reactions The major adverse effect of mitomycin is a cumulative, delayed myelosuppression. Infrequently, renal failure with microangiopathic hemolytic anemia may be seen. Interstitial pneumonitis is rare, but may be fatal. Mitomycin may potentiate doxorubicin cardiotoxicity. Drug extravasation may cause significant local tissue injury.

PLANT DERIVATIVES

Some of the most effective chemotherapeutic agents are derived from natural plant products.

These include the *Vinca* alkaloids (vincristine and vinblastine), the podophyllotoxins (etoposide and teniposide), a taxane (paclitaxel), and topotecan.

Vinblastine and Vincristine

Mechanism of Action Vinblastine and vincristine are *Vinca* alkaloids derived from the periwinkle plant (*Vinca rosea*). These agents cause the arrest of cell division in metaphase and inhibit the assembly of microtubules and, thus, the failure of the mitotic spindle. Cells in S phase appear to be most sensitive to the effects of these alkaloids.

Pharmacokinetics Both vinblastine and vincristine are administered intravenously. The drugs are approximately 75 percent bound to plasma proteins. Both are metabolized by the liver. The plasma half-life of both drugs is triphasic: the initial, middle, and terminal half-lives of vincristine are 5 min, 2.3 h, and 85 h, respectively; for vinblastine these half-lives are 4 min, 1.6 h, and 25 h, respectively. Vincristine is partially metabolized by the liver and is excreted in the bile. Vinblastine is partially metabolized to deacetyl vinblastine, a more active form of the drug, then eliminated in the bile. The remainder of the drugs is excreted unchanged in the bile. Dose modification is advisable for both compounds in the presence of liver disease.

Therapeutic Uses Vincristine is extremely effective in combination with other chemotherapeutic agents in the treatment of acute lymphatic leukemia, non-Hodgkin's lymphoma, and Hodgkin's disease. It is also useful in multiple myeloma, neuroblastoma, Ewing's sarcoma, and Wilms' tumor. Vinblastine has found its major use in Hodgkin's disease, choriocarcinoma, breast cancer, testicular cancer, and lymphoma.

Adverse Reactions A significant and often dose-limiting effect of vincristine is neurotoxicity or peripheral neuropathy, which can manifest itself as muscular weakness or sensory impairment. Constipation and paralytic ileus can also occur. An advantage of vincristine for combination chemotherapy is its relative lack of severe, dose-limiting myelosuppression. The syndrome of inappropriate antidiuretic hormone secretion (as with cyclophosphamide) may occur.

Vinblastine has as its major toxicity profound myelosuppression (leukopenia, anemia, and granulocytopenia). Neurotoxicity is rarely seen.

Podophyllotoxins

Mechanism of Action Etoposide (VP-16) and teniposide (VM-26) are two synthetic derivatives of the American mandrake plant (*Podophyllum pelatum*). Their structures differ by the substitution of a methyl group (VP-16) for a thenylidine moiety (VM-26). Both agents arrest cells in late S phase or early G_2 phase. This effect is believed to be due to stabilization of the topoisomerase II cleavable enzyme-DNA complex, with resultant double-strand DNA breaks. Both compounds also inhibit topoisomerase II from disentangling DNA during replication and transcription. Etoposide also inhibits transport of nucleosides across the plasma membrane.

Pharmacokinetics Etoposide is administered either orally or by intravenous infusion. The oral bioavailability is approximately 50 percent, with marked inter- and intra-patient variability. About 97 percent of etoposide is bound to plasma proteins. Its plasma disposition is biphasic with a terminal half-life ranging from 4 to 11 h. The drug is metabolized to inactive products. Renal excretion accounts for about 35 percent of the total body clearance, so etoposide dosages should be adjusted for renal impairment. Dosage modifications are not necessary for hepatic dysfunction.

Teniposide is available only for intravenous use. Plasma clearance has been described as either biphasic or triphasic in various studies, while the terminal half-life has been reported to range from 6 to 48 h. Teniposide is highly bound to plasma proteins (99 percent). It is metabolized more extensively than etoposide with less than 15 percent appearing unchanged in the urine.

Therapeutic Uses Etoposide has shown significant activity against testicular and small-cell lung cancers, lymphoma, leukemia, and Kaposi's sarcoma. Prolonged oral administration has shown promising activity against non-small-cell lung cancer. Teniposide is an active antitumor agent which has been approved for use in childhood leukemias.

Adverse Reactions The principle toxicity of etoposide and teniposide is dose-related myelosuppression. Other side effects include mild nausea and vomiting, reversible alopecia, and stomatitis. Acute hypersensitivity reactions have also been described characterized by fever, chills, bronchospasm, flushing, and hypotension. These reactions occur more frequently with teniposide and may be related to the polyoxyethylated castor oil vehicle used to enhance solubility. High doses of etoposide are associated with severe mucositis and hepatic toxicity.

Drug Interactions The podophyllotoxins have demonstrated synergistic interactions with a wide range of antineoplastic agents, including cisplatin, cyclophosphamide, antimetabolites, and hydroxyurea. They also enhance cellular accumulation of methotrexate.

Paclitaxel

Mechanism of Action Paclitaxel is derived from the bark of the Pacific yew tree, *Taxus brevifolia*. Its structure is a complex 15-membered taxane ring system. It exerts its antitumor activity by promotion of microtubule assembly from tubulin dimers and microtubule stabilization by preventing depolymerization. These actions result in the formation of bundles of disorganized microtubules in cells in all phases of the cell cycle which decrease interphase and mitotic functions. In addition, it appears to promote premature cell division.

Pharmacokinetics Paclitaxel is administered intravenously, usually as a 24 h continuous infusion. Due to its poor aqueous solubility, it is formulated in a diluent with polyoxyethylated castor oil and ethanol. It has a biphasic half-life, with an initial half-life of 16 to 19 min and a terminal half-life of approximately 5 h. It is metabolized in the liver and excreted in the bile.

Therapeutic Uses Paclitaxel has shown significant activity in cisplatin-resistant ovarian cancer, metastatic breast cancer, malignant melanoma, and acute myelogenous leukemia. Used alone in breast cancer, it has activity approaching that of doxorubicin.

Adverse Reactions The primary toxicity is dose-dependent neutropenia occurring 7 to 10 days following therapy. In addition, hypersensitivity reactions, including urticaria, bronchospasm, and hypotension are common. Whether this is due to the vehicle or to the drug itself is unclear. These reactions can be diminished by premedication with corticosteroids, antihistamines, and H_2-receptor antagonists. Mild sensory neuropathy and transient myalgias and arthalgias are also common. Rare instances of bradyarrhythmias have been reported.

Topotecan

Topotecan is an experimental heterocyclic alkaloid and a semi-synthetic water-soluble analog of camptothecin. It is the first of several closely related compounds to enter clinical trials.

Mechanism of Action This drug is a potent inhibitor of DNA topoisomerase I. This enzyme transiently breaks a single strand of DNA to reduce torsional strain during replication or transcription. Topotecan stabilizes the topoisomerase-cleaved DNA complex and prevents re-ligation of the DNA strands. Although initially felt to be highly specific for the S phase, it is now known that topoisomerase I is active in cells in G_0 as well as mitotically active cells.

Pharmacokinetics Topotecan is administered intravenously. When given as a bolus injection, it has a biphasic half-life, with an average distribution (α) half-life of 9 min and an elimination (β) half-life of 103 min.

Therapeutic Uses Phase I trials have shown activity against a broad range of tumors including ovarian, non-small-cell lung, colorectal, esophageal, breast, and head and neck carcinomas. Responses have also been noted in lymphoma and leukemia. Significantly, topotecan is effective against tumors which express the P-glycoprotein multi-drug resistance gene.

Adverse Reactions The primary toxicity of topotecan is myelosuppression. Other toxicities include alopecia, mild nausea and vomiting, and occasional fever. Elevations of serum hepatic transaminases and alkaline phosphatase levels have also been described.

MISCELLANEOUS COMPOUNDS

There are a number of miscellaneous antineoplastic drugs including asparaginase, hydroxyurea, and a few interferons (i.e., interferon alfa-2a, alfa-2b, and alfa-n3). Asparaginase and hydroxyurea are discussed below; the pharmacology of the interferons are covered in depth in Chapter 44.

Asparaginase

Mechanism of Action Asparagine is a nonessential amino acid which can be synthesized by a reaction catalyzed by the enzyme L-asparagine synthetase. Asparaginase is an enzyme which can hydrolyze L-asparagine to L-aspartic acid and cause depletion of L-asparagine. Asparaginase derived from *Escherichia coli* can be highly effective against acute lymphocytic leukemia by intracellular depletion of L-asparagine and subsequent inhibition of protein and nucleic acid synthesis.

Pharmacokinetics Asparaginase can be given by the intravenous route, but the intramuscular route is preferred because of a decreased frequency of hypersensitivity reactions. Intramuscular peak plasma levels are approximately 50 percent of intravenous levels. Systemic absorption is slow. The half-life ranges from 11 to 22 h. Minimal urinary or biliary excretion occurs.

Therapeutic Uses Asparaginase is particularly effective in the treatment of acute lymphocytic leukemia primarily in combination with other antineoplastic drugs.

Adverse Reactions Asparaginase is an unusual chemotherapeutic agent in that it does not cause significant bone marrow or gastrointestinal toxicity. Nausea and vomiting may occur but are usually transitory and easily managed. Asparaginase inhibits protein synthesis and can cause liver toxicity in the form of hypoalbuminemia, decreased production of clotting factors and subsequent bleeding, and elevated bilirubin and transaminases. Dysfibrinogenemia can occur on the basis of a shortened fibrinogen survival due to the production of an intrinsically abnormal fibrinogen. Hypersensitivity reactions such as urticaria, bronchospasm, and hypotension may occur. Less frequent side effects include acute pancreatitis and encephalopathy.

Hydroxyurea

Mechanism of Action Hydroxyurea is a substituted derivative of urea which inhibits ribonucleotide reductase. This enzyme reduces ribonucleotides to deoxyribonucleotides, a necessary step prior to their insertion into DNA. Hydroxyurea thereby inhibits DNA synthesis.

Pharmacokinetics Hydroxyurea is well absorbed orally, achieving peak plasma levels within 2 h. The serum half-life is 5.5 h. Fifty percent of an oral dose is metabolized in the liver and excreted in the urine as urea. The remainder is excreted in the urine unchanged. Hydroxyurea has substantial penetration into the CNS, reaching peak levels in about 3 h.

Therapeutic Uses Hydroxyurea is useful for treatment of the myeloproliferative disorders. It can also be used to rapidly decrease the white blood cell count in acute myelogenous leukemia. When combined with other agents, it also has activity against renal, ovarian, colon, and head and neck cancers.

Adverse Reactions Mild gastrointestinal side effects and reversible myelosuppression are its only common toxicities.

HORMONES

The hormones commonly used as adjuncts in cancer chemotherapy are listed in Table 43-1. Their pharmacology is not discussed in this chapter, as it is covered in other chapters: estrogens, antiestrogens, and progestins (Chapter 40), the adrenocorticoids (Chapter 42), androgens and antiandrogens, and gonadotropin analogs (Chapter 41). A brief description of the therapeutic use of these drugs is discussed below.

Estrogens including diethylstilbestrol, estradiol, and estramustine, are available for use in advanced breast cancer in receptor-positive postmenopausal females and in men with advanced prostate carcinoma. The presence of estrogen and progesterone receptor positivity in breast cancer tissue will predict those women most likely to benefit from estrogen therapy. The antiestrogens have largely replaced estrogens for the treatment of advanced breast cancer. In prostatic carcinoma, the estrogens will antagonize the androgen effect.

Side effects of estrogens include gastrointestinal upset, phebitis, hypercalcemia flare, and gynecomastia in men.

Tamoxifen is an oral antiestrogen which blocks the activity of estrogen by competitively inhibiting estradiol binding to the estrogen receptor. Tamoxifen was the first antiestrogen for clinical use because of its low toxicity profile. It is a frontline drug in the treatment of receptor-positive postmenopausal females with breast cancer where it has been shown to increase both disease-free and overall survival. Since 1992, a chemoprevention trial to evaluate the role of tamoxifen to prevent the development of breast cancer in women at high risk has been underway.

The side effects, though infrequent, are nearly always manageable and include mild nausea, fluid retention, thrombocytopenia, skin rash, and vaginal bleeding. Ocular side effects have been seen when given in high doses.

Progestational agents may be helpful in certain advanced breast and endometrial malignancies. In patients with endometrial carcinoma, progestins may inhibit luteinizing hormone as well as DNA and RNA synthesis. Side effects include fluid retention and weight gain.

Adrenocorticosteroids can be quite effective in the treatment of neoplastic disorders as well as in the palliation of a variety of complications of malignancy. The exact mechanisms involved in their antitumor activity are not completely understood, but glucocorticoid receptors have been shown to be present on the malignant cells in some breast cancers.

Side effects include fluid retention, muscle weakness, glucose intolerance, and immunosuppression. The major uses of glucocorticoids in the treatment of cancer include acute lymphatic leukemia, non-Hodgkin's lymphoma, Hodgkin's disease, and breast cancer. Steroids are also helpful in treatment of hypercalcemia, cerebral or spinal cord edema, nausea, fever, and anorexia.

Androgens are occasionally effective for hormone-responsive advanced breast cancer. They are believed to act through inhibition of gonadotropin-releasing hormone with consequent suppression of estrogen production. In general, the response to androgens is no better than to estrogens, but greater toxicity is seen. Common side effects are cholestatic jaundice, alteration of libido, virilization, and hypercalcemia.

Antiestrogens are commonly employed in the treatment of advanced prostate cancer. One such agent, flutamide, is a toluidine derivative which binds to dihydrotestosterone receptors on the nuclear membrane, thereby suppressing nuclear androgen binding. It is administered orally and is usually well-tolerated. The most frequent adverse reactions are diarrhea, abdominal cramps, and "gas pains."

Several **gonadotropin analogs** are now available for treatment of metastatic prostate and breast cancers. Initially, these compounds cause the release of gonadotropin stores from the pituitary gland. This can lead to a flare up of the disease with an increase in bone pain. Continued doses cause inhibition of pituitary/gonadal function. **Leuprolide acetate**, a synthetic gonadotropin releasing hormone is administered as a monthly intramuscular injection. Side effects include hot flashes (seen in 50 to 60 percent) and a decrease in libido and impotence.

BIBLIOGRAPHY

Ackland, S.P., and R.L. Schilsky: "High-Dose Methotrexate: A Critical Reappraisal," *J. Clin. Oncol.* **5**: 2017-2031 (1987).

Bohr, V.A., D.H. Phillips, and P.C. Hanawalt: "Heterogeneous DNA Damage and Repair in the Mammalian Genome," *Cancer Res.* **47**: 6426-6436 (1987).

Brodsky, I.: "Busulfan: Effect on Platelet RNA Dependent DNA Polymerase — Implications in the Treatment of Polycythemia Vera, Thrombosis and Atherosclerosis," *Biomed. Pharmacother.* **36**: 125-127 (1982).

Calabrese, P., P.S. Schein, and S.A. Rosenberg: *Medical Oncology: Basic Principles and Clinical Management of Cancer*, MacMillan, New York, 1985.

Capizzi R.L., B.L. Powell, M.R. Cooper, et al.: "Dose-Related Pharmacologic Effects of High Dose Ara-C and Its Use in Combination with Asparaginase for the Treatment of Patients with Acute Nonlymphocytic Leukemia," *Scand. J. Haematol. Suppl.* **44**: 17-39 (1986).

Chabner, B.A.: *Pharmacologic Principles of Cancer Treatment*, Saunders, Philadelphia, 1982.

Chabner, B.A.: "Taxol," *PPO Updates* **5**: 1-10 (1991).

Clark, P.I., and M.L. Slevin: "The Clinical Pharmacology of Etoposide and Teniposide," *Clin. Pharmacokinet.* **12**: 223-252 (1987).

Cohen, N.A., M.J. Egorin, S.W. Snyder, B. Ashar, B.E. Wietharn, S.S. Pan, D.D. Ross, and J. Hilton: "Interaction of N,N',N''-Triethylenethiophosphoramide and N,N',N''-Triethylenephosphoramide with Cellular DNA," *Cancer Res.* **51**: 4360-4366 (1991).

DeVita, V.T., S. Hellman, and S. A. Rosenberg: *Cancer Principles and Practice of Oncology*, J.B. Lippincott, Philadelphia, 1993.

Faulds, D., J.A. Balfour, P. Chrisp, and H.D. Langtry: "Mitoxantrone. A Review of Its Pharmacodynamic and Pharmacokinetic Properties and Therapeutic Potential in the Chemotherapy of Cancer," *Drugs* **41**: 400-449 (1991).

Forastiere, A.A., R.B. Natale, B.J. Takasugi, M.P. Goren, W.C. Vogel, and V. Kudia-Hatch: "A Phase I-II Trial of Carboplatin and 5-Fluorouracil Combination Therapy for Small-Cell Lung Cancer," *J. Clin. Oncol.* **5**: 190-196 (1987).

Gordon, J.A., and V.H. Gattone: "Mitochondrial Alterations in Cisplatin-Induced Acute Renal Failure," *Am. J. Physiol.* **250**: F991-F998 (1986).

Hagen, B.: "Pharmacokinetics of Thio-TEPA and TEPA in the Conventional Dose-Range and Its Correlations to Myelosuppressive Effects," *Cancer Chemother. Pharmacol.* **27**: 373-378 (1991).

Hainsworth, J.D., D.H. Johnson, S.R. Fazier, and F.A. Greco: "Chronic Daily Administration of Oral Etoposide — A Phase I Trial," *J. Clin. Oncol.* 7: 396-401 (1989).

Kiang, D.T., and B.J. Kennedy: "Tamoxifen (Antiestrogen) Therapy in Advanced Breast Cancer," *Ann. Intern. Med.* **87**: 687-690 (1977).

Lieschke, G.J., and A.W. Burgess: "Granulocyte Colony-Stimulating Factor and Granulocyte-Macrophage Colony Stimulating Factor (First of Two Parts)," *N. Engl. J. Med.* **327**: 28-35 (1992).

Lieschke, G.J., and A.W. Burgess: "Granulocyte Colony-Stimulating Factor and Granulocyte-Macrophage Colony-Stimulating Factor (Second of Two Parts)," *N. Engl. J. Med.* **327**: 99-106 (1992).

Ludlum, D.B.: "Alkylating Agents and the Nitrosureas," in Becker, T.T.F. (ed.), *Cancer: A Comprehensive Treatise, Vol. 5*, Plenum Press, New York, 1977: pp. 285-307.

O'Dwyer, P.J., B. Leyland-Jones, M.T. Alonzo, S. Marsoni, and R.E. Wittes: "Etoposide (VP-16-213) Current Status of an Active Anticancer Drug," *N. Engl. J. Med.* **312**: 692-700 (1985).

O'Dwyer, P.J., B. Wagner, B. Leyland-Jones, R.E. Wittes, B.D. Cheson, and D.F. Hoth: "2-Deoxycoformycin (Pentostatin) for Lymphoid Malignancies. Rational Development of An Active New Drug," *Ann. Intern. Med.* **108**: 733-743 (1988).

Osborne, C.K., D.H. Boldt, G.M. Clark, and J.M. Trent: "Effects of Tamoxifen on Human Breast Cancer Cell Kinetics: Accumulation of Cells in Early G_1 Phase," *Cancer Res.* **43**: 3583-3585 (1983).

Perry, M.C.: "*The Chemotherapy Source Book,*" Williams and Wilkins, Baltimore, 1992.

Pinto, A.L., and S.J. Lippard: "Sequence-Dependent Termination of *in vitro* DNA Synthesis by Cis-and Trans-diamminedichloroplatinum (II)," *Proc. Natl. Acad. Sci. USA* **82**: 4616-4619 (1985).

Plunkett, W., P. Huang, and V. Ghandi: "Metabolism and Action of Fludarabine Phosphate," *Semin. Oncol.* **17 (5 Suppl. 8)**: 3-17 (1990).

Reid, J.M., T.W. Pendergrass, M.D. Krailo, G.D. Hammond, and M.M. Ames: "Plasma Pharmacokinetics and Cerebrospinal Fluid Concentrations of Idarubicin and Idarubicinol in Pediatric Leukemia Patients: A Children's Cancer Study Group Report," *Cancer Res.* **50**: 6525-6528 (1990).

Safirstein, R., J. Winston, M. Goldstein, D. Moel, S. Dikman, and J. Guttenplan: "Cisplatin Nephrotoxicity," *Am. J. Kidney Dis.* **8**: 356-367 (1986).

Saven, A., and S.A. Piro: "2-Chlorodeoxyadenosine: A New Nucleoside Agent Effective in the Treatment of Lymphoid Malignancies," *Leuk. Lymphoma* **10 (Suppl.)**: 43-49 (1993).

Shenkenberg, T.D., and D.D. Von Hoff: "Mitoxantrone: A New Anticancer Drug with Significant Clinical Activity," *Ann. Intern. Med.* **105**: 67-81 (1986).

Slichenmyer, W.J., E.K. Rowinsky, R.C. Donehower, and S.H. Kaufmann: "The Current Status of Camptothecin Analogues as Antitumor Agents," *J.N.C.I.* **85**: 271-291 (1993).

Smith, J.A., Jr.: "Luteinizing Hormone-Releasing Hormone (LH-RH) Analogs in Treatment of Prostatic Cancer," *Urology* **27 (Suppl. 1)**: 9-15 (1986).

Tucker, M.A., C.N. Coleman, R.S. Cox, A. Varghese, and S.A. Rosenberg: "Risk of Second Cancers After Treatment for Hodgkin's Disease," *N. Engl. J. Med.* **318**: 76-81 (1988).

Von Hoff, D.D.: "Whither Carboplatin? — A Replacement for or an Alternative to Cisplatin?," *J. Clin. Oncol.* **5**: 169-172 (1987).

Weinstein, G.D.: "Methotrexate," *Ann. Intern. Med.* **86**: 199-204 (1977).

Wiley, J.S., J. Taupin, G.P. Jamieson, M. Snook, W.H. Sawyer, and L.R. Finch: "Cytosine Arabinoside Transport and Metabolism in Acute Leukemias and T Cell Lymphoblastic Lymphoma," *J. Clin. Invest.* **75**: 632-642 (1985).

CHAPTER 44

Immunopharmacologic Drugs

Eric M. Scholar

The immune system is vital to the protection of the host against invaders, both organic and inorganic. It also is the disposal system for sick, dead, or unwanted cells and the major defense against cancer. What is regarded as inflammation is in reality a major part of the immune reaction. In this sense all the drugs and mechanisms involved in inflammation which have been described in other chapters, such as histamine and antihistamines, prostaglandins and non-steroidal antiinflammatory agents, kinins, serotonin and many others belong to immunopharmacology. It would be impractical to discuss the interrelationship of these agents to the immune process in this chapter. The focus will be on those drugs which have a direct effect on the cells that have immune functions such as lymphocytes, polymorphonuclear leukocytes, basophils, eosinophils, macrophages and subtypes of these cells. The products of these cells (such as tumor necrosis factor, colony stimulating factors, interferons and interleukins), are also important as drugs in their own right. Based on these considerations, a reasonable classification of immunopharmacologic drugs is shown in Table 44-1.

In this chapter immunopharmacology has been divided into two major areas: the *immunosuppressive agents* and the *immunostimulants*. The clinical usefulness of the latter group will become increasingly important in the next few years as more compounds become approved for use and the number of their therapeutic uses expand.

IMMUNOSUPPRESSIVE AGENTS

Agents that suppress the immune response have assumed an increasing importance in medicine in recent years. These agents have two important uses. One is for inhibiting organ transplant rejection; in this situation, immunosuppressives are needed because of the difficulty in obtaining a perfect tissue type match with the transplanted tissue. The second use of these drugs is in the treatment of autoimmune and inflammatory diseases. In these conditions there is some abnormality in immune regulation, so that there is a loss in the ability to discriminate between self and foreign.

There are several limitations to immunosuppressive therapy. First, immunosuppression is often nonspecific in that many immune responses are affected. The immunosuppression makes the patient susceptible to multiple infections; therefore, patients must be carefully monitored for viral, fungal and bacterial infections. Reduction of dosage of the immunosuppressive drug and rigorous antimicrobial therapy is often necessary. Thus an ideal immunosuppressant would be selective against one particular immune response. Second, many of the immunosuppressive agents can produce serious toxic effects. This could, for example, include toxicity to the bone marrow, reproductive system and gastrointestinal tract. This should be expected since many immunosuppressives have been taken from the anticancer field. Finally, there is an increased incidence of malignancies in patients taking these drugs for long periods of time.

The major drugs used as immunosuppressives can be subdivided into several categories. Corticosteroids are the drugs that have been most widely used over the years. They have now been replaced to a large extent by the cytotoxic agents, a group of drugs used mostly for cancer chemotherapy. More recently, a new class of immunosuppressives have been developed which are more specific for certain aspects of the immune system than any other compounds. This group includes cyclosporine and, more recently, FK506.

TABLE 44-1 Classification of immunopharmacologic drugs

Drug class	Specific Agents	FDA approved indications	Unlabeled and experimental uses
IMMUNOSUPPRESSIVE AGENTS			
Corticosteroids	Prednisone, prednisolone, [others]	Many autoimmune diseases, including rheumatic disorders, collagen diseases, respiratory diseases	Transplants of all types, often in conjunction with other agents. All auto-immune disorders
Cytotoxic Agents	Azathioprine	Renal transplantation and rheumatoid arthritis	Cardiac and other transplants, chronic ulcerative colitis, and other autoimmune diseases
	Cyclophosphamide	Cancer chemotherapy of lymphomas, multiple myeloma, leukemias, nephrotic syndrome	Wegener's granulomatosis, systemic lupus erythematosus, polyarthritis nodosa, multiple sclerosis, bone marrow transplants, rheumatoid arthritis
	Methotrexate	Rheumatoid arthritis, cancer chemotherapy	Several autoimmune diseases including Reifer's syndrome, pemphigus, inflammatory bowel disease, graft vs. host disease
Specific T cell Inhibitors	Cyclosporine	Rejection crisis, prophylaxis of organ rejection in renal, liver, and heart transplants	Other transplants such as bone marrow, pancreas, and heart/lung. Various auto-immune diseases such as uveitis, aplastic anemia, psoriasis, sarcoidosis, rheumatoid arthritis, myasthenia gravis
Antibodies	Anti-thymocyte globulin	Renal allograft rejection and prophylaxis, aplastic anemia	Multiple sclerosis, myasthenia gravis, pure red cell aplasia
	Muromonab-CD3	Treatment of acute allograft rejection	Psoriasis, organ transplant rejection

TABLE 44-1 (continued) Classification of immunopharmacologic drugs

Drug class	Specific Agents	FDA approved indications	Unlabeled and experimental uses
IMMUNOSTIMULANTS			
Cytokines	Interferon alpha	Hairy cell leukemia, hepatitis B and C, Kaposi's sarcoma	Many carcinomas, including bladder, leukemias, and lymphomas. Many viral infections, including AIDS
	Interferon gamma	Chronic granulomatous disease	AIDS, several cancers including breast carcinoma and leukemia, rheumatoid arthritis, venereal warts
	Interferon beta	Multiple sclerosis	
	Aldesleukin	Renal cell carcinoma	Therapy of melanoma and other chemotherapy-resistant cancers, Epstein Barr virus infections, atopic dermatitis
Growth Factors	Sargramostim	Bone marrow transplantation	Agranulocytosis, AIDS, aplastic anemia, cancer chemotherapy, myelodysplasia, peripheral blood stem cell transfusion
	Filgrastim	Chemotherapy-induced neutropenia	Agranulocytosis, AIDS, leukemia, infections
Miscellaneous Agents	Levamisole	Colon carcinoma (with 5-fluorouracil)	
	BCG vaccine	Bladder cancer	Several cancers, including breast, gastric, ovarian

Corticosteroids

The adrenal corticosteroids have been extensively used to suppress many different kinds of the immune response. They were first reported to be effective in 1949, when hydrocortisone was discovered to inhibit manifestations of rheumatoid arthritis. Since then they have been found to be effective in the treatment of several autoimmune disorders.

All of the corticosteroids have similar mechanisms of action. They bind to specific corticosteroid binding receptors in the cytoplasm. These complexes are then transported into the nucleus where they bind to discrete portions of the cell's DNA. This binding results in depression of regulatory genes and the subsequent transcription of new messenger RNA. New regulatory proteins are then formed which can enhance or suppress specific cellular functions.

Corticosteroids inhibit the consequences of the immune response. They have several different actions in this regard. One of their most important effects is to transiently alter the number of circulating leukocytes. There is a rapid increase in the number of neutrophils and a concomitant decrease in the number of lymphocytes, monocytes, eosinophils and basophils.

Corticosteroids also alter important functional activities of lymphocytes and monocytes. This effect is mainly on T lymphocytes and is at least partly due to a decrease in interleukin 2 (IL-2) production. The effect on B lymphocytes is less prominent. These drugs also profoundly impair the function of monocytes/macrophages by decreasing the phagocytic ability of these cells. Corticosteroids can also effect the production of soluble mediators that regulate both inflammatory and immune responses.

The complete pharmacology of corticosteroids is discussed in Chapter 42. Of the many drugs available, prednisone and prednisolone have been found to be the most useful in immune therapy. Prednisone therapy attenuates, but does not cure, practically all autoimmune diseases. Especially satisfactory responses are obtained in rheumatoid arthritis, idiopathic, thrombocytopenic purpura, lupus erythematosus and many other less common autoimmune and collagen diseases. In transplantation, prednisone has an important effect, but by itself does not ensure successful engraftment. Prednisone is therefore used as an adjunct, which has a valuable sparing effect on the dose of more toxic, but more effective, drugs such as azathioprine and cyclosporine.

Prolonged therapy with the corticosteroids is not innocuous. Were it not for the unacceptable toxicity of prednisone in long-term high-dose therapy, it would, in effect, be acceptable for palliative therapy. These drugs have numerous and potentially serious adverse reactions such as psychoses, Cushing's syndrome and cataracts.

Cytotoxic Agents

Cytotoxic agents were originally introduced into medicine as anticancer agents. They are able to kill cells that are capable of self-replication, including both normal and neoplastic cells. In the process of responding to an antigen, immunologically competent lymphocytes are transformed from resting cells to actively proliferating cells. Thus they are susceptible to the action of the cytotoxic agents. Several different cytotoxic agents have proved highly active as immunosuppressive agents.

Azathioprine

One of a series of analogs of mercaptopurine, azathioprine has been shown to be more effective as an immunosuppressive than as a cytotoxic drug for the treatment of cancer (see Chapter 43). Chemically it is an imidazolyl derivative of 6-mercaptopurine.

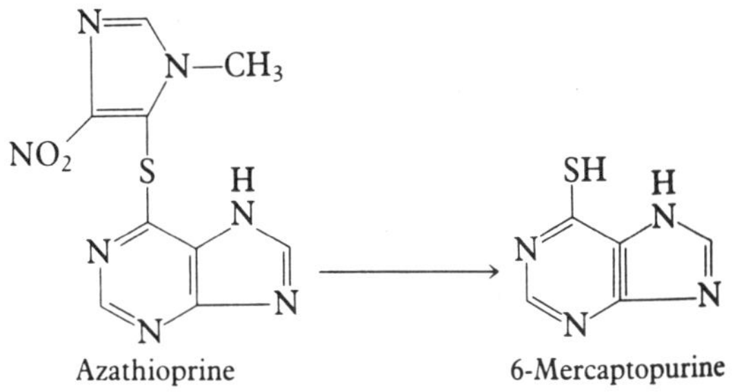

N—CH_3 NO_2 S H N N N N SH H N N N N

Azathioprine → 6-Mercaptopurine

Actually azathioprine is a prodrug in that it is converted in the body to mercaptopurine. This reaction can occur in a nonenzymatic fashion with the aid of glutathione or other sulfhydryl-containing compounds. Perhaps it is this attribute that makes azathioprine superior to mercaptopurine as an immunosuppressant. After conversion to 6-mercaptopurine, its mechanism of action is similar to other purine antimetabolites. The compound interferes with nucleic acid synthesis through enzyme inhibition and it may be incorporated into DNA after conversion to the nucleotide form. Therefore, its action in suppression of the growth of lymphoid cells is not selective. Although both cell-mediated and humoral responses are suppressed, the drug does appear to have a preferential effect to inhibit T cell responses.

Azathioprine is well absorbed from the gastrointestinal tract, with a peak level at 1 to 2 h after administration. The half-life of 5 h, measured by radioactive technology, does not reflect the duration of action of azathioprine, which is much longer. This is because after being cleaved into 6-mercaptopurine, further conversion into inactive 6-thiouric acid occurs, a reaction catalyzed by xanthine oxidase. Clearance is via the kidney and patients with poor renal function may need to have a reduction in dosage.

Azathioprine has been a mainstay drug in all types of transplantation but especially in renal allografts. Prior to the widespread use of cyclosporine, azathioprine along with corticosteroids, were standard therapy for the prevention and inhibition of transplant rejection. It still has an important role in this area but is used less than it was previously. Under the best circumstances it can achieve 50 to 70 percent engraftment of 1 year or more. With respect to renal allograft survival, azathioprine must be given in advance or at least simultaneously with the graft transplant. It has little effect on initiated graft rejections. Cyclosporine has replaced azathioprine in most circumstances. Azathioprine, however, is useful in combinations with cyclosporine or may replace it in selected cases.

Azathioprine is also widely used in the treatment of many immune mediated disorders. For example, it has been used in classical rheumatoid arthritis which is severe, erosive and nonresponding to conventional therapy. Other uses include Wegener's granulomatosis, systemic lupus erythematosus and ulcerative colitis. Other thiopurines, e.g., 6-mercaptopurine and 6-thioguanine, have also been used occasionally as immunosuppressives, but are not as effective as azathioprine.

Azathioprine has all the potential toxicities associated with cytotoxic drugs. This includes the induction of severe leukopenia and thrombocytopenia secondary to bone marrow depression. Periodic blood counts are thus necessary during therapy. As with other cytotoxic drugs the risk of malignancy is increased by immunosuppressive therapy with azathioprine. Renal transplant patients maintained on azathioprine have shown an increased incidence of skin cancers and reticulum cell and lymphomatous tumors. Azathioprine must be avoided in pregnant patients because it is teratogenic.

Xanthine oxidase inhibitors, such as allopurinol, inhibit the biotransformation of azathioprine to the inactive 6-thiouric acid and hence increase its action. Patients on both drugs need to have the dose of azathioprine reduced to one-third to one-half the usual dose.

Cyclophosphamide

The alkylating agent cyclophosphamide is widely used in cancer chemotherapy. Its complete pharmacology (including mechanism of action) is discussed in Chapter 43 and will not be repeated here. As an immunosuppressive drug, cyclophosphamide is highly potent. It destroys proliferating cells and also appears to alkylate a portion of the DNA in resting cells. Comparatively, cyclophosphamide has a greater effect on humoral antibody responses than on cellular reactions. Its effect on cell mediated immunity is variable. Some reactions are inhibited while others are augmented. The inhibition is due to the effect of the drug on T-suppressor lymphocytes.

Cyclophosphamide has been successfully used in renal allotransplants as an alternative to azathioprine especially in developing countries; this is a result of its low cost and ready availability. In relatively small doses cyclophosphamide has been effective in autoimmune disorders, including systemic lupus erythematosus, severe rheumatoid arthritis, polyarthritis nodosa, Wegener's granulomatosis and certain cases of aplastic anemia. An advantage of cyclophosphamide is that it can be given either orally or by IV injection.

Large doses of cyclophosphamide cause pancytopenia. Gastrointestinal symptoms are usually severe. Cystitis occurs in about 25 percent of all cases, including the hemorrhagic variety in a lesser percentage. Alopecia, pulmonary fibrosis and cardiac toxicity (hemorrhagic myocarditis) add to the adverse reactions. Thus the benefits of cyclophosphamide must be balanced against the risks of therapy. In addition, there is also the risk of the induction of cancer and teratogenicity.

Methotrexate

Methotrexate is a folic acid analog. The mechanism of action of this drug has been discussed in the chapter on cancer chemotherapeutic agents. In lower doses it has often been used as an immunosuppressive drug for several indications. Methotrexate has recently gained favor for and is approved for the treatment of rheumatoid arthritis in adults who have severe active classical rheumatoid arthritis. It is an investigational agent for juvenile rheumatoid arthritis. It also has some use in other autoimmune diseases such as polymyositis and dermatomyositis. This folic acid analogue also has been used to prevent both acute and chronic graft vs. host disease in bone marrow recipients.

The most common adverse reactions are associated with the gastrointestinal tract and include ulcerative stomatitis, nausea, abdominal distress, and liver toxicity. This latter effect is most common when large doses or prolonged therapy is employed. Pneumonitis is also seen on occasion.

Specific T Cell Inhibitors

Cyclosporine (Cyclosporine A)

With the discovery and development of cyclosporine, a new era in immunopharmacology was born. Cyclosporine is the first agent that affects a specific cell line of the body's immune defenses. It is suppressive mainly to T cells, in contrast to the cytotoxic agents which affect all cell lines at the same time. The fact that it has markedly improved the engraftment of transplants and increased the potential of treating autoimmune diseases has amplified the interest of scientists and clinicians. Cyclosporine is the forerunner of a group of immunosuppressive drugs that are active against specific components of the immune system.

Chemistry Cyclosporine was originally isolated from the cultural broths of the fungus *Tolypocladium inflatum Gams*. Cyclosporine is composed of 11 amino acids arranged in a cyclic fashion. All are known aliphatic amino acids except number 1, which has never been isolated before. N-Methyl- is in position 5; alanine in position 7; D-alanine in leucine occupies positions 4, 6, 9 and 10; valine position 8; α-aminobutyric acid in position 2; sarcosine in position 3; and N-methylvaline in position 11. All are levo with the exception of alanine at position 8. The structure lends itself to hydrogen bonding and is, therefore, quite rigid. There are many analogs of cyclosporine, and some structure-activity relationships have been found. For example, it is believed that the amino acid in the number 1 position is an important factor in the drug's activity.

Mechanism of Action The exact molecular mechanism of action is unclear, but the drug appears to act on several aspects of the immune response of T cells. For example, it has been reported to inhibit the production of the interleukins and interferon gamma as a result of blocking transcription of lymphokine genes. Of most importance is the inhibition of IL-2.

Although a relatively large molecule, cyclosporine passes through cell membranes easily. Apparently there are no surface recognition receptors, but there is a cytosolic cyclosporine-binding protein known as *cyclophilin A* with a molecular weight of about 15,000 daltons. Cyclophilins are present especially in T lymphocytes, but they are also in other tissues such as brain and kidney. Cyclophilins and similar binding proteins are now referred to collectively as *immunophilins* and their

Cyclosporine

enzymatic activities are relevant to the actions of immunosuppressants such as cyclosporine and FK506. Cyclophilin A has now been purified, the gene encoding it has been cloned, and the sequence was found to match the sequence of an enzyme, peptidyl-prolyl *cis-trans* isomerase. This enzyme speeds up the isomerization of proline peptide bonds in polypeptides, and thereby facilitates protein folding. According to the current model, cyclosporine works by binding to and inhibiting the normal cellular function of the peptidyl-prolyl isomerase. This enzyme is apparently intimately involved in T cell signalling that leads to transcription of the IL-2 gene upon antigen recognition.

While the mechanism of action of cyclosporine is still under intense investigation, it is important to point out that cyclosporine is not cytotoxic in the ordinary sense and hence does not depress bone marrow. Because it does not encourage (in fact, it suppresses) graft vs. host immune reactions, it is especially useful in bone marrow transplants. Cyclosporine also has antiparasitic actions against schistosoma and malarial parasites. It also appears to be effective in reducing multidrug resistance in patients receiving cancer chemotherapy. The mechanism of action of these effects is unknown.

Pharmacokinetics The oral absorption of cyclosporine is quite variable. Based on patient studies, oral bioavailability is about 30 percent of that obtained by IV administration. Peak blood levels are achieved in about 3.5 h. Although highly bound to lipoproteins in the blood (approximately 90%), cyclosporine is largely distributed outside the blood volume. Cyclosporine is extensively biotransformed, but no major pathway appears to exist. Hydroxylation of some of the amino acids by the microsomal mixed-function oxidase system constitutes one of the major metabolic pathways. Only 0.1 percent appears in the urine unchanged. Most of the drug is excreted in the bile after biotransformation in the liver. The terminal half-life is approximately 19 h.

Therapeutic Uses Although in clinical use for only a decade, cyclosporine has established itself as the prime drug for organ transplantation. In renal allotransplants it has improved graft acceptance in most centers to 95 percent. Cyclosporine has also significantly improved the initial and long term survival of renal allografts. It has also mitigated the impact of immunologic risk factors such as HLA mismatching and the absence of pretransplantation blood transfusions. In addition it has reduced morbidity, the incidence of graft rejection, the period of initial hospitalization, and the rate of readmission.

The effects of cyclosporine are even more dramatic in the field of heart, liver and lung transplants. Results are generally better in heart transplantations than was the previous combination of prednisone, azathioprine, and other immune modulators. One year survival for heart transplants is now more than 75 percent. One of the most notable successes of cyclosporine has been in liver transplantation; survival of liver transplants is now about 75 percent, a dramatic improvement over the previous figures. Cyclosporine is investigational for treating graft vs. host disease in bone marrow transplant patients and to prevent bone marrow transplant rejection. For the purposes of transplantation, the drug has been used alone successfully in some cases. Experience has, however, indicated that the dose and hence the toxicity of cyclosporine can be reduced by the simultaneous use of prednisone. Cyclosporine must be continued indefinitely to prevent rejection and attempts to reduce its long-term toxicity have included replacement by other immunosuppressants.

Usually the clinical response to cyclosporine does not correlate well with the administered dose. This is because there is a pronounced interpatient variation in pharmacokinetics, a fluctuating bioavailability and an interference of several drugs with the biotransformation of cyclosporine. Therefore, the measurement of cyclosporine concentrations in the blood is essential in order to optimize the immunosuppressive therapy with this drug.

Cyclosporine is being investigated for the treatment of a number of autoimmune diseases. As might be anticipated, cyclosporine is most effective in those autoimmune diseases, which are T cell mediated. These include several forms of psoriasis, rheumatoid arthritis refractive to all other therapy, uveitis, nephrotic syndrome and Type I (insulin-dependent) diabetes mellitus. The last deserves mention, since for the first time it is possible to prevent the development of insulin-dependent diabetes by inhibiting the self-destruction of the beta cells of the pancreas. Treatment must be started early, preferably even before insulin dependence begins, and must be continued indefinitely.

In antibody-mediated autoimmune diseases such as myasthenia gravis, systemic lupus erythematosus, autoimmune thrombocytopenic purpura and Crohn's disease, the role of cyclosporine is less clear, although promising results have been reported. Trials with multiple sclerosis show a lack of efficacy.

Adverse Reactions Cyclosporine is a very toxic drug, although perhaps not more so than other immunosuppressants. Nephrotoxicity is the most consistent and significant risk. Other frequent adverse reactions include hypertension, hirsutism, gum hyperplasia and neurotoxicity (e.g., tremors and headaches). Thromboembolism, convulsions, diabetogenesis, and hepatitis are less common.

The mechanism of the cyclosporine-induced nephrotoxicity is unknown. Pathologists have difficulty distinguishing between a kidney which is undergoing graft rejection or one with cyclosporine toxicity. In all cases, including normal kidneys, there is some degree of reduction of creatinine clearance and constant monitoring of renal function is required to avoid serious kidney damage. Reduction of the dosage often reduces the renal toxicity, but sometimes the cyclosporine therapy has to be terminated.

Like all immunosuppressants, cyclosporine increases the risk of development of lymphoproliferative disease. These neoplasms do not appear to be specific to cyclosporine therapy but probably are a result of immunosuppression in general. Cyclosporine renders the individual susceptible to all kinds of infections, but the incidence is lower than after most other immunosuppressants.

Drug Interactions Several different agents can affect the action of cyclosporine as well as its toxicity. Cyclosporine is biotransformed by the microsomal mixed-function oxidase system; consequently, any drug that induces this system may increase the elimination of cyclosporine and an increase in the dose of cyclosporine may be required. Included in this list are phenobarbital, carbamazepine, phenytoin, and rifampin. In contrast, diltiazem, erythromycin, ketoconazole, danazol, methyltestosterone, and oral contraceptives, which tend to depress the microsomal liver enzyme system, may increase the blood level of cyclosporine.

The nephrotoxicity of cyclosporine may be increased by the simultaneous use of aminoglycosides and nonsteroidal anti-inflammatory drugs. Since cyclosporine already causes some potassium retention, potassium-sparing diuretics should not be given simultaneously in order to avoid the occurrence of dangerous hyperkalemia.

Several cyclosporine analogs are being investigated because they have equal efficacy to cyclosporine but may have reduced toxicity.

FK506

FK506 is one of several new investigational immunosuppressants that are in various stages of development. It is 100 times more potent than cyclosporine *in vitro*, but is at least as toxic. There are many similarities in the mechanism of action of FK506 and cyclosporine. As with cyclosporine there is an initial interaction with a binding protein called FK506-binding protein. Like cyclophilin A, FK506-binding protein is a peptidyl-prolyl isomerase.

Antibodies

The production of antisera against a cell type is one of the oldest effective methods of achieving a specific immune action. Ideally this methodology is particularly suited to homologous organ transplantation. The technology ranges from the old method of injecting large animals with human lymphoid cells and collecting the serum to the more modern hybridoma techniques for the generation of monoclonal antibodies. These antibodies can be divided into two groups: polyclonal antisera that react with multiple antigenic determinants (or epitopes) and monoclonal antibodies that are directed at only a single epitope.

The hybridoma technique is particularly useful for the production of anti-T cell antibodies. Such antibodies are now being produced and are being clinically evaluated. Of special value to prevent graft vs. host syndrome is the procedure of "purging" the donor marrow *in vitro* with one or more monoclonal anti-T cell antibodies prior to marrow infusion in the recipient.

Anti-Thymocyte Globulin (Equine)

Currently available among polyclonal antibodies is anti-thymocyte globulin (lymphocyte immune globulin). It is prepared by immunizing horses with human thymocytes. Clinically this antisera is used primarily to treat organ graft rejections in combination with other immunosuppressants. More recently it has been used to promote remissions in some patients with aplastic anemia. Precise methods of determining potency have not been developed with this and other polyclonal antibodies. This reagent is not specific for T cells and will cross react with other cell types. It will also react with foreign proteins causing an immune response. Anaphylactic and serum sickness do occur, especially when prednisone and azathioprine are stopped, and may require cessation of therapy. Patients need to be skin-tested for horse-serum sensitivity. The exact effectiveness of anti-thymocyte globulin cannot be predicted because it is used in conjunction with azathioprine and prednisone. With the advent of cyclosporine the need for anti-thymocyte globulin has declined.

Muromonab-CD3 (Murine Monoclonal Antibody, Anti-CD3)

This is a monoclonal antibody to the T-3 (CD3) antigen of human T cells. It functions as an immunosuppressant, blocking graft rejection especially in renal transplants. It is indicated in the treatment of acute allograft rejection in renal transplant patients. T cell function is blocked by interfering with CD3, a molecule in the membrane of these cells that is associated with antigen recognition and signal transduction. The number of circulating CD3 positive, CD4 positive and CD8 positive T cells is decreased within minutes of administration of muromonab-CD3. Complement apparently is not involved in this reaction and T cell removal probably results from phagocytic activity of the reticuloendothelial system that follows opsonization by the monoclonal antibody. This is believed to play a major role in the clinical efficacy of this antibody.

Recent evidence indicates that other mechanisms also play a role. There is evidence that this antibody induces apoptosis or programmed cell death in certain T cells. Apoptosis is characterized by the cleavage of DNA into small fragments and is initiated by signals that activate calcium-dependent endonucleases. A third mechanism is that this antibody may mediate T cell cytolysis by inter-T cell bridging.

Monoclonal antibodies like muromonab-CD3 have the advantage over polyclonal antibodies of being more selective in their action and of being able to be more precisely administered. In addition they can be more accurately quantified.

Administered intravenously as a bolus (not infused), muromonab-CD3 is usually given in conjunction with azathioprine and prednisone. Pyrexia, chills, dyspnea, chest pain and vomiting are complications. Infections may be precipitated. Lymphoma, has on rare occasion, followed this treatment.

IMMUNOSTIMULATING AGENTS

Since many diseases other than primary immunodeficiencies are associated with cellular immunodeficiency, there is an important need for immunostimulants. They have potential use as vaccine adjuvants and in patients with cancer, human immunodeficiency virus infection and in certain other infections. Presently they are probably best known for their use in the treatment of cancer. When used for this purpose, their effect is due to more than one mechanism. For example, in addition to their ability to augment the immune system, these drugs may have direct cytotoxic effects as well as effects to induce differentiation of the cancer cells. As with the immunosuppressives, the immunostimulating agents can also be categorized into different subgroups. These would include cytokines (such as interferons and interleukins), growth factors (such as granulocyte-macrophage colony stimulating factor) and miscellaneous agents (such as levamisole and BCG vaccine).

Cytokines

Interferons

It is now known that there are many growth stimulants and growth inhibitors which are manufactured by various tissues under the appropriate conditions. Among these are interferons, which were first characterized as antiviral proteins produced by host cells. Later it was found that interferons had antiproliferative activity and also served as modulating agents for macrophages and natural killer cells.

Interferons consist of three families of protein molecules, designated alpha (alfa), beta, and gamma, whose production can be induced in most cells by several different stimuli (Table 44-2). Interferon alpha is induced in several types of leukocytes by foreign cells, virus-infected cells, tumor cells, bacterial cells and products, and virus envelopes. Interferon beta is produced in fibroblasts, epithelial cells and macrophages by viral and other foreign nucleic acids. Interferon gamma is induced in T lymphocytes by foreign antigens to which the T cells are sensitized. Natural killer cells also produce this interferon under certain conditions. Recent technology allows interferons to be produced by recombinant DNA techniques, usually by using a genetically engineered *Escherichia coli*

TABLE 44-2 Classification of human interferons

Type	Cells of origin	Inducing agents
Alpha	B lymphocytes, null lymphocytes, macrophages, lymphoblastoid cell lines	Foreign cells, virus-infected cells, tumor cells, bacterial cells and products, viral envelopes
Beta	Fibroblasts, epithelial cells, macrophages	Viral and other foreign nucleic acids, synthetic polyribonucleotides
Gamma	T lymphocytes	Foreign antigens to which the T cells are sensitized, T cell mitogens (e.g., concanavalin A, phytohemagglutinin)

bacterium containing DNA coded for human interferon. The interferons are all polypeptides with 145 to 166 amino acids and with molecular weights of 17 to 25 kD. There are at least 17 different human alpha interferon genes. In contrast, there is only one beta interferon gene and one gamma interferon gene. The different roles for the multiple alpha interferons are being studied.

The precise mechanism of action of the interferons is not known. The interferons must bind to a specific receptor on the cell surface. This immediately activates a transcription factor (probably through tyrosine phosphorylation) inside the cell where it moves into the nucleus. Inside the cell, interferon affects various biochemical processes by altering the expression of several genes.

The anticancer activity of these compounds has been mainly studied *in vitro* by the use of clonogenic cell assays and *in vivo* by studying the regression of tumors implanted in nude mice. Unfortunately, the laboratory predictions do not always agree with clinical experience. Nevertheless, there is sufficient evidence to state that interferon alpha may induce remissions in 90 percent of cases of hairy cell leukemia. It is also effective against Kaposi's sarcoma, and certain cases of chronic myelogenous leukemia seem to respond well. A few cases of multiple myeloma, malignant lymphoma and breast cancer have shown complete or partial responses to interferons. Interferons are seldom used as the sole therapeutic agent, so it is difficult to assign exact values to effectiveness. Indeed, their efficacy seems to be enhanced when they are used in conjunction with other cancer chemotherapeutic agents, with other cytokines, or with surgery or radiation.

Interferons also enhance the host's defenses against tumor cells. For example, natural killer cells (large granular lymphocytes) which can kill tumor cells have their activity enhanced by interferons. The activity of these cells can also be increased by double-stranded RNAs, which can induce the production of endogenous interferons. The use of interferon in viral diseases has been disappointing for the most part. Some viral diseases which respond are chronic non-A, non-B/C hepatitis; herpes keratoconjunctivitis; rhinoviruses; varicella zoster; and viral hepatitis B.

Adverse reactions to interferons are common. Flu-like symptoms of fever, fatigue, myalgias, headache and chills occur in the majority of patients. Gastrointestinal symptoms (mainly anorexia, nausea and diarrhea) are fairly common, while CNS symptoms such as dizziness and confusion seem to occur early in therapy and tend to disappear with continued drug use. More serious are skin rashes and alopecia. There is usually leukopenia and decreased hemoglobin and some rise in liver function tests and proteinuria. Hypocalcemia is also induced. These toxicities discourage the use of interferon except where the benefit is clearly greater than the risk.

Purified single-species-derived interferons are now produced by recombinant DNA techniques in *Escherichia coli*. Two of the commercial forms of interferon alfa available in the United States differ by a single amino acid at the number 23 position: lysine in interferon alfa-2a and arginine in interferon alfa-2b.

Interferon alfa-2a is indicated for use in hairy cell leukemia and Kaposi's sarcoma. In addition to the above therapeutic uses, **Interferon alfa-2b** is indicated for use chronic hepatitis B and in chronic non-A, non B/C hepatitis. **Interferon gamma** is approved for use as an immunomodulatory drug for the treatment of chronic granulomatous disease. This is an inherited immune disease characterized by severe recurrent infections of the skin, lymph nodes, liver, lung and bones due to phagocyte dysfunction. **Interferon beta** has been recently approved for the treatment of multiple sclerosis.

Aldesleukin (Interleukin-2, IL-2)

IL-2 is a lymphokine produced by activated T-helper lymphocytes. It induces the proliferation of T cells and promotes the differentiation of lymphocytes into cytotoxic cells. IL-2 also induces interferon gamma production. Activation of peripheral leukocytes with the drug produces lymphokine-activated killer cells (LAK) that lyse a variety of tumor cells *in vitro*. IL-2 has been cloned in bacteria through recombinant DNA technology, thus allowing the production of large amounts. IL-2 alone or with LAK cells can cause regression of several established metastatic tumors in animals.

Aldesleukin has been approved for the treatment of metastatic renal cell carcinoma, but also has shown good activity in malignant melanoma. Both of these tumors are refractory to chemotherapy. Complete or partial responses have occurred with IL-2 in 6 to 20 percent of patients. The majority have lasted less than a year. It has also been used as an investigational agent, both alone and in combination with LAK cells, with chemotherapy and with other biologic response modifiers to treat a variety of different cancers (e.g., head and neck carcinoma, colorectal cancer, central nervous system cancer). The results have varied with the type of cancer being treated.

Adverse reactions are frequently encountered with aldesleukin and many may be serious. Drug administration commonly results in fever, chills, fatigue, weakness, malaise, pruritus, and gastrointestinal effects (e.g., nausea, vomiting, diarrhea, anorexia, and stomatitis); these may be self-limiting after a few days of therapy. Other adverse effects with a rather high incidence in patients given aldesleukin include sinus tachycardia; pulmonary congestion and dyspnea; anemia, thrombocytopenia, and leukopenia; and erythema and rash.

Aldesleukin increases capillary permeability and promotes the extravasation of plasma proteins and fluids into the extravascular space, resulting in a loss of vascular tone. Within 12 hours of initiation of drug administration, clinically significant hypotension, reduced organ perfusion, edema and effusions may occur. This condition (known as the *capillary leak syndrome, CLS*) may also be associated with other severe adverse effects of aldesleukin including supraventricular and ventricular arrhythmias, angina, myocardial infarction, pulmonary insufficiency, renal insufficiency, and changes in mental status. The CLS can be managed effectively with careful monitoring of the patient's fluid and perfusion status and treatment with pressor agents and oxygen if necessary. Recovery from the CLS begins within a few hours after aldesleukin therapy is stopped.

Aldesleukin may also cause alterations in laboratory test results, including elevations in serum bilirubin, BUN, serum creatinine, transaminase, and alkaline phosphatase. Reduced electrolyte concentrations, and acidosis or alkalosis are less commonly observed.

Growth Factors

Sargramostim

Sargramostim is a human granulocyte macrophage colony stimulating factor (GM-CSF); it is produced in a yeast by recombinant DNA technology. It supports the growth and differentiation of stem cells into granulocytes and macrophages. In addition to triggering proliferation, GM-CSF acts on mature neutrophils and monocytes to increase cellular functions. For example, it can enhance the chemotactic, antifungal and antiparasitic activity of granulocytes and monocytes. It can also increase the cytotoxicity of monocytes for neoplastic cells and activates the inhibition of tumor growth by polymorphonuclear leukocytes. The action of GM-CSF like that of G-CSF (see below) is mediated by binding to specific receptors on the surface of the target cells. These receptors also share homology with receptors for a number of other hematopoietic growth factors and are members of a newly recognized growth factor receptor superfamily.

Sargramostim is used to accelerate myeloid recovery in patients who are undergoing bone marrow transplantation as well as patients who are undergoing myelotoxic anticancer therapy. It is also beneficial in increasing neutrophil counts in people with congenital and idiopathic chronic neutropenia. Sargramostim will also elevate neutrophil, monocyte and eosinophil counts in patients with AIDS. In these patients, it increases neutrophils and other myeloid cells following zidovudine therapy. In both adults and children with aplastic anemia, sargramostim has increased neutrophils and decreased infectious complications.

With this drug, transient fever and bone pain may occur and fluid accumulation, including pleural and pericardial effusions can be troublesome. Transient elevations of serum creatinine and aminotransferase activity have also occurred, as they do with filgrastim.

Filgrastim

Natural human granulocyte-colony stimulating factor (G-CSF) is a glycoprotein produced by monocytes, fibroblasts and endothelial cells and regulates the production of neutrophils within the bone marrow. It has minimal effects on the production of other cell types. Unlike GM-CSF, G-CSF is lineage specific but species nonspecific. It primarily affects the proliferation and differentiation of neutrophil progenitors as well as the functional activities of mature neutrophils such as enhanced phagocytosis and antigen dependent cell killing. It has also been reported to enhance the phagocytic and bactericidal activity of normal and defective human neutrophils.

The drug filgrastim is produced in *E. coli* by recombinant DNA technology and is used to increase neutrophil counts after a number of different cancer chemotherapeutic regimens (e.g., cyclophosphamide, doxorubicin and etoposide). Patients given this compound have had a lower incidence of febrile neutropenia, hospitalization and antibiotic treatment after receiving myelosuppressive drugs. Patients given filgrastim also had accelerated recovery of neutrophils after autologous bone marrow transplantation. Filgrastim, like sargramostim, is used in the treatment of congenital neutropenia and idiopathic chronic neutropenia, aplastic anemia, and AIDS to increase the levels of neutrophils and to decrease infectious complications.

The main adverse effect associated with this drug has been bone pain. Splenomegaly and abnormalities in uric acid concentrations, and LDH and alkaline phosphatase activities may also occur. Transient elevations of serum creatinine and aminotransferase activity have occurred after filgrastim therapy.

It is still not known if either one of these colony stimulating factors has any advantage over the other and how broad the indications should be for use of these expensive drugs. It should be noted that sargramostim seems to have significantly more toxicity as compared to filgrastim.

Levamisole

This is an established anthelminthic drug that was first reported to be an immunostimulant in 1972. It appears to act as an immunostimulant, although it can be an immunodepressant depending on the dose and time of administration. The drug appears to act directly on lymphocytes, macrophages and granulocytes to modify their proliferation, mobility and secretion. The maturation and proliferation of T cells are enhanced but natural killer cells do not appear to be affected. Several investigators consider that facilitation of monocyte chemotaxis is its principal action. It has been shown to enhance monocyte phagocytosis and to increase neutrophil mobility, adherence and chemotaxis.

Levamisole is indicated as adjuvant treatment in combination with 5-fluorouracil after surgical resection in patients with advanced colon cancer. The combination decreases recurrences and possibly prolongs survival in these patients. In the doses used toxicity has been minimal with levamisole alone and no more severe than the usual toxicity with 5-fluorouracil when the two drugs are used together. However, levamisole can cause nausea, vomiting, flu-like symptoms, rash, dizziness, somnolence, or insomnia, confusion, blurred vision, irritability, convulsions and agranulocytosis. A characteristic reaction to levamisole is an unusual taste generally described as metallic and occasionally associated with an altered sense of smell.

BCG Vaccine

This is an attenuated strain of *Mycobacterium bovis*. It has been known to be an immunostimulant for many years and has been used in the past to induce immunity against tuberculosis but the results have been variable. BCG vaccine has recently been used to stimulate the immune response in patients with bladder cancer. It has been most successful when the tumor is small and localized and the patient has a normal immune system. Also the vaccine works best when there is close contact between BCG and the tumor cells. It has been approved by the FDA for intravesicular use in bladder cancer.

BCG vaccine apparently acts through a nonspecific stimulation of the reticuloendothelial system. However, it is not known if this is a primary effect or if it is secondary to T cell activation and lymphokine production. BCG vaccine activates natural killer cells and enhances the production of hematopoietic stem cells. Macrophages affected by BCG become more active killer cells and more efficiently clear antigen and immune complexes. These macrophages will also recruit other cells that are involved in the destruction of cancer cells.

When instilled intravesically, local reactions are common. These include difficult and frequent urination, hematuria, cystitis and urinary tract infection.

BIBLIOGRAPHY

Assan, R., G. Fleutren, and J. Sirmai: "Cyclosporine Trials in Diabetes: Update Results of the French Experience," *Transplant Proc.* **20 (Supp. 4)**: 178-183 (1988).

Baron, S., S.K. Tyring, W.R. Fleischmann Jr., D.H. Coppenhauer, D.W. Niesel, G.R. Klimpel, G.J. Stanton, and T.K. Hughes: "The Interferons. Mechanisms of Action and Clinical Applications," *J. Amer. Med. Assn.* **266**: 1375-1383 (1991).

Barry, J.M.: "Immunosuppressive Drugs in Renal Transplantation," *Drugs* **44**: 554-566 (1992).

Borel, J.F.: "Immunosuppression: Building on Sandimmune (Cyclosporine)," *Transplant Proc.* **20 (1, Suppl. 1)**: 149-153 (1988).

Borel, J.F.: "Basic Science Summary," *Transplant Proc.* **20 (2, Suppl. 2)**: 722-730 (1988).

Brodsky, I., and H.R. Hubbell: "Interferons as Anticancer Agents," *Am. Fam. Physician* **29**: 146-428 (1984).

Dale, M.M., and J.C. Foreman (eds.): *Textbook of Immunopharmacology*, Blackwell Scientific, Boston, 1984.

DiPalma, J.R.: "Cyclosporine: An Immunologic Breakthrough," *Am. Fam. Physician* **36**: 245-247 (1987).

Dorr, R.T.: "Interferon-α in Malignant and Viral Diseases. A Review," *Drugs* **45**: 177-211 (1993).

Drug Evaluations Annual 1993, prepared by the Division of Drugs and Toxicology, American Medical Association, Chicago, 1993, pp. 1791-1829.

Ferguson, R.M., and B.G. Sommer (eds.): *The Clinical Management of the Renal Transplant Recipient with Cyclosporine*, Grune and Stratton, New York, 1986.

Fries, D., C. Hiesse, J.P. Santelli, *et al.*: "Triple Therapy with Low-Dose Cyclosporine, Azathioprine, and Steroids: Long-Term Results of a Randomized Study in Cadaver Donor Renal Transplantation," *Transplant Proc.* **20 (Suppl. 3)**: 130-135 (1988).

Hadden, J.W., and D.L. Smith: "Immunopharmacology-Immunomodulation and Immunotherapy," *J. Amer. Med. Assn.* **268**: 2964-2969 (1992).

Hess, A.D., A.H. Esa, and P.M. Colombani: "Mechanisms of the Action of Cyclosporine. Effects on Cells of the Immune System and on Subcellular Events in T Cell Activation," *Transplant Proc.* **20 (2, Suppl. 2)**: 29-40 (1988).

Kahan, B.D. (ed.): *Cyclosporine. Vol. I. Biological Activity and Clinical Applications*, Grune and Stratton, New York, 1983.

Kahan, B.D. (ed.): *Cyclosporine. Vol. III. Diagnosis and Management of Associated Renal Injury*, Grune and Stratton, New York, 1985.

Penn, I., and M.E. Brunson: "Cancers after Cyclosporine Therapy," *Transplant Proc.* **20 (3, Suppl. 3)**: 885-892 (1988).

Tilney, N.L., T.B. Strom, and J.W. Kupliec-Weglinski: "Pharmacologic and Immunologic Agonists and Antagonists of Cyclosporine," *Transplant Proc.* **20 (3, Suppl. 3)**: 13-22 (1988).

PART X

Anti-Infective Agents

SECTION EDITOR

G. John DiGregorio

CHAPTER 45

Antimicrobials I: General Concepts, Beta-Lactam Antibiotics, and Glycopeptides

Abdolghader Molavi

GENERAL CONCEPTS

An antibiotic is a chemical substance, produced by a microorganism, which in low concentrations can kill or inhibit the growth of other microorganisms. This definition distinguishes between antimicrobial agents produced by microorganisms and those that are totally synthetic. The distinction is rather academic, and the words *antibiotic* and *antimicrobial* are now used interchangeably.

The central concept of antimicrobial action is that of *selective toxicity* — that is, the growth of the infecting organism is inhibited or the organism is killed without damage to the cells of the host. All clinically useful antimicrobials are selectively toxic to microorganisms. The nature and the degree of this selectivity determine whether an antimicrobial is essentially nontoxic for mammalian cells or exhibits potential toxicity for certain mammalian tissues.

The antimicrobial agents exert their antibacterial effects through one of the following mechanisms: (1) inhibition of cell wall synthesis (beta-lactam antibiotics, glycopeptides, and cycloserine), (2) inhibition of protein synthesis (aminoglycosides, macrolides, clindamycin, chloramphenicol, and tetracyclines), (3) inhibition of nucleic acid synthesis or function (sulfonamides, trimethoprim, metronidazole, quinolones, and rifampin), and (4) inhibition of cytoplasmic membrane function (polymyxins).

The use of antimicrobial drugs falls into three categories: (1) *specific therapy* — when the infecting organism *and* its antimicrobial susceptibility are known; (2) *empiric therapy* — when the infecting organism or its antimicrobial susceptibility is unknown, but can reasonably be predicted based on previous studies; and (3) *prophylaxis* — when the aim is to prevent either a specific infection in some individuals or a postoperative infection following certain surgical procedures.

In choosing an antimicrobial agent for therapy of a given infection, a number of important factors must be considered. First, the identity of the infecting organism must be known or can reasonably be predicted on the basis of clinical information, tissue tropism, and bacteriologic statistics. Second, the antimicrobial susceptibility (or potential susceptibility) of the infecting organism should be known. Third, the drug chosen must achieve therapeutic concentrations at the site of infection. Finally, a series of host factors including age, history of allergic reactions, renal and/or hepatic dysfunction, and pregnancy should be taken into consideration.

Antimicrobial Susceptibility

Since different organisms, including strains of a given species, vary in their susceptibility to antimicrobial agents, the antimicrobial susceptibility of the infecting organism must be determined. Antimicrobial susceptibility is usually determined by either the disk-diffusion or the broth-dilution method. In the disk-diffusion method, paper disks containing specific amounts of antimicrobials are applied to an agar surface that has been freshly inoculated with a suspension of the bacterium. After an overnight incubation, the diameters of clear zones around the disks (zones of growth inhibition) are measured. These diameters are interpreted as *susceptible*, *intermediate*, or *resistant* for the individual drugs by referring to standardized values. The limitation of the disk-diffusion method is that it provides only qualitative data on the inhibitory activity of antimicrobial agents.

Quantitative susceptibility testing is usually performed by the broth-dilution method. Serial two-fold dilutions of the drug in broth are inoculated with a standardized suspension of the organism. The results are expressed as the *minimum inhibitory concentration* (MIC), which is the lowest concentration of the drug that inhibits visible growth after 18 to 24 hours incubation. The efficacy with which an antibiotic kills an organism is indicated by the *minimum bactericidal concentration* (MBC), defined as the lowest concentration of the drug that kills at least 99.9 percent of the original bacterial inoculum. MBC is determined by subculturing the tubes that show no growth onto agar plates and reincubating overnight. The results of quantitative susceptibility tests, MIC and MBC, should be correlated with the concentrations of the drug achieved in the blood and various tissues and body fluids.

Bactericidal versus Bacteriostatic Activity

Antimicrobials can be classified on the basis of their *in vitro* action as either bactericidal or bacteriostatic. A bactericidal agent causes microbial cell death at concentrations that are achieved clinically. For these agents the MBCs are identical or very close to the corresponding MICs. Bactericidal agents include beta-lactam antibiotics, glycopeptides, aminoglycosides, quinolones, and metronidazole. A bacteriostatic agent inhibits bacterial growth but does not kill the organism at concentrations that are achieved clinically. As might be expected, the MBCs of such an agent are substantially higher than the corresponding MICs. Bacteriostatic antibiotics include clindamycin, macrolides, sulfonamides, trimethoprim, tetracyclines, and chloramphenicol.

Treatment with a bacteriostatic drug stops bacterial growth, thereby allowing neutrophils and other host defenses to eliminate the pathogen. In cases where almost total reliance must be placed on a chemotherapeutic effect that is unaided by host defenses, such as infective endocarditis and infection in neutropenic hosts, bactericidal agents are more effective than bacteriostatic compounds. This difference, however, is nonexistent when the host defense mechanisms (local and systemic) are intact.

The bactericidal agents can be divided into two groups based on their patterns of bactericidal activity. The first group (aminoglycosides, quinolones, and metronidazole) exhibit marked *concentration-dependent bactericidal activity*. For these agents the rate and extent of bacterial killing increase with increasing drug concentrations above the MBC. The second group (beta-lactam antibiotics and glycopeptides) exhibit *time-dependent bactericidal activity*. Bacterial killing with these agents does not increase with increasing drug concentrations above the MBC.

Short exposures to inhibitory concentrations of antimicrobials may result in continued suppression of bacterial replication for a few hours. This phenomenon occurs in the absence of the drug and assumes clinical importance by extending the antimicrobial effect on the organism. The term *postantibiotic effect* is used to describe this recovery period or persistent suppression of bacterial growth. When the postantibiotic effect ends, residual organisms will start multiplication. Factors that affect the duration of postantibiotic effect include the type of organism, the class of antimicrobial, the drug concentration, and the duration of antimicrobial exposure. Inhibitors of protein and nucleic acid synthesis produce the postantibiotic effect against susceptible gram-positive cocci and gram-negative bacilli. However, antibiotics that act on the cell wall induce the postantibiotic effect only against gram-positive cocci. The postantibiotic effect provides theoretical rationale for some dosing schedules used to treat infections.

Resistance to Antimicrobial Drugs

Bacterial resistance to antimicrobial agents can be either *intrinsic* or *acquired*. Intrinsic resistance of an organism is a stable genetic property encoded in the chromosome and shared by all strains of the species. Acquired resistance implies that certain strains of a species have developed the ability to resist an antimicrobial drug to which the species as a whole is naturally susceptible. Acquired resistance results from a change in the DNA of the bacteria such that a new phenotypic trait is expressed. This resistance may develop by either a mutation in the bacterial chromosome or acquisition of new DNA sequences (plasmids) that encode a resistance function.

The biochemical mechanisms of intrinsic and acquired resistance are similar and can be divided into four basic categories: (1) drug inactivation or modification by bacterial enzymes, (2) permeability barrier so that the drug cannot reach the target site of its action, (3) alteration of the target so that it no longer binds or is affected by the drug, and (4) development of an altered metabolic pathway that bypasses the reaction inhibited by the drug.

Antimicrobial Combinations

When an organism is exposed simultaneously to two antimicrobial agents, the effect of the combination may fall into one of three patterns: additive effect, synergism, or antagonism. Two drugs are said to be additive when the activity of the drugs in combination is equal to the sum of their independent activities. The combined antimicrobial effect of two drugs may be less than (antagonism) or greater than (synergism) the additive effect. Several different mechanisms of antimicrobial synergism are known: (1) enhancement by one drug of the entry of a second drug into microbial cells, (2) inhibition by one drug of a microbial enzyme that inactivates the second drug, and (3) inhibition of successive steps in a metabolic sequence.

Despite the availability of antibiotics that provide highly potent activity against specific organisms or that possess activity against an extremely broad spectrum of bacteria, the simultaneous use of two or more agents in combination is common in the hospital setting. Such combinations are used in the following situations: (1) treatment of polymicrobial infections for which one antibiotic may not be sufficient, (2) initial treatment of life-threatening infections prior to the isolation of the etiologic agent, (3) to prevent selection of resistant mutants leading to the emergence of resistant strains, and (4) when there is synergism between two antimicrobials against a specific infecting organism.

Antimicrobial Chemoprophylaxis

Chemoprophylaxis is the use of antibiotics for preventing infection. Prophylaxis is most effective when it is directed against a specific microorganism with known antimicrobial susceptibility. When chemoprophylaxis is aimed at preventing all possible organisms from initiating infection, it is not likely to be successful.

The current uses of chemoprophylaxis fall into four categories. First, prevention of infection following exposure to a specific pathogen. An example of this type of prophylaxis is the administration of rifampin to household contacts of a patient with meningococcal meningitis. Second, prevention of disease by a dormant pathogen that is already infecting the host. An example is the administration of isoniazid to a person with recent tuberculin conversion to prevent active tuberculosis. Third, prevention of a specific infection in highly susceptible individuals. An example is the administration of antibiotics to a person with rheumatic heart disease prior to dental procedures in order to prevent infective endocarditis. Finally, prevention of postoperative infective complications after certain surgical procedures.

Protein Binding

Most antimicrobials bind to serum proteins, primarily albumin; the extent of binding varies from 0 to 97 percent. Only the unbound (free) drug can pass through capillary pores into the interstitial fluid. However, free drug that passes into the interstitial fluid can also bind to tissue fluid proteins. Protein binding is a rapidly reversible process; an equilibrium exists between the antibiotic-protein complex and the free drug, not only in the plasma but also in the interstitial fluid. Only the free drug exerts antibacterial activity; the bound drug cannot enter the bacterial cell to reach its target. The protein-bound antimicrobial is essentially inactive and unable to diffuse between plasma and interstitial fluid; however, it serves as a constant reservoir, releasing more drug as the free drug is excreted or metabolized.

BETA-LACTAM ANTIBIOTICS

Beta-lactam antibiotics include penicillins, cephalosporins, monobactams, and carbapenems. All have a four-membered beta-lactam ring (Fig. 45-1), which is essential for their antibacterial activity. The beta-lactam ring is fused to a five-membered thiazolidine ring in the penicillins and to a six-membered dihydrothiazine ring in the cephalosporins. In carbapenems, the beta-lactam ring is attached to a five-membered ring, as in penicillins. Substitution of carbon for sulfur and the presence of a double bond in the five-membered ring account for the name *carbapenem*. The monobactams lack the bicyclic structure characteristic of the other beta-lactam antibiotics; a sulfonic acid group is attached to the nitrogen of the beta-lactam ring.

Mechanism of Action

The basic mechanism of action of beta-lactam antibiotics is inhibition of cell wall synthesis. This primary action triggers bacterial autolytic enzymes, which then disrupt the cell wall and cause lysis of the organism.

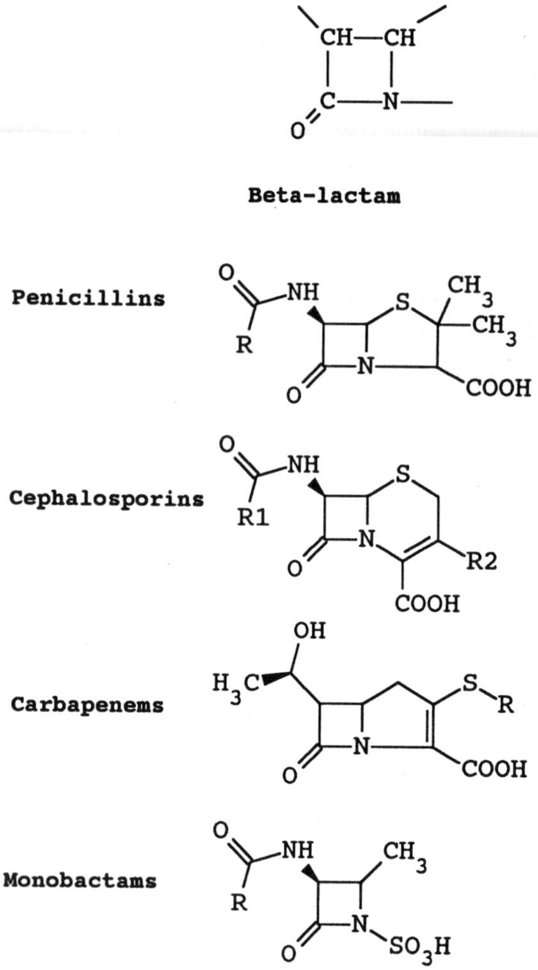

Beta-lactam

Penicillins

Cephalosporins

Carbapenems

Monobactams

FIGURE 45-1 *Comparative structural formulas of beta-lactam antibiotics.*

The bacterial cytoplasmic membrane encases the cytoplasm which is hypertonic to the environment. Although this membrane is critical to the maintenance of the osmotic gradient between the bacterium and its environment, it is not strong enough to keep the hypertonic sac from rupturing by osmotic shock. The cell wall is a relatively rigid structure that encases the cytoplasmic membrane, protecting the bacterial cell against lysis due to the osmotic pressure difference between the cytoplasm and the external environment.

The basic component of the cell wall is a mixed polymer, known as *murein* or *peptidoglycan*. The peptidoglycan is composed of long polysaccharide chains (called *glycan* chains), that are cross linked by short interconnecting peptides. A glycan chain consists of two alternating amino sugars, N-acetylglucosamine and N-acetylmuramic acid. A tetrapeptide (composed of L-alanine, D-glutamic acid, L-lysine, and D-alanine in *Staphylococcus aureus*) is attached to each N-acetylmuramic acid unit, forming side branches to the glycan chains. Many of the tetrapeptides on adjacent glycan chains are cross-linked to one another either directly or via short peptide chains (a pentaglycine in *S. aureus*, Fig. 45-2). The resulting structure forms a single, bag-shaped macromolecule that surrounds the cytoplasmic membrane — countering the osmotic pressure exerted by the cytoplasm and conferring the bacterium its shape. The peptidoglycan layer of gram-negative bacteria is thinner than that of gram-positive bacteria and contains fewer cross-links.

Inhibition of Cell Wall Synthesis The biosynthesis of peptidoglycan can be divided into three stages according to where the reactions take place. The first-stage reactions take place in the cytoplasm and result in the synthesis of the

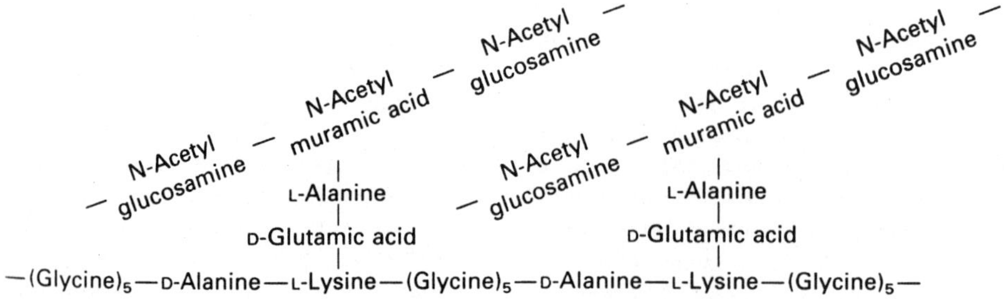

— N-Acetyl glucosamine — N-Acetyl muramic acid — N-Acetyl glucosamine —

L-Alanine

D-Glutamic acid

— N-Acetyl glucosamine — N-Acetyl muramic acid — N-Acetyl glucosamine —

L-Alanine

D-Glutamic acid

—(Glycine)$_5$—D-Alanine—L-Lysine—(Glycine)$_5$—D-Alanine—L-Lysine—(Glycine)$_5$—

FIGURE 45-2 *The structure of a portion of peptidoglycan in Staphylococcus aureus.*

precursor unit, uridine diphospho-N-acetylmuramyl pentapeptide. The last reaction sequence involves the racemization of L-alanine to D-alanine and incorporation of D-alanyl-D-alanine into the pentapeptide. Cycloserine, an antibiotic which is used occasionally for the treatment of tuberculosis (Chapter 48), blocks cell wall synthesis at this stage by competitive inhibition of alanine racemase and alanine synthetase. The second-stage reactions take place while the precursor unit is translocated across the cytoplasmic membrane. First, the N-acetylmuramyl pentapeptide moiety is linked, by a pyrophosphate bridge (P-P) to a carrier lipid bound to the cytoplasmic membrane. Then, N-acetylglucosamine is added to form a lipid-P-P-disaccharide-pentapeptide. Further modifications of the pentapeptide chain (depending on the species) may follow, such as addition of pentaglycine in *S. aureus*. The modified disaccharide-pentapeptide is then translocated from the carrier lipid to a growing point on the existing peptidoglycan. Vancomycin inhibits cell wall synthesis at this stage; it binds to the D-alanyl-D-alanine terminus of the pentapeptide and prevents the transfer of the disaccharide-pentapeptide unit from the lipid carrier to the peptidoglycan.

The third and final stage of cell wall synthesis takes place outside the cytoplasmic membrane. During this process, the linear glycopeptide polymers become cross-linked to each other by means of a transpeptidation reaction. Peptidoglycan transpeptidase, a membrane-bound enzyme, links the pentapeptide side chains by displacing a terminal D-alanine. Beta-lactam antibiotics inhibit the transpeptidation reaction, initiating events that eventually lead to bacterial cell death.

Since beta-lactam antibiotics interfere with peptidoglycan biosynthesis and such synthesis does not occur in the cells of humans, these agents are nontoxic for human cells.

Autolytic Enzyme Activity Inhibition of cell wall synthesis does not alone account for the bactericidal action of beta-lactam antibiotics. The lysis of bacteria that follows exposure to these agents is ultimately dependent on the activity of autolysins, the endogenous peptidoglycan hydrolyzing enzymes. Autolysins are required to make nicks in the peptidoglycan lattice so that new subunits can be inserted during growth. They are also necessary for the separation of daughter cells during division. It is thought that the inhibition of cell wall synthesis "triggers" autolytic enzymes by inactivating their endogenous inhibitors. These enzymes then disrupt the covalent bonds in the cell wall and cause lysis of the organism.

Certain bacterial strains that are "autolysin-deficient" have been identified. These organisms do not lyse in the presence of beta-lactam antibiotics, although their growth is inhibited. The term *tolerance* has been used to describe the dissociation between inhibition and killing of bacteria by agents that inhibit peptidoglycan synthesis. Tolerant organisms differ from those which are resistant in that they are still susceptible to the growth-inhibiting effect of the antibiotic but are tolerant with respect to its lytic action.

The bactericidal effects of beta-lactam antibiotics are observed only in growing organisms. If growth is prevented by the omission of a nutrient or by the addition of a bacteriostatic agent, there will be no peptidoglycan synthesis and the organism would survive in the presence of beta-lactam antibiotics.

Penicillin-Binding Proteins Beta-lactam antibiotics bind specifically to a number of proteins bound to the cytoplasmic membrane, known as *penicillin-binding proteins* (PBPs). The PBPs of a given organism are numbered by convention in the order of decreasing molecular weight. A number of these PBPs are the enzymes that are involved in the third stage of cell wall synthesis and in reshaping the cell wall during growth and division.

Escherichia coli has six PBPs. PBP-1a and PBP-1b are the transpeptidases involved in peptidoglycan synthesis associated with cell elongation. Inhibition of these enzymes results in spheroplast formation and rapid lysis. PBP-2 is required for the maintenance of the "rod" shape of the bacterium. Selective inhibition of this enzyme is associated with loss of rod shape and formation of large ovoid cells which eventually lyse. PBP-3 is required for septum formation during division; it catalyzes a reaction needed for the special peptidoglycan synthesis that ensues when cells divide. Selective inhibition of this enzyme results in formation of filamentous forms containing multiple rod-shaped units that cannot separate and eventually die. Different beta-lactam antibiotics have selective affinities for one or more of these PBPs. Inactivation of high molecular weight PBPs (PBP-1a, -1b, -2, or -3) causes bacterial cell death. Low molecular weight PBPs (PBP-4, -5, and -6) are not essential for bacterial vitality and their inactivation does not lead to cell death.

The rate of killing of bacteria by beta-lactam antibiotics is not concentration-dependent. Maximal killing rates are observed at concentrations of four times the minimal inhibitory concentrations.

Mechanisms of Resistance

Bacterial resistance to a beta-lactam antibiotic may be due to one or more of the following mechanisms: (1) inability of the drug to reach the target site of its action, (2) altered PBP target resulting in reduced affinity for the drug, and (3) inactivation of the drug by bacterial enzymes.

Permeability Barrier The beta-lactam antibiotics must penetrate through the outer cell envelope to reach their PBP targets on the cytoplasmic membrane. In gram-positive bacteria, the cell wall, occasionally covered by a polysaccharide capsule, is the only layer external to the cytoplasmic membrane. Neither of these structures presents a barrier to the passage of small molecules like the beta-lactams. Therefore, inability to reach the PBP targets is unlikely to be a mechanism of resistance in gram-positive species.

Gram-negative bacteria have a more complex envelope structure. Exterior to the peptidoglycan layer, there is an outer membrane usually covered with a polysaccharide capsule. The outer membrane, which is composed of lipopolysacharide and lipoprotein, constitutes a significant barrier to the passage of hydrophilic molecules. Penetration through this membrane occurs through transmembrane hydrophilic channels, formed by proteins called *porins*, which allow diffusion of solutes into the interior of the bacterium. The ease with which beta-lactam antibiotics diffuse through the porin channels varies according to their size, electrical charge, and hydrophilic properties. Mutational changes in porins may affect porin channel properties and consequently the outer membrane permeability, resulting in decreased susceptibility to beta-lactam antibiotics.

Altered PBP Targets A second mechanism of resistance to beta-lactam antibiotics is an alteration of PBP targets, resulting in reduced affinity for the beta-lactam molecule. Alterations in the binding characteristics of PBPs for beta-lactam compounds are responsible for the development of resistance in some organisms that are usually sensitive to these agents.

Beta-Lactamase Production The most common and the most important mechanism of resistance to beta-lactam antibiotics is bacterial production of beta-lactamases. The beta-lactamases cleave the C-N bond in the beta-lactam ring of the antibiotic. Since an intact beta-lactam ring is an absolute requirement for interaction with the PBPs, the cleavage of this ring destroys the antibacterial activity of the compound.

Beta-lactamases are produced by both gram-positive and gram negative species. The genes for these enzymes may be on chromosomes, on plasmids that can transfer from one species to another, or on transposons. Some beta-lactamases are constitutive, that is they are produced continuously. Others are inducible; that is their production is normally repressed by one or more regulatory genes. Enzyme production begins when the organism is exposed to a beta-lactam antibiotic (acting as an inducer) and declines to the basal state after the inducing agent is removed.

The beta-lactamases of *S. aureus* and coagulase-negative staphylococci are plasmid-mediated and inducible with activity directed principally against penicillins. The enzyme is released in large amounts into the surrounding medium, where it carries out its protective role by destroying the penicillins in the environment. In gram-negative bacteria (aerobic and anaerobic), beta-lactamases are produced in smaller amounts and retained in the periplasmic space (between the cytoplasmic and the outer membranes). The enzyme is thus strategically located to destroy the beta-lactam molecules before they reach the cytoplasmic membrane-bound PBP targets. These beta-lactamases are encoded either on the chromosome or on plasmids. They may be inducible or constitutively produced and possess affinity for penicillins and/or cephalosporins.

A number of gram-negative species, including *Enterobacter cloacae, Serratia marcescens, Citrobacter freundii, Proteus vulgaris,* and *Pseudomonas aeruginosa,* have inducible beta-lactamase (chromosomal). Populations of these organisms usually contain mutants in which the repressor mechanism for beta-lactamase production has been lost. Selection of these mutants by a beta-lactam antibiotic results in the emergence of strains that are stably derepressed and constitutively produce large amounts of beta-lactamase. These strains usually exhibit resistance to most beta-lactam antibiotics. This mechanism of resistance, namely the selection of mutants excessively producing a chromosomally determined beta-lactamase, occurs only in species that have the capacity to produce large quantities of the enzyme but that do not express this potential because they also possess a set of regulatory genes. It is mutation in regulatory genes that results in this excessive production.

PENICILLINS

Penicillin G was discovered in 1928, when Alexander Fleming noted that a contaminating mold in one of his cultures had caused the bacteria in its vicinity to undergo lysis. Because the mold belonged to the genus *Penicillium*, he named the antibacterial substance *penicillin*.

Almost a decade later, a group of investigators at Oxford University isolated a crude preparation of penicillin, which was introduced for clinical trials in 1941. This early penicillin was a mixture of several penicillin compounds designated as F, G, X, and K. Penicillin G (benzylpenicillin), the most active of these, was later purified and subsequently introduced into clinical medicine.

Major progress in the development of penicillins occurred in 1959, when the penicillin nucleus, 6-aminopenicillanic acid, was isolated from *Penicillium chrysogenum* grown in a broth medium devoid of precursors for a side chain. Addition of various side chains to the nucleus led to the development of semisynthetic penicillins.

Chemistry

The basic penicillin structure is composed of a beta-lactam ring attached to a five-membered thiazolidine ring and a side chain (Fig. 45-3). Modifications of the penicillin molecule take place only on the acyl side chain (R). The side chain determines the antimicrobial spectrum, stability to beta-lactamases, and the pharmacokinetic properties of a particular penicillin.

Since a free carboxyl group is required for antimicrobial activity, most penicillins are available as either sodium or potassium salts. Carboxylester formulations require hydrolysis by nonspecific esterases in serum and tissues for *in vivo* activity.

Classification

Penicillins can be divided into four groups on the basis of their antimicrobial spectra (Table 45-1). Differences within a group are usually of a pharmacologic nature, although one compound in a group may be more active than another against some organisms.

Natural penicillins include penicillin G and penicillin V. Penicillin G has a narrow antimicrobial spectrum. It is active against gram-positive bacteria and *Neisseria* species, but gram-negative bacilli are generally resistant. Penicillin G is degraded by gastric acid and destroyed by staphylococcal penicillinase. Penicillin V is acid-resistant and used for oral administration.

Penicillinase-resistant penicillins (methicillin, nafcillin, oxacillin, cloxacillin, and dicloxacillin) are active against penicillin G-resistant staphylococci. Their antimicrobial spectrum is limited to gram-positive organisms.

The antimicrobial spectrum of *aminopenicillins* (ampicillin, bacampicillin, and amoxicillin) resembles that of penicillin G except that it also includes a limited number of gram-negative species. The *extended-spectrum penicillins*, which include carboxypenicillins (carbenicillin and ticarcillin) and ureidopenicillins (mezlocillin, azlocillin, and piperacillin), are active against a much broader spectrum of gram-negative organisms. Both aminopenicillins and extended-spectrum penicillins are destroyed by staphylococcal penicillinase (beta-lactamase).

The addition of a *beta-lactamase inhibitor* (clavulanic acid, sulbactam, or tazobactam) to an aminopenicillin or an extended-spectrum penicillin broadens the antimicrobial spectrum to include penicillin G-resistant staphylococci and many beta-lactamase-producing gram-negative bacilli.

Pharmacokinetics

There are marked differences in the oral absorption of various penicillins (Table 45-1). Except for penicillin G, all penicillins available for oral administration are acid-stable. Peak serum levels are obtained 1 to 2 h after ingestion. When ingested with food, absorption is delayed and peak serum levels are achieved in 2 to 3 h.

Penicillins bind to plasma proteins in varying degrees, ranging from 20 percent for ampicillin to 97 percent for dicloxacillin. They diffuse readily into all tissues and body fluids except the brain, cerebrospinal fluid (CSF), eye, and prostate. In the presence of inflammation, therapeutic concentrations are attained in the CSF and the brain.

Penicillins are rapidly eliminated from the body with half-lives ranging from 30 to 70 min. Most penicillins are excreted primarily by the kidneys in unchanged form. Excretion occurs by glomerular filtration and by tubular secretion, which can be blocked with probenecid. Metabolism plays a major role in the elimination of nafcillin, oxacillin, cloxacillin, and dicloxacillin. Biliary excretion is important only for nafcillin (8 percent) and for mezlocillin, azlocillin, and piperacillin (20 to 30 percent). The daily dose of most penicillins has to

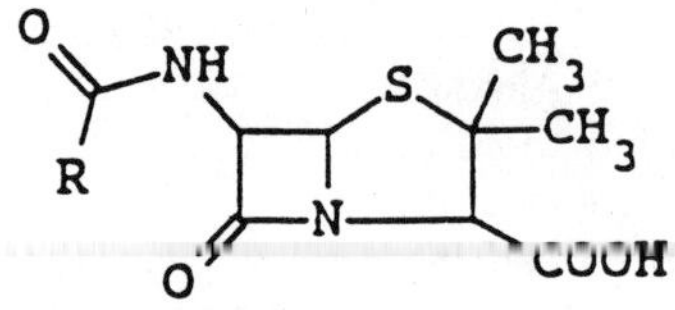

O, NH, R, S, CH_3, CH_3, N, O, COOH

BASIC STRUCTURE

R Side Chain	Generic Name	R Side Chain	Generic Name
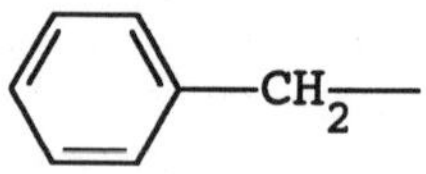 $-CH_2-$	Penicillin G	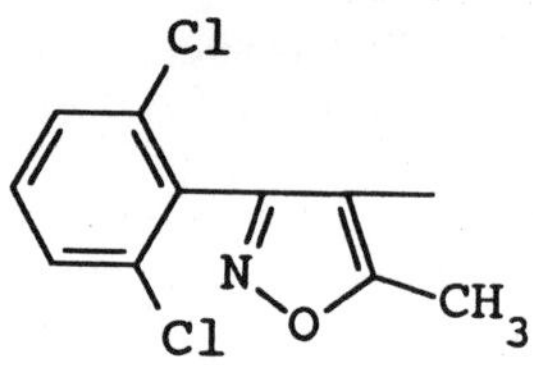 Cl, N, O, CH_3, Cl	Dicloxacillin
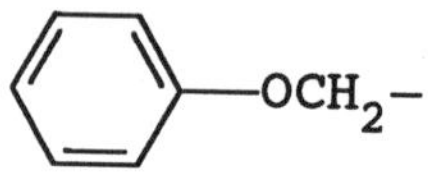 $-OCH_2-$	Penicillin V	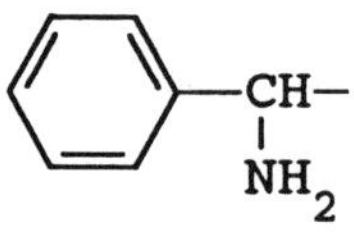 $-CH-$, NH_2	Ampicillin
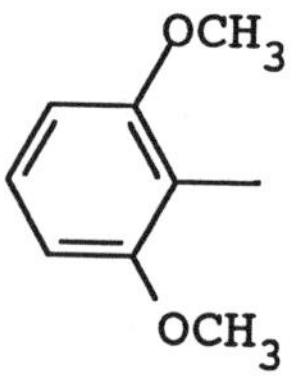 OCH_3, OCH_3	Methicillin	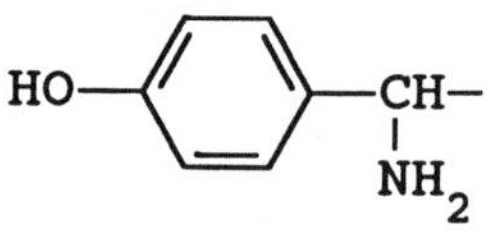 HO, $-CH-$, NH_2	Amoxicillin
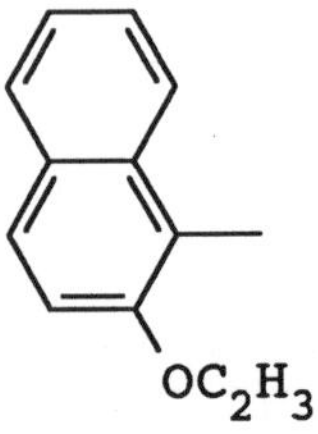 OC_2H_3	Nafcillin	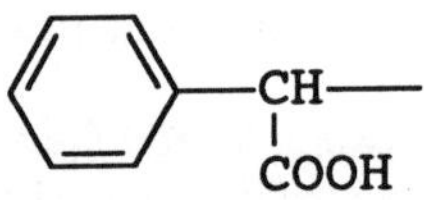 $-CH-$, COOH	Carbenicillin
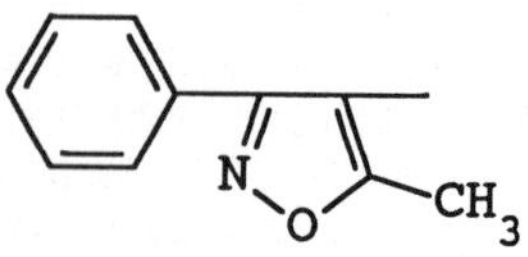 N, O, CH_3	Oxacillin	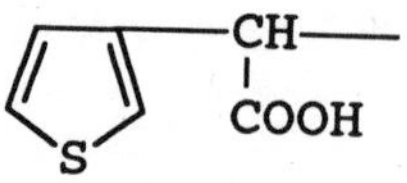 S, $-CH-$, COOH	Ticarcillin
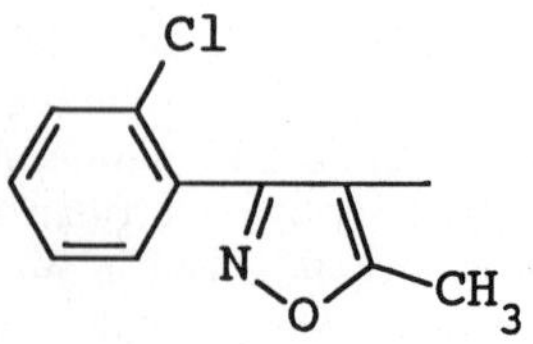 Cl, N, O, CH_3	Cloxacillin	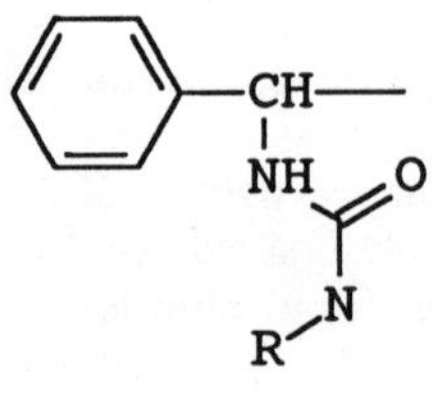 $-CH-$, NH, O, N, R	Azlocillin Mezlocillin Piperacillin

FIGURE 45-3 *Chemical structures of penicillins.*

TABLE 45-1 Classification and pharmacokinetic properties of penicillins

Generic name	Oral absorption, %	Plasma protein binding, %	Elimination half-life, h	Elimination half-life, h (anuria)
NATURAL PENICILLINS				
Penicillin G	20	55	0.5	4.0
Penicillin V	30	80	0.5	2.0
PENICILLINASE-RESISTANT				
Methicillin	—[a]	35	0.5	4.0
Nafcillin	10 to 20	88	0.5	1.0
Oxacillin	30	92	0.5	1.0
Cloxacillin	50	94	0.6	1.5
Dicloxacillin	70	97	0.7	2.2
AMINOPENICILLINS				
Ampicillin	30 to 50	20	1.0	8.0
Amoxicillin	75 to 90	20	1.0	8.0
EXTENDED-SPECTRUM PENICILLINS				
Carbenicillin indanyl sodium	30 to 40	50	1.1	15
Ticarcillin	—	50	1.2	15
Mezlocillin	—	30	1.0	3.6
Azlocillin	—	30	1.0	5.2
Piperacillin	—	20	1.0	4.0

[a] Not used by the oral route.

be reduced in patients with renal impairment. The degree of modification depends on the creatinine clearance and the extent to which the individual compound is excreted by the kidneys.

Adverse Effects

Since beta-lactam antibiotics interfere with peptidoglycan biosynthesis and such synthesis does not occur in the cells of humans and other mammals, these agents are relatively nontoxic for human cells.

Hypersensitivity reactions are the main adverse effects encountered with the use of penicillins. Sensitization is usually the result of previous treatment with a penicillin. The penicillin molecule or its breakdown products may evoke allergy by acting as haptens, combining with body proteins to form antigenic compounds. It is difficult to estimate the degree of cross allergy from one penicillin derivative to another, but allergy to one should be considered as allergy to all penicillins.

Immediate reactions occur within the first hour after penicillin administration and are immunoglobulin E-mediated. These reactions include anaphylaxis (fatal in 10 percent), urticaria, bronchospasm, and angioedema. Accelerated reactions occur 1 to 72 hours after penicillin administration; they include urticaria (most cases), angioedema and bronchospasm. Late or delayed hypersensitivity reactions occur in 1 to 10 percent of patients receiving these drugs. Maculopapular skin rashes are the most common delayed reactions and occur more frequently with ampicillin. These can be treated symptomatically and may subside despite continuation of the drug. Serum sickness, Stevens-Johnson syndrome, exfoliative dermatitis, and allergic vasculitis are rare forms of allergic reactions that require discontinuation of the compound. Drug fever can occur with or without eosinophilia; the elevation of body temperature is usually low-grade but may occasionally be high-grade. Eosinophilia is an occasional accompaniment of other allergic reactions but may be the sole manifestation.

The majority of patients who give a history of allergy to penicillin should be treated with a different type of antibiotic. In the unusual instance where treatment with a penicillin is essential, skin tests should be performed. A negative skin test to major and minor antigenic determinants of penicillin makes it unlikely that the patient will develop an immediate reaction to penicillin.

Penicillins are not nephrotoxic; however, allergic interstitial nephritis may occur, particularly with methicillin. It manifests itself by fever, occasional rashes, eosinophilia, the presence of eosinophils in the urine, and a rise in serum creatinine. Discontinuation of the penicillin will result in the return of renal function to normal in the majority of situations.

Hematologic reactions caused by penicillins are rare. Coombs-positive hemolytic anemia, immune thrombocytopenia, leukopenia, or neutropenia may occur. The white blood cell counts return to normal rapidly when the offending agent is discontinued. Neutropenia has been reported more frequently with nafcillin and oxacillin than with other penicillins. All penicillins at high concentrations, particularly carbenicillin and ticarcillin, impair platelet function, resulting in prolongation of the bleeding time and, rarely, a clinically significant bleeding episode.

Diarrhea may occur in 1 to 5 percent of patients taking penicillin; it is more common with oral ampicillin. *Clostridium difficile* colitis can develop with any of these agents. Transient elevations of transaminases may occur with most penicillins, especially oxacillin and carbenicillin. They are benign and reversible.

High doses of some penicillins can produce fluid overload because of their sodium content. The sodium content of ticarcillin (5.1 mEq/g) and carbenicillin (4.7 mEq/g) obligates the patient to receive 90 to 170 mEq of sodium per day. The sodium overload can exacerbate congestive heart failure. Ureidopenicillins (mezlocillin, azlocillin, and piperacillin) contain less sodium (approximately 2 mEq/g). Administration of large doses of any penicillin, but most often carbenicillin and ticarcillin, may result in hypokalemia due to the large quantity of nonreabsorbable anions presented to the distal renal tubules.

Myoclonic jerks, hyperreflexia, and seizures may develop when high doses of penicillins are given in the presence of renal insufficiency.

All the penicillins used at high doses for prolonged periods will alter the indigenous bacterial flora resulting in colonization with resistant gram-negative bacilli and/or fungi. Occasionally superinfection due to these organisms may occur.

Jarisch-Herxheimer reaction may occur when patients with syphilis are treated with penicillin G. It consists of fever, headache, myalgia, and malaise, which start abruptly (a few hours after therapy) and last up to 24 h. Herxheimer reaction occurs in 50 to 70 percent of patients with early syphilis and a small proportion of those with later stages of syphilis. Its pathogenesis is unclear.

Injection of penicillin G procaine may result in an immediate reaction characterized by dizziness, tinnitus, headache, and hallucinations. This reaction is due to the rapid release of procaine into the circulation.

Natural Penicillins

Natural penicillins, produced biosynthetically, include penicillin G (benzylpenicillin) and penicillin V (phenoxymethylpenicillin). Only penicillin G is available for parenteral administration. The structures of these compounds are shown in Fig. 45-3.

Antimicrobial Spectrum

Penicillin G is highly active against all *Streptococcus* species, including groups A, B, C, D, and G streptococci, *Streptococcus pneumoniae*, and viridans streptococci. Approximately 5 percent of clinically significant isolates of *S. pneumoniae* in the U.S. show intermediate resistance to penicillin G (MICs of 0.1 to 1.0 μg/mL). Although this level of resistance can be overcome by using increased doses of penicillin G, it is difficult to achieve CSF levels adequate to treat meningitis due to these organisms. Strains of pneumococci with high-level penicillin resistance (MIC over 1.0 μg/mL) have been detected, but are rare in the U.S.

Most strains of *Enterococcus* species (*E. faecalis* and *E. faecium*) are sensitive to penicillin G. However, penicillin G is bacteriostatic against these organisms. Combinations of penicillin G and an aminoglycoside (gentamicin or streptomycin) usually exhibits a synergistic bactericidal effect against enterococci. Exposure to penicillin enhances the intracellular uptake of the aminoglycoside which exerts a lethal effect.

When penicillin G was first introduced, staphylococci were mostly sensitive. Within a few years, penicillin-resistant strains were encountered with increasing frequency, particularly among the hospital isolates. The resistance was due to the acquisition of plasmids coding for penicillinase (a beta-lactamase) which hydrolyzed penicillin G. Today nearly all strains of *S. aureus* and coagulase-negative staphylococci produce penicillinase and are resistant to penicillin G.

Penicillin G is active against most aerobic gram-positive bacilli, including *Listeria monocytogenes*, *Corynebacterium diphtheriae,* and *Bacillus anthracis*. However, *Nocardia* species and diphtheroids are resistant.

Neisseria meningitidis is highly sensitive to penicillin G. *Neisseria gonorrhoeae* is also susceptible, but its continued exposure to the drug has led to a gradual decrease in sensitivity. This appears to be due to the additive effects of mutations affecting the binding affinity of PBPs and/or the permeability of the outer membrane. Strains of *N. gonorrhoeae* that do not produce penicillinase, but are completely resistant to penicillin G, have been detected in recent years. However, most resistant strains produce penicillinase, which is plasmid-mediated. Penicillinase-producing *N. gonorrhoeae* account for a significant proportion of isolates in some parts of the U.S.

Penicillin G has very limited activity against aerobic gram-negative species. It is active against *Pasteurella multocida*, a common cause of infection in animal bite wounds, and *Eikenella corrodens*, a common cause of infection in human bites. All *Enterobacteriaceae* and *Pseudomonas* species are resistant to the drug.

Penicillin G is active against most anaerobic bacteria, including *Peptococcus*, *Peptostreptococcus*, *Clostridium*, *Actinomyces*, *Fusobacterium*, and non-beta-lactamase-producing strains of *Bacteroides*. *Bacteroides fragilis* is resistant to penicillin G.

Treponema pallidum, *Leptospira*, and *Borrelia* species are consistently sensitive to penicillin G. Penicillin G is ineffective against mycobacteria, *Chlamydia*, *Rickettsia*, *Mycoplasma*, fungi, and protozoa.

The antibacterial spectrum of penicillin V is generally similar to that of penicillin G; but it is less active against meningococci and gonococci.

Pharmacokinetics

Penicillin G is acid-labile and destroyed by gastric acid; therefore absorption after oral administration is irregular and variable. In order to achieve adequate absorption, it should be given 1 h before, or 2 to 3 h after, a meal. Penicillin V is acid-stable and is preferred for oral use since it achieves blood levels 2 to 5 times higher than the same dose of penicillin G.

Penicillin G is 55 percent bound to plasma proteins. It is widely distributed throughout the body but does not enter the CSF when the meninges are normal. In the presence of meningeal inflammation, the concentrations attained in the CSF are approximately 5 percent of those in the serum.

Over 70 percent of penicillin G administered parenterally is excreted unchanged by the kidneys, predominantly via tubular secretion. Approximately 25 percent is metabolized in the liver, and a small amount is secreted into the bile in the unchanged form. The elimination half-life of penicillin G, which is 30 min with normal renal function, increases to 4.0 h in anuric patients.

Crystalline penicillin G is available as the potassium or sodium salt and may be given either intravenously or intramuscularly. The sodium salt is more expensive than the potassium salt and rarely needs to be used. The dose of penicillin G is usually expressed in units. One unit of activity is equivalent to 0.625 mg of pure potassium penicillin G. Administration of 4 million units (2.5 g) of crystalline penicillin G intravenously every 4 h results in a mean serum concentration of 20 units/mL. One million units of potassium penicillin G contains 1.7 mEq of potassium.

Given intramuscularly as an aqueous solution, penicillin G is rapidly cleared from the body; it is therefore preferable to use a repository form. Repository penicillins provide tissue depots from which the drug is absorbed over hours in the case of penicillin G procaine (procaine penicillin) or over days in the case of penicillin G benzathine (benzathine penicillin). Repository penicillins are for intramuscular use only and cannot be used intravenously or subcutaneously. After intramuscular injection of 600,000 units of procaine penicillin, the peak serum level is reached in about 2 h and detectable levels are maintained for 24 h. An intramuscular injection of 1.2 million units of benzathine penicillin G provides detectable serum levels for up to 30 days.

Therapeutic Uses

Penicillin G is the drug of choice for infections caused by *Streptococcus* species, including *S. pneumoniae*, viridans streptococci, and groups A,

B, C, and D streptococci. Penicillin G combined with an aminoglycoside is the treatment of choice for enterococcal endocarditis and other serious enterococcal infections when the infecting strain is sensitive to penicillin.

Since all *N. meningitidis* strains are sensitive, penicillin G remains the drug of choice for meningococcal infections. Penicillin G is no longer the agent of choice for gonococcal infections, as an increasing number of resistant strains have emerged.

Penicillin G is the drug of choice for infections caused by non-beta-lactamase-producing anaerobes, such as periodontal infections, gas gangrene, community acquired aspiration pneumonia, and actinomycosis. It is the agent of choice for syphilis and for infections caused by *Pasteurella multocida* and *Eikenella corrodens*.

Penicillin V can be substituted for penicillin G in situations in which oral administration is suitable. Penicillin V is most commonly used for the treatment of group A streptococcal pharyngitis. Benzathine penicillin is used for the treatment of syphilis and group A streptococcal pharyngitis and for the prevention of group A streptococcal pharyngitis in patients with previous rheumatic fever.

Penicillinase-Resistant Penicillins

Methicillin was the first penicillinase-resistant semisynthetic penicillin to be derived from the penicillin nucleus, 6-aminopenicillanic acid. Subsequently nafcillin and isoxazolyl penicillins (oxacillin, cloxacillin, and dicloxacillin) were developed (Fig. 45-3). These agents are of interest only because of their activity against staphylococci which are resistant to penicillin G.

Antimicrobial Spectrum

Penicillinase-resistant penicillins are highly active against both penicillin G-sensitive and penicillin G-resistant *S. aureus* and coagulase-negative staphylococci. *In vitro*, methicillin is four- to eight-fold less active than nafcillin and isoxazolyl penicillins; the activities of the latter agents are comparable. Combinations of penicillinase-resistant penicillins and aminoglycosides exhibit synergy against staphylococci.

A variable proportion of *S. aureus* strains, depending on geographic area and the hospital, and most coagulase-negative staphylococci are resistant to penicillinase-resistant penicillins. These strains, referred to as *methicillin-resistant*, are also resistant to cephalosporins and carbapenems. The resistance is mediated through the production of an altered PBP-2 (PBP-2′) that has a much lower affinity for beta-lactam antibiotics than does PBP-2. Methicillin-resistant *S. aureus* has become an important cause of nosocomial infections in some parts of the U.S.

Penicillinase-resistant penicillins are active against all *Streptococcus* species. They are, however, less active than penicillin G against these organisms. Anaerobic gram-positive organisms, including *Peptococcus, Peptostreptococcus,* and *Clostridium* species, are also sensitive. These agents are inactive against enterococci, *N. meningitidis, N. gonorrhoeae*, and gram-negative bacilli (aerobic or anaerobic).

Pharmacokinetics

Methicillin is acid-labile and therefore not useful for oral administration. Nafcillin is poorly and inconsistently absorbed from the gastrointestinal tract. Isoxazolyl penicillins are acid-stable and absorbed when administered orally. Food delays absorption, resulting in lower peak levels. After oral administration of equivalent doses, the serum concentrations of cloxacillin are twice those of oxacillin, and the serum levels of dicloxacillin are twice those of cloxacillin. Variations in serum levels are due to differences not only in absorption but also in the clearance of these drugs.

With the exception of methicillin, which is 35 percent bound to serum proteins, all penicillinase-resistant penicillins are highly bound to plasma proteins: nafcillin, 88 percent; oxacillin, 92 percent; cloxacillin, 94 percent; and dicloxacillin, 97 percent. Methicillin is excreted primarily into the urine in active, unchanged form. Metabolism and biliary secretion play important roles in the excretion of nafcillin and isoxazolyl penicillins. Approximately 60 percent of an administered dose of nafcillin is inactivated in the liver. The elimination half-lives of nafcillin and oxacillin, which are 30 min with normal renal function, increase only to 1.0 h in anuric patients. Dosage adjustments, therefore, are not necessary for either of these agents in patients with renal failure.

Therapeutic Uses

Penicillinase-resistant penicillins are the drugs of choice for infections caused by *S. aureus* or coagulase-negative staphylococci, except for strains that are methicillin-resistant. Although indicated only for those infections, they are also effective in infections caused by *Streptococcus* species, including groups A, B, C, and G streptococci and pneumococci. These agents, either alone or combined with an aminoglycoside, are ineffective in enterococcal infections.

Cloxacillin and dicloxacillin are available only for oral use and are the preferred agents for administration by this route. Oxacillin and nafcillin are available for both oral and parenteral use. Because of poor absorption, nafcillin is not recommended for oral administration. Methicillin is available only for parenteral administration. Because of a higher incidence of adverse effects (i.e., interstitial nephritis) and lower *in vitro* activity, methicillin is seldom used today.

Aminopenicillins

Ampicillin (2-aminobenzylpenicillin) differs from penicillin G by the presence of an amino group on the acyl side chain (Fig. 45-3). It is available for both oral and parenteral administration. Bacampicillin is a carboxyl ester of ampicillin, available only for oral administration. Amoxicillin differs from ampicillin by the presence of a hydroxyl group in the para-position of the benzyl side chain. In the United States, amoxicillin is available only for oral administration.

Antimicrobial Spectrum

The antibacterial activities of ampicillin and amoxicillin are identical. Bacampicillin has no antimicrobial activity; it is a prodrug that is rapidly hydrolyzed to ampicillin after absorption from the intestine.

The activities of ampicillin and amoxicillin against gram-positive organisms are nearly identical to that of penicillin G. Like penicillin G, these agents are destroyed by staphylococcal penicillinase. Therefore, penicillinase-producing strains of *S. aureus* and coagulase-negative staphylococci are resistant to these drugs. Ampicillin and amoxicillin are highly active against *Streptococcus* species, including groups A, B, C, D, and F streptococci, *S. pneumoniae*, and viridans streptococci. These agents are slightly more active than penicillin G against enterococci and *Listeria monocytogenes*.

Ampicillin and amoxicillin are identical to penicillin G in activity against *Neisseria* species. They are also active against a few gram-negative species that are resistant to penicillin G. *Haemophilus influenzae* is susceptible except for strains that produce beta-lactamase (plasmid mediated). These strains account for 10 to 30 percent of the isolates in many parts of the U.S. Approximately 80 percent of *Escherichia coli* strains isolated from community-acquired infections are sensitive to aminopenicillins. Resistance is plasmid mediated and is more common in hospital isolates. *Proteus mirabilis* is almost always sensitive to these agents. Most *Salmonella* and some *Shigella* strains are also susceptible, but other aerobic gram-negative species are resistant.

The activity of aminopenicillins against anaerobes is comparable to that of penicillin G.

Pharmacokinetics

Approximately 30 to 50 percent of ampicillin that is administered orally is absorbed from the gastrointestinal tract. Peak serum levels occur in 1 to 2 h after ingestion. The peak serum levels are delayed and lower if the drug is ingested with food. Amoxicillin is more completely absorbed (75 to 90 percent); the serum concentrations are twice those attained with an equivalent dose of ampicillin. Absorption of amoxicillin is not altered when it is ingested with food. Bacampicillin is absorbed rapidly after oral administration (80 to 95 percent) and hydrolyzed immediately to ampicillin by esterase enzymes present in the serum. The serum levels of ampicillin after an oral dose of bacampicillin are twice those attained with an equimolar dose of ampicillin. The presence of food in the stomach does not decrease or delay absorption of bacampicillin.

Ampicillin and amoxicillin are the least protein bound (20 percent) penicillins. Both are excreted primarily (75 to 80 percent) by the kidneys in active, unchanged form. A small fraction is inactivated, chiefly in the liver, and 2 to 3 percent is excreted unchanged into the bile. The elimination half-life of ampicillin, which is 1.0 h with normal renal function, increases to 8.0 h in anuric patients.

Therapeutic Uses

Ampicillin is effective in a variety of infections caused by susceptible organisms, including bacteremia, meningitis, endocarditis, respiratory tract infections, urinary tract infections, otitis media, sinusitis, and enteric fever. It is the drug of choice for infections caused by beta-lactamase-negative strains of *H. influenzae*, *L. monocytogenes*, and susceptible strains of *Enterococcus* species. For enterococcal endocarditis, it is given in combination with an aminoglycoside in order to provide bactericidal activity against the organism.

Because of better absorption and a lower incidence of side effects (i.e., diarrhea), amoxicillin is preferred to ampicillin for oral administration. Bacampicillin is more expensive than ampicillin. On a molar basis, 400 mg of bacampicillin is equivalent to 278 mg of ampicillin.

Extended-Spectrum Penicillins

Extended-spectrum penicillins are a group of semisynthetic penicillins that have a significantly wider range of activity against aerobic gram-negative bacilli than aminopenicillins. These agents can be divided into two subgroups: the carboxypenicillins (carbenicillin and ticarcillin) and the ureidopenicillins (mezlocillin, azlocillin, and piperacillin). Carbenicillin and ticarcillin have a carboxyl group on the acyl side chain (Fig. 45-3). Mezlocillin, azlocillin, and piperacillin are derivatives of ampicillin; they all have a ureido group (NH-CO-N-R), in place of the amino group (NH_2) of ampicillin, on the acyl side chain. The presence of a carboxyl group or a ureido group on the acyl side chain leads to increased activity against gram-negative species primarily because of greater penetration through the outer membrane. The extended-spectrum penicillins are available only for parenteral administration, except for an ester of carbenicillin, carbenicillin indanyl sodium, which is available for oral administration.

Antimicrobial Spectrum

All extended-spectrum penicillins are susceptible to staphylococcal penicillinase and thus inactive against penicillin G-resistant staphylococci. Carboxypenicillins (carbenicillin and ticarcillin) do not have clinically significant activity against *Enterococcus* species and are less potent than ampicillin against *Streptococcus* and *L. monocytogenes*. The activities of ureidopenicillins against these organisms are comparable to those of ampicillin.

Extended-spectrum penicillins are active against aerobic gram-negative organisms that are sensitive to ampicillin (*Neisseria* species, *E. coli*, *Proteus mirabilis*, *H. influenzae*, and *Salmonella* species). They are also active against most strains of *Enterobacter*, *Proteus vulgaris*, *Providencia*, *Morganella*, *Serratia marcescens*, *Citrobacter*, *Pseudomonas aeruginosa*, and *Acinetobacter*. There are some differences in the activities of these agents against specific organisms. *Klebsiella* species are uniformly resistant to carbenicillin and ticarcillin, whereas 50 to 60 percent of strains are susceptible to ureidopenicillins. The activities of mezlocillin and piperacillin against enteric gram-negative bacilli (*Enterobacteriaceae*) are slightly superior to those of carbenicillin, ticarcillin, and azlocillin. Piperacillin and azlocillin are two- to four-fold more active than mezlocillin and ticarcillin and eight- to sixteen-fold more active than carbenicillin against *Pseudomonas aeruginosa*. Ureidopenicillins are more active than carboxypenicillins against *H. influenzae*, however, ampicillin-resistant strains (beta-lactamase positive) are also resistant to these agents.

Extended-spectrum penicillins combined with an aminoglycoside exhibit synergistic activity against many isolates of *P. aeruginosa* and against some strains of enteric gram-negative species.

Extended-spectrum penicillins are active against most anaerobes, including the *Bacteroides fragilis* group. Approximately 80 percent of *B. fragilis* isolates are susceptible to these agents.

Pharmacokinetics

The extended-spectrum penicillins are not absorbed from the gastrointestinal tract and must be given parenterally, except for an ester of carbenicillin, carbenicillin indanyl sodium, which is acid-stable and rapidly, but incompletely (30 to 40 percent), absorbed following oral administration. After absorption, the ester is rapidly hydrolyzed to free carbenicillin. Serum and tissue concentrations of carbenicillin attained after oral administration of carbenicillin indanyl sodium are inadequate for the treatment of systemic infections; however, unless renal function is impaired, high concentrations are attained in the urine.

Approximately 85 percent of ticarcillin administered intravenously is excreted unchanged into the urine. Some ticarcillin (10 to 15 percent) is inactivated in the body, chiefly in the liver. The elimination half-life of this agent (1.1 h with normal renal function) increases to 15 h in anuric patients.

Mezlocillin, azlocillin, and piperacillin are also excreted primarily (55 to 70 percent) by the kidneys in unchanged form. Twenty to 30 percent of the administered dose is excreted unchanged into the bile, and small fractions are inactivated in the body. The elimination half-lives of mezlocillin, piperacillin, and azlocillin, which are 1.0 h with normal renal function, increase to 3.6, 4.0, and 5.0 h, respectively, in anuric patients.

Piperacillin, mezlocillin, and azlocillin exhibit nonlinear pharmacokinetics — that is, a 4 g dose produces serum levels that are greater than 4 times the 1 g dose. They are therefore administered in larger doses at intervals of 6 h rather than the 4 h interval used for carbenicillin and ticarcillin.

Therapeutic Uses

The extended-spectrum penicillins are most useful for infections caused by aerobic gram-negative bacilli and anaerobes. For the treatment of serious *Pseudomonas* infections, these agents should be combined with an aminoglycoside to prevent emergence of resistance during therapy. In compromised hosts, especially those with neutropenia, and in patients with intraabdominal infections, pelvic infections, or nosocomial aspiration pneumonia, these antibiotics are usually used in combination with an aminoglycoside.

Piperacillin, mezlocillin, and ticarcillin are the most commonly used extended-spectrum penicillins. Azlocillin is used primarily for infections caused by *P. aeruginosa*.

Carbenicillin indanyl sodium is indicated only for the treatment of urinary tract infections particularly those caused by *P. aeruginosa*.

Combinations with Beta-Lactamase Inhibitors

Beta-lactamases are responsible for the resistance of many bacteria to beta-lactam antibiotics. To overcome this type of resistance, a beta-lactam antibiotic may be combined with a beta-lactamase inhibitor, clavulanate, sulbactam, or tazobactam. Clavulanate is a naturally occurring beta-lactamase inhibitor, which was isolated from *Streptomyces clavuligerus*. Sulbactam and tazobactam are semisynthetic compounds derived from 6-aminopenicillanic acid.

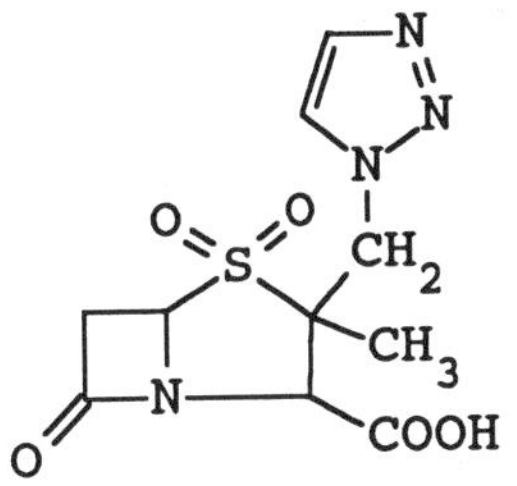

The beta-lactamase inhibitors (Fig. 45-4) contain a beta-lactam ring, but exhibit poor antibacterial activity. They bind irreversibly to many beta-lactamases and function as "suicide" inhibitors. These agents cross the outer membrane of most enteric gram-negative bacilli and interact with the beta-lactamase in the periplasmic space. The beta-lactamases that are readily inhibited include those produced by *Staphylococcus* species, *B. fragilis*, and most beta-lactamases of enteric gram-negative species. All three compounds inhibit approximately the same range of beta-lactamases.

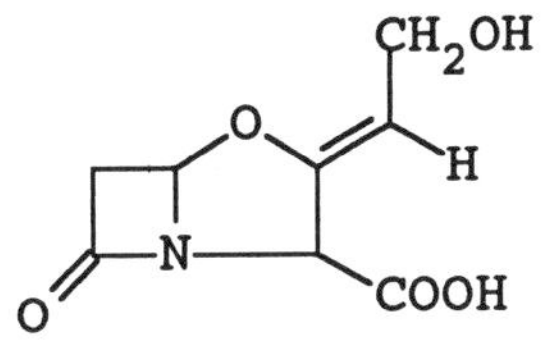

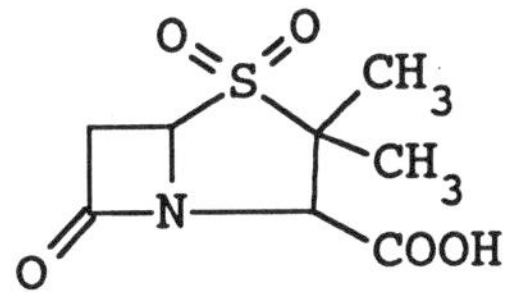

FIGURE 45-4 *Chemical structures of the beta-lactamase inhibitors.*

Clavulanate is available in combination with amoxicillin for oral use and in combination with ticarcillin for intravenous administration. Sulbactam is available in combination with ampicillin for parenteral use. Tazobactam is available in combination with piperacillin for parenteral use.

Antimicrobial Spectrum

The beta-lactamase inhibitors do not influence the intrinsic activity of the penicillin component of the combination against susceptible organisms. They do, however, expand its antimicrobial spectrum to include beta-lactamase-producing strains of *S. aureus*, coagulase-negative staphylococci, *H. influenzae*, *Haemophilus ducreyi*, *N. gonorrhoeae*, *Moraxella catarrhalis*, *E. coli*, *Proteus*, *Klebsiella*, and *Bacteroides*. All anaerobes including 100 percent of *B. fragilis* strains are sensitive to these combinations. Clavulanate and tazobactam do not inhibit beta-lactamases produced by *P. aeruginosa*; the activities of ticarcillin or piperacillin against this organism are unaffected by the addition of these compounds.

Pharmacokinetics

Approximately 60 percent of orally administered clavulanate is absorbed from the gastrointestinal tract. The absorption is unaffected when it is taken with food. Clavulanate, sulbactam, and tazobactam are widely distributed into tissues and body fluids. Both clavulanate and sulbactam are approximately 30 percent bound to plasma proteins; sulbactam is 40 percent protein bound.

Approximately 50 percent, 75 percent, and 80 percent of administered clavulanate, sulbactam, and tazobactam, respectively, are excreted unchanged into the urine. A small fraction is excreted into the bile, and the remainder is inactivated in the body. The elimination half-life of each of these agents in the presence of normal renal function is 1.0 h.

Therapeutic Uses

Amoxicillin-clavulanate is useful for the treatment of infections caused by susceptible beta-lactamase-producing organisms. It is the oral drug of choice for human-bite or animal-bite infections in which *S. aureus*, *Streptococcus* species, anaerobes, *Pasteurella multocida* (animal bite), and *Eikenella corrodens* (human bite) are the potential etiologic agents.

Ticarcillin-clavulanate and piperacillin-tazobactam are useful for treating mixed infections in which *S. aureus*, gram-negative aerobes, and beta-lactamase-producing anaerobes (especially *B. fragilis*) may be present. Ampicillin-sulbactam is a drug of choice for the treatment of community-acquired pneumonia. It is used either alone or combined with an aminoglycoside for mixed infections involving *S. aureus*, *Enterococcus*, enteric bacilli, and/or anaerobes.

CEPHALOSPORINS

The first cephalosporin, known as *cephalosporin C*, was isolated from the fermentation products of a fungus, *Cephalosporium acremonium*. Hydrolysis of this compound produced 7-aminocephalosporanic acid, which was subsequently modified with different side chains to produce the family of cephalosporin antibiotics.

Chemistry

The cephalosporin nucleus consists of a beta-lactam ring fused to a six-membered dihydrothiazine (cephem) ring (Fig. 45-5). In contrast to the penicillin nucleus, the cephalosporin nucleus is inherently more resistant to beta-lactamases. It also provides more sites for potential manipulation. Modifications of the acyl side chain at position R1 alter antimicrobial activity, whereas substitutions at position R2 are associated with changes in pharmacokinetics and metabolic parameters of the drug. Representative chemical structures of cephalosporins are shown in Fig. 45-6. The substitution of an acetoxy group (-CH_2-O-CO-CH_3) at R2 (as in cephalothin, cephapirin, and cefotaxime) is associated with significant metabolism to a desacetyl derivative. The presence of an N-methylthiotetrazole group at this position (as in cefamandole, cefmetazole, cefotetan, and cefoperazone) is associated with disulfiram-like reactions and hypoprothrombinemia. The presence of a methoxy group at position 7 (as in cefoxitin, cefmetazole, and cefotetan) enhances stability to many beta-lactamases, especially those produced by *Bacteroides* species.

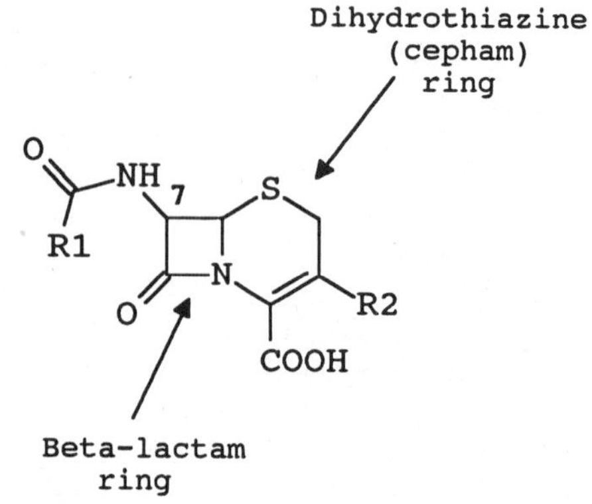

Dihydrothiazine (cepham) ring

O NH 7 S R1 N R2 O COOH

Beta-lactam ring

FIGURE 45-5 *The cephalosporin nucleus.*

FIRST GENERATION

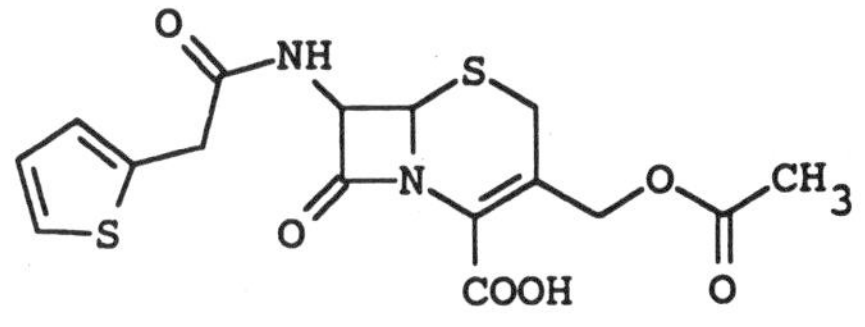

Cephalothin

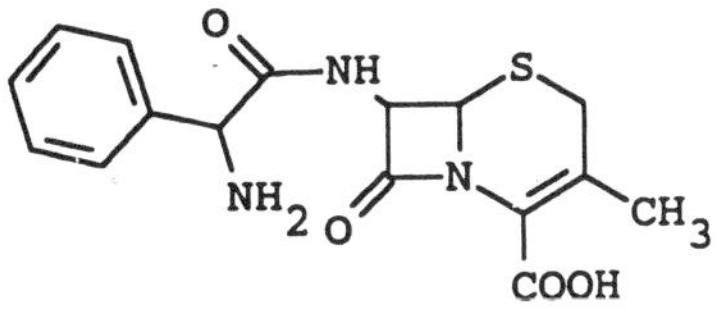

Cephalexin

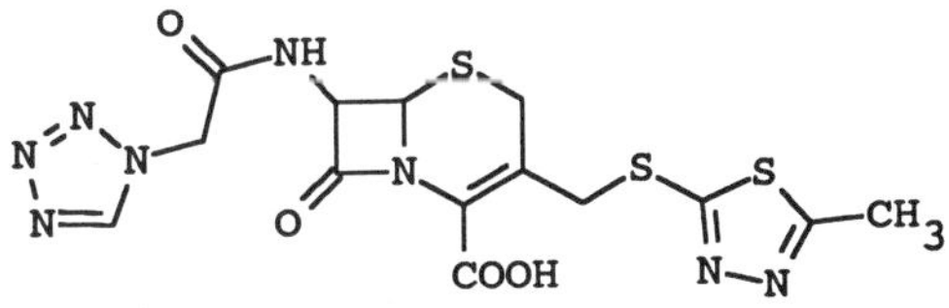

Cefazolin

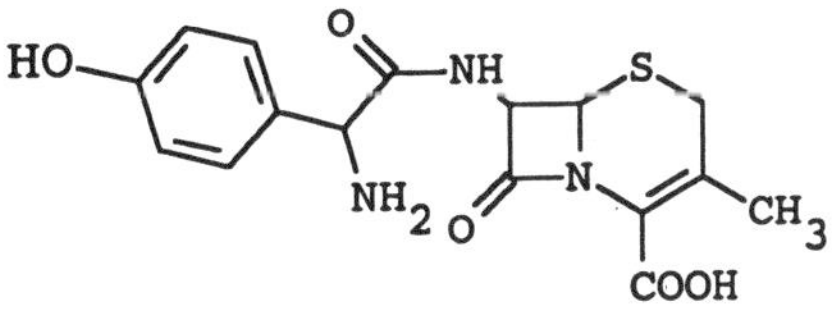

Cefadroxil

SECOND GENERATION

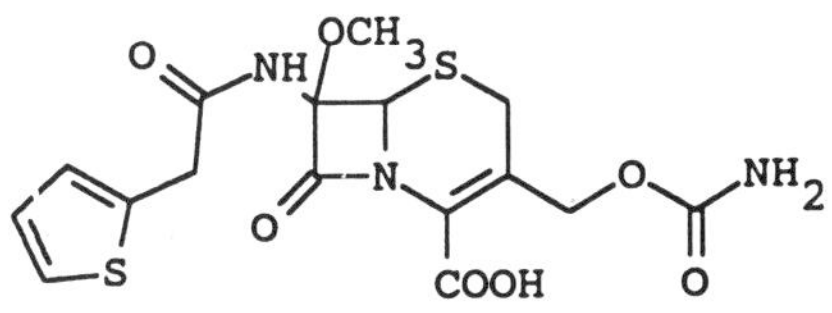

Cefoxitin

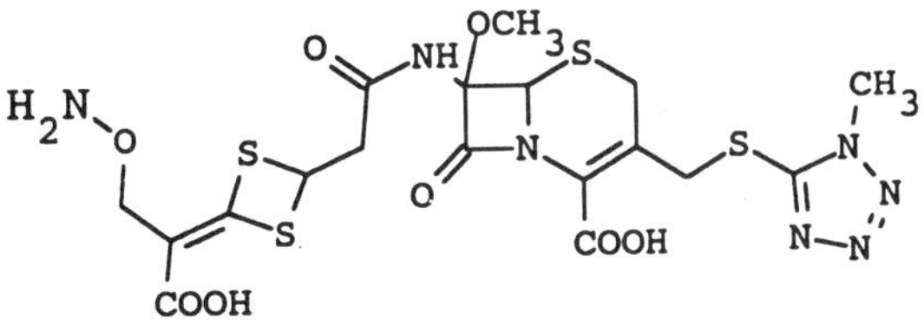

Cefotetan

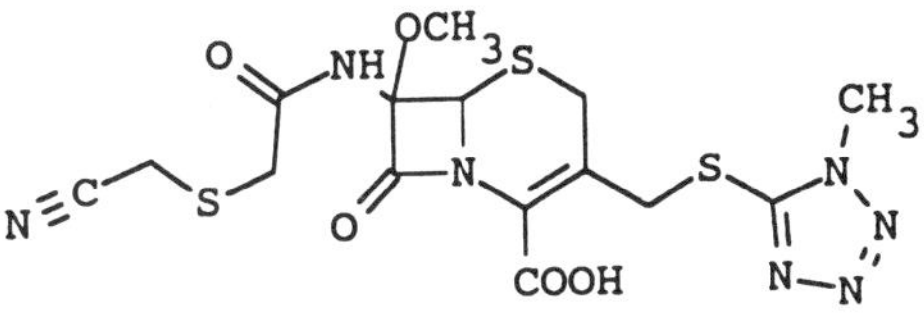

Cefmetazole

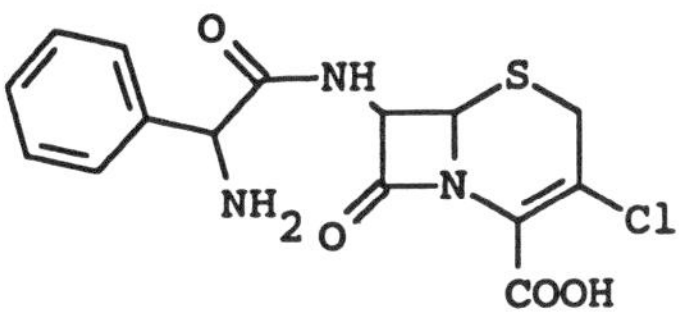

Cefaclor

THIRD GENERATION

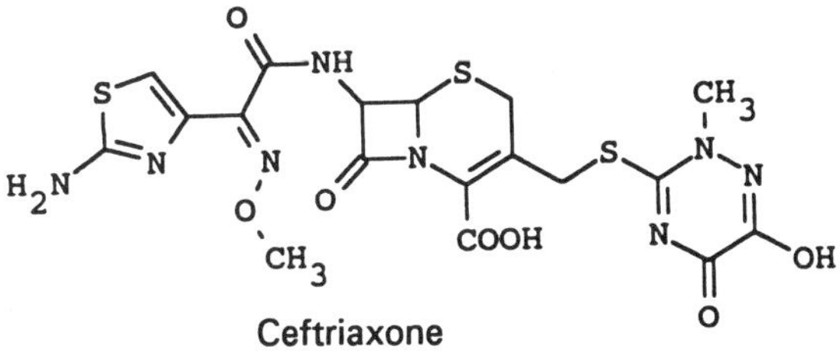

Ceftriaxone

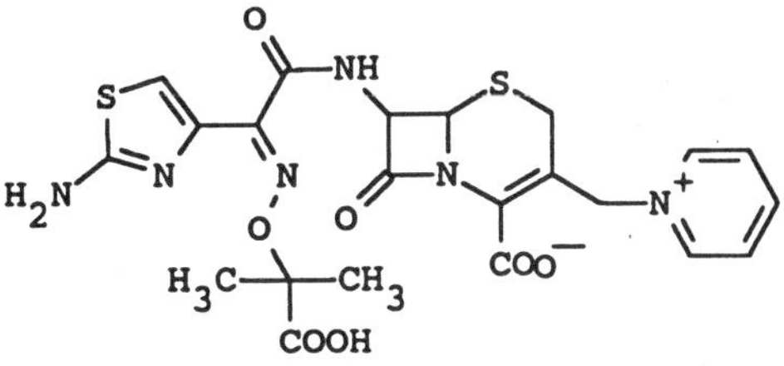

Ceftazidime

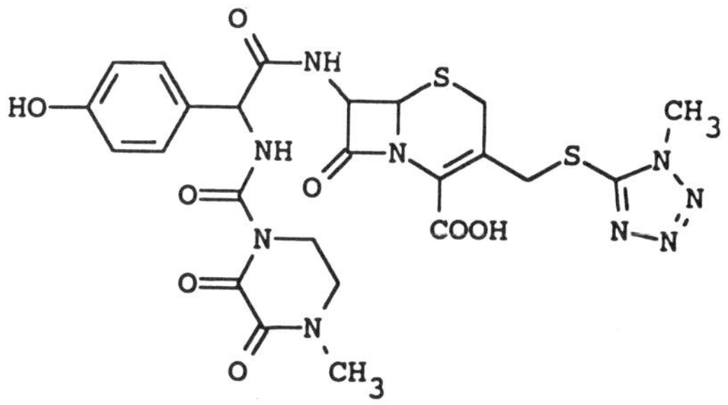

Cefoperazone

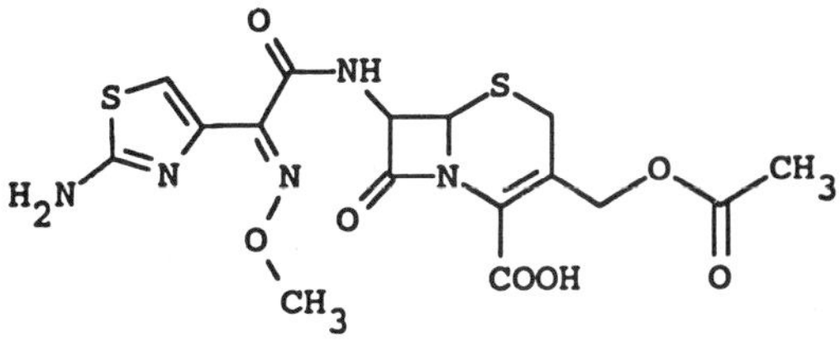

Cefotaxime

FIGURE 45-6 *Chemical structures of representative cephalosporins.*

Classification

Cephalosporins are classified into three groups, or *generations*, on the basis of their spectrum of activity against gram-negative bacilli (Table 45-2). Compounds within a generation differ from one another primarily in pharmacokinetic properties, although there may be significant differences in activity against certain organisms. The first generation compounds (cephalothin, cefazolin, cephapirin, cephalexin, cefadroxil, and cephradine) are hydrolyzed by many beta-lactamases produced by gram-negative organisms and therefore have a relatively narrow gram-negative spectrum. The second generation cephalosporins (cefuroxime, cefamandole, cefonicid, cefoxitin, cefmetazole, cefotetan, cefaclor, cefprozil, and loracarbef) have greater beta-lactamase stability and a broader spectrum of activity against gram-negative organisms. The third generation drugs (cefotaxime, ceftizoxime, cefoperazone, ceftriaxone, ceftazidime, cefixime, and cefpodoxime) are relatively resistant to hydrolysis by beta-lactamases and have the broadest gram-negative spectrum.

Pharmacokinetics

Three first generation cephalosporins (cephalexin, cephradine, and cefadroxil), four second generation cephalosporins (cefaclor, cefuroxime axetil, cefprozil and loracarbef), and two third generation cephalosporins (cefixime and cefpodoxime) are acid-stable and absorbed after oral administration. The other cephalosporins are suitable only for parenteral administration.

The cephalosporins penetrate well into most body tissues and fluids. The first and second generation cephalosporins, with the exception of cefuroxime, do not penetrate the CSF in high enough concentrations to treat meningitis. By contrast, the third generation cephalosporins produce therapeutic levels in the CSF when the meninges are inflamed.

Most cephalosporins are excreted unchanged into the urine by glomerular filtration and/or tubular secretion. Cephalothin, cephapirin, and cefotaxime are 20 to 30 percent metabolized and the desacetyl metabolites are excreted into the urine. Desacetylcephapirin and desacetylcefotaxime are active antibacterial compounds. Cefpodoxime proxetil is a prodrug that is deesterified in the liver to the active metabolite cefpodoxime. Cefoperazone and ceftriaxone are excreted chiefly into the bile in active, unchanged form.

Adverse Effects

The adverse effects of cephalosporins are generally similar to those of penicillins. Allergic reactions including skin rash, drug fever, eosinophilia, urticaria, angioedema, anaphylaxis, and allergic interstitial nephritis may occur with cephalosporins as with penicillins. Approximately 3 to 7 percent of patients allergic to penicillins will also prove allergic to cephalosporins. Cephalosporins should not be used in patients who have a history of immediate hypersensitivity reaction to penicillins or in patients with skin test reactivity to antigenic determinants of penicillin G.

Cephalosporins that possess an N-methylthiotetrazole side chain (cefamandole, cefmetazole, cefotetan, and cefoperazone) may produce hypoprothrombinemia by inhibiting vitamin K metabolism. Parenteral vitamin K, administered once or twice weekly, will prevent this complication. Granulocytopenia, thrombocytopenia, or hemolytic anemia are rare complications of therapy with cephalosporins.

Diarrhea may occur with any of the cephalosporins. It is more common with cefoperazone and ceftriaxone, which are predominantly excreted into the bile, and orally-administered cefixime and cefpodoxime. *Clostridium difficile* colitis, manifested occasionally as pseudomembranous colitis, has been reported with all cephalosporins. A disulfiram-like reaction, characterized by flushing, sweating, headache, and tachycardia, may occur when alcohol is ingested a few hours after administration of cephalosporins containing an N-methylthiotetrazole side chain (cefamandole. cefmetazole, cefotetan, and cefoperazone).

Superinfection with resistant organisms may occur during therapy with third generation cephalosporins. These include *Enterococcus* species, *Acinetobacter calcoaceticus*, *Pseudomonas* species, *Enterobacter* species, *Xanthomonas maltophilia* and *Candida* species.

First Generation Cephalosporins

Currently available first generation cephalosporins for parenteral administration (intramuscular and intravenous) include cefazolin, cephalothin, and cephapirin (Table 45-2). Cephalexin and cephadroxil are available for oral administration and cephradine is used orally, as well as by intramuscular and intravenous injection.

TABLE 45-2 Classification and pharmacokinetic properties of cephalosporins

Generic name	Oral absorption, %	Plasma protein binding, %	Elimination half-life, h	Elimination half-life, h (anuria)
FIRST GENERATION				
For Parenteral Use				
Cefazolin		80	1.8	24
Cephalothin		60	0.6	3
Cephapirin		60	0.6	2
For Oral Use				
Cephalexin	95	15	1.0	20
Cefadroxil	95	20	1.5	20
Cephradine	95	15	1.0	15
SECOND GENERATION				
For Parenteral Use				
Cefuroxime		50	1.5	21
Cefamandole		70	0.6	11
Cefonicid		95	4.5	65
Cefoxitin		70	0.9	15
Cefmetazole		65	1.2	20
Cefotetan		90	3.5	35
For Oral Use				
Cefaclor	90	25	0.7	2.5
Cefuroxime axetil	50	50	1.5	21
Cefprozil	95	35	1.3	5.9
Loracarbef	90	25	1.0	32
THIRD GENERATION				
For Parenteral Use				
Cefotaxime		30	1.0	2.6
Ceftizoxime		30	1.7	20
Cefoperazone		90	2.1	2.2
Ceftriaxone		90	6.4	12
Ceftazidime		15	2.0	20
Cefepime		18	2.0	14
For Oral Use				
Cefixime	45	65	3.0	11.5
Cefpodoxime proxetil	50	27	2.3	9.8

Antimicrobial Spectrum

The activity of the first generation cephalosporins against gram-positive bacteria is almost identical to that of penicillinase-resistant penicillins. These agents are active against *S. aureus* and coagulase-negative staphylococci including strains that produce penicillinase. Methicillin-resistant strains, however, are uniformly resistant. The first generation cephalosporins are active against *Streptococcus* species including *S. pneumoniae*. They are, however, less potent than penicillin G against these organisms. *Enterococcus* species and *L. monocytogenes* are uniformly resistant to all cephalosporins.

The first generation cephalosporins have a narrow spectrum of activity against gram-negative organisms. Most strains of *E. coli*, *Klebsiella*, *P. mirabilis*, and *Citrobacter diversus* are susceptible. Other gram-negative species, including *H. influenzae*, are resistant. These agents do not have clinically useful activity against *N. meningitidis* and *N. gonorrhoeae*.

The first generation cephalosporins are active against anaerobic bacteria with the exception of *B. fragilis*. Their activity against these organisms, however, is inferior to that of penicillin G.

Although the first generation cephalosporins have identical antimicrobial spectra, there are some differences in their *in vitro* potencies. Cefazolin, cephalothin, and cephapirin are virtually identical, whereas the oral agents (cephradine, cephalexin, and cefadroxil) are two- to four-fold less potent against most bacterial species. The *in vitro* potencies of the latter three agents are comparable.

Pharmacokinetics

Cephalexin, cephradine, and cefadroxil are almost completely absorbed after oral administration. Food delays absorption, resulting in lower peaks and more prolonged serum levels. These agents are excreted into the urine in active, unchanged form. Cefadroxil is eliminated more slowly than others; it can therefore be administered at less frequent intervals.

The pharmacokinetics of cephalothin and cephapirin are similar. Approximately 70 percent of the administered dose is excreted unchanged into the urine. The remainder is metabolized to desacetyl derivatives. Because of metabolism, the half-lives of these agents are only modestly increased in anuric patients. Cefazolin is excreted totally by the kidneys in active, unchanged form. The elimination half-life of cefazolin (1.8 h) is longer than the those of cephalothin or cephapirin (0.6 h) and increases substantially in anuric patients (24 h).

Therapeutic Uses

The first generation cephalosporins are alternatives to penicillins for treating staphylococcal and streptococcal infections in patients who cannot tolerate penicillins. They are also effective in infections caused by susceptible strains of *E. coli*, *Klebsiella* species, or *P. mirabilis*. Cefazolin is usually the preferred first generation cephalosporin because it can be administered less frequently and it is relatively well tolerated after intramuscular injection.

The first generation cephalosporins, especially cefazolin, are widely used for prophylaxis in cardiovascular, orthopedic, biliary, pelvic, and gastric surgeries. In this regard, they are preferable to second generation cephalosporins because they are effective, they cost less, and they have a narrower spectrum.

Second Generation Cephalosporins

Currently available second generation cephalosporins for parenteral administration include cefuroxime, cefamandole, cefonicid, cefoxitin, cefmetazole, and cefotetan (Table 45-2). Cefoxitin, cefmetazole, and cefotetan are 7-methoxy cephalosporins and, strictly speaking, cephamycins. Despite this difference, these agents are usually considered to be "cephalosporins". The 7-methoxy group enhances activity against beta-lactamase-producing strains of *Bacteroides*. This advantage is, to a degree, offset by a moderate loss of intrinsic activity against gram-positive organisms. The orally administered second-generation agents include cefaclor, cefuroxime axetil, cefprozil, and loracarbef (Table 45-2). Loracarbef is a carbacephem; it differs from cephalosporins by the substitution of a carbon for sulfur in the six-membered dihydrothiazine ring.

Antimicrobial Spectrum

Cefuroxime and cefamandole compare favorably with the parenteral first generation cephalosporins in activity against *Streptococcus* species, but are slightly less active against staphylococci. Other second-generation cephalosporins, especially the cephamycins, are significantly less active against these organisms.

The second generation cephalosporins are active against *N. meningitidis*, *N. gonorrhoeae*, and *Moraxella catarrhalis*, including strains that produce beta-lactamase. Cefuroxime and cefonicid are highly active against *H. influenzae*, including strains that produce beta-lactamase. Cefoxitin, cefmetazole, and cefotetan are less potent against this organism. Cefamandole is relatively inactive against beta-lactamase-producing strains of *H. influenzae*. The oral second generation cephalosporins are all active against *H. influenzae*, including strains that produce beta-lactamase.

The second generation cephalosporins are more potent than the first generation compounds against *E. coli*, *Klebsiella*, and *P. mirabilis*. A variable percentage of strains of *Proteus vulgaris*, *Morganella morganii*, *Providencia stuartii*, *Serratia marcescens*, and *Enterobacter* species are also susceptible to the second generation cephalosporins. There are differences in the susceptibility of these organisms to the individual agents; however, cefotetan is generally more active than others against these species.

Cefoxitin, cefmetazole, and cefotetan (i.e., the cephamycins) are the most active cephalosporins against anaerobes, especially the *B. fragilis* group. Approximately 80 percent of strains of *B. fragilis* are susceptible. The activities of other second generation cephalosporins against anaerobic bacteria are comparable to those of the first generation agents.

Pharmacokinetics

Cefaclor and loracarbef are rapidly absorbed after oral administration; peak serum levels are lower and occur late if they are taken with food. Cefprozil is well absorbed after oral administration; the rate and extent of absorption is unchanged when the drug is taken with food. Cefuroxime axetil, an ester of cefuroxime, does not have antimicrobial activity. It is a prodrug that is rapidly hydrolyzed to cefuroxime after absorption. Absorption of cefuroxime axetil is enhanced when it is taken with food.

Except for cefaclor, which undergoes some metabolism, all second generation cephalosporins are excreted predominantly into the urine in unchanged form. The elimination half-lives of these agents in persons with normal renal function varies from 0.6 h (cefoxitin) to 4.5 h (cefonicid).

Among the second generation cephalosporins, only cefuroxime penetrates into the CSF in concentrations adequate to treat meningitis.

Therapeutic Uses

Cefuroxime is commonly used for the treatment of community-acquired pneumonia. The potential pathogens, including pneumococcus and *H. influenzae*, are all sensitive to the drug. Other infections, such as bacteremia, urinary tract infections, and soft tissue infections due to susceptible organisms can also be treated with this agent. Because of its longer half-life and better activity against *H. influenzae*, cefuroxime has replaced cefamandole in most clinical situations. Cefonicid, because of its long half-life, is used in a once-daily regimen to treat a variety of mild to moderate infections, due to susceptible organisms.

Cefoxitin, cefmetazole, and cefotetan are useful as monotherapy for mild to moderately severe community-acquired mixed aerobic-anaerobic infections, including intraabdominal infections, infected decubiti, pelvic infections, and foot infections in diabetic patients. These agents should not be used for life-threatening mixed infections if *B. fragilis* is thought to be a significant component, for empiric therapy of serious nosocomial infections, and for infections that are caused primarily by gram-positive organisms.

Third Generation Cephalosporins

Currently available third generation cephalosporins for parenteral use include cefotaxime, ceftizoxime, ceftriaxone, cefoperazone, and ceftazidime (Table 45-2). Another parenteral compound, cefepime, will soon become available. The orally administered agents include cefixime and cefpodoxime.

The third generation cephalosporins differ from each other primarily in pharmacokinetic properties. There are also some differences in their antimicrobial activity, especially with respect to *S. aureus* and *P. aeruginosa*.

Antimicrobial Spectrum

The third generation cephalosporins vary in their activity against *Staphylococcus* species. Cefotaxime, ceftizoxime, and cefepime are the most active of these agents against *S. aureus* and coagulase-negative staphylococci, yet they are two-fold less potent than the first generation cephalosporins against these organisms. Ceftriaxone, cefoperazone, and cefpodoxime are slightly less active. Ceftazidime and cefixime have poor antistaphylococcal activity. The third generation cephalosporins are as active as the first generation compounds against *Streptococcus* species. However, they lack activity against enterococci and *L. monocytogenes*.

The third generation cephalosporins are highly active against *N. meningitidis*, *N. gonorrhoeae*, *M. catarrhalis*, and *H. influenzae*, including strains that produce beta-lactamase. Ceftriaxone has the greatest activity against *N. gonorrhoeae*. All of these drugs have a broader spectrum of activity combined with a greater potency against aerobic gram-negative species than the second generation compounds and extended-spectrum penicillins. Most enteric gram-negative organisms, including *E. coli*, *Klebsiella*, *Proteus*, *Providencia*, *Morganella*, *Serratia marcescens*, and *Citrobacter*, are highly susceptible to these agents. Strains of *Enterobacter* show variable susceptibility. Cefepime has a broader spectrum of activity and a greater potency against enteric gram-negative organisms than other third generation cephalosporins. The factors responsible include its greater resistance to degradation by beta-lactamases, its higher affinity for multiple essential PBPs, and its better penetration through the outer membrane.

Based on their activity against gram-negative organisms, the third generation cephalosporins can be divided into two subgroups: those with activity against *P. aeruginosa* (ceftazidime, cefepime, and cefoperazone) and those without clinically significant anti-pseudomonal activity (cefotaxime, ceftizoxime, ceftriaxone, cefixime, and cefpodoxime). Ceftazidime and cefepime, the most active third generation cephalosporins against *P. aeruginosa*, are two- to four-fold more active than cefoperazone against this organism. *Xanthomonas maltophilia*, *Pseudomonas cepacia*, and *Acinetobacter* species are frequently resistant to the third generation cephalosporins.

The third generation cephalosporins are active against anaerobes; however, 20 to 60 percent of *B. fragilis* strains are resistant. Ceftizoxime is more active than others against this organism.

Pharmacokinetics

Approximately 45 percent of orally administered cefixime is absorbed; the presence of food does not affect the extent of absorption. Peak serum levels occur 4 h after oral administration. Cefpodoxime proxetil is a prodrug that is hydrolyzed to cefpodoxime after absorption. Approximately 50 percent of orally administered cefpodoxime is absorbed. Peak serum levels occur 2 to 3 hours after administration. Food increases the bioavailability of cefpodoxime.

The third generation cephalosporins penetrate well into all body tissues and fluids, including the central nervous system. In the presence of meningitis, the CSF concentrations of the parenterally administered agents are in the therapeutic range for susceptible organisms. The plasma protein binding of these agents ranges from 15 percent (ceftazidime) to 90 percent (cefoperazone and ceftriaxone).

Ceftizoxime, ceftazidime, and cefepime are excreted almost entirely by the kidneys in active, unchanged form. Therefore, significant dosage adjustments are required in patients with renal failure. Metabolism and biliary excretion play important roles in the elimination of other third generation agents. Twenty to 30 percent of administered cefotaxime is metabolized to a desacetyl derivative that has antimicrobial activity; the remainder is excreted unchanged in the urine. Approximately 40 percent of ceftriaxone and 70 percent of cefoperazone administered parenterally are excreted into the bile in active, unchanged form. Neither of these two agents requires dosage adjustment in patients with renal failure. Approximately 50 percent of the absorbed cefixime and 80 percent of the absorbed cefpodoxime are excreted unchanged in the urine.

The elimination half-lives of the third generation cephalosporins vary widely. Cefotaxime has a relatively short half-life (1.0 h), whereas ceftriaxone has a long half-life (6.4 h), allowing once-a-day administration. Ceftizoxime, ceftazidime, cefoperazone, and cefepime have intermediate half-lives, ranging from 1.7 to 2.1 h. The elimination half-lives of cefpodoxime and cefixime are 2.3 and 3.0 h, respectively (Table 45-2).

Therapeutic Uses

Infections caused by multidrug resistant gram-negative bacilli are the main indication for the use of third generation cephalosporins. For infections involving *P. aeruginosa*, ceftazidime is the third generation agent of choice.

The third generation cephalosporins are useful

agents for the treatment of meningitis caused by susceptible bacteria. Ceftriaxone (or cefotaxime) is the drug of choice for the empiric therapy of bacterial meningitis in children and for *H. influenzae* meningitis. The combination of cefotaxime and ampicillin is the regimen of choice for neonatal meningitis. In adults over 50 years of age, ceftriaxone combined with ampicillin is the recommended empiric therapy for bacterial meningitis. The third generation cephalosporins are the drugs of choice for meningitis caused by susceptible gram-negative bacilli including *P. aeruginosa*.

Ceftazidime alone is an effective monotherapy for the empiric treatment of febrile neutropenic patients. Ceftriaxone is the drug of choice for gonococcal infections. Cefixime is also a drug of choice for uncomplicated urethral and cervical gonorrhea.

Some gram-negative species, particularly *Enterobacter cloacae*, and to a lesser extent, *Serratia marcescens*, *Citrobacter freundii*, and *P. aeruginosa*, may develop resistance to the third generation cephalosporins during therapy. This is due to selection of stably derepressed mutants that produce large amounts of chromosomally mediated beta-lactamase.

CARBAPENEMS

The term carbapenem denotes similarity with the 4:5 fused ring structure of penicillins, the substitution of carbon for sulfur, and the presence of a double bond in the five-membered ring. Imipenem (N-formimidoyl thienamycin) is the only carbapenem currently available for clinical use. It is derived from thienamycin, which was isolated form *Streptomyces cattleya*.

In contrast with penicillins and cephalosporins, which have an acyl amino side chain attached to the beta-lactam ring, imipenem has a hydroxyethyl side chain. Marked resistance to hydrolysis by beta-lactamases is provided by the *trans*-configuration of the side chain which contrasts with the *cis*-configuration of the penicillins and the cephalosporins (see Fig. 45-1).

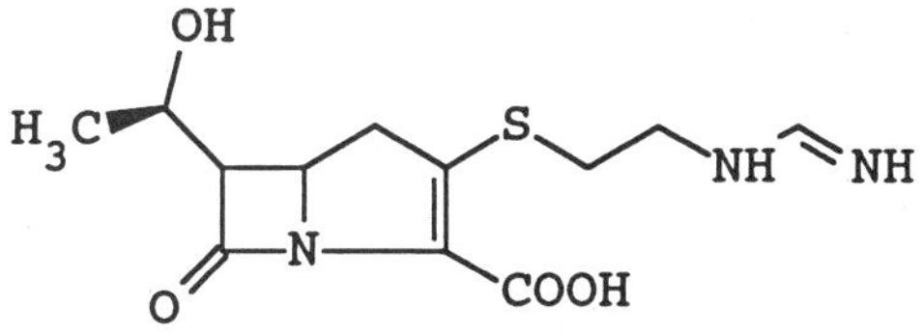

OH
H_3C
S
NH
NH
N
O
COOH

Imipenem

Imipenem binds primarily to PBP-2 and PBP-Ib. Its high affinity for PBP-2 contrasts with other beta-lactam antibiotics. Bacteria exposed to imipenem assume a spherical shape which is rapidly followed by lysis.

Antimicrobial Spectrum

Imipenem has the widest antimicrobial spectrum of any currently available beta-lactam antibiotic. It is highly active against *S. aureus* and coagulase-negative staphylococci; its level of activity against *S. aureus* is superior to that displayed by penicillinase-resistant penicillins. Methicillin-resistant strains are also resistant to imipenem.

Imipenem is highly active against *Streptococcus* species. Enterococci exhibit variable susceptibility, depending on the species. *E. faecalis* is usually sensitive, whereas *E. faecium* is commonly resistant. Like penicillin G and ampicillin, imipenem has bacteriostatic activity against susceptible enterococci. The combination of imipenem and aminoglycosides has synergistic bactericidal activity against these organisms. Imipenem is active against *L. monocytogenes* and *Nocardia*; however, diphtheroids (*Corynebacterium JK*) are usually resistant.

Imipenem is highly active against *N. meningitidis*, *N. gonorrhoeae* (including strains that produce beta-lactamase), *H. influenzae*, and *M. catarrhalis*. Enteric gram-negative species are generally susceptible to imipenem, although occasional resistant strains are encountered. With few exceptions, the level of activity of imipenem against these organisms is comparable to that of third generation cephalosporins. The third generation cephalosporins are substantially more active than imipenem against *Proteus*, *Providencia*, and *Morganella*. Imipenem-resistant strains among these organisms are not uncommon; and resistance may develop during therapy. Imipenem, however, is more active than the third generation cephalosporins against *Enterobacter* and, in contrast to cephalosporins, is highly active against *Acinetobacter calcoaceticus*.

Organisms that possess inducible beta-lactamase (chromosomal) often contain mutants that constitutively produce large amounts of beta-lactamase. Imipenem, in contrast to cephalosporins, does not provide a selective growth advantage for these mutants, reflecting the high resistance of the drug to degradation by beta-lactamases.

An important feature of imipenem is its activity against *P. aeruginosa*, which is comparable to that of ceftazidime. Resistance, however, may develop during therapy. It is usually due to altered porin proteins which result in reduced permeability of the outer membrane. *Xanthomonas maltophilia* and *Pseudomonas cepacia* are usually resistant to imipenem.

Imipenem is highly active against anaerobes, including the *B. fragilis* group. It is the most potent beta-lactam antibiotic against *B. fragilis* and other penicillin G-resistant anaerobes. Occasional *Fusobacterium* strains are resistant to imipenem.

Pharmacokinetics

Imipenem penetrates well into all body tissues and fluids, including the CSF if the meninges are inflamed. Only 20 percent of the drug is bound to plasma proteins.

Approximately 75 percent of administered imipenem is excreted unchanged by the kidneys via glomerular filtration (50%) and tubular secretion (25%). A renal dipeptidase, dehydropeptidase I (DHP-I), located in the luminal brush border of the proximal tubular epithelium, hydrolyzes the drug after it is cleared from the plasma. This post-excretory metabolism is a unique phenomenon that does not occur with other beta-lactam antibiotics. Degradation of imipenem by DHP-I results in loss of antibacterial activity in the urine and the formation of a product that exhibits slight nephrotoxicity in animals. To overcome this problem, imipenem is combined with cilastatin, a compound that inhibits DHP-I. Imipenem is available only in a fixed 1:1 combination with cilastatin for parenteral use. Cilastatin is devoid of antimicrobial activity and does not affect the activity of imipenem. Approximately 25 percent of administered imipenem is metabolized outside the kidneys.

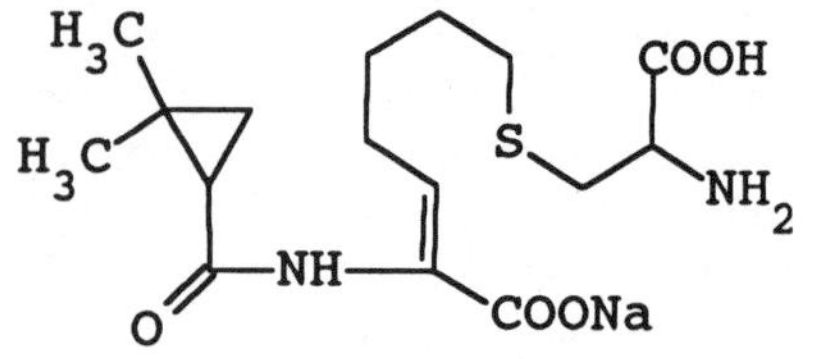

Cilastatin

In persons with normal renal function, the elimination half-lives of imipenem and cilastatin are 1.0 h. Cilastatin is less subject to extrarenal metabolism. In anuric patients, the half-life of imipenem is 3.5 h whereas that of cilastatin is extended to 13 h.

Adverse Effects

Allergic reactions described with penicillins may occur with imipenem. Cross-allergy with other beta-lactam antibiotics can occur; imipenem-cilastatin should not be used in patients who give a history of immunoglobulin E-mediated reactions to penicillins or cephalosporins.

Nausea and vomiting occur more commonly with imipenem-cilastatin than with other parenteral beta-lactam antibiotics. Diarrhea, occasionally due to *C. difficile* colitis, may also occur. Seizures have been reported in 0.3 to 1.0 percent of patients who receive imipenem-cilastatin. These generally occur in the elderly and in patients with predisposing factors such as head trauma, underlying abnormalities of the central nervous system, and renal functional impairment. Superinfection with resistant organisms (mainly *Candida* species and resistant *Pseudomonas* species) may occur during therapy with imipenem.

Therapeutic Uses

Infections caused by multidrug resistant gram-negative species (mostly nosocomial) and complicated polymicrobial infections involving *S. aureus*, gram-negative bacilli, and anaerobes are the main indications for imipenem-cilastatin. Because of its potent activity against anaerobes, imipenem-cilastatin is effective therapy for intraabdominal infections. Similar to ceftazidime, imipenem-cilastatin is effective monotherapy for the empiric treatment of febrile neutropenic patients. For *P. aeruginosa* infections, imipenem-cilastatin should be used in combination with an aminoglycoside in order to decrease the emergence of resistance.

MONOBACTAMS

Monobactams do not have the two-ringed structure of other beta-lactam antibiotics. Side chain substitutions on the core beta-lactam ring confer beta-lactamase stability and a high affinity for penicillin-binding proteins. Aztreonam, the only currently available monobactam, is a totally synthetic compound. The methyl group on the beta-lactam ring enhances the stability of the ring to beta-lactamases. The amino acyl side chain, identical to that of ceftazidime, is responsible for the potent activity of the drug against aerobic gram-negative bacteria.

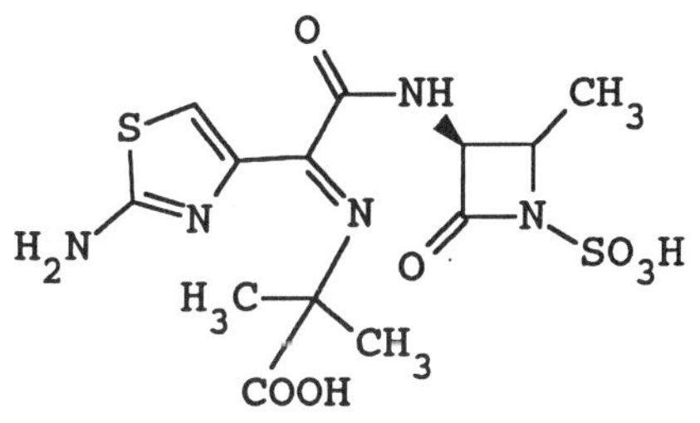

Aztreonam binds primarily to PBP-3 of susceptible gram-negative bacteria, resulting in the formation of filamentous cells that ultimately lyse. It does not bind to the essential penicillin-binding proteins of gram-positive bacteria and has poor affinity for the penicillin-binding proteins of anaerobic bacteria.

This drug is highly resistant to hydrolysis by most bacterial beta-lactamases. Despite this stability, it does not induce the production of chromosomally mediated beta-lactamases, as do the cephalosporins and imipenem.

Antimicrobial Spectrum

Aztreonam has no activity against gram-positive organisms and anaerobes. Its antimicrobial spectrum is limited to aerobic gram negative species.

Aztreonam is highly active against *N. meningitidis*, *N. gonorrhoeae*, *H. influenzae*, *M. catarrhalis*, and enteric gram-negative species, including *E. coli*, *Klebsiella*, *Proteus*, *Morganella*, *Serratia marcescens*, *Providencia*, *Enterobacter*, and *Citrobacter*. Its potency against these organisms is comparable to that of third generation cephalosporins. Aztreonam is slightly less active than ceftazidime and imipenem against *P. aeruginosa*. *In vitro* synergy with aminoglycosides occurs in 30 to 60 percent of susceptible strains. *Acinetobacter*, *Xanthomonas maltophilia*, and *Pseudomonas cepacia* are usually resistant to aztreonam.

Pharmacokinetics

Aztreonam is not absorbed from the gastrointestinal tract and, therefore, can only be used parenterally. It is 55 percent bound to plasma proteins and penetrates into all body tissues and fluids, including CSF if the meninges are inflamed.

Approximately 70 percent of administered aztreonam is excreted unchanged by the kidneys via glomerular filtration and tubular secretion. A small fraction is excreted unchanged into the bile, and 25 to 30 percent is inactivated in the body. The elimination half-life of aztreonam, which is 1.6 h with normal renal function, increases to 6.0 h in anuric patients.

Adverse Effects

Allergic skin reactions occur in about 1 percent of patients treated with aztreonam. Cross-reactivity with other beta-lactam antibiotics is rare; therefore, aztreonam can be used in patients allergic to penicillins or cephalosporins. Diarrhea occurs infrequently, and *C. difficile* colitis is less commonly reported with aztreonam than with other beta-lactam antibiotics.

Therapeutic Uses

Aztreonam is a useful agent for infections caused by aerobic gram-negative bacilli. In patients with documented or suspected mixed infections, it should be used in combination with other agents such as clindamycin, metronidazole, nafcillin, or vancomycin. Aztreonam has a similar antimicrobial spectrum to aminoglycosides; it is a potential substitute for these agents in most instances.

GLYCOPEPTIDES

Glycopeptides are a group of antibiotics that are composed of a heptapeptide nucleus attached to two or more sugars and aminosugars. Vancomycin is the only glycopeptide currently available in the United States. Teicoplanin, another glycopeptide, is widely used in Europe; it is expected to be available soon in the United States.

Mechanism of Action

The mechanism of action of glycopeptides is inhibition of cell wall synthesis. In contrast to beta-lactam antibiotics, which inhibit the third stage of peptidoglycan synthesis, glycopeptides interfere with the second stage. Glycopeptides bind to the D-alanyl-D-alanine terminus of the pentapeptide moiety in the membrane-bound lipid-disaccharide pentapeptide complex and prevent the transfer of disaccharide-pentapeptide from the lipid carrier to the existing peptidoglycan. As with beta-lactam antibiotics, autolysins mediate the lethal action of glycopeptides after inhibition of peptidoglycan synthesis.

Glycopeptides have a bactericidal effect against susceptible organisms. Their bactericidal action, like that of beta-lactam antibiotics, is not concentration dependent.

Vancomycin

Vancomycin was isolated in 1956 from *Streptomyces orientalis* (currently designated as *Nocardia orientalis*). It is a tricyclic glycopeptide with a molecular weight of 1449 daltons, considerably higher than that of any other antibiotic.

Antimicrobial Spectrum

Vancomycin is a narrow-spectrum antibiotic which is active primarily against gram-positive bacteria. It does not have clinically significant activity against gram-negative organisms.

Vancomycin is active against both methicillin-susceptible and methicillin-resistant strains of *S. aureus* and coagulase-negative *Staphylococcus* species. Although rare strains of vancomycin-resistant coagulase-negative staphylococci have been reported, vancomycin-resistant *S. aureus* has not yet been encountered. The combination of vancomycin and rifampin exhibits synergism against coagulase-negative staphylococci. All *Streptococcus* species, including groups A, B, C, D, and G streptococci, *S. pneumoniae*, and viridans streptococci, are sensitive to vancomycin. Occasional strains of viridans streptococci and *Streptococcus bovis* are autolysin deficient and exhibit tolerance to the bactericidal activity of the drug. Most enterococci (*E. faecalis* and *E. faecium*) are sensitive to vancomycin. However, like penicillin G and ampicillin, vancomycin is bacteriostatic against these organisms. A synergistic bactericidal effect is obtained when vancomycin is combined with an aminoglycoside (gentamicin or streptomycin). Diphtheroids (*Corynebacterium JK*), *Bacillus* species, and *L. monocytogenes* are sensitive to vancomycin.

Anaerobic gram-positive bacteria including *Peptococcus*, *Peptostreptococcus*, *Clostridium* species (including *C. difficile*), and most strains of *Actinomyces* are sensitive to vancomycin. Anaerobic gram-negative bacilli (*Bacteroides* and *Fusobacterium*), chlamydiae, and rickettsiae are resistant.

Mechanisms of Resistance

Resistance of gram-negative organisms to vancomycin is due to the permeability barrier provided by the outer membrane. Until 1988, resistance among gram-positive species was extremely rare. During the past few years, vancomycin-resistant enterococci have been encountered with increasing frequency, particularly among *E. faecium* strains. Two patterns of resistance, both inducible, have been identified: high-level resistance (VanA) which is plasmid-mediated, and low-level resistance (VanB) which is encoded in chromosomes. High-level resistance is due to the synthesis of enzymes, induced by exposure to vancomycin, that allow cell wall synthesis in the presence of vancomycin.

Pharmacokinetics

Vancomycin is poorly absorbed from the gastrointestinal tract. Intramuscular injections are very painful; therefore, it is administered intravenously.

Vancomycin is approximately 55 percent bound to plasma proteins. It diffuses readily into most tissues and body fluids. Penetration into the CSF is poor when the meninges are intact. However, therapeutic levels are obtained if the meninges are inflamed. Vancomycin is not concentrated in the bile; the biliary concentrations are generally in the subtherapeutic range.

Virtually all of the administered vancomycin is excreted unchanged by the kidneys, primarily by glomerular filtration. The elimination half-life of vancomycin in persons with normal renal function is 6 h; in functionally anephric patients it is extended to several days. In patients with impaired renal function, the dosage of vancomycin must be reduced, guided by peak (obtained one hour after completion of the intravenous infusion) and trough (obtained within 30 min of a dose) serum levels. Vancomycin is not cleared by either peritoneal dialysis or hemodialysis.

Adverse Effects

When vancomycin was first introduced for clinical use, the commercial preparations contained greater than 20 percent impurities and adverse effects were reported at a high rate. Current preparations contain less than 10 percent impurities and adverse effects are much less frequent.

Hypersensitivity reactions to vancomycin,

including skin rash and drug fever, are uncommon. Rapid intravenous infusion of the drug may cause the so-called "red neck" or "red man" syndrome. This is an infusion rate-dependent, non-immunologic reaction related to histamine release. It consists of tingling and erythematous flushing of the face, neck, and upper thorax, occasionally associated with hypotension, that usually subsides within minutes after the infusion is terminated. To minimize the occurrence of this reaction, vancomycin should be administered by slow intravenous infusion over a period of 60 min.

Nephrotoxicity was relatively common with early impure preparations of vancomycin and was usually reversible. With current preparations, nephrotoxicity is uncommon. However, concomitant use of vancomycin with an aminoglycoside may enhance the nephrotoxicity associated with aminoglycoside use. Renal function should be monitored during therapy with vancomycin.

Although occasional cases of auditory toxicity and rare cases of vestibular toxicity have been reported in patients receiving vancomycin, the ototoxic potential of vancomycin is in doubt. Most cases of hearing loss attributed to vancomycin have occurred in patients who have received other ototoxic agents. As with nephrotoxicity, the concomitant use of vancomycin with an aminoglycoside may enhance the ototoxicity of the aminoglycoside.

Therapeutic Uses

Vancomycin is the drug of choice for: (1) infections caused by methicillin-resistant strains of *S. aureus*, and coagulase-negative staphylococci, (2) endocarditis caused by *Staphylococcus* species or streptococci in patients allergic to penicillins and cephalosporins, (3) enterococcal infections caused by strains that are resistant to ampicillin, (4) enterococcal infections in patients with allergy to penicillin, (5) diphtheroids infections, (6) endocarditis prophylaxis for selected procedures in patients allergic to penicillins, and (7) seriously ill patients with *C. difficile* colitis (administered orally).

In patients with end-stage renal disease vancomycin is given once every 5 to 7 days and is often the preferred agent for the treatment of infections caused by susceptible bacteria.

Teicoplanin

Teicoplanin was isolated from the fermentation products of *Actinoplanes teichomyceticus*. It is a tetracyclic glycopeptide antibiotic that, in contrast to vancomycin, has a fatty acid side chain. Teicoplanin is a complex of six analogs which differ only in fatty acid side chains. Owing to the presence of fatty acid moiety, teicoplanin is far more lipophilic than vancomycin, which accounts for its greater tissue and cellular penetration.

Teicoplanin has an antimicrobial spectrum similar to that of vancomycin. It is slightly more active than vancomycin against *S. aureus* and *Streptococcus* species, including *S. pneumoniae*. Vancomycin-resistant enterococci of the VanB phenotype (low-level resistance) are susceptible to teicoplanin; however, those of VanA phenotype are also resistant to teicoplanin. Like vancomycin, teicoplanin combined with an aminoglycoside exhibits synergistic bactericidal activity against enterococci. Some strains of coagulase-negative staphylococci are relatively resistant to teicoplanin but sensitive to vancomycin.

Teicoplanin is not absorbed from the gastrointestinal tract. It is 90 percent bound to plasma proteins and widely distributed in the body. About 80 percent of the administered intravenous dose is excreted unchanged into the urine. The elimination half-life is 40 hours, which permits once-a-day dosing.

The adverse effects of teicoplanin appear to be less than those of vancomycin. Intramuscular injections are well tolerated; there is only mild pain at the injection site. Phlebitis is uncommon with intravenous administration and infusion-related red-man syndrome does not seem to occur. The nephrotoxicity and ototoxicity of teicoplanin are similar to those of vancomycin. The indications for the use of teicoplanin are essentially the same as those for vancomycin.

BIBLIOGRAPHY

Adkinson N.F.: "Immunogenicity and Cross-Allergenicity of Aztreonam," *Am. J. Med.* **88 (Suppl. 3C)**: 12S-15S (1990).

Arthur, M., and P. Courvalin: "Genetics and Mechanisms of Glycopeptide Resistance in Enterococci," *Antimicrob. Agents Chemother.* **37**: 1563-1571 (1993).

Bauernifeind, A: "Classification of Beta-Lactamases," *Rev. Infect. Dis.* **8 (Suppl. 3)**: S470-S481 (1986).

Brummett, R.E., and K.E. Fox: "Vancomycin- and Erythromycin-Induced Hearing Loss in Humans," *Antimicrob. Agents Chemother.* **33**:

791-796 (1989).

Bush, L.M., J. Calmon, and C.C. Johnson: "Newer Penicillins and Beta-Lactamase Inhibitors," *Infect. Dis. Clin. N. Amer.* **3**: 571-594 (1989).

Cohen, M.L.: "Epidemiology of Drug Resistance: Implications for a Post-Antimicrobial Era," *Science* **257**: 1050-1056 (1992).

Craig, W.A.: "Penicillins," In: S.L. Gorbach, T.G. Bartlett, and N.R. Blacklow (eds.), *Infectious Diseases*, W.B. Saunders Company, Philadelphia, 1992, pp. 160-171.

Craig, W.: "Pharmacodynamics of Antimicrobial Agents as a Basis for Determining Dosage Regimens," *Eur. J. Clin. Microbiol. Infect. Dis.* **12 (Suppl. 1)**: 6-8 (1993).

Donowitz, G.R.: "Third Generation Cephalosporins," *Infect. Dis. Clin. N. Amer.* **3**: 595-612 (1989).

Dever, L.A., and T.S. Dermody: "Mechanisms of Bacterial Resistance to Antibiotics," *Arch. Intern. Med.* **151**: 886-895 (1991).

Drusano, G.L.: "Role of Pharmacokinetics in the Outcome of Infections," *Antimicrob. Agents. Chemother.* **32**: 289-297 (1988).

Eliopoulos, G.M.: "Synergism and Antagonism," *Infect. Dis. Clin. N. Amer.* **3**: 399-406 (1989).

Georgopapadakou, N.H.: "Penicillin-Binding Proteins and Bacterial Resistance to Beta-Lactams," *Antimicrob. Agents Chemother.* **37**: 2045-2053 (1993).

Glew, R.: "Vancomycin," In: S.L. Gorbach, T.G. Bartlett, and N.R. Blacklow (eds.), *Infectious Diseases*, W.B. Saunders Company, Philadelphia, 1992, pp. 231-238.

Greenwood, D: "An Overview of the Response of Bacteria to Beta-Lactam Antibiotics," *Rev. Infect. Dis.* **8 (Suppl. 5)**: S487-S495 (1986).

Hessen, M.T., and D. Kaye: "Principles of Selection and Use of Antibacterial Agents," *Infect. Dis. Clin. N. Amer.* **3**: 479-489 (1989).

Ingerman, M.J., and J. Santoro: "Vancomycin. A New Agent," *Infect. Dis. Clin. N. Amer.* **3**: 641-651 (1989).

Jacoby, G.A., and G.L. Archer: "New Mechanisms of Bacterial Resistance to Antimicrobial Agents," *N. Engl. J. Med.* **324**: 601-612 (1991).

Johnson, A.P., A.H.C. Uttley, N. Woodford, and R.C. George: "Resistance to Vancomycin and Teicoplanin: An Emerging Clinical Problem," *Clin. Microbiol. Rev.* **3**: 280-291 (1990).

Kucers, A., and N.M. Bennett: *The Use of Antibiotics*, J.B. Lippincott, Philadelphia; 1987.

Levison, M.E., and L.M. Bush: "Pharmacodynamics of Antimicrobial Agents Bactericidal and Postantibiotic Effects," *Infect. Dis. Clin. N. Amer.* **3**: 415-421 (1989).

Lin, R.Y.: "A Perspective on Penicillin Allergy," *Arch. Intern. Med.* **152**: 930-937 (1992).

Livermore, D.M.: "Determinants of the Activity of Beta-Lactamase Inhibitor Combinations," *J. Antimicrob. Chemother.* **31 (Suppl. A)**: 9-21 (1993).

Moellering, R.C.: "The Enterococcus: A Classic Example of the Impact of Antimicrobial Resistance on Therapeutic Options," *J. Antimicrob. Chemother.* **28**: 1-12 (1991).

Molavi, A., and J.L. LeFrock: "Antistaphylococcal Penicillins," In: B.A. Cunha and A.M. Ristuccia (eds.), *Antimicrobial Therapy*, Raven Press, New York, 1984, pp. 183-195.

Mulligan, M.J., and C.G. Cobbs: "Bacteriostatic Versus Bactericidal Activity," *Infect. Dis. Clin. N. Amer.* **3**: 389-398 (1989).

Nathwani, D., and M.J. Wood: "Penicillins. A Current Review of Their Clinical Pharmacology and Therapeutic Use," *Drugs* **45**: 866-894 (1993).

Neu, H.C.: "Aztreonam: The First Monobactam," *Med. Clin. North Am.* **72**: 555-566 (1988).

Neu, H.C.: "The Crisis in Antibiotic Resistance," *Science* **257**: 1064-1072 (1992).

Okamoto, M.P., R.K. Nakahiro, A. Chin, and A. Bedikian: "Cefepime Clinical Pharmacokinetics," *Clin. Pharmacokinet.* **25**: 88-102 (1993).

Rolinson, G.N.: "Evolution of Beta-Lactamase Inhibitors," *Rev. Infect. Dis.* **13: (Suppl. 9)**: S727-732 (1991).

Sanders, C.C.: "Cefepime: The Next Generation," *Clin. Infect. Dis.* **17**: 369-379 (1993).

Sattler, F.R., M.R. Weitekamp, A. Sayegh, and J. O. Ballard: "Impaired Hemostasis Caused By Beta-Lactam Antibiotics," *Am. J. Med.* **155 (Suppl. 5A)**: 30-39 (1988).

Sobel, J.D.: "Imipenem and Aztreonam," *Infect. Dis. Clin. N. Amer.* **3**: 613-624 (1989).

Sorgel, F., and M. Kinzig: "The Chemistry, Pharmacokinetics, and Tissue Distribution of Piperacillin/Tazobactam," *J. Antimicrob. Chemother.* **31 (Suppl. A)**: 39-60 (1993).

Tomasz, A: "Penicillin-Binding Proteins and the Antibacterial Effectiveness of Beta-Lactam Antibiotics," *Rev. Infect. Dis.* **8 (Suppl. 3)**: S260-S278 (1986).

CHAPTER 46

Antimicrobials II: Aminoglycosides and Quinolones

Abdolghader Molavi

The two classes of antibiotics discussed in this chapter, aminoglycosides and quinolones, are used primarily for the treatment of infections caused by aerobic gram-negative bacteria. They both have a bactericidal action against susceptible organisms, and their bactericidal action is concentration dependent. In contrast to beta-lactam antibiotics, both aminoglycosides and quinolones exhibit post-antibiotic effect against gram-negative bacteria. The bacterial replication is inhibited for a few hours after the antibiotic concentration falls below the minimum inhibitory concentration (MIC).

AMINOGLYCOSIDES

Chemistry

Aminoglycosides are a group of antibiotics that consist of a central six-membered aminocyclitol ring attached to two or more aminosugars by glycosidic bonds. The aminocyclitol of streptomycin is streptidine, whereas all other available aminoglycosides contain 2-deoxystreptamine.

Of the eight aminoglycosides currently available in the United States, five are derived from *Streptomyces* species: streptomycin (isolated in 1943 from *Streptomyces griseus*), neomycin (isolated in 1949 from *Streptomyces fradiae*), paromomycin (isolated in 1956 from *Streptomyces rimosus*), kanamycin (isolated in 1957 from *Streptomyces kanamyceticus*), and tobramycin (isolated in 1967 from *Streptomyces tenebrarius*). Gentamicin was isolated in 1963 from *Micromonospora purpurea*. Amikacin and netilmicin are both semisynthetic. Amikacin is produced through chemical modification of kanamycin; netilmicin is a semisynthetic derivative of sisomicin, an investigational aminoglycoside isolated from *Micromonospora inyoensis*. The spelling of gentamicin and netilmicin with *micin* rather than *mycin* denotes origin from *Micromonospora* rather than *Streptomyces* species.

Neomycin and paromomycin are too toxic for parenteral administration. Kanamycin, the most commonly used aminoglycoside in the 1960s, is seldom employed today. The discussion that follows focuses on streptomycin, gentamicin, tobramycin, amikacin, and netilmicin. Gentamicin consists of a mixture of roughly equal amounts of three individual components: gentamicin C_1, C_{1a}, and C_2 (Fig. 46-1).

Mechanism of Action

The aminoglycoside antibiotics have a rapid bactericidal action against susceptible organisms. An essential element in the process leading to lethality is the active transport of the aminoglycoside from an external milieu into the bacterial cell. The transport mechanism results in the accumulation of the drug inside the bacterial cell to concentrations far above those in the external milieu.

Aminoglycosides diffuse readily through the porin channels in the outer membrane of gram-negative bacteria and enter the periplasmic space. Transport across the cytoplasmic (inner) membrane is energy-dependent and occurs in two energy-dependent phases. The first phase (termed *energy-dependent phase I*) is dependent upon the electrical potential across the cytoplasmic membrane, which is generated by aerobic metabolism. In this phase, the strongly cationic aminoglycoside binds to anionic transporters and is driven across the cytoplasmic membrane by the membrane potential which is negative on the interior. This phase of transport, which is rate limiting, is inhibited by both a reduction in pH and anaerobiosis,

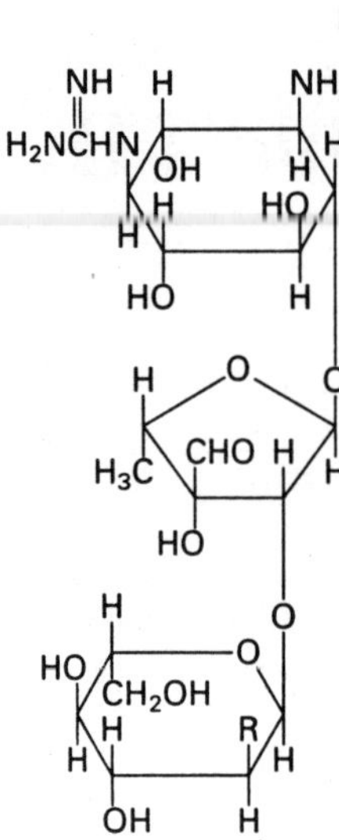

FIGURE 46-1 *Structural formulas of representative aminoglycosides.*

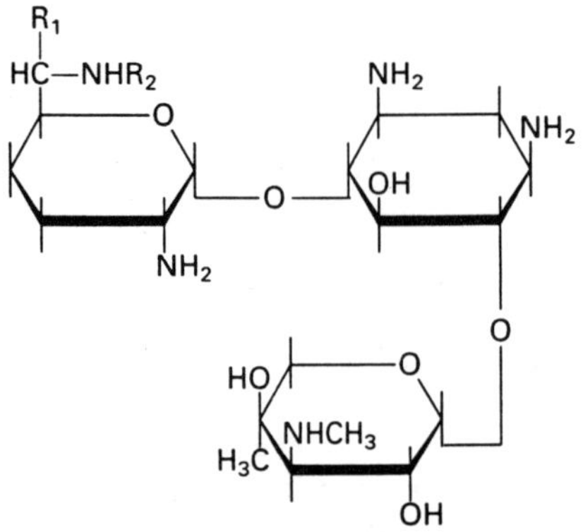

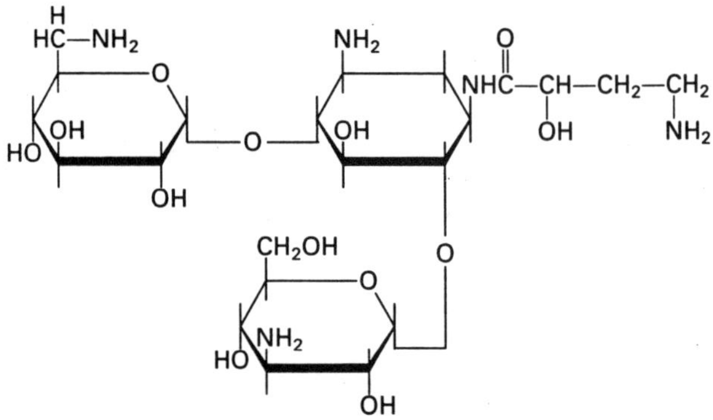

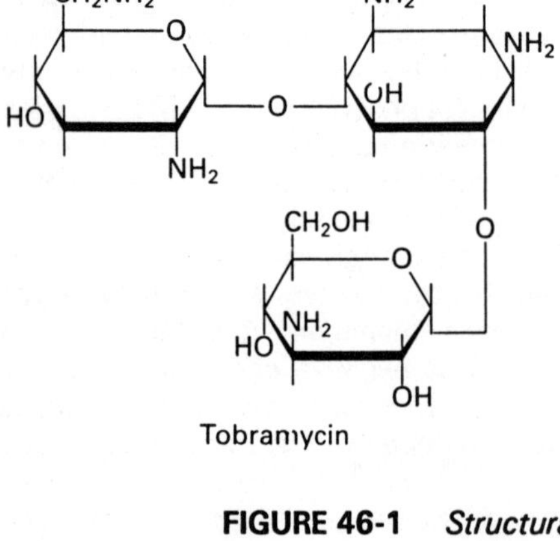

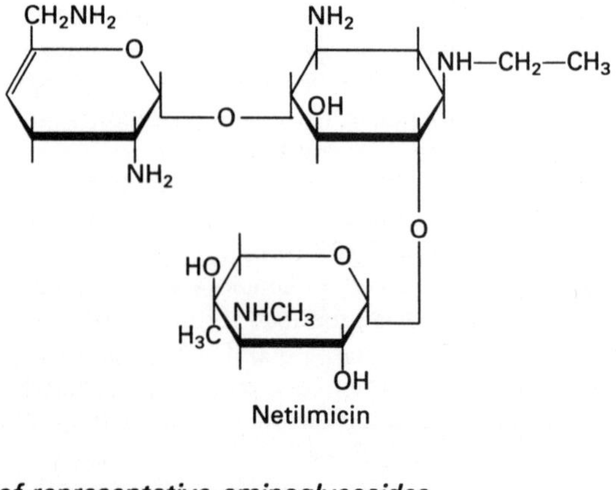

which impair the ability of bacteria to maintain the necessary membrane potential. A faster rate of aminoglycoside uptake (termed *energy-dependent phase II*) starts after the aminoglycoside interacts with the ribosome.

The primary intracellular site of action of aminoglycosides is the bacterial ribosome. There appears to be at least two different types of ribosomal binding: one unique to streptomycin and one shared by other aminoglycosides. Streptomycin binds to the 30S ribosomal subunit. Other aminoglycosides bind to multiple sites on both 30S and 50S ribosomal subunits and fail to compete with streptomycin binding to the 30S ribosomal subunit.

The binding of aminoglycosides to the ribosome results in (1) inhibition of protein synthesis and (2) misreading of the genetic code of the messenger RNA template with resultant incorporation of incorrect amino acids into the growing polypeptide chains. However, neither of these effects explains the bactericidal effect of aminoglycosides. Some other antibiotics inhibit protein synthesis as effectively as do the aminoglycosides and yet fail to cause a lethal event, that is, they produce only bacteriostasis. The mechanism of rapid lethal action of aminoglycosides remains unclear, although effects on the energy-dependent transport mechanism have been proposed.

Aminoglycosides have a concentration-dependent bactericidal activity against susceptible bacteria. They also exhibit a significant postantibiotic effect against these organisms.

Antimicrobial Spectrum

The antimicrobial spectrum of aminoglycosides includes aerobic and facultative gram-negative bacilli, *Staphylococcus aureus*, and mycobacteria. These antibiotics have no activity against anaerobic microorganisms, chlamydiae, or rickettsiae.

Gram-Positive Bacteria *S. aureus* and coagulase-negative staphylococci are usually quite susceptible, especially to the 2-deoxystreptamine-containing aminoglycosides (gentamicin, tobramycin, netilmicin, and amikacin). *Listeria monocytogenes* is also generally susceptible to those agents. *Streptococcus* species are resistant to the clinically achievable concentrations. However, combination of penicillin G, ampicillin, or vancomycin with an aminoglycoside exhibits synergistic bactericidal activity against viridans streptococci and groups B, C, and G streptococci.

Enterococci are generally resistant to the concentrations of aminoglycosides achieved clinically. Enterococcal strains exhibit two patterns of aminoglycoside resistance: (1) *Low-level resistance* related to decreased intracellular transport; the MICs of streptomycin and gentamicin for these strains are equal to or less than 2,000 g/mL and 500 g/mL, respectively, and (2) *high-level resistance* due to production of an aminoglycoside-modifying enzyme, or in case of streptomycin, an altered ribosomal binding site. The MICs of streptomycin and gentamicin for these strains are greater than 2,000 g/mL and 500 g/mL, respectively. The combination of an aminoglycoside and either penicillin G, ampicillin, or vancomycin has synergistic bactericidal action against enterococcal strains that exhibit low-level resistance to the aminoglycoside. High-level resistance to an aminoglycoside correlates with the lack of synergistic activity of the combination.

Gram-Negative Bacteria Gentamicin, tobramycin, netilmicin, and amikacin are active against aerobic and facultative gram-negative bacteria, including *Escherichia coli*, *Klebsiella*, *Proteus*, *Providencia*, *Morganella*, *Enterobacter*, *Serratia*, *Citrobacter*, *Franciscella tularensis*, *Yersinia pestis*, *Brucella*, *Acinetobacter*, *Pseudomonas aeruginosa*, *Pseudomonas cepacia*, *Xanthomonas maltophilia*, *Haemophilus influenzae*, *Neisseria meningitidis*, and *Neisseria gonorrhoeae*. The antibacterial activities of gentamicin and tobramycin are nearly identical except that gentamicin is more potent against *Serratia marcescens* whereas tobramycin is 2 to 4 times more potent against *P. aeruginosa*. Netilmicin shares the spectrum of gentamicin and tobramycin, but some strains of *E. coli*, *Klebsiella*, *Enterobacter*, and *Citrobacter* that are gentamicin-resistant are susceptible to netilmicin. Amikacin is active against many strains of gram-negative species that are resistant to other aminoglycosides. The gram-negative spectrum of streptomycin is similar to other aminoglycosides; however, resistant strains are common in most species, and *P. aeruginosa* is usually resistant.

Mycobacteria Streptomycin is the most active aminoglycoside against *Mycobacterium tuberculosis*. Amikacin and kanamycin are also active against this organism. Amikacin is also active against *Mycobacterium fortuitum*. The activities of gentamicin, tobramycin, and netilmicin against mycobacteria are not clinically significant.

Mechanisms of Resistance

Bacterial resistance to the aminoglycosides can occur by one of the following mechanisms: (1) inactivation of the drug by microbial enzymes (aminoglycoside-modifying enzymes), (2) altered ribosomal binding site, and (3) impaired intracellular transport.

The most common mechanism of resistance to aminoglycosides in clinical isolates is enzymatic modification of a substituent group on the aminoglycoside: acetylation of an amino group, adenylation of a hydroxyl group, or phosphorylation of a hydroxyl group. The modified drug competes with the unaltered drug for intracellular transport but fails to bind to ribosomes. As a consequence, the second energy-dependent phase of aminoglycoside uptake does not occur. Over 20 aminoglycoside-modifying enzymes have been identified. The genes for these enzymes are located on plasmids; this allows transfer of the enzyme-mediated resistance between strains of a species or from one species to another. Different aminoglycosides vary in their ability to resist enzymatic inactivation. Gentamicin and tobramycin are both susceptible to the same enzymes; netilmicin is more resistant to such modifications. Amikacin is least vulnerable to the enzymes that are currently prevalent.

Streptomycin binds to a specific protein (S_{12}) on the 30S subunit of the ribosome. Alteration of this protein by mutation eliminates the binding affinity of streptomycin and makes the organism totally resistant to the drug. Such mutations occur with a relatively high frequency and result in the emergence of resistance during therapy. The 2-deoxystreptamine aminoglycosides (gentamicin, tobramycin, netilmicin, and amikacin) bind to multiple sites on both ribosomal subunits. Due to the requirement for multiple mutational events, mutational resistance to these agents is exceedingly uncommon.

A third mechanism of resistance is impaired intracellular transport which leads to resistance to all aminoglycosides. This type of resistance is uncommon among gram-negative aerobic or facultative bacilli. Since the transport of aminoglycosides across the cytoplasmic membrane is an oxygen-dependent active process, strictly anaerobic bacteria are invariably resistant to these drugs.

Pharmacokinetics

Aminoglycosides are very poorly absorbed from the intestinal tract (less than 1 percent) and must be given parenterally. Streptomycin is 35 percent bound to plasma proteins; other aminoglycosides have negligible protein binding (0 to 5 percent). The aminoglycosides penetrate into various tissues except the brain and the prostate. High concentrations are found in the renal cortex and in the endolymph and perilymph of the inner ear. Penetration into bronchial secretions is poor, and the biliary concentrations are lower than the concurrent serum levels. Penetration into the cerebrospinal fluid (CSF) and ocular fluids is poor even in the presence of inflammation. Therapeutic CSF levels are obtained in the neonates with meningitis, perhaps because of immaturity of the blood-brain barrier.

The aminoglycosides are totally excreted unchanged by the kidneys. Less than 1 percent of a parenterally administered dose appears in feces. The elimination half-lives of gentamicin, tobramycin, netilmicin, amikacin, and streptomycin in persons with normal renal functions are identical, 2.0 to 2.5 h. In functionally anephric patients, the half-lives are prolonged to 40 to 60 h. Dosage adjustment is essential with any degree of renal impairment. The aminoglycosides are removed from the body by either hemodialysis or peritoneal dialysis.

Adverse Effects

The incidence of allergic reactions to aminoglycosides is very low. The principal toxicities are ototoxicity, nephrotoxicity, and neuromuscular blockade.

Ototoxicity All aminoglycosides are capable of causing ototoxicity. Their toxic effect on the neuroepithelial cells of the inner ear may produce cochlear damage, vestibular impairment, or both. Although relatively uncommon, ototoxicity is especially worrisome because of its irreversibility and its cumulative nature with repeated courses of aminoglycosides.

The auditory toxicity of aminoglycosides is manifest clinically as neurosensory hearing loss. The initial manifestations are tinnitus and/or high-frequency hearing loss (usually bilateral). Since the latter is outside the conversational range, it can only be detected by audiometry. Loss of low-tone hearing occurs if exposure is continued. Vestibular toxicity is manifest clinically by vertigo, dizziness, and/or ataxia, especially in the dark. The occurrence and the severity of both auditory toxicity and vestibular toxicity correlate with high serum levels and prolonged therapy with aminoglycosides.

The auditory toxicity of aminoglycosides is due to selective destruction of the hair cells of the organ of Corti. The hair cells located in the basal turn of the cochlea are affected first, with destruction progressing toward the apex. The progression is consistent with clinical experience, since the basal region corresponds to high-frequency and the apex to low-frequency tones. The vestibular system is affected primarily by damage to type I hair cells of the summit of the ampullar cristae. Neither cochlear nor ampullar cells can regenerate once they have been destroyed, thus accounting for irreversibility of ototoxicity.

The cellular damage in the inner ear is due to the high concentrations of aminoglycosides in the perilymph and endolymph that bathe the cells. Aminoglycosides enter the perilymph and the endolymph when concentrations in plasma are high. Diffusion back into the blood stream is slow, and their half-lives in these fluids (10 to 12 h) are much longer than the plasma half-lives.

The incidence of aminoglycoside-induced auditory and vestibular toxicity is less than 0.5 percent if clinically detectable hearing loss or vestibular dysfunction is used to determine the incidence, but it is higher if more sensitive measures of auditory or vestibular function are employed.

Nephrotoxicity All aminoglycosides are capable of causing nephrotoxicity. The toxicity is due to marked accumulation and avid retention of these drugs in the renal cortex by the proximal tubular cells.

Nephrotoxicity manifests itself initially by proteinuria, cylindruria, and inability to concentrate the urine. This is followed by a reduction in glomerular filtration rate with a rise in serum creatinine and blood urea nitrogen (nonoliguric acute renal failure). The impairment in renal function is almost always reversible, since the proximal tubular cells have the capacity to regenerate.

Streptomycin does not concentrate much in the renal cortex; it is the least nephrotoxic aminoglycoside. The nephrotoxic potentials of gentamicin, amikacin, and netilmicin are similar. Tobramycin may be less nephrotoxic, but this is controversial. The reported incidence of aminoglycoside-induced nephrotoxicity varies depending upon the criteria used to define toxicity; it is generally in the range of 5 to 10 percent.

Risk factors for development of nephrotoxicity from aminoglycosides include advanced age, preexisting renal disease, and concurrent use of vancomycin, amphotericin B, cephalothin, cisplatin, and cyclosporine.

Neuromuscular Blockade All aminoglycosides are capable of producing neuromuscular blockade resulting in respiratory paralysis. This effect is associated with plasma concentrations significantly above therapeutic levels. Susceptibility to neuromuscular blockade is enhanced by hypocalcemia, myasthenia gravis, and neuromuscular blocking agents used with general anesthesia.

The mechanism responsible for aminoglycoside-induced neuromuscular blockade involves both an inhibition of the presynaptic release of acetylcholine and a reduction in sensitivity of the postsynaptic receptor for acetylcholine. Calcium overcomes the effect of the aminoglycoside at the neuromuscular junction, and the intravenous administration of a calcium salt is the preferred treatment of this toxicity.

Therapeutic Uses

The principle uses of aminoglycosides are for the treatment of gram-negative bacillary infections (gentamicin, tobramycin, amikacin, and netilmicin) and in synergistic combinations for the treatment of gram-positive coccal infections (gentamicin and streptomycin). Because of its low cost, gentamicin is the preferred agent for most indications. Tobramycin is most commonly used for the treatment of infection caused by *P. aeruginosa*. Amikacin and netilmicin are used primarily to treat infections caused by nosocomial pathogens resistant to gentamicin. For infections caused by *P. aeruginosa*, aminoglycosides are used in combination with an extended-spectrum penicillin, ceftazidime, imipenem, or aztreonam.

Streptomycin is the drug of choice for the treatment of tularemia (*Franciscella tularensis*), plague (*Yersinia pestis*), and brucellosis (in combination with tetracycline). It is not used for other gram-negative bacillary infections because high-level resistance may develop during therapy due to a single-step mutation.

Combination of streptomycin or gentamicin with penicillin G or ampicillin (vancomycin in patients allergic to penicillin) is the treatment of choice for enterococcal endocarditis, other serious enterococcal infections, and viridans streptococcal endocarditis if the infecting strain requires greater than 0.1 g/mL of penicillin G for inhibition. For the treatment of *S. aureus* endocarditis, gentamicin is usually added to a penicillin effective against staphylococci or vancomycin during the first 3 to 5 days of therapy.

In patients treated with aminoglycosides, a loading dose is administered in order to achieve therapeutic concentrations quickly. The loading dose is the same regardless of the kidney function. The initial maintenance dose is determined by calculating the patient's creatinine clearance. Subsequently, the serum levels (peak and trough) are monitored, and the maintenance dose is adjusted, if necessary, to avoid toxic levels as well as subtherapeutic concentrations. The aim is to achieve peak (obtained 30 min after a 30-min infusion) and trough (drawn within 30 min of the next dose) serum levels which are within the accepted ranges. For gentamicin and tobramycin, a reasonable goal for peak serum levels is between 5 and 8 μg/mL; the trough levels should be greater than 2 μg/mL.

Spectinomycin

Spectinomycin, isolated from *Streptomyces spectabilis*, is an aminocyclitol antibiotic. It is not an aminoglycoside, because it contains neither an amino sugar nor a glycosidic bond.

Similar to streptomycin, spectinomycin binds to the 30S ribosomal subunit and inhibits protein synthesis. However, misreading of the genetic code does not occur.

Although spectinomycin has a wide spectrum of activity, it is used only for gonococcal infections. Other gram-negative bacteria develop resistance during therapy. Resistance to spectinomycin is rarely encountered in *N. gonorrhoeae*.

Spectinomycin does not enter saliva and is not effective in gonococcal pharyngitis. It is totally excreted into the urine in unchanged form and has a half-life of 1.0 h.

Spectinomycin is neither ototoxic nor nephrotoxic. It is used for the treatment of penicillinase-producing gonococcal infections. Spectinomycin is administered only by intramuscular injection.

QUINOLONES

Quinolones are a rapidly expanding class of antimicrobial drugs that may become as large as the cephalosporins. The first quinolone, nalidixic acid, was developed in 1962 and a few analogues were subsequently introduced. However, because of narrow spectra of activity and the rapid development of resistance during therapy, none achieved a wide usage.

The fluoroquinolones, a new generation of quinolones developed in 1980's, have greatly improved microbiologic and pharmacologic properties. These agents differ from the older compounds in that they have a fluorine at the C-6 position and a piperazinyl moiety at the C-7 position of the bicyclic quinolone nucleus (Fig. 46-2). The 6-fluoro modification increases potency against gram-negative bacteria and broadens the spectrum to include gram-positive organisms. The 7-piperazinyl group provides activity against *P. aeruginosa*. Substituents at the N-1 position of the quinolone ring and the para-position of the piperazine ring vary from one agent to another. The fluoroquinolones currently marketed in the U.S. include norfloxacin, ciprofloxacin, ofloxacin, enoxacin, and lomefloxacin, all available for oral administration. Ciprofloxacin and ofloxacin are also available for parenteral administration. Another quinolone, fleroxacin, will soon be available for oral and parenteral administration.

Mechanism of Action

The fluoroquinolones are potent bactericidal agents that alter the structure and function of bacterial DNA by interfering with the activities of the enzyme DNA gyrase (topoisomerase II). DNA gyrase is a tetramer composed of two A subunits and two B subunits that are the products of genes referred to as *gyr*A and *gyr*B, respectively. This enzyme is responsible for the insertion of negative superhelical twists (negative supercoils) into the covalently closed circular DNA. The A subunits induce transient breaks at specific sites on the double-stranded DNA, the B subunits introduce negative supercoils (ATP-dependent), and then the A subunits seal the breaks they initially produced. DNA gyrase is essential to accommodate the bacterial DNA, approximately 1100 μm in *E. coli*, within a cell which is only 2 to 3 μm in length. This enzyme is required for DNA replication, DNA repair, recombination, transposition, and transcription of certain operons. Quinolones inhibit the DNA supercoiling by interfering with the action of the A subunits, thereby interrupting the DNA breakage and resealing steps. The DNA gyrase of eukaryotic cells is much more resistant to the quinolones than is the bacterial enzyme.

Quinolones have a concentration-dependent bactericidal action against susceptible organisms.

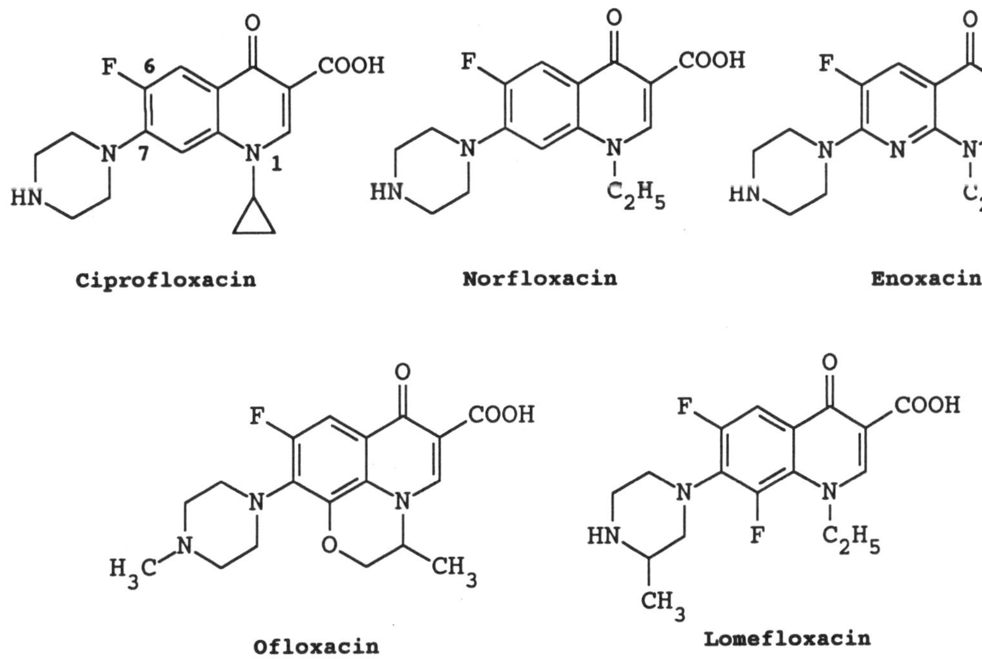

FIGURE 46-2 *Chemical structures of fluoroquinolones.*

They also exhibit a significant postantibiotic effect for both gram-negative bacteria and *S. aureus*.

Antimicrobial Spectrum

The antimicrobial spectra of the quinolones are similar. However, there are differences in their activities against some organisms.

Gram-Negative Bacteria. Quinolones are highly active against *N. gonorrhoeae*, *N. meningitidis*, and *Moraxella catarrhalis* including strains that produce beta-lactamase. They have excellent activity against *Enterobacteriaceae*, including *E. coli*, *Klebsiella*, *Enterobacter*, *Proteus*, *Morganella*, *Providencia*, *Citrobacter*, *Serratia*, *Salmonella*, *Shigella*, and *Yersinia enterocolitica*. Other gram-negative species including *Eikenella corrodens*, *Pasteurella multocida*, *Aeromonas hydrophila*, *Campylobacter jejuni*, *Vibrio*, *Helicobacter pylori*, *Haemophilus influenzae*, *Haemophilus ducreyi*, and *Legionella* are also sensitive to quinolones. The activities of different quinolones against these organisms vary by two- to four-fold; ciprofloxacin is the most potent agent. *P. aeruginosa* is highly susceptible to ciprofloxacin; other quinolones are less active against this organism. Most strains of *Acinetobacter calcoaceticus*, *Xanthomonas maltophilia*, and *Pseudomonas cepacia* are resistant to quinolones.

Gram-Positive Bacteria Quinolones have good activity against methicillin-susceptible *S. aureus* and coagulase-negative staphylococci. However, resistant strains have become increasingly prevalent in the past few years, particularly among methicillin-resistant strains. Most quinolones do not have adequate activity against *Streptococcus* species (including groups A, B, C, D, and G streptococci and *S. pneumoniae)* and *Corynebacterium* species. Ciprofloxacin and ofloxacin are the most active quinolones against gram-positive bacteria.

Other Organisms Ciprofloxacin and ofloxacin are active against *Mycobacterium tuberculosis*, *M. kansasii*, *M. fortuitum*, and *M. xenopi*, but their activity against *M. avium-intracellulare* is only fair to poor. Ofloxacin is active against *Chlamydia trachomatis*, *Ureaplasma urealyticum*, and *Mycoplasma hominis*; other quinolones are less potent against these organisms. Quinolones are also active *in vitro* against species of *Rickettsia*, *Coxiella burnetii*, and *Plasmodium falciparum* but they lack activity against *Treponema pallidum*. The quinolones do not have clinically significant activity against anaerobic bacteria.

Mechanisms of Resistance

Two mechanisms of bacterial resistance to quinolones have been identified: (1) altered DNA gyrase secondary to mutations in the *gyr*A gene and (2) altered outer membrane protein, resulting in decreased permeability. Destruction or modification of these agents by bacterial enzymes have not been described. Resistance to quinolones is encoded on chromosomes; no plasmid-mediated resistance has been demonstrated in clinical isolates.

Spontaneous single-step mutations to quinolone resistance tends to be infrequent (less than 10^{-9}), and when it occurs the resistance is of a low level for many bacterial species. Higher frequencies (10^{-7} to 10^{-8}) are seen in *P. aeruginosa* and mycobacteria. Emergence of resistance to quinolones has been a problem primarily in *P. aeruginosa*, *S. aureus* (particularly methicillin-resistant strains), coagulase-negative staphylococci, and, to a lesser extent, *Serratia marcescens*. When the quinolones were first introduced, *S. aureus* and coagulase-negative staphylococci, including methicillin-resistant strains, were uniformly sensitive to these agents. Within a few years, resistant strains emerged. Subsequent transmission of these strains within hospitals has led to an increasing prevalence of quinolone resistance among staphylococci.

Pharmacokinetics

All quinolones are absorbed from the gastrointestinal tract. The extent of absorption varies from 40 percent with norfloxacin to 98 percent with ofloxacin (Table 46-1). Peak serum concentrations are achieved 1 to 2 h after the drugs are ingested after a meal). Quinolones form chelates with metal cations. Therefore, concurrent administration of antacids containing magnesium, aluminum, or calcium, causes a marked reduction (up to 90 percent) in the absorption of quinolones and results in insufficient serum and tissue concentrations. Similarly sucralfate (which contains aluminum), ferrous sulfate, and multivitamins containing zinc interfere with the absorption of these agents. Since absorption of quinolones is virtually complete two hours after oral administration, the use of antacids or sucralfate two hours after the quinolone dose eliminates this interaction.

Quinolones are widely distributed within the tissues (including prostate) and body fluids (including salivary secretions). They enter macrophages and polymorphonuclear leukocytes, attaining high intracellular concentrations. Penetration into the CSF is low (except for ofloxacin), higher levels are achieved when the meninges are inflamed. Binding to plasma proteins of various quinolones ranges from 15 to 40 percent.

Quinolones differ in their elimination pathways. Ofloxacin is almost totally excreted by the

TABLE 46-1 Pharmacokinetic properties of quinolones

Drug	Oral bioavailability, %	Plasma protein binding, %	Elimination half-life, h	Elimination half-life, h (anuria)
Ciprofloxacin	75	30	3.5	9
Ofloxacin	98	30	5.0	30
Fleroxacin	95	23	10.0	21
Lomefloxacin	98	12	7.5	27
Enoxacin	90	40	5.0	9
Norfloxacin	40	15	3.5	9

kidneys in unchanged form. Other quinolones are eliminated through renal excretion and hepatic metabolism. Renal excretion of quinolones occurs by both glomerular filtration and tubular secretion, with glomerular filtration being the major component. Hepatic metabolism occurs via glucuronidation, hydroxylation, and oxidation, depending on the particular compound. Biliary excretion of quinolones is not significant.

The elimination half lives of quinolones in persons with normal renal function ranges from 3.5 h (ciprofloxacin and norfloxacin) to 10 h (fleroxacin). In the presence of renal failure, the half-lives are increased by about two- to three-fold for ciprofloxacin, fleroxacin, norfloxacin, enoxacin, and lomefloxacin and by six-fold for ofloxacin (Table 46-1).

Adverse Effects

The adverse effects of the quinolones are fairly similar among the various agents. Gastrointestinal symptoms are the most common and account for most of the reactions seen. These include nausea, abdominal discomfort, vomiting, and less frequently diarrhea. *Clostridium difficile* colitis has been rare with quinolone therapy. Central nervous system symptoms, including insomnia, dizziness, confusion, anxiety, tremors, restlessness, headache, and very rarely convulsions, have occurred with all quinolones.

Acute hypersensitivity (anaphylactic) reactions may occur in patients receiving quinolones, even following the first dose. Other allergic reactions including rashes, exfoliative dermatitis, and Stevens-Johnson Syndrome may occur. Photosensitivity reactions have been observed in patients exposed to sunlight or artificial ultraviolet light while receiving quinolones, particularly lomefloxacin and fleroxacin, although the overall number of patients with this reaction is extremely low.

In juvenile animals, quinolones produce cartilage erosion in weight bearing joints. There have been no reports of joint damage in adult patients taking these drugs for long periods of time. Nonetheless, the concern over arthropathy has led to the recommendation that quinolones should not be used in children whose skeletal growth is incomplete, nor should they be administered to pregnant women.

Crystalluria is infrequent with quinolones, although it has been reported with high doses of ciprofloxacin and norfloxacin. It is important to avoid alkalization of the urine because that will increase the crystalluria. Other adverse effects associated with the use of quinolones include transient elevations of serum transaminases, lactate dehydrogenase, and alkaline phosphatase, and hematologic abnormalities including thrombocytopenia and leukopenia.

Drug Interactions

A number of quinolones, including enoxacin, ciprofloxacin, and norfloxacin inhibit some isozymes of the cytochrome P-450 hepatic microsomal enzyme system responsible for the metabolism of methylxanthines (theophylline and caffeine). These agents interfere with the metabolism of theophylline, resulting in a dose-related decrease in theophylline clearance and a subsequent increase in serum theophylline levels. Enoxacin inhibits theophylline clearance by 60 percent, ciprofloxacin by 20 to 30 percent, and norfloxacin by 10 to 15 percent. In patients receiving these drugs, serum theophylline levels should be monitored and the dosage be adjusted. Ofloxacin, fleroxacin, and lomefloxacin have negligible effects on the elimination of theophylline. The effect of quinolones on the clearance of caffeine is similar to that of theophylline.

Administration of quinolones with cyclosporine may result in elevated serum levels of cyclosporine.

Therapeutic Uses

Although effective in a variety of infections caused by susceptible organisms, quinolones should be used only when a definite advantage exists over alternative antibiotics with respect to pharmacokinetics, toxicity, efficacy, or cost. Since quinolones are not nephrotoxic, they are suitable alternatives to aminoglycosides in patients with renal insufficiency and those in whom potential aminoglycoside toxicity is a major concern. Quinolones are used for: (1) complicated urinary tract infections, particularly those caused by *P. aeruginosa* and other multiply resistant gram-negative bacteria; (2) lower respiratory tract infections caused by gram-negative organisms; (3) bacterial prostatitis; (4) bone and joint infections caused by susceptible gram-negative bacilli; (5) uncomplicated urethral and cervical gonorrhea; (6) chlamydia infections (ofloxacin only); (7) enterocolitis due to bacterial pathogens, including travelers' diarrhea; (8) gram-negative bacteremia; (9) typhoid fever; and (10) multiple-drug resistant tuberculosis (ofloxacin and ciprofloxacin). Only a few of these indications are approved for some of the available quinolones. Quinolones are also effective in gonococcal infections, intraabdominal infections (used in combination with a drug active against anaerobes), and soft tissue infections caused by susceptible organisms.

Ciprofloxacin and ofloxacin, the most commonly used quinolones, are considered alternatives to each other. Ciprofloxacin is more active against *P. aeruginosa* whereas ofloxacin is more effective against *Chlamydia trachomatis*. Ofloxacin is more completely absorbed and has a longer elimination half-life than ciprofloxacin, resulting in higher serum concentrations. However, this difference is offset by the greater potency of ciprofloxacin against most gram-negative bacteria.

BIBLIOGRAPHY

Appel, G.B.: "Aminoglycoside Nephrotoxicity," *Am. J. Med.* **88 (Suppl. 3C)**: 16S-20S (1990).

Brummett, R.E., and K.E. Fox: "Aminoglycoside-Induced Hearing Loss in Humans," *Antimicrob. Agents Chemother.* **33**: 797-800 (1989).

Cunha, B.A.: "Aminoglycosides: Current Role in Antimicrobial Therapy," *Pharmacotherapy* **8**: 334-350 (1988).

Davis, B.D.: "The Lethal Action of Aminoglycosides," *J. Antimicrob. Chemother.* **22**: 1-3 (1988).

Davis, B.D.: "Mechanism of Bactericidal Action of Aminoglycosides," *Microbiol. Rev.* **51**: 341-350 (1987).

Dudley, M.N.: "Pharmacodynamics and Pharmacokinetics of Antibiotics with Special Reference to the Fluoroquinolones," *Am. J. Med.* **91 (Suppl. A)**: 45S-50S (1991).

Edson, R.S., and C.L. Terrell: "The Aminoglycosides," *Mayo Clin. Proc.* **66**: 1158-1164 (1991).

Gadebusch, H.H., and D.L. Shungu: "Norfloxacin, the First of a New Class of Fluoroquinolone Antimicrobials, Revisited," *Intern. J. Antimicrob. Agents* **1**: 3-28 (1991).

Guay, D.R.: "The Role of the Fluoroquinolones," *Pharmacotherapy* **12**: 71S-85S (1992).

Hooper, D.C., and J.S. Wolfson: "Fluoroquinolone Antimicrobial Agents," *N. Engl. J. Med.* **324**: 384-394 (1991).

John, J.F.: "What Price Success? The Continuing Saga of the Toxic: Therapeutic Ratio in the Use of Aminoglycoside Antibiotics," *J. Infect. Dis.* **158**: 1-6 (1988).

Just, P.M.: "Overview of the Fluoroquinolone Antibiotics," *Pharmacotherapy* **13**: 4S-17S (1993).

Lamp, K.C., E.M. Bailey, and M.J. Rybak: "Ofloxacin Clinical Pharmacokinetics," *Clin. Pharmacokinet.* **22**: 32-46 (1992).

Marchbanks, C.R.: "Drug-Drug Interactions with Fluoroquinolones," *Pharmacotherapy* **13**: 23S-28S (1993).

Neu, H.C.: "Quinolone Antimicrobial Agents," *Ann. Rev. Med.* **43**: 465-486 (1992).

Neu, H.C.: "Use of Fluoroquinolones," *Infect. Dis. Clin. Pract.* **1**: 1-10 (1992).

Nightingale, C.H.: "Pharmacokinetic Considerations in Quinolone Therapy," *Pharmacotherapy* **13**: 34S-38S (1993).

Nightingale, C.H.: "Overview of the Pharmacokinetics of Fleroxacin," *Am. J. Med.* **94 (Suppl. 3A)**: 38S-43S (1993).

Sanders, C.C.: "Ciprofloxacin: In Vitro Activity, Mechanism of Action, and Resistance," *Rev. Infect. Dis.* **10**: 516-525 (1988).

Sorgel, F., and M. Kinzig: "Pharmacokinetics of Gyrase Inhibitors, Part 2: Renal and Hepatic Elimin. Pathways and Drug Interactions," *Am. J. Med.* **94 (Suppl. 3A)**: 56S-69S (1993).

Stein, G.E.: "Drug Interactions with Fluoroquinolones," *Am. J. Med.* **91 (Suppl. A)**: 81S-86S (1991).

Stuck, A.E., D.S. Kim, and F.J. Frey: "Fleroxacin Clinical Pharmacokinetics," *Clin. Pharmacokinet.* **22**: 116-131 (1992).

Taber, H.W., J.P. Mueller, P.F. Miller, and A.S. Arrow: "Bacterial Uptake of Aminoglycoside Antibiotics," *Microbiol. Rev.* **51**: 439-456 (1987).

Trucksis, M., D.C. Hooper, and J.S. Wolfson: "Emerging Resistance to Fluoroquinolones in Staphylococci: An Alert," *Ann. Intern. Med.* **114**: 424-426 (1991).

Walker, R.C., and A.J. Wright: "The Fluoroquinolones," *Mayo Clin. Proc.* **66**: 1249-1259 (1991).

Wolfson, J.S., and D.C. Hooper: "Norfloxacin: A New Targeted Fluoroquinolone Antimicrobial Agent," *Ann. Intern. Med.* **108**: 238-251 (1988).

Wolfson, J.S., and D.C. Hooper: "Comparative Pharmacokinetics of Ofloxacin and Ciprofloxacin," *Am. J. Med.* **87 (Suppl. 6C)**: 31S-36S (1989).

CHAPTER 47

Antimicrobials III: Macrolides, Clindamycin, Metronidazole, Sulfonamides, Trimethoprim, Chloramphenicol, and Tetracyclines

Abdolghader Molavi

MACROLIDES

Macrolides are a group of antibiotics that contain a 14- to 16-membered lactone ring attached to one or two sugar moieties. The currently available macrolides include erythromycin, clarithromycin, and azithromycin. All are available for oral administration but only erythromycin is available for parenteral use. The chemical structures of macrolides are shown in figure 47-1.

Erythromycin is a 14-membered macrolide which was isolated in 1952 from *Streptomyces erythreus*. Clarithromycin and azithromycin, both semisynthetic derivatives of erythromycin, were introduced in 1992. Clarithromycin is 6-O-methylerythromycin; it differs from erythromycin only by methylation of the hydroxyl group at position 6 of the lactone ring. Azithromycin differs from erythromycin in that a methyl-substituted nitrogen atom is incorporated into the lactone ring, resulting in a 15-membered ring; it is also referred to as an azalide antibiotic.

Mechanism of Action

The macrolides inhibit bacterial protein synthesis by binding to the 50S ribosomal subunit at a site located in the peptidyl-tRNA binding region (P site). This attachment blocks translocation by interfering with the association of peptidyl-tRNA with its binding site after peptide bond formation. Macrolides do not bind to mammalian 80S ribosomes; this accounts for their relative lack of toxicity in humans.

Macrolides have a bacteriostatic action against susceptible organisms. They may, however, have a bactericidal action against some microbial species at achievable serum concentrations.

Antimicrobial Spectrum

The antimicrobial spectra of erythromycin, clarithromycin, and azithromycin are similar. There are, however, significant differences in their activities against some organisms.

Gram-Positive Bacteria Macrolides are highly active against *Streptococcus* species, including groups A, B, C, D, and G streptococci, *Streptococcus pneumoniae*, and viridans streptococci; occasionally, resistant strains are encountered. Methicillin-susceptible *Staphylococcus aureus* is frequently sensitive to macrolides; resistant strains are more common among hospital isolates. Methicillin-resistant strains of *S. aureus* and coagulase-negative staphylococci are usually resistant to macrolides. Clarithromycin is slightly more active than erythromycin against susceptible *Streptococcus* and *Staphylococcus* species; by contrast azithromycin is two- to four-fold less active than erythromycin. However, erythromycin-resistant strains of any of these organisms are resistant to the other macrolides.

Most strains of *Listeria monocytogenes* and *Corynebacterium diphtheriae* are sensitive to macrolides. Approximately 50 percent of strains of enterococci are sensitive to erythromycin and clarithromycin.

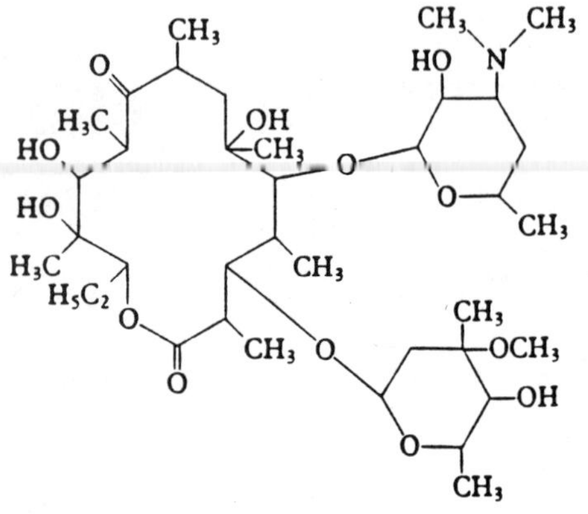

Erythromycin

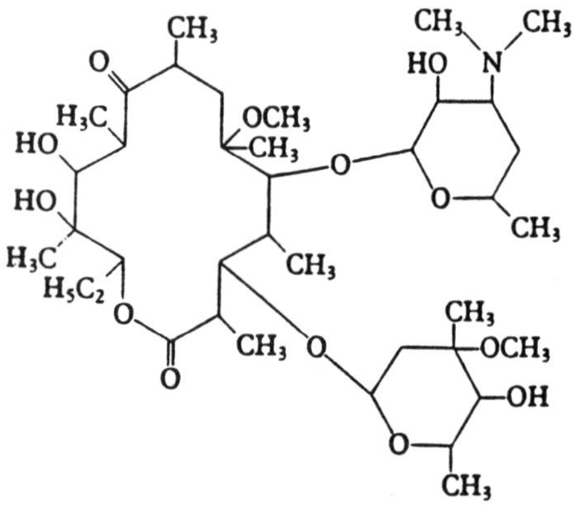

Clarithromycin

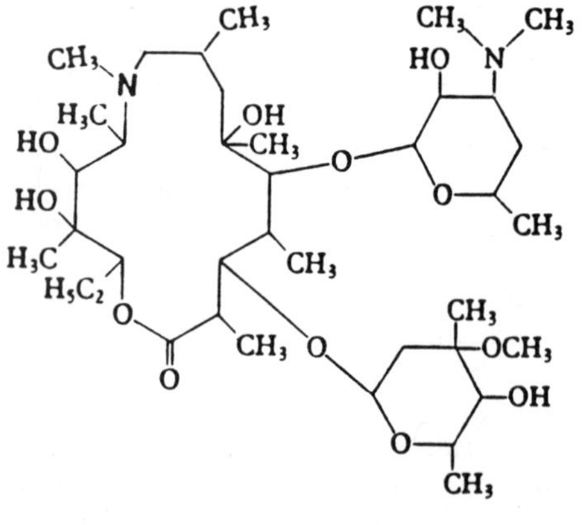

Azithromycin

FIGURE 47-1 *Chemical structures of macrolides.*

Gram-Negative Bacteria Macrolides are active against *Neisseria* species, *Moraxella catarrhalis*, *Legionella* species, *Campylobacter jejuni*, *Helicobacter pylori*, *Bordetella pertussis*, *Haemophilus ducreyi*, and *Haemophilus influenzae*. Azithromycin is four- to eight-fold more active than erythromycin and clarithromycin against *Haemophilus influenzae*, *M. catarrhalis*, and *Neisseria gonorrhoeae*. Clarithromycin is two- to four-fold more active than erythromycin against *Legionella*. *Enterobacteriaceae* and other gram-negative bacilli are resistant to all macrolides.

Anaerobic Bacteria Gram-positive anaerobic bacteria, including *Peptococcus*, *Peptostreptococcus*, *Clostridium*, *Propionibacterium acne*, and *Actinomyces* are sensitive to macrolides. *Bacteroides fragilis* group and *Fusobacterium* species are usually resistant, but other *Bacteroides* species are susceptible.

Mycobacteria Clarithromycin and azithromycin are active against *Mycobacterium avium* complex, *Mycobacterium chelonei*, and *Mycobacterium fortuitum*. Clarithromycin is approximately four-fold more potent than azithromycin against these organisms. Erythromycin does not have clinically useful activity against mycobacteria.

Other Organisms Macrolides are active against *Mycoplasma pneumoniae*, *Chlamydia pneumoniae*, *Chlamydia trachomatis*, *Ureaplasma urealyticum*, *Mycoplasma hominis*, *Rickettsia*, *Treponema pallidum*, and *Borrelia burgdorferi* (the agent of Lyme diseases). Clarithromycin and azithromycin are four- to eight-fold more active than erythromycin against *C. trachomatis* and *U. urealyticum*. Similarly, they are more active than erythromycin against *M. pneumoniae* and *Mycoplasma hominis*. Azithromycin and clarithromycin have excellent activity against *Toxoplasma gondii*.

Mechanisms of Resistance

Bacterial resistance to macrolides is due to either inability of the drug to penetrate the cell envelope or altered ribosomal binding site. Enzymatic inactivation of these agents is rare and clinically insignificant.

The outer membrane of enteric gram-negative bacilli is relatively impermeable to macrolides; this accounts for the resistance of these organisms. Macrolide resistance in gram-positive organisms, such as *S. aureus*, is due to altered ribosomal binding site, which is usually plasmid mediated. Plasmids from resistant strains contain the gene for RNA methylase. This enzyme methylates adenine groups in 23S ribosomal subunits, resulting in decreased binding of macrolides to the 50S ribosomal subunit. The methylating enzyme may be constitutive (i.e., produced continuously) or inducible (i.e., produced only when exposed to erythromycin).

Pharmacokinetics

Erythromycin Erythromycin base is poorly soluble in water, has a very bitter taste, and is rapidly inactivated by gastric acid. In order to prevent degradation by gastric acid and improve absorption, the preparations of erythromycin base are made with an acid-resistant coating, which delays drug dissolution until the drug reaches the small bowel (enteric-coated tablets, enteric-coated pellets in capsules, and "film"-coated tablets). Several salts and esters of erythromycin have also been prepared with the aims of eliminating the bitterness (important in pediatric preparations) and improving the absorption. These include erythromycin stearate (a salt), erythromycin ethylsuccinate (an ester), and erythromycin estolate (lauryl sulfate salt of the propionyl ester of erythromycin). The stearate salt dissociates in the duodenum, releasing the base, which is subsequently absorbed in the upper small intestine. The two ester derivatives are absorbed intact and partially hydrolyzed to the free base in the blood; the esters do not have significant antibacterial activity. With erythromycin ethylsuccinate, 45 percent of the drug in the serum is in ester form and 55 percent in the bioactive base form. With erythromycin estolate, 70 to 80 percent of the drug in the serum is in propionate ester form and 20 to 30 percent in the bioactive base form. The serum concentrations of erythromycin base after oral administration of various enteric-coated preparations, salts or esters of the drugs are approximately the same.

Erythromycin gluceptate and erythromycin lactobionate are soluble salts of erythromycin that can be administered intravenously. The serum concentrations of erythromycin after intravenous administration of these compounds are substantially higher than those achieved with the oral preparations.

Erythromycin is 65 percent bound to plasma proteins. It is widely distributed in the tissues (including prostate) and body fluids. It does not penetrate the normal meninges, but low levels are detectable in the cerebrospinal fluid (CSF) when the meninges are inflamed. Erythromycin is actively concentrated intracellularly in both macrophages and polymorphonuclear leukocytes.

Approximately 2.5 percent of an orally administered dose and 15 percent of a parenteral dose of erythromycin are excreted unchanged in the urine. A considerable proportion is excreted unchanged into the bile, and a large proportion is inactivated in the body, mostly in the liver.

The elimination half-life of erythromycin in persons with normal renal function is 1.4 h, it increases to 5.0 to 6.0 h in anuric patients. Only minor, if any, dosage reduction is necessary in patients with end stage renal disease. However, in patients with severe hepatic disease the drug may accumulate and dosage reduction may be necessary.

Clarithromycin Approximately 55 percent of orally administered clarithromycin is absorbed from the gastrointestinal tract. Food delays the absorption but does not affect the bioavailability.

The serum protein binding of clarithromycin ranges from 65 to 75 percent. Clarithromycin penetrates well into tissues and body fluids; the tissue concentrations are usually higher than the simultaneous serum levels. Clarithromycin readily enters into macrophages and leukocytes and attains high intracellular concentrations.

Clarithromycin is eliminated by hepatic metabolism and renal excretion. Approximately 20 to 30 percent of an orally administered dose is excreted unchanged in the urine. The remainder of the drug undergoes metabolism. The major metabolite, 14-hydroxyclarithromycin, is excreted in the urine and accounts for an additional 10 to 15 percent of the dose. Because of hepatic metabolism, dosage adjustment is necessary only in patients with severe renal impairment.

Clarithromycin has a nonlinear pharmacokinetics which results in elimination half-lives ranging from 3 to 6 h, depending upon the dosage. The elimination half-life increases with higher doses, which result in saturation of its metabolic pathways.

Azithromycin Approximately 37 percent of orally administered azithromycin is absorbed from the gastrointestinal tract. Food decreases the absorption by 50 percent.

Azithromycin is widely distributed in the body. It has a unique pharmacokinetic profile characterized by low serum levels and high tissue concentrations. The intracellular/extracellular concentration ratio in macrophages and polymorphonuclear leukocytes exceeds 100. The serum protein binding of azithromycin varies with the concentration of the drug and is less than 50 percent in achievable concentrations.

Azithromycin is eliminated by hepatic metabolism and biliary and renal excretion. Biliary excretion, predominantly as unchanged drug, is the major route of elimination. Approximately 12 percent of the administered dose is excreted unchanged in the urine. Azithromycin is released slowly from tissues, maintaining a tissue half-life of approximately 70 h. The serum half-life is 11 to 14 h, allowing for once daily administration.

Adverse Effects

Allergic reactions (skin rash, fever, and eosinophilia) may occur with any of the macrolides but they are uncommon. The most frequent adverse effect of macrolides is gastrointestinal upset. Epigastric pain, nausea, and vomiting are common after oral administration of erythromycin. The incidence varies with the dose, formulation, patient's age, and time of administration in relation to meals. Gastrointestinal disturbances may also occur, though less frequently, with intravenous administration of the drug. Degradation of erythromycin in the stomach, under acidic conditions, produces products which may be responsible for the gastrointestinal symptoms. Clarithromycin and azithromycin are not degraded in the stomach. As a consequence, the frequency of gastrointestinal adverse effects with these agents is significantly less than that of erythromycin. Diarrhea may occur with any of the macrolides; however, it is uncommon and *Clostridium difficile* colitis is rare.

The most serious adverse effect of erythromycin is cholestatic hepatitis, manifested by fever, abdominal pain, elevated serum transaminases, and hyperbilirubinemia. This complication occurs chiefly in adults and almost always with the estolate preparation. It appears to be a hypersensitivity reaction to the specific structure of the estolate compound. Since erythromycin estolate does not provide higher serum levels of the bioactive erythromycin and it is uniquely associated with cholestatic hepatitis, its use is not recommended.

Bilateral neurosensory hearing loss may occur in patients receiving high doses of intravenous erythromycin and is associated with high serum concentrations of the compound. The hearing loss usually disappears 1 to 2 weeks after therapy is discontinued.

Therapeutic Uses

Erythromycin is an alternative to penicillin for the treatment of infections caused by group A streptococci and *S. pneumoniae*. It is the drug of choice for pneumonia caused by *Mycoplasma pneumoniae*, *Legionella pneumophila* and other *Legionella* species, *Chlamydia pneumoniae*, and *Chlamydia psittaci*. It is also the drug of choice for empiric therapy of atypical pneumonia. Erythromycin is the drug of choice for *Campylobacter enterocolitis*, pertussis, diphtheria, prostatitis caused by *Chlamydia trachomatis* or *Ureaplasma urealyticum*, and *Chlamydia trachomatis* infections during pregnancy and childhood. It is also an effective drug for the treatment of chancroid. In patients allergic to penicillin, erythromycin is the drug of choice for endocarditis prophylaxis after oropharyngeal procedures.

Clarithromycin and azithromycin may be used for the treatment of pharyngitis and tonsillitis due to *Streptococcus pyogenes* and of community acquired pneumonia of mild severity due to *S. pneumoniae* in patients appropriate for outpatient oral therapy. Azithromycin is a drug of choice for the treatment of chlamydial genital infections. A single 1 g dose of azithromycin is as effective for the treatment of chlamydial urethritis and cervicitis as a standard seven day course of tetracycline.

Clarithromycin and azithromycin are the drugs of choice for the treatment of *Mycobacterium avium* complex infections in patients with acquired immunodeficiency syndrome (AIDS). Either may be included in the two-drug or three-drug regimens which are used for this infection. Toxoplasma encephalitis in AIDS patients who are intolerant of both sulfadiazine and clindamycin is treated with azithromycin combined with pyrimethamine.

CLINDAMYCIN

Lincosamides are a group of antibiotics which consist of an amino acid attached to a sugar moiety. Lincomycin, the first lincosamide available for clinical use, was isolated in 1962 from *Streptomyces linconensis*, an organism derived from soil collected near Lincoln, Nebraska. Clindamycin is the 7-chloro-7-deoxy derivative of lincomycin. It is superior to the parent compound in both antimicrobial activity and antimicrobial potency as well as gastrointestinal absorption. Lincomycin has no therapeutic advantage; it has virtually been replaced by clindamycin and will not be discussed.

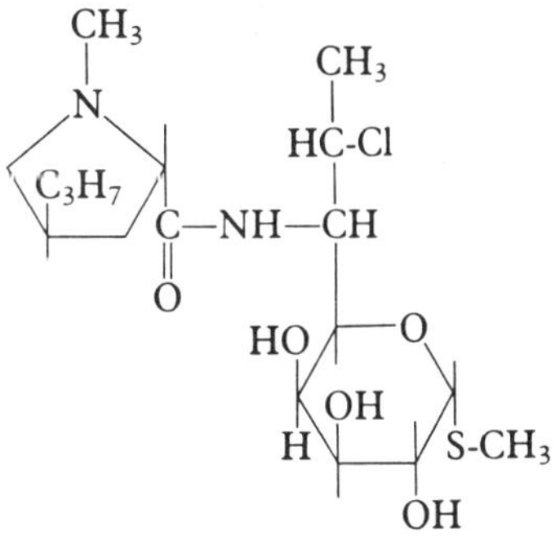

CH_3 CH_3
N HC-Cl
C_3H_7 C—NH—CH
O
HO O
OH
H S-CH_3
OH

Mechanism of Action

Clindamycin inhibits protein synthesis by binding to the 50S ribosomal subunit in susceptible organisms. It interacts with ribosomes that are free of nascent peptides and interferes with the binding of the aminoacyl-tRNA to its ribosomal attachment site. In contrast to macrolides which prevent extension of the growing peptide chain on the ribosome, clindamycin inhibits initiation of peptide chain formation.

Clindamycin is a bacteriostatic antibiotic. It may, however, have a bactericidal action against some bacteria at achievable serum concentrations.

Antimicrobial Spectrum

Aerobic Bacteria Clindamycin is active against *Streptococcus* species, including groups A, B, C, D, and G streptococci, *S. pneumoniae*, and viridans streptococci; however, *Enterococcus* species are invariably resistant. Most strains of *S. aureus* are sensitive to clindamycin; methicillin-resistant isolates and coagulase-negative staphylococci are frequently resistant. The *in vitro* potency of clindamycin against *S. aureus* is comparable to that of erythromycin.

All aerobic gram-negative bacteria are resistant to clindamycin. Unlike erythromycin, clindamycin is not active against *Mycoplasma* pneumonia and *Treponema pallidum*, and has only moderate activity against *Chlamydia trachomatis*.

Anaerobic Bacteria Clindamycin has excellent activity against anaerobic bacteria. *Peptococcus*, *Peptostreptococcus*, *Actinomyces*, *Propionibacterium*, *Clostridium perfringens*, *Bacteroides* species, including *B. fragilis*, and *Fusobacterium* are sensitive. Approximately 10 percent of *Peptococcus* strains, 10 to 20 percent of clostridial strains other than *C. perfringens*, and 4 to 10 percent of *B. fragilis* strains are resistant to clindamycin.

Other Organisms Clindamycin is active against *Toxoplasma gondii*, *Babesia microti*, and *Plasmodium* species.

Mechanisms of Resistance

Resistance to clindamycin is due to either inability of the drug to penetrate the cell envelope or altered ribosomal binding site. Enzymatic inactivation of clindamycin is rare and clinically insignificant.

Inability of clindamycin to penetrate the cell envelope of aerobic gram-negative bacilli accounts for the resistance of these organisms. Resistance in gram-positive species is due to an altered ribosomal binding site, accomplished by methylation of adenine groups in the 23S ribosomal RNA. It is mediated by plasmids that contain genes for the methylating enzymes and confer resistance to both clindamycin and macrolides.

Pharmacokinetics

Clindamycin is available in two formulations for oral administration. Clindamycin hydrochloride is bitter tasting and poorly soluble in water. Available as capsule, it is rapidly and virtually completely (90 percent) absorbed from the gastrointestinal tract. Food does not significantly affect the rate or the amount of the drug absorbed. For children and elderly patients unable to swallow capsules, clindamycin palmitate (a water-soluble ester) is available as an oral solution. This ester has no antibacterial activity but is rapidly hydrolyzed in the blood to the active drug. Clindamycin phosphate, another water-soluble ester of clindamycin, is available for parenteral administration. Clindamycin phosphate has no antimicrobial activity but is hydrolyzed rapidly in the blood to the active parent compound.

Clindamycin is 60 percent bound to plasma proteins. It is widely distributed in the tissues and body fluids. High levels are achieved in bone and synovial fluid, but passage into the CSF is very poor even when the meninges are inflamed. Like erythromycin, clindamycin is actively transported into polymorphonuclear leukocytes and macrophages.

About 10 percent of administered clindamycin is excreted unchanged in the urine, and a fraction is eliminated unchanged in the bile. Most of the drug is metabolized, mainly in the liver, to products which are excreted into the urine and bile.

The elimination half-life of clindamycin is 2.4 h in persons with normal renal function and increases to 6.0 h in functionally anephric patients. Dosage adjustment is usually not necessary in functionally anephric patients if hepatic function is normal. In patients with severe hepatic disease, the elimination half-life of clindamycin is prolonged significantly and dosage adjustment is necessary.

Adverse Effects

The most frequent adverse effects of clindamycin are gastrointestinal reactions. Nausea, vomiting, and epigastric pain may occur with either oral or parenteral administration. Diarrhea occurs in 5 to 15 percent of patients; it is more common with oral administration. The diarrhea is occasionally due to *Clostridium difficile*, which is resistant to clindamycin and produces toxins that cause colitis. *C. difficile* colitis may present clinically as pseudomembranous colitis, manifested by fever, abdominal cramps, and diarrhea, which may be bloody.

Hypersensitivity reactions, including skin rashes and drug fever, are infrequent with clindamycin. Reversible elevations of transaminases (aspartate aminotransferase and alanine aminotransferase) may occur and are usually due to interference by clindamycin with the colorimetric measurements of these enzymes. However, rare cases of hepatotoxicity have been reported. Clindamycin may potentiate the action of neuromuscular blocking agents.

Therapeutic Uses

Clindamycin is used most commonly for the treatment of anaerobic infections, particularly those below the diaphragm, such as intra-abdominal sepsis and female pelvic infections, that commonly involve *B. fragilis*. Most of these infections are polymicrobial, involving gram-negative aerobes as well as anaerobes. Therefore clindamycin is frequently administered in combination with an another agent, such as an aminoglycoside or aztreonam. Clindamycin is also an alternative to penicillin G for the treatment of anaerobic infections above the diaphragm, such as aspiration pneumonia, lung abscess, and empyema in patients allergic to penicillin. Because of increasing prevalence of beta-lactamase-producing strains of *Bacteroides* species, clindamycin may be superior to penicillin G in some of these infections.

Clindamycin is a therapeutic alternative to beta-lactam antibiotics for the treatment of infections due to *S. aureus* or streptococci. It is particularly useful for osteomyelitis and septic arthritis because of the high concentrations which are achieved in the bone.

Clindamycin combined with pyrimethamine is an alternative to the pyrimethamine-sulfadiazine combination for the treatment of *Toxoplasma* encephalitis in patients with AIDS. Clindamycin combined with quinine is used for the treatment of babesiosis. Clindamycin combined with primaquine is an alternative to trimethoprim-sulfamethoxazole for the treatment of *Pneumocystis carinii* pneumonia.

Lastly, topical application of clindamycin is useful in reducing the inflammatory lesions of acne vulgaris caused by *Propionibacterium acne*.

METRONIDAZOLE

Metronidazole is a synthetic antimicrobial agent that was initially introduced into clinical medicine in 1960 for the treatment of vaginal trichomoniasis. It is a nitroimidazole compound and has a low molecular weight (170). Metronidazole is available for both oral and parenteral administration.

N
CH_3
O_2N N
CH_2CH_2OH

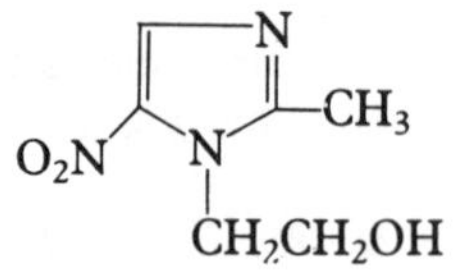

Mechanism of Action

Metronidazole has a potent bactericidal action that is specific for obligate anaerobes. The bactericidal action of metronidazole occurs in the following sequence: (1) entry of the drug into the bacterial cell, (2) reductive activation, and (3) toxic effect of the reduced intermediate products resulting in cell death.

Metronidazole diffuses readily into both aerobic and anaerobic bacteria. Activation of the drug requires a reduction process that occurs only in anaerobic organisms and in facultative bacteria under anaerobic conditions. Reduction occurs at the nitro group of the drug by the low-redox-potential electron-transport proteins. This decreases the intracellular concentration of unchanged metronidazole and produces a gradient that promotes further entry of the drug into the cell. Short-lived intermediate products of metronidazole reduction or free radicals interact with bacterial DNA, resulting in cell death.

Antimicrobial Activity

Metronidazole has excellent activity against strict anaerobes but is inactive against aerobic organisms.

Anaerobic Bacteria Metronidazole is highly active against *Peptococcus, Peptostreptococcus, Clostridium, Bacteroides* (including *B. fragilis*), and *Fusobacterium*; resistant strains are extremely rare. The drug is much less active against anaerobic, non-spore-forming, gram-positive bacilli (*Actinomyces, Eubacterium,* and *Propionibacterium*); 40 to 60 percent of strains are resistant.

Anaerobic Protozoa Metronidazole is highly active against anaerobic protozoa, including *Trichomonas vaginalis, Entamoeba histolytica, Giardia lamblia,* and *Balantidium coli.* Occasional strains of *T. vaginalis* may be resistant (see Chapter 50).

Mechanisms of Resistance

The precise mechanisms of resistance to metronidazole are unknown. Resistance may be due to decreased intracellular reduction of the drug to active intermediate compounds, resulting in slow cellular uptake.

Pharmacokinetics

Metronidazole is well absorbed (85 percent) after oral administration. The presence of food in the stomach delays absorption, but the bioavailability remains unchanged.

Metronidazole is 10 percent bound to plasma proteins. The small size of the molecule, lipid solubility, and the low plasma protein binding account for its wide distribution in tissues and body fluids. Metronidazole penetrates well into the brain and the CSF even when the meninges are normal. In patients with meningitis, the concentrations in the CSF are equal to those in the serum.

Approximately 10 to 15 percent of administered metronidazole is excreted unchanged in the urine. Most of the drug is metabolized in the liver, and the metabolites are excreted in the urine. The elimination half-life of metronidazole, which is 7.0 h in persons with normal renal function, increases only to 10.0 h in anuric patients. In the presence of impaired renal function, dosage reduction is not required and although some metabolites may accumulate, they have not been associated with adverse effects. In patients with severe liver disease, the plasma clearance of metronidazole is decreased, and the dose should be adjusted to avoid toxicity.

Adverse Effects

The incidence of untoward effects associated with the use of metronidazole is low. An unpleasant metallic taste, anorexia, nausea, and vomiting are occasionally experienced. Neurotoxicity manifested by sensory neuropathy, ataxia, and rarely encephalopathy and seizures are rare complications which may occur after prolonged treatment with high doses of the drug.

In persons ingesting alcohol, metronidazole may produce a reaction similar to that produced by disulfiram. Patients should be advised not to drink alcohol when taking the drug. Metronidazole inhibits the metabolism of warfarin by the liver. In patients taking both agents, the dose of the anticoagulant should be decreased.

Therapeutic Uses

Metronidazole is effective in the therapy of a wide variety of anaerobic infections, including those involving *B. fragilis*, such as intra-abdominal and female pelvic infections. Since most of these infections are mixed, involving both aerobes and anaerobes, the drug is usually combined with another agent active against aerobic bacteria.

Because of its excellent penetration into the central nervous system, metronidazole is usually included in regimens used to treat brain abscess. Metronidazole is the drug of choice for bacterial vaginosis. It is an alternative to oral vancomycin for the therapy of *C. difficile* colitis in patients who are not severely ill.

Metronidazole is the drug of choice for amebiasis (intestinal and extra-intestinal), giardiasis, and vaginal trichomoniasis (see Chapter 50). In addition, metronidazole has been used in the Mexican cutaneous form of leishmaniasis; however, it is considered investigational in the U.S. for this purpose.

SULFONAMIDES

Sulfonamides are synthetic antimicrobial agents derived from sulfanilamide (para-aminobenzenesulfonamide). They are structural analogs of para-aminobenzoic acid (PABA), an essential precursor for folic acid synthesis in bacteria (Table 47-1). The nature of substitutions at the sulfonyl group (SO_2) determines the antimicrobial potency and the pharmacokinetic properties of the individual compound.

The sulfonamides currently available include sulfisoxazole, sulfamethoxazole, sulfadiazine, sulfacetamide, sulfamethizole, and trisulfapyrimidines (a mixture of sulfamerazine, sulfamethazine, and sulfadiazine); the first two are most commonly used. A long-lasting sulfonamide, sulfadoxine, is available only in fixed combination with pyrimethamine (as Fansidar) for prophylaxis and treatment of *Plasmodium falciparum* malaria. Sulfacetamide is only used topically in the eye.

Mechanism of Action

The sulfonamides are bacteriostatic compounds that inhibit bacterial growth by interfering with folic acid synthesis. They competitively inhibit dihydropteroate synthetase, an enzyme that catalyzes the conversion of PABA to folic acid (Fig. 47-2).

Folic acid is essential for purine and ultimately DNA synthesis in both bacterial and mammalian cells. Bacteria are unable to use folic acid from external sources, due to impermeability of the cell envelope, and must synthesize it. On the other hand, mammalian cells are unable to synthesize folic acid and require preformed folic acid. Folic acid, obtained largely through dietary sources, enters mammalian cells by an active transport mechanism. This difference between the bacterial and mammalian cells is the basis for the selective toxicity of sulfonamides.

Antimicrobial Spectrum

Sulfonamides have a wide range of antimicrobial activity that includes *S. aureus*, *Streptococcus* species, *Nocardia*, *Listeria monocytogenes*, *Neisseria*, *Haemophilus influenzae*, enteric gram-negative species (especially *E. coli* and *Proteus mirabilis*), and some anaerobic bacteria. Resistance, however, is widespread and may be found in 10 to 50 percent of strains of various species. Sulfonamides are active against *Chlamydia trachomatis*.

Sulfonamides, particularly when combined with pyrimethamine or trimethoprim, are active against some protozoa, including *Toxoplasma*, *P. falciparum*, and *Pneumocystis carinii*.

Mechanisms of Resistance

Bacterial resistance to sulfonamides may develop by mutation, resulting in either microbial overproduction of PABA or an altered dihydropteroate synthetase that is less readily inhibited by the drug. Resistance also may be mediated by plasmids that may code for the production of drug-resistant dihydropteroate synthetase or may result in decreased permeability of the cell envelope to sulfonamides.

Pharmacokinetics

Sulfonamides are generally well absorbed from the gastrointestinal tract (70 to 100 percent). Administration with food delays, but does not affect, the total amount absorbed. Sulfonamides are bound to plasma proteins to varying degrees, depending on the agent, and readily penetrate into various tissues and body fluids including the eye and the CSF. The CSF concentrations vary depending on the individual drug, and may be as high as 60 percent of the concurrent serum levels when the meninges are inflamed. High levels are also attained in saliva and breast milk. Sulfonamides readily cross the placenta and enter the fetal circulation.

Sulfonamides are metabolized to varying degrees, primarily in the liver, by acetylation on the para-amino moiety or by conjugation. The acetylated metabolites have no antibacterial activity and yet retain the toxic potentialities of the parent compound.

Sulfonamides are excreted into the urine as unchanged drug and the acetylated and conjugated metabolites. Biliary excretion is not significant. The elimination half-lives of sulfonamides vary widely, ranging from 6 h (sulfisoxazole) to 6 to 8 days (sulfadoxine).

TABLE 47-1 Chemical structures and pharmacokinetic properties of selected sulfonamides

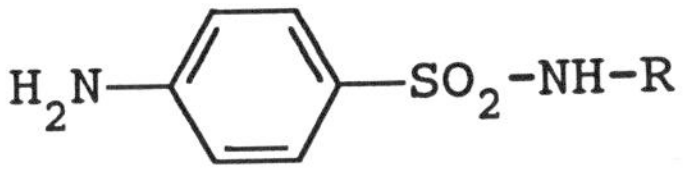

H_2N— —SO_2-NH-R

Drug	Chemical structure at R	Plasma protein binding, %	Elimination half-life, h	Percent excreted unchanged
Sulfisoxazole	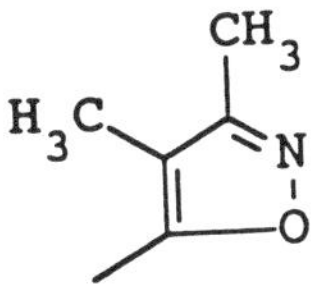 CH_3, H_3C, N, O	85	6	40 to 70
Sulfamethoxazole	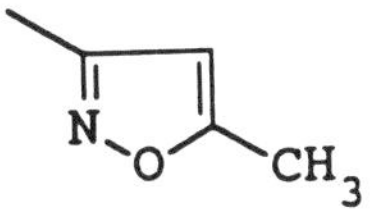 N, O, CH_3	65	10	30
Sulfadiazine	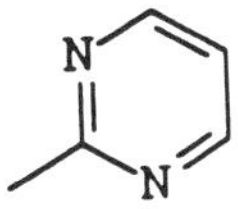 N, N	40	10	65
Sulfamethizole	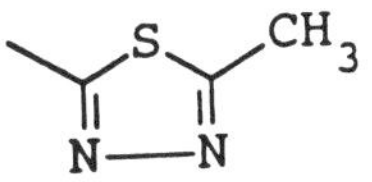 S, CH_3, N, N	90	1 to 2	95
Sulfamerazine	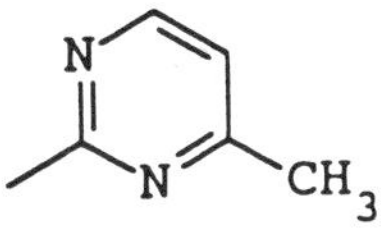 N, N, CH_3	75	10	
Sulfamethazine	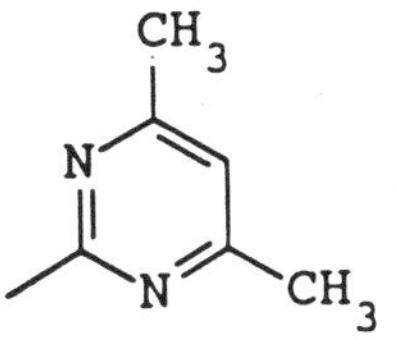 CH_3, N, N, CH_3	80	10	20 to 40
Sulfadoxine	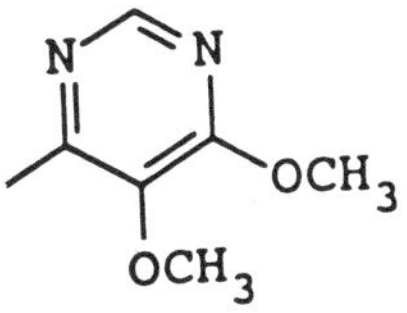 N, N, OCH_3, OCH_3	80	170	80

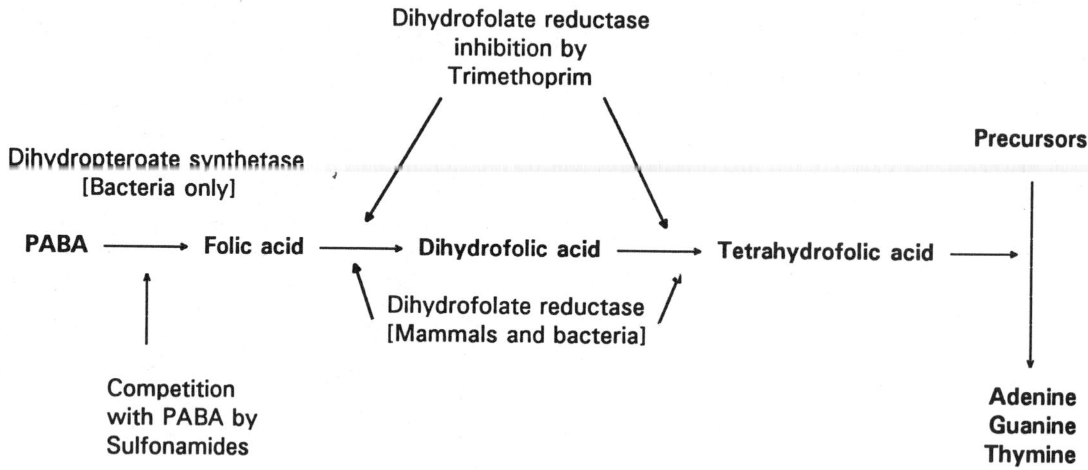

FIGURE 47-2 *The diagram shows the site of action of competitors of para-aminobenzoic acid (PABA) and inhibitors of dihydrofolate reductase in the synthesis and utilization of folic acid by bacteria and mammals.*

Adverse Effects

Nausea, vomiting, and diarrhea may occur but are uncommon. Hypersensitivity reactions are the most common adverse effects. These include a variety of rashes, erythema multiforme (including Stevens-Johnson syndrome), erythema nodosum, vasculitis resembling periarteritis nodosa, drug fever, and a serum sickness-like syndrome. Rashes seem to occur more frequently in patients with AIDS who are given sulfonamides than among the population at large.

Adverse hematologic effects including leukopenia, agranulocytosis (reversible), acute hemolytic anemia (sometimes related to a glucose-6-phosphate dehydrogenase deficiency), and thrombocytopenia are among the serious complications of sulfonamide therapy.

Renal damage, manifested by hematuria, proteinuria, and elevated creatinine, may occur as a result of crystalluria caused by precipitation of sulfonamides and/or their metabolites in the renal tubules. This complication occurs rarely, if at all, with sulfisoxazole, which is highly soluble in urine, and sulfamethoxazole, which is slightly less soluble. Sulfadiazine has a lower solubility and therefore it is important to maintain a high fluid intake when the drug is used. Alkalization of the urine may also be desirable, since the solubility of sulfonamides increases greatly with slight elevations of pH. Since the solubility of one agent is independent of another, trisulfapyrimidines (a mixture of sulfadiazine, sulfamerazine, and sulfamethazine) is associated with a lower incidence of crystalluria than are the individual components.

Sulfonamides should not be administered during the last month of pregnancy because they compete for bilirubin binding sites on plasma albumin and increase fetal levels of unconjugated bilirubin, increasing the risk of kernicterus.

Sulfonamides inhibit the metabolism of warfarin, phenytoin, tolbutamide, and chlorpropamide. Dosage adjustment may be necessary when a sulfonamide is given concurrently.

Sulfacetamide, the topical ophthalmic agent, may cause local adverse effects including blurred vision, local irritation, and transient stinging. As with all sulfonamides, hypersensitivity reactions may occur.

Therapeutic Uses

The clinical use of sulfonamides is limited by the high prevalence of resistance that has developed among susceptible organisms. Currently, these agents are used primarily for the treatment of uncomplicated urinary tract infections. Most organisms (*E. coli* and *Proteus mirabilis*) responsible for urinary tract infections acquired in the community are sensitive to sulfonamides. Sulfonamides are the drugs of choice for *Nocardia* infections.

Sulfonamides are effective in preventing streptococcal pharyngitis and recurrences of rheumatic fever (used in patients allergic to penicillins). They are effective in eradication of meningococci from the nasopharynx of asymptomatic carriers and in preventing meningococcal disease in close contacts of patients with meningococcal meningitis if the infecting organism is susceptible.

Sulfadiazine combined with pyrimethamine is the regimen of choice for the treatment of toxoplasmosis. The combination of quinine, a sulfonamide, and pyrimethamine is the regimen of choice for the treatment of chloroquine-resistant *P. falciparum* malaria.

TRIMETHOPRIM AND TRIMETHOPRIM-SULFAMETHOXAZOLE

Trimethoprim is a synthetic antimicrobial compound which is available as a single agent for oral administration and in a fixed combination with sulfamethoxazole, trimethoprim-sulfamethoxazole (TMP-SMX), for oral and parenteral administration. The chemical structure of trimethoprim is:

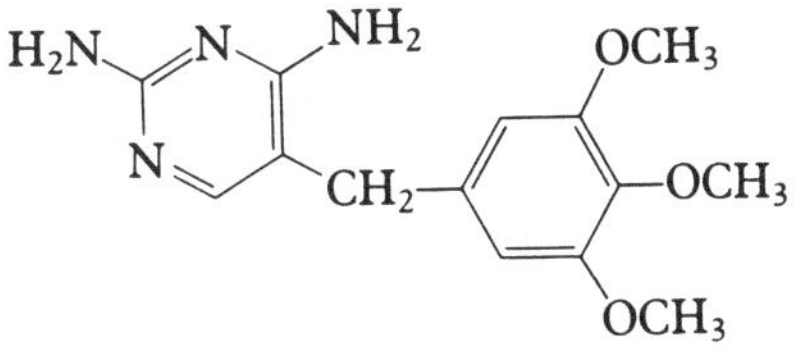

H_2N N NH_2 OCH_3
N CH_2 OCH_3
OCH_3

Mechanism of Action

Trimethoprim interferes with the action of dihydrofolate reductase, the enzyme that reduces folic acid and dihydrofolic acid to tetrahydrofolic acid, an essential step in purine and, ultimately, DNA synthesis (Fig. 47-2). Sulfonamides inhibit an earlier reaction in the same biosynthetic pathway (i.e., the incorporation of para-aminobenzoic acid into folic acid). The sequential blockade of the same biosynthetic pathway by these agents results in a high degree of synergistic activity against a wide spectrum of microorganisms.

The reduction of folates to tetrahydrofolic acid in humans is also catalyzed by dihydrofolate reductase. However, trimethoprim has at least 10,000 times more inhibitory effect on the bacterial enzyme than on the corresponding mammalian enzyme. This difference in intrinsic sensitivity of the enzyme is the primary basis for the selective toxicity of trimethoprim.

Trimethoprim has a bacteriostatic action on susceptible bacteria. In combination with sulfamethoxazole, a bactericidal effect is obtained against many organisms.

Antimicrobial Spectrum

Trimethoprim has a wide range of antimicrobial activity. It is 20 to 100 times more potent than sulfamethoxazole against most bacterial species. The combination of trimethoprim and sulfamethoxazole exhibits synergism against susceptible organisms. Although the optimal concentration ratio of these agents for synergism varies for different bacteria, the most effective ratio for the greatest number of organisms is 20 parts of sulfamethoxazole to one part of trimethoprim. Synergism, however, occurs over a wide ratio of drug concentrations, with trimethoprim susceptibility being the most important predictor of susceptibility to the drug combination.

Gram-Positive Bacteria Trimethoprim is active against *S. aureus* (including some methicillin-resistant strains), coagulase-negative staphylococci, *Streptococcus* species, and *Listeria monocytogenes*. Enterococci are often resistant, and resistance may develop during therapy. The activity of trimethoprim against *Nocardia* is inferior to that of the sulfonamides.

Gram-Negative Bacteria Most strains of enteric gram-negative bacilli including *E. coli, Enterobacter, Proteus, Klebsiella, Providencia, Morganella, Serratia marcescens, Citrobacter, Salmonella, Shigella,* and *Yersinia enterocolitica* are sensitive to trimethoprim. Trimethoprim is active against *Legionella, Acinetobacter, Vibrio, Aeromonas, Xanthomonas maltophilia* and *Pseudomonas cepacia*, but *Pseudomonas aeruginosa* is invariably resistant.

H. influenzae (including ampicillin-resistant strains) and *H. ducreyi* are susceptible to trimethoprim. *Neisseria meningitidis, N. gonorrhoeae,* and *Moraxella catarrhalis* are moderately resistant to trimethoprim but often sensitive to TMP-SMX.

Other Organisms Anaerobic bacteria are generally resistant to trimethoprim. The activity of TMP-SMX against these organisms is due to the sulfamethoxazole component. *Pneumocystis carinii* is sensitive to TMP-SMX.

Mechanisms of Resistance

Bacterial resistance to trimethoprim may be due to any of the following mechanisms: (1) inability of the drug to penetrate through the cell envelope (e.g., in *P. aeruginosa*); (2) the production of an altered dihydrofolate reductase that is resistant to trimethoprim inhibition (the most common mechanism); (3) overproduction of dihydrofolate reductase; and (4) mutation resulting in thymine dependence, whereby the organism requires exogenous thymine (found in purulent material) for DNA synthesis, thus bypassing the metabolic blockade produced by trimethoprim.

Trimethoprim-resistant bacteria may arise by mutation. However, resistance is often associated with acquisition of plasmids that code for altered dihydrofolate reductases.

Pharmacokinetics

Trimethoprim is absorbed almost completely from the gastrointestinal tract. The administration of sulfamethoxazole does not affect the rate of absorption of trimethoprim.

Trimethoprim is 45 percent bound to plasma proteins. It is lipid-soluble and penetrates readily into tissues (including the prostate) and body fluids. The volume of distribution of trimethoprim is significantly larger than that of sulfamethoxazole. The ratio of trimethoprim to sulfamethoxazole in the available oral and intravenous preparations of TMP-SMX is 1:5. After the components have been distributed throughout the body, the concentration ratio of the bioactive forms in blood and tissues is about 1:20, which is optimal for synergy.

Trimethoprim penetrates well into the CSF. The CSF concentrations are approximately 20 percent of the concurrent serum levels and increase to 40 percent when the meninges are inflamed. Sulfamethoxazole attains CSF concentrations that are 12 percent of the serum levels and increase to 25 percent when the meninges are inflamed.

Approximately 80 percent of trimethoprim is excreted unchanged into the urine. The remainder is biotransformed in the liver and the metabolites are excreted into the urine. The principal metabolites are 1- and 3-oxides and 3′- and 4′-hydroxy derivatives which have some antibacterial activity. The elimination half-life of trimethoprim is 10 h in persons with normal renal function; it increases to 24 to 30 h in functionally anephric patients.

Approximately 30 percent of an administered dose of sulfamethoxazole is excreted unchanged in the urine; the remainder is inactivated in the liver, and the metabolites are excreted into the urine. The elimination half-life of sulfamethoxazole is 10 h in persons with normal renal function; it increases to 24 to 30 h in functionally anephric patients.

Adverse Effects

Nausea, diarrhea, and hypersensitivity reactions are the most frequent adverse effects of trimethoprim. The drug can interfere with human folate metabolism if large doses are given over prolonged periods. In persons with suboptimal folate nutrition, megaloblastosis, granulocytopenia, and thrombocytopenia may occur. The administration of folinic acid (N^5-formyl tetrahydrofolic acid) usually prevents or treats effectively the antifolate effects of trimethoprim, without affecting its antibacterial efficacy, except possibly against enterococci.

The side effects of TMP-SMX are a summation of those due to the sulfonamide component and those caused by trimethoprim; most are caused by the former. The frequency of rash due to TMP-SMX in persons with human immunodeficiency virus infection is significantly higher than the general population.

Therapeutic Uses

Although trimethoprim is available as a single agent, it is most commonly used in combination with sulfamethoxazole.

TMP-SMX is effective in the therapy of urinary tract infections, prostatitis, epididymo-orchitis, and other infections caused by susceptible organisms. It is the therapy of choice for *Pneumocystis carinii* pneumonia.

TMP-SMX is a therapy of choice for *Nocardia* infections, shigellosis, travelers' diarrhea, and *Yersinia enterocolitica* enteritis. It is a second-line drug for *Listeria* meningitis, *Legionella* infection, and typhoid fever.

TMP-SMX is effective in meningitis due to susceptible gram-negative bacteria. It is most useful when meningitis is caused by *Acinetobacter*, *Xanthomonas maltophilia*, and *Enterobacter*, organisms that are frequently resistant to the third-generation cephalosporins.

CHLORAMPHENICOL

Chloramphenicol was originally isolated in 1947 from *Streptomyces venezuelae*. It has a simple structure and is now manufactured by chemical synthesis.

$$O_2N-C_6H_4-CH(OH)-CH(CH_2OH)-NH-C(=O)-CHCl_2$$

Mechanism of Action

Chloramphenicol inhibits protein synthesis in bacteria and, to a lesser extent, in eukaryotic cells. The drug binds reversibly to the 50S ribosomal subunit and prevents attachment of aminoacyl-tRNA to its binding site. As a consequence, the amino acid substrate is unavailable for peptidyl transferase and peptide bond formation is inhibited.

Protein synthesis in mammalian cells occurs on 80S ribosomes and is not inhibited by chloramphenicol. The drug, however, inhibits mitochondrial protein synthesis in mammalian cells, perhaps because mitochondrial ribosomes resemble bacterial ribosomes; both are 70S ribosomes.

Chloramphenicol has a bacteriostatic action against susceptible organisms. It has, however, bactericidal activity against *H. influenzae*, *S. pneumoniae*, and *N. meningitidis* at concentrations that can be achieved clinically.

Antimicrobial Spectrum

Chloramphenicol has a broad spectrum of antimicrobial activity that includes gram-positive and gram-negative aerobic and anaerobic bacteria, spirochetes, mycoplasmas, chlamydiae, and rickettsiae.

Aerobic Bacteria Chloramphenicol is active against methicillin-sensitive *S. aureus*, *Streptococcus* species (including *S. pneumoniae*), and *Listeria monocytogenes*. *Enterococcus* species and methicillin-resistant staphylococci are usually resistant.

Many gram-negative bacteria, including *N. meningitidis*, *N. gonorrhoeae*, *H. influenzae*, *Salmonella*, *E. coli*, *P. mirabilis*, *Klebsiella*, and *Brucella* are susceptible to chloramphenicol. *Enterobacter*, *Proteus vulgaris*, and *Serratia marcescens* have varying sensitivities. *P. aeruginosa* and *Acinetobacter* are almost always resistant to chloramphenicol.

Anaerobic Bacteria Chloramphenicol is one of the most active antimicrobials against anaerobic bacteria. *Peptococcus*, *Peptostreptococcus*, *Clostridium*, *Actinomyces*, *Bacteroides* (including *B. fragilis*), *Fusobacterium*, and other anaerobic bacteria are all susceptible to chloramphenicol.

Other Organisms Chloramphenicol is active against spirochetes, *Mycoplasma* species, chlamydiae, and rickettsiae.

Mechanisms of Resistance

Drug inactivation by bacterial enzymes (chloramphenicol acetyltransferase) is the major mechanism of resistance to chloramphenicol among gram-positive and gram-negative organisms. Acetylation of the drug by chloramphenicol acetyltransferase makes it unable to bind to the 50S ribosomal subunit. The enzyme is plasmid mediated and may be either constitutive or inducible.

Another mechanism of chloramphenicol resistance is impaired outer membrane permeability. This is caused by altered membrane proteins and is chromosomally mediated.

Pharmacokinetics

Chloramphenicol administered orally is rapidly and completely absorbed from the intestinal tract. Since the drug is exceedingly bitter, a suspension of tasteless chloramphenicol palmitate (an ester) is available for children. The ester is a prodrug with no antimicrobial activity. It is rapidly hydrolyzed in the intestine by pancreatic enzymes to active chloramphenicol which is then absorbed. The bioavailability of chloramphenicol palmitate is slightly lower than that of chloramphenicol.

Chloramphenicol is poorly soluble in water. A soluble ester of the drug, chloramphenicol sodium succinate, is available for parenteral administration. The ester has no antimicrobial activity and must be hydrolyzed in the liver to produce active chloramphenicol. Hydrolysis is incomplete and, therefore, the serum levels of active chloramphenicol following intravenous administration of the succinate ester are lower than those obtained with the equivalent doses of oral chloramphenicol.

Chloramphenicol is approximately 60 percent bound to plasma proteins. It is lipid-soluble and diffuses well into tissues and body fluids, and it also crosses the placenta. The CSF concentrations are 50 to 65 percent of the concurrent serum levels in the presence or absence of meningeal inflammation.

About 10 percent of orally administered

chloramphenicol is excreted unchanged in the urine. The remaining 90 percent is conjugated with glucuronic acid in the liver. The glucuronide conjugate has no antibacterial activity and is excreted into the urine.

Approximately 70 percent of intravenously administered chloramphenicol succinate is hydrolyzed to active chloramphenicol, which is eliminated by hepatic metabolism and renal excretion. The remainder of the dose is excreted into the urine in unchanged ester form.

The elimination half-life of chloramphenicol in persons with normal renal and hepatic function is 3.0 h. In patients with renal failure, the half-life is not altered significantly and dosage adjustment is not necessary. Inactive metabolites accumulate in these patients, but they are not associated with adverse effects. Patients with hepatic insufficiency metabolize chloramphenicol at a slower rate, resulting in increased levels of active drug. The dosage should be reduced in such patients.

Adverse Effects

Hematologic toxicity is by far the most important adverse effect of chloramphenicol. This can be divided into two types. The first is a reversible depression of bone marrow due to a direct toxic effect of the drug on mitochondria. Chloramphenicol inhibits the activity of ferrochelatase, an enzyme that catalyzes hemoglobin synthesis within the mitochondria. This toxicity is manifested by reticulocytopenia that occurs after 5 to 7 days of therapy, rising serum iron concentrations due to underutilization, and anemia. Leukopenia and/or thrombocytopenia may also occur. The dose-related marrow depression is common and occurs during therapy, particularly when serum levels exceed 25 μg/mL. It is reversible when the antibiotic is discontinued.

The second type of toxicity is a rare but generally fatal aplastic anemia, which occurs in one of 25,000 to 40,000 patients who receive chloramphenicol. Aplastic anemia usually develops weeks to months after administration of the drug but may develop during the course of therapy. It appears to occur more commonly in individuals who receive prolonged therapy and those who are exposed to the drug on more than one occasion. The pathogenesis of this idiosyncratic reaction is unknown.

A complete blood count should be obtained twice weekly in all patients receiving chloramphenicol. If the white blood cell count decreases below 2500 per mm^3, the antibiotic should be discontinued if the clinical condition allows.

Chloramphenicol can produce a potentially fatal toxic reaction, called the *gray syndrome*, in newborn infants, especially premature babies. Gray syndrome begins 3 to 8 days after the initiation of therapy and is characterized by abdominal distention, vomiting, cyanosis, lethargy, ashen-gray color, hypotension, and death. It is due to diminished ability of neonates to conjugate chloramphenicol and to excrete the active drug in the urine, resulting in high concentrations which inhibit mitochondrial function. Reduced dosing and careful monitoring of serum levels are required in this age group.

Allergic reactions including skin rash and drug fever are rare with chloramphenicol. Nausea, vomiting, and diarrhea may occur but are uncommon. Hemolytic anemia may develop in persons with severe glucose-6-phosphate dehydrogenase deficiency (Mediterranean type) who are treated with chloramphenicol.

Chloramphenicol inhibits the activity of certain hepatic microsomal enzymes and interferes with the metabolism of warfarin, phenytoin, phenobarbital, tolbutamide, and chlorpropamide. Toxicity due to these drugs may occur if they are administered in usual doses to a patient who is also receiving chloramphenicol.

Therapeutic Uses

Chloramphenicol is a potentially toxic agent that has very few clinical indications. It is a drug of first choice for the treatment of typhoid fever and is often included in regimens used to treat brain abscess. Chloramphenicol is an effective alternative in a number of infections when the drug of first choice cannot be used. These include rickettsial infections and meningitis caused by *S. pneumoniae*, *N. meningitidis*, or *H. influenzae*.

The risk of aplastic anemia does not contraindicate the use of chloramphenicol in situations in which it is necessary. However, the drug should never be employed in infections which can be safely and effectively treated with other antimicrobial agents. Chloramphenicol should never be used for prophylaxis or for treatment of minor infections. Prolonged use and repeated exposure should be avoided.

Chloramphenicol is used topically for infections of the skin and in the eye for infections caused by microorganisms that are sensitive to the compound.

TETRACYCLINES

The tetracyclines are a family of chemically related compounds that share in common a fused four-ring structure. The first of these compounds, chlortetracycline, isolated from *Streptomyces aureofaciens* and introduced in 1948, is now only available for topical use. Six congeners, introduced later, are currently available in the United States. Oxytetracycline (isolated from *Streptomyces rimosus*) became available in 1950, tetracycline (semisynthetic) in 1952, demeclocycline (isolated from a mutant strain of *Streptomyces aureofaciens*) in 1959, methacycline (semisynthetic) in 1961, doxycycline (semisynthetic) in 1966, and minocycline (semisynthetic) in 1972 (see Table 47-2). Although there are some differences among these agents in terms of pharmacokinetic properties and antimicrobial activity, they are very much alike.

Tetracycline can be divided into three groups based upon their pharmacologic properties: (1) short-acting compounds, tetracycline and oxytetracycline; (2) an intermediate group consisting of demeclocycline and methacycline; and (3) long-acting compounds, doxycycline and minocycline. All are available for oral administration. Doxycycline and minocycline are also available for intravenous administration.

TABLE 47-2 Structures of the tetracyclines

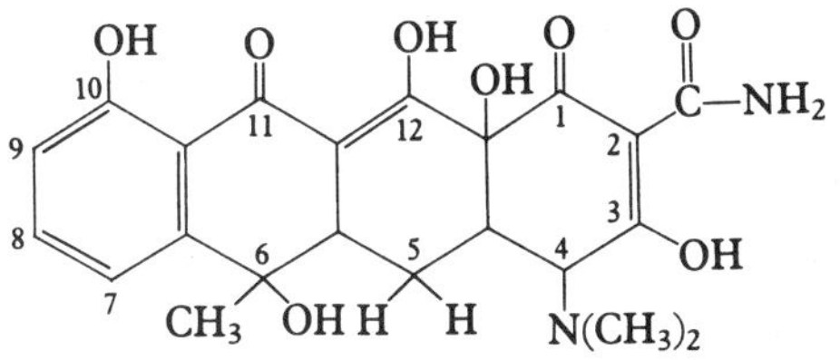

OH O OH O O
10 OH 1 ‖
11 12 C—NH_2
9 2
3
8 6 5 4 OH
7 CH_3 OH H H $N(CH_3)_2$

Tetracycline

Drug	Substituents	Position(s)
Oxytetracycline	-OH, -H	5
Demeclocycline	-OH, -H	6
	-Cl	7
Methacycline	-OH, -H	5
	$=CH_2$	6
Doxycycline	-OH, -H	5
	$-CH_3$, -H	6
Minocycline	-H, -H	6
	$-N(CH_3)_2$	7

Mechanism of Action

The tetracyclines inhibit protein synthesis by binding to the 30S ribosomal subunit in susceptible bacteria. An essential element in this process is the active transport of the drug across the cytoplasmic membrane. This energy-dependent transport mechanism results in the accumulation of the antibiotic inside the bacterial cell. Once within the cell, the drug binds reversibly to the 30S ribosomal subunit. This blocks the attachment of the aminoacyl-tRNA to the A site on the ribosome and prevents the addition of new amino acids into the growing peptide chain. Tetracyclines have a bacteriostatic action against susceptible organisms.

At higher concentrations, tetracyclines inhibit protein synthesis in mammalian cells to a small extent. The selective toxicity of these agents resides in their differential entry into bacterial cells; mammalian cells lack the active transport system found in bacteria.

Antimicrobial Spectrum

The antimicrobial spectra of all tetracyclines are almost identical. However, differences in activity against some organisms do exist among the congeners. In general, doxycycline and minocycline are the most potent analogues; whereas, tetracycline and oxytetracycline are two- to fourfold less active against many bacteria and are the least active.

Gram-Positive Bacteria The activity of tetracyclines against *Staphylococcus aureus* and coagulase-negative staphylococci is variable, and the prevalence of resistant strains varies considerably. *Streptococcus pneumoniae* and *S. pyogenes* are usually sensitive, but resistant strains are occasionally encountered. Resistance is more frequent among other *Streptococcus* species. Minocycline is the most active tetracycline against *S. aureus* and streptococci, followed closely by doxycycline. Both are active against a proportion of strains that are resistant to other congeners. Enterococci are usually resistant to tetracyclines.

Gram-Negative Aerobic Bacteria Tetracyclines are active against *N. gonorrhoeae*, *N. meningitidis*, *H. influenzae*, *Moraxella catarrhalis*, *Legionella*, *Brucella*, *Vibrio cholerae*, *Vibrio vulnificus*, *Yersinia pestis*, *Yersinia enterocolitica*, *Franciscella tularensis*, and *Pasteurella multocida*. Enteric gram-negative species, except for a small proportion of *E. coli*, *Enterobacter*, and *Klebsiella* strains, are resistant.

Anaerobes Tetracyclines are active against many anaerobic bacteria; their activity against *Actinomyces* is particularly relevant clinically. Most strains of anaerobic species, including 75 percent of *B. fragilis* strains, are sensitive to doxycycline, the most active congener against these organisms.

Other Organisms Tetracyclines are active against *Mycoplasma* species, *Ureaplasma urealyticum*, *Chlamydia trachomatis*, *Chlamydia pneumoniae*, *Chlamydia psittaci* (psittacosis), *Rickettsia*, *Coxiella burnetii*, *Ehrlichia canis*, *Treponema pallidum*, *Borrelia recurrentis* (the agent of relapsing fever), *Borrelia burgdorferi* (the agent of Lyme disease), *Leptospira*, and *Plasmodium falciparum*. Doxycycline is active against *Mycobacterium fortuitum* and *Mycobacterium marinum*.

Mechanisms of Resistance

Resistance to tetracyclines is due to either altered ribosomal binding site or inability of the drug to accumulate within the bacterial cell. The latter is mediated by plasmids that contain genes for tetracycline efflux. These genes produce a cytoplasmic membrane protein that pumps tetracycline out of the cell at a rate equal to its uptake. This keeps the intracellular concentrations low enough to allow protein synthesis to proceed. Resistance to one tetracycline usually implies resistance to all, except for *S. aureus*, which is more sensitive to minocycline and doxycycline, and *B. fragilis*, which is more sensitive to doxycycline.

Pharmacokinetics

All the tetracyclines are absorbed from the gastrointestinal tract. The bioavailability of an oral dose varies from 60 percent for oxytetracycline to 95 percent for doxycycline and minocycline (Table 47-3). The presence of food in the stomach does not affect the absorption of doxycycline or minocycline but reduces the absorption of other tetracyclines. All the tetracyclines form stable chelates with divalent or trivalent cations. Absorption is markedly decreased when these drugs are administered simultaneously with milk (which contains calcium), antacids (which contain magnesium, aluminum, or calcium), or iron preparations (including multiple vitamins with minerals).

The amount of tetracyclines bound to plasma proteins varies; the degree of binding is greater for the intermediate and long-acting compounds. Tetracyclines penetrate well into various tissues and body fluids. Penetration into the CSF is highest for minocycline, followed by doxycycline, and correlates with lipid solubility. The concentrations in CSF are approximately 10 to 25 percent of the concurrent serum levels. Minocycline penetrates well into salivary secretions; this accounts for its efficacy in eradicating meningococcal carrier state. All tetracyclines cross the placenta and are excreted in breast milk in concentrations that are usually a fraction of maternal serum levels.

Except for minocycline, tetracyclines are excreted unchanged in the urine and the feces. A proportion of the dose, depending upon the agent, is excreted in the urine (Table 47-3). The remainder is eliminated in the feces as a result of drug secretion into the intestinal tract, unabsorbed drug (oral administration), and biliary excretion (a small fraction). Cationic chelation in the intestine prevents reabsorption in the lower intestine. More than 70 percent of administered minocycline is metabolized; the remainder is excreted in the urine (10 percent) and feces. Metabolism does not play a significant role in the elimination of other tetracyclines. The elimination half-lives of tetracyclines range from 6 to 12 h (tetracycline and oxytetracycline) to 12 to 24 h (minocycline and doxycycline).

In persons with renal failure, the elimination half-life of doxycycline remains unchanged (due to increased excretion in the feces) and dosage reduction is not necessary. This drug is the tetracycline of choice in patients with renal failure.

Adverse Effects

Allergic reactions including skin rash and drug fever are infrequent with tetracyclines. When a person is allergic to one tetracycline, he or she should be considered allergic to all. Photosensitivity reactions, consisting of a red rash over areas exposed to sunlight, are more common in patients receiving demeclocycline, but may occur with any tetracycline derivative.

TABLE 47-3 Pharmacokinetic features of the tetracyclines

Drug	Oral Bioavailability, %	Plasma protein binding, %	Elimination half-life, h	Excreted unchanged in urine, %
Short-acting				
Tetracycline	75	65 to 70	6 to 12	60
Oxytetracycline	60	20 to 40	6 to 12	60
Intermediate				
Demeclocycline	65	65 to 90	12 to 16	40
Methacycline	60	80 to 90	14 to 16	50
Long-acting				
Doxycycline	95	80 to 95	15 to 24	35
Minocycline	95	70 to 80	12 to 18	10

Epigastric pain, nausea, and vomiting are relatively common with tetracyclines. Diarrhea may occur; it is rarely due to *Clostridium difficile* colitis.

Tetracyclines, administered to children early in life or to pregnant women during the second and third trimester of pregnancy, may be deposited in the deciduous teeth, causing a yellow-brown color. These drugs may also produce a lifelong discoloration of the permanent teeth if they are administered to children under 8 years of age. Hence, tetracyclines should not be administered to pregnant women and to children under 8 years of age.

Vestibular toxicity is a side effect unique to minocycline. It is manifested by dizziness, tinnitus, vertigo, and ataxia which may begin on the second or third day of therapy. The symptoms are reversible after discontinuation of the drug. Vestibular toxicity has significantly limited the use of minocycline.

Except for doxycycline, tetracyclines aggravate preexisting renal failure, possibly by inhibiting protein synthesis which increases azotemia from amino acid metabolism. Only doxycycline can be used safely in patients with renal insufficiency. Other side effects associated with tetracyclines include hepatic toxicity (with high doses especially in pregnant women) and superinfection with *Candida* and resistant bacteria.

Therapeutic Uses

Tetracyclines are the drug of choice for a wide variety of infections, including sexually transmitted diseases caused by *Chlamydia* species (urethritis, pelvic inflammatory disease, and lymphogranuloma venereum), other chlamydial infections (psittacosis and pneumonia caused by *Chlamydia pneumoniae*), *Mycoplasma* pneumonia (many prefer erythromycin), rickettsial infections (Rocky Mountain spotted fever, Q fever, etc.), Lyme disease, leptospirosis, relapsing fever, brucellosis (in combination with streptomycin or rifampin), ehrlichiosis, plague, cholera, *Vibrio vulnificus* infections, granuloma inguinale (caused by *Calymmatobacterium granulomatis*), chloroquine-resistant *Plasmodium falciparum* malaria (in combination with quinine), and infections caused by *Mycobacterium fortuitum* (only doxycycline). In addition, these drugs are effective alternatives in a number of infections when the drug of first choice cannot be used. These include syphilis, actinomycosis, tularemia, *Yersinia enterocolitica* enteritis, and rat-bite fever. Long-term low-dose tetracycline therapy is frequently used to control severe acne. For persons who cannot take mefloquine, doxycycline is the drug of choice for prophylaxis of chloroquine-resistant *P. falciparum*.

Doxycycline and tetracycline are the oral preparations which are most commonly used. Doxycycline is the preferred agent when intravenous administration is required.

Tetracycline and chlortetracycline are used on the skin for prophylaxis of abrasions, minor cuts, wounds, and burns and for the treatment of superficial skin infections due to susceptible organisms. These two compounds are also used topically for ocular infections.

BIBLIOGRAPHY

Bahal, N., and M.C. Naheta: "The New Macrolide Antibiotics: Azithromycin, Clarithromycin, and Roxithromycin," *Ann. Pharmacother.* **26**: 46-55 (1992).

Calia, F.M.: "Erythromycin," In: Gorbach S.L., J.G. G. Bartlett, and N.R. Blacklow (eds): *Infectious Diseases*, W.B. Saunders, Philadelphia, 1992, pp. 223-231.

Calia, F.M. "Clindamycin" In: Gorbach S.L., J.G. Bartlett, and N.R. Blacklow (eds): *Infectious Diseases*, W.B. Saunders, Philadelphia, 1992, pp. 214-222.

Dever, L.A., and T.S. Dermody: "Mechanisms of Bacterial Resistance to Antibiotics," *Arch. Intern. Med.* **151**: 886-895 (1991).

Dhawan, V.K., and H. Thadepalli: "Clindamycin: A Review of Fifteen Years of Experience," *Rev. Infect. Dis.*, **4**: 1133-1153 (1982).

Drew, R.H., and H.A. Gallis: "Azithromycin — Spectrum of Activity, Pharmacokinetics, and Clinical Applications," *Pharmacotherapy* **12**: 161-173 (1992).

Edwards, D.I.: "Nitroimidazole Drugs—Action and Resistance Mechanisms. II. Mechanisms of Action," *J. Antimicrob. Chemother.* **31**: 201-210 (1993).

Kucers, A., and N.McK. Bennett: *The Use of Antibiotics*, J.B. Lippincott, Philadelphia, 1987.

Mathisen G.E., and S.M. Finegold: "Metronidazole and Other Nitroimidazoles". In: Gorbach S.L., J.G. Bartlett, and N. R. Blacklow (eds): *Infectious Diseases*, W.B. Saunders, Philadelphia, 1992, pp. 261-265.

Mazzei, T., E., Mini, A. Novelli, and P. Periti: "Chemistry and Mode of Action of Macrolides," *J. Antimicrob. Chemother.* **13 (Suppl. C)**: 1-9 (1993).

Neu, H.C.: "The Developments of Macrolides: Clarithromycin in Perspective," *J. Antimicrob. Chemother.* **27**: 1-9 (1991).

Piscitelli, S.C., L.H. Danziger, and K.A. Rodvold: "Clarithromycin and Azithromycin: New Macrolide Antibiotics," *Clin. Pharm.* **11**: 137-152 (1992).

Speer, B.S., N.B. Shoemaker, and A.G. Salyers: "Bacterial Resistance to Tetracyclines: Mechanisms, Transfer, and Clinical Significance," *Clin. Microbiol. Rev.* **5**: 387-399 (1992).

Standiford, H.C.: "Tetracyclines and Chloramphenicol," In: Mandel, G.L., R.G. Douglas, Jr., and J.E. Bennett (eds): *Principles and Practice of Infectious Diseases, Third Edition*, Churchill Livingstone Inc., New York, 1990, pp. 284-295.

Swanson, D.J., R.J. Sung, M.J. Fine, J.J. Orloff, S.U. Chu, and V.L. Yu: "Erythromycin Ototoxicity, Prospective Assessment with Serum Concentrations and Audiograms in a Study of Patients with Pneumonia," *Am. J. Med.* **92**: 61-68 (1992).

Williams, J.D. and A.M. Sefton: "Comparison of Macrolide Antibiotics," *J. Antimicrob. Chemother.* **31 (Suppl. C)**: 11-26 (1993).

Zinner, S.H. and K.H. Mayer: "Sulfonamides and Trimethoprim," In: Mandel, G.L., R.G. Douglas, Jr., and J.E. Bennett (Eds): *Principles and Practice of Infectious Diseases, Third Edition*, Churchill Livingstone Inc., New York, 1990, pp. 325-334.

CHAPTER 48

Antimicrobials IV: Antimycobacterial Drugs

Abdolghader Molavi

ANTITUBERCULOSIS DRUGS

The drugs used for the chemotherapy of tuberculosis are divided into two groups: the "first-line drugs", which have the greatest level of efficacy with relatively low toxicity, and the "second-line drugs" which have inferior efficacy and/or greater toxicity. The first-line drugs include isoniazid, rifampin, ethambutol, pyrazinamide, and streptomycin. All except for ethambutol are bactericidal against *Mycobacterium tuberculosis*. Isoniazid and rifampin are the two most effective drugs for treating tuberculosis. A great majority of patients with tuberculosis can be successfully treated with the first-line drugs. Occasionally, because of microbial resistance and/or patient-related factors, it may be necessary to use the second-line drugs. These agents, which include ethionamide, cycloserine, para-aminosalicylic acid, capreomycin, kanamycin, and amikacin, have important limitations that interfere with their usefulness in treating tuberculosis. The quinolones are also active against *M. tuberculosis* and occupy a position between the first- and the second-line drugs in the treatment of tuberculosis.

Isoniazid

Isoniazid (isonicotinic acid hydrazide or INH), is a synthetic compound which was introduced in 1953 for the treatment of tuberculosis. It is available for both oral and parenteral administration.

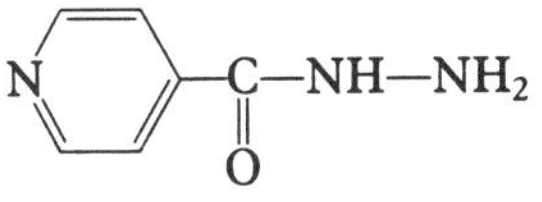

$$\text{N}\langle\text{C}_5\text{H}_4\rangle\text{—C(=O)—NH—NH}_2$$

Mechanism of Action Isoniazid has a bactericidal action against *M. tuberculosis*. It inhibits the synthesis of mycolic acid, an important constituent of the mycobacterial cell wall. Since mycolic acid is unique to mycobacteria, isoniazid is selectively toxic for these organisms.

Antimicrobial Activity Isoniazid is highly active against *M. tuberculosis*. It is more effective against organisms that are extracellular than those which reside within macrophages. Most strains of *M. kansasii* are sensitive to the drug but at higher concentrations than those effective for *M. tuberculosis*. Other atypical mycobacteria are resistant to isoniazid.

Mechanisms of Resistance Naturally occurring isoniazid-resistant mutants occur at random and spontaneously in growing populations of tubercle bacilli at a rate of one per 10^5 to 10^6 organisms. These mutants exhibit decreased isoniazid uptake. Large populations of the organism, like the 10^9 to 10^{10} bacilli in open pulmonary cavities, contain significant numbers of resistant mutants. If isoniazid is used alone for treatment of tuberculosis, the sensitive organisms are killed while the resistant mutants multiply and eventually emerge as the dominant phenotype. The shift from primarily sensitive to mainly insensitive microorganisms during therapy is termed *acquired* (or *secondary*) *resistance*; it occurs within a few weeks.

Strains of isoniazid-resistant *M. tuberculosis* may be isolated from patients who have not received previous treatment with this drug (*primary resistance*). The primary isoniazid resistance occurs with an average frequency of 5.3 percent in the United States. The incidence is higher in certain populations, including Asians and Hispanics.

Pharmacokinetics Isoniazid is well absorbed from the gastrointestinal tract. It diffuses into all tissues and body fluids, including the central nervous system and the cerebrospinal fluid (CSF), and enters readily into macrophages. The CSF concentrations are approximately 20 percent of the serum levels but reach the serum concentrations when the meninges are inflamed. Isoniazid passes readily across the placenta and enters the fetal circulation. It is 10 percent bound to plasma proteins.

Most of the administered isoniazid is metabolized in the liver to inactive products which are excreted in the urine. Inactivation occurs primarily via acetylation by the hepatic enzyme N-acetyl transferase, which converts isoniazid to acetyl isoniazid. The rate at which humans acetylate isoniazid is genetically determined. There is a bimodal distribution of slow and rapid inactivators of the drug due to differences in the activity of the enzyme acetyl transferase. Slow inactivators are autosomal homozygous recessives; rapid inactivators are either heterozygous or homozygous dominants. The frequency of the two phenotypes varies in populations of different racial origin. Fifty eight percent of Caucasians in the United States are slow inactivators. The mean elimination half-life of isoniazid is 80 min in rapid inactivators, whereas it is 180 min in slow inactivators. The average serum concentration of isoniazid in rapid inactivators is 30 to 50 percent of that in slow inactivators. There is, however, no evidence that therapeutic efficacy of isoniazid is affected by the rate of acetylation in patients who receive the drug every day.

Some unchanged, active isoniazid is excreted into the urine; the amount depends on the rate of acetylation. Approximately 3 percent of the administered dose is excreted this way in rapid inactivators. The fraction excreted unchanged in the urine is several times higher in patients who are slow inactivators.

Adverse Effects Peripheral neuropathy, manifested by paraesthesia, is a relatively common adverse effect of isoniazid. It occurs more frequently if high doses of the drug are used. Peripheral neuropathy is due to the effects of isoniazid on pyridoxine metabolism and can be prevented by prophylactic administration of pyridoxine.

Asymptomatic transaminase elevation occurs in 10 to 20 percent of patients receiving isoniazid. Severe hepatitis is much less frequent. Age appears to be the most important factor in determining the risk of hepatotoxicity. Hepatitis is rare in persons less than 20 years old, but it occurs in 0.3 percent of those 20 to 34 years old. The incidence increases to 1.2 percent in persons 35 to 49 years old and 2.3 percent in those 50 to 65 years old. Hepatitis can occur at any time during treatment; it is more common within the first 2 months. Routine monitoring of serum transaminases is not necessary during isoniazid therapy. However, the patient should be monitored clinically, and if symptoms suggesting hepatitis occur, appropriate laboratory tests should be performed.

Other adverse effects of isoniazid include hypersensitivity reactions, drug fever, and agranulocytosis. Isoniazid inhibits the metabolism of phenytoin and carbamazepine; toxicity due to these agents may occur if they are co-administered with isoniazid.

Therapeutic Uses The use of isoniazid for the treatment of tuberculosis is discussed later in this chapter. In order to prevent peripheral neuropathy, pyridoxine is usually administered with isoniazid, especially in malnourished patients, the elderly, pregnant women, alcoholics, and patients with end-stage renal disease.

Isoniazid, administered alone, is the drug of choice for chemoprophylaxis in persons at risk of developing tuberculosis. These include household contacts of persons with active disease, persons with known recent tuberculin conversion (within two years), and tuberculin skin-test reactors under 35 years of age.

Rifampin

Rifampin (also known as rifampicin) is a semisynthetic derivative of rifamycin B, produced by *Streptomyces mediterranei*. It was introduced for clinical use in 1968. Rifampin is available for both oral and parenteral administration. It has a complex macrocyclic structure.

Mechanism of Action Rifampin inhibits DNA-dependent RNA polymerase by binding to the beta subunit of the enzyme in susceptible microorganisms. This interferes with protein synthesis by preventing chain initiation. Selective toxicity of rifampin is due to relative lack of affinity for RNA polymerase in mammalian cells. Rifampin has a bactericidal action against susceptible organisms.

Antimicrobial Activity Rifampin is highly active against *M. tuberculosis*, including both intracellular and extracellular organisms. Among atypical

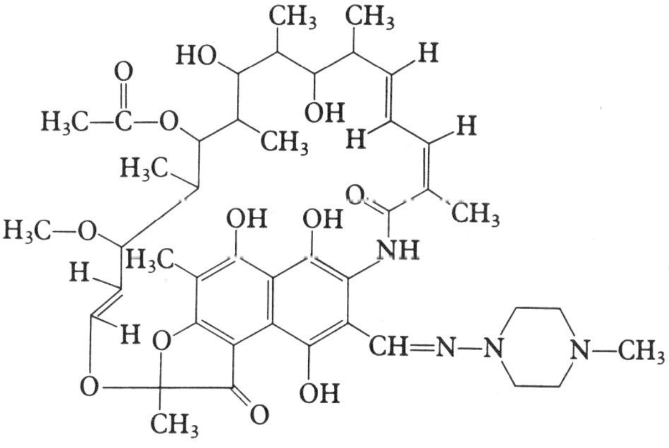

Rifampin

mycobacteria, *Mycobacterium kansasii*, *Mycobacterium marinum*, and most strains of *Mycobacterium scrofulaceum* and *Mycobacterium xenopi* are sensitive; the susceptibility of others is variable. Rifampin is bactericidal against *Mycobacterium leprae*.

In addition to mycobacteria, rifampin exhibits bactericidal activity against a wide range of organisms. Among the gram-positive bacteria, rifampin is most active against *Staphylococcus aureus* and coagulase-negative staphylococci, including some methicillin-resistant strains. It is also active against *Streptococcus* species and *Listeria monocytogenes*. Enterococci are usually resistant to rifampin.

Among gram-negative bacteria, *Neisseria meningitidis*, *Neisseria gonorrhoeae*, *Moraxella catarrhalis*, and *Haemophilus influenzae* (including ampicillin-resistant strains) are highly sensitive to rifampin. Rifampin is also active against *Legionella*, *Brucella*, and *Chlamydia*. Enteric gram-negative bacilli are usually resistant.

Rifampin is active against most anaerobic bacteria, including *Peptococcus*, *Peptostreptococcus*, *Clostridium*, and *Bacteroides* species.

Mechanisms of Resistance The rapid emergence of resistance has been a common problem for monotherapy with rifampin. Susceptible bacteria contain naturally occurring mutants that are resistant to rifampin. Resistance is due to single-step mutations that alter the beta subunit of the RNA polymerase. In a population of susceptible bacteria, approximately one of every 10^6 to 10^8 organisms is resistant to the drug. When rifampin is used alone for the treatment of tuberculosis or other infections, the sensitive organisms are killed while the resistant mutants multiply and emerge as the dominant phenotype. Acquired resistance can be prevented if rifampin is used with another effective chemotherapeutic agent. Rifampin should not be used alone for the treatment of any infection.

Primary resistance of *M. tuberculosis* to rifampin occurs with a frequency of less than 1 percent in the United States. The incidence is significantly higher in developing countries.

RNA polymerases of gram-negative and gram-positive bacteria are equally sensitive to rifampin; resistance of gram-negative species is due to impaired penetration of the drug through the outer membrane.

Pharmacokinetics Rifampin is rapidly and virtually completely absorbed from the gastrointestinal tract. Serum levels are slightly lower if the drug is taken immediately after food.

Rifampin is 80 percent bound to plasma proteins. It penetrates readily into tissues and body fluids, including CSF and saliva. The CSF concentrations are approximately 50 percent of the concurrent serum levels when the meninges are inflamed. Rifampin is lipid soluble and penetrates well into leukocytes, macrophages, and peripheral nerves. It passes readily across the placenta and enters fetal circulation.

Rifampin is metabolized in the liver by deacetylation to desacetylrifampin, which is also biologically active but less so than the parent compound. The unchanged drug and the desacetyl metabolite are both excreted into the bile. The unchanged drug is reabsorbed from the intestine in an enterohepatic cycle, but the metabolite is very poorly reabsorbed. Eventually, most of the administered dose is eliminated in the feces. A small fraction (10 to 20 percent) of the dose is excreted in the urine, mostly in the form of desacetylrifampin. The dosage of rifampin need not be modified in patients with renal failure. However, when hepatic function is impaired, the dosage should be adjusted.

The elimination half-life of rifampin shortens progressively during the first 7 to 10 days of therapy. The drug induces hepatic microsomal enzymes which increase its own rate of metabolism. The half-life of rifampin, which is 3.5 h at the onset of therapy, decreases to 2.0 h after daily administration for 1 to 2 weeks and remains constant thereafter.

Adverse Effects Allergic reactions including skin rashes and drug fever may occur. Nausea, vomiting, and abdominal pain are uncommon. Asymptomatic elevation of transaminase may occur during the first few weeks of therapy; however, the incidence of overt hepatitis is less than 1 percent. Other adverse effects of rifampin include rare instances of thrombocytopenia, leukopenia, hemolytic anemia, and acute renal failure.

Rifampin is a potent inducer of the hepatic cytochrome P-450 enzyme system and, therefore, decreases the elimination half-lives of a number of drugs including methadone, warfarin, glucocorticoids, estrogens, propranolol, quinidine, phenytoin, digoxin, cyclosporine, and sulfonylureas. Proper management of these drug-drug interactions is essential to avoid therapeutic failures on initiating rifampin therapy and potential toxic reactions after discontinuing rifampin. By accelerating estrogen metabolism, rifampin may interfere with the effectiveness of oral contraceptives.

Rifampin and its metabolite give a red-orange color to urine, saliva, sweat, and tears. Patients should be warned of this and of possible permanent discoloration of soft contact lenses.

Therapeutic Uses The use of rifampin for the treatment of tuberculosis is discussed later in this chapter. Rifampin is an important component of regimens used to treat leprosy.

Rifampin is effective in eliminating meningococci and *H. influenzae* from the nasopharynx of asymptomatic carriers. It is the drug of choice for chemoprophylaxis in close contacts of patients with meningococcal disease and *H. influenzae* meningitis. Short-term chemoprophylaxis is usually associated with very few side effects except for the red discoloration of urine and permanent staining of soft contact lenses.

Rifampin combined with nafcillin or vancomycin is the treatment of choice for prosthetic valve endocarditis due to coagulase-negative staphylococci. In patients with *S. aureus* endocarditis, rifampin may be a useful addition to nafcillin or vancomycin if there are myocardial, splenic, or brain abscesses. Similarly, in patients with *S. aureus* meningitis, addition of rifampin to nafcillin or vancomycin may improve clinical outcome. In patients with brucellosis, doxycycline combined with rifampin is as effective as tetracycline plus streptomycin.

Ethambutol

Ethambutol was discovered in 1961 among synthetic compounds being screened for antimycobacterial activity. It is available only for oral administration.

$$
\begin{array}{ccccccc}
 & CH_2OH & & & & C_2H_5 & \\
 & | & & & & | & \\
H- & C & -NH-CH_2-CH_2-HN- & & & C & -H \\
 & | & & & & | & \\
 & C_2H_5 & & & & CH_2OH &
\end{array}
$$

Mechanism of Action Ethambutol has a bacteriostatic action against *M. tuberculosis*, but the precise mechanism is not known. It appears to inhibit RNA synthesis, however, its selective toxicity for mycobacteria is unexplained.

Antimicrobial Activity Ethambutol is active only against mycobacteria; all other bacteria are completely resistant. It is active against *M. tuberculosis, M. kansasii*, and most strains of *M. avium* and *M. scrofulaceum*. Both intracellular and extracellular tubercle bacilli are inhibited by ethambutol.

Mechanism of Resistance The incidence of primary resistance to ethambutol is less than 1 percent in the United States. Secondary resistance develops when the drug is used without a companion, effective agent for the treatment of tuberculosis. The mechanism of resistance to ethambutol is not known. There is no cross-resistance between ethambutol and other antimycobacterial agents.

Pharmacokinetics Approximately 80 percent of orally administered ethambutol is absorbed from the gastrointestinal tract. Following absorption, the drug is widely distributed throughout the body and enters into macrophages. Penetration through normal meninges is poor; however, when the meninges are inflamed, the CSF concentrations are approximately 25 to 50 percent of the concurrent serum levels. Ethambutol penetrates into pulmonary parenchyma and caseous tuberculous lesions, where the levels achieved are 5 to 10 times and 3 times the simultaneous serum concentrations, respectively. It also passes across the placenta and enters the fetal circulation. Ethambutol is 20 to 30 percent bound to plasma proteins.

Approximately 65 percent of administered ethambutol is excreted unchanged into the urine. Up to 15 percent is converted into inactive metabolites which are also excreted in the urine. The elimination half-life of ethambutol is 4.0 h; it increases to 18 h in patients with renal failure.

Adverse Effects Ethambutol is generally well tolerated and produces very few adverse reactions. Retrobulbar neuritis is the most important adverse effect; symptoms include decreased visual acuity, central scotoma, and color blindness, but sometimes the only change is constriction of visual fields. Vision may be unilaterally or bilaterally affected, and the degree of impairment is related to the duration of therapy after the symptoms first become apparent. Retrobulbar neuritis is completely reversible if ethambutol is promptly withdrawn; permanent impairment of vision may result if the drug is continued long after the onset of symptoms. Visual toxicity of ethambutol is dose related; the incidence is 1 to 2 percent with the currently recommended doses. Patients receiving ethambutol should be instructed to report any visual disturbances. Testing of visual acuity, visual fields, and color discrimination is recommended every 4 to 6 weeks.

Other adverse effects include allergic reactions, drug fever, gastrointestinal upset, hyperuricemia, arthralgia, and peripheral neuritis. The latter manifests itself by numbness and tingling in the extremities, which disappear when the drug is withdrawn.

Therapeutic Uses In addition to its use in the treatment of tuberculosis, ethambutol is also used as part of a multidrug regimen for the treatment of *M. avium* complex infection in patients with acquired immunodeficiency syndrome.

Pyrazinamide

Pyrazinamide is a derivative of nicotinamide. It was synthesized in 1952. Its chemical structure is

[Structure: pyrazine ring (N, N) bearing $CONH_2$]

Pyrazinamide has a bactericidal action against *M. tuberculosis in vitro*, when the pH of the growth medium is slightly acidic (pH 5.0 to 5.5); it has little or no activity at neutral pH. Pyrazinamide is highly active against intracellular tubercle bacilli which reside within phagosomes in an acid environment. It has no activity against extracellular organisms which reside in cavitary pulmonary lesions at a neutral pH. The precise mechanism of action of pyrazinamide is not known.

Pyrazinamide is completely absorbed from the gastrointestinal tract. It is widely distributed throughout the body and readily penetrates into macrophages. Therapeutic CSF concentrations are attained when the meninges are inflamed. Most of the absorbed pyrazinamide is metabolized in the liver, and the metabolites are excreted in the urine. Only 4 to 10 percent of the dose is excreted unchanged in the urine. The elimination half-life of pyrazinamide is approximately 9 h.

Hepatotoxicity is the most serious adverse effect of pyrazinamide. Asymptomatic elevations of transaminases are relatively common, but overt hepatitis is infrequent. Hepatotoxicity of pyrazinamide is dose-related; with the currently recommended doses it is quite uncommon. Another adverse effect of pyrazinamide is hyperuricemia, occasionally progressing to symptomatic gout. It is due to the interference of pyrazinoic acid (a metabolite of pyrazinamide) with the tubular secretion of uric acid.

Pyrazinamide is the most active agent against intracellular tubercle bacilli. Eradication of these organisms is necessary to prevent relapse after the completion of therapy. Pyrazinamide is used only for the first two months of therapy. Continuing pyrazinamide beyond the initial 2 months does not seem to improve the outcome. In contrast to other first-line drugs, pyrazinamide has little ability to prevent emergence of drug resistance.

Streptomycin

Streptomycin was the first clinically effective drug to become available for the treatment of tuberculosis. It is an aminoglycoside antibiotic discussed in

Chapter 46. The following brief comments pertain to its antimycobacterial activity and its role in the treatment of tuberculosis.

Streptomycin is active against *M. tuberculosis* and *M. kansasii*; other atypical mycobacteria are only occasionally susceptible. It has a bactericidal effect against extracellular organisms, but it does not enter macrophages and, therefore, has no effect against intracellular mycobacteria.

There are naturally occurring mutants in any large population of tubercle bacilli that are resistant to streptomycin. Such resistant mutants occur with a frequency of one in 10^6 to 10^7 organisms. Use of streptomycin alone for the treatment of tuberculosis leads to the development of secondary resistance. Primary resistance to streptomycin is found in 2 to 3 percent of isolates of *M. tuberculosis* in the United States.

The most serious adverse effect of streptomycin is ototoxicity. This usually results in vertigo and ataxia, but hearing loss may also occur. Streptomycin is significantly less nephrotoxic than other aminoglycosides. The risks of ototoxicity and nephrotoxicity are related both to the cumulative dose and to serum concentrations.

The use of streptomycin for the treatment of tuberculosis is discussed later in this chapter. The drug is usually administered daily as a single intramuscular injection. A total dose of no more than 120 g over the course of therapy should be given. Streptomycin should be used with extreme caution in the elderly and in patients with renal insufficiency.

Quinolones

The quinolones were discussed in Chapter 46. Ofloxacin and ciprofloxacin are active *in vitro* against *M. tuberculosis* and have proved effective in re-treatment regimens with remarkably good tolerance and relatively little toxicity. These agents are preferable to oral second-line drugs with regard to both antimycobacterial activity and safety. Their use for the treatment of tuberculosis is discussed later in this chapter.

Second-Line Drugs

The second-line antituberculosis drugs include three agents available only for oral administration (ethionamide, cycloserine, and para-aminosalicylic acid) and three drugs available for parenteral administration (capreomycin, amikacin, and kanamycin). All these agents have significant potential toxicity and/or weak antimycobacterial activity which limit the usefulness in treating tuberculosis.

Ethionamide Ethionamide is a derivative of isonicotinic acid. It is active against *M. tuberculosis* and *M. leprae*. Ethionamide is 80 percent absorbed from the gastrointestinal tract. It is widely distributed in tissues and body fluids, including CSF where the concentrations equal those in the blood. Ethionamide is metabolized in the liver to active and inactive metabolites which are excreted in the urine. Only 1 to 5 percent of a dose is excreted unchanged in the urine.

Ethionamide is the most poorly tolerated antituberculosis agent. Gastrointestinal distress (nausea, vomiting, and abdominal pain) is almost universal and typically quite severe, often necessitating discontinuation of the drug. Other adverse effects include diarrhea and a bitter metallic taste (that causes profound anorexia), hepatotoxicity (which occurs in 5 percent of patients), and neurotoxicity (mental disturbances, and peripheral neuropathy). The neurotoxicity may be alleviated by the administration of pyridoxine.

Cycloserine Cycloserine is an antibiotic isolated from *Streptomyces orchidaceus*. It interferes with the first stage of cell wall synthesis (see Chapter 45). Cycloserine is well absorbed when administered orally. It is distributed widely in tissues and body fluids, including CSF. Approximately 65 percent of the dose is excreted unchanged in the urine, and the remainder is metabolized to unknown substances.

Cycloserine is well tolerated in terms of gastrointestinal side effects, but it has substantial potential central nervous system toxicity. High serum concentrations may precipitate focal or tonic-clonic seizures. Psychic disturbances such as excitement, aggression, confusion, and depression are not infrequent. The serum concentrations of cycloserine should be monitored during therapy.

Para-Aminosalicylic Acid (PAS) PAS has a weak bacteriostatic activity against *M. tuberculosis*. It is 85 percent absorbed from the gastrointestinal tract. PAS is excreted in unchanged active form (20 percent) and as metabolites (80 percent) in the urine. The usual dose of the drug (10 to 12 g daily) is associated with a high frequency of gastrointestinal intolerance, which often causes poor patient compliance. In addition, hypersensitivity reactions occurs in 5 to 10 percent of patients.

Capreomycin Capreomycin is a macrocyclic polypeptide antibiotic isolated from *Streptomyces capreolus*. It is active only against mycobacteria. Capreomycin is not absorbed after oral administration and must be administered intramuscularly. Approximately 60 to 80 percent of a dose is excreted unchanged in the urine; the remainder is inactivated in the body. The elimination half-life of capreomycin (2 to 3 h in persons with normal renal function) is extended to over 50 h in functionally anephric patients. Nephrotoxicity and ototoxicity (vertigo, tinnitus, and deafness) are the most serious adverse effects of the drug. Capreomycin should not be given in combination with streptomycin or other aminoglycosides.

Amikacin and Kanamycin Amikacin and kanamycin are aminoglycoside antibiotics discussed in Chapter 46. Both are active against *M. tuberculosis*, but amikacin is more potent. The pharmacokinetics and toxicities of these two drugs are similar.

CHEMOTHERAPY OF TUBERCULOSIS

Two characteristics of tubercle bacilli, their slow rate of growth and their high rate of mutation to resistant forms, have important implications for the therapy of tuberculosis. The doubling time of tubercle bacilli *in vitro* is 18 to 24 hours compared with 30 minutes for *Staphylococcus aureus* and enteric gram-negative organisms. The slow rate of growth accounts for the very long duration of chemotherapy ($\geq$ 6 months) needed to cure tuberculosis.

Tubercle bacilli have spontaneous, predictable rates of mutation that confer resistance to antimycobacterial agents. Populations of tubercle bacilli never exposed to any drug will all contain mutants spontaneously resistant to one or another agent at a rate of 1 in 10^6 to 10^8 organisms. Large populations of tubercle bacilli which exist in pulmonary cavities (10^9 to 10^{11}) contain a significant number of organisms resistant to any one drug. When a single agent is used to treat tuberculosis, the sensitive organisms are killed while the resistant mutants multiply and eventually emerge as the dominant phenotype.

Mutations that confer resistance to various antimycobacterial agents are not linked; hence, resistance to one drug is not associated with resistance to an unrelated drug. For example, isoniazid-resistant mutants occur with a frequency of 1 in 10^6 organisms while mutations causing resistance to rifampin occur with a frequency of 1 in every 10^7 to 10^8 organisms. The likelihood of spontaneous mutations causing resistance to both isoniazid and rifampin is the product of these probabilities, i.e., 1 in 10^{13} to 10^{14}. Because the total number of bacilli in an infected person, even with advanced cavitary disease, does not approach 10^{13}, the development of spontaneous dual resistance is highly improbable. That the mutations are not linked is the basis for using multidrug regimens in the treatment of tuberculosis so that resistant mutants would not be selected. The regimen used must contain at least two drugs to which the infecting organism is susceptible; each helps prevent the emergence of resistance to the other.

Successful treatment of tuberculosis requires eradication of two different subpopulations of tubercle bacilli. The first subpopulation, extracellular tubercle bacilli, is large and includes drug-resistant mutants. Eradication of this subpopulation requires administration of at least two agents to which the organism is susceptible. Failure to eradicate these organisms results in acquired resistance and treatment failure. The second subpopulation, intracellular tubercle bacilli, is small ($< 10^4$ organisms) and does not contain resistant mutants. These organisms, however, multiply slower than extracellular bacilli and are, therefore, killed very slowly by the chemotherapeutic agents. Eradication of this subpopulation requires a long course of therapy. Failure to eradicate these organisms results in persistence of tubercle bacilli and relapse after therapy is completed. Established regimens which have proven to be effective in drug-sensitive infections include: (1) isoniazid and rifampin administered for 9 months, and (2) isoniazid, rifampin, and pyrazinamide administered for 2 months followed by isoniazid and rifampin for an additional 4 months. Pyrazinamide is active only against intracellular tubercle bacilli. Its inclusion in the chemotherapeutic regimens permits shortening the length of therapy from 9 months to 6 months.

The prevalence of drug-resistant organisms in the United States has steadily increased in the past three decades. Currently 9 percent of the isolates exhibit resistance to one of the first-line drugs. Furthermore, multidrug-resistant strains, defined as *M. tuberculosis* resistant to both isoniazid and rifampin, with or without resistance to other agents, have been reported in some areas. In order to provide at least two effective agents until the *in vitro* susceptibilities become available, a four-drug regimen with isoniazid, rifampin, pyrazinamide, and ethambutol or streptomycin is currently recommended for the initial, empiric treatment of tuberculosis. If susceptibility to isoniazid and rifampin is documented, ethambutol is discontinued. Pyrazinamide is continued for 2 months and isoniazid and rifampin are continued for a full 6 months (9 months in patients with human immunodeficiency virus infection, and those with disseminated disease, or disease involving bones or joints).

In areas with high frequency of multidrug-resistant strains, initial empiric treatment of tuberculosis should include at least five drugs to protect against additional acquired resistance. For patients with HIV infection in these areas, a six-drug regimen based on local patterns of resistance may be indicated until the susceptibility pattern of the patient's organism becomes available.

DRUGS ACTIVE AGAINST *MYCOBACTERIUM AVIUM* COMPLEX AND *MYCOBACTERIUM LEPRAE*

Rifabutin

Rifabutin is a semisynthetic derivative of rifamycin S, an antibiotic produced by *Streptomyces mediterranei*. Its chemical structure is

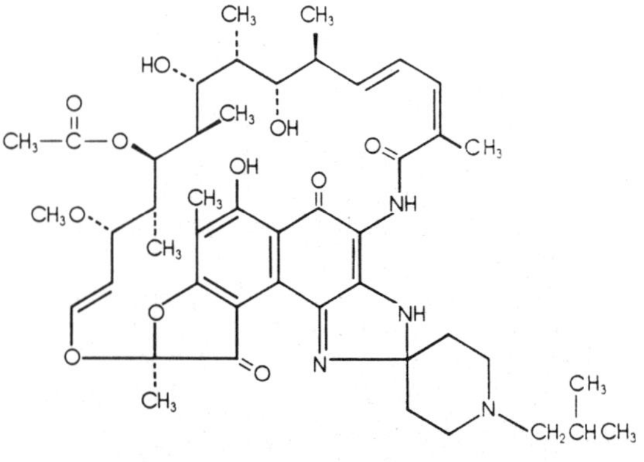

The mechanism of action of rifabutin is similar to that of rifampin. Rifabutin is more potent than rifampin against *Mycobacterium avium* complex. Their activities against *M. tuberculosis* are similar.

Approximately 53 percent of administered rifabutin is absorbed from the gastrointestinal tract. The drug is lipophilic and concentrates in tissues (such as lung and liver) and macrophages. The serum levels are relatively low; with equal doses, the serum concentrations of rifampin exceed those of rifabutin by more than 8 fold. Rifabutin is 85 percent bound to plasma proteins.

Rifabutin is metabolized in the liver to desacetyl rifabutin, which is only slightly less active than the parent compound and is excreted into the urine. The elimination half-life of rifabutin is 48 h.

The adverse effects of rifabutin are similar to those of rifampin. The drug is used for the prevention of *M. avium* complex infection in patients with acquired immunodeficiency syndrome.

Macrolides

Clarithromycin and azithromycin, discussed in Chapter 47, are the most potent currently available drugs against *M. avium* complex. The preferred regimen for *M. avium* infection in patients with acquired immunodeficiency syndrome consists of either clarithromycin or azithromycin combined with ethambutol. Usually a third agent (rifabutin or clofazimine) is added to the regimen. Therapy should continue for the lifetime of the patient if clinical and microbiological improvement is observed.

Clofazimine

Clofazimine, a synthetic agent, is a substituted iminophenazine. Its chemical structure is

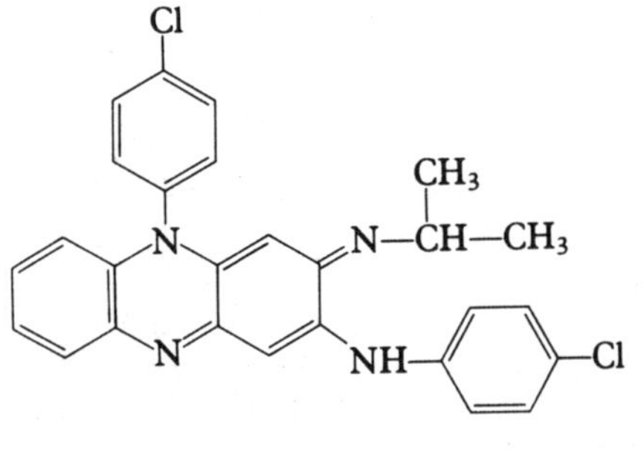

Clofazimine is weakly bactericidal against *M. leprae*. In addition, it is active against *M. avium* complex. It acts by inhibiting transcription resulting from direct binding to DNA.

Approximately 45 to 62 percent of orally administered clofazimine is absorbed. The drug is widely distributed in the body and retained for a long time. Clofazimine is lipophilic and is deposited in the adipose tissue, the skin, the reticuloendothelial system, and the distal small intestine at the site of absorption. It is taken up by macrophages but does not penetrate into the central nervous system. Clofazimine is not excreted in the urine or metabolized to any significant extent, biliary excretion appears to be the major route of disposition. It is eliminated very slowly with a half-life that is at least 70 days. A daily dose of 100 mg eventually results in total accumulation of at least 10 g of the drug in tissues.

The principle adverse effects of clofazimine are related to the skin and the gastrointestinal tract. The compound is a dye and the skin and body fluids, including urine, sputum, and sweat, acquire a dark-reddish hue after a few weeks of treatment, due to the deposition of red crystals. The pigmentation increases with time and is accompanied by dryness and itching of the skin. When clofazimine is given at high doses for extended periods, it is deposited in the small intestinal wall, causing segmental thickening which may be associated with abdominal discomfort and a variety of gastrointestinal disturbances.

Clofazimine is used in a triple drug combination (dapsone, rifampin, and clofazimine) for the treatment of multibacillary forms of leprosy. It is also used, as part of a multidrug regimen, for the treatment of *M. avium* complex infection in patients with acquired immunodeficiency syndrome.

Dapsone

Dapsone (4,4-diaminodiphenyl sulfone, DDS) is a synthetic compound which was first introduced for the therapy of leprosy in 1941.

NH_2— —SO_2— —NH_2

Dapsone is a structural analog of para-aminobenzoic acid. Like sulfonamides, it blocks the synthesis of folic acid by competitive inhibition of the enzyme dihydropteroate synthetase. Dapsone is weakly bactericidal for *M. leprae*. Secondary resistance may develop particularly in patients with multibacillary disease. Primary resistance to dapsone occurs with a varying frequency, depending on geographic location.

Dapsone is slowly and nearly completely absorbed from the gastrointestinal tract. It is 70 percent bound to plasma proteins and penetrates readily into tissues and body fluids. Dapsone is acetylated by N-acetyl transferase, the same enzyme that acetylates isoniazid. There are large differences in the rate of clearance of dapsone from the body as the result of genetic polymorphism in acetylating enzyme. As a consequence the half-life of the drug varies widely from 20 to 44 h, with an average of 28 h. Although the serum concentration of dapsone is higher in slow acetylators than in rapid acetylators, the acetylation phenotype does not affect the efficacy of the drug. Dapsone is ultimately excreted in the urine, predominantly as glucuronide and sulfate conjugates.

The most common adverse reactions of dapsone are anemia and methemoglobinemia. Hemolysis is a dose-related effect and occurs more commonly in persons with glucose-6-phosphate dehydrogenase deficiency. The most serious hematologic side effect is marrow suppression which is rare, but deaths due to agranulocytosis and aplastic anemia have been reported. Other adverse effects of dapsone include allergic reactions, drug fever, nausea, vomiting, vertigo, tinnitus, blurred vision, and peripheral neuropathy (predominantly motor).

The major indication for dapsone is leprosy. Multibacillary disease is treated for a minimum of two years with the triple drug combination of dapsone, rifampin, and clofazimine. Paucibacillary disease is treated with a 6 month course of dapsone combined with rifampin. Dapsone is also used for the treatment (combined with trimethoprim) and prophylaxis of *Pneumocystis carinii* pneumonia in patients with HIV infection who are allergic to sulfonamides.

BIBLIOGRAPHY

Alexander, M.R., S.G. Louie, and B.G. Guernsey: "Isoniazid-Associated Hepatitis," *Clin. Pharmacol.* **1**: 148-153 (1982).

Barnes, P.F., and S.A. Barrows: "Tuberculosis in the 1990's," *Ann. Intern. Med.* **119**: 400-410 (1993).

Bass, J.B., Jr., L.S. Farer, P.C. Hopewell, and R.F. Jacobs: "Treatment of Tuberculosis and Tuberculosis Infection in Adults and Children," *Am. Rev. Resp. Dis.* **134**: 355-363 (1986).

Borcherding, S.M., A.M. Baciewicz, and T.H. Self: "Update on Rifampin Drug Interactions II," *Arch. Intern. Med.* **152**: 711-716 (1992).

Combs, D.L., R.J. O'Brien, and L.J. Geiter: "USPHS Tuberculosis Short-Course Chemotherapy Trial 21: Effectiveness, Toxicity, and Acceptability," *Ann. Intern. Med.* **112**: 397-406 (1990).

Davidson, P.T. and H.Q. Le: "Drug Treatment of Tuberculosis - 1992," *Drugs* **43**: 651-673 (1992).

Grosset, J.: "Bacteriologic Basis of Short-Course Chemotherapy for Tuberculosis," *Clin. Chest Med.* **1**: 231-241 (1980).

Hastings, R.C., and S.G. Franzblau: "Chemotherapy of Leprosy," *Ann. Rev. Pharmacol. Toxicol.* **28**: 231-245 (1988).

Horsburgh, C.R., Jr.: "*Mycobacterium avium* Complex Infection in the Acquired Immunodeficiency Syndrome," *N. Engl. J. Med.* **324**: 1332-1338 (1991).

Initial Therapy for Tuberculosis in the Era of Multidrug Resistance. Recommendations of the Advisory Council for the Elimination of Tuberculosis, *MMWR.* **42 (RR-7)**: 1-8 (1993).

Iseman, M.D.: "Treatment of Multidrug-Resistant Tuberculosis," *N. Engl. J. Med.* **329**: 784-791 (1993).

Kamper, C.A., T.C. Meng, J. Nussbaum, J. Chiu, et al.: "Treatment of Mycobacterium avium Complex Bacteremia in AIDS with a Four-Drug Oral Regimen," *Ann. Intern. Med.* **116**: 466-472 (1992).

Nightingale, S.D., D.W. Cameron, F.M. Gordin, et al.: "Two Controlled Trials of Rifabutin Prophylaxis Against *Mycobacterium avium* Complex Infection in AIDS," *N. Engl. J. Med.* **329**: 828-833 (1993).

CHAPTER 49

Antifungal and Antiviral Drugs

Henry W. Hitner

ANTIFUNGAL AGENTS

The development of antifungal drugs has not been as successful as that of the antibiotics. Unlike bacteria that are prokaryotic, both fungal and mammalian cells are eukaryotic. Consequently, targets of selective toxicity for drug development are more difficult to identify. The main target of currently available drugs is the fungal cell membrane that utilizes ergosterol, rather than cholesterol, as the primary membrane sterol. Amphotericin B, nystatin, flucytosine, and griseofulvin are drugs that have been available for many years. Newer additions to the antifungal drug armamentarium include a number of azole ring derivatives that are divided into imidazole and triazole subclasses.

For therapeutic purposes, fungal infections are divided into three categories: cutaneous, mucocutaneous, and systemic. Cutaneous fungal infections are the most common and involve the skin, hair, and nails; common infections include athlete's foot, ringworm, and *Tinea cruris*. Most infections can be treated with over-the-counter or prescription topical agents such as tolnaftate, undecylenic acid, clotrimazole, and miconazole. For deep infection, particularly of the nail beds, griseofulvin (administered orally) is the drug of choice. Ketoconazole, an imidazole derivative, is administered orally for cutaneous infections that do not respond to topical treatment or to griseofulvin.

Mucocutaneous infections, mostly *Candida albicans*, involve the moist skin and mucous membranes (e.g., gastrointestinal tract, perianal, and vulvovaginal areas). Agents used topically include amphotericin B, nystatin, miconazole, and clotrimazole. Ketoconazole and fluconazole are administered orally for treatment of chronic infections.

Systemic fungal infections occur less frequently, but are a serious problem because they are usually chronic in nature and difficult to diagnose. Systemic infections also occur more frequently in immunocompromised individuals. Many patients with acquired immune deficiency syndrome (AIDS) require antifungal maintenance therapy to prevent recurrence. In addition, chemoprophylaxis can be initiated to prevent or delay the development of infection. Amphotericin B is usually indicated for severe, life-threatening infections. Azole ring derivatives that include ketoconazole, fluconazole, and itraconazole provide alternative therapy to amphotericin B; they are also generally preferred for nonlife-threatening infections, maintenance therapy and chemoprophylaxis.

Amphotericin B

Amphotericin B is a large polyene antibiotic derived from *Streptomyces nodosus*. The compound has a broad spectrum of antifungal activity, including *Candida albicans*, *Leishmania brasiliensis*, *Mycobacterium leprae*, *Histoplasma capsulatum*, *Blastomyces dermatitidus*, and *Coccidioides immitis*. It has both fungistatic and fungicidal activity, dependent on the dose used. Its chemical structure is shown in Fig. 49-1.

Mechanism of Action The antifungal activity of amphotericin B is due to its binding to sterols, particularly ergosterol, in the cell membrane of sensitive fungi (see Table 49-1). This interaction creates pores in the membrane and increases membrane permeability to small molecules, thus reducing the function of the membrane as an osmotic barrier and making the cell more susceptible to destruction. Amphotericin B is active in growing and resting cells. However, the drug is

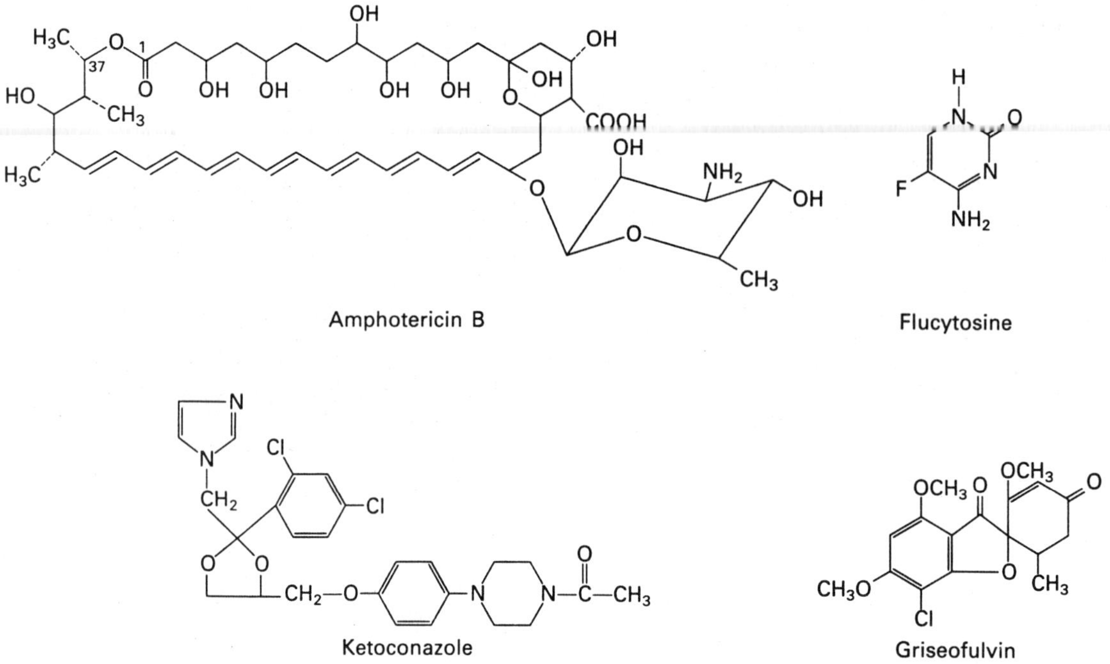

FIGURE 49-1. *Structures of a few common antifungal drugs.*

TABLE 49-1. Mechanisms of action of antifungal agents

Drugs	Mechanism of action
Polyene antifungals Amphotericin B Nystatin	Bind to sterols (e.g., ergosterol) in the cell membrane, forming pores or channels that increase membrane permeability and susceptibility to destruction.
Flucytosine	Converted to 5-fluorouracil and 5-fluorodeoxyuridylic acid in sensitive fungi. 5-Fluorodeoxyuridylic acid inhibits thymidylate synthetase. The triphosphate of 5-fluorouracil is incorporated into RNA.
Griseofulvin	Inhibits fungal cell mitosis by disrupting the mitotic spindle.
Imidazole antifungals Ketoconazole Miconazole Clotrimazole Econazole Butoconazole Oxiconazole Sulconazole	Inhibit ergosterol biosynthesis which increases fungal cell membrane permeability and susceptibility to destruction.
Triazole antifungals Fluconazole Itraconazole Terconazole	Same mechanism as the imidazoles.

not highly selective and will interfere with membrane function of the mammalian host cell.

Pharmacokinetics Amphotericin B is poorly absorbed from the gastrointestinal tract due to its large, bulky structure. When given by intravenous infusion, peak plasma levels are attained very rapidly. The plasma half-life is 24 h, though active drug can be detected in the plasma for up to 7 weeks after the last administered dose. The persistence of the drug in the body is consistent with its uptake into tissue reservoirs from which the drug is later slowly released.

Only 2 to 5 percent of the drug is excreted in the urine unchanged. The distribution of amphotericin B is limited; it crosses the blood-brain barrier poorly, although this may increase in the presence of inflammation. Thus the drug may have to be administered by intrathecal or intraventricular routes for fungal meningitis. It is also available for topical administration. Several new formulations of amphotericin B are under development. These include intravenous liposomal suspensions that allow higher dosages to be administered without additional toxicity, and a nasal spray that provides high intrapulmonary concentrations in respiratory infections.

Adverse Reactions Most patients receiving intravenous amphotericin B exhibit the side effects associated with this form of administration. Within 3 h after infusion is begun, an acute hypersensitivity reaction may occur. Symptoms include fever, headache, nausea, vomiting, abdominal pain, hypotension, flushing, sweating, and delirium. Hydrocortisone, added to the infusion, may reduce this reaction. Renal impairment is probably the most prevalent adverse reaction in patients receiving amphotericin B. This effect is time- and dose-dependent; it is reversible if recognized early enough and the dose of the drug reduced. Other adverse reactions may include fatigue, enteritis, thrombocytopenia, hypokalemia, and phlebitis at the injection site. Intrathecal administration may also produce paresthesias, vomiting, urinary retention, vertigo, and nerve palsies.

Therapeutic Uses Despite its many adverse reactions, amphotericin B remains the primary drug for therapy of acute, severe, systemic fungal infections. Amphotericin B is given for life-threatening infections of blastomycoses, histoplasmoses, and paracoccidioidomycoses. It is useful topically for both local cutaneous and mucocutaneous infections.

Nystatin

Nystatin was isolated in 1949 from *Streptomyces* and was the first antimycotic antibiotic to be discovered. It is a polyene antibiotic, structurally similar to amphotericin B. Nystatin has a fairly broad spectrum of activity including yeast and various fungi. The mechanism of nystatin's antifungal activity is similar to that of amphotericin B in that it binds to sterols in fungal cell membranes (Table 49-1). This increases membrane permeability, making the cell more susceptible to destruction.

Nystatin is available for topical or oral administration. When used topically, the drug does not cross the skin or mucous membranes. Absorption from the gastrointestinal tract is negligible following oral administration. Therefore, nystatin has few adverse reactions when given by either route. Used topically, the only potential problem is local burning and itching. Nystatin is given orally to treat local infections of the gastrointestinal tract. Large doses, administered orally, can produce gastrointestinal upset, including nausea, vomiting, and diarrhea. Nystatin is not available for systemic administration due to its severe renal toxicity. Therapy with nystatin is limited to the prevention and topical treatment of superficial candidal infections of the skin and mucous membranes including gums, gastrointestinal tract, rectum, and vagina.

Flucytosine

Flucytosine is a fluorinated pyrimidine derivative (see Fig. 49-1). Its spectrum of activity is narrower than that of amphotericin B; it includes *Candida*, *Cryptococcus*, and *Chromomycosis*. Clinical use has been disappointing due to a high incidence of resistance. It does, however, have a synergistic effect when used in combination with amphotericin B. The drug is given orally to treat systemic infections.

Mechanism of Action Flucytosine is converted in sensitive fungi to 5-fluorouracil by a fungal enzyme, diaminase. 5-Fluorouracil is further biotransformed to 5-fluorodeoxyuridylic acid, an inhibitor of thymidylate synthetase and thus DNA synthesis. The triphosphate of 5-fluorouracil can also be incorporated into RNA and will produce defective RNA. This mechanism is fairly selective, since mammalian cells do not biotransform large amounts of flucytosine to 5-fluorouracil.

Pharmacokinetics Flucytosine is well absorbed from the gastrointestinal tract and is therefore used by the oral route. It is well distributed throughout the body including the central nervous system (CNS). The plasma half-life is 3 to 6 h. Approximately 80 percent of the drug is excreted in the urine unchanged. Therefore the drug must be used with extreme caution in patients with renal impairment. The physician should also be aware that amphotericin B, which can reduce renal function, may increase the toxicity of flucytosine when they are used in combination.

Adverse Reactions The most common adverse reactions of flucytosine include nausea, vomiting, diarrhea, and rash. Anemia, leukopenia, thrombocytopenia, and elevation of hepatic enzymes, BUN, and creatinine have been reported. Therefore frequent monitoring of hepatic function and hematologic status is indicated during therapy. Less common reactions include sedation, vertigo, headache, and confusion.

Therapeutic Use Flucytosine is used primarily in combination with amphotericin B for treatment of selected systemic fungal infections. The agent is rarely used alone.

Griseofulvin

The spectrum of antimycotic activity of griseofulvin includes infections of the skin, nails, and scalp. It is fungistatic. The compound is inactive against yeast and fungi that cause deep, systemic infections. Resistance to its effectiveness can develop.

Mechanism of Action The mechanism of action of griseofulvin appears to be its ability to inhibit fungal cell mitosis, thus producing multinucleated defective cells (Table 49-1). It acts by binding to microtubules, disrupting the mitotic spindle. It can be classified as a spindle inhibitor.

Pharmacokinetics Griseofulvin, administered orally, undergoes variable absorption from the gastrointestinal tract. Due to its lipid solubility, absorption is enhanced when taken with a fatty meal. The drug distributes to growing nails and skin, binding to keratin and making the cells resistant to fungal infection. Therefore, only new growth is protected against the fungal infection. The drug is biotransformed in the liver, mostly to 6-methyl griseofulvin, which is slowly excreted in the urine. The plasma half-life of the parent compound is approximately 24 h.

Adverse Reactions Serious adverse reactions to griseofulvin are rare. Common side effects include headache, lethargy, fatigue, blurred vision, insomnia, and gastrointestinal upset. Hepatotoxicity has been reported. Griseofulvin reduces the effectiveness of oral anticoagulants by enhancing their metabolism. Concomitant use of barbiturates enhances the metabolism of griseofulvin and may require an increase in dose.

Therapeutic Use Griseofulvin is administered orally for treatment of cutaneous fungal infections. Since it does not destroy the fungal cells, but only inhibits new growth, the compound must be given for prolonged periods of time, usually several months or more.

Imidazole Derivatives

Several imidazole analogs are available for treatment of fungal infections. Those agents used for systemic administration include ketoconazole and miconazole; those used topically include miconazole, clotrimazole, econazole, butoconazole, oxiconazole, and sulconazole.

Mechanism of Action The antifungal activity of the imidazoles is due to their ability to selectively inhibit the activity of the fungal cytochrome P-450 system that catalyzes 14α-demethylation of lanosterol, the precursor of ergosterol. Reduction of ergosterol synthesis increases fungal cell membrane permeability and susceptibility to destruction. Only at high concentrations do imidazole antifungals interfere with the biosynthesis of cholesterol in humans. The imidazoles are generally fungistatic, but may exert fungicidal activity at higher doses.

Ketoconazole

Ketoconazole has broad antifungal activity including many candidal infections. The chemical structure is shown in Fig. 49-1.

Pharmacokinetics Ketoconazole is readily absorbed from the gastrointestinal tract under acidic conditions. Agents that reduce gastric acidity (e.g., anticholinergics, H_2-receptor blockers, and antacids) reduce absorption and decrease the therapeutic effectiveness of ketoconazole. Peak plasma levels occur approximately 2 h after oral administration. The drug is extensively biotransformed in the liver; metabolites are excreted largely in the bile and feces, with smaller amounts in the urine. Ketoconazole does not penetrate well into the cerebrospinal fluid which limits its effectiveness in treatment of CNS infections.

Adverse Reactions The most frequent side effects of ketoconazole are nausea, vomiting, and diarrhea. Other untoward effects include rash, itching, dizziness, constipation, fever, chills, and headache. Ketoconazole can inhibit the biosynthesis of sex hormones and, less frequently, adrenal steroids. Reduced levels of testosterone may cause gynecomastia and impotency in males; females may experience menstrual irregularities. Hepatocellular toxicity, including fatalities, has been associated with ketoconazole. Hepatic function should be monitored during drug therapy.

Therapeutic Uses Ketoconazole has been shown to be most effective in chronic suppressive therapy. It is also very effective in treatment of chronic mucocutaneous candidiasis and cutaneous infections when administered by the oral route. Therapy may be for up to 1 year. Slow improvement makes ketoconazole less useful for acute, severe systemic mycoses. A topical preparation is also available.

Drug Interactions The ability of ketoconazole to inhibit human P-450 enzymes can interfere with drug metabolism. Reduced clearance of chlordiazepoxide, theophylline, cyclosporine, and warfarin have occurred. Rifampin, isoniazid, and cimetidine can reduce ketoconazole concentrations.

Miconazole

Miconazole is another synthetic imidazole derivative designed initially for topical treatment of candidal and other cutaneous infections of the skin and for vaginal candidiasis. Its primary use is still topical. Miconazole, administered intravenously, is highly toxic and therefore only used for severe systemic fungal infections in which patients do not respond or cannot tolerate amphotericin B. All other systemic use has been taken over by ketoconazole. Adverse reactions to topically administered miconazole include local burning, itching, and rash. Intravenous administration can cause nausea, vomiting, and anemia. Anaphylactoid reactions, CNS toxicity, hyponatremia, and phlebitis have been reported.

Clotrimazole

Clotrimazole is closely related to miconazole. It has broad antifungal activity and is very effective when applied topically to the skin and vaginal mucosa. Clinical improvement from vulvovaginal candidiasis usually occurs within 1 week. Other dermatophytes may take longer. Clotrimazole is also available as a topical oral form (troche) for treatment of oropharyngeal candidiasis. Adverse reactions from topical administration are local and include erythema, blistering, edema, pruritus, and urticaria. Used topically, less than 0.5 percent is absorbed through the intact skin, 5 to 10 percent from the vagina.

Econazole

Econazole is a derivatives of miconazole that is useful topically for the treatment of tinea pedis, tinea cruris, tinea corporis, tinea versicolor, and cutaneous candidiasis. When applied topically, less than 1 percent is absorbed systemically. Therefore, adverse reactions are local, consisting of burning, itching, and rash.

Butoconazole

Butoconazole is an imidazole derivative particularly effective against vulvovaginal infections produced by *Candida albicans* and *Candida tropicalis*. It is only used topically, and therefore only local adverse reactions have been reported.

Oxiconazole and Sulconazole

These two drugs are structurally related to other imidazoles; sulconazole contains sulfur. Both drugs are primarily indicated for the topical treatment of fungal skin infections. The efficacy of both drugs is similar to that of other antifungal imidazoles.

Triazoles

The antifungal triazoles demonstrate greater effectiveness, tissue penetration, and elimination half-life, and reduced toxicity when compared to the imidazoles. The antifungal action of the triazoles is similar to that of the imidazoles; however, triazoles bind more selectively to fungal P-

450 enzymes than to the mammalian counterpart; this may account for the reduced toxicity usually observed with triazoles as compared to imidazole drugs. Triazoles that are indicated for systemic administration include fluconazole and itraconazole; terconazole is only available for topical administration.

Fluconazole

Fluconazole was the first triazole to be approved; indications are for the treatment of cryptococcal meningitis and serious mucocutaneous or systemic candidal infections.

Pharmacokinetics Fluconazole is well absorbed from the gastrointestinal tract (the bioavailability is approximately 90 percent) and, unlike the absorption of ketoconazole, is independent of gastric acidity. The plasma half-life is 22 to 30 h; approximately 80 percent of fluconazole is eliminated unchanged in the urine. Consequently, the dosage should be adjusted in patients with reduced renal function. Initial loading doses allow for a more rapid achievement of the steady state. Drug concentrations in cerebrospinal fluid (CSF) are 60 to 90 percent of plasma concentrations.

Adverse Effects Fluconazole is generally well tolerated. Nausea, vomiting, and abdominal discomfort are the most common complaints; headache, rash, elevated hepatic enzymes, and thrombocytopenia are less frequently reported. Unlike ketoconazole, fluconazole does not usually affect the biosynthesis of sex hormones or adrenal steroids.

Therapeutic Uses Fluconazole is orally effective in the initial treatment of serious mucocutaneous candidal infections and in chronic suppressive therapy of cryptococcal meningitis. In the treatment of acute cryptococcal meningitis or serious systemic candidal infections, fluconazole is used alternatively in patients who fail to respond to, or are intolerant of, amphotericin B. Although less toxic than amphotericin B, fluconazole is also less effective during the initial treatment period.

Drug Interactions Fluconazole can inhibit the drug metabolizing enzymes associated with the cytochrome P-450 system and drug-drug interactions are similar to those reported with ketoconazole. The drug can increase the prothrombin time after warfarin administration. Fluconazole will increase the plasma concentration and reduce the biotransformation of tolbutamide, glyburide, and glipizide.

Itraconazole

The pharmacologic actions of itraconazole are similar to those of fluconazole; however, itraconazole has a broader spectrum of antifungal activity.

The oral absorption of itraconazole is increased by food and administration with meals is recommended. Tissue concentrations are often higher than those of plasma; however, penetration into the CSF is low. The elimination half-life increases with dosage and usually ranges from 17 to 30 h. Itraconazole is highly protein bound (99.8 percent). The compound undergoes extensive hepatic metabolism to a large number of inactive products, including hydroxyitraconazole, the major metabolite. Fecal excretion of the parent drug is between 3 and 18 percent; urinary elimination of the metabolites accounts for over 40 percent of an administered dose.

Nausea, vomiting, and headache are the most common side effects. Hypokalemia, elevation of hepatic enzymes, hypertension, and adrenal insufficiency may occur at higher dosages.

Itraconazole has demonstrated oral effectiveness in a wide variety of fungal infections including blastomycosis, histoplasmosis, aspergillosis, and sporotrichosis. The drug is considered alternative therapy to amphotericin B in serious life-threatening infections; however, itraconazole is usually preferred for nonlife-threatening infections and chronic therapy.

Itraconazole can interfere with P-450 drug metabolizing enzymes similar to other azole derivatives. Life-threatening ventricular tachycardia and torsade de pointes have been reported in patients taking both itraconazole and the antihistamine terfenadine. Therefore, this combination is contraindicated.

Terconazole

Terconazole is only available for topical treatment of vulvovaginal candidiasis. Vulvovaginal burning, irritation, and itching are possible local reactions. Although only 0.8 percent of a topical dose is absorbed, transient headache, fever, and chills (flu-like syndrome) have been reported during the initial treatment period.

Additional Antifungal Compounds: Topically Applied Agents

Although orally administered griseofulvin is very useful in the treatment of cutaneous infections, many mild or superficial infections can be treated effectively with topical agents, thus causing less adverse reactions. Such compounds shown to be effective include undecylenic acid, tolnaftate, haloprogin, and ciclopirox olamine in addition to the imidazole and triazole derivatives, which have previously been mentioned.

ANTIVIRAL AGENTS

The chemotherapy of viral infections has been approached by three different modalities. These include (1) prophylactic immunization, (2) use of an endogenous antiviral substance (i.e., interferon), and (3) antiviral drugs. Immunization has made great strides in the prevention of many viral infections; among those for which vaccines have been produced include measles, mumps, polio, rubella, smallpox, and specific types of influenza. Interferons are a group of endogenous antiviral substances produced by lymphocytes and viral-infected cells. Interferons and inducers of endogenous synthesis are discussed in greater detail in Chapter 44.

Progress in the development of clinically useful antiviral drugs has recently accelerated. This is primarily due to the increased effort expended in the search for effective treatments of human immunodeficiency virus (HIV) infection that is associated with acquired immunodeficiency syndrome (AIDS). AIDS patients are also more susceptible to other viral infections as immune function becomes impaired.

There are three stages to multiplication of viruses: (1) adsorption, penetration, and uncoating as the virus enters the host cell and sheds its protective coat; (2) synthesis of viral components; and (3) assembly and release of the virus which can destroy or permanently change the cell (Fig. 49-2). Viruses contain either DNA or RNA. DNA viruses that cause infections include Herpes simplex virus (HSV) types 1 and 2, varicella-zoster (VZ), cytomegalovirus (CMV), and Epstein-Barr virus. RNA virus-induced infections include HIV, influenza, and respiratory syncytial infections. Acyclovir, ganciclovir, foscarnet, vidarabine, trifluridine, and idoxuridine are used to treat infections caused by DNA viruses. Amantadine, zidovudine, didanosine, and zalcitabine are indicated for infections caused by RNA viruses. Ribavirin is effective against several DNA and RNA viruses. Table 49-2 summarizes the treatment of viral infections.

Acyclovir

Acyclovir (acycloguanosine) is a nucleoside analog of the pyrimidine, guanosine. It has the following chemical structure, which includes a linear (acyclic) side chain instead of a cyclic sugar:

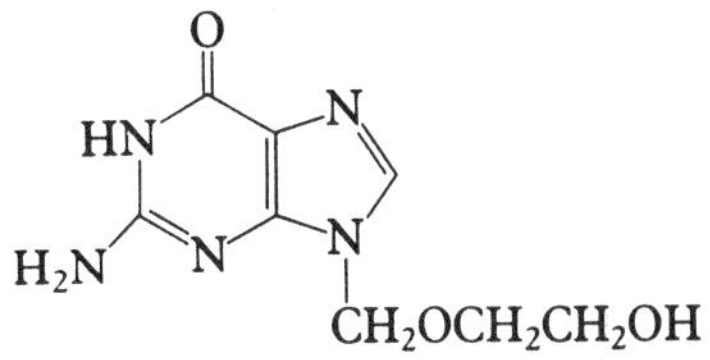

O
HN N
H_2N N N
$CH_2OCH_2CH_2OH$

Mechanism of Action The mechanism of action of acyclovir involves its conversion to the triphosphate and subsequent inhibition of viral DNA synthesis; its activity is highly selective (Fig. 49-2). The compound enters herpes virus-infected cells and is phosphorylated to the monophosphate by herpes virus-induced thymidine kinase; uninfected cells do not use acyclovir as a substrate. The monophosphate is further converted into the diphosphate and to the triphosphate (acycloguanosine triphosphate, acyclo-GTP). Acyclo-GTP is a competitive inhibitor of herpes viral DNA polymerase and is also incorporated into viral DNA, where it functions as a chain terminator, thus preventing the further elongation of the DNA molecule and therefore viral replication. Other antiviral mechanisms may be involved against cytomegalovirus (CMV) and Epstein-Barr virus.

Pharmacokinetics Acyclovir is available for topical, oral, and intravenous administration. Transcutaneous absorption is limited; therefore, no drug is detectable in blood or urine following topical use. Absorption of acyclovir from the gastrointestinal tract is limited (15 to 30 percent); the concentration of drug in the blood is much lower than following intravenous administration. Acyclovir is widely distributed in tissues and in body fluids; concentration in CSF is approximately 50 percent of plasma values. Plasma protein binding is relatively low. The major route of elimination of acyclovir is renal excretion of unchanged drug by glomerular filtration and tubular secretion; this accounts for 60 to 90 percent of

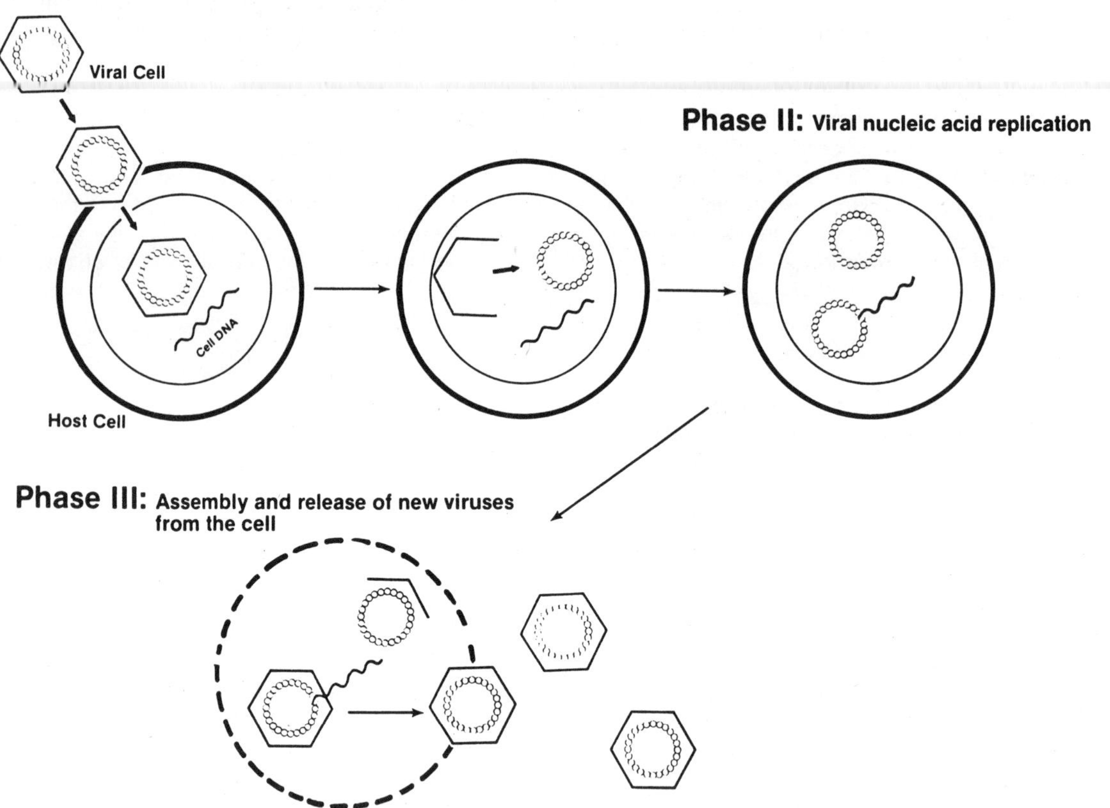

Phase I Inhibitors

Amantadine Rimantadine	Blocks adsorption, penetration, and assembly of virus.

Phase II Inhibitors

Acyclovir Ganciclovir	Triphosphate competitively inhibits viral DNA polymerase. It also incorporates into DNA, acting as a chain terminator.
Trifluridine Vidarabine Idoxuridine	Triphosphate inhibits viral DNA polymerase.
Zidovudine Didanosine Zalcitabine	Inhibits viral reverse transcriptase (RNA-dependent DNA polymerase) and acts as a chain terminator.
Ribavirin	May block synthesis of viral RNA.
Foscarnet	Inhibits DNA polymerase and reverse transcriptase.

FIGURE 49-2. *The phases of viral cell multiplication and mechanisms of action of drugs that inhibit them.*

TABLE 49-2. Summary of treatment of viral infections

Viral infection	Drugs available
Herpes simplex	
Keratitis	Trifluridine, vidarabine, idoxuridine
Genital	Acyclovir
Encephalitis	Acyclovir, vidarabine
Neonatal	Acyclovir, vidarabine
Disseminated, adult	Acyclovir, vidarabine
Acyclovir-resistant	Foscarnet
Varicella zoster	Acyclovir, vidarabine,
Acyclovir-resistant	Foscarnet
Cytomegalovirus	
Retinitis	Ganciclovir, foscarnet
Respiratory syncytial virus	Ribavirin
Influenza A	Amantadine, rimantadine
Human immunodeficiency virus	Zidovudine, didanosine, zalcitabine

the intravenous dose. The only major urinary metabolite is 9-carboxymethoxymethylguanine, which may account for up to 14 percent of the dose. Plasma half-life in a patient with normal renal function is 2.5 to 3.5 h. Probenecid, which alters the tubular secretion of acyclovir, reduces urinary excretion and increases its plasma half-life.

Adverse Reactions Only local adverse reactions occur with acyclovir ointment. These include mild pain, transient burning and stinging, pruritus, and rash. The most common adverse reactions to oral administration are nausea, vomiting, and headache. Less frequent reactions include diarrhea, dizziness, anorexia, fatigue, edema, skin rash, leg pain, adenopathy, and sore throat. Acyclovir may also cause fever, cardiac palpitations, acne, and depression.

The most frequent adverse reactions to intravenous acyclovir are inflammation or phlebitis at the injection site, reversible renal dysfunction (as shown by transient elevations of serum creatinine and BUN), and itching, rash or hives. Less frequent reactions include diaphoresis, hematuria, hypotension, headache, and nausea and vomiting. Administered systemically, the drug is generally well tolerated.

Therapeutic Uses Acyclovir administered by intravenous injection is the drug of choice for treatment of serious infections caused by Herpes simplex virus (HSV) and varicella-zoster (VZ) virus. Intravenous use of acyclovir is indicated in HSV encephalitis, severe initial herpes genitalis, and in immunocompromised patients with cutaneous and mucocutaneous infections with HSV or infection with varicella-zoster (shingles).

Oral acyclovir is indicated in the treatment of initial episodes and treatment or suppression of recurrent episodes of genital herpes infection and in varicella (chicken pox) and herpes zoster (shingles).

Acyclovir ointment is indicated in the management of initial herpes genitalis and in nonlife-threatening mucocutaneous HSV infections in immunocompromised patients. The compound produces a decrease in healing time, duration of viral shedding, and pain. There is no evidence of clinical benefit in patients with recurrent herpes genitalis or herpes labialis.

Ganciclovir

Ganciclovir is a nucleoside analog of guanine that is structurally similar to acyclovir. The mechanism of action of the drug is the same as acyclovir and the antiviral activity of ganciclovir triphosphate is similar to acyclovir; however, this compound is significantly more active against cytomegalovirus

(CMV). The main indications for ganciclovir are CMV retinitis and other life-threatening CMV infections in immunocompromised patients.

Ganciclovir is administered only by intravenous injection. Plasma protein binding is very low (1 to 2 percent) and the drug is widely distributed throughout the body. Biotransformation is insignificant and over 90 percent of the compound is excreted by the kidneys in an unchanged form. The elimination half-life is normally between 2 and 4 h and is increased in patients with impaired renal function.

The adverse effects of ganciclovir are usually more serious than those caused by acyclovir. Dose-limiting toxicities are usually due to granulocytopenia and thrombocytopenia. Concurrent therapy with zidovudine can cause severe myelosuppression. Other adverse reactions include anemia, fever, confusion, abnormal liver function, phlebitis, and rash. Ganciclovir is teratogenic, carcinogenic, and causes aspermatogensis in laboratory animals.

Vidarabine

Chemically, vidarabine (adenine arabinoside) is a stereoisomer of adenosine in which arabinose substitutes for the ribose sugar. Like acyclovir, vidarabine is converted to the triphosphate in virus-infected cells. Vidarabine triphosphate inhibits DNA polymerase, thus reducing DNA synthesis. It is fairly selective for viral DNA polymerase.

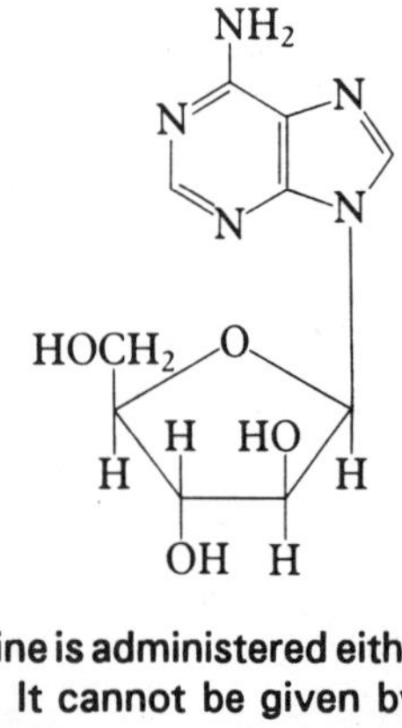

NH_2
N N
N N
$HOCH_2$ O
H HO
H H
OH H

Vidarabine is administered either intravenously or topically. It cannot be given by subcutaneous or intramuscular routes due to its low solubility and poor absorption. When given intravenously, the drug is infused for 12 to 24 h; the plasma elimination half-life is approximately 4 h. The compound is deaminated to an active metabolite, arabinosylhypoxanthine, which is primarily excreted into the urine; only 1 to 3 percent appears in the urine as parent compound.

Vidarabine is used as an ophthalmic preparation for topical treatment of HSV keratitis. Although vidarabine is indicated for the treatment of herpes simplex virus encephalitis, neonatal herpes simplex infections, and herpes zoster, its use in these infection has largely been replaced by acyclovir. It is also available for intravenous administration in the treatment of HSV encephalitis, other severe systemic herpes infections.

Used systemically, the most common adverse reactions include anorexia, nausea, vomiting, and diarrhea. Occasionally, the drug may cause tremors, dizziness, hallucinations, confusion, psychosis, and ataxia. Reductions in red and white blood cells, and platelets may occur. In addition, the drug may cause liver dysfunction, weight loss, pruritus, rash, and hematemesis. Topical reactions are usually limited to localized burning and itching.

The drug is contraindicated in patients who develop hypersensitivity reactions to it. The drug should not be given to patients susceptible to fluid overloading, cerebral edema, or with impaired renal function. Those patients with reduced renal function may require a lower dose of the drug.

Trifluridine

Trifluridine (trifluorothymidine) is a halogenated thymidine derivative used as an ophthalmic solution for HSV-induced keratoconjunctivitis. Its mechanism of action is similar to acyclovir, ganciclovir, and vidarabine (Fig. 49-2); it is converted to the triphosphate, which inhibits DNA polymerase. Adverse reactions include local burning or stinging; no systemic effects have been reported following topical use. The drug appears to be effective, yet better tolerated than idoxuridine.

Idoxuridine

Idoxuridine is a halogenated derivative of deoxyuridine. The primary action of idoxuridine is the inhibition of DNA viral replication by inhibition of DNA polymerase. The major use of this drug is in the treatment of HSV keratitis.

Because of severe adverse reactions, the drug is only used topically on the eye. When applied topically to the eye, idoxuridine may cause the following adverse reactions: inflammatory edema of the eyelids, photophobia, lacrimal duct occlusion, and contact dermatitis.

Foscarnet

Foscarnet is a pyrophosphate analog of phosphonoacetic acid that has demonstrated potent antiviral activity against a variety of viruses. This includes HSV types 1 and 2, CMV, VZ, HIV, and influenza A virus. Foscarnet inhibits DNA polymerase and the reverse transcriptases of retroviruses by blocking the pyrophosphate binding site; this prevents viral chain elongation.

Foscarnet is administered by intravenous infusion and is distributed throughout the body; it accumulates to some extent in bone. The drug does not appear to be metabolized and is excreted primarily in the urine.

Fever, nausea, diarrhea, anemia, nephrotoxicity, vomiting, and headache are the most frequent adverse reactions. Granulocytopenia, genital ulceration, and seizures occur less frequently. Electrolyte disturbances involving magnesium, phosphate, calcium, and potassium may occur. Foscarnet chelates divalent cations, and ionized serum calcium should be measured if symptoms of hypocalcemia are evident. Renal function should also be monitored; adequate hydration can reduce the extent of renal damage. Use with other nephrotoxic drugs should be avoided.

Foscarnet is currently indicated for the treatment of CMV retinitis in patients with AIDS. The drug is active against acyclovir- and ganciclovir-resistant CMV. Other uses are currently under investigation.

Ribavirin

Ribavirin is a synthetic nucleoside analog that has shown to be effective *in vitro* against several DNA and RNA viruses, including respiratory syncytial virus (RSV), HSV, and influenza A and B viruses. It is approved for aerosol treatment of infants and young children with severe RSV infections. The compound may act by interfering with viral messenger RNA synthesis. Adverse reactions may include rash, headache, and fatigue. The drug may precipitate on the valves and tubing of a mechanical respirator, causing malfunctions. This may limit its use in those individuals who would benefit most from it. The drug has been used experimentally in AIDS patients with mixed results.

Amantadine

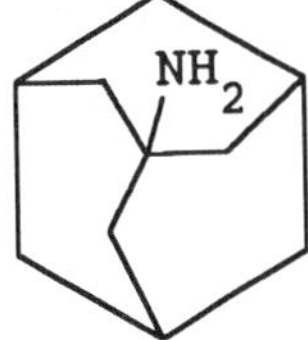

Amantadine is a synthetic stable amine with an unusual structure. The compound has a very narrow spectrum of antiviral activity and is only indicated in the treatment or prophylaxis of influenza A virus. The prophylactic use of amantadine is considered in high-risk patients, such as elderly persons in nursing homes, during influenza A epidemics. It is also used for treatment of Parkinson's disease (see Chapter 22).

The exact mechanism of action responsible for the antiviral activity of amantadine is not fully understood. Amantadine is believed to inhibit the adsorption of viral particles to host cell, resulting in delayed penetration of the virus into the cell and/or inhibition of uncoating which prevent the release of viral nucleic acid into the cell. (Fig. 49-2). Recent studies have demonstrated that the drug may inhibit virus assembly.

Amantadine is rapidly and completely absorbed following oral administration. The elimination half-life is 12 to 36 h, with peak levels occurring within 2 to 4 h. Amantadine is not significantly biotransformed; approximately 90 percent is eliminated unchanged in the urine.

Amantadine is fairly well tolerated. The major adverse reactions when used as a antiviral drug primarily involve the CNS and include confusion, ataxia, sleep disorders, tremors, and hallucinations. Anticholinergic effects have also been reported. Anorexia, nausea, vomiting, and orthostatic hypotension may also occur. Occasionally, amantadine may cause livedo reticularis, edema, and slurred speech. Generally, the adverse reactions are dose-related and reversible. The drug increases susceptibility to rubella and is therefore contraindicated in patients exposed to this virus. Amantadine is excreted in breast milk and thus should not be given to nursing mothers. Animal studies have shown teratogenic effects associated with this compound.

Rimantadine is a recently approved analog of amantadine that is also active against influenza A. It is reported to have a lower incidence of adverse CNS effects.

TREATMENT OF AIDS

Although a wide variety of compounds are being tested worldwide to treat human immunodeficiency virus (HIV)-infected patients, at this writing only three drugs are available and approved for use in the U.S.: zidovudine, didanosine, and zalcitabine. None of these can eradicate the infection; all are considered palliative therapy.

Zidovudine

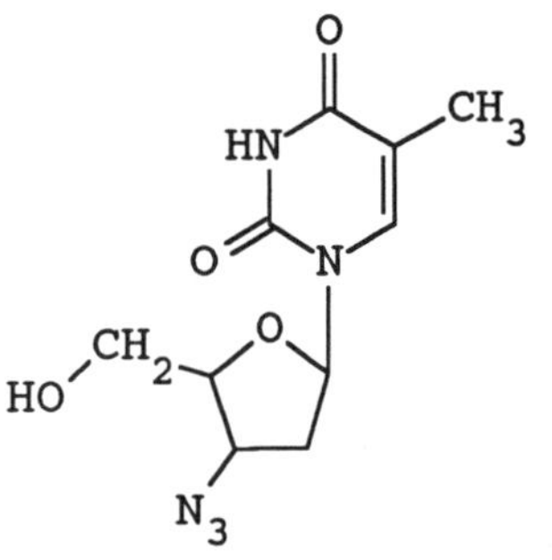

Zidovudine (formerly azidothymidine or AZT) is currently the drug of choice for initial treatment of AIDS. Zidovudine prolongs survival in patients with AIDS, and reduces the frequency and severity of opportunistic infections. Drug treatment is generally indicated when CD_4 lymphocyte (T-helper cell) counts fall below 500/mm^3. Zidovudine treatment increases CD_4 counts and reduces HIV p24 antigen levels that reflect the severity of infection. Some resistance to zidovudine usually develops after 6 months or more of treatment.

Mechanism of Action Zidovudine is inactive until it enters an infected cell, whereupon it is activated to the triphosphate form by the same enzymes that normally catalyze the phosphorylation of thymidine and thymidine nucleosides. Zidovudine triphosphate inhibits HIV viral RNA-dependent DNA polymerase, also known as *reverse transcriptase*. This action reduces viral replication and delays progression of the disease. Viral DNA polymerase is inhibited to a greater degree than human DNA polymerase. Zidovudine can also be incorporated into the DNA chain where it functions as a chain terminator.

Pharmacokinetics Zidovudine is well absorbed after oral administration. The drug is subject to first-pass metabolism and subsequently undergoes rapid liver biotransformation. Zidovudine can also be administered by slow intravenous infusion. The plasma half-life is about one hour; excretion is primarily in the urine as the glucuronide. Zidovudine is widely distributed and attains adequate levels in the CSF.

Adverse Reactions Bone marrow suppression is usually the most serious adverse effect. Anemia and neutropenia are the usual dose-limiting toxicities. Gastrointestinal complaints consist of nausea, anorexia, and vomiting. Neurologic disturbances include headache; insomnia; confusion; and less frequently, agitation or seizures. Muscular complaints include myalgia and myositis, the latter is associated with long-term treatment and may involve muscle wasting and elevations of creatinine kinase.

Drug Interactions Administration of zidovudine with other drugs that suppress bone marrow will increase hematologic toxicity. The toxicity of zidovudine and of other drugs that are metabolized by glucuronidation (e.g., aspirin, acetaminophen) may be increased with concomitant therapy. Probenecid and other drugs that decrease renal excretion may also increase zidovudine toxicity.

Didanosine

Didanosine (dideoxyinosine or DDI) is the second antiretroviral drug approved for the treatment of AIDS. The drug is a nucleoside analog of deoxyadenosine and is activated by cellular enzymes to the triphosphate form. The mechanism of action of didanosine is similar to that of zidovudine, i.e., the compound is an HIV reverse transcriptase inhibitor.

Didanosine is indicated for treatment of advanced HIV infection in patients who cannot tolerate zidovudine or who are experiencing deterioration during zidovudine therapy. Some didanosine-resistant isolates of HIV have been identified.

Didanosine is administered orally; however, it is rapidly degraded by gastric acid. Consequently, all formulations include a buffering agent to raise gastric pH. Bioavailability averages 20 to 50 percent and is significantly decreased in the presence of food. The drug is fairly well distributed and does penetrate the CSF, although to a lesser extent than with zidovudine. The plasma half-life is between 1 and 2 h; however, the intracellular half-life ranges between 12 and 24 h and allows less frequent daily dosing than with zidovudine. The metabolism of didanosine appears to be similar to that of endogenous purines; three metabolites identified in the urine were hypoxanthine, xanthine, and uric acid. Excretion of didanosine is primarily renal, but also involves the biliary and gastrointestinal tract.

Peripheral neuropathy is a frequent adverse reaction to didanosine. Symptoms usually include numbness, tingling, burning, and pain in the distal extremities. Pancreatitis is another dose-limiting effect that can be fatal. Other complaints include headache, confusion, insomnia, gastrointestinal disturbances, rash, and hyperuricemia. Although didanosine causes minimal suppression of bone marrow, some leukopenia or thrombocytopenia may occur.

Zalcitabine

Zalcitabine (dideoxycytidine or DDC) is a pyrimidine nucleoside analog of deoxycytidine. It is activated to the triphosphate form by cellular enzymes, inhibits HIV reverse transcriptase, and is also incorporated into the viral DNA chain where it functions as a chain terminator. Zalcitabine is indicated for the treatment of advanced AIDS; in addition, combination therapy with zidovudine provides additive and possibly synergistic effects.

Zalcitabine has good oral bioavailability, but this is significantly reduced when administered with food. Drug distribution is not as extensive as with zidovudine and CSF penetration is relatively low. The plasma half-life is between 1 and 3 h. Drug metabolism appears to be minimal; excretion is primarily renal.

Serious adverse reactions are similar to those of didanosine and include peripheral neuropathy and, to a lesser degree, pancreatitis. Other untoward reactions include gastrointestinal disturbances, rash, headache, dizziness, and myalgia.

BIBLIOGRAPHY

Antifungal Drugs

------- "Antifungal Drugs Used in Ear, Skin, and Mucous Membrane Infections," in *Drug Evaluations Annual 1993*, prepared by the Division of Drugs and Toxicology, American Medical Association, Chicago, 1993, pp. 1549-1592.

------- "Drugs Used for Systemic Mycoses," in *Drug Evaluations Annual 1993*, prepared by the Division of Drugs and Toxicology, American Medical Association, Chicago, 1993, pp. 1625-1647.

Benson, J.M., and M.C. Nahata: "Clinical Use of Systemic Antifungal Agents," *Clin. Pharmacol.* **7**: 424-438 (1988).

Blatchford, N.R.: "Treatment of Oral Candidosis with Itraconazole: A Review," *J. Am. Acad. Dermatol.* **23**: 565-567 (1990).

Bodey, G.P.: "Topical and Systemic Antifungal Agents," *Med. Clin. North Am.* **72**: 637-658 (1988).

Brajtburg, J., W.G. Powderly, G.S. Kobayashi, and G. Medoff: "Amphotericin B: Delivery Systems," *Antimicrob. Agents Chemother.* **34**: 381-384 (1990).

Cleary, J.D., J.W. Taylor, and S.W. Chapman: "Itraconazole in Antifungal Therapy," *Ann. Pharmacother.* **26**: 502-508 (1992).

Grant, S.M., and S.P. Clissold: "Itraconazole: A Review of its Pharmacodynamics and Pharmacokinetic Properties, and Therapeutic Use in Superficial and Systemic Mycoses," *Drugs* **37**: 310-344 (1989).

Grant, S.M., and S.P. Clissold: "Fluconazole: A Review of its Pharmacodynamic and Pharmacokinetic Properties, and Therapeutic Potential in Superficial and Systemic Mycoses," *Drugs* **39**: 877-916 (1990).

Larsen, R.A.: "Azoles and AIDS," *J. Infect. Dis.* **162**: 727-730 (1990).

Musial, C.E., F.R. Cockerill 3rd, and G.D. Roberts: "Fungal Infections of the Immunocompromised Host: Clinical and Laboratory Aspects," *Clin. Microbiol. Rev.* **1**: 349-364 (1988).

Sugar, A.M., J.J. Stern, and B. Dupont: "Overview: Treatment of Cryptococcal Meningitis," *Rev. Infect. Dis.* **12 (Suppl. 3)**: S338-S348 (1990).

Antiviral Drugs

------- "Antiviral Drugs," in *Drug Evaluations Annual 1993*, prepared by the Division of Drugs and Toxicology, American Medical Association, Chicago, 1993, pp. 1723-1753.

Betts, R.F., J.J. Treanor, P.S. Graham, D.W. Bentley, and R. Dolin: "Antiviral Agents to Prevent or Treat Influenza in the Elderly," *J. Respir. Dis.* **8 (Suppl. 11A)**: S56-S59 (1987).

Buhles, W.C., B.J. Mastre, A.J. Tinker, U. Strand, S.H. Koretz, and the Syntex Collaborative Ganciclovir Treatment Study Group: "Ganciclovir Treatment of Life- or Sight-Threatening Cytomegalovirus Infection: Experience in 314 Immunocompromised Patients," *Rev. Infect. Dis.* **10 (Suppl. 3)**: 495-506 (1988).

Fischl, M.A., D.D. Richman, N. Hansen, A.C. Collier, J.T. Carey, M.F. Para, W.D. Hardy, R. Dolin, W.G. Powderly, and J.D. Allan: "The Safety and Efficacy of Zidovudine (AZT) in the Treatment of Subjects with Mildly Symptomatic Human Immunodeficiency Virus Type 1 (HIV) Infection: A Double-Blind, Placebo-Controlled Trial," *Ann. Intern. Med.* **112**: 727-737 (1990).

Fletcher, C.V., J.A. Englund, B. Bean, B. Chinnock, D.M. Brundage, and H.H. Balfour Jr.: "Continuous Infusion of High-Dose Acyclovir for Serious Herpesvirus Infections," *Antimicrob. Agents Chemother.* **33**: 1375-1378 (1989).

Huff, J.C., B. Bean, H.H. Balfour Jr., O.L. Laskin, J.D. Connor, L. Corey, Y.J. Bryson, and P. McGuirt: "Therapy of Herpes Zoster with Oral Acyclovir," *Am. J. Med.* **85 (2A)**: 85-89 (1988).

Jabs, D.A., C. Enger, and J.G. Bartlett: "Cytomegalovirus Retinitis and Acquired Immunodeficiency Syndrome," *Arch. Ophthalmol.* **107**: 75-80 (1989).

Konig, H., E. Behr, J. Lower, and R. Kurth: "Azidothymidine Triphosphate is an Inhibitor of Both Human Immunodeficiency Virus Type 1 Reverse Transcriptase and DNA Polymerase Gamma," *Antimicrob. Agents Chemother.* **33**: 2109-2114 (1989).

Larder, B.A., G. Darby, and D.D. Richman: "HIV with Reduced Sensitivity to Zidovudine (AZT) Isolated During Prolonged Therapy," *Science* **243**: 1731-1734 (1989).

Laskin, O.L., C.M. Stahl-Bayliss, C.M. Kalman, and L.R. Rosecan: "Use of Ganciclovir to Treat Serious Cytomegalovirus Infections in Patients with AIDS," *J. Infect. Dis.* **155**: 323-327 (1987).

Laskin, O.L., D.M. Cederberg, J. Mills, L.J. Eron, D. Mildvan, S.A. Spector, et al.: "Ganciclovir for Treatment and Suppression of Serious Infections Caused by Cytomegalovirus, *Am. J. Med.* **83**: 201-207 (1987).

Richman, D.D.: "Antiviral Therapy of HIV Infection," *Annu. Rev. Med.* **42**: 69-90 (1991).

Shelton, M.J., A.M. O'Donnell, and G.D. Morse: "Didanosine," *Ann. Pharmacother.* **26**: 660-670 (1992).

Shepp, D.H., et al.: "Treatment of Varicella-Zoster Virus Infection in Severely Immunocompromised Patients: Randomized Comparison of Acyclovir and Vidarabine," *N. Engl. J. Med.* **314**: 208-212 (1986).

Spruance, S.L., J.C. Stewart, N.H. Rowe, M.B. McKeough, and G. Wenerstrom: "Treatment of Recurrent Herpes Simplex Labialis with Oral Acyclovir," *J. Infect. Dis.* **161**: 185-190 (1990).

Whitley, R.J., C.A. Alford, M.S. Hirsch, R.T. Schooley, J.P. Luby, F.Y. Aoki, D. Hanley, A.J. Nahmias, and S.J. Soong: "Vidarabine Versus Acyclovir Therapy for Mucocutaneous Herpes Simplex Encephalitis," *N. Engl. J. Med.* **314**: 144-149 (1986).

CHAPTER 50

Drugs Used in Protozoan Infections

Joseph R. DiPalma

The most common protozoan infections in the United States are trichomoniasis, amebiasis, giardiasis, and toxoplasmosis. Malaria, leishmaniasis, and trypanosomiasis are more prevalent in subtropical and tropical zones (Table 50-1). Because of immigration, returning armed forces personnel, and widespread travel, all protozoan diseases are of economic, medical, and societal importance worldwide.

Protozoa are unicellular organisms with a much more versatile and adaptable metabolism than bacteria. They have complex life cycles and thus exist in several different forms which may require different chemotherapeutic approaches. In addition, some have insect vectors and animal reservoirs which may require chemical measures to eliminate this source of infection. It is, therefore, not surprising that numerous chemotherapeutic agents have been and are being employed to combat these parasites (Table 50-1).

This chapter discusses the chemotherapy of malaria in some detail as the prime example of antiprotozoan chemotherapy. Then the other agents useful today in the therapy of other protozoan infections are discussed mainly from the viewpoint of their pharmacologic properties and usefulness in other protozoan diseases.

MALARIA

Although now uncommon in most parts of the world, malaria remains the most devastating disease in many tropical "third world" countries (see Table 50-1). This disease is particularly fatal to young children, who typically experience mortality in excess of 15 percent.

Many factors contribute to the success of the malaria parasite despite significant efforts to remove the *Anopheles* mosquito, which carries the parasite. Sanitary measures such as isolation of cases and screening of windows are not feasible in poverty zones. War and poverty in areas where malaria is endemic, e.g., Vietnam, have favored a recrudescence of the disease. An increase in air travel has also caused its reintroduction into areas previously freed. Constant vigilance is necessary even in temperate zone countries because the *Anopheles* mosquito is ubiquitous.

Life Cycle of the Malaria Parasite

Malaria is the result of infestation with protozoa belonging to the genus *Plasmodium*. Of the many species which exist, only four infect humans: *Plasmodium falciparum*, *Plasmodium vivax*, *Plasmodium malariae*, and *Plasmodium ovale*. Infestation by the first two organisms is by far more common. *P. falciparum*, because some of its many strains have acquired resistance to antimalarial drugs, is the most problematic species from a therapeutic standpoint.

A proper understanding of the chemotherapy of malaria can best be achieved by examining the life cycle of the parasite in the female *Anopheles* mosquito and in humans. This is shown in Fig. 50-1. The female *Anopheles* mosquito requires a blood meal prior to laying her eggs. When the female bites an infected host (whose blood contains male and female sexual forms of the malarial parasite) fertilization occurs in the stomach of the mosquito. The resulting zygote penetrates the stomach wall and forms a cyst on its outer surface. After many cell divisions, this oocyst bursts, releasing thousands of sporozoites into the body cavity. Sporozoites migrate to the salivary glands and are injected when the mosquito bites a suitable host. Once injected, these sporozoites disappear rapidly from the blood and appear within

TABLE 50-1 The most common protozoan infections and the indicated drug therapy

Disease	Worldwide distribution	Drugs
Malaria	USA: 1000 to 2000 cases/year. Tropical regions: at least 200 million infected; 1 million deaths annually.	Quinine Mefloquine Chloroquine Hydroxychloroquine Halofantrine Primaquine Proguanil[a] Pyrimethamine Chloroguanide[b] Doxycycline Sulfadoxine[c]
Amebiasis	USA: 3 to 5% of the population infected. Tropical regions: 10% of the population infected.	Metronidazole Diloxanide furoate Tinidazole[a, d] Dehydroemetine Iodoquinol Paromomycin Chloroquine
Leishmaniasis	USA: uncommon. Tropical regions: 12 million new cases/year.	Sodium stibogluconate Meglumine antimonate[e] Amphotericin B Metronidazole Pentamidine
Trypanosomiasis	USA: uncommon. South American and Caribbean: 10 million cases (Chagas' disease). Africa: many millions in the tropical belt.	Eflornithine Pentamidine Melarsoprol Nifurtimox Suramin
Giardiasis	USA: 2 to 10% of the population infected, mainly nonsymptomatic. Worldwide: very common.	Quinacrine Metronidazole Furazolidone
Trichomoniasis	Worldwide: pandemic proportions.	Metronidazole
Toxoplasmosis	Worldwide: serological evidence of infection in 50% of the population.	Pyrimethamine-sulfadiazine
Pneumonia caused by *P. carinii*	Worldwide: high incidence in immunodeficiency states such as AIDS.	Trimethoprim-sulfamethoxazole Pentamidine Dapsone

[a] Not available in the USA.
[b] Although widely used in Africa and the safest of the folate antagonists, it is not available in the USA.
[c] Usually combined with pyrimethamine in a preparation known as Fansidar®.
[d] A nitro-imidazole similar to metronidazole.
[e] The French equivalent of sodium stibogluconate.

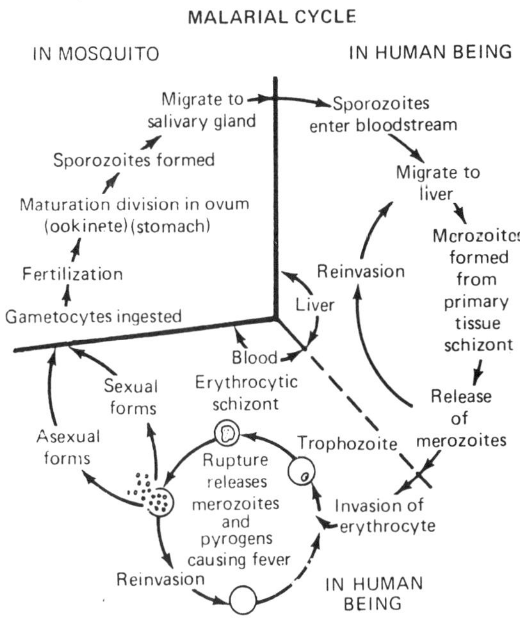

FIGURE 50-1 *Life cycle of the malarial parasite. [Schematic diagram after W.B. Pratt: Fundamentals of Chemotherapy, Oxford, New York, 1973.]*

liver parenchymal cells and elsewhere. In the liver, the sporozoites divide asexually and mature to form a hepatic (exoerythrocytic) schizont containing many merozoites. When this schizont ruptures, merozoites are released into the blood and may reinvade parenchymal cells to form secondary hepatic schizonts or may invade red blood cells where they multiply asexually to form erythrocytic schizonts. At this point, the patient is asymptomatic and will remain so until these erythrocytic schizonts rupture, releasing merozoites and pyrogens into the blood. Clinically this event is marked by the first in a series of febrile episodes. Some of the merozoites released will reinvade red blood cells to form new (secondary erythrocytic) schizonts, others will undergo sexual division and become male and female gametocytes. These sexual forms are ingested when a new female *Anopheles* bites the infected host, and the process begins again.

Based on the complex life cycle of the malarial parasite in humans, there are certain terms describing more accurately the goals and purposes of chemotherapy. These are listed in Table 50-2. **Suppressive therapy** only affects the asexual, erythrocytic forms. This type of therapy will ensure that clinical symptoms do not appear, but it does not affect the infectivity of the host from the mosquito, nor does it ensure that a relapse will not occur when chemotherapy is terminated. Therapy with a **radical curative agent** will eliminate secondary-tissue schizonts and thus ensure that no relapse can occur at a later date. **Causal prophylaxis** refers to action on primary-tissue schizonts, which may be achieved by some drugs which attack both erythrocytic and primary-tissue (exoerythrocytic) schizonts. *Plasmodium falciparum* does not form secondary-tissue schizonts; thus causal prophylaxis achieves a radical cure in this case, but not for the other plasmodia which infect humans.

Chemotherapeutic Agents

The chemotherapy of malaria is designed to interfere with specific stages of the life cycle of the parasite. The drugs presented here are divided into three groups: those that affect the erythrocytic stage of the life cycle, those that disrupt the exoerythrocytic (or hepatic) stage, and those that attack both stages simultaneously.

Drugs Effective Against Erythrocytic Stages of *Plasmodium* Infestation

Three classes of drugs are particularly useful in the erythrocytic stage of malarial infections: these are the 4-aminoquinolines (e.g., chloroquine and hydroxychloroquine), the quinoline methanols (e.g., quinine, quinidine, and mefloquine), and the phenanthrene methanols (e.g., halofantrine).

Chloroquine and Hydroxychloroquine

These 4-aminoquinoline derivatives are synthetic compounds in which the substitution of an amino group at position 4 of the quinoline ring is the most important structural characteristic. The composition of the side chain may vary, but this is not as critical as the presence of a chlorine atom at position 7 of the ring.

The prototype compound in this group is chloroquine, and its pharmacology will be considered representative of the entire group.

Mechanism of Action Chloroquine selectively concentrates in parasitized red blood cells. As a

TABLE 50-2 Major antimalarial drugs classified in relation to the different stages of the malarial parasite

Stage	Type of therapy	Effective drugs	Purpose
Sporozoites	True causal prophylaxis	None	If effective drugs were available to destroy sporozoites, malarial infection could be prevented.
Exoerythrocytic (primary)	Causal prophylaxis[a]	Primaquine Chloroguanide[b]	Drugs are effective against primary tissue schizonts. Therapy prevents erythrocytic infection.
Exoerythrocytic (secondary)	Radical (antirelapse therapy)	Primaquine	Only this drug is active against the secondary tissue schizonts, and thus it eliminates the source of recurrent invasion of the blood cells.
Erythrocytic	Suppressive[a] (schizonticidal)	Quinine Chloroquine Hydroxychloroquine Mefloquine Halofantrine Pyrimethamine Chloroguanide[b]	Used for the temporary prevention of clinical symptoms. The tissue schizonts are not destroyed, and upon stoppage of therapy relapse frequently occurs.
Sexual	Gametocidal	Primaquine	Used to prevent the spread of infection from man to the mosquito and thus back to the animal reservoir. Important only in endemic and epidemic areas.
Mosquito	Sporontocidal (antisporogenic, gametostatic)	Pyrimethamine Primaquine	At best, gametocytes are resistant, and those escaping destruction in the host may still be inhibited from developing in the mosquito by treatment of the host.

[a] Other terms which apply are *clinical cure* and *clinical prophylaxis*.
[b] Not available in the U.S.

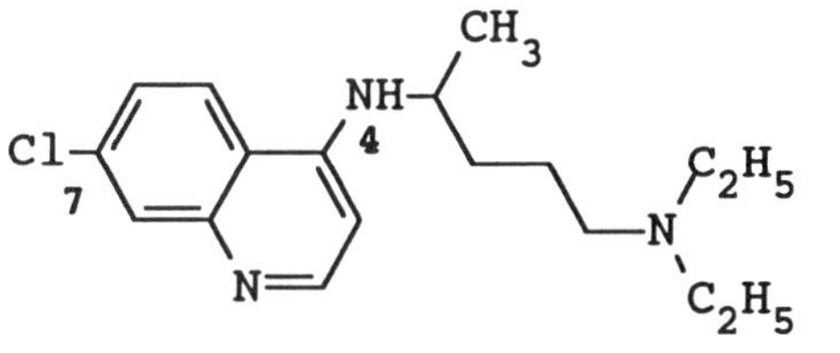

Chloroquine

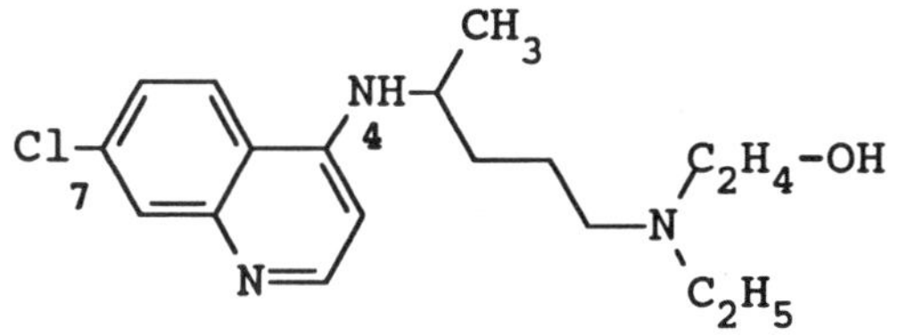

Hydroxychloroquine

weak base it accumulates in the acid vesicle of the parasite. This effect cannot be completely explained on a physicochemical basis. Nevertheless, the alkalinizing effect of chloroquine on the acid vesicle effectively destroys the viability of the parasite, although the mechanism by which this occurs is not clear. There is considerable evidence that development of resistance by the parasite is associated with the ability to pump chloroquine out of the acid vesicle.

Another mechanism of action may involve the binding of chloroquine to aggregates of ferriprotoporphyrin IX which are released from parasitized erythrocytes during plasmodium-induced degradation of hemoglobin. The chloroquine-protein complex appears to cause lysis of the membranes of the parasite and infected erythrocyte. Another method for *P. falciparum* to acquire resistance to chloroquine may reside in its ability of affect this ferriprotoporphyrin IX mechanism.

The latest proposed mechanism of action of chloroquine involves inhibition of the enzyme heme polymerase present in the lysosomes of *P. falciparum* trophozoites. This enzyme joins heme molecules remaining from hemoglobin destruction into an inert brownish pigment called hemozoin. This protects the plasmodium trophozoites from the toxic effects of free heme which would, when oxidized, disrupt membranes, inhibit proteases and damage DNA.

Pharmacokinetics The oral bioavailability of chloroquine is in the range of 90 percent. After an oral dose, maximum blood levels are achieved in 6 h. Approximately 55 percent of the total plasma concentration is bound to plasma proteins. Extensive tissue binding, however, contributes to a large apparent volume of distribution. Normal red blood cells concentrate this drug at levels twice that found in plasma; liver, lung, kidney, and heart concentrate it at 10 times plasma levels. The elimination half-life is 5 days. Twenty-five percent of an oral dose appears unchanged in the urine, the rest as the N-desethyl derivative. The parent compound appears in greater concentration in acidic urine.

Effects Chloroquine has a slight quinidine-like effect on the heart and depresses cardiac function in higher doses, especially when administered parenterally. In larger doses, chloroquine has unique actions apart from its antimalarial activity. It has anti-inflammatory activity, especially against inflammatory diseases such as rheumatoid arthritis and chronic discoid lupus erythematosus. This action is believed to be due to the suppression of the immune process. At such doses, however, toxicity is greatly increased and may outweigh clinical benefit.

Other actions include enzyme inhibition; binding of melanin, porphyrin, and nucleic acids; and antihistaminic effects.

Therapeutic Uses Chloroquine is effective against acute attacks of malaria and for prophylactic suppression of malaria due to *P. vivax*, *P. ovale*, *P. malariae* and susceptible strains of *P. falciparum*. For prophylaxis, oral treatment should start 1 to 2 weeks before entering the endemic area and continue for 4 weeks after returning. To prevent relapses from *P. vivax* and *P. ovale*, primaquine is the preferred drug.

A much larger oral doses of chloroquine must be employed in inflammatory diseases; hydroxychloroquine is more commonly used in this regard. A level of 10 ng/mL of chloroquine clears the blood of malaria parasites, but a plasma concentration of 250 to 280 ng/mL is required to achieve therapeutic results in rheumatoid arthritis.

The therapy of amebic abscess of the liver may also include chloroquine.

Adverse Reactions Other than mild gastrointestinal complaints (anorexia, nausea, vomiting, diarrhea, and abdominal cramps), side effects are almost unknown with doses of chloroquine used to treat malaria. However, the high doses required as anti-inflammatory medication lead to a variety of severe reactions. Generalized loss of hair pigment and a blue-black pigmentation of the skin and mucous membranes may occur. More important are the keratopathy and retinopathy resulting in constriction of the visual fields and loss of central vision. Early changes are reversible, but later the visual changes become permanent. Prolonged therapy should be attended by periodic ophthalmologic examinations. Mothers receiving high doses during pregnancy may give birth to children with sensorineural deafness. Lichen planus skin eruption and even exfoliative dermatitis have occurred. Intravenous doses, especially in children, may cause fatal cardiorespiratory collapse. Deaths have been associated with blood levels as low as 1 μg/mL.

Quinine and Quinidine

The second group of drugs useful against the erythrocytic stages of malarial infection is the quinoline methanols. This group includes the cinchona alkaloids, among which only quinine and quinidine are still used in the therapy of malaria. Quinine is obtained from the bark of the cinchona tree, which grows in South America and in the plantations of the East Indies. Quinine is the levorotatory isomer of quinidine and consists of a quinoline ring substituted in the 4 position with a methylene bridge to a quinuclidine ring structure.

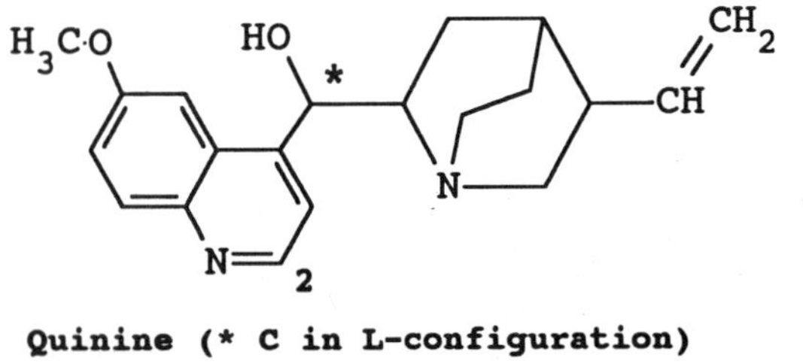

Quinine (* C in L-configuration)

Quinidine (* C in D-configuration)

Quinine has other physical properties of importance. It fluoresces easily, polarizes light, and screens out ultraviolet light. Its bitter taste gives it the property of a stomachic, and it finds use in proprietary products such as quinine water.

Mechanism of Action Although not completely understood, it is believed that the mechanism of action of quinine and quinidine are similar to chloroquine; i.e., the drugs concentrate in the acid vesicle of the parasite and produces an alkalinity which destroys its function. Quinine also depresses many enzyme systems and has been characterized as a generalized protoplasmic poison.

Effects Quinine has analgesic and antipyretic properties similar to the salicylates. When injected locally, quinine has a local anesthetic action in which it briefly stimulates and then paralyzes sensory neurons. Because of its nature as a protoplasmic poison, local tissue destruction often results, which prolongs its action for weeks or months. Quinine may also cause a quinidine-like depression of myocardial excitability and conduction velocity.

Quinine inhibits cholinesterases, and it has a weak curare-like effect and may aggravate the muscular weakness of myasthenia gravis. On the other hand, quinine is quite useful in relieving the excessive tone of muscle in myotonia congenita and in the night cramps of peripheral vascular disease.

Pharmacokinetics Quinine is rapidly and completely absorbed from the gastrointestinal tract, reaching a maximum plasma concentration in 1 to 2 h. The drug is widely distributed, achieving its highest concentrations in the liver, lung, kidney, and spleen. Leukocytes concentrate quinine, but erythrocytes contain less of the compound than does the plasma. Plasma protein binding is approximately 70 percent. Biotransformation occurs by hydroxylation at position 2 of the quinoline ring in the liver drug-metabolizing microsomal system. About 5 percent is found unchanged in the urine. The plasma level falls rapidly to negligible levels in 6 to 8 h, and hence daily doses are required.

Therapeutic Uses Administered by the oral route, quinine is effectively combined with pyrimethamine, sulfadiazine, and/or tetracycline in treating an uncomplicated attack of chloroquine-resistant *P. falciparum* malaria. When parenteral therapy is necessary, quinidine gluconate administered by intravenous drip is the drug of choice for all strains of chloroquine-resistant malaria. Because of adverse reactions, its use is fairly limited. It is, however, occasionally prescribed for night cramps.

Adverse Reactions Quinine has many toxicities because of its complex pharmacology. All persons who must take quinine chronically may eventually suffer from *cinchonism*, a syndrome similar to salicylism. In mild cases it consists of tinnitus, headache, nausea, and disturbances of vision. More advanced cases show changes in color vision, photophobia, constriction of visual fields, and scotomas; *quinine amblyopia* is a term applied to severe cases. Confusion, excitement, and delirium may eventually result.

Skin reactions occasionally occur. These usually consist of a scarlatiniform rash; more often it is urticarial in nature. Angioneurotic edema and asthmatic attacks may occur. Purpura is not uncommon and is caused by thrombocytopenia. Recovery is rapid as soon as the drug is stopped.

Mefloquine

This is an antimalarial drug developed for treatment and prevention of chloroquine-resistant strains of *P. falciparum* malaria. Chemically, mefloquine is an analog of quinine. It differs from quinine in that the side chain is a piperidyl ring rather than a quinuclidine ring. In addition, there are trifluoromethyl groups substituted at positions 2 and 8 of the quinoline ring. The trifluoromethyl group at position 2 blocks ring hydroxylation, which is a major site of biotransformation for quinine.

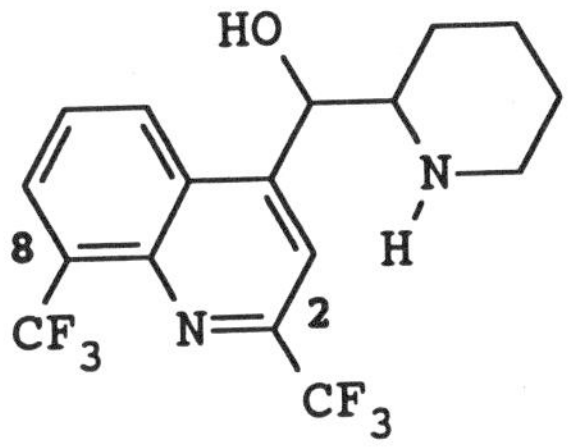

HO, N, H, 8, 2, CF_3, N, CF_3

Mechanism of Action and Effects The mechanism of action is unknown; it is believed to affected the acid vesicle of the parasite similar to chloroquine. As might be expected, mefloquine shows similarities to quinine in its pharmacologic effects.

Pharmacokinetics The pharmacokinetics of mefloquine are quite variable among patients. There is a delay in absorption of several hours. The drug is highly bound to plasma proteins (98 percent) and it concentrates in erythrocytes, the target cells in malaria. Most of the compound is biotransformed prior to elimination. Mefloquine appears to have a long duration of action; the mean elimination half-life is about 3 weeks.

Adverse Effects Single oral doses of mefloquine up to 2 g are generally well tolerated. Common adverse effects include nausea, vomiting, diarrhea, dizziness, and myalgia. Skin rashes, vertigo, tinnitus, central nervous system disturbances, and visual disturbances have also occurred.

Therapeutic Uses Mefloquine has been widely used, both as a prophylactic and therapeutic drug in infections caused by *P. vivax* and especially in cases of drug resistant *P. falciparum* infections. Many investigators believe this drug to be the most effective single-dose agent for chloroquine-resistant *P. falciparum*. However, some strains of *P. falciparum* resistant to mefloquine have already been reported.

Halofantrine

This drug was developed along with mefloquine by the Walter Reed Army Institute of Research; however, it was not tested clinically until more recently and is available now in the U.S. It has many of the attributes of mefloquine but appears to have less adverse reactions. It is effective in the erythrocytic stage of malaria and in chloroquine-resistant *P. falciparum* infections. Halofantrine is a completely synthetic drug; it differs from quinine and mefloquine by having a phenanthrene ring structure instead of a quinoline ring. The trifluoromethyl and chlorine substitutions on the phenanthrene ring enhance its activity.

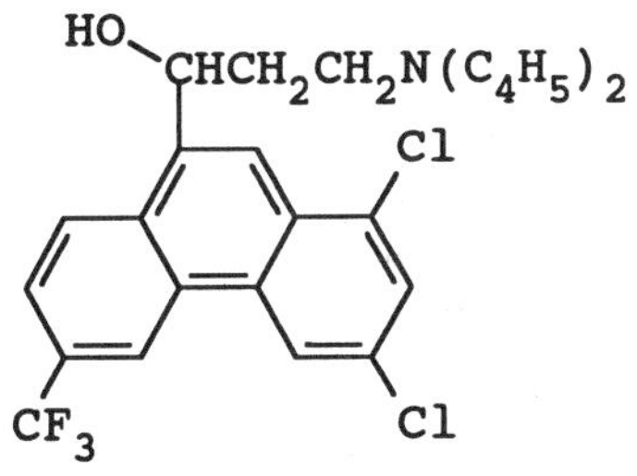

HO, $CHCH_2CH_2N(C_4H_5)_2$, Cl, CF_3, Cl

Mechanism of Action It is believed that the mechanism of action of halofantrine involves inhibition of the proton pump present at the host-parasite interface. At a very low concentrations (10 μmol/L), halofantrine inhibits glucose-dependent proton efflux from erythrocytes infected with *P. bergliei*.

Pharmacokinetics Oral absorption of halofantrine is poor, possibly because of the low water solubility of the compound. For this reason, the drug is administered in a 3-dose regimen at 6 hour intervals. Absorption may be even less in malaria patients as compared to healthy volunteers. Food may enhance the oral absorption of halofantrine.

After oral administration of a single dose, peak plasma drug concentrations are reached in 5 to 7.5 hours. The volume of distribution is large in patients with malaria (73.2 L/kg). A major metabolite of halofantrine is an N-desbutyl derivative. Following the usual 3-dose regimen, the total body clearance is 0.58 L/h/kg. Its elimination half-life is approximately 3 months.

Adverse Effects The most common adverse effects in order of frequency are abdominal pain, pruritus, vomiting, diarrhea, headache, and rash. Generally halofantrine is well tolerated. Pruritus induced by chloroquine in African patients is especially severe; that induced by halofantrine is less in incidence and severity.

Therapeutic Uses Clinical experience with halofantrine is still limited. It is effective against both drug-resistant and nonresistant types of *P. falciparum* infections. It is also quite effective in *P. vivax* infectious. The question of whether it is effective against strains of *P. falciparum* which are resistant to mefloquine is not yet settled. In all, halofantrine appears to be a useful addition to the array of drugs for malaria.

Drugs Effective Against Hepatic (Exoerythrocytic) Forms of *Plasmodium* Infestation

The only group of drugs considered effective against the hepatic forms of the malaria parasite is the 8-aminoquinoline derivatives. These are synthetic compounds first introduced in Germany in 1926. After World War II, further investigation in the U.S. led to the development of primaquine, a compound with a good therapeutic index.

Primaquine

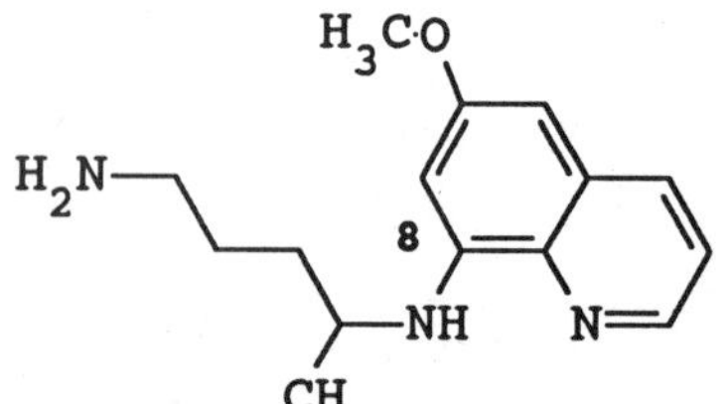

H_3CO, H_2N, 8, NH, N, CH_3

The shift of the side chain from position 4 of the quinoline nucleus to position 8 completely changes the spectrum of activity of primaquine. In contrast to the 4-aminoquinolines, primaquine has virtually no effect on erythrocytic forms of the malarial parasite: its activity is restricted to the tissue forms of the parasite in humans and in the mosquito (Table 50-2). This makes primaquine an extremely valuable aid because it permits a radical cure and causal prophylaxis which cannot be achieved with the purely erythrocytic drugs.

Mechanism of Action The site of action of primaquine is within the mitochondria of the malaria parasite. Here primaquine is believed to interfere with electron transport, causing oxidative damage to mitochondrial enzyme systems. This results in swelling and vacuolation of the parasite's mitochondria. Host mitochondria are not affected. In addition, primaquine attacks the sexual forms of the parasite in human blood and renders them incapable of maturation division in the mosquito. This is probably accomplished by causing oxidative damage to electron-rich nucleic acids within the gametocytes. Primaquine, therefore, can be used to prevent the spread of malaria in endemic areas.

Pharmacokinetics Primaquine is rapidly and completely absorbed from the gastrointestinal tract, achieving maximum plasma concentrations within 2 h of an oral dose. Primaquine is not as extensively tissue-bound as are the 4-aminoquinolines but is somewhat concentrated in the liver and, in descending order, the lung, brain, heart, and skeletal muscle.

Primaquine is rapidly biotransformed in the liver to active quinoline products which are potent oxidizing agents. After 8 to 10 h, following an oral dose, the plasma level of the parent compound is very low; only 1 percent of the original dose is excreted unchanged in the urine. One of the major biotransformation products, the 6-hydroxyl derivative, undergoes conjugation prior to urinary excretion.

Effects In the usual therapeutic doses primaquine has only minor effects. In some respects, it is similar to quinine because intravenous injection may produce a fall in blood pressure, cardiac arrhythmias, and electrocardiographic changes; its use by this route is not recommended.

Therapeutic Uses Primaquine is used alone for the radical cure or causal prophylaxis of malaria caused by *P. vivax* or *P. ovale*. More commonly the drug is given concomitantly or consecutively with chloroquine or a comparable drug for the prophylaxis of malaria regardless of the species of *Plasmodium*. Typically, therapy is started at least 1 day prior to entering an endemic area and continued for several weeks after leaving the malarious area.

Adverse Reactions Much is now known about the phenomenon called *primaquine sensitivity*, a form of intravascular hemolysis accompanied by the formation of methemoglobin. The mechanism by which this sensitivity arises is common to a number of drugs which are capable of acting as oxidants and is believed to be intimately related to the mechanism by which primaquine exerts its schizonticidal and gametocidal actions.

Red blood cells contain many components which are particularly sensitive to oxidative damage, notably, hemoglobin and the cell membrane. Normal erythrocytes which are exposed to oxidants, e.g., primaquine, neutralize these offensive agents via reduced cofactors (NADH and NADPH), which permit the reduction of oxidized glutathione (GSSG) to reduced glutathione (GSH). Reduced glutathione in turn gives up its electrons to the oxidant, neutralizing it, and in this process is, itself, oxidized to GSSG. As long as reduced cofactors are available, this protective cycle continues (see Fig. 50-2). The hexose monophosphate shunt serves a homeostatic role by producing reduced cofactors in direct response to the levels of GSSG present in the erythrocyte, using the enzyme glucose-6-phosphate dehydrogenase (G6PD).

Primaquine and certain other drugs, including sulfones, menadiol, and sulfonamides, are converted to oxidant products in the blood. These metabolites consume electrons and, in the absence of protective GSH, do oxidative damage to hemoglobin, forming methemoglobin, and to the red blood cell membrane, causing hemolysis.

Primaquine sensitivity is most common in persons who belong to ethnic groups originating in the Mediterranean basin and is linked closely to a genetic defect: a deficiency of G6PD, which leads to increased fragility of the red blood cells. Old cells are affected first, and the hemolysis is dose-dependent. Using small doses of primaquine, few patients experience hemolysis; with larger doses, hemolysis is apt to occur in sensitive individuals. Because the hemolysis can be severe and because the procedure is easily accomplished, it is worthwhile to screen patients for G6PD deficiency prior to the initiation of primaquine therapy.

Primaquine may also cause abdominal discomfort, nausea, headache, changes in visual accommodation, and pruritus. The predisposition for intravascular hemolysis in susceptible individuals is its principal side effect. Some methemoglobinemia is frequently attendant with its use but rarely requires cessation of therapy.

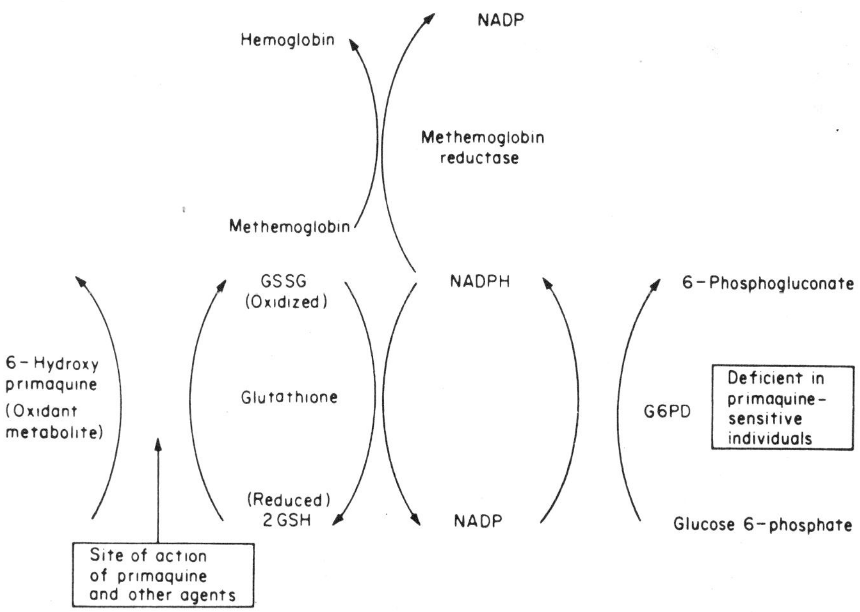

FIGURE 50-2 *A schema showing the complex cycle which renders the red blood cell susceptible to hemolysis in primaquine-sensitive individuals. The deficiency in glucose-6-phosphate dehydrogenase (G6PD) makes it possible for primaquine to oxidize glutathione because of inadequate production of NADPH. An added complication is failure of conversion of methemoglobin to hemoglobin, which also requires NADPH.*

Drugs Effective Against Erythrocytic and Hepatic Forms of *Plasmodium* Infestation

Early studies showed that sulfonamides and sulfones had some curative value in malarial infections. However, it was not until compounds such as chloroguanide and pyrimethamine became available that a new class of drugs with a different mechanism of action in malaria were discovered. Experimental studies showed a marked synergism between sulfonamides and pyrimethamine. In field studies it was shown that these new agents alone were prophylactic and curative in malaria. It was later learned that all strong inhibitors of dihydrofolate reductase such as trimethoprim could destroy the malarial parasite with relatively little damage to the human host. The scheme shown in Figure 47-2 serves to illustrate the synergistic relationship between sulfonamides, which compete for para-aminobenzoic acid (PABA), and the inhibitors of dihydrofolate reductase.

Pyrimethamine

Chloroguanide was introduced in England in 1945, the result of work on a long series of biguanide compounds. A few years later pyrimethamine was discovered as the culmination of intensive study of antimetabolites of folic acid. Trimethoprim was a still later development (see Chapter 47). The close structural resemblance of these compounds is shown below.

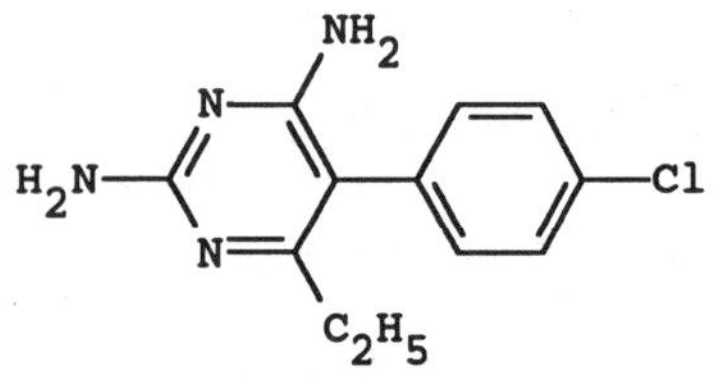

Pyrimethamine

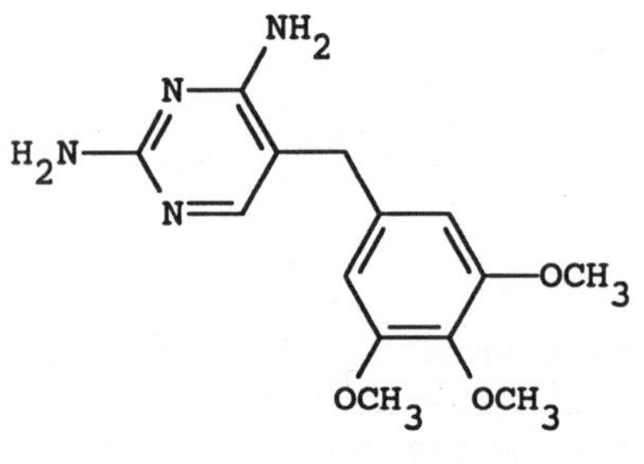

Trimethoprim

One may perceive similarities between the pteridine ring of folic acid and the diaminopyrimidine structure of pyrimethamine. Undoubtedly this contributes to the affinity of this compound for a receptor site of dihydrofolate reductase (DHFR).

Mechanism of Action Pyrimethamine and other diaminopyrimidine derivatives are inhibitors of DHFR in bacteria, plasmodia, and humans. Fortunately, they have a relatively high affinity for bacterial and protozoal DHFR; pyrimethamine, for example, inhibits parasitic DHFR at a level several hundred times lower than that required to inhibit human DHFR. This serves as a basis for a selective toxicity which favors the host against the parasite.

Pyrimethamine is active against both the exoerythrocytic and the erythrocytic forms of plasmodia. They are most useful in suppressive therapy, but a causal cure may be obtained when treating *P. falciparum* infections. It also has an effect on gametocytes such that they are unable to undergo maturation, thus preventing sporogony in the mosquito's gut sporozoite formation. The major disadvantage of pyrimethamine is the rapidity with which the parasite develops resistance to it. This includes *P. falciparum* and *P. vivax*, as well as many experimental strains.

Pharmacokinetics Pyrimethamine is well absorbed in the gastrointestinal tract. Peak plasma levels occur in 2 to 6 h. Plasma protein binding is approximately 87 percent. The plasma half-life is about 4 days; concentrations that suppress the parasite are maintained for about 2 weeks. Tissue concentrations are high; even the cerebrospinal fluid has significant levels. Pyrimethamine is secreted in maternal milk at concentrations high enough to provide chemosuppression of malaria in a breast-fed infant. Several products of the biotransformation of pyrimethamine are found in the urine.

Effect As might be expected, pyrimethamine exhibits no special organ effects. The action of the drug is restricted to those metabolic systems affected by folate metabolism, including the reticuloendothelial system and gastrointestinal tract (see "Adverse Reactions," below).

Therapeutic Uses Pyrimethamine administered alone may be used for the prophylaxis of malaria. However, used alone, it is not very effective in the treatment of a primary attack of malaria. When pyrimethamine is combined with the sulfonamide, sulfadoxine, in a preparation known as Fansidar, it has been used successfully in treating chloroquine-resistant *P. falciparum* malaria, providing a 95 to 98 percent cure with only minor host toxicities. Combination therapy also significantly reduces the dosage required and the development of resistance.

Given simultaneously with a sulfonamide (e.g., sulfadiazine), pyrimethamine has had considerable use in the therapy of toxoplasmosis, another parasitic infection. In this application, it is usually advisable to supplement with leucovorin (folinic acid).

Adverse Reactions The toxicity of pyrimethamine resides in its ability to inhibit dihydrofolate reductase. The usual dosages used for malaria do not have appreciable effects on the host enzyme. However, larger dosages for prolonged periods can cause the symptoms of folic acid deficiency. These include bone marrow depression and megaloblastosis, and they are readily reversible by the administration of leucovorin or by cessation of treatment. In endemic areas, where continual use is expected, the simultaneous administration of leucovorin is recommended. Because of its teratogenic effect in animals, the use of pyrimethamine in pregnant women is not advisable.

The sulfonamides and sulfones commonly used with pyrimethamine have their own toxicity (see Chapter 47). Skin rashes which occur may be due to either ingredient, but the sulfonamides are more culpable.

Other Drugs

The malaria parasite is susceptible to many different types of drugs. The major problem is the development of resistance, especially in the case of *P. falciparum* infections. As a consequence, different drugs are used in combination as the occasion requires.

Quinacrine Quinacrine is an acridine derivative closely related to the 4-aminoquinolines chemically and in clinical use. It was the main drug for prophylaxis and therapy during World War II. It is now rarely used as an antimalarial, but it finds use in amebiasis and giardiasis. It is also used as a sclerosing agent by intrapleural administration for the prevention of recurrence of pneumothorax.

Tetracycline and Doxycycline These antibiotics (described in Chapter 47) are quite active against most malarial species. Tetracycline is seldom used as the sole agent; it is an alternative drug most often combined with another drug such as quinine for use in cases of resistant strains. At present, the use of tetracycline for malaria is considered investigational.

Doxycycline is the tetracycline derivative most frequently used. It is indicated for use in the prophylaxis of malaria due to *P. falciparum* in areas where pyrimethamine-sulfadoxine or chloroquine resistant strains exist.

Dapsone Dapsone is 4,4-diaminodiphenylsulfone and is also known as DDS. As a sulfone it has much the same characteristics as sulfonamides with somewhat greater toxicity. Dapsone has been widely used for the therapy of leprosy. It also finds utility in the prophylaxis of malaria. Because of the easy development of resistance, it is combined with pyrimethamine.

AMEBIASIS

Entamoeba histolytica, the causative agent of amebiasis, has a very complicated life cycle in its human host. It may exist as an asymptomatic infection, as a mild to moderate intestinal infection (nondysenteric colitis), much more severe intestinal infection causing dysentery and invasion of the wall of the intestine, or as a systemic stage with abscesses usually in the liver but also in late stages appearing in other parts of the body, such as the brain. As shown in Table 50-1, many drugs are utilized to treat amebiasis in its various stages. None are completely effective because the cystic form of the organism is extremely resistant to chemotherapy. In addition, chemotherapeutic agents cannot penetrate the heavily walled abscesses, which in most cases must be surgically drained and removed.

Metronidazole

Originally introduced about 35 years ago for the treatment of trichomoniasis, metronidazole has proven to be a remarkably effective chemotherapeutic agent not only for amebiasis but also for leishmaniasis, trichomoniasis, and giardiasis. It is also effective in bacterial anaerobic infections.

Metronidazole is amebicidal for *Entamoeba histolytica* in both the intestinal (luminal) and tissue stages. At the present time, it is the preferred drug for amebiasis except for asymptomatic cyst carriers (use iodoquinol or paromomycin). Since oral doses are completely absorbed, another luminal amebicide must be given, usually iodoquinol, to eradicate intestinal ameba and thus prevent relapse. The complete pharmacology of metronidazole is described in Chapter 47.

Diloxanide Furoate

Since the late 1950s, diloxanide furoate has been used mainly outside the U.S. to treat the intestinal phase of amebiasis. Although not clearly more effective than luminal amebicides, it has fewer side effects.

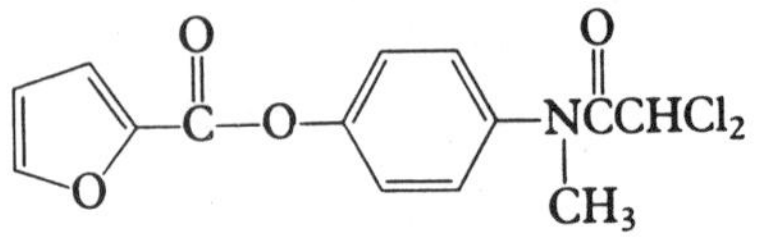

Diloxanide is a dichloroacetamide derivative that is insoluble in water and must be protected from light. There are no major pharmacologic effects from ordinary doses. Diloxanide is rapidly absorbed in the intestine, reaching a peak blood level in about 1 h. After conjugation to the glucuronide, it is excreted in the urine in about 6 h.

Diloxanide is available from the Centers for Disease Control and Prevention (CDC) and may be used alone in the asymptomatic early stage of amebiasis. Combined with metronidazole, it is usually curative in the purely luminal stage of amebiasis. It has no effect on the cystic form of the ameba. Except for gastrointestinal complaints, there are few adverse reactions.

Dehydroemetine

Traditionally and historically, emetine, an alkaloid extracted from ipecac (Brazil root), has been a major drug in the therapy of amebiasis. A very toxic alkaloid, its use was restricted to severe cases of bowel wall infestation by the ameba resistant to other amebicides. Although the use of ipecac alkaloids for amebiasis has been largely replaced by metronidazole, dehydroemetine is available from the CDC as an alternative drug for treating severe intestinal disease and hepatic abscesses.

Dehydroemetine is thought to act by inhibiting polypeptide chain elongation; hence protein synthesis in parasites and mammalian cells is arrested. As a general irritant and protoplasmic poison, dehydroemetine has effects on the gastrointestinal tract, cardiovascular, neuromuscular, and central nervous systems; these effects are generally considered adverse effects and often preclude use of the drug. Dehydroemetine is used by intramuscular injection and affects ameba in the bowel wall and liver; by this route it has no effect on intraluminal parasites. When necessary to resort to the use of dehydroemetine, it is best to closely watch the patient in a hospital setting.

Iodoquinol

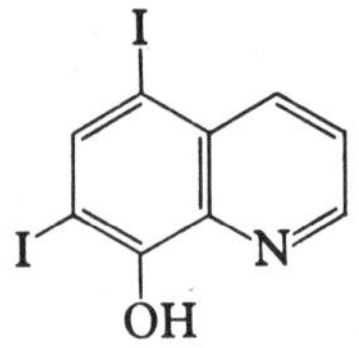

This agent is useful in amebal intraluminal infections only. As such it is indicated in mild infections. The mechanism of action is unknown.

Absorption is poor from the gastrointestinal tract, and this is advantageous because it is the focus of action of the drug. Some is absorbed, however; metabolic studies indicate a half-life of 11 to 14 h. Thyroid function tests are unreliable in patients taking iodoquinol. Adverse reactions consist of rashes (acneform, papular, and pustular iododerma), gastrointestinal disturbances, fever, and enlargement of the thyroid gland. Iodoquinol in large doses over a long period of time can also cause optic neuritis, atrophy, and peripheral neuropathy.

In addition to its use s an amebicide, iodoquinol is also used as a powder which is insufflated intravaginally for trichomonal infections. By this route it is generally a safer drug because absorption is minimized.

Paromomycin

As an aminoglycoside antibiotic, paromomycin is a close relative of neomycin and streptomycin. It is active against the intestinal stage of amebiasis. It is also effective against enteric bacteria *Salmonella* and *Shigella*.

Only a very small portion of orally administered paromomycin is absorbed. Nearly 100 percent of the drug is recovered in the stool. As a result, paromomycin is effective only in the intraluminal stage of amebiasis.

The side effects are usually restricted to nausea, vomiting, abdominal cramps, and diarrhea. In an ulcerated bowel, considerable absorption can occur, which may result in renal toxicity and ototoxicity, effects commonly associated with the aminoglycosides. Super infection is another complication which requires vigilance.

Chloroquine

This antimalarial drug is also very useful in amebiasis. It is effective against the trophozoite stage and does prevent and eradicate liver abscess. Chloroquine is not used and is ineffective in the luminal stage of amebiasis. Chloroquine may be used when ulceration of the mucosa is present and the danger of invasion of the intestinal wall and metastatic liver abscess is probable. (See under "MALARIA" for a complete description of the pharmacology of chloroquine.)

LEISHMANIASIS

A group of trypanosome protozoal parasites of the genus *Leishmania* cause a variety of diseases which are known generally as leishmaniasis. The insect vector is a biting sandfly, which transmits the infection from human to human or from rodents and canines to humans. Kala-azar in India is caused by *L. donovani*. This is a serious chronic systemic disease with splenomegaly and hepatomegaly with dysentery, which if untreated is usually fatal. *L. tropica* and *L. mexicana* cause only a cutaneous lesion, and spontaneous recovery is the rule. *L. braziliensis* infection results in destructive ulcers of mucous membranes, which require treatment for recovery.

Sodium Stibogluconate

```
CH2OH                HOH2C
|                        |
CHOH                 HOHC
|                        |
CHO\  OH        O-  /OHC
|    \ |        |  /     |
CHO-->Sb--O--Sb<--OHC      3Na+
|    /             \     |
CHO/                \OHC
|                        |
COO                  -OOC
```

Antimony trivalent organic salts have been the traditional and effective therapy for kala-azar or visceral leishmaniasis. More recently a pentavalent compound, sodium stibogluconate, has been found to be more convenient to use.

In the body sodium stibogluconate is probably converted to the trivalent form of antimony. Although the mechanism of action is unknown, antimony, like other metals, is known to react with sulfhydryl groups. Intestinal absorption is poor, and the drug must be given intramuscularly or intravenously. Excretion is 80 to 90 percent complete via the kidneys in 6 h. Sodium stibogluconate is available in the U.S. only from the CDC. Meglumine antimonate is the French equivalent of sodium stibogluconate.

Other drugs have been used successfully in various forms of leishmaniasis. These include amphotericin B and pentamidine for the visceral form resistant to antimony. Metronidazole has been used in the Mexican cutaneous form. At present, the use of these drugs in leishmaniasis is considered investigational in the U.S.

TRYPANOSOMIASIS

In Africa, trypanosomiasis is transmitted by the tsetse fly and is commonly known as sleeping sickness. The parasite *T. brucei* exists in two subspecies, *rhodesiense* and *gambiense*. The former causes a progressive fatal form of the disease with early central nervous system involvement. The latter has late central nervous system invasion, which gives rise to the symptoms of sleeping sickness.

American trypanosomiasis (Chagas' disease) is common in South America. It is transmitted by *T. cruzi* through bloodsucking triatomid insects. The main pathology is cardiomyopathy and hypertrophy of the esophagus and colon, which is eventually fatal.

Eflornithine

This drug is an antiprotozoal agent that is a drug of choice for *T. brucei gambiense* infections.

Mechanism of Action Eflornithine is a fluorinated derivative of ornithine and acts as an irreversible inhibitor of ornithine decarboxylase, an enzyme found in all mammalian and many non-mammalian cells that is necessary for the biosynthesis of polyamines such as putrescine, spermidine, and spermine. These compounds are believed to be

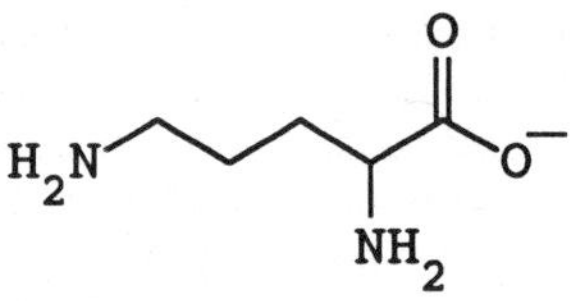

Ornithine

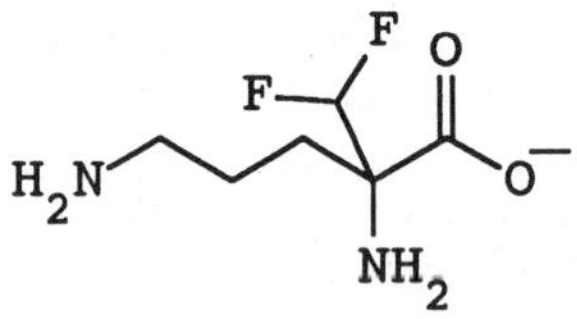

Eflornithine

involved in DNA packaging, cell division, and cellular differentiation.

In mammalian cells, ornithine decarboxylase has a rapid turn-over and new enzyme is synthesized continuously to replace it. The enzyme in the parasite is stable and not readily replaced by new synthesis. Consequently, inhibition of the enzyme affects the protozoa more than the host.

Eflornithine, like ornithine, binds to pyridoxal phosphate, the co-factor for the enzyme. When this complex binds to the enzyme, a fluoride is lost, and a covalent bond is formed between the enzyme and the eflornithine-pyridoxal phosphate complex. This is an example of the action of a "suicide inhibitor".

Pharmacokinetics After an intravenous dose, most of the drug (80 percent) is eliminated unchanged in the urine. There is no significant binding to plasma proteins. The elimination half-life is about 3 hours.

Therapeutic Use Eflornithine is used for the treatment of both the hemolymphatic and central nervous system stages of *T. brucei gambiense* infections (sleeping sickness). Intravenous infusion of the drug is given every 6 hours for 14 days. Although a very effective drug, the toxicities may be severe.

Adverse Effects There is a high incidence of adverse reactions associated with the hematopoietic system that occur with eflornithine; anemia (55 percent incidence), leukopenia (37 percent), and thrombocytopenia (14 percent) are the most common. Other untoward effects include diarrhea, seizures, hearing impairment, vomiting, alopecia, abdominal pain, anorexia, headache, and eosinophilia.

Pentamidine

Pentamidine is a aromatic diamidine that has a selective spectrum of activity against trypanosomes.

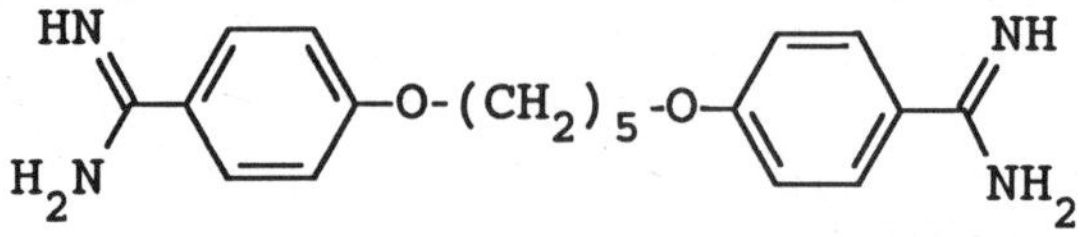

It is particularly effective against *T. brucei gambiense* infections both for prevention and treatment. Pentamidine is less effective, but still useful, in *T. brucei rhodesiense* infections. Other trypanosomes which are susceptible are *L. donovani* and *P. carinii*.

There are several possible chemotherapeutic actions. Uptake by the parasite is energy dependent and in susceptible organisms is very rapid. Pentamidine is highly positively charged and may react with DNA and inhibit the synthesis of DNA, RNA, phospholipids, and proteins. The activity of pentamidine is antagonized by glucose, and thus the drug may interfere with glycolysis.

Adverse reactions include, but are not limited to, elevated serum creatinine, elevated liver function tests, leukopenia, hypotension, hypoglycemia, fever, and skin rashes. In addition, there is a high incidence of pain, sterile abscess, or induration at the site of intramuscular injection.

The clinical use of pentamidine in the U.S. is for *P. carinii* infections resistant to other agents. It is especially useful in HIV-infected patients. The investigational use of pentamidine in trypanosomiasis is preventive and also for the early stages without central nervous system involvement. Pentamidine is administered by intramuscular and intravenous injection and by inhalation.

Nifurtimox

In acute Chagas' disease with *T. cruzi*, nifurtimox, a nitrofurazone derivative, is a drug of choice.

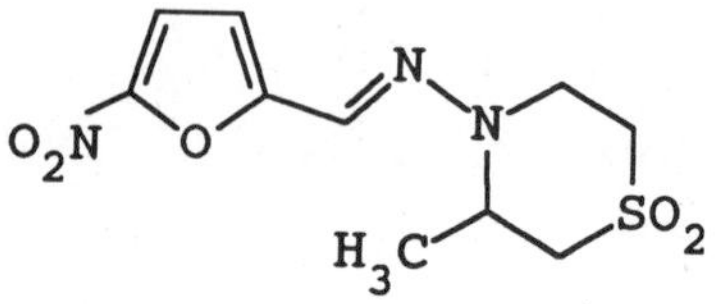

Nifurtimox is apparently is capable of forming chemically reactive radicals (superoxide, hydrogen peroxide, hydroxyl, etc.) in the parasite. The parasite *T. cruzi* lacks catalase and glutathione peroxidase, thus increasing the susceptibility of the organism to hydrogen peroxide. The same effect probably causes toxicity in the host. The drug can cause serious gastrointestinal disturbances, allergic reactions, and neurologic syndromes; therefore, its use in the chronic form of Chagas' disease is impractical. Nifurtimox is obtainable from the CDC.

Melarsoprol

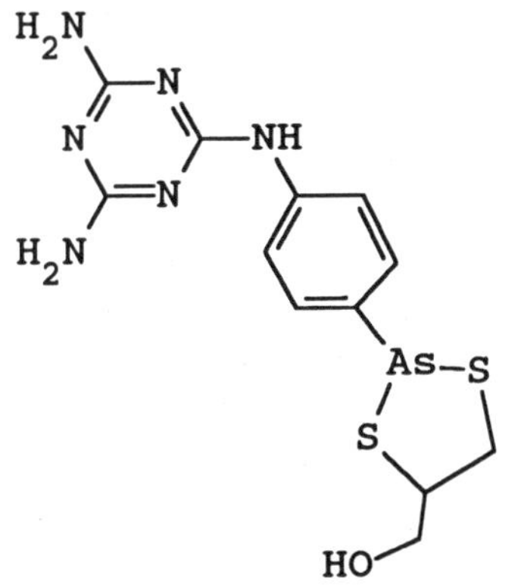

The later stages of trypanosomiasis with central nervous system involvement are treated with melarsoprol, an organic arsenical. Chemically, the drug is a condensation product of melarsen oxide with dimercaprol, an arsenical antagonist. This arrangement lowers the toxicity of the arsenic, while retaining its trypanosomicidal activity.

The mechanism of action is probably due to the reaction of arsenic with sulfhydryl groups and inactivation of sulfhydryl-containing enzymes. Melarsoprol is given only intravenously (as slowly as possible to avoid acute toxicity). A severe adverse reaction is a reactive encephalopathy, which may occur by the end of the first week of therapy. Unfortunately, the more severe the disease, the more likely is the encephalopathy to occur. Melarsoprol is available only from the CDC.

Suramin

An older drug, suramin is interesting because it is derived from the observation that certain dyes (trypan red and blue and afridol violet) had trypanosomicidal activity. Chemically suramin consists of two large organic dye molecules which are joined by a urea linkage. Now less used than previously, it is still a drug of choice in the early stages of African trypanosomiasis. Suramin is of no value in South American trypanosomiasis. It is given intravenously, and the patient must be watched for adverse reactions such as shock, loss of consciousness, colic, acute urticaria, and seizures. Late toxicity may consist of albuminuria and peripheral neuritis. Rarely, blood dyscrasias have been reported.

GIARDIASIS

This protozoan intestinal disease caused by *Giardia lamblia* is quite common and has occurred in endemic form in the United States. Often asymptomatic, it can invade the intestinal wall, causing ulceration and severe, foul diarrhea. The cystic form is very resistant to therapy and may cause abscesses in the liver and other organs.

Quinacrine has been the main therapy, but metronidazole, with much lower toxicity, is probably just as active and is replacing the former drug. In especially resistant cases, the two drugs may be used together.

Furazolidone, a broad-spectrum antibacterial compound, is also active against the organism. Since it is relatively less toxic than metronidazole, it has been recommended for use in children.

OTHER PROTOZOAN DISEASES

Other protozoan diseases are toxoplasmosis, trichomoniasis, and pneumonia caused by *P. carinii*. Toxoplasmosis is caused by *Toxoplasma gondii* and responds best to a combination of pyrimethamine and sulfadiazine. Trichomoniasis due to *Trichomonas vaginalis* is best treated with metronidazole (see Chapter 47). The *P. carinii* pneumonia is of particular importance because it is a frequent complication of AIDS and is treated with pentamidine, the trimethoprim-sulfamethoxazole combination, or dapsone (see Chapter 48).

BIBLIOGRAPHY

Barrett-Connor, E.: "Drugs for the Treatment of Parasitic Infection," *Med. Clin. North Am.* **66**: 245 (1982).

Bryson, H.M. and K.L. Goa: "Halofantrine: A Review of its Antimalarial Activity, Pharmacokinetic Properties and Therapeutic Potential," *Drugs* **43**: 236-258 (1992).

Fairlamb, A.H.: "Future Prospects for the Chemotherapy of Human Trypanosomiasis, 1. Novel Approaches to the Chemotherapy of Trypansomiasis," *Transact. Royal Soc. Trop. Med. Hyg.* **84**: 613-617 (1990).

Goldman, P.: "Metronidazole," *N. Engl. J. Med.* **303**: 1212-1218 (1980).

Jiang, J.B., et al.: "Antimalarial Activity of Mefloquine and Qinghaosu," *Lancet,* **2**:285-288 (1982).

Krogstad, D.J., H.C. Spencer, Jr., and G.R. Healy: "Amebiasis," *N. Engl. J. Med.* **298**: 262-265 (1978).

LeFrock, J.L.: "Drugs for Protozoan Infections," *Am. Fam. Physician* **35**: 247-251 (1987).

Lehninger, A.L., D.L. Nelson, and M.M. Cox: *Principles of Biochemistry, Second Edition,* Worth Publishers, New York, 1993, pp. 716-717.

Lerman, S.J., and R.A. Walker: "Treatment of Giardiasis. Literature Review and Recommendation," *Clin. Pediatr.* **21**: 409-414 (1982).

Lister, G.D.: "Delayed Myocardial Intoxication Following the Administration of Dehydroemetine Hydrochloride," *J. Trop. Med. Hyg.* **71**: 219 (1986).

Lossick, J.G.: "Treatment of *Trichomonas vaginalis* Infection," *Rev. Infect. Dis.* **4 (Suppl.)**: S801 (1982).

Marsden, P.D.: "Current Concepts in Parasitology Leishmaniasis," *N. Engl. J. Med.* **300**: 350-352 (1979).

Panisko, D.M., and J.S. Keystone: "Treatment of Malaria-1990," *Drugs* **39**: 160-189 (1990).

Phillips, R.E., D.A. Warrell, N.J. White, S. Looareesuwan, and J. Karbwang,: "Intravenous Quinidine for the Treatment of Severe *Falciparum* malaria: Clinical and Pharmacokinetic Studies," *N. Engl. J. Med.* **312**: 12-73 (1985).

Pratt, W.B.: Fundamentals of Chemotherapy, Oxford, New York, 1973.

Reed, S.L.: "Amebiasis, an Update," *Clin. Infect. Dis.* **14**: 385-393 (1992).

Sattler, F.R., R. Cowan, D.M. Nielseu, and J. Ruskin: "Trimethoprim-sulfamethoxazole Compared with Pentamidine for Treatment of *Pneumocystis carinii* Pneumonia in the Acquired Immunodeficiency Syndrome: A Prospective, Non Conserver Study," *Ann. Intern. Med.* **109**: 280-287 (1988).

Scott, J.A., R.N. Davidson, A.H. Moody, H.R. Grant, D. Felmingham, G.M. Scott, P. Olliaro, and A.D. Bryceson: "Aminosidine (Paromomycin) in the Treatment of Leishmaniasis Imported into the United Kingdom, " *Transact. Royal Soc. Trop. Med. Hyg.* **86**: 61-67 (1992).

Slater, A.F.G.: "Chloroquine: Mechanism of Drug Action and Resistance in *Plasmodium falciparum,"* *Pharmacol. Ther.* **57**: 203-235 (1993).

Wolfe, M.S.: "The Treatment of Intestinal Protozoan Infections," *Med. Clin. North Am.* **66**: 707 (1982).

Wyler, D.J.: "The Ascent and Decline of Chloroquine," *J. Am. Med. Assoc.* **251**: 2420-2422 (1984).

CHAPTER 51

Chemotherapy of Helminthiases

Benjamin Z. Ngwenya

Helminthic infections represent a major problem to the health of millions of people throughout the world, especially in the subtropics and the tropics. The anthelmintic drugs are utilized to eradicate and control human intestinal helminthiases and may improve the health of the individual by alleviating the parasite-related suffering. The anthelmintic drugs covered in this chapter are listed in Table 51-1. It is advisable that before a drug is prescribed, a diagnosis and identification of the parasite must be made. This can be accomplished by finding the adult parasites and their characteristic eggs or larvae in feces, urine, sputum, blood, and tissues of the infected host. The anthelminthic of choice (Table 51-1) for the treatment of a parasitic infection is usually the most active agent against the pathogenic parasite or the least toxic alternative among relatively effective anthelmintics. As a group, the anthelmintics are the least studied of all drugs in current clinical use. There is insufficient information on the disposition of anthelmintics in children. Most treatments are recommended either empirically or by extrapolation from observations in adults. This chapter provides some basic information for effective and safe anthelmintic drug treatment required by the prescriber to understand the essential pharmacology of the drugs used.

DIETHYLCARBAMAZINE

Chemistry

Diethylcarbamazine, a piperazine derivative, is an effective drug for the treatment of filariasis. It is available as the citrate salt containing 51 percent of the active base. The drug is highly soluble in water. It should be stored in airtight containers and protected from light. Its structure is as follows:

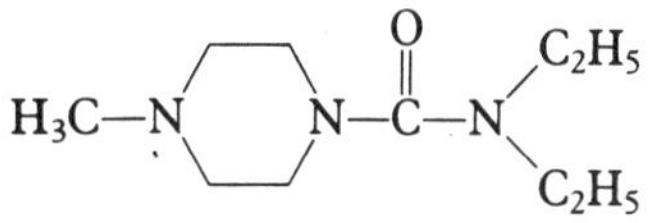

$$H_3C-N\langle\text{piperazine}\rangle N-\overset{O}{\overset{\|}{C}}-N\begin{matrix} C_2H_5 \\ C_2H_5 \end{matrix}$$

Mechanism of Action

The exact mechanism of antimicrofilarial activity of diethylcarbamazine has not been fully elucidated. The drug causes rapid sensitization of the microfilariae, and they become trapped in the reticuloendothelial system. The drug also causes a rapid disappearance of microfilariae of *Brugia malayi*, *Loa loa*, and *Wuchereria bancrofti* from the circulatory system.

Pharmacokinetics

Orally administered diethylcarbamazine is rapidly absorbed from the gastrointestinal tract. In adults, a single dose produces a peak plasma level within 1 to 3 h. The drug is rapidly distributed and equilibrated with all tissues, except fat. Its half-life is about 2 to 3 h in the presence of acidic urine and 10 h in alkaline urine. Diethylcarbamazine is completely excreted, primarily in the urine, within 30 h, either as unchanged drug or as an N-oxide metabolite. Less than 10 percent of the drug is excreted in feces.

Adverse Effects

At therapeutic levels, diethylcarbamazine is relatively safe. However, mild transient malaise, headache, joint pains, anorexia, nausea, and vomiting may occur 2 to 4 h posttreatment. There

TABLE 47-1 Treatment of helmintic infections

Infecting agent and disease	Treatment of choice	Alternative treatment
Cestodes (tapeworms)		
Cysticercus cellulosae (pork tapeworm larval stage) Cysticercosis	Praziquantel or Albendazole	Surgery
Diphyllobothrium latum (fish tapeworm) Diphyllobothriasis	Niclosamide or Praziquantel	None
Dipylidium caninum (dog tapeworm) Dipylidiasis	Niclosamide or Praziquantel	None
Echinococcus granulosus (hydatid worm) Echinococcosis	Surgery or Albendazole	None
Echinococcus multilocularis (hydatid worm) Echinococcosis	Surgery	Albendazole or Mebendazole
Hymenolepis nana (dwarf tapeworm) Hymenolepiasis	Praziquantel or Niclosamide	None
Taenia saginata (beef tapeworm) Taeniasis	Niclosamide or Praziquantel	None
Taenia solium (pork tapeworm) Taeniasis	Niclosamide or Praziquantel	None
Nematodes (roundworms)		
Ancylostoma braziliense (dog and cat hookworm) Anclyostomiasis (cutaneous larva migrans, creeping eruption)	Thiabendazole	Albendazole
Ancylostoma caninum (dog hookworm) Ancylostomiasis (cutaneous larva migrans, creeping eruption)	Thiabendazole or Albendazole	Diethylcarbamazine
Ancylostoma duodenale (human hookworm) Ancylostomiasis	Mebendazole or Pyrantel pamoate	Albendazole
Angiostrongylus cantonensis Angiostrongyliasis	Mebendazole	None
Anisakis sp. Anisakiasis	Surgery	None

TABLE 47-1 (continued) Treatment of helmintic infections

Infecting agent and disease	Treatment of choice	Alternative treatment
	Nematodes (roundworms) (continued)	
Ascaris lumbricoides (roundworm) Ascariasis	Pyrantel pamoate or Mebendazole	Albendazole
Brugia malayi (Malayan filarial worm) Malayan filariasis	Diethylcarbamazine	None
Dracunculus medinensis (guinea worm) Dracunculiasis	Metronidazole	Thiabendazole
Enterobius vermicularis (pinworm) Enterobiasis	Pyrantel pamoate or Mebendazole	Albendazole
Intestinal capillariasis	Mebendazole	Albendazole
Loa loa (eyeworm) Loiasis	Diethycarbamazine	None
Necator americanus (human hookworm) Necatoriasis	Mebendazole or Pyrantel pamoate	Albendazole
Onchocerca volvulus (filarial worm) Onchocerciasis	Ivermectin	None
Strongyloides stercoralis (threadworm) Strongyloidiasis	Thiabendazole	Ivermectin
Toxocara canis (dog ascarid) Toxocariasis (viceral larva migrans)	Diethylcarbamazine	Thiabendazole
Toxocara cati (cat ascarid) Toxocariasis (visceral larva migrans)	Diethylcarbamazine	Thiabendazole
Trichinella spiralis Trichinosis	Steroids for severe symptoms plus mebendazole	None
Trichostrongylus sp. Trichostrongyliasis	Pyrantel pamoate	Mebendazole or Albendazole
Trichuris trichiura (whipworm) Trichuriasis	Mebendazole or Albendazole	Pyrantel pamoate

TABLE 47-1 (continued) Treatment of helmintic infections

Infecting agent and disease	Treatment of choice	Alternative treatment
Nematodes (roundworms) (continued)		
Wuchereria bancrofti (filarial worm) Bancroft's filariasis	Diethylcarbamazine	None
Trematodes (flukes)		
Clonorchis sinensis (liver fluke) Clonorchiasis	Praziquantel	None
Fasciola hepatica (sheep liver fluke) Fascioliasis	Bithionol	None
Fasciolopsis buski (large intestinal fluke) Fasciolopsiasis	Praziquantel	Niclosamide
Heterophyes heterophyes Heterophyiasis	Praziquantel	None
Metagonimus yokogawai (Yokogawa's fluke) Metagonimiasis	Praziquantel	None
Opisthorchis sp. (liver fluke) Opisthorchiasis	Praziquantel	None
Paragonimus westermani (lung fluke) Paragonimiasis	Praziquantel	Bithionol
Schistosoma haematobium (vesical blood fluke) Vesical schistosomiasis Urinary bilharziasis	Praziquantel	None
Schistosoma japonicum (Oriental blood fluke) Oriental schistosomiasis Katayama disease	Praziquantel	None
Schistosoma mansoni (Manson's blood fluke) Schistosomal dysentery Intestinal bilharziasis	Praziquantel	Oxamniquine
Trematodes (roundworms)		
Schistosoma mekongi (Mekong schistosome)	Praziquantel	None

are a number of specific adverse effects seen only in filarial-infected patients.

Parasite-induced Reactions These reactions are assumed to be caused by the release of foreign proteins (antigens) from dying microfilariae or adult worms in sensitized patients. Usually the reactions are associated with intensified eosinophilia and leukocytosis. In lymphatic filariasis, the reactions may be very severe in heavy infections, producing a syndrome known as the *Mazzotti reaction*. It is characterized by generalized pruritus, rash, edema of the skin, erythema, lymphangitis, chills, conjunctiva, tearing, photophobia, and sweating. Respiratory distress, tachycardia, and hyperpyrexia have also been reported. The severity of the Mazzotti reaction is directly related to the microfilarial burden in the skin. Treating the patient with serotonin antagonists, antihistamines, or prostaglandin synthesis inhibitors will not diminish the Mazzotti reaction. However, the severity of the Mazzotti reaction may be alleviated by systemic administration of corticosteroids; but this reduces the efficacy of diethylcarbamazine. In loiasis, treatment may aggravate ocular lesions and result in blindness due to reaction against the dying microfilariae.

Clinical Uses

Diethylcarbamazine is indicated for the treatment of *W. bancrofti*, *B. malayi*, *L. loa*, *T. canis* and *T. cati*. The drug has a high therapeutic efficacy against these parasites. It is used as an alternate treatment to thiabendazole for *A. caninum* infestations. It is also used in *Mansonella streptocerca* infections and in tropical eosinophilia. Diethylcarbamazine has been used for mass treatment to reduce transmission of *W. bancrofti*. The drug may be given in low doses as a medicated salt, which is stable in cooking and seems to be free of adverse effects but still active against the microfilariae. The drug has also been recommended for prophylactic measures against *L. loa*, *W. bancrofti*, and *B. malayi* infections.

Although there are no absolute adverse effects, diethylcarbamazine should be used with caution in patients with hypertension and renal disease. Dosage should be adjusted in patients with high urinary pH, because renal function and pH are critical factors associated with the excretion of the drug. In patients with mixed filariasis, the dosage of diethylcarbamazine should be increased gradually.

MEBENDAZOLE

Chemistry

Mebendazole is a synthetic benzimidazole derivative with broad-spectrum anthelmintic activity. Two derivatives, thiabendazole and albendazole, are discussed later in the chapter.

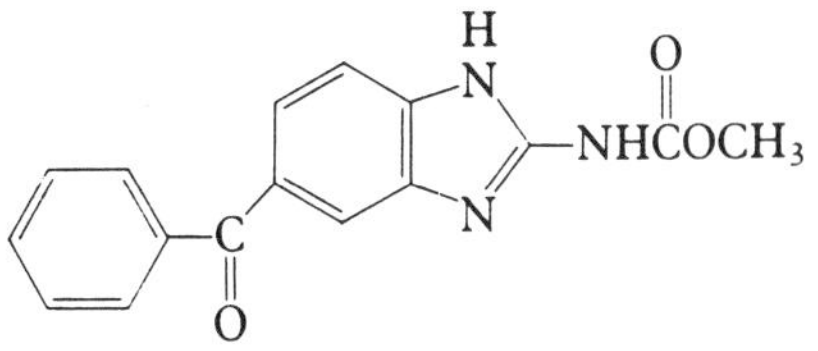

H N, O, NHCOCH$_3$, N, C, O

Mechanism of Action

The exact mechanism of anthelmintic action of mebendazole has not been completely elucidated. The drug inhibits the formation of the microtubules in the helminth and selectively and irreversibly inhibits glucose uptake by the parasites, resulting in glycogen depletion which leads to the ultimate death of the parasites. Mebendazole does not affect blood glucose concentrations in humans.

Pharmacokinetics

Orally administered mebendazole is minimally absorbed from the gastrointestinal tract and a high first-pass biotransformation results in a low bioavailability (5 to 10 percent); peak plasma concentrations of the drug occur about 2 to 4 h after administration. Plasma protein binding of the drug is approximately 95 percent. The drug is rapidly metabolized via decarboxylation to methyl 5-(α-hydroxybenzyl)-2-benzimidazole and 2-amino-5-benzoylbenzimidazole. The elimination half-life of mebendazole is between 3 and 9 h, and the drug is eliminated slow in the urine and the bile over a 24 to 48 h period.

Adverse Effects

At recommended dosage for a short-term (1 to 3 days) use, mebendazole appears to be remarkably free of adverse effects. Few cases of transient nausea, vomiting, abdominal pain, and diarrhea have been reported in patients with massive infections. High doses of mebendazole have been shown to induce bone marrow toxicity.

Clinical Uses

Mebendazole is indicated as a drug of choice for the treatment of ancylostomiasis, ascariasis, enterobiasis, intestinal capillariasis, necatoriasis, and trichuriasis. It is also effective in the treatment of echinococcosis and trichostrongylosis. A dose of 100 mg twice daily for 3 days produces 90 to 100 percent cure rates for ascariasis and trichostrongylosis. In trichuriasis and ancylostomiasis infections, cure rates of 60 to 90 percent and 70 to 95 percent are obtained, respectively. A single day therapy with mebendazole can cure 90 to 100 percent of pinworm infestations. The cure rates of mebendazole compare favorably with that of other drugs, however, mebendazole has the added advantage of fewer adverse effects.

Mebendazole is contraindicated in patients who are pregnant or hypersensitive to the drug. Mebendazole should be used with caution in patients with severe hepatic parenchymal disease because the drug is poorly detoxified in such patients.

NICLOSAMIDE

Chemistry

Niclosamide is a halogenated salicylanilide derivative that has proven to be very effective in the treatment of a variety of cestode infections.

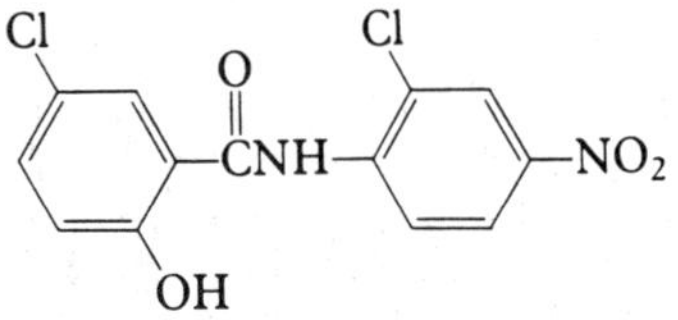

Mechanism of Action

Niclosamide exerts its effect against cestodes by inhibition of mitochondrial oxidative phosphorylation in the parasites. The mechanism of action of niclosamide is also related to its inhibition of glucose and oxygen uptake in the parasite. The scolex and proximal segments of the worm are killed on contact with the drug and drug-induced alteration of the parasite integument may render the cestodes susceptible to digestion by the host intestinal proteolytic enzymes and may become unrecognizable. At therapeutic doses, the drug appears to have no pharmacologic effect on human cells.

Pharmacokinetics

The absorption of niclosamide from the gastrointestinal tract following oral administration is minimal. Therefore, only trace amounts of an oral dose of niclosamide reach the circulatory system. Although the exact metabolic fate of the drug has not been elucidated, limited evidence indicates that the drug is metabolized in the gastrointestinal tract and excreted in feces.

Adverse Effects

Niclosamide is generally well tolerated and therapy may be associated with transient, mild to severe side effects. The infrequent adverse effects are abdominal discomfort, nausea, vomiting, and diarrhea; rarely reported adverse effects associated with niclosamide treatment include fever, headache, pruritus ani, skin rash, and urticaria, some of which may be attributed to a hypersensitivity reaction to massive antigens absorbed from disintegrating tapeworms.

Consumption of alcohol is contraindicated on the day of treatment and for one day past treatment. The drug is also contraindicated in patients who are hypersensitive to the drug. Niclosamide safety in children under 2 years of age has not been established.

Clinical Uses

Niclosamide is effective against adult intestinal cestodes such as *D. latum* (fish tapeworm), *T. saginata* (beef tapeworm), *T. solium* (pork tapeworm), *D. caninum* (cat and dog tapeworm), *H. diminuta* (rat tapeworm), and *H. nana* (dwarf tapeworm).

A single 2 g oral dose of the drug results in cure rates of 85 and 95 percent for adult *D. latum, T. saginata*, and *T. solium*. The drug is ineffective for the treatment of cysticercosis (an invasive larval disease) acquired by humans via the ingestion of the eggs of *T. solium*. Niclosamide is effective against the adult *H. nana* tapeworms but not against tissue-embedded cysticercoides. The cure rate for *H. nana* is about 75 percent for a treatment regimen of 5 to 7 days. Niclosamide is also considered as an effective alternative treatment for intestinal fluke (*F. buski*) infection.

Niclosamide exerts its effect against intestinal cestodes and should not be used in the treatment of invasive larval disease (cysticercosis). Some authorities advise not to use niclosamide for the treatment of *T. solium*, because the drug causes disintegration of proglottids (worm segments) and the release of infective eggs. The presence of the eggs in the intestinal tract is correlated with a serious theoretical risk of the development of cysticercosis. To avoid this possibility, some clinicians consider praziquantel the drug of choice for the treatment of *T. solium* infections.

OXAMNIQUINE

Chemistry

Oxamniquine is a derivative of 2-aminomethyl-tetrahydroquinoline and the most active of an entire series of compounds with anthelmintic activity. The structure is as follows:

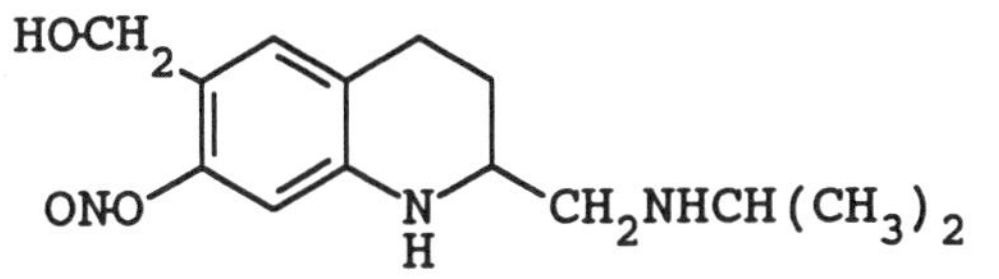

Mechanism of Action

Although its mechanism of action is unknown the compound possesses anticholinergic activity which may play a part in its ability to kill various helminths. Another possible mechanism is the ability of the drug to alkylate DNA molecules thus rendering the organism inactive. Male schistosomes concentrate oxamniquine more than the females and are therefore more sensitive to the drug. Surviving females do not lay eggs.

Pharmacokinetics

Oxamniquine can be given orally with peak plasma concentrations occurring within 0.5 to 3 h; the bioavailability is approximately 60 percent. The drug is metabolized in the intestines to a 6-carboxyl metabolite which reaches high concentrations in the plasma prior to excreted in the urine.

Adverse Effects

The most common adverse effects of oxamniquine are headaches, dizziness, drowsiness, nausea, and diarrhea. Other less common untoward effects reported are convulsions, transient elevations in liver transaminases, and eosinophilia (probably a host reaction to the dead and dying worms).

Clinical Uses

The only use of oxamniquine is for the treatment of infections with *S. mansoni*. Usually a single day's therapy is sufficient to eradicate this worm. *S. haematobium* and *S. japonicum* are resistant to the drug.

PRAZIQUANTEL

Chemistry

Praziquantel, a synthetic pyrazinoisoquinoline derivative, is a broad-spectrum anthelmintic agent. It is structurally unrelated to other anthelmintic agents currently available. The (−) isomer is responsible for most of the compounds anthelmintic activity.

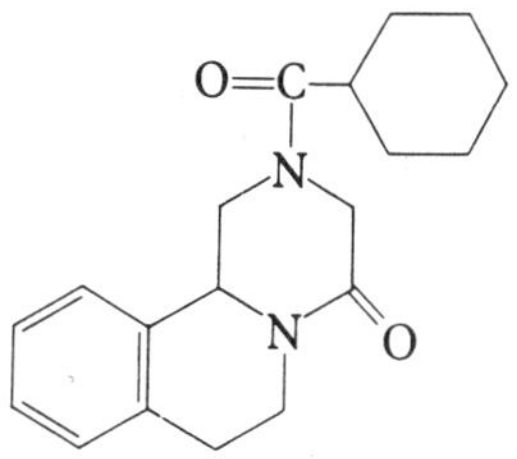

Mechanism of Action

The precise mechanism of action of praziquantel has not been fully elucidated. Praziquantel appears to kill the adult schistosome by increasing the permeability of the cell membrane of the parasite to calcium and consequent influx of calcium ions. This results in drug-induced muscular contraction and subsequent paralysis of the parasite's muscles. This causes immobilization of their suckers, resulting in detachment of the parasite from their sites of residence in the mesenteric veins or vesical plexus. The worms are then carried to the liver, where they elicit tissue reaction with subsequent phagocytosis. The drug appears also to be active against the schistosomal infective stage (cercaria) for humans and animals.

Praziquantel has also been shown to cause irreversible focal vacuolization and subsequent disintegration of the trematodes and cestodes.

Pharmacokinetics

Praziquantel is well absorbed (about 80 percent) after oral administration. A small portion of the drug reaches the blood unchanged since it undergoes a high first-pass biotransformation. Although the precise metabolic fate of praziquantel is unclear, most of the drug is quickly and extensively metabolized in the liver via hydroxylation to monohydroxylated and polyhydroxylated products. Peak plasma drug concentration is reached 1 to 2 h after a single oral dose. The concentration of the drug in cerebrospinal fluid is reported to be 14 to 20 percent of the plasma concentration.

Praziquantel has a serum half-life of between 0.8 and 1.5 h in normal adults. The serum half-life of the metabolites is about 4 to 5 h. The drug and its metabolites are mostly excreted in urine. Approximately 70 to 80 percent of the orally administered dose is excreted in urine as metabolites within 24 h.

Adverse Effects

At recommended dosage, praziquantel is generally well tolerated. The drug is associated with frequent occurrence of transient and mild to moderate side effects such as malaise, headache, abdominal pain, and dizziness, which occur in a high percent of patients. Diarrhea, anorexia, and vomiting have also been reported. Other adverse effects are pruritus, skin rashes, low-grade fever, and elevated eosinophilia. Heavily infected patients are associated with increased frequency of adverse effects. The intensity and frequency of the adverse effects appear to be dose-related.

Clinical Uses

Praziquantel is indicated for, and is the drug of choice for, the treatment of all forms of human schistosomiasis (*S. haematobium*, *S. japonicum*, *S. mansoni*, and *S. mekongi*). The drug is highly effective, has low toxicity, and is easily administered orally. Praziquantel is well tolerated by patients in the chronic stage (hepatosplenic stage) of advanced schistosomiasis. The drug produces cure rates of 75 to 95 percent and/or 80 to 98 percent egg reduction in infected patients.

Praziquantel is also considered the drug of choice for its effectiveness against many cestode infections, including those caused by *T. solium*, *T. saginata*, *D. latum*, *D. caninum*, and *H. nana*. Some clinicians consider praziquantel the drug of choice for *T. solium* because paromomycin and niclosamide cause disintegration of proglottids and the release of eggs which may produce *Cysticercus cellulosae* infection.

Praziquantel should not be administered in patients who are hypersensitive to the drug. Preferably the drug should not be taken during pregnancy. Patients should be advised not to drive because praziquantel causes dizziness and drowsiness on the day of and the day after therapy.

PYRANTEL PAMOATE

Chemistry

Pyrantel is a pyrimidine derivative, administered as the pamoate salt. It has antihelmintic activity against a broad range of nematodes, including pinworms, hookworms, and roundworms. The drug has the following structure:

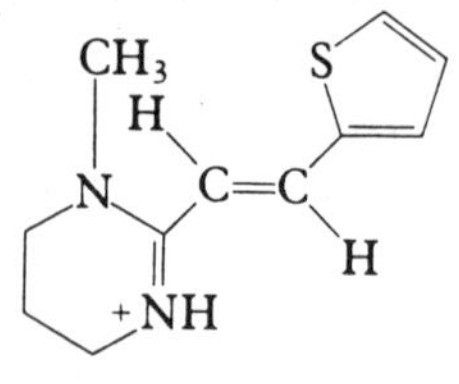

Mechanism of Action

Pyrantel pamoate exerts its anthelmintic effect via the inhibition of neuromuscular transmission; the drug is a depolarizing neuromuscular blocker. In susceptible worms, a spastic neuromuscular paralysis occurs, resulting in the expulsion of the worms from the intestinal tract of the host. Pyrantel also exerts its effect against parasites via release of acetylcholine and inhibition of cholinesterase.

Pharmacokinetics

Since it is a positively charged molecule, orally administered pyrantel pamoate is poorly absorbed from the gastrointestinal tract. Peak plasma concentrations are attained in 1 to 3 h. The drug is partially metabolized in the liver, and about 7 percent is excreted in urine unchanged or as metabolites. The major portion of an oral dose of the drug is excreted unchanged in the feces.

Adverse Effects

Adverse effects of pyrantel pamoate occur in 4 to 20 percent of patients and are usually mild and transient. They include abdominal cramps, nausea, diarrhea, vomiting, headache, insomnia, drowsiness, rash, fever, and weakness.

Pyrantel does not appear to produce any clinically significant alterations in urinary values at therapeutic dosages. However, minimal transient increases in serum concentrations of liver transaminases have been reported in a few patients.

Clinical Uses

Pyrantel is administered orally. It is used for the treatment of ascariasis, enterobiasis, trichuriasis, and several hookworm diseases and is considered the drug of choice for some of these (see Table 51-1). The drug has cure rates of 85 to 100 percent in patients infected with ascariasis and 90 to 100 percent in patients with enterobiasis.

THIABENDAZOLE

Chemistry

Thiabendazole is a benzimidazole derivative and is effective against a broad range of nematodes that infect the gastrointestinal tract, including pinworm, roundworm, threadworm, hookworm, and whipworm. It is structurally related to mebendazole and albendazole.

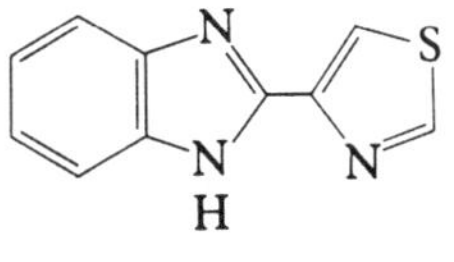

Mechanism of Action

The exact mechanism of action associated with the anthelmintic activity of thiabendazole is not clearly elucidated. The drug has been shown to inhibit the mitochondrial enzyme, fumarate reductase, a helminth-specific enzyme. In *Strongyloides stercoralis*, the drug may suppress the assembly of microtubules and inhibit the secretion of acetylcholinesterase in the parasite leading to dislodgement of the worm. In animal studies, thiabendazole has been shown to have analgesic, anti-inflammatory, and antipyretic activity.

Pharmacokinetics

Thiabendazole is administered orally and is rapidly absorbed from the gastrointestinal tract. Peak plasma concentrations are achieved within 1 to 2 h. The drug is extensively metabolized in the liver to 5-hydroxythiabendazole and then is conjugated with glucuronic or sulfuric acid. About 90 percent of orally administered drug is eliminated in urine within 48 h as glucuronic or sulfate conjugates of the metabolite. Approximately 5 percent of an oral dose of thiabendazole is eliminated in feces over the first 24 h.

Adverse Effects

At the recommended dosage, 7 to 50 percent of patients experience mild and transient side effects. The commonly observed side effects include headache, nausea, vomiting, abdominal pain, and dizziness; side effects occur 3 to 4 h post-administration of thiabendazole and last up to 2 to 8 h. The incidence of these side effects increases with the administration of higher doses and length of treatment. Occasionally, epigastric distress, skin reactions, diarrhea, fatigue, and drowsiness may occur. Hypersensitivity reactions such as chills, fever, anaphylaxis, angioedema, erythema multiforme, and lymphadenopathy have been reported in thiabendazole-treated patients.

Clinical Uses

Thiabendazole is a broad-spectrum anthelmintic, active against many human intestinal nematode infections, including *Ancylostoma braziliense*, *A. caninum*, *A. duodenale*, *Ascaris lumbricoides*, *Dracunculus medinensis*, *Enterobius vermicularis*, *Necator americanus*, *Strongyloides stercoralis*, *Toxocara canis*, *T. cati*, and *Trichuris trichiura*. The drug is both ovicidal and larvicidal.

Although, thiabendazole has been reported to be larvicidal against *Trichinella spiralis* in animals and active against the intestinal phase in human infections, its activity against migrated and encysted larvae in human infections has not been established. The effect of the drug on the intestinal phase of trichinosis is limited. Its use may ameliorate the signs and symptoms of the infection without subsequent changes in laboratory finding.

Thiabendazole is presently considered the drug of choice against *A. braziliense*, *A. caninum*, and *S. stercoralis* and an alternate treatment against *D.*

medinesis, *T. canis* and *T. cati*. Its activity against other parasites is more variable. Despite the fact that thiabendazole is a broad-spectrum drug, it is no longer recommended for treatment of many nematode infections due to its potential toxicity.

Warnings and Precautions

Thiabendazole should be given with caution and careful monitoring to patients with a history of renal dysfunction and drug hypersensitivity. If hypersensitive reactions develop during treatment, the use of the drug should be discontinued immediately. Supportive therapy is indicated for dehydrated, malnourished, or anemic patients before administration of thiabendazole. Since the drug can induce adverse effects on the CNS, it should not be given during the day for patients requiring mental alertness, such as driving a motor vehicle and operating machinery. Ideally, such activities should be avoided.

INVESTIGATIONAL DRUGS

The following drugs are not presently available in the United States, and are therefore considered investigational but are recommended as drugs of choice or alternative therapies for many helminth infestations.

ALBENDAZOLE

Chemistry

Albendazole, a synthetic benzimidazole derivative that is structurally related to mebendazole and thiabendazole, is a broad-spectrum anthelmintic agent.

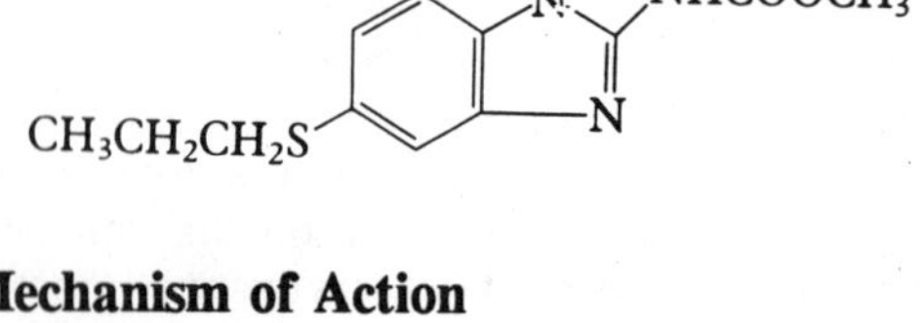

H
N NHCOOCH$_3$
$CH_3CH_2CH_2S$ N

Mechanism of Action

Albendazole exerts an anthelmintic effect against susceptible cestodes and nematodes by blocking glucose uptake of adult and larval stages, resulting in the depletion of glycogen stores and the subsequent decrease of adenosine triphosphate (ATP). Consequently, the parasites are immobilized and die. The drug is ovicidal against *Ascaris lumbricoides*, *Ancylostoma braziliense*, *A. caninum*, *A. duodenale*, *Necator americanus*, and *Trichuris trichiura* and larvicidal against *Necator americanus* and *Cysticercus cellulosae*.

Pharmacokinetics

Orally administered albendazole is rapidly absorbed from the gastrointestinal tract and is metabolized to yield mainly albendazole sulfoxide and other metabolites. Large amounts of the metabolites formed by hydroxylation and hydrolysis of albendazole sulfoxide are mainly excreted in the urine, and only a trace amount is excreted in the feces. The plasma elimination half-life of the sulfoxide is about 8 to 9 h. Albendazole itself is not detected in plasma due to its rapid metabolism. The sulfoxide metabolite appears to mediate most of the anthelmintic effect of albendazole.

Adverse Effects

When used at recommended dosage for 1 to 3 days, albendazole appears to be practically free of adverse effects. However, mild transient headache, nausea, diarrhea, epigastric distress, lassitude, insomnia, and dizziness have been reported in about 6 percent of the patients. Controlled experiments suggest that the incidence of side effects attributed to the drug is similar to that in the control group. A few cases of transient abdominal pain, low-grade elevations in hepatic transaminase, mild transient neutropenia, and fever have been reported during albendazole treatment. Further evaluation of the type and severity of the adverse effects of the drug after both single and repeated treatment is warranted.

Clinical Uses

Albendazole has been used effectively and is considered as a drug of choice against *A. caninum*, *T. trichiura* and *C. cellulosae*. The drug is presently judged as an alternative treatment against *A. braziliense*, *A. duodenale*, *A. lumbricoides*, *N. americanus*, *Enterobius vermicularis*, and *Trichostrongylus* species. A single dose of orally administered albendazole can result in cure rates of 70, 80, 88, and 100 percent for trichuriasis, ascariasis, necatoriasis, and enterobiasis, respectively. To attain a satisfactory reduction in worm burden in patients with heavy trichuriasis and necatoriasis and high cure rates in ascariasis may require a higher initial single dose or repeated treatment for several days (2 to 3 days). The cure rates of the drug in patients who attain low plasma concentrations of the sulfoxide metabolite remains to be elucidated. Recent reports suggest that albendazole is a useful adjunct in the management of cerebral hydatid diseases. It can, in some cases, replace surgery as the treatment of choice.

Contraindications

Albendazole has been shown to be teratogenic and embryotoxic in some experimental animals. Therefore, it is not recommended during pregnancy and lactation. The drug should be used with caution in patients with history of hematologic and liver diseases.

BITHIONOL

Chemistry

Bithionol is a dichlorophenol derivative that is structurally similar to hexachlorophene. It is the anthelmintic of choice for the treatment of human infection by *Fasciola hepatica* (sheep liver fluke) and is an alternative to praziquantel for the treatment of pulmonary paragonimiasis (lung fluke) and acute cerebral paragonimiasis. This drug is not marketed in the United States; it is distributed by the Centers for Disease Control (CDC), Atlanta, Georgia.

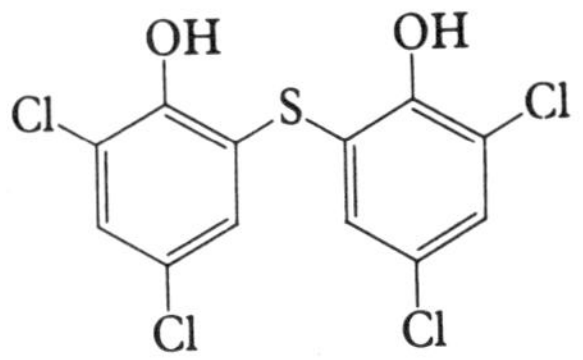

Mechanism of Action

Although the exact mechanism of anthelmintic action of bithionol has not been fully elucidated, the drug appears to inhibit oxidative phosphorylation in *Paragonimus westermani*. Morphological alterations in *F. hepatica* have been attributed to the drug.

Pharmacokinetics

Little is known about the pharmacokinetics of bithionol. The drug is readily absorbed from the gastrointestinal tract and glucuronidated in the liver. Excretion of bithionol appears to be mainly through the kidney.

Adverse Effects

Side effects have been reported in about one-third of the patients. Usually the effects are mild and transient. The most common side effects are abdominal cramps and diarrhea. Diarrhea may be accompanied by anorexia, nausea, and vomiting. Some patients receiving long-term therapy may develop pruritic, urticaria, or papular skin rashes. Since the onset of skin rashes occurs after a latent period of a week or more of therapy, they could be due to allergic reactions resulting from massive release of antigens from the dying parasites. Other infrequent adverse effects are leukopenia, proteinuria, and hepatitis.

Clinical Uses

Bithionol is the anthelmintic of choice for the treatment of fascioliasis (sheep liver fluke) and as an alternative to praziquantel for the treatment of human infections by *Paragonimus* species. A treatment regimen with 10 to 50 mg/kg on alternate days for a total of 15 doses resulted in a cure rate of 91 to 97 percent in patients with pulmonary paragonimiasis. However, in patients with combined pulmonary and cerebral paragonimiasis, the results were less satisfactory. In patients with acute cerebral paragonimiasis, the effectiveness of bithionol may be enhanced by administering more than one course of treatment. The drug effectiveness is minimal in patients with long-term cerebral paragonimiasis.

Contraindications

There is limited experience with bithionol treatment during pregnancy and lactation. Therefore, its use in such patients is not recommended. The development of toxic hepatitis and leukopenia should be evaluated by liver function and hematologic tests, respectively. Evidence is inconclusive concerning the neurological toxicity in patients with cerebral paragonimiasis.

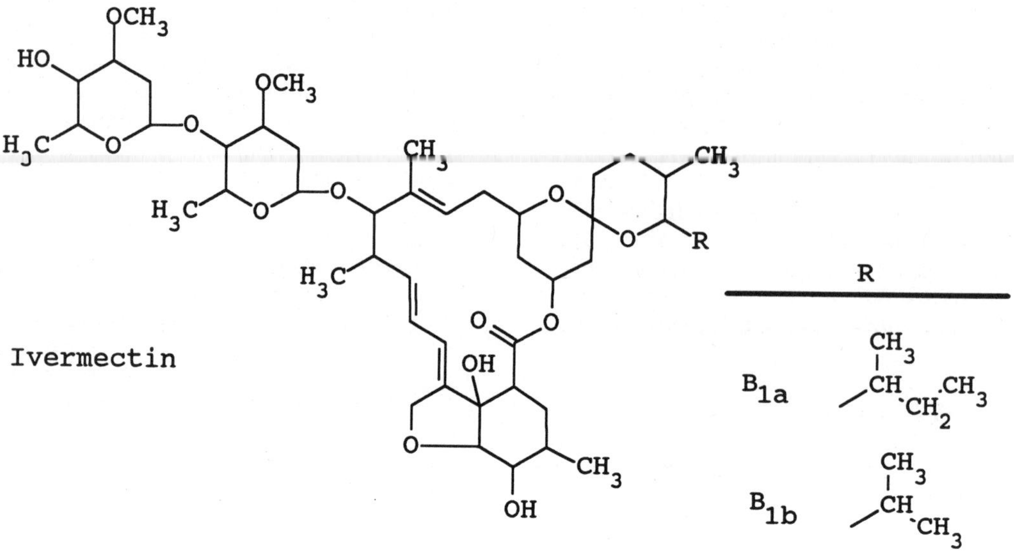

Ivermectin

R

B_{1a} — $CH(CH_3)CH_2CH_3$

B_{1b} — $CH(CH_3)CH_3$

IVERMECTIN

Chemistry

Ivermectin is a complex macrocyclic lactone formed by the catalytic hydrogenation of avermectin B_1. Ivermectin is comprised of 80 percent B_{1a} (sec-butyl) and 20 percent B_{1b} (isopropyl) derivatives of avermectin.

Mechanism of Action

The compound produces toxic paralysis of the peripheral musculature of the helminth, thus immobilizing the organism. One explanation proposed for this effect is the release and potentiation of GABA (γ-aminobutyric acid) by ivermectin.

Pharmacokinetics

Peak blood levels of ivermectin occur within 4 h of administration. The elimination half-life is approximately 10 h. The majority of the compound is excreted in the urine unchanged.

Adverse Effects

Major adverse effects of ivermectin include pruritus, dizziness, and postural hypotension.

Clinical Uses

Ivermectin is used to control onchocerciasis in man. The drug is also effective against strongyloidiasis, ascariasis, trichuriasis, and enterobiasis.

BIBLIOGRAPHY

Awadzi, K., K.K. Adjepon-Yamoah, G. Edwards, M.L'E. Orme, A.M, Breckenridge, and H.M. Gilles: "The Effects of Moderate Urine Alkalinisation on Low Dose Diethylcarbamazine Therapy in Patients with Onchocerciasis," *Br. J. Clin. Pharmacol.* **21**: 669-676 (1986).

Bruce, S.I.: "New Anthelmintics," in Howell, M.S. (ed.), *Parasitology — Quo Vadis*, Proceedings of the Sixth International Congress of Parasitology, Australian Academy of Science, 1986, pp. 131-140.

Chan, L., S.P. Kan, and D.A. Bundy: "The Effect of Repeated Chemotherapy on the Prevalence and Intensity of *Ascaris lumbricoides* and *Trichuris trichiura* Infection," *Southeast Asian J. Trop. Med. Publ. Health* **23**: 228-234 (1992).

Geary, T.G., R.D. Klein, L. Vanover, J.W. Bowman, and D.P. Thompson: "The Nervous Systems of Helminths as Targets for Drugs," *J. Parasitol.* **78**: 215-230 (1992).

Goa, K.L., D. McTavish, and S.P. Clissold: "Ivermectin: A Review of its Antifilarial Activity, Pharmacokinetic Properties and Clinical Efficacy in Onchocerciasis," *Drugs*

42: 640-658 (1991).

Greene, B.M.: "Modern Medicine Versus an Ancient Scourge: Progress Toward Control of Onchocerciasis," *J. Infect. Dis.* **661**: 15-21 (1992).

Gustofsson, L., L. Beerman, and Y. A. Abdi: *Handbook of Drugs for Tropical Parasitic Infections*, Taylor and Francis, Inc., New York, 1987.

Johnson, R.J., E.C. Jong, S.B. Dunning, W.L. Carberry, and B.H. Minshew: "Paragonimiasis: Diagnosis and the Use of Praziquantel in Treatment," *Rev. Infect. Dis.* **7**: 200-206 (1985).

Katiyar, J.C., S. Gupta, and S. Sharma: "Experimental Models in Drug Development for Helminthic Diseases," *Rev. Infect. Dis.* **2**: 638-654 (1989).

Pearson, R.D., and E.L. Hewlett: "Niclosamide Therapy for Tapeworm Infections," *Ann. Intern. Med.* **102**: 550-551 (1985).

Shekhar, K.C.: "Schistosomiasis: Drug Therapy and Treatment Considerations," *Drugs* **43**: 379-405 (1991).

Shu-hua, X., Y. Ji-Qing, G. Hui-Fang, and B.A. Catto: "Plasma Pharmacokinetics and Therapeutic Efficacy of Praziquantel and 4-Hydroxypraziquantel in *Schistosoma Japonicum*-Infected Rabbits After Oral, Rectal, and Intramuscular Administration," *Am. J. Trop. Med. Hyg.* **46**: 582-588 (1992).

Singounas, E.G., A.S. Leventis, D.E. Sakas, D.M. Hardley, D.A. Lampadarios, and P.C. Karvounis: "Successful Treatment of Intracerebral Hydatid Cyst with Albendazole: Case Report and Review of the Literature," *Neurosurgery* **31**: 571-574 (1992).

White, N.J.: "Antiparasitic Drugs in Children," *Clin. Pharmacokin.* **17**: 138-155 (1989).

PART XI

Toxicology

SECTION EDITOR

Joseph R. DiPalma

CHAPTER 52

Toxicology

Thomas L. Pazdernik

This chapter will deal with definitions and terms, toxicokinetics, toxicodynamics, factors that modify toxicity, incidence of acute poisoning, prevention of acute poisoning, treatment of acute poisoning and specific drugs used in the management of poisoning. Chapter 53 will summarize some important non-metallic toxicants and Chapter 54 will focus on heavy metals and antagonists.

DEFINITIONS AND TERMS

Toxicology is the science which relates hazardous effects of chemicals, including drugs, to biological systems. A *poison* is a substance which when introduced into a living organism in sufficient amounts may have an injurious or deadly effect. Virtually all substances are poisonous if given in sufficient quantities. Poisons are sometimes referred to as *toxins. Toxicity* is the capacity of a substance to produce injury under defined conditions (e.g., dose, duration of exposure, rate of exposure, time course). Therefore, toxicity is a qualitative term in that whether or not injury occurs depends on the conditions of exposure to the toxin. *Hazard*, on the other hand, is the probability that injury will result from the use of a substance in a proposed quantity and manner. Humans can safely use toxic substances as long as they minimize absorption. *Risk* is the expected frequency of occurrence of an undesirable effect arising from the exposure to a toxic substance. *Acute toxicity* arises from a single or multiple exposure of a toxin over 1 to 2 days, whereas *subacute toxicity* occurs from repeated exposures to a toxin for a period of no greater than 3 months and *chronic toxicity* occurs from repeated exposure to a toxin for a period of greater than 3 months. The appearance of an injurious effect after an acute exposure to a toxin may occur rapidly or at a much later time period, i.e., *delayed toxicity*. The *lethal dose-50* (LD_{50}) is the computed dose which produces death in 50 percent of test animals. The *lethal concentration-50* (LCT_{50}) is the air concentration calculated to produce death in 50 percent of animals inhaling the substance for a given time period. In inhalation toxicology, *maximal allowable concentration* (MAC) or *threshold limit value* (TLV) is the maximum concentration that can be in the air and yet be considered safe to breathe.

TOXICOKINETICS

Toxicokinetics is the term used to describe the absorption, distribution, biotransformation and elimination of toxic substances and their metabolites. The basic pharmacokinetic principles discussed in earlier chapters apply to toxicokinetics; however, a few points require special consideration when considering toxic substances.

The *absorption* of toxic substances depends on the route of exposure. For the toxic effects of drugs, the route of exposure is usually related to their therapeutic route of administration. Air pollutants usually gain entry by inhalation, whereas oral ingestion is the principle route of exposure for pollutants of water and soil. For toxins in the industrial setting, inhalation and transdermal routes are both of major importance.

The *apparent volume of distribution* (V_d) of a toxin is an important consideration in the management of a poisoned patient. When a toxicant is highly tissue-bound, the V_d is large and the plasma concentration is low. Therefore, compounds with high V_d are not readily removed by hemodialysis or hemoperfusion.

The *biotransformation* of lipophilic toxicants usually makes them less toxic (*detoxification*) and more easily excreted. However, some substances have to be *biologically activated* to exert their toxic effects. Some notable examples include: acetaminophen, benzene, carbon tetrachloride, cyclophosphamide, furosemide, halothane, isoniazid, and parathion, just to name a few.

Clearance (CL) is another important determinant in the toxicity of chemicals. Clearance is a measure of the plasma volume that is totally cleared of a chemical per unit of time. Chemicals are cleared from the body by various organs (e.g., kidneys, liver, intestine, lungs). *Total body clearance* (CL_{total}) is the sum of individual clearances such that:

$$CL_{total} = CL_r + CL_h + CL_i + CL_l \ldots\ldots$$

where subscripts are r = renal; h = hepatic; i = intestine and l = lung.

Some chemicals that are mainly cleared by hepatic clearance may be cleared more rapidly if biotransformation processes are enhanced by treatment with inducers (e.g., phenobarbital). Likewise, renal clearance of some weak organic acids (e.g., phenobarbital) may be enhanced by alkalinization of the urine, whereas renal clearance of weak organic bases (e.g., amphetamine) may be enhanced by acidification of the urine. Thus, for detoxification strategies, it is important to know which organs significantly contribute to total clearance of a chemical. Moreover, artificial clearance processes can be introduced via the techniques of peritoneal dialysis, hemodialysis or hemoperfusion. Most drugs are cleared at a rate proportional to plasma concentration (i.e., first-order kinetics), but with overdose, biotransformation processes may be saturated and the rate of elimination may become fixed (i.e., zero-order kinetics). Furthermore, the toxic effects of a drug may alter normal physiological function of organs which in turn can alter clearance of a toxic substance. See Chapter 4 for a complete discussion of these pharmacokinetic parameters.

TOXICODYNAMICS

The dose-response principles described for pharmacodynamics in Chapter 2 also apply to toxicodynamics. The definitions of *therapeutic index* and *margin of safety* were given in Chapter 2. For many drugs, some of their toxic effects may be distinct from their therapeutic actions. However, for other drugs, the major toxic effects may be just an overextension of their therapeutic actions (i.e., an exaggerated response).

Chemicals produce their toxic effects by alterations in normal biochemical and physiological cellular processes. For details, consult any of the toxicology texts cited in the Bibliography. Some general mechanisms of toxic actions include:

1. Interference with normal receptor-ligand interactions (e.g., strychnine).
2. Interference with membrane function (e.g., DDT).
3. Interference with cellular energy production (e.g., cyanide).
4. Binding to biomolecules (e.g., organophosphates).
5. Oxidative stress (e.g., paraquat).
6. Perturbation in calcium homeostasis (e.g., oxalates).
7. Toxicity from selective cell loss (e.g., MPTP or 1-methyl-4-phenyl-1,2,3,6-tetrahydropyridine).
8. Nonlethal genetic alterations in somatic cells (e.g., carcinogens).

Several examples of chemicals that exert their toxic actions via these mechanisms will be cited in the following two chapters.

FACTORS THAT MODIFY TOXICITY

There are a number of biological factors that may modify the toxicity of a chemical. These include:

1. Biotransformation: For example, methanol is converted to formaldehyde (a toxic metabolite).
2. Genetic factors: The peripheral neurotoxicity of isoniazid is greater in "slow" metabolizers than "fast" metabolizers.
3. Immune function: A classical example is penicillin-induced anaphylactic shock in a penicillin sensitive individual.
4. Phototoxic effects: Systemic tetracyclines, especially demeclocycline can induce skin photosensitization in individuals exposed to sunlight.
5. Species differences: Malaoxon is rapidly metabolized by mammals but very slowly by insects; thus, it has selective toxicity for insects.
6. Age: Both toxicodynamic and toxicokinetic parameters change with age.

Many chemicals are cleared much slower in geriatric patients than younger patients due to decreased biotransformation capacity and decreased glomerular filtration.

7. Gender: Hormonal status affects several toxicokinetic and toxicodynamic processes.
8. Nutritional status: There is now developing considerable evidence that diet markedly influences the incidence of different cancers.
9. Drug interactions: Just as drug interactions can modify pharmacodynamic actions of drugs, they can also modify toxicodynamic actions of chemicals.
10. Environmental factors: "Safe" chemicals may interact with substances in air, water or soil to form toxins. In order to predict the environmental impact of a chemical, it is essential to have knowledge about the following properties of chemicals: ability of the substance to be degraded; mobility of the substance through air, water and soil; bioaccumulation and its transport and biomagnification through the food chain.

INCIDENCE OF POISONING

Incidence of poisoning is given each year in the annual report of the American Association of Poison Control Centers National Data Collection System published in the *American Journal of Emergency Medicine*. The Centers for Disease Control also report information on poisoning in *Morbidity and Mortality Weekly Report*. As an example, Table 52-1 shows a list of substances most frequently involved in human exposure. The classes of poisons which cause the largest number of deaths are given in Table 52-2.

Poisoning is the second leading cause of suicide and the third leading cause of accidental deaths. Accidental exposure to poisons occur most frequently in children under 5 years of age and in the elderly. Sixty percent of all poisonings occur in children under 6 years of age and 46% occur in children under the age of 3. Although the invention of child-resistant caps in 1972 has markedly reduced pediatric poisoning fatalities, the unintentional ingestion of drugs and household products by children continues to result in significant morbidity and mortality.

TABLE 52-1 Substances most frequently involved in human exposure

Substance	Number of cases	%
Cleaning substances	191,830	10.4
Analgesics	183,013	10.0
Cosmetics	153,424	8.3
Plants	112,564	6.1
Cough and cold preparations	105,185	5.7
Bites/envenomizations	76,941	4.2
Pesticides (including rodenticides)	70,523	3.8
Topicals	69,096	3.8
Antimicrobials	64,805	3.5
Foreign bodies	64,472	3.5
Hydrocarbons	63,536	3.5
Sedative-hypnotics and antipsychotics	58,450	3.2
Chemicals	53,666	2.9
Alcohols	50,296	2.7
Food poisoning	46,482	2.5
Vitamins	40,883	2.2

Adapted from Litovitz, T.L., K.C. Holm, K.M. Bailey, and B.F. Schmitz: "1991 Annual Report of the American Association of Poison Control Centers National Data Collection System," *Am. J. Emerg. Med.* **10**: 452-505 (1992).

PREVENTION OF ACCIDENTAL POISONING

Health care personnel play a very important role in the education of the general public with respect to the safeguards which can prevent many cases of accidental poisonings. Parents of young children are in special need of such guidance. The following rules for prevention of accidental poisonings are recommended:

TABLE 52-2 Classes of poisons causing the largest number of deaths

Category	No. of cases	% of all exposures in category
Analgesics	190	0.104
Antidepressants	188	0.525
Sedative-hypnotics	97	0.166
Stimulants and street drugs	90	0.434
Cardiovascular drugs	87	0.348
Alcohols	72	0.143
Gases and fumes	49	0.188
Asthma therapies	39	0.229
Chemicals	37	0.069
Hydrocarbons	36	0.057
Cleaning substances	26	0.014
Pesticides (including rodenticides)	18	0.026

Adapted from Litovitz, T.L., K.C. Holm, K.M. Bailey, and B.F. Schmitz: "1991 Annual Report of the American Association of Poison Control Centers National Data Collection System," *Am. J. Emerg. Med.* 10: 452-505 (1992).

1. Medicines should be stored in high or locked cabinets.
2. Patients should be told not to save unused prescription medicines.
3. Children should not be coaxed into taking medications by comparing them to candy.
4. Do not store poisons in the same cabinets as foodstuffs.
5. Do not store poisons in cups, soft drink bottles or other food containers.
6. Label all stored material carefully.
7. Write down emergency phone numbers before the need arises.
8. If occupational exposure is a hazard, follow the manufacturer's cautions.

TREATMENT OF ACUTE POISONING

When not in attendance:

1. Warn patients to avoid hysteria.
2. Obtain important information such as name, age, weight, address, phone number and when possible, time of ingestion, substance ingested and amount ingested.
3. Determine severity of exposure. *Nonserious ingestion* (e.g., small amount of ink from a pen) requires only a telephone conversation. If *serious symptomatology* is reported, phone emergency services (such as an ambulance) immediately, have the container from which the poison was attained brought with patient as well as all bottles of medication in the area either empty or full, and alert personnel to set up appropriate equipment.
4. Suggested immediate home treatment. Remove the individual from continued exposure (i.e., especially true for corrosives) and remove contaminated clothing. Acid or alkali burns should be flooded with *water* for at least 5 minutes. If eyes have been exposed to caustic substances, they should be washed with *water* while the lids are held open, acids for 5 minutes and alkali for 20 minutes. In case of carbon monoxide or other inhalation poisons, immediately remove to open air. Give artificial respiration if needed. Dilute and absorb poison but keep in mind that fluids (except in the case of ingested caustic or irritant poisons) may increase gastric emptying time and once the poison passes out of the stomach it can no longer be removed by emesis or lavage. In certain cases emesis can be suggested but it is usually better to rush the patient to the hospital. If syrup of ipecac is available, it should be given immediately.

When in attendance:

1. Immediately check and support vital signs since breathing is of primary importance and then terminate further exposure. Obtain a brief history and do a cursory physical examination. It is important to obtain sufficient information to decide whether or not lavage should be performed, when to remove contents

from the stomach or intestinal tract and the conditions under which the stomach should be emptied are not always clearly defined:

Gastric lavage is of no value once the material has left the stomach. Gastric lavage usually is not recommended if more than 4 hours have elapsed since the last exposure (the exception is for poisons which delay gastric emptying time). Contraindications to performance of gastric lavage include: (1) if more than 30 minutes have elapsed since ingestion of a corrosive alkaline or acid poison, (2) ingestion of volatile petroleum distillates (which may induce chemical pneumonitis), (3) coma, stupor or delirium (hazard of aspiration). Gastric lavage can be used if a cuffed endotracheal tube is put in place to prevent aspiration.

Induced emesis. Contraindications are essentially the same as described for gastric lavage. Emesis is best induced by a central acting emetic such as ipecac syrup. Emesis is contraindicated for patients who have swallowed corrosive substances with pH far from neutral, such as Lysol (an acid) and Drano (an alkali); in comatose patients; in patients who are convulsing or have ingested a convulsant; and in patients who have ingested hydrocarbons.

Activated charcoal will adsorb many toxins (see list below) and is usually given immediately before or after lavage.

Cathartics will help remove toxins from the intestinal tract. Do not use oil base cathartics if convulsions are present.

2. Provide symptomatic and supportive treatment as appropriate.
3. Use specific antidote(s), if available, and under conditions indicated.
4. Increase the rate of excretion when appropriate: catharsis, altered urinary pH, osmotic diuretics, and dialysis.

SPECIFIC DRUGS USED IN THE MANAGEMENT OF POISONS

Some of the specific drugs used in the management of poisons is given below. All should be available in emergency rooms. For specific details and doses see Olson, K.R.: *Poisoning and Drug Overdose, First Edition*, 1990.

Activated charcoal Use 5 to 10 times the estimated weight of the poison; the usual dose is 5 grams in a water slurry orally. Charcoal is inert and non-toxic; there are no contraindications for its use. Charcoal is especially useful to adsorb the following compounds.

alcohol	muscarine
amphetamine	nicotine
antimony	opium
antipyrine	oxalates
atropine	parathion
arsenic	penicillins
barbiturates	phenol
camphor	phenolphthalein
cantharides	phenothiazines
cocaine	phosphorous
digitalis	potassium permanganate
glutethimide	quinine
iodine	salicylates
ipecac	selenium
malathion	silver
mercuric chloride	stramonium
methylene blue	strychnine
morphine	sulfonamides

Ammonium chloride The dose is 75 mg/kg four times a day, to a maximum of 2 to 6 grams, IV or orally for acidification of the urine in forced diuresis to pH 4.5 - 5.5.

Acetylcysteine This is used in acetaminophen poisoning. The dose is 140 mg/kg orally as a loading dose, followed by 70 mg/kg orally every 4 hours for 17 doses or until the serum acetaminophen level is zero.

Ascorbic acid For acidification of the urine, use 500 mg to 1 g IV or orally as needed to achieve a pH of 4.5 - 5.5. Give slowly IV.

Atropine In organophosphate poisonings, a test dose of 2 mg is given IV. It may be required to go much higher; the goal is to stop secretions: use that as an absolute end point rather than pupil dilation. The *pediatric dose* is 0.05 mg/kg IV, repeated every 5 to 10 minutes as needed.

Bicarbonate, sodium This is used for membrane depressant cardiotoxic drugs (e.g., tricyclic antidepressants, quinidine). The usual dose of 1 to 2 mg/kg as an IV bolus usually reverses cardiotoxic effects.

Cyanide Antidote Package For the treatment of cyanide poisoning, a kit is available that consists of sodium nitrate, sodium thiosulfate, and amyl nitrite. Follow instructions sequentially packed with drug in the kit. See Chapter 53 for further information on cyanide toxicity and its treatment.

Deferoxamine mesylate This is used for iron poisoning by giving 15 mg/kg/h IV, not to exceed 6 g daily. The pharmacology of this drug is discussed in Chapter 34.

Dimercaprol Administer IM for arsenic, gold or mercury poisoning and for acute lead encephalopathy. Doses vary depending on the heavy metal poison; see Chapter 54.

Flumazenil Flumazenil is a benzodiazepine receptor antagonist that is indicated for the management of benzodiazepine overdose. The initial dose is 0.2 mg IV (given over 30 seconds); a second 0.2 mg dose may be given, if necessary. Further doses of 0.5 mg IV can be given at 1 minute intervals to a maximum cumulative dose of 3 mg.

Digoxin-specific FAB antibodies This is used for toxicity to digoxin and other cardiac glycosides. One vial (40 mg) binds 0.6 mg of digoxin.

Edetate calcium disodium (calcium EDTA) Use this compound (not edetate disodium (EDTA)) for lead poisoning. The dosage is variable depending on the route of administration (IM or IV) and the severity of the toxicity.

Ethanol For methanol or ethylene glycol poisoning, a solution containing 10% ethanol in 5% dextrose is used for IV administration. Any blended whiskey or plain ethanol (less than 20%) is recommended for oral use.

Glucagon Glucagon has been used for poisoning with β-adrenoceptor blockers. A bolus IV injection of 2 to 5 mg may reverse bradycardia and hypotension resistant to β-adrenergic agonists.

Ipecac syrup For children, 15 mL orally is used and repeated in 20 minutes if no emesis occurs. Stimulate the hypopharynx, give copious fluids orally and keep the patient ambulatory. In adults, the dose is 30 mL followed by fluids, ambulation and stimulation.

Magnesium sulfate 5 grams orally or 50 mL of a 10% solution orally is used for catharsis. Children should receive 250 mg/kg.

Mannitol This drug is given IV in a 25% solution to maintain diuresis.

Naloxone hydrochloride For suspected opioid-induced coma, give 0.4 to 2 mg IV; repeat at 2 to 3 minute intervals, but do not exceed a total dose of 10 mg. The dosage used in children is 0.01 mg/kg IV, IM or SC; may repeat as described above.

Penicillamine Penicillamine is a copper chelator that is given orally to promote copper excretion. See Chapter 54 for a more complete discussion of this compound.

Physostigmine salicylate This drug is used to reverse toxic CNS effects of anticholinergic compounds. Do not use neostigmine or pyridostigmine which do not cross into the CNS. The usual adult dose is 2 mg IM or by slow IV administration. Repeat at 10 to 30 minute intervals until the desired response is obtained. For *pediatric patients*, the dose is 0.02 mg/kg IM or by slow IV injection; repeat at 5 to 10 minute intervals, if necessary, to a maximum dose of 2 mg.

Pralidoxime chloride This is given IV for organophosphate poisoning. It is not effective against carbamate cholinesterase inhibitors. Dosage varies in adults and children and also depends upon the route of administration (oral, IV).

BIBLIOGRAPHY

Amdur, M.O., J. Doull, and C.D. Klaassen (eds): *Casarett and Doull's Toxicology, 4th Ed.*, Pergamon Press, New York, 1991.

Becker, C.E., and K.R. Olson: "Management of the Poisoned Patient," in Katzung, B.G. (ed.), *Basic and Clinical Pharmacology, 5th Ed.*, Appleton and Lange, Norwalk, 1992.

Bryson, P.D.: *Comprehensive Review in Toxicology," 2nd Ed.*, An Aspen Publication, Rockville, MD, 1989.

Centers for Disease Control: "Unintentional Ingestions of Prescription Drugs in Children under Five Years Old," *Morb. Mort. Week. Rep.*, **36**: 124 (1987).

Centers for Disease Control: "Unintentional Poisoning Mortality — U.S. 1980-1986," *Morb. Mort. Week. Rep.*, **38**: 153 (1989).

Ellenhorn, M.J., and D.G. Barceloux: *Medical Toxicology: Diagnosis and Treatment of Human Poisoning, 2nd Ed.*, Elsevier, New York, 1991.

Ferguson, J.A., C. Sellar, and M.J. Goldacre: "Some Epidemiological Observations on Medicinal and Non-medicinal Poisoning in Preschool Children," *J. Epidem. Commun. Health*, **46**: 207-210 (1992).

Goldfrank, L.R.: *Toxicologic Emergencies, 4th Ed.*, Appleton-Century-Crofts, New York, 1990.

Gossel, T.A, and J.D. Bricker: *Principles of Clinical Toxicology*, Raven Press, New York, 1984.

Gosselin, R.E., R.P. Smith, and H.C. Hodge: *Clinical Toxicology of Commercial Products 5th Ed.*, Williams and Wilkins, New York, 1984.

Haddad, L. M., and J.F. Winchester: *Clinical Management of Poisoning and Drug Overdose*," W.B. Saunders, Philadelphia, 1990.

Hodgson, E., and P.E. Levi: *A Textbook of Modern Toxicology*, Elsevier, New York, 1987.

Klaassen, C.D.: "Principles of Toxicology," in Gilman, A.G., T.W. Rall, A.S. Nies, and P. Taylor, (eds.) *Goodman and Gilman's The Pharmacological Basis of Therapeutics, 8th Ed.*, Pergamon Press, New York, 1990, pp. 49-61.

Litovitz, T.L., K.C. Holm, K.M. Bailey and B.F. Schmitz: "1991 Annual Report of the American Association of Poison Control Centers National Data Collection System," *Am. J. Emerg. Med.* **10**: 452-505, 1992.

Lu, F.C.: *Basic Toxicology: Target Organs, and Risk Assessment*, Hemisphere, 1991.

Olson, K.R.: *Poisoning and Drug Overdose, 1st Ed.*, Appleton and Lange, Norwalk, 1990.

Ottobon, M.A.: *The Dose Makes the Poison*, van Nostrand Reinhold, New York, 1979.

Plaa, G.L.: "Introduction to Toxicology: Occupational and Environmental Toxicology," in Katzung, B.C. (ed.) *Basic and Clinical Pharmacology, 5th Ed.*, Appleton and Lange, Norwalk, 1992, pp. 821-830.

Proctor, N.H., and J.P. Hughes: *Chemical Hazards of the Workplace, 3rd Ed.*, J.B. Lippincott Company, Philadelphia, 1991.

Skoutakis, V.A.: *Clinical Toxicology of Drugs*, Lea and Febiger, Philadelphia, 1982.

Zeckhauser, R.J., and W.K. Viscusi: "Risk Within Reason," *Science*, **248**: 559-564, 1990.

CHAPTER 53

Non-Metallic Toxicants

Thomas L. Pazdernik

Industrialization and urbanization have markedly contributed to the pollution of air, water, and soil. The production and use of energy, the use of chemicals in agriculture and the production and use of industrial chemicals are major causes of pollution.

HOUSEHOLD POISONS

There are numerous products in the home that contain a variety of potentially toxic substances that individuals can be exposed to accidentally or intentionally. This section will deal only with the more common household hazards. Product formulations change frequently, but fortunately, labels are becoming more complete and accurate and antidote information on labels is improving. However, in most cases it is still advisable to contact the local Poison Control Center when questions occur.

Soaps and Detergents

The largest quantity of household poisons found in the home are soaps and detergents. They include *anionic, non-ionic* and *cationic detergents*, each differ in their toxic effects.

Anionic detergents are sulfonated or polyphosphorylated hydrocarbons. Soaps are made of sodium, potassium or ammonium salts of these fatty acids. Laundry compounds have added water softeners such as sodium carbonate, sodium phosphate or sodium silicate. The anionic detergents can irritate the skin. Ingestion of anionic detergents cause diarrhea, intestinal distention and occasional vomiting if large amounts have been swallowed. Additives, including deodorants, may be skin sensitizers.

The non-ionic detergents include sorbitan monostearate, polyethylene glycol, alkyl aryl ethers and alkyl aryl polyether sulfates, alcohols or sulfonates. These chemicals are only slightly irritating to the skin and are relatively harmless if swallowed. No treatment is necessary.

Cationic detergents such as benzalkonium chloride, benzethonium chloride, methyl benzethonium chloride and cetyl pyridinium chloride are used in numerous products for the destruction of microbes. Ingestion of 1 to 3 grams is estimated to be lethal. The clinical findings from ingestion are nausea, vomiting, corrosive damage to the esophagus, collapse, hypotension, convulsions and coma. Death can occur within 24 hours. Treatment requires the establishment of an airway and the maintenance of respiration. Give milk or activated charcoal and remove by catharsis. Lavage and emesis are contraindicated with the presence of esophageal injury.

Bleach

Most bleaching solutions are 3 to 6% aqueous solutions of sodium hypochlorite. Clinical findings of ingestion of bleach are severe irritation and corrosion of mucous membranes with pain and vomiting. Since bleach has a bad taste, most individuals don't swallow large amounts. With severe intoxication, there may be a fall in blood pressure with delirium and coma. Edema of the larynx and pharynx may be severe. Skin irritation occurs with prolonged contact with bleaching solutions. Treatment consists of flooding the skin with water. If swallowed, dilute by giving milk, melted ice cream or beaten eggs. Do not use lavage, emesis or acid antidotes. Aluminum hydroxide gel or magnesium hydroxide may be useful.

Oxalic Acid and Oxalates

Oxalic acid and oxalates are in bleaches and metal cleaners used in industrial and household products. Rhubarb leaves also contain high amounts of oxalate. Ingestion of 5 to 15 grams is estimated to be fatal. Oxalic acid is a corrosive acid, whereas oxalates bind calcium to form insoluble calcium oxalates. Lowering of free calcium in the body may lead to violent muscle stimulation with convulsions and collapse. At autopsy, calcium oxalate crystals are found in kidneys and other tissues; corrosive effects are common on mouth, esophagus, and stomach; and cerebral edema is often noted. Treatment consists of precipitating oxalate in the gastrointestinal tract by giving some form of oral calcium. Do not use emesis or lavage if tissue corrosion is present. Give 10 mL of 10% calcium gluconate solution by slow IV injection as an antidote, repeat if symptoms persist.

AIR POLLUTION

Carbon monoxide (52%), sulfur oxides (18%), hydrocarbons (12%), particulate matter (10%), and nitrogen oxides (6%) account for 98% of air pollution. Transportation (60%), industry (18%), electric-power generation (13%), space heaters (6%), and refuse disposal (3%) account for 90% of the pollutants that are emitted annually. The "reducing-type" of air pollution that comes from sulfur dioxide and smoke from incomplete combustion of coal and by conditions of fog and cool temperatures gives rise to the most serious adverse health effects. These effects are particularly prominent in individuals with pre-existing cardiac or respiratory diseases and in the elderly. The "oxidizing" or "photochemical" type of air pollution comes from hydrocarbons, oxides of nitrogen, and photochemical oxidants produced by automobile exhaust where intense sunlight (e.g., the Los Angeles basin) induces photochemical reactions in polluted air masses that are trapped by layers of air inversion. Adverse health effects other than severe eye irritation have not been associated with photochemical oxidant air pollution. Ambient air pollution is a contributing factor to allergic disorders, bronchitis, obstructive ventilatory disease, pulmonary emphysema, bronchial asthma, and lung cancer.

Carbon Monoxide

The most common cause of accidental and suicidal poisoning in the United States is carbon monoxide (CO), with an estimate of 4000 deaths annually. In addition, at least twice as many people suffer from partial poisoning, resulting in disability and absence from work. Persons with pre-existing heart or brain damage are more susceptible. Victims of CO poisoning of some severity who recover are subject to various and subtle neurologic sequelae.

Sources

The body itself produces a significant amount of CO from hemoglobin catabolism. CO has recently been reported to serve as a gaseous neurotransmitter in the brain, similar to that of nitric oxide. The normal carboxyhemoglobin (COHb) level seldom exceeds 0.4 to 0.7 percent. Hemoglobin destruction, as in hemolytic anemia, may raise levels of COHb to as much as 8 percent. Heavy smokers (at least a pack of cigarettes a day) have a COHb blood level of up to 6 percent.

In today's society, automobile exhaust provides the greatest source of environmental CO. However, catalytic converters have reduced the amount of CO emitted to about 1 percent. Nevertheless, because of the large number of cars on highways, the CO air levels can reach 25 to 100 ppm, enough to cause symptoms, especially in persons with pre-existing cardiovascular disease. Running the automobile engine in a closed garage is still one of the most common causes of accidental or suicidal poisoning.

The second most common source of CO is faulty heating equipment. This includes all types of stoves, whether fueled by wood, coal, gas, or oil. The rise in use of kerosene space heaters has increased the incidence of CO poisoning. All combustible material gives rise to a certain amount of CO. Therefore, the space occupied by the heating equipment must be vented at all times not only to allow a fresh and adequate oxygen supply but also to eliminate the CO produced by the heating equipment.

Deaths from fire are largely caused by inhalation of CO. Levels of this gas in fires may reach as high as 10 percent. This produces an atmosphere which can kill within minutes.

Industrial causes of CO poisoning occur in the smelting of metals, welding, ceramics working, glass-blowing, and in many processes using metal carbonyls. Methylene chloride (CH_2Cl), a constituent of some paint removers, is converted by the body to CO. This type of paint remover must be used in a vented room.

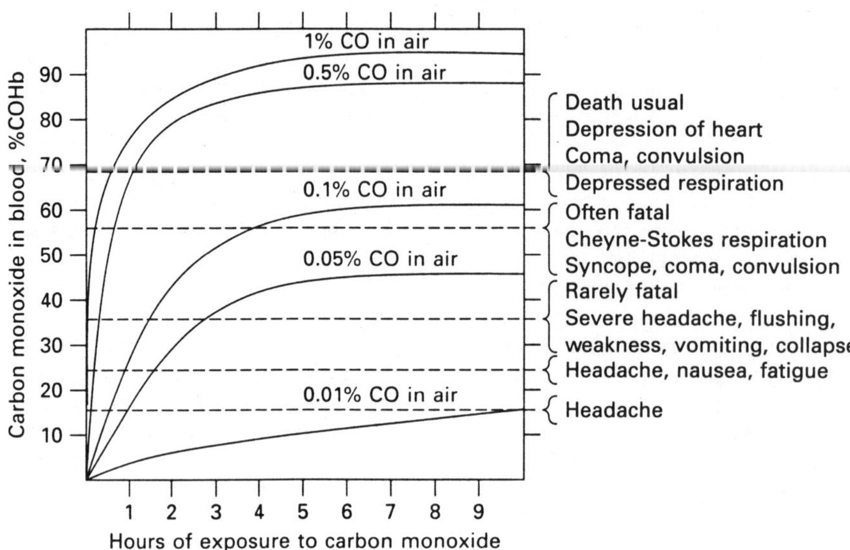

FIGURE 53-1 *The effect of the concentration of carbon monoxide in the air on the rate of uptake, expressed as a percent of carboxyhemoglobin (COHb). The relationship to time of exposure and the symptoms to be expected is also shown.*

Mechanism of Action

CO has an affinity for hemoglobin that is approximately 220 times greater than oxygen, resulting in the formation of COHb which cannot carry oxygen. Structural changes in the COHb molecule has an inhibitory influence on the dissociation of any oxyhemoglobin available, i.e., it causes the oxyhemoglobin curve to shift to the left. In addition, the reduction of red blood cell 2,3-diphosphoglycerate further accentuates the left shift. This causes a severe reduction in the oxygen-carrying capacity of blood. CO has an affinity for other heme compounds, including hydroperoxidase, myoglobin, cytochrome oxidase, guanylate cyclase, and cytochrome P-450. Although these are considerably less important, they do add to the general toxicity, and at low blood oxygen tension they assume a greater influence.

The effects of CO depend entirely on the concentration in inspired air and the duration of exposure. A brief exposure to a high concentration is less dangerous than a long exposure to a lower concentration. Another critical factor is the partial pressure of CO relative to the partial pressure of oxygen. High partial pressures of oxygen will tend to impede the uptake of CO, and vice versa. This is the basis of therapy with 100 percent oxygen and the use of the hyperbaric chamber.

Clinical Findings and Treatment

CO is a nonirritating, colorless, odorless gas that is slightly lighter than air. Because of these features, the individual is not aware of poisonous concentrations of CO in inspired air.

The organ systems affected by CO are the central nervous system (CNS), cardiovascular, respiratory, and musculoskeletal systems. The most common CNS symptoms are headache and dizziness and, in severe cases, convulsions and coma. CNS lesions are mainly restricted to the white matter. Pathologic changes range from mild inflammation to myelin necrosis. In severe poisoning cerebral edema occurs. The most common cardiovascular disorder noted is hypertension. Chronic exposure to low concentrations of CO (as in smokers) accelerates the development of atherosclerosis. Endothelial hypertrophy, subintimal edema, and increased vascular permeability are observed in experimental animals. The cardiac output is increased along with minute ventilation. Shortness of breath is not often felt, but a tight feeling in the chest is experienced by some. Profound weakness and inability to perform routine tasks are a dominant symptom. Over 5 percent of victims with a concentration of 50 percent COHb who survive have permanent sequelae; concentrations of COHb of over 50 percent is often fatal. The duration of exposure is of critical importance, and this is illustrated in Fig. 53-1. An exposure to 0.01 percent of CO in inspired air for as long as 9 h results in nothing more than a headache. Contrast this to exposure to a concentration of 1 percent of CO in inspired air for 10 min, which is uniformly fatal. All gradations exist in between, as shown in Fig. 53-1. The fetus may be more susceptible to the effects of CO.

Removal of the individual from the contaminated environment is the most important step. Establishment of an airway and administration of 100 percent oxygen by a tight-fitting mask or an endotracheal tube, if required, is the next step.

The half-life of COHb is about 5 to 6 h with no treatment. Administration of 100 percent oxygen reduces this to 0.5 to 1 h. Hyperbaric oxygen (3 atmospheres) further reduces the half-life of COHb to 20 to 30 min. This is illustrated in Fig. 53-2.

The actual value of hyperbaric oxygen is somewhat controversial. Once a degree of tissue damage has occurred, there is doubt that more rapid elimination of CO with the use of hyperbaric oxygen has a significant advantage over 100 percent oxygen. The situation is made difficult by the scarcity of hyperbaric oxygen units. Usually the patient must be transported over long distances to a suitable facility.

There is no other specific antidote. Supportive therapy (especially for acidosis), cardiovascular support, and hydration, where indicated, are important.

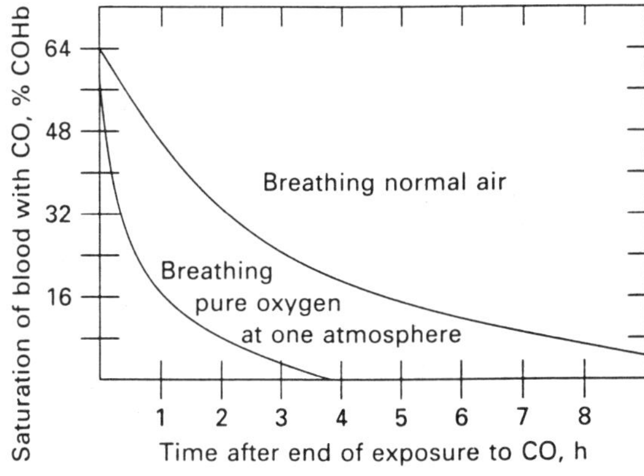

FIGURE 53-2 *Rates of elimination of carbon monoxide from blood when room air, as compared to 100 percent oxygen, is respired.*

Sulfur Dioxide

Sulfur dioxide (SO_2) is a gas generated by the combustion of fossil fuels. Sulfur dioxide forms sulfurous acid on contact with moist membranes which gives rise to its irritant effects on eyes, mucous membranes and skin. Inhaled sulfur dioxide (90%) is absorbed in the upper respiratory tract. Inhalation of sulfur dioxide causes bronchial constriction that is dependent on intact parasympathetic innervation. Asthmatics are especially sensitive to sulfur dioxide.

Signs and symptoms of sulfur dioxide exposure are irritation of the eyes, nose and throat and reflex bronchoconstriction. There is no specific treatment for sulfur dioxide exposure other than management of respiratory tract problems.

Nitrogen Dioxide

Nitrogen dioxide (NO_2) is a brownish irritant gas that may cause pulmonary edema. It forms from fires and is particularly abundant from silage. Pulmonary damage, referred to as "silo-fillers disease", occurs in farmers exposed to nitrogen dioxide in the confines of a silo.

The Type I cells of the alveoli appear to be most affected by nitrogen dioxide exposure. Exposure to 50 ppm produces substantial pain after 1 minute and causes pulmonary edema and chronic pulmonary lesions after 1 hour. Higher concentrations have been fatal. Acute exposure to nitrogen dioxide produces irritation to the eyes and nose, dyspnea and chest pain. Treatment consists of giving oxygen for dyspnea and cyanosis and management of the pulmonary edema.

Ozone

Ozone (O_3) is a bluish gas found several miles above the earth's surface where it is an important absorbent of ultraviolet light. Ozone is also one of the major components of air pollution which is responsible for lung injury. It may cause irritation of mucous membranes, pulmonary edema, and death.

Pulmonary edema due to ozone may be from the formation of free radicals. Ozone-induced free radicals may be derived from oxidative decomposition of unsaturated fatty acids or from interaction with sulfhydryl groups. The interaction of free radicals with unsaturated fatty acids leads to lipid peroxidation. Treatment consists of management of the pulmonary edema.

SOLVENTS

Halogenated Aliphatic Hydrocarbons

The halogenated aliphatic hydrocarbons include carbon tetrachloride, chloroform, trichloroethylene, tetrachloroethylene, and 1,1,1-trichloroethane. These compounds are used as industrial solvents, degreasers, and cleaning agents.

All of the halogenated aliphatic hydrocarbons can depress the CNS in humans; chloroform is the most potent. Acute or chronic exposure to these compounds can also produce hepatotoxicity; carbon tetrachloride is the most potent. Carbon tetrachloride, trichlorethylene and chloroform sometimes cause nephrotoxicity in humans. Lifetime exposure studies in rats and mice have indicated that carbon tetrachloride, chloroform, trichlorethylene and tetrachloroethylene can produce an increase incidence of tumors; it is not known whether an increased incidence of tumors occur in humans exposed to these compounds for long periods of time. Treatment of halogenated aliphatic hydrocarbon intoxication requires management of the organ system involved.

Aromatic Hydrocarbons

Benzene, toluene, xylene and other aromatic hydrocarbons are widely used in the chemical industry. Toluene is found in many commercial glue products. Acute poisoning from mild exposure to these aromatic hydrocarbons results in dizziness, weakness, euphoria, nausea and vomiting. More severe exposure progresses to visual blurring, tremors, shallow and rapid respiration, ventricular arrhythmias, paralysis, unconsciousness, and convulsions. Violent excitement and delirium may precede coma. Treatment of acute poisoning consists of complete bed rest until respiration is normal and administration of diazepam to control excitement or convulsions. Avoid epinephrine or related drugs, they may induce fatal ventricular fibrillation.

Chronic benzene exposure may cause aplastic anemia, leukopenia, thrombocytopenia, and possibly an increased incidence of leukemia.

ALCOHOLS

The pharmacology of ethanol, methanol, and ethylene glycol are discussed in Chapter 18.

PESTICIDES

Pesticides include insecticides, rodenticides, fungicides, herbicides and fumigants. These compounds are specifically designed tc cause selective toxicity to pests, but all can produce some toxicity to humans.

Organochlorine Insecticides

The organochlorine insecticides are classified in 4 groups: DDT (chlorophenothane) and its analogs (methoxychlor, tetrachlorodiphenylethane (TDE)), cyclodienes (aldrin, chlordane, dieldrin, heptachlor), toxaphene, and benzene hexachloride (BHC, lindane). These compounds were extensively used from the mid 1940s to the mid 1960s. The degradation of these compounds is slow and there is marked bioaccumulation, particularly in the aquatic ecosystem. The use of organochlorine insecticides has been reduced in North America and Europe because of their environmental impact. DDT was banned in the United States in 1972 for most uses. The chlorinated cyclodienes produce dose-related hepatomas in mice and, thus, the use of aldrin and dieldrin was banned in the United States in 1974, followed by chlordane and heptachlor in 1976.

These compounds differ greatly in their toxicokinetic properties and in their acute toxicity. In general, they can be absorbed through the skin and by inhalation and oral ingestion; however, DDT is very poorly absorbed through the skin.

The organochlorine insecticides interfere with the inactivation of sodium channels in excitable membranes and thereby cause rapid repetitive firing in many neurons. DDT first produces tremors followed by convulsions, whereas with the other compounds, convulsions may occur immediately after intoxication without the presence of tremors. Treatment consists of the management of symptoms and the use of IV diazepam to control convulsions. The use of epinephrine is to be avoided, since these agents sensitize the myocardium to catecholamines and ventricular fibrillation may occur.

Organophosphorus Insecticides

The organophosphorus insecticides have largely replaced the organochlorine insecticides since they do not persist in the environment and they have an extremely low carcinogenic potential. The pharmacology of this general class of agents is discussed in Chapter 10. These agents are used to combat a large variety of pests. Some of the organophosphorus insecticides are: azinophos-methyl, chlorfenvinphos, diazinon, dichlorovos, dimethoate, fenitrothion, leptophos, malathion, parathion, parathion-methyl and trichlorfon. The organophosphorus compounds are absorbed through the skin and the respiratory and gastrointestinal tracts. Their biotransformation is rapid in comparison to the organochlorine insecticides.

Mechanism of Action

These compounds exert their effect through the inhibition of cholinesterases by phosphorylation of the serine hydroxyl group at the esteratic site of these enzymes. Some sulfur analogs have to be biologically activated to their oxygen analogs to inhibit cholinesterases. Notable examples are the conversion of parathion and malathion to paraoxon and malaoxon, respectively.

In addition to inhibition of cholinesterases, some organophosphorus compounds phosphorylate another enzyme called "neurotoxic esterase". This results in the development of a delayed neurotoxicity characterized by paralysis and axonal degeneration. In humans, triorthocresyl phosphate (TOCP) has been shown to produce this delayed neurotoxicity. Some organophosphorus insecticides such as merphos, mipafox, trichlorfon and leptophos have been suggested to also cause delayed neurotoxicity.

Clinical Findings and Treatment

The following symptoms and signs occur after poisoning with cholinesterase inhibitors. Symptoms begin within 30 to 60 minutes and are maximum in 2 to 8 hours. Mild symptoms include anoxia, headaches, dizziness, weakness, anxiety, tremors of the tongue and eyelids, miosis and impairment of visual acuity. Moderate symptoms consist of nausea, salivation, tearing, abdominal cramps, vomiting, sweating, slow pulse and muscular fasciculation. Severe symptoms include diarrhea, pinpoint and nonreactive pupils, respiratory difficulty, pulmonary edema, cyanosis, loss of sphincter control, convulsions, coma, and death.

Treatment includes maintenance of respiration, diazepam to control convulsions, atropine in large doses to block cholinomimetic effects associated with muscarinic receptor activation, and removal of the poison by decontamination of the skin and/or lavage or emesis. In the presence of symptoms, give atropine, 2 mg IM, and repeat every 3 to 8 minutes until signs of atropinization appear (e.g., flushed face, dry mouth, widely dilated pupils, fast pulse). Repeat atropine (2 mg) frequently to maintain signs of atropinization. Pralidoxime is used as a cholinesterase reactivator for organophosphorus poisoning but is contraindicated for carbamate poisoning; give 1 gram IV slowly in aqueous solutions and repeat after 30 minutes if respiration does not improve.

Mono-Carbamate Insecticides

These compounds inhibit acetylcholinesterase by carbamylation of the esteratic site. Their pharmacology is discussed in Chapter 10 and their toxicity is similar to the organophosphorus insecticides except that the reactivation of acetylcholinesterase occurs more rapidly. Mono-carbamate insecticides include aldicarb, aminocarb, carbaryl, carbofuran, dimetan, dimetilan, isolan, methomyl, propoxur, pyramal, pyrolan and zectran. Treatment is the same as for organophosphorus insecticides except pralidoxime is contraindicated.

Botanical Insecticides

Botanical insecticides are derived from natural sources and include nicotine, rotenone and pyrethrum.

Nicotine reacts with nicotinic receptors in ganglia, brain and the neuromuscular junction. The effects of nicotine are described in Chapters 10 and 11. Treatment of nicotine toxicity includes maintenance of vital signs and suppression of convulsions.

Rotenone is obtained from roots of plants from *Derris* and *Zonchocarpus*. Human poisoning is rare with rotenone. Oral ingestion of rotenone produces gastrointestinal irritation, nausea and vomiting. Conjunctivitis, dermatitis, and rhinitis have been reported. Treatment is symptomatic.

Pyrethrums are derived from the flowers of the pyrethrum plants, *chrysanthemum* and *cincerariaefolinium*. Pyrethrum contains 6 known insecticidal esters. The greatest activity resides in pyrethrin I. Pyrethrum and synthetic derivatives (pyrethroids) are used in many household insecticides because of their rapid action. These compounds may be absorbed after inhalation or ingestion. Their toxicity is similar to DDT with convulsions being the most serious problem. Treatment is with IV diazepam to control convulsions. These compounds produce a high frequency of allergies in humans, contact dermatitis is prominent.

Fumigants

Fumigants are used to control insects, rodents and soil nematodes. Agents used include hydrogen cyanide, acrylonitrile, carbon disulfide, carbon tetrachloride, ethylene oxide, methyl bromide, and phosphine. Cyanide requires special discussion since it is one of the deadliest and most easily available poisons.

CYANIDE

Endogenously cyanide is part of vitamin B_{12} metabolism. It is taken in as food especially in certain plants such as *Prunus* species (cherry, almonds, and peaches), bamboo sprouts, cassava, and *Sorghum* species. Tobacco smoke also contains cyanide. Ordinarily the amount of cyanide for endogenous sources is too small to cause significant toxicity. However, it is possible to ingest enough almonds or peach pits to cause poisoning. The bitter taste is attractive to some palates. Tobacco amblyopia is probably caused by the cyanide content of smoke.

Industrial sources are many and include the industries involved in electroplating, extraction of ores, photography, synthetic rubber, and manufacture of plastics. Many chemical synthetic processes utilize cyanide; thus chemists are particularly subject to accidental poisoning. Cyanide has also been used as a fumigant for rodents and insects.

Mechanism of Action

Cyanide forms a stable coordination complex with ferric iron, thus keeping this metal in a higher oxidation state (Fe^{3+}). Thus it greatly diminishes its activity as an electron carrier in reactions involving $Fe^{3+} + e \longrightarrow Fe^{2+}$ transitions. Numerous enzymes may be involved, but the main one is ferricytochrome oxidase, which is changed to ferricytochrome oxidase-cyanide. This seriously impairs cellular oxygen utilization. Consequently, the many pathways which converge at the cytochrome system to utilize oxygen are arrested, and aerobic metabolism ceases. This histotoxic hypoxia results in a shift to anaerobic metabolism, which in turn causes the accumulation of lactate and pyruvate.

Cells are unable to utilize the oxygen in oxyhemoglobin. Venous blood becomes bright red and has almost the same oxygen saturation as arterial blood. Physiologically the most sensitive cells in the body to tissue hypoxia are the carotid and aortic bodies. A small amount of cyanide injected intravenously will upon reaching the carotid body cause an inspiratory gasp.

Tissues most sensitive to hypoxia are first affected. Obviously the CNS and the heart are organs which are critically first disturbed in cyanide poisoning. All cells eventually are affected; those with the lowest metabolism tend to survive the best.

Other hematin compounds which complex with cyanide are catalase, peroxidase, cytochrome c peroxidase, and methemoglobin. Some metal-bearing enzymes that complex with cyanide are tyrosinase, ascorbic acid oxidase, xanthine oxidase, succinic acid, lactic acid, and formic acid dehydrogenase. The role of cyanide in hydroxocobalamin metabolism is described in Chapter 34.

Toxicokinetics

Cyanides can be absorbed by all routes, although fatalities by skin absorption are rare. Most instances of poisoning are either by inhalation of hydrogen cyanide or oral absorption of cyanide salts such as potassium or sodium cyanide. Distribution is very rapid, since cyanide is water-soluble and carried by blood to every organ. The concentration in blood is the highest except for the spleen, salivary glands, thyroid, and stomach. In survivors, cyanide is converted to the much less toxic thiocyanate ion, which is excreted in the urine. The enzyme mitochondrial sulfurtransferase (rhodanese) catalyzes this reaction (Fig. 53-3). Other minor pathways of excretion and biotransformation are also shown in Fig. 53-3.

The liver and kidneys contain large amounts of sulfurtransferase, but a limiting factor is the amount of intracellular reducing sulfur which can serve as a substrate. *In vivo*, suitable sulfur is found in thiosulfate, cystine, and cysteine. To effectively combat poisoning, exogenous reducing sulfur must be provided.

Acute Toxicity

Inhaled cyanide acts as rapidly as intravenous

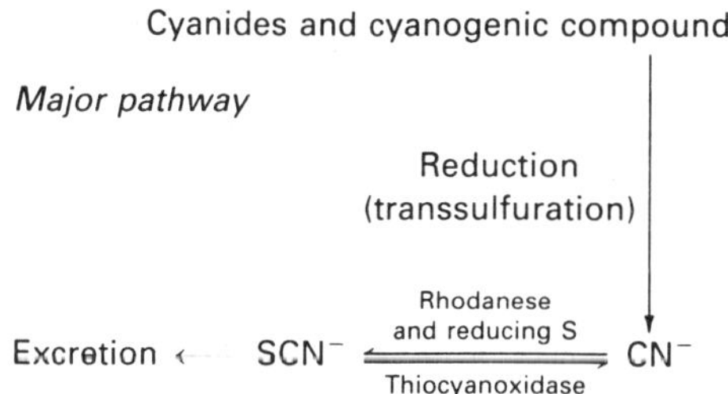

Minor pathways

1. Direct excretion
   a. As HCN in breath
   b. As CN^- in secretion
2. Oxidation
   a. ⟶ HCOOH ⟶ Excretion

   Metabolic pool of one-carbon compounds

   b. —HCNO ⟶ CO_2 ⟶ Excretion
3. Metal coordination

   $\xrightleftharpoons[h]{B_{12a}} B_{12}$
4. Condensation

   $\xrightarrow{\text{Cystine}}$ HOOC—HC—NH—C(=NH)—S—H_2C (ring) ⟶ Excretion

   2-Iminothiazolidine-4-carboxylic acid

FIGURE 53-3 *The fate of absorbed cyanide: detoxication and excretion pathways.*

cyanide. Immediate symptoms are flushing, headache, dizziness, and tachypnea. This is followed by stridorous breathing, coma, and death within 10 min. Oral exposures are less rapid because of a slower rise in blood levels and some first-pass biotransformation in the liver. Death may occur in 30 min to 1 h. The absence of cyanosis despite intensive respiratory distress should suggest cyanide poisoning.

Five parts of hydrogen cyanide per million of air (5 ppm) is the threshold limit for continual occupational exposure. One hundred ppm of hydrogen cyanide in air endangers life in 1 h exposure. Any higher concentration is likely to be fatal with immediate symptoms.

The minimum lethal dose of the salts of cyanide is 0.2 g for adults. Persons attempting suicide usually take a teaspoonful (2 to 6 g).

Chronic Toxicity

Headache, dizziness, nausea, sometimes vomiting, and a bitter or abnormal taste have been reported as symptoms of chronic exposure to sublethal doses of cyanide. This usually occurs in industrial occupations such as metal smelting. Certain clinical syndromes have been attributed to chronic cyanide poisoning. These include tobacco amblyopia, Leber's hereditary optic atrophy, and Nigerian nutritional ataxic neuropathy. The last syndrome is associated with elevated plasma thiocyanate levels and reduced levels of sulfur-containing amino acids. It is caused by the consumption of large amounts of cassava containing cyanogenic glycosides. Thus nutritional factors and genetic defects must be considered in cases of chronic toxicity.

Treatment

The absolute necessity for immediate institution of therapy as soon as symptoms appear cannot be over-emphasized. Of first importance is support of respiration and circulation. Institution of 100 percent oxygen, assistance of respiration as needed, insertion of intravenous lines, and cardiac monitoring are the first steps. Correction of metabolic acidosis (pH below 7.15) is also necessary. Hemodialysis and hemoperfusion are ineffective measures. The effectiveness of hyperbaric oxygen therapy has not been proven and should be resorted to only in the most extreme cases. Decontamination should be carried out where indicated. Removal of contaminated clothing and washing affected skin with a strong soap are important measures.

Institution of antidote therapy should be next; then gastrointestinal decontamination should be done if less than 2 h have passed since ingestion. Gastric lavage, charcoal, and cathartics can all be used. While some patients may survive with supportive care alone, antidote therapy is usually very effective.

Antidotes

The principles of combating cyanide poisoning are, first, to induce the formation of methemoglobin, which has a high affinity for cyanide, and, second, to provide reducing sulfur in the form of thiosulfate so that the body can excrete cyanide as thiocyanate.

The three-step cyanide kit is the approved preparation in the United States. It contains sodium nitrite, 300 mg in 10 mL (2 amps); sodium thiosulfate, 12.5 g in 50 mL (2 amps); amyl nitrite inhalant, 0.3 mL (12 aspirols). In practice, amyl nitrite is given by crushing the aspirol and inhaling the vapor. This will produce a 3 to 5 percent methemoglobinemia. Sodium nitrite 300 mg is then administered by slow intravenous injection over 4 min and will produce a 20 percent methemoglobinemia. After sodium nitrite is given, sodium thiosulfate is administered intravenously as a 25 percent solution (12.5 g) at a rate of 3 to 5 mL/min.

Cyanide poisoning, especially that caused by sodium nitroprusside, has been successfully treated with hydroxocobalamin (vitamin B_{12a}). This provitamin combines with cyanide to form cyanocobalamin (vitamin B_{12}), which is excreted in the urine. There is now a preparation with sodium thiosulfate that is FDA approved. A suggested dose is 50 times the estimated cyanide dose. At present there is not sufficient evidence to recommend hydroxocobalamin therapy in preference to the standard nitrite-thiosulfate treatment.

HERBICIDES

Chlorophenoxy Herbicides

2,4-Dichlorophenoxyacetic acid (2,4-D) and 2,4,5-trichlorophenoxyacetic acid (2,4,5-T) are the major compounds used for the destruction of weeds. In large doses, 2,4-D can cause coma and generalized muscle hypotonia in humans. Marked myotonia may last for weeks. 2,4,5-T may also produce coma, but muscle dysfunction is less prominent. Reports of poisoning in humans are rare. These compounds do not accumulate in animals because they are extensively excreted in the urine. The chlorophenoxy compounds produce contact dermatitis, including chloracne in humans. The dermatitis effects may be due to contaminations with 2,3,7,8-tetrachlorodibenzo-p-dioxin (TCDD) formed in the manufacturing of chlorophenoxy herbicides. TCDD is an exquisitely toxic substance in some species (i.e., LD_{50} of 0.6 μg/kg in guinea pigs). Humans appear to be much less sensitive to TCDD from observations of individuals accidentally exposed. Chloracne, porphyria, hypocholesterolemia and psychiatric disturbances have been reported in humans accidentally exposed to relatively large dose of TCDD. Epidemiological studies do not support the hypothesis that TCDD is a troublesome teratogen or carcinogen in humans.

Bipyridyl Herbicides

Paraquat has been reported to produce several hundred cases of accidental or suicidal fatalities. Many samples of illegal marijuana are contaminated with paraquat. Early symptoms are attributed to gastrointestinal irritations but within a few days damage to lungs, liver, kidneys and myocardium occur; these effects are delayed. The most notable pathology is widespread proliferation of fibrocytic cells in the lung. The onset of respiratory problems which may eventually lead to death may be delayed for several days. Paraquat is proposed to undergo redox cycling thereby converting oxygen to superoxide which in turn initiates lipid peroxidation. Because paraquat can produce serious delayed pulmonary toxicity prompt removal from the gastrointestinal tract is necessary. Gastric lavage catharsis, the oral administration of adsorbents and the removal of absorbed paraquat by hemodialysis or hemoperfusion has been advocated.

Polychlorinated Hydrocarbons

The polychlorinated biphenyls (PCBs) were widely used as dielectric and heat transfer fluids, plasticisers and flame retardants. They were banned in the United States in 1977 but they still persist in the environment. These compounds are highly lipophilic, very stable, poorly metabolized and resistant to environmental degradation. They accumulate in the food chain, and thus, food is the major source of PCB exposure to humans. These compounds are relatively non-toxic but may be contaminated with more toxic polychlorinated hydrocarbons (e.g., polychlorinated dibenzofurans, PCDFs). Dermatological problems, including chloracne, some hepatotoxic involvement and elevated plasma triglycerides have been reported in workers occupationally exposed to high concentrations of PCBs. Most evidence suggest that PCBs in the environment pose minimal hazard to human health.

BIBLIOGRAPHY

Abou-Donia, M.B., and D.M. Lapadula: "Mechanisms of Organophosphorus Ester-induced Delayed Neurotoxicity: Type I and Type II," *Annu. Rev. Pharmacol. Toxicol.* **30**: 405-440 (1990).

Amdur, M.O., J. Doull, and C.D. Klaassen (eds.): *Casarett and Doull's Toxicology, 4th Ed.*, Pergamon Press, New York, 1991.

Austin, H., E. Delzell, and P. Cole: "Benzene and Leukemia: A Review of The Literature and a Risk Assessment," *Am. J. Epidemiol.* **127**: 419-439 (1988).

Beamer, W.C., R.M. Shealy, and D.S. Prough: "Acute Cyanide Poisoning from Laetrile Ingestion," *Ann. Emerg. Med.* **12**: 449-451 (1983).

Bertazzi, P.A., C. Zocchetti, A.C. Pesatori, S. Guercilena, M.Sanarico, and L. Radice: "Ten-year Mortality Study of the Population Involved in the Seveso Incident in 1976," *Am. J. Epidemiol.* **129**: 1187-1200 (1989).

Bertazzi, P.A., C. Zocchetti, A.C. Pesatori, S. Guercilena, D. Consonni, A. Tironi, and M.T. Landi: "Mortality of a Young Population after Accidental Exposure to 2,3,7,8-Tetrachlorodibenzo-p-dioxin," *Int. J. Epidemiol.* **21**: 118-123 (1992).

Blanc, P., M. Hogan, K. Mallin, D. Hryhorczuk, S. Hessi, and B. Bernard: "Cyanide Intoxication among Silver-Reclaiming Workers," *J. Amer. Med. Assoc.* **253**: 367-371 (1985).

Borowitz, J.L., A.G. Kanthasamy, and G.E. Isom: "Toxicodynamics of Cyanide," Somani, S.M. (ed.), *Chemical Warfare Agents*, Academic Press, San Diego, 1992, pp. 209-236.

Bruckner, J.V., B.D. Davis, and J.N. Blancato: "Metabolism Toxicity and Carcinogenicity of Trichloroethylene," *CRC Crit. Rev. Toxicol.* **20**: 31-50 (1989).

Caplan, Y.H., B.C. Thompson, B. Levine, and W. Masemore: "Accidental Poisonings Involving Carbon Monoxide, Heating Systems and Confined Spaces," *J. Forensic Sci.*, **31**: 117-121 (1986).

Dreisbach, R.H., and W.O. Robertson: *Handbook of Poisoning: Prevention, Diagnosis and Treatment," 15th Ed.*, Appleton and Lange, Norwalk, 1990.

Drew, R.H.: "The Use of Hydroxocobalamin in the Prophylaxis and Treatment of Nitroprusside-Induced Cyanide Toxicity," *Vet. Hum. Toxicol.* **25**: 342-345 (1983).

Ellenhorn, M.J., and D.G. Barceloux: *Medical Toxicology: Diagnosis and Treatment of Human Poisoning, 2nd Ed.*, Elsevier, New York, 1991.

Eriksson, M., L. Hardell, and H.-O. Adami: "Exposure to Dioxins as a Risk Factor for Soft Tissue Sarcoma: A Population-based Case-control Study," *J. Natl. Cancer Inst.*, **82**: 486-490 (1990).

Ginsberg, M.D.: "Carbon Monoxide Intoxication. Clinical Features, Neuropathology and Mechanisms of Injury," *Clin. Toxicol.* **23**: 281-288 (1985).

Gossel, T.A, and J.D. Bricker: *Principles of Clinical Toxicology*, Raven Press, New York, 1984.

Gosselin, R.E., R.P. Smith, and H.C. Hodge: *Clinical Toxicology of Commercial Products 5th Ed.*, Williams and Wilkins, New York, 1984.

Hayes, W.J., Jr.: *Pesticides Studied in Man*, Williams and Wilkins, 1982.

Hodgson, E., and P.E. Levi: *A Textbook of Modern Toxicology*, Elsevier, New York, 1987.

Huber, J.A.: "Do Awake Patients with High Carboxyhemoglobin Levels Need Hyperbaric Oxygen?," *J. Emerg. Med.*, **1**: 555-556 (1984).

Kizer, K.W.: "Hyperbaric Oxygen and Cyanide Poisoning," *Am. J. Emerg. Med.* **2**. 113 (1984).

Klaassen, C.D.: "Nonmetallic Environmental Toxicants, Air Pollutants, Solvents and Vapors, and Pesticides," in Gilman, A.G., T.W. Rall, A.S. Nies, and P. Taylor, (eds.) *Goodman and Gilman's The Pharmacological Basis of Therapeutics, 8th Ed.*, Pergamon Press, New York, 1990, pp. 1615-1639.

Marcus, W.L.: "Chemical of Current Interest: Benzene," *Toxicol. Ind. Health* **3**: 205-266 (1987).

Mosier, D., and R. Baldwin: "Carbon Monoxide Poisoning," South Dakota, *MMWR* **34**: 113 (1985).

Myers, R.A., S.K. Snyder, and T.A. Emhoff: "Subacute Sequelae of Carbon Monoxide Poisoning," *Am. Emerg. Med.* **14**: 1163-1167 (1985).

NIOSH: "Recommendations for Occupational Safety and Health Standards," *MMWR*, **37** **(Suppl. 7)**: 1 (1988).

Olson, K.R.: "Carbon Monoxide Poisoning: Mechanism, Presentation and Controversies in Management" *J. Emerg. Med.* **1**: 233-243 (1984).

O'Sullivan, B.P.: "Carbon Monoxide Poisoning in an Infant Exposed to a Kerosene Heater." *J. Pediatr.* **103**: 249-251 (1983).

Plaa, G.L.: "Introduction to Toxicology: Occupational and Environmental Toxicology," in Katzung, B.C. (ed.) *Basic and Clinical Pharmacology, 5th Ed.*, Appleton and Lange, Norwalk, 1992, pp. 821-830.

Proctor, N.H., and J.P. Hughes: *Chemical Hazards of the Workplace, 3rd Ed.*, J.B. Lippincott Company, Philadelphia, 1991.

Rieders, F.: "Noxious Gases and Vapors. I: Carbon Monoxide, Cyanides, Methemoglobin and Sulphemoglobin," in J. R. DiPalma (ed.) *Drill's Pharmacology in Medicine*, McGraw-Hill, New York, 1971, pp. 1180-1205.

Seinfeld, J.H.: "Urban Air Pollution: State of the Science," *Science*, **243**: 745 (1989).

Snyder, S.H.: "Nitric Oxide: First in New Class of Neurotransmitters?", *Science*, **257**: 494-496 (1992).

Sullivan, J.B., and C.K. Krieger: *Hazardous Materials Toxicology*, Williams and Wilkins, Baltimore, 1992.

Way, J.L.: "Cyanide Intoxication and Its Mechanism of Antagonism," *Annu. Rev. Pharmacol. Toxicol.* **24**: 451-481 (1984).

Wright, E.S., D. Dziedzic, and C.S. Wheeler: "Cellular, Biochemical, and Functional Effects of Ozone: New Research and Perspectives on Ozone Health Effects," *Toxicol. Lett.* **51**: 125-145 (1990).

CHAPTER 54

Heavy Metals and Antagonists

Thomas L. Pazdernik

Since life began, heavy metals in the environment have produced a hazard to biologic organisms. Some diseases of humans can be traced to heavy metal poisoning associated with the development of metal mining, refining, and use. Even with the present recognition of the hazards of heavy metals (see Table 54-1), the incidence of intoxication remains significant and the need for effective therapy remains high.

Heavy metals are not metabolized and therefore they persist in the body and accumulate. Most often they combine with sulfhydryl groups present in many key enzymes, and thus, cell function is severely disrupted. Some metals such as iron, zinc, cobalt, copper, and a few trace elements perform vital cellular functions, usually as cofactors or even as electron donors (hemoglobin, for example).

Since this is a vast subject and cannot be covered in depth, the plan for this chapter is as follows: the toxicology of lead, mercury, gold, and arsenic as primary examples of heavy metal toxicity is discussed in some detail. Next the main antagonists (chelating agents) which have proven to be useful in therapy are described.

LEAD

Lead forms two well-defined series of compounds in which the metal is bivalent and tetravalent, respectively. Lead is found in practically all foods as well as in the air, and can therefore be both ingested and inhaled. Industrial uses of lead, such as the manufacture of batteries, cables, automotive body paints, and ceramics, provide potential sources of lead exposure. Some paint pigments contain lead: white lead (basic lead carbonate) and red lead (lead oxide). Formerly, paints used for interior and exterior surfaces contained lead pigments. Even though this application of lead has largely been discontinued, the hazard still remains, especially in dilapidated dwellings where peeling of multicoated walls and woodwork constitutes the most important single source of lead poisoning in young children.

Toxicokinetics

The average daily American intake of lead may vary from 0.1 to 0.4 mg, this is primarily from food. About 0.04 mg of lead is inhaled daily. Of this amount, 30 to 50 percent is retained by the lung and readily absorbed. Only about 10 percent of ingested lead is absorbed in an adult. In contrast to this low absorption in adults, the absorption of dietary lead in normal infants and young children is approximately 50 percent. Thus, lead ingestion is more of a hazard to children than to adults. Inorganic lead does not readily penetrate intact skin; however, lipid-soluble forms such as tetraethyllead are significantly absorbed. Some of the absorbed lead is excreted via the bile into the gastrointestinal tract and passes out in the feces with the unabsorbed portion. Thus, the fecal excretion of lead approximates that which is ingested with food. The remainder of the absorbed lead is excreted in the urine. Therefore, the daily intake of lead is equal to the daily output under normal conditions.

Lead is a bone-seeker. Over 90 percent of the human body burden of lead is found in bone. Of the soft tissues, liver, muscle, skin, dense connective tissues, and hair contain the largest amounts, in that order. Of major concern is the distribution of lead into the brain, kidney, and hematopoietic system, where it produces toxicologic effects.

Blood and urinary lead levels have been

TABLE 54-1 Summary of heavy metal toxicology

Metal	Chemical form absorbed	Distribution	Target organs
Lead	Inorganic lead oxides and lead salts	Bone (90%), teeth, hair, red blood cells, liver, kidneys	Hematopoietic tissues and liver, CNS, kidneys, neuromuscular junction
	Organic (tetraethyl lead)	Liver	CNS
Mercury	Elemental mercury	CNS (where it is trapped as Hg^{2+}), kidneys (following conversion of elemental Hg to Hg^{2+})	CNS (neuropsychiatric due to elemental Hg and its Hg^{2+} metabolite), kidneys (substantial due to conversion of elemental Hg to Hg^{2+})
	Inorganic: Hg^{+} (less toxic); Hg^{2+} (more toxic)	Kidneys (predominant); blood, brain (minor)	Kidneys, gastrointestinal tract
	Organic: alkyl	Kidneys, brain, blood	CNS
Arsenic	Inorganic arsenic salts	Red blood cells (95 - 99% bound to globin) (24 h); then to liver, lungs, kidneys, wall of gastro-intestinal tract, spleen, muscle, nerve tissues (2 weeks); then to skin, hair, and bone (years)	Increased vascular permeability leading to vasodilation and vascular collapse. Uncoupling of oxidative phosphorylation resulting in impaired cellular metabolism
Zinc	Elemental zinc	Red blood cells and plasma proteins; prostate, liver, and choroid plexus	Bone, brain, skeletal muscle, eye tissue
Aluminum	Inorganic aluminum oxides and salts	Intestine, liver, spleen	Brain
Cadmium	Inorganic cadmium salts	Gastrointestinal tract, lungs	Lungs, kidneys, intestine
Manganese	Inorganic manganese oxides and salts	Liver, kidneys, intestine, and pancreas	Basal ganglia, cerebellum
Gold	Gold salts	Liver, kidneys, spleen, pancreas, intestine	Skin, kidneys, and liver

determined in people from all parts of the world. The worldwide "average" urinary and blood lead levels are 35 μg/L and 10 to 25 μg per 100 mL, respectively. The urinary level of lead indicative of a hazardous exposure is 150 μg per liter of urine, while 80 μg per 100 mL of blood indicates dangerous exposure. Recent reports have indicated that even very low levels of lead in the plasma may alter normal physiologic functions.

TABLE 54-2 Toxic effects of lead on hemoglobin synthesis

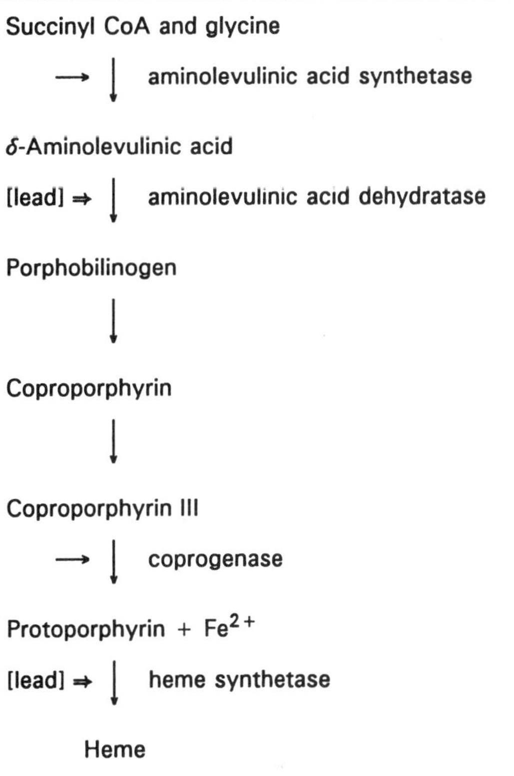

[lead] ⇒, steps inhibited by lead
→, steps at which lead is thought to act, but evidence is inconclusive

Acute Lead Poisoning

Acute lead poisoning is rare; it may result from the massive inhalation of large quantities of finely divided lead or lead fumes. The symptoms include sweet metallic taste, salivation, vomiting, abdominal pain, intestinal colic, lowered body temperature, and cardiovascular collapse. Death may result in 1 or 2 days.

Chronic Lead Poisoning

The signs and symptoms of chronic lead poisoning can be divided into five categories: (1) hematologic, (2) neurologic, (3) renal, (4) gastrointestinal, and (5) other.

Hematologic Signs One sign of lead intoxication is the appearance of stippled cells in the peripheral blood. These juvenile forms of erythrocytes are not in themselves diagnostic since basophilic stippling can occur in a variety of blood dyscrasias. Furthermore, stippling is observed in only 60 percent of childhood lead intoxications. Basophilic stippling, however, is an indication that lead interferes with hemoglobin synthesis. An important chemical clue to the effects of lead on the hematopoietic system is the appearance of coproporphyrin III in the urine. Inconclusive evidence reveals lower activity of coprogenase with increasing blood lead levels (see Table 54-2). This finding alone may be misleading, since coproporphyrinuria occurs in a large variety of other diseases and poisonings. An excellent correlation exists, however, between the amount of lead in the urine and the appearance of urinary coproporphyrins.

Another consistent finding in lead poisoning is the appearance of δ-aminolevulinic acid in the urine. This results from an inhibition by lead of the enzyme aminolevulinic acid dehydratase, which converts δ-aminolevulinic acid to porphobilinogen (see Table 54-2). Urinary lead and coproporphyrin levels correlate well with the appearance of δ-aminolevulinic acid. A raised urinary δ-aminolevulinic acid level provides an earlier sign of lead exposure than a raised coproporphyrin level.

Lead also interferes with the incorporation of iron into protoporphyrin by the activity of heme synthetase to form heme. Protoporphyrin levels rise in bone narrow and erythrocytes. The anemia associated with lead poisoning is of the hypochromic, normocytic type and is seldom severe. Hemoglobin values rarely fall below 60 percent, or the red blood cell count below 4 x 10^6 per mL.

Neurologic Signs The neurotoxic effects of lead at high doses is well documented. The central nervous system manifestations of lead poisoning are termed *lead encephalopathy*. Today, these symptoms occur rarely in adults, and only after very high doses of lead; they are of more importance and of higher frequency in children. The early symptoms include irritability, headache, insomnia, restlessness, and ataxia. Later, confusion, delirium, convulsions, and coma may develop. Morphologic changes appear as nonspecific lesions in the cerebrum and cerebellum. Accumulations of serous fluid which distort the normal architecture, and capillary damage and hemorrhages of the meninges, are evident. It is believed that these changes are secondary to increased cranial pressure due to edema.

Children with blood lead levels considered subclinical intoxication may have mild neurologic dysfunction. Therefore, permissible exposure levels of lead in children are being revised downward by the Centers for Disease Control. Lead at extremely low concentrations has an inhibitory effect on brain and aminolevulinic acid dehydratase, adenylyl cyclase, and on mitochondrial function. In addition, there are peripheral neurologic effects known as *lead palsy*. This peripheral neuropathy leads to muscle paralysis which involves primarily the extensor muscles of the wrist and foot. In advanced cases the antigravity muscles may atrophy. Contraction of the flexors produces a limb which is immovable and extremities with a clawlike appearance.

Renal Signs The effects of lead on the kidney occur only at very high doses and occur in both adults and children. One effect is proximal tubular damage, which is readily reversible by chelation therapy. The second major effect involves reduced glomerular function associated with vascular damage and fibrosis. These effects occur at levels of lead above that affecting hemoglobin formation and brain function.

Gastrointestinal Signs Lead stimulates the smooth muscle of the gut, giving rise to intestinal symptoms such as distention after meals, constipation, nausea, and vomiting. Appetite loss leads to loss of body weight and easy fatigability. Dull pains in various parts of the abdomen precede colic. Colic is important diagnostically, since it constitutes a symptom for which the patient seeks relief. Characteristically, the onset of lead colic is sudden and usually occurs at night with severe pain.

Other Signs Another nonspecific sign of lead intoxication is the appearance of a lead line at the margin of the gums. Today, the lead line is infrequent because of better dental hygiene. A black or purplish line is formed when lead sulfide is precipitated at the gingival borders; sulfides produced by bacteria react with lead in the saliva. Other metals, for example, bismuth, mercury, tin, and arsenic, produce similar precipitates at the gingival border, illustrating the nonspecificity of the lead line in diagnosing lead intoxication.

Lead poisoning invariably produces changes in skin coloration known as *lead hue* or *lead pallor*. The patient takes on a pale or ashen-gray appearance.

Treatment of Lead Intoxication

The mainstay for treatment of lead poisoning in both adults and children is chelation therapy. The three drugs primarily used are edetate calcium disodium, dimercaprol, and succimer. Therapy in children usually involves intramuscular injections of edetate calcium disodium combined with dimercaprol. Alternatively, oral administration of succimer can be used. (The individual agents are discussed below.) Supportive measures include continuous intravenous infusion of 10 percent dextrose in water to increase urine flow before administration of the chelating agent.

MERCURY

Mercury exists in three states of oxidation: as the element, in a monovalent (mercurous) form, and in a divalent (mercuric) form. Divalent mercury can form covalent bonds with carbon atoms: mercury in this form is usually referred to as *organic* mercury. The organomercurial compounds that were used as diuretics and many of the mercurial fungicides contain mercury covalently bound to carbon.

Elemental or metallic mercury is a highly toxic, somewhat volatile liquid. Human exposure to mercury vapor is mainly occupational and has been noted since antiquity. Mercurous chloride (calomel) is the best known of the mercurous compounds. It is still used in some skin creams as an antiseptic and was once frequently employed as a cathartic. The mercuric salts are the most irritating and acutely toxic forms of mercury. Mercuric salts have wide application in industry as catalysts in the production of vinyl plastics and to suppress the growth of slime molds in the manufacturing of paper pulp. Microorganisms in river water can synthesize methylmercury from the inorganic forms of mercury such as those discharged in industrial waste. Therefore, discharge of mercury into rivers from industries has led to problems of environmental pollution in Japan, Sweden, and the United States.

All the organomercurial compounds in use today contain mercury having only one covalent link to a carbon atom. Methoxyethylmercury chloride belongs to a new group of mercury fungicides. The alkylmercury salts are by far the most dangerous of all the compounds of mercury. The simple salts such as methylmercury chloride and ethylmercury chloride are sufficiently volatile to produce serious toxic effects by inhalation. Methylmercury dicyandiamide is less volatile. All the alkyl mercurials produce characteristic and usually irreversible damage to the central nervous system (CNS). They have had extensive use as fungicides.

Mechanism of Action

Mercury has a specific affinity for the sulfur atom in thiol groups of enzymes and other proteins, inactivating these substances. This uniquely high affinity for sulfur is ultimately responsible for the toxicity of all mercury compounds. The organic moiety of the organomercurials and the dissociable anion in the mercuric salts undoubtedly account for the differences found between the compounds, such as the degree and type of toxic symptoms, and the differences in hazardous properties associated with volatility and solubility.

Toxicokinetics

Mercury may be absorbed into the body via the respiratory and gastrointestinal tracts, and the skin. In general, most compounds of mercury, both organic and inorganic, are well absorbed except mercurous chloride (HgCl). Mercurous chloride is poorly absorbed from the gastrointestinal tract because of its low solubility.

The pattern of deposition of mercury is an important consideration in its toxicology. Both organic and inorganic mercury compounds, if present at a sufficient concentration, will produce toxic effects in any cell with which they come in contact. Irrespective of the route of administration, mercury is distributed within a few hours to all organs of the body. The mercury in plasma is protein-bound, and the mercury present in red blood cells is bound to the cysteine residues of hemoglobin.

Mercury is excreted in the urine, bile, feces, sweat, and saliva. Urinary and fecal routes of excretion are the most important for elimination.

The biological half-life in humans for methylmercury is close to 70 days, corresponding to an excretion of about 1 percent per day of the body burden. The decrease in blood mercury follows a similar time course. The half-life of clearance from the brain is about 20 percent longer than the clearance from the whole body.

Normal Levels of Mercury

For mercury, the intake rate roughly balances the total urinary and fecal excretion. A statistical analysis of over 800 samples from 15 countries indicates that 84 percent of the general population have urinary concentrations of less than 5 μg/L. A zero value, that is, less than 0.5 μg/L, was found in 79 percent of the samples. The 95 percent confidence limit indicates an upper limit for "normal" mercury in urine of 20 to 25 μg/L and for blood, 4 μg per 100 mL. Fecal excretion was reported to average 10 μg of mercury per day.

Chronic and Acute Poisoning from Inorganic Mercury

No clinical distinction has been made between symptoms associated with exposure to mercury vapor and to mercuric salts. The experimental findings of higher brain levels associated with the vapor suggest that CNS disturbances would be more pronounced following exposure to this form of mercury.

Symptoms involving the CNS are the most frequently seen, the principal features being tremor and psychologic disturbances (erethismus mercurialis). Proteinuria and progressing renal damage may occur. Symptoms related to the mouth such as gingivitis, stomatitis, and excessive salivation often occur. These symptoms may be connected with the secretion of mercury in the saliva. Dermatitis has been observed in some workmen exposed to mercury. Mercurialentis (a colored reflex from the lens) is seen in chronic exposure, but does not indicate intoxication. A number of nonspecific symptoms such as anorexia, weight loss, anemia, and muscular weakness are also associated with chronic exposure.

The symptoms associated with acute oral intake of inorganic mercury salts are acute gastroenteritis with abdominal pain, vomiting, and some bloody diarrhea. Anuria and uremia are associated with severe kidney damage and may appear a day or more after exposure and frequently precede a fatal outcome. The approximate lethal dose to humans of mercuric chloride is 1 g. Acute exposure to high concentrations of mercury vapor may give rise to a condition characterized by a metallic taste, nausea, abdominal pain, vomiting, diarrhea, headache, and sometimes albuminuria. A few days later the salivary glands swell, stomatitis and gingivitis develop, and a dark line of mercurous sulfide (HgS) forms on the inflamed gums. The teeth may loosen and ulcers may form on the lips and cheeks.

Chronic and Acute Poisoning from Organomercurial Compounds

The symptoms of chronic and acute exposure to organomercurial compounds are the same. Symptoms may appear weeks to months after an acute exposure, and include ataxia; slurring of speech; numbness and tingling of the lips, hands, and feet; concentric restriction of the visual fields; impairment of hearing; and emotional disturbances. The symptoms are irreversible in cases of severe poisoning.

Mothers ingesting large amounts of methylmercury give birth to babies suffering from palsy, convulsions, and mental retardation. Experimental work indicates that methylmercury compounds are potent inhibitors of cell division and chromosome segregation.

Treatment of Mercury Poisoning

The treatment of mercury poisoning aims at the removal of mercury from the gastrointestinal tract and the inactivation with subsequent excretion of mercury which has been absorbed. Although edetate calcium disodium, penicillamine, and dimercaprol all increase the excretion of mercury, dimercaprol has greater efficacy. Therefore, it remains the drug routinely used in the treatment of acute mercury poisoning (see section on dimercaprol, below).

ARSENIC

Arsenic is readily available in inorganic and organic forms. Inorganic arsenic is an active constituent in many fungicides, herbicides, and pesticides. It is used in the paint and dye industry and was at one time used extensively in cosmetics. Organic arsenical compounds are used today to treat protozoan infestations such as trypanosomiasis and amebiasis. Arsanilic acid is fed to poultry and livestock to enhance growth rate.

Arsenic exists in the elemental form, and in salts where it is trivalent or pentavalent. The arsenites, for example, potassium arsenite, $KAsO_2$, and salts of arsenous acid, $H_2As_2O_4^{2-}$, contain trivalent arsenic. The pentavalent oxidation state is found in the arsenates such as lead arsenate, $PbHAsO_4$. These are salts of arsenic acid. The arsenates have a high affinity for thiol groups and are considerably more toxic than the arsenates. The latter have properties similar to those of phosphate and have no affinity for thiol groups.

The organic arsenicals contain arsenic linked to a carbon atom by a covalent bond, where arsenic exists in the trivalent or pentavalent state. Arsphenamine contains trivalent arsenic; sodium arsanilate contains the element in the pentavalent form.

Arsine, AsH_3, is a colorless gas with a garlic-like odor and is produced by the action of nascent hydrogen on the elemental form of arsenic. It produces toxic effects which are different from those of the other compounds of arsenic.

Mechanism of Action

Trivalent arsenical compounds, both the inorganic arsenic salts and the monosubstituted organic arsenicals, possess a high affinity for vicinal thiol groups. Thus, reactions with thiol functional groups lead to the formation of stable five-membered rings.

$$R{-}As{=}O + \begin{array}{l} HS{-}CH_2 \\ HS{-}CH \\ HO{-}CH_2 \end{array} \longrightarrow R{-}As\begin{array}{l} S{-}CH_2 \\ S{-}CH \\ HO{-}CH_2 \end{array} + H_2O$$

It is likely that this affinity of trivalent arsenic for thiol groups of enzymes and other proteins in tissues is ultimately responsible for the toxicity of this class of arsenic compounds.

Toxicokinetics

Systemic poisoning can be produced by absorption from the lungs, the gastrointestinal tract, and through the skin. After acute exposure, arsenic is deposited in tissues such as the liver, kidney, intestine, spleen, and lungs, in that order. Arsenic appears in hair about 2 weeks after the first exposure, where it is bound to the sulfide linkages in keratin. Chronic exposure leads to accumulation in hair, bone, and skin. Arsenic may be found in high concentrations in the hair years after cessation of exposure and after most of the metal has been removed from the soft tissues.

Arsenic passes the blood-brain barrier slowly. Brain levels are among the lowest in the body. Arsenic readily crosses the placental barrier, and fetal damage has been reported. The pathways and products of biotransformation of arsenic are not well defined. Excretion occurs by all physiologic routes—feces, urine, sweat, and milk. In general, the arsenite salts are lost mainly via the feces, and the arsenates via the urine. Arsenate excretion is more rapid than arsenite excretion and probably occurs via the phosphate excretory mechanisms.

Symptoms of Acute Toxicity

Acute arsenic poisoning occurs because arsenic, especially in the form of As_2O_3 (arsenic trioxide, arsenous acid) is readily available, practically tasteless, has the appearance of sugar, and is quickly absorbed from the gastrointestinal tract. Oral intake is followed by an asymptomatic period of about 30 min. The victim then experiences a tightness in the throat, difficulty in swallowing, and stomach pains. Projectile vomiting may ensue, which can be lifesaving. Other effects quickly follow, such as intensive diarrhea with watery feces containing shreds of mucus. Depressed urine flow is characteristic of acute arsenic intoxication. Symptoms of shock due to hypovolemia may develop. Death usually results in 1 to 3 days, with the victim in a state of collapse. Deaths which occur up to 14 days after poisoning are caused by nephritis.

Inhalation of arsine gas leads to rapid hemolysis, which gives rise to anemia, reduced red blood cell count, and hemoglobin in the urine. The released hemoglobin causes jaundice and may block the kidney tubules. Death usually results from anoxemia in 2 to 9 days after exposure. Some symptoms of typical arsenic poisoning may also appear.

Symptoms of Chronic Poisoning

Nausea, vomiting, and diarrhea occur but are less pronounced than in cases of acute poisoning. The mucous membranes are affected, giving rise to symptoms of the common cold. The horny layer of the skin is stimulated, leading to the appearance of dark brown scales. Peripheral neuritis similar to that associated with chronic alcoholism is observed in approximately 5 percent of the cases of chronic arsenic poisoning. The afferent motor nerves and sensory fibers are affected, especially in the legs. The ankle jerk disappears and the leg muscles atrophy. Tremors have been reported in 10 percent of the cases of chronic exposure. Renal cortical necrosis has also been reported.

Continued exposure to arsine gas generally results in symptoms similar to the picture of arsenic poisoning. Arsine binds to red blood cells, making them susceptible to hemolysis. This results in a steady level of anemia.

Skin keratoses result from prolonged exposure to arsenic, and may become malignant. Arsenic has been reported as an industrial carcinogen implicated in producing lung and skin carcinomas.

The Action of Arsenic on Capillaries

Arsenic produces dilatation of capillaries, and an increase in permeability of the capillary walls. This results in a fall in blood pressure and tissue edema leading to a state of shock.

Capillary damage is especially pronounced in the splenic area. The loss of plasma proteins into the intestinal areas causes blisters under the mucosal layer. Stimulated intestinal peristalsis leads to diarrhea and the shedding of epithelial cells.

Capillary and epithelial cell damage also occurs in the kidneys. Protein and red blood cells appear in the urine. The depression in urine flow results from both the vascular damage to kidney and the loss of fluid in the capillary beds.

Treatment of Arsenic Poisoning

Although sodium thiosulfate has been used in to treat arsenic poisoning, dimercaprol is the primary agent. This compound is used in the treatment of mild to severe arsenic poisoning. For mild poisoning, dimercaprol (2.5 mg/kg) is given by deep IM injection every 4 hours for 2 days, every 6 hours on the third day, and then every 12 hours for 10 days. For severe poisoning, 3 mg/kg is used in the dosage regimen described. (See under "Dimercaprol," below.)

GOLD

At present, gold compounds (e.g., gold sodium thiomalate, aurothioglucose, and auranofin) have a therapeutic usefulness limited to the treatment of rheumatoid arthritis of the peripheral joints and of certain rare skin diseases such as discoid lupus.

Toxicokinetics

Gold compounds administered by intramuscular injection, either in an aqueous solution (gold sodium thiomalate) or as an oil suspension (aurothioglucose), are absorbed slowly from the site of injection. Auranofin is used orally and has a low bioavailability (about 25%). The compounds are carried in the plasma in a nondialyzable form, with little in the cells, and are distributed throughout the soft tissues of the body. Even after a single injection, gold appears in the blood and urine for days to weeks. Of the gold that is absorbed, about 20 percent is rapidly excreted (mostly in the urine, in the case of the more water-soluble compounds, and in the feces in the case of the lipid-soluble drug) and about 80 percent is fixed for long periods in the tissues. With therapeutic doses, the levels in plasma and urine in humans contain about 1 to 2 mg per 100 mL.

Use of Gold Compounds in Treatment of Rheumatoid Arthritis

The principal therapeutic use of gold compounds is in the treatment of adult or juvenile rheumatoid arthritis. Gold, certainly no miracle drug, nevertheless offers considerable benefit to many individuals subjected to a painful and prolonged disease. Gold compounds are most efficacious in the early stages of the arthritic disease, reducing the inflammatory process but without inducing any repair process in the joints. Although the exact mechanism of its anti-inflammatory action is unknown, gold is taken up by macrophages, inhibits phagocytosis and lysosomal enzyme activity. There are two disadvantages associated with chrysotherapy (use of gold in treating disease). One is that patients who show improvement as a result of treatment may relapse after treatment is discontinued. The second disadvantage is the toxicity: gold compounds should be used with great caution, especially in elderly patients. These drugs should only be used as part of a complete therapeutic course, not alone.

Adverse Reactions

The most frequent toxic reaction to gold is dermatitis—an erythema urticaria, or rash—often accompanied by gastrointestinal disturbances. These reactions are usually preceded by pruritus. The skin lesions may last for some time but will eventually disappear after gold therapy has been discontinued. In some cases, severe exfoliative dermatitis results. Gold may be toxic to the kidney, producing a nephropathy or glomerulosis. Gastrointestinal damage (gastritis, colitis, or stomatitis) and hepatitis have been rarely observed. Blood dyscrasias (such as leukopenia, agranulocytosis, thrombocytopenia, or aplastic anemia) are rare but are very serious when they occur. Anaphylactoid reactions have been reported. Symptoms include flushing, fainting, dizziness, sweating, and gastrointestinal upset. Toxic effects may occur immediately or at any time during therapy.

Contraindications to the use of gold are impaired renal or hepatic function, skin lesions, or abnormalities of the hematopoietic system. The drugs should be used in pregnancy only when essential.

Treatment of Gold Toxicity

Treatment consists primarily of topical or systemic administration of corticosteroids. Severe cases of toxicity respond well to treatment with dimercaprol.

ZINC

Zinc is an element necessary for normal growth and development of plants and animals. It is omnipresent in the environment and is found in water, air, and living organisms. It functions as an cofactor for a number of enzymes and therefore is important in many types of syntheses in the body, including DNA and RNA.

Millions of tons of zinc metal are used commercially, principally to galvanize iron and to manufacture brass. Exposure to zinc fumes is the main industrial hazard. Many zinc salts have industrial, agricultural, and medical uses. Zinc can be found in adhesive plaster (containing zinc oxide) used to prevent dialysis coils from unwinding, water used for dialysis fluid, and galvanized iron pipes or tanks. Welders, smelter workers, and solderers are exposed to aerosolized zinc.

The normal adult body zinc content is 1.5 to 3.0 g. Daily intake ranges from 5 to 35 mg. Zinc is bound to metallothionines synthesized in the liver and is excreted by both the urine and the gastrointestinal tract, choroid plexus, and prostate; substantial amounts are also found in the bone, brain, eyes, skeletal muscle, and other tissues. Zinc has a strong affinity for red blood cells and plasma proteins.

Two human zinc-deficiency syndromes have been described, *hypogonadal dwarf syndrome* and *acrodermatitis enteropathica*. Parakeratosis and impaired wound healing are also associated with zinc deficiency. The manifestations of zinc toxicity do not necessarily correlate well with plasma or whole blood zinc levels. Nausea, vomiting, anorexia, lethargy, irritability, abdominal pain, and anemia are the most frequent manifestations. Fever may accompany zinc toxicity, along with diarrhea, muscle pain, hyperamylasemia (with or without pancreatitis), intestinal bleeding, thrombocytopenia, oliguria, hypotension, and renal failure with tubular necrosis.

Toxicities caused by aerosolized zinc may be zinc fume fever, chills, myalgias, metallic taste, cough, nausea, lethargy, and, occasionally, hemoptysis. Ordinarily, all toxicities disappear after cessation of exposure. Zinc tablets are now sold in health food stores, and excessive intake may result in toxicity. There is no specific chelator for the treatment of zinc toxicity; calcium supplements have been used as a protection against zinc toxicity.

ALUMINUM

Aluminum is widely used as a building material and for other uses where light weight and corrosion resistance are important. Aluminum oxide has industrial uses as an abrasive and catalyst. Medically, various soluble salts of aluminum have been used as astringents, styptics, and antiseptics. The insoluble salts are used as antacids and as antidiarrheal agents. Inhalation of aluminum hydroxide is used as a preventive and curative agent for silicosis.

Orally, aluminum salts are converted to the phosphate salt in the gastrointestinal tract and excreted in the feces and in the milk of nursing females. Parenteral injection of aluminum salts results in excretion in both the feces and urine as well as slight increase in the concentration of aluminum in the liver and spleen.

Early toxic effects of aluminum include malaise, memory loss, and a characteristic speech disturbance. As the disease progresses, dysarthria, asterixis, myoclonic twitches, dementia, somnolence, and seizures occur. The electroencephalogram shows slowing, together with bursts of delta-wave activity and high voltage, symmetric spikes. Postmortem examinations show that aluminum levels are markedly increased in the gray matter.

Other toxic effects include anemia, myopathy, and severe pain caused by profound osteodystrophy. It has been suggested that Alzheimer's disease and other types of senile dementia may be related to brain aluminum deposition, possibly caused by improper use of aluminum utensils.

Although frequently lethal, in some cases encephalopathy has regressed after intake of oral aluminum is stopped; sometimes deferoxamine, which complexes with aluminum, as well as iron, may be beneficial.

CADMIUM

Cadmium ranks close to lead and mercury as a metal of current toxicologic concern. Over 10 million pounds of cadmium are used industrially every year in the United States. It is used in the manufacture of electrical conductors and in electroplating; and it is present in ceramics, pigments, dental prosthetics, plastic stabilizers, and storage batteries. It is also a by-product of zinc smelting, and it is used in the photographic, rubber, motor, and aircraft industries. Smelters, metal-processing furnaces, and the burning of coal and oil are responsible for much of the cadmium in the air.

Cadmium is used as various inorganic salts. The most important are cadmium stearate, which is used as a heat stabilizer in PVC plastics, and cadmium sulfide and cadmium sulfoselenide, used as yellow and red pigments in plastics and colors. Cadmium sulfide is also used in photocells and solar cells. Cadmium chloride is used in the production of certain photographic films.

Acute intoxication by cadmium fumes exceeding 0.1 mg/m^3 produces a characteristic clinical picture. Four to 10 h after exposure dyspnea, cough, and substernal discomfort supervene, often accompanied by prominent myalgias, fatigue, headache, and vomiting. In more severe cases wheezing, hemoptysis, and progressive dyspnea caused by pulmonary edema may occur and may be accompanied by hypotension and renal failure.

In most cases, the pulmonary manifestations resolve rapidly but pulmonary function abnormalities may not disappear for months; in these cases vital capacity is reduced and there is a restrictive defect.

Ingestion of large amounts of cadmium results in nausea, vomiting, and abdominal pain, often accompanied by weakness, prostration, and myalgias. The onset of gastroenteritis occurs 1.5 to 5 h after ingestion and lasts for less than 24 h.

Chronic exposure to cadmium aerosol for years has resulted in emphysema; this is not accompanied by bronchitis and may appear many years after industrial exposure has stopped. It is reported that workers exposed for years to work-room concentrations of respirable cadmium greater than 0.01 mg/m^3 also suffer olfactory nerve damage, which in some cases progresses to total anosmia. The most frequent systemic long-term consequence of aerosol or oral exposure is protein-uria. After prolonged and heavy contact, cadmium urinary excretion continues for years and is associated with damage to the proximal tubule. The major urinary protein is a low-molecular weight β-macroglobulin.

On occasion, the proteinuria may be accompanied by glycosuria and aminoaciduria. Only infrequently are the proteinuria and tubular damage followed by progressive renal failure. An exception to the relatively benign course of renal damage is the disease in Japan known as *itai-itai* (ouch-ouch), which affected almost exclusively multiparous women of ages 40 to 70 who lived in an area contaminated by industrial cadmium waste. Manifestation included back and joint pain, a waddling gait, osteomalacia, bone deformities, and fractures, all presumably secondary to cadmium-induced renal tubular damage.

Persons who have ingested cadmium salts should be made to vomit or given gastric lavage; persons exposed to acute inhalation should be removed from exposure and given oxygen therapy as necessary. No specific treatment for chronic cadmium poisoning is available and symptomatic treatment must be relied upon. Administration of chelating agents is contraindicated, since they are nephrotoxic in combination with cadmium.

MANGANESE

Manganese is a cofactor in a number of enzymatic reactions, particularly those involved in phosphorylation, cholesterol, and fatty-acids syntheses. While it is present in urban air and in most water supplies, the principal portion of the intake is derived from food, especially vegetables, the germinal portions of grains, fruits, nuts, tea, and some spices.

Manganese and its compounds are used in making steel alloys, dry cell batteries, electrical coils, ceramics, matches, glass, dye, fertilizers, and welding rods and are used as oxidizing agents and animal food additives. In medicine, potassium permanganate is applied topically as an antiseptic and for its slight astringent activity. This is the only manganese compound of medical use at the present time.

The body burden of manganese has been estimated at 20 mg. The liver, kidney, intestine, and pancreas contain the highest concentrations. No significant changes in tissue concentration occur with age, except that tissues that have low manganese amounts in adults tend to contain higher amounts in the newborn. The lungs do not accumulate manganese with age despite significant concentrations in urban air. The turnover of manganese is rapid.

Manganese toxicity occurs primarily in miners who have been exposed to aerosolized manganese dioxide for prolonged periods. The manifestions, known as *manganic madness*, concentrate primarily in the basal ganglia and cerebellum, accounting for the extrapyramidal Parkinson-like reactions. Other manifestations include compulsive behavior (including singing, dancing, fighting, and running), explosive and involuntary laughter, headache, muscular weakness, tremors, somnolence, dystonia, hypotonia, retropulsion, propulsion, dementia, speech disturbances, irritability, hypersomnia, and memory defects. In some cases psychosis may be the dominant feature.

There is no effective therapy. After removal from manganese exposure, followed by attempts to reduce the body manganese load by treatment with edetate calcium disodium, the patients are treated with levodopa. The mental aberrations improve, but the neurologic abnormalities tend to persist.

BISMUTH

Widely used in industry in the manufacture of alloys, ceramics, magnets, and radiographic contrast media, bismuth is also much in demand as a medicinal agent. Exposure to this metal is as common as that to lead and mercury. For example, bismuth is one of the contaminants found in urban air. Yet bismuth is not considered a serious industrial hazard, possibly because few cases of poisoning from this source are reported.

The advent of more effective agents has displaced bismuth for the systemic therapy of syphilis and amebiasis. Today it is the insoluble salts of bismuth (bismuth subgallate and bismuth subsalicylate) that are widely used for gastrointestinal complaints such as nausea and diarrhea.

There is the possibility that intestinal bacteria might methylate bismuth and form a soluble salt. In animals, trimethyl bismuth is highly toxic, causing an encephalopathic syndrome. Blood levels of bismuth should not exceed 20 μg/L. Urinary excretion is less than 1 μmol per day.

Like the other heavy metals, bismuth forms strong covalent double bonds with sulfhydryl groups of cellular proteins, including many enzymes. It also coagulates and denatures protein. Similar to gold, mercury, and lead, bismuth has an affinity for renal and central nervous tissues. Thus encephalopathy and renal damage might be expected. Bismuth can also cause hepatitis and various skin disorders such as a lichen planus-like lesion.

Fever, diarrhea, weakness, stomatitis, black oropharynx and gum line, dermatitis, jaundice, and nephritis, so often seen when soluble salts of bismuth were used, are no longer seen. The reported cases today present as encephalopathy. At higher risk are patients who chronically take insoluble bismuth salts for gastrointestinal complaints for months and years. In Europe and Australia there is an incidence of bismuth encephalopathy due to the practice of using a bismuth subgallate powder daily to dust a colostomy to control odor and stool consistency.

Therapy of bismuth encephalopathy involves discontinuation of use of the bismuth compound; recovery takes place slowly over a period of months. Attempts to remove the bismuth more rapidly by use of chelates are not recommended.

The subsalicylate salt of bismuth can be dissociated and cause salicylate poisoning. Aspirin should not be given with remedies containing bismuth subsalicylate.

OTHER METALS

Practically all metals have important toxicities when a certain exposure level is exceeded. The route of exposure is pivotal to the degree and type of toxicity. When metals are inhaled as a fine powder, lung toxicity is the dominant picture. Oral absorption may lead to rapid toxicity, as contrasted to skin absorption which usually results in chronic symptoms. Other texts should be consulted for the less common metalic poisonings. Note that iron toxicity is discussed in Chapter 34, along with the use of deferoxamine, the specific antidote for iron toxicity.

HEAVY METAL ANTAGONISTS

The basis for treatment of heavy metal toxicity is chelation therapy. Heavy metals produce their toxic effects by binding with endogenous ligands, forming complexes which block or inhibit some physiologic or biochemical process. Chelating agents bind to the metal ions, thus competitively inhibiting the binding of the metals to endogenous ligands. The chelates, being more water-soluble, are readily excreted in the urine. In some heavy metal toxicity, such as that produced by cadmium and gold, present chelating agents are contraindicated, since these chemical complexes may increase the risk of renal toxicity.

Edetate Calcium Disodium

Chemistry Edetate calcium disodium is the calcium chelate of the disodium salt of ethylenediaminetetraacetic acid (EDTA). EDTA binds cations generally. Sodium and potassium are held most weakly. Calcium, magnesium, and barium are bound more tightly but can be displaced by cobalt, chromium, cadmium, copper, nickel, and lead, whose chelates have higher stability constants.

$$(HO{-}\overset{O}{\overset{\|}{C}}{-}H_2C)_2N{-}CH_2{-}CH_2{-}N(CH_2{-}\overset{O}{\overset{\|}{C}}{-}OH)_2$$

Ethylenediaminetetraacetic acid (EDTA)

$$NaO{-}\overset{O}{\overset{\|}{C}}{-}H_2C{-}N{-}CH_2{-}CH_2{-}N{-}CH_2{-}\overset{O}{\overset{\|}{C}}{-}ONa;\quad H_2C{-}C(=O){-}O\cdots Ca\cdots O{-}C(=O){-}CH_2$$

Edetate calcium disodium (calcium disodium EDTA)

Mechanism of Action The therapeutic action of edetate calcium disodium in heavy metal intoxication is due to the ability of the heavy metals such as lead to displace the sodium and calcium to form stable, soluble metal chelates. It is generally held that edetate calcium disodium mobilizes lead from the soft tissues. Subsequently, the soft tissue stores are replenished by the redistribution of lead from bone. The lead chelate formed by EDTA is represented structurally as:

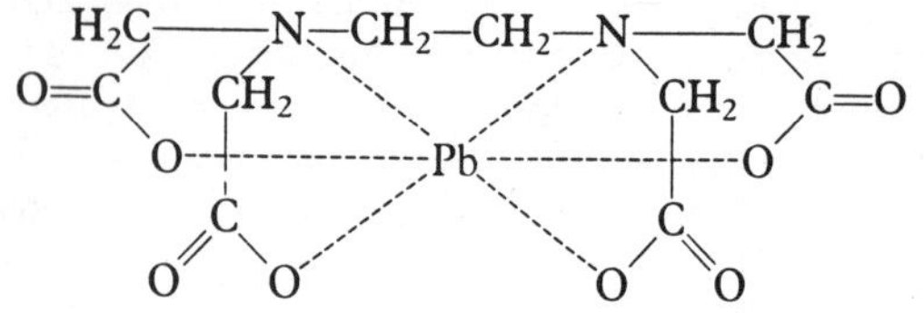

```
  H2C———N—CH2—CH2—N———CH2
  /      \              /      \
O=C    CH2          CH2    C=O
  \      |              |      /
   O--+---------Pb---------+---O
          |                  |
          C                  C
        //  \              /  \\
       O     O            O     O
```

Pharmacokinetics The absorption of edetate calcium disodium from the gastrointestinal tract after oral administration is poor. Following parenteral administration, 50 percent of a dose is excreted unchanged in the urine within 1 h; almost 100 percent is excreted in the urine within 24 h. The drug is distributed exclusively in body fluids. In blood, all of the drug is found in the plasma.

Therapeutic Uses Edetate calcium disodium is primarily used in the diagnosis and treatment of lead intoxication. It is ineffective in the treatment of arsenic and mercury toxicity and has questionable activity against other heavy metals.

Routes of Administration and Dosage As a diagnostic agent for lead poisoning, edetate calcium disodium is given IV (over 1 hour) or IM and urine is collected in a lead free container for 24 hours. If the number of micrograms of lead excreted is greater then the number of milligrams of EDTA given, the test is considered positive. For the treatment of lead intoxication, the intravenous route of administration is preferred in adults. The therapeutic dosage is determined by the concentration of lead in the blood, the size of the patient, and reactions to the drug. The average dose for adults is 3 to 5 g/day for 3 to 5 days in two daily doses, each given in saline or 5 percent dextrose solution. For greater convenience and safety in treating children, the drug is usually administered intramuscularly at a dose of 50 mg/kg daily. In children with acute lead encephalopathy, the mortality rate is reduced to about 25 percent when they are treated with edetate calcium disodium alone. However, administration of the drug alone to an individual with a relatively high concentration of lead (>60 μg per 100 mL) can intensify the toxic effects of lead. For this reason it is often given in combination with dimercaprol.

Adverse Reactions The most common adverse reactions are pain at the site of intramuscular injection. The principal toxic effect is renal tubular necrosis. An excessive chelation syndrome may be produced by large doses or prolonged administration. This is an acute febrile state with marked myalgia, headache, nasal congestion, nocturia, and chills. The symptoms subside upon removal of the drug. Deaths have been reported rarely. The drug is contraindicated in patients with severe renal disease. Safety in pregnancy has not been established; therefore, the drug should not be used in women of childbearing age unless potential benefit outweighs the risk.

Dimercaprol

Dimercaprol (2,3-dimercaptopropanol) has the following structure:

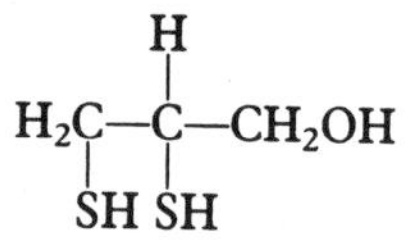

```
          H
          |
  H2C—C—CH2OH
    |    |
   SH SH
```

Mechanism of Action Dimercaprol forms stable chelates with arsenic, gold, and mercury, thus enhancing the excretion of these metals. In the case of mercury, the drug may form two different complexes:

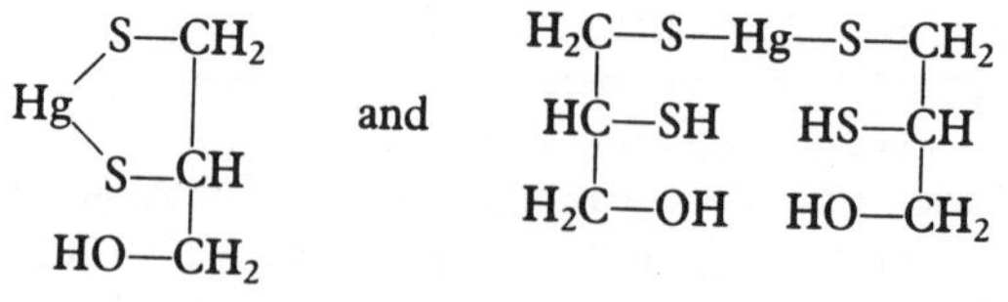

```
     S—CH2                  H2C—S—Hg—S—CH2
    /    |                    |            |
 Hg      |        and       HC—SH     HS—CH
    \    |                    |            |
     S—CH                   H2C—OH    HO—CH2
        |
   HO—CH2
```

At a molar ratio of dimercaprol to Hg^{2+} of 1, a chelate is formed. When the molar ratio is 2, a complex forms containing two dimercaprol molecules to one atom of mercury. This compound is water-soluble at pH 7.5 and binds mercury more tightly than does the chelate. The drug prevents the inhibition of sulphydryl enzymes by the heavy metal and also reactivates the enzymes.

Pharmacokinetics When administered intramuscularly as a 10 percent solution of dimercaprol in oil, the drug reaches a peak plasma level within 1 h. The drug is biotransformed very rapidly by the liver and almost completely excreted in the urine within 4 h.

Therapeutic Uses Dimercaprol is highly effective in the treatment of arsenic, gold, and mercury poisoning. It is effective in acute mercury poisoning when administered within 1 to 2 h following ingestion. It is not effective in treatment of chronic mercury poisoning. Dimercaprol is also used in combination with edetate calcium disodium for use in lead poisoning in children.

Route of Administration and Dosage Dimercaprol is given only by deep intramuscular injection. For therapy of arsenic and gold intoxication, it is given for approximately 10 days as follows: 2.5 mg/kg, four times daily for 2 days, two times on the third day, and once on days 4 to 10. For acute mercury toxicity, the drug is given at 5 mg/kg initially, followed by 2.5 mg/kg once or twice on days 2 to 10. For treatment of lead toxicity, dimercaprol is given at 4 mg/kg intramuscularly initially, followed by the same dose of dimercaprol combined with 12.5 mg/kg of edetate calcium disodium, every 4 hours.

Adverse Reactions At therapeutic doses, side effects to dimercaprol are generally mild. At larger doses, adverse reactions such as nausea and vomiting, headache, burning sensation in mouth and throat, salivation, lacrimation, and anxiety and restlessness have been reported. These untoward effects are usually relieved by the administration of an antihistamine. The most prominent toxic effect reported has been hypertension and tachycardia. High doses can produce convulsions or coma. The drug is potentially nephrotoxic. Because the drug-metal complex breaks down easily under acid conditions, producing an alkaline urine protects the kidney during therapy. Iron should not be given to the patient taking dimercaprol because iron will complete with the toxic metal for complexing.

SUCCIMER

This drug is an orally active heavy metal chelating agent. Succimer has been shown to be effective in mercury and arsenic poisoning; however, presently it is only indicated for the treatment of lead intoxication in children with blood levels over 45 μg/dL.

A course of treatment lasts 19 days. The usual dosage is 10 mg/kg orally every 8 hours for 5 days, followed by the same dose given every 12 hours for 14 days. Depending on lead blood level, repeated courses of therapy may be given after a minimum of 2 weeks without drug therapy. Patient who have used edetate calcium disodium, with or without dimercaprol, may use succimer after an interval of 4 weeks.

The most common adverse effects are gastrointestinal upset and increases in serum transaminases. Skin rashes, sore throat, rhinorrhea, nasal congestion, and cough are less common.

Penicillamine

Penicillamine is D-3-mercaptovaline.

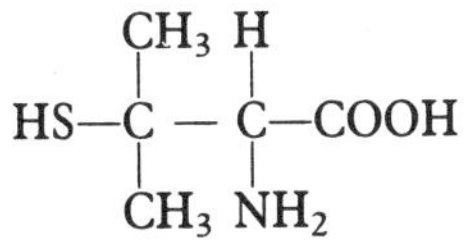

$$\begin{array}{ccccc} & CH_3 & & H & \\ & | & & | & \\ HS— & C & — & C & —COOH \\ & | & & | & \\ & CH_3 & & NH_2 & \end{array}$$

Mechanism of Action Penicillamine acts by binding to copper, iron, mercury, and lead, producing chelates which are readily excreted in the urine. It is superior to other heavy metal antagonists in chelating copper and is used therapeutically to remove excess copper. It also interacts with cystine, increasing its excretion in cystinuria.

Pharmacokinetics Penicillamine is well absorbed from the gastrointestinal tract following oral administration. The drug is relatively stable to biotransformation and is excreted unchanged primarily in the urine.

Therapeutic Uses The major use of penicillamine is to eliminate excess copper in patients with Wilson's disease (hepatolenticular degeneration due to an abnormality in copper metabolism). Penicillamine is sometimes used in adjunct therapy in the treatment of lead, mercury and arsenic poisoning.

Route of Administration and Dosage As mentioned above, penicillamine has the advantage of being effective following oral administration. In Wilson's disease, penicillamine is given at a dosage of 250 mg four times daily to adults and 250 mg/day to infants and small children. In cystinuria, the drug is given at 1 to 4 g daily in divided doses. Dosages for treatment of all these syndromes must be individualized.

Adverse Reactions The most common adverse effects are allergic reactions manifested by maculopapular or erythematous rash occasionally accompanied by fever, arthralgia, or lymphadenopathy. Urticaria has also been reported. Adrenal corticosteroids and antihistamines may be given to relieve these reactions. Cross-sensitivity to penicillin may exist; therefore, the drug is contraindicated in patients with penicillin hypersensitivity. Other adverse reactions include gastrointestinal irritation, hepatic dysfunction, thrombocytopenia, leukopenia, and purpura. Severe glomerulonephritis and intraalveolar hemorrhage has been rarely reported. Penicillamine increases the need for pyridoxine, and patients should receive this vitamin along with the drug. The patient must be closely observed to determine liver function and to prevent nephrotic syndrome and proteinuria.

BIBLIOGRAPHY

Calesnick, B., and A.M. Dinan: "Zinc Deficiency and Zinc Toxicity," *Am. Fam. Phys.* **37**: 267-270 (1988).

Charhon, S.A., P.M. Chavassieux, P.J. Meunier, and M. Accominotti: "Serum Aluminum Concentration and Aluminum Deposits in Bone in Patients Receiving Haemodialysis," *Br. Med. J.* **290**: 1613-1614 (1985).

DiPalma, J.R.: "Bismuth Toxicity," *Am. Fam. Phys.* **38**: 244-246 (1988).

Ellenhorn, M.J., and D.G. Barcalrix: *Medical Toxicology, Diagnosis and Treatment of Human Poisoning, 2nd Ed.*, Elsevier, New York, 1991.

Friberg, L.: "Cadmium," *Annu. Rev. Public Health* **4**: 367-373 (1983).

Goyer, G.A.: "Toxic Effects of Metals," In Amdur, M.O., J. Doull, and C.D. Klaassen (eds.): *Casarett and Doull's Toxicology, 4th Ed.*, Pergamon Press, New York, 1991, pp. 623-680.

Hassan, J., J. Hanly, B. Bresnihan, C. Feighery, and C.A. Whelan: "The Immunological Consequences of Gold Therapy: A Prospective Study in Patients with Rheumatoid Arthritis," *Clin. Exp. Immunol.* **63**: 614-620 (1986).

Hurst, N.P., A.L. Bell, and G. Nuki: "Studies of the Effect of D-Penicillamine and Sodium Aurothiomalate Therapy on Superoxide Anion Production by Monocytes from Patients with Rheumatoid Arthritis: Evidence for in vivo Stimulation of Monocytes," *Ann. Rheum. Dis.* **45**: 37-43 (1986).

Jones, M.M.: "New Developments in Therapeutic Chelating Agents as Antidotes for Metal Poisoning," *Crit. Rev. Toxicol.* **21**: 209-233 (1991).

Kark, R.A., D.C. Poskanzer, J.D. Bullock, and G. Boylen: "Mercury Poisoning and Its Treatment with N-Acetyl--D,L-Penicillamine," *N. Engl. J. Med.* **285**: 10-16 (1971).

Khandelwal, S., D.N. Kachru, and S.K. Tandon: "Influence of Metal Chelators on Metalloenzymes," *Toxicol. Lett.* **37**: 213-219 (1987).

Klaassen, C.D.: "Nonmetallic Environmental Toxicants, Air Pollutants, Solvents and Vapors, and Pesticides," in Gilman, A.G., T.W. Rall, A.S. Nies, and P. Taylor, (eds.) *Goodman and Gilman's The Pharmacological Basis of Therapeutics, 8th Ed.*, Pergamon Press, New York, 1990, pp. 1615-1639.

Landrigan, P.J.: "Toxicity of Lead at Low Dose," *Br. J. Med.* **46**: 593-596 (1989).

Manton, W.I.: "Total Contribution of Airborne Lead to Blood Lead," *Br. J. Ind. Med.* **42**: 168-172 (1985).

Moel, D.I., H.K. Sachs, and M.A. Drayton: "Slow, Natural Reduction in Blood Lead Level after Chelation Therapy for Lead Poisoning in Childhood," *Am. J. Dis. Child.* **140**: 905-908 (1986).

Nadig, R.J.: "Treatment of Lead Poisoning," *J. Amer. Med. Assoc.* **263**: 2181-2182 (1990).

Nightingale, S.L.: "Oral Chelation Products," *Am. Fam. Phys.* **33**: 325 (1986).

Plunkett, E.R.: *Handbook of Industrial Toxicology, 3d Ed.* Chemical Publishing, New York, 1987.

Schneitzer, L., H.H. Osborn, A. Bierman, A Mezey, and B. Kaul: "Lead Poisoning in Adults from Renovation of an Older Home.", *Ann. Emerg. Med.* **19**: 415-420, 1990.

Szeliga-Cetnarska, M., and J.S. Zbrojkiewicz: Chronic Manganese Poisoning," *Med. Pracy.* **36**: 382-386 (1985).

Takahashi, W., K. Pfenninger, and L. Wong: "Urinary Arsenic, Chromium and Copper Levels in Workers Exposed to Arsenic-Based Wood Preservatives," *Arch. Environ. Health.* **38**: 209-214 (1983).

United States Pharmacopeial Convention, Inc.: *Drug Information for the Health Care Professional, 8th Ed.*, Rockville, Maryland, 1988.

Weigel, H.J., D. Ilge, I. Elmadia, and H.J. Jager: "Availability and Toxicological Effects of Low Levels of Biologically Bound Cadmium," *Arch. Environ. Contam. Toxicol.* **16**: 85-93 (1987).

INDEX

A

Absorbable gelatin, 536
Absorption, 43-50, 803
Absorption sites:
  alimentary canal, 46-48
  injection routes, 48-49
  respiratory tract, 49
  skin, 49-50
Acarbose, 609
Acceptor, definition of, 20
ACE inhibitors, *see* Angiotensin converting enzyme inhibitors
Acebutolol (*see also* β-Adrenergic blocking agents):
  classification, 130, 133, 137
  compliance, 474
  pharmacodynamic properties, 133, 134, 473, 474
  pharmacokinetics, 135, 137
  physicochemical properties, 135, 474
  structure, 132
  uses, 137-138, 419, 474
Acetaldehyde, 69-70, 240, 255-256
Acetaminophen:
  adverse reactions, 360-361, 804
  drug interactions, 79, 258, 575, 768
  mechanism of action, 360
  pharmacokinetics, 72, 360
  poisoning, 807
  structure, 360
  treatment of toxicity, 360, 808
  uses, 334, 360, 361, 362
Acetazolamide:
  adverse reactions, 465
  chemistry, 465
  classification, 306, 455
  drug interactions, 287
  effects on urinary electrolytes, 466
  mechanism of action, 465
  pharmacokinetics, 465
  uses, 306, 313, 465
Acetohexamide, (*see also* Sulfonylurea derivatives):
  classification, 604
  disulfiram-like reaction, 259
  pharmacokinetics, 605-606
  structure, 605
2-Acetylaminofluorene, 67
Acetylcholine:
  adverse reactions, 149
  biotransformation, 72, 147
  chemistry, 147, 148
  cholinergic mechanisms, 82
  history of, 5
  in neurohumoral transmission, 104-106, 148
  in peptic ulcer disease, 560
  pharmacodynamics, 147-149, 150
  receptors, 109-111
  structure, 148
  use, 149
Acetylcholinesterase:
  chemistry, 153
  hydrolysis of cholinomimetic drugs, 149, 153-154, 176
  inhibition by drugs, 153-161
  in neurohumoral transmission, 104, 106, 147, 175
Acetylcysteine (N-Acetylcysteine):
  pharmacologic properties, 496
  uses, 360, 495, 807
N-Acetyl-p-benzoquinone, 258
Acetylsalicylic acid, *see* Aspirin
Acquired immunodeficiency syndrome (AIDS):
  drug dependence, 377
  treatment of, 768-769
Acrylonitrile, 816
ACTH, *see* Adrenocorticotropic hormone
Actinomycin D, *see* Dactinomycin
Acute toxicity, definition of, 803
Acyclo-GTP, *see* Acyclovir
Acycloguanosine, *see* Acyclovir
Acyclovir (Acycloguanosine):
  adverse reactions, 765
  history of, 9
  mechanism of action, 763, 764
  pharmacokinetics, 763, 765
  structure, 763
  uses, 765
Addiction, 376 (*see also* Drug dependence)
Adenosine:
  adverse reactions, 422
  as a neurotransmitter, 323, 492
  classification, 401
  mechanism of action, 401
  pharmacokinetics, 422
  pharmacologic effects, 401, 422
  receptors, 492
  structure, 422
  uses, 394, 422, 423
Adrenaline, *see* Epinephrine
Adrenergic agonists (*also see Individual Agents*):
  chemistry, 116-117
  classification, 113-114
  pharmacokinetics, 120
  structure-activity relationships, 116-117
  uses, 468
Adrenergic blockade, definition of, 130
Adrenergic receptors, 102-103, 105, 110-112, 114, 115

α-Adrenergic blocking agents (*also see Individual Agents*):
  classification, 130
  effects on blood pressure, 142
  history of, 8
  nonselective drugs, 139-143
  selective drugs, 143
  structures, 475
  uses, 267, 269, 397, 398, 468, 475
β-Adrenergic agonists (*also see Individual Agents*):
  adverse reactions, 491
  classification, 490
  history of, 8
  mechanism of action, 490
  pharmacologic effects, 116-128, 490
  uses, 490, 491, 498-500
β-Adrenergic blocking agents (*also see Individual Agents*):
  adverse reactions, 136
  classification, 133, 137, 401
  chemistry, 131
  compliance, 474
  drug interactions, 136, 412, 416, 418, 435, 447, 607, 750
  mechanism of action, 131, 133, 473
  pharmacokinetics, 135-136, 137
  pharmacologic effects, 133-135, 401, 429-430, 473-475
  physicochemical properties, 135, 474
  sites of action, 131
  structures, 132
  treatment of poisoning, 808
  uses, 130, 137, 138, 252, 269, 401, 419, 422, 423, 425, 429-430, 468, 473, 475, 477, 478, 482
Adrenergic neuronal blockade, definition of, 130
Adrenergic neuronal blocking drugs:
  classification, 130
  drug monographs, 143-145
  uses, 468, 476
Adrenocorticosteroids, *see* Corticosteroids
Adrenocorticotropic hormone (ACTH):
  adverse reactions, 639
  chemistry, 638
  formation of, 321
  opioid release of, 330
  pharmacokinetics, 639
  physiologic effects, 638-639
  regulation of secretion, 638
  source, 638
  structure, 639
  uses, 639
Aflatoxin, 67
Agonist, definition of, 29
Air pollution, 811
Albendazole: 788, 789, 796-797
Albuterol:
  adverse reactions, 123, 491
  classification, 123, 490
  mechanism of action, 115, 119
  pharmacokinetics, 123, 491
  pharmacologic effects, 123
  structure, 117, 123
  use, 123, 490, 491
Alclometasone dipropionate, 648
Alcohol, *see* Ethanol
Alcohol dehydrogenase, 71, 72, 255-256
Alcohols, 253, 807
Aldesleukin, 678, 686
Aldicarb, 815
Aldosterone, 640, 641, 643-644, 646, 647
Aldrin, 814
Alfentanil:
  chemistry, 335, 336
  classification, 219, 325
  pharmacokinetics, 328, 336
  uses, 230-231, 336
Alkyl aryl compounds, 810
Alkylating agents (*see also Individual Agents*):
  adverse reactions, 664-665
  chemistry, 663-664
  classification, 657, 664
  mechanism of action, 663, 664
  pharmacokinetics, 664
  site of action, 654
  structures, 665
Alkylmercury salts, 825
Allopurinol:
  adverse reactions, 363
  drug interactions, 363, 532, 607, 660, 680
  mechanism of action, 363, 660
  pharmacokinetics, 363
  structure, 362, 659
  uses, 363
Alprazolam:
  adverse reactions, 249
  chemistry, 244
  contraindications and precautions, 250
  dependence, 249, 378
  pharmacokinetics, 246, 247, 248
  structure, 245
  uses, 247, 250
  withdrawal, 249
Alprostadil, 215, 350
Alteplase (t-PA), 533, 534
Aluminum, 565, 822, 829
Aluminum hydroxide:
  adverse reactions, 568
  drug interactions, 412
  effects, 567
  uses, 567, 568, 810
Aluminum oxide, 829
Amantadine:
  adverse reactions, 767-768
  classification, 763
  history of, 9, 11
  mechanism of action, 317, 764, 767
  pharmacokinetics, 767
  structure, 317, 767
  uses, 317, 381, 763, 765

Ambenonium:
classification, 154
pharmacological effects, 159
structure, 155
uses, 159
Amcinonide, 648
Amebiasis, 772, 781
Amikacin:
adverse reactions, 722 723
antimicrobial spectrum, 721
chemistry, 719, 720
mechanism of action, 719, 721
mechanism of resistance, 722
pharmacokinetics, 722
uses, 723-724, 752, 753
Amiloride:
adverse reactions, 464-465
classification, 455, 470
mechanism of action, 464
pharmacokinetics, 463-464, 470
structure, 464
uses, 465
Aminocaproic acid, 535
Aminocarb, 815
Aminoglutethimide, 647, 648-649
Aminoglycosides:
adverse reactions, 85, 722-723
antimicrobial spectrum, 721
drug interactions, 176, 462, 683, 753
mechanism of action, 719
mechanism of resistance, 722
pharmacokinetics, 85, 722
structures, 720
uses, 723-724
Aminophylline:
classification, 490
drug interactions, 287
pharmacokinetics, 493
uses, 490, 494
4-Aminoquinolines, 773, 778
8-Aminoqinolines, 87, 778
5-Aminosalicylic acid (5-ASA), 577
Amiodarone:
adverse reactions, 420
chemistry, 419
classification, 401
drug interactions, 420
inhibition of throid function, 584
mechanism of action, 401
pharmacokinetics, 420
pharmacologic effects, 401, 419-420
structure, 419
uses, 420, 423
Amitriptyline:
chemistry, 289
drug interactions, 225, 258, 296, 566
mechanism of action, 291
pharmacokinetics, 294-295
pharmacologic effects, 293
structure, 290
Amlodipine:
adverse reactions, 435, 436
classification, 430, 478
pharmacologic effects, 432, 434
pharmacokinetics, 435
structure, 431
uses, 434, 478
Ammonium chloride, 807
Amobarbital:
adverse reactions, 237
classification, 234
controlled substance schedule, 376
pharmacokinetics, 235
sedative effects, 235
structure, 234
uses, 238
Amoxapine:
adverse reactions, 297
mechanism of action, 291, 297
pharmacokinetics, 295, 297
pharmacologic effects, 293, 297
Amoxicillin:
adverse reactions, 704
antimicrobial spectrum, 697, 703
chemistry, 698, 703
classification, 697
pharmacokinetics, 699, 703
structure, 698
uses, 562, 704
Amoxicillin-clavulanate, 705, 706
Amphetamine:
adverse reactions, 268-269
antidepressant effects, 292
classification as a psychotomimetic, 262
contraindications, 127
controlled substance schedule, 376
drug interactions, 220, 568
history of, 8
mechanism of action, 114, 267
pharmacodynamics, 126, 127, 267-268, 292
pharmacokinetics, 80, 127, 268
structure, 117, 265
tolerance and dependence, 268, 380
toxicity, treatment of, 268-269, 807
uses, 127, 128, 380
Amphotericin B:
adverse reactions, 77, 85, 759
mechanism of action, 757-759
pharmacokinetics, 759
spectrum of activity, 757
structure, 758
uses, 757, 759, 760, 772, 783
Ampicillin:
adverse reactions, 699, 700, 704
antimicrobial spectrum, 703
chemistry, 703
classification, 697
pharmacokinetics, 697, 699, 703
structure, 698
uses, 567, 703-704, 713

Ampicillin-sulbactam, 705, 706
Amrinone:
  adverse reactions, 397
  cardiovascular effects, 396
  history of, 10
  mechanism of action, 396
  pharmacokinetics, 396-397
  structure, 396
  uses, 387, 389, 396
Amyl nitrite:
  adverse reactions, 428
  classification, 425
  pharmacokinetics, 428
  pharmacologic effects, 428
  structure, 426
  uses, 429, 808, 818
Anabolic steroids:
  abuse of, 630
  adverse reactions, 635
  controlled substance schedule, 630, 635
  history of, 9
  relative activity of, 633
  structures, 631
  uses, 630, 635-636
Anadamide, 382
Androgen receptor antagonists, 636-637
Androgens:
  abuse of, 635
  adverse reactions, 634, 674
  chemistry, 630
  classification as antineoplastic drugs, 657
  effects on organ systems, 632-633
  mechanism of action, 630-631
  pharmacokinetics, 631-632
  physiologic effects, 632
  physiologic regulation of, 630
  precautions, 634
  relative activity of, 633
  structures, 631
  uses, 630, 633-634, 674
Androgen synthesis inhibitors, 637
Δ^4-Androstenedione:
  biotransformation, 613, 614
  endogenous formation, 613, 614, 632
Anemia:
  Description of, 503
  Hypoproliferative Normocytic anemias, 504, 517-518
  Megaloblastic anemias:
    folate deficiency, 504, 511-514
    vitamin B_{12} deficiency, 504, 515-517
  Microcytic anemia (iron deficiency), 503-511
Anesthetics, General (*see also Individual Agents*):
  classification, 219
  definition, 219
  drug interactions, 237, 282
  inhaled anesthetics, 223-228
  intravenous anesthetics, 228-232
  principles of use, 219-223
    minimum alveolar concentration (MAC), 219-220
    uptake and distribution, 219, 220-222
    mechanism of action, 219, 222-223
Anesthetics, Local (*see also Individual Agents*):
  adverse reactions, 369-370
  chemistry, 365-366
  classification, 365
  mechanism of action, 366-367
  pharmacodynamics, 369-370
  pharmacokinetics, 367-369
  structure-activity relationships, 365-366
  structures, 366
  types, 371-372
  uses, 371
Angiotensin-converting enzyme (ACE), 3, 468, 478-479
Angiotensin converting enzyme inhibitors (*see also Individual Agents*):
  adverse reactions, 481
  chemistry, 479
  cardiovascular effects, 479, 481
  history of, 8, 10
  mechanism of action, 479
  pharmacokinetics, 481, 482
  pharmacologic effects, 398, 479, 481
  structures, 480
  uses, 387, 397, 398, 468, 481, 482
Angiotensin, 3, 473, 478-479
Anistreplase, 10, 534
Antacids:
  adverse reactions, 568
  drug interactions, 78, 136, 307, 350, 395, 412, 568
  history of, 5, 13
  pharmacologic effects, 567
  types, 567
  uses, 562, 568-569
Antagonist, 26, 29
Anterior pituitary hormone, 5, 630
Anthelmintic agents, 787-798
Anthracyclines, 669
Anthraquinones, 572
Antiandrogens, 636
Antianginal drugs, 425-438 (*see also Individual Agents*):
Antianxiety drugs, 244-252 (*see also Individual Agents*)
Antiarrhythmic drugs (*see also Individual Agents*):
  classification, 401, 409
  clinical aspects of therapy, 422-423
  mechanism of action, 404
  pharmacologic effects, 409-423
Antibiotic, definition of, 691
Antibiotics (*see also Individual Agents*):
  drug interactions, 15
  as antineoplastic drugs, 654, 657, 668-670
Anticholinergic, definition of, 109
Anticholinergic agents (*see also* Antimuscarinic Drugs):
  adverse reactions, 317

classification, 562
drug interactions, 78-79, 282, 575
mechanism of action, 316, 564
pharmacodynamics, 82, 316, 494
treatment of poisoning, 808
uses, 315, 316-317, 491, 494, 562, 563
Anticoagulants:
Oral, 528-532 (*see also Individual Agents*)
Injectable, 526-528 (*see also Individual Agents*)
Antidepressants (*see also Individual Agents*):
Monoamine oxidase inhibitors:
adverse reactions, 296, 300, 806
chemistry, 299
drug interactions, 121, 298, 300, 316, 343, 607
mechanism of action, 299
pharmacologic effects, 293
pharmacokinetics, 295, 299-300
structures, 290
uses, 301
Other cylic antidepressants:
adverse reactions, 299, 806
mechanism of action, 291, 298
pharmacodynamics, 293, 298
pharmacokinetics, 295
structures, 290
uses, 301
Serotonin uptake blockers:
adverse reactions, 298, 806
chemistry, 290, 297
drug interactions, 298
mechanism of action, 291, 297
pharmacodynamics, 293
pharmacokinetics, 295, 297-298
structures, 290
uses, 301
Tricyclic antidepressants:
adverse reactions, 294-296, 806
chemistry, 289, 290
drug interactions, 258, 296-297, 471, 476, 550
mechanism of action, 289, 291
pharmacodynamics, 291-294
pharmacokinetics, 294, 295
treatment of poisoning, 807-808
Antidiarrheal agents, 568-571
adsorbents, 570
fluid and electrolyte control, 568-570
octreotide, 571
opioids, 570
Antiemetics, 574
Antiepileptic drugs (*see also Individual Agents*), 305-314
Antiestrogens 615, 619-620, 674 (*see also Individual Agents*)
Antifungal agents, 757-763
Antihemophilic factor (Factor VIII), 12, 521-523, 534, 535
Antihistamines, *see* H_1 receptor antagonists
Antihypertensive drugs (*see also Individual Agents*):
Adverse reactions, 83
Angiotensin converting enzyme inhibitors, 478-482
Direct-acting vasodilators, 476-478
Diuretics, 469-470
Drug interactions, 414
Sympatholytic agents:
centrally-acting drugs, 470-473
peripherally-acting drugs, 473-476
Uses, 482-484
Antimalarial drugs, 550, 773-781
Antimetabolites (*see also Individual Agents*):
classification, 656
folate antagonists, 656-659
purine derivatives, 659-661
pyrimidine derivatives, 662-663
site of action, 654
Antimicrobials (*see also Individual Categories and Agents*):
Antifungal agents, 757-763
Aminoglycosides, 719-724
Antimycobacterial drugs, 747-755
Antiviral drugs, 763-769
Beta-lactam antibiotics, 693-715
Definition of, 691
General concepts:
antimicrobial susceptibility, 691-692
bactericidal vs. bacteriostatic activity, 692
combinations, 693
chemoprophylaxis, 693
protein binding, 693
resistance to antimicrobial drugs, 692
Drug interactions, 550
Glycopeptides, 715-717
Macrolides, 729-732
Miscellaneous drugs, 732-736, 740-742
Quinolones (Fluoroquinolones), 724-728
Sulfonamides, 736-740
Tetracyclines, 743-745
Antimony, 807
Antimuscarinic drugs (*see also Individual agents*):
antagonist effects, 82
atropine and scopolamine, 163-168
synthetic derivatives, 168-170
definition of, 163
sources, 163
Antimycobacterial drugs (*see also Individual Agents*):
antituberculosis drugs, 747-754
drugs against *M. avium* complex and *M. leprae*, 754-755
Antineoplastic drugs, *see* Cancer chemotherapy
Antiparkinsonian agents, 6, 314-318
α-Antiplasmin, 524
Antiplatelet drugs, 532-533
Antiprotozoal drugs, 771-785
Antipsychotic drugs (*see also Individual Agents*):
Benzisoxazole derivative, 285
Binding to sigma sites, 323

Butyrophenone derivatives:
adverse reactions, 628
drug interactions, 575
mechanism of action, 277
pharmacokinetics, 283
pharmacologic effects, 278, 283
uses, 283
Classification, 275
Dibenoxazepine derivative, 278, 284
Dibenzodiazepine derivative, 278, 284-285
Dihydroindolene derivative, 278, 283-284
Diphenylbutylpiperidine derivative, 278, 285
Drug interactions, 249, 550
History of, 6
Phenothiazine derivatives:
adverse reactions, 280-282, 628
chemistry, 275
contraindications, 282
drug interactions, 282, 476, 550, 575
mechanism of action, 275-277
pharmacokinetics, 279
pharmacologic effects, 275, 277-279
uses, 269, 270, 279-280
Poisoning, treatment of, 805
Selection of an antipsychotic, 285-286
Thioxanthene derivatives, 278, 282-283
Antipyrine, 807
Antisecretory agents (*see also Individual Agents*):
anticholinergics, 562, 563-564
omeprazole, 562-563
H_2 receptor antagonists, 561-562
Antispasmodics, *see* Anticholinergic agents
Antithrombin III, 526, 527, 533
Anti-thymocyte globulin, 677, 683-684
Antiviral drugs, 9, 763-769 (*see also Individual Agents*)
Anxiety, definition of, 244
Apparent volume of distribution, 58-60, 803
Arsenic:
mechanism of action, 826
pharmacologic effects, 827
pharmacokinetics, 822, 826-827
poisoning, 808, 824, 827
sources, 826
treatment of poisoning, 807, 808, 827, 833
Arsenic trioxide, 827
Arsenous acid, 826, 827
Arsine, 826, 827
Arsphenamine, 5, 826
Ascorbic Acid:
adverse reactions, 555-556
biochemistry, 553-554
classification, 539
deficiency syndrome, 554
history of, 5
role in metabolism, 554
uses, 554-555, 807
Asparaginase, 657, 672-673
Aspirin (Acetylsalicylic acid):
adverse reactions, 486, 351-353
chemistry, 346
classification, 346
drug interactions, 79, 258, 349, 362, 532, 607, 768
history of, 5, 8, 10, 13
mechanism of action, 209, 213, 346-347
pharmacokinetics, 72, 87, 346, 350-351
pharmacologic effects, 85, 347-350
sources, 345
structure, 346
treatment in bismuth toxicity, 831
uses, 347, 351, 437
Astemizole (*see also* H_1-receptor antagonists):
adverse reactions, 195
pharmacokinetics, 194-195
pharmacologic properties, 194, 497
structural class, 192
uses, 196, 496, 497
Atenolol (*see also* β-Adrenergic blocking agents):
classification, 130, 133, 137
compliance, 474
pharmacodynamic properties, 133-134, 473, 474
pharmacokinetics, 135, 137
physicochemical properties, 135, 474
structure, 132
uses, 137-138, 430, 474
Atracurium:
history of, 12
mechanism of action, 175
pharmacokinetics, 178
release of histamine, 177
structure, 174
Atropine:
adverse reactions, 166-167, 347, 564
chemistry, 163
classification as a psychotomimetic, 262
drug interactions, 82
mechanism of action, 163-164, 265
pharmacologic effects, 110, 111, 164-166, 265-266, 561, 564
pharmacokinetics, 166
source, 163
structure, 164
treatment of poisoning, 807
uses, 167-169, 170, 315, 337, 395, 564, 570, 807, 815
Attapulgite, 570
Auranofin, 828
Aurothioglucose, 828
Autacoid, definition of, 185
Autonomic nervous system:
anatomy, 99-101
cotransmitters, 109
physiology, 101
receptors, 102-103, 109-113
responses, 102-103
synaptic transmission, 101, 104-109
Azathioprine:
adverse reactions, 680, 684
drug interactions, 363, 680

  history of, 9
  mechanism of action, 679
  pharmacokinetics, 679
  structure, 679
  uses, 578, 677, 679, 680, 682, 684
Azidothymidine, *see* Zidovudine
Azinophosmethyl, 815
Azithromycin:
  adverse reactions, 732
  antimicrobial spectrum, 729-730
  chemical structure, 730
  mechanism of action, 729
  pharmacokinetics, 731-732
  uses, 732, 754
Azlocillin:
  adverse reactions, 700
  antimicrobial spectrum, 704, 705
  classification, 697, 704
  pharmacokinetics, 697, 699, 704-705
  structure, 698
  uses, 705
AZT, *see* Zidovudine
Aztreonam, 714-715

B

Bacampicillin, 703-704
Baclofen, 181
Barbital, 4, 233, 376
Barbiturate receptor, 254
Barbiturates:
  abuse, 379-380
  adverse reactions, 236-238
  biotransformation, 74, 80, 87
  chemistry, 233
  contraindications, 238
  drug interactions, 237, 258, 282, 395, 412, 532, 607, 626
  gender factors, 84
  hypersensitivity, 237
  idiosyncratic reactions, 237
  mechanism of action, 233-234
  pharmacodynamics, 84, 85, 235-236
  pharmacokinetics, 235, 236
  structural classification, 234
  toxicity, treatment of, 237, 807
  uses, 228, 238, 244, 309, 314, 509
Barbituric acid, 233
Barley malt extract, 572
BCG vaccine, 678, 687-688
BCNU, *see* Carmustine
Beclomethasone diproprionate, 489, 499
Belladonna alkaloids, 163, 169, 170, 315, 316
Benazepril: 479, 480, 482
Bendroflumethiazide, 458, 470
Benzalkonium chloride, 810
Benzene, 804, 814
Benzene hexachloride (BHC), 814
Benzethonium chloride, 810
Benzocaine:
  mechanism of action, 367
  pharmacokinetics, 368
  structure, 374
  uses, 371, 374
Benzodiazepines:
  adverse reactions, 249
  chemistry, 244
  contraindications and precautions, 250
  drug interactions, 249-250, 258, 282, 296, 626
  history of, 6, 8
  mechanism of action, 238, 244-246
  pharmacodynamics, 247-249
  pharmacokinetics, 238, 246-248
  receptors, 239, 254
  structures, 245
  tolerance, 379
  treatment of overdose, 808
  uses, 219, 231-232, 250-251, 257, 312, 509
  withdrawal and dependence, 249, 378, 379
  withdrawal, treatment of, 379
Benzopyrene, 66-67, 74
Benzopyrene epoxide, 66
Benzphetamine, 120
Benzthiazide, 470
Benztropine, 169, 280, 316
Bepridil:
  adverse reactions, 436
  chemistry, 430
  pharmacokinetics, 435
  pharmacologic effects, 432, 434
  structure, 431
  uses, 434
Beta-lactam antibiotics (*see also Individual agents*):
  carbapenems, 694, 713-714
  cephalosporins, 694, 706-713
  inhibition of cell wall synthesis, 694-695
  mechanism of action, 693-695
  mechanism of resistance, 696
  monobactams, 694, 714-715
  penicillin combinations, 705-706
  penicillins, 694, 697-705
  structural classification, 693, 694
Betamethasone, 642, 644
Betamethasone benzoate, 648
Betamethasone dipropionate, 648
Betaxolol (*see also* β-Adrenergic blocking agents):
  classification, 130, 133, 137
  compliance, 474
  pharmacodynamic properties, 133, 134, 137, 473, 474
  pharmacokinetics, 135, 137
  physicochemical properties, 135, 474
  uses, 137-138, 474
Bethanechol:
  adverse reactions, 150, 575
  chemistry, 149, 575
  pharmacodynamics, 149-150, 575
  structure, 148
  uses, 149-150, 575

Benzodiazepine receptors, 246
Biguanides, *see* Oral hypoglycemic agents
Bile acid binding resins, 441, 446-447, 452
(*see also* Colestipol and Cholestyramine)
Bioavailability, definition of, 77
Bioequivalence, definition of, 77-78
Biotransformation, *see* Drug biotransformation
Biperiden, 169, 316
Bipyridyl herbicides, 818
Bis(β-chloroethyl)sulfide, 663
Bisacodyl, 572
Bismuth:
adverse reactions, 566-567, 824, 831
chemistry, 566
classification, 562
pharmacokinetics, 566
pharmacologic effects, 566, 571
sources, 830
uses, 562, 567, 570, 571, 831
Bismuth subcitrate, *see* Bismuth
Bismuth subnitrate, *see* Bismuth
Bismuth subsalicylate, *see* Bismuth
Bisoprolol (*see also* β-Adrenergic blocking agents):
classification, 130, 133, 137
compliance, 474
pharmacodynamic properties, 134, 473, 474
pharmacokinetics, 135, 137
physicochemical properties, 135, 474
uses, 137-138, 474
Bithionol, 790, 797
Bitolterol:
classification, 490
mechanism of action, 115
pharmacokinetics, 124
use, 119, 124, 490
Bleach, 810
Bleomycin sulfate, 657, 668-669
Blood coagulation:
coagulation pathways, 520-524
factors, 521-523
fibrinolytic pathway, 523-525
Boric acid, 550
Botanical insecticides, 815-816
Bradykinin, 213, 323, 347, 348, 494
Bretylium: 8, 401, 420-421, 423
BREVICON, 625
Bromhexine, 496
Bromocriptine:
adverse reactions, 317, 628
history of, 8
mechanism of action, 317, 628
pharmacokinetics, 317
structure, 317
uses, 281, 317, 628, 636
Brompheniramine, *see* H_1 receptor antagonists
Bulk laxatives, 572
α-Bungarotoxin, 31
Bumetanide:
adverse reactions, 461-462
chemistry, 460
classification, 455
drug interactions, 462
pharmacokinetics, 461-462
structure, 461
uses, 462
Bupivacaine:
adverse reactions, 370, 373
history of, 365
pharmacokinetics, 366, 368, 369, 373
structure, 366
uses, 371, 372, 373
Buprenorphine:
chemistry, 340
classification, 325
controlled substance schedule, 376
mechanism of action, 341
pharmacokinetics, 327, 328
pharmacologic effects, 338-339
receptor binding, 326, 338
structure, 341
tolerance and dependence, 339
uses, 339, 341
Bupropion:
adverse reactions, 299
mechanism of action, 291, 298
pharmacokinetics, 295
pharmacologic effects, 293
structure, 290
Buspirone, 251
Busulfan, 656, 657, 667
Butabarbital:
classification, 234
pharmacokinetics, 235
sedative effects, 235
structure, 234
Butamben, 368, 371, 374
Butoconazole, 758, 761
Butorphanol:
classification, 325, 338
pharmacokinetics, 327, 328, 340
pharmacologic effects, 340
receptor binding, 326, 338
structure, 340

C

Cadmium, 822, 829-830
Caffeine:
adverse reactions, 349
biotransformation, 69
drug interactions, 282
pharmacologic effects, 492
sources, 491
structure, 492
uses, 491
Calcifediol, 594
Calcitonin:
administration, 592

adverse reactions, 592
in calcium homeostasis, 583, 590, 591-592
mechanism of action, 592
preparations (human and salmon), 592
uses, 592
Calcitonin gene-related peptide, 323
Calcitriol, 544, 545, 594
Calcium, 395, 435, 589-590
Calcium carbonate, 567, 568
Calcium-channel blockers (*see also Individual Agents*):
adverse reactions, 435, 436
chemistry, 430
classification, 430, 478
drug interactions, 435-436
history of, 10
mechanism of action, 432-433
pharmacokinetics, 387, 434-435
pharmacologic effects, 428, 432, 434, 476
structures, 431
uses, 394, 425, 430, 434, 435, 468, 478, 482, 486, 497
Calcium channels, 430, 599
Calcium gluconate, 811
Calcium leucovorin, 514
Calcium polycarbophil, 570, 572
Camphor, 495, 807
Cancer Chemotherapy:
Cell cycle, 653-655
Drug classification, 656-674 (*see also Individual Categories and Agents*):
alkylating agents, 654, 663-668
antibiotics, 654, 668-670
antimetabolites, 654, 656-663
hormones, 654, 673-674
miscellaneous compounds, 672-673
plant derivatives, 670-672
General toxicities to normal tissues, 655-656
Cannabinols, 271-272 (*see* Tetrahydrocannabinols)
Cantharides, 807
Capreomycin, 753
Captopril:
adverse reactions, 481
chemistry, 479
classification, 479
history of, 3
mechanism of action, 479
pharmacokinetics, 481, 482
pharmacologic effects, 398, 479, 481
structure, 480
uses, 397, 398, 481
Carbachol, 147-150
Carbamazepine:
adverse reactions, 309
classification, 305
drug interactions, 436, 626, 683, 748
history of, 10
pharmacokinetics, 305, 309
structure, 308
uses, 303, 305, 308-309
Carbamylcholine, 147-150
Carbapenems, 713-714 (*see also Individual Agents*)
Carbaryl, 155, 815
Carbenicillin:
adverse reactions, 700
antimicrobial spectrum, 704
classification, 697, 704
pharmacokinetics, 699, 704-705
structure, 698
uses, 705
Carbenicillin indanyl sodium, *see* Carbenicillin
Carbidopa, 316
Carbofuran, 815
Carbon disulfide, 816
Carbon monoxide, 811-813
Carbon tetrachloride, 69-70, 804, 814, 816
Carbonic anhydrase inhibitors, 465, 466
Carboplatin, 657, 663, 667
Carboprost, 214, 215
S-Carboxymethylcysteine, 495, 496
Cardiac arrhythmias:
cardiac electrophysiology, 400-405, 406
pathophysiology of, 405-407, 410
types, 407-409
Cardiac glycosides, *see* Digitalis glycosides, Digoxin, and Digitoxin
Carisoprodol, 181
Carmustine (BCNU), 657, 665, 666-667
β-Carotene, 312
biochemistry, 540
cancer link, 542-543
toxicity, 541, 542
use in coronary disease, 453
Carteolol (*see also* β-Adrenergic blocking agents):
classification, 130, 133, 137
compliance, 474
pharmacodynamic properties, 133, 134, 473, 474
pharmacokinetics, 135, 137
physicochemical properties, 135, 474
uses, 137-138, 474
Casanthranol, 572
Cascara sagrada, 572
Castor oil, 572
Catecholamines:
adrenergic mechanisms, 81, 106-109
adverse reactions, 121, 409
binding sites, 114
biotransformation, 69
pharmacodynamics, 119, 120
pharmacokinetics, 120
uses, 121
CCNU, *see* Lomustine
Cefaclor:
antimicrobial spectrum, 710
pharmacokinetics, 709, 711
structure, 707
uses, 711
Cefadroxil:

antimicrobial spectrum, 708
pharmacokinetics, 709-710
structure, 707
uses, 710
Cefamandole:
antimicrobial specturm, 710
pharmacokinetics, 709, 711
Cefazolin:
antimicrobial spectrum, 708
pharmacokinetics, 709-710
structure, 707
uses, 710
Cefepime:
antimicrobial spectrum, 711
pharmacokinetics, 709, 712
uses, 712
Cefixime:
antimicrobial spectrum, 711
pharmacokientics, 709, 712
uses, 713
Cefmetazole:
antimicrobial spectrum, 710
pharmacokinetics, 709, 711
structure, 707
uses, 711
Cefonicid:
anatimicrobial spectrum, 710
pharmacokinetics, 709, 711
uses, 711
Cefoperazone:
antimicrobial spectrum, 711
disulfiram-like reaction, 259
pharmacokinetics, 709, 712
structure, 707
uses, 711
Cefotaxime:
antimicrobial spectrum, 711
pharmacokinetics, 709, 712
structure, 707
uses, 711
Cefotetan:
antimicrobial spectrum, 710
pharmacokinetics, 709, 711
structure, 707
uses, 711
Cefoxitin:
antimicrobial spectrum, 710
pharmacokinetics, 709, 711
structure, 707
uses, 711
Cefpodoxime proxetil:
adverse reactions, 708
antimicrobial spectrum, 712
classification, 708, 711
pharmacokinetics, 708, 709, 712
uses, 713
Cefprozil:
antimicrobial spectrum, 710
pharmacokientics, 709, 711
uses, 711
Ceftazidime:
antimicrobial spectrum, 711
pharmacokinetics, 709, 712
structure, 707
uses, 713
Ceftizoxime:
antimicrobial spectrum, 711
pharmacokinetics, 709, 712
uses, 713
Ceftriaxone:
antimicrobial spectrum, 711
difulfiram-like reaction, 259
pharmacokinetics, 709, 712
structure, 707
uses, 713
Cefuroxime:
antimicrobial spectrum, 710
pharmacokinetics, 709, 711
uses, 711
Cefuroxime axetil, *see* Cefuroxime
Cephalexin:
antimicrobial spectrum, 708
pharmacokientics, 709, 710
structure, 707
uses, 710
Cephalosporins (*see also Individual Agents*):
adverse reactions, 708
chemistry, 706
classification, 708
drug interactions, 362
first generation, 708, 710
history of, 6, 9, 11
pharmacokinetics, 708-709
second generation, 710-711
structures, 707
third generation, 711-713
Cephalothin:
antimicrobial spectrum, 708
pharmacokinetics, 709-710
structure, 707
uses, 710
Cephapirin, 708-710
Cephradine, 708-710
Cetyl pyridinium chloride, 810
Charcoal, activated, 351, 396, 807, 810, 818
Chloral hydrate:
adverse reactions, 240
biotransformation, 70-71, 87, 240
chemistry, 239
controlled substance schedule, 376
drug interactions, 258, 532
pharmacodynamics, 239, 240
pharmacokinetics, 240
precautions, 240-241
uses, 241
Chlorambucil, 657, 664, 665
Chloramphenicol:
adverse reactions, 259, 742
antimicrobial spectrum, 741
biotransformation, 69-70, 72, 87

disulfiram-like reaction, 259
drug interactions, 307, 532
history of, 6
mechanism of resistance, 741
mechanism of action, 741
pharmacodynamics, 85
pharmacokinetics, 741-742
structure, 741
uses, 742
Chlordecone, 447
Chlordane, 814
Chlordiazepoxide:
controlled substance schedule, 376
drug interactions, 626, 761
history of, 13
pharmacokinetics, 246, 247, 248
structure, 245
uses, 247, 250, 257
Chlorfenvinphos, 815
2-Chlorodeoxyadenosine, *see* Cladribine
Chloroform, 814
Chloroguanide, 772, 774, 780
Chlorophenothane, *see* DDT
Chlorophenoxy herbicides, 818
p-Chlorophenylalanine, 200
Chloroprocaine:
adverse reactions, 371
pharmacokinetics, 368, 369
structure, 366
uses, 371, 372, 373
Chloroquine:
adverse reactions, 775-776
chemistry, 773
mechanism of action, 773, 775
pharmacologic effects, 85, 775
pharmacokinetics, 87, 775
structure, 775
uses, 772, 775, 783
Chlorothiazide,
adverse reactions, 458
classification, 455, 470
drug interactions, 81
mechanism of action, 457
pharmacokinetics, 458, 470
pharmacologic effects, 457, 466
structure, 458
uses, 470
Chlorotrianisene, 615, 619
Chlorphenesin, 181
Chlorpheniramine (*see also* H_1 receptor antagonists):
pharmacologic effects, 188
structure, 191, 192
Chlorpromazine:
adverse reactions, 280-282
drug interactions, 81, 282, 316, 550
history of, 6
mechanism of action, 275
pharmacokinetics, 67, 279
pharmacologic effects, 277-278
structure, 276
uses, 270, 279-280
Chlorpropamide (*see also* Sulfonylurea derivatives):
adverse reactions, 606
classification, 604
disulfiram-like reaction, 259
pharmacokinetics, 605-606
structure, 605
uses, 608
Chlorpyrifos, 161
Chlorthalidone:
adverse reactions, 460
classification, 455, 459, 470
mechanism of action, 459
pharmacokinetics, 460, 470
structure, 460
uses, 460, 471
Chlorzoxazone, 181
Cholecalciferol (Vitamin D_3), 544, 593
Cholestyramine:
adverse reactions, 446-447
classification, 446
drug interactions, 307, 395, 447
history of, 8
mechanism of action, 446
pharmacologic effects, 446
uses, 447, 451
Choline magnesium trisalicylate: 346, 353, 354
Cholinergic drugs, (*see* Cholinomimetic agents)
Cholinergic receptors, 31-32, 102-103, 109-112
Cholinesterase, 82, 106, 776
Cholinesterase inhibitors:
chemical classes, 154
irreversible, 160-
reversible, 154-159
structures, 155
Cholinomimetic drugs:
definition of, 147
direct acting, 147-153
indirect acting, 153-162
irreversible, 160-162
reversible, 154-160
Chronic obstructive pulmonary diseases, 485-487
Chronic toxicity, definition of, 803
Ciclopirox olamine, 763
Cilastatin, 714
Cimetidine:
adverse reactions, 198, 562
biotransformation, 80
chemistry, 197
drug interactions, 79, 199, 258, 297, 307, 416, 418, 436, 493, 566, 575, 576, 761
history of, 8
mechanism of action, 197, 562
pharmacokinetics, 198
pharmacologic effects, 188, 197-198, 562
structure, 197
uses, 199, 561, 562
Cinchona alkaloids, 776
Cinchonism, 351
Ciprofloxacin:

adverse reactions, 727
antimicrobial spectrum, 725, 752
drug interactions, 493, 566
history of, 11
mechanism of resistance, 726
mechanism of action, 724
pharmacokinetics, 726-727
structure, 725
uses, 727-728, 752

Cisapride: 11, 575-576

Cisplatin:
adverse reactions, 667
classification, 657
history of, 12
mechanism of action, 663, 667
pharmacokinetics, 664, 667
structure, 665
uses, 667

Cladribine, 656, 657, 659, 661

Clarithromycin:
adverse reactions, 732
antimicrobial spectrum, 729-730
mechanism of action, 729
pharmacokinetics, 732
structure, 730
uses, 732, 754

Clavulanate, 705-706

Clearance, 60-61, 804

Clemastine, *see* H_1 receptor antagonists

Clidinium, 168

Clindamycin:
adverse reactions, 734
antimicrobial spectrum, 733
mechanism of resistance, 733
mechanism of action, 733
neuromuscular blockade, 176
pharmacokinetics, 733-734
structure, 733
uses, 734

Clobetasol propionate, 648

Clofazimine, 754-755

Clofibrate,:
adverse reactions, 448-449
drug interactions, 447, 532
history of, 8
mechanism of action, 448
pharmacokinetics, 448
structure, 448
uses, 448, 449

Clomiphene:
history of, 9
mechanism of action, 619
pharmacokinetics, 619
pharmacologic effects, 619-620
structure, 615
uses, 619-620, 636

Clomoxir, 609

Clonazepam:
adverse reactions, 313
biotransformation, 70
classification, 305
controlled substance schedule, 376
pharmacokinetics, 247, 248, 305, 313
structure, 313
uses, 247, 250, 306, 312-313

Clonidine:
adverse reactions, 471
drug interactions, 81, 220, 436, 471
history of, 6
mechanism of action, 115, 122, 470-471
pharmacokinetics, 471
pharmacologic effects, 471
structure, 470
uses, 252, 377-378, 383, 471, 482, 734

Clorazepate:
contraindications and precautions, 250
controlled substance schedule, 376
pharmacokinetics, 246, 247, 248
structure, 245
uses, 247, 250, 312

Clotrimazole, 757, 758, 761

Cloxacillin:
classification, 697
pharmacokinetics, 697, 699, 702
structure, 698
uses, 702-703

Clozapine, 278, 284-285

Cocaine:
adrenergic mechanisms, 81
adverse reactions, 380-381
chemistry, 269
classification, 262
controlled substance schedule, 376
detoxification, 380
drug interactions, 220
history of, 5, 8, 365
intoxication, 270
mechanism of action, 267
pharmacokinetics, 269-270
pharmacologic effects, 269, 270, 292, 365, 371, 380
preparations of, 269, 380
sources, 269
structure, 269, 366
tolerance and dependence, 270, 380
treatment of toxicity, 270, 381, 807
uses, 365, 371, 373

Codeine:
classification, 325
chemistry, 325, 333
controlled substance schedule, 376
pharmacokinetics, 67, 87, 326-328, 333
pharmacologic effects, 330, 333
structure, 333
structure-activity relationship, 325
source, 325
uses, 333, 570

Colchicine, 361, 497

Colistin, 176

Colestipol, 8, 446-447, 451

Congestive heart failure, 387-399
Conjugated estrogens, 617, 618
Contraception, methods of, 627
Contraceptive steroids, 553
Copper:
adverse reactions, 821
deficiency, ascorbic acid use, 553
treatment of poisoning, 808
Corticosteroids (*see also Individual Agents*):
adverse reactions, 489, 648, 674, 679
anti-inflammatory actions, 643
biosynthetic pathways, 641
chemistry, 639-640
classification, 644, 648, 676, 677
dosage, 648
drug interaction, 238
functional tests, 646-647
immunosuppressive actions, 643, 679
mechanism of action, 209, 487, 578, 640, 678-679
pharmacokinetics, 640
pharmacologic effects, 207, 209, 487, 488, 643-646
relative potencies, 644
structure-activity relationships, 640
structures, 641, 642
uses, 487, 491, 499, 578, 647-648, 672, 674, 677, 679, 789, 828, 834
Corticotropin, *see* Adrenocorticotropic hormone
Cortisol (hydrocortisone), 638-641, 644, 645
Cortisone, 644
Cosyntropin, 638
Cotransmitters, 109
Cromakalim, 497
Cromolyn sodium:
chemistry, 489
inhibition of histamine release, 187
mechanism of action, 486, 489
pharmacokinetics, 489
pharmacologic effects, 489, 490
structure, 489
uses, 485, 489, 499
Crystalline zinc insulin, 601
Curare, 173 (*see also* Tubocurarine)
Curariform drugs, 173, 180, 412 (*see also Individual Agents*)
Cyanide:
adverse reactions, 816-817
antidotes, 808, 818
formation from sodium nitroprusside, 484
mechanism of action, 804, 816
pharmacokinetics, 816, 817
sources, 816
treatment of toxicity, 818
uses, 816
Cyanocobalamin, *see* Vitamin B_{12}
Cyclizine, *see* H_1 receptor antagonists
Cyclobenzaprine:
adverse reactions, 181
drug interactions, 259
pharmacodynamics, 181
structure, 181
uses, 181
Cyclodienes, 814
Cyclopentolate, 169-170
Cyclophosphamide:
adverse reactions, 664, 666, 680, 804
classification, 657
pharmacodynamics, 665-666, 680
structure, 665
uses, 656, 666, 677, 680
Cyclopropane, 5
Cycloserine, 752
Cyclosporine:
adverse reactions, 452, 683
chemistry, 681
drug interactions, 452, 683, 761
mechanism of action, 681-682
pharmacokinetics, 682
structure, 681
uses, 497, 677, 680, 682-683
Cyproheptadine (*see also* H_1 receptor antagonists):
adverse reactions, 203
pharmacologic properties, 203
structure, 192, 203
uses, 193, 203
Cytarabine:
adverse reactions, 663
classification, 656, 657
mechanism of action, 662-663
pharmacokinetics, 663
structure, 658, 663
uses, 663
Cytochrome B_5, 68
Cytochromes P-450, 17-22, 25-26, 66, 206, 207, 255-256, 505
Cytokines, 678, 684-686
Cytosine arabinoside, *see* Cytarabine

D

Dacarbazine (DTIC), 657, 667
Dactinomycin, 657, 668
Danazol, 620, 634, 683
Dantrolene:
adverse reactions, 180
mechanism of action, 180
pharmacokinetics, 180
structure, 180
uses, 180, 226, 281
Dapsone:
adverse reactions, 755
chemistry, 755
mechanism of action, 755
pharmacokinetics, 87, 755
structure, 755
uses, 755, 772, 781, 785
Daunorubicin, 657, 669
DDT (chlorophenothane), 69-70, 804, 814

Debrisoquine, 75
Deferoxamine:
  adverse reactions, 510
  chemistry, 509
  contraindications, 510
  pharmacokinetics, 510
  uses, 509, 511, 808, 829
Dehydroemetine, 772, 782
Delayed toxicity, definition, 803
Delirium tremens, 257
Demecarium:
  adverse reactions, 159
  classification, 154
  structure, 155
  use, 159
Demeclocycline, 743-745, 804
DEMULEN 1/35, 625
DEMULEN 1/50, 625
Deoxycoformycin, *see* Pentostatin
Deoxyadenosylcobalamin, 515
Deoxycytidine, 769
Deoxyuridine, 766
Dependence, 375 (*see also* Drug dependence)
L-Deprenyl, 318
DES, *see* Diethylstilbestrol
Desensitization, 24, 112, 115
Desflurane,
  chemistry, 227
  classification, 219
  drug interactions, 228
  pharmacodynamics, 228
  physicochemical properties, 220, 227
  structure, 227
Designer drugs, 336, 383-384
Desipramine,
  chemistry, 289
  mechanism of action, 291
  pharmacologic effects, 293
  pharmacokinetics, 294-295
  structure, 290
  uses, 270, 301, 381
Desmethyldoxepin, 294
Desmopressin, 534, 535
DESOGEN, 625
Desogestrel, 623, 625
Desonide, 648
Desoximetasone, 648
Dessicated thyroid, 587
Detergents, 810
Detoxification, definition of, 803
Dexamethasone, 642, 644, 646-647, 648
Dexamethasone sodium phosphate, 489
Dexchlorpheniramine, *see* H_1 receptor antagonists
Dextroamphetamine, 127, 268, 376
Dextromethorphan, 330, 335
Dextropropoxyphene, *see* Propoxyphene
Dextrothyroxine, 452, 587
Dezocine,
  classification, 325
  pharmacokinetics, 327, 328
  pharmacologic effects, 340
  receptor binding, 338, 340
  structure, 340
Diabetes mellitus, 596-597, 607-609
cis-Diaminedichloroplatinum, *see* Cisplatin
Diazepam:
  adverse reactions, 249
  biotransformation, 66-67, 72, 248
  contraindications and precautions, 250
  controlled substance schedule, 376
  drug interactions, 298, 626
  mechanism of action, 244
  pharmacodynamics, 85, 248-249
  pharmacokinetics, 246, 247
  structure, 245
  uses, 181, 219, 231, 247, 250, 251, 257, 270, 312, 313-314, 814, 815, 816
Diazinon, 815
Diazoxide, 476, 483, 607
Dibenzodiazepines, 275, 278, 284
Dibucaine, 371, 373
2,4-Dichlorophenoxyacetic acid, 818
Dichlorovos, 815
Diclofenac potassium, 346, 359
Diclofenac sodium, 346, 359
Dicloxacillin:
  classification, 697
  pharmacokinetics, 697, 699, 702
  structure, 698
  uses, 702-703
Dicumarol:
  chemistry, 529
  drug interactions, 307
  pharmacokinetics, 80, 530
  structure, 529
Dicyclomine, 168-169
Didanosine:
  adverse reactions, 769
  history of, 11
  mechanism of action, 764, 768
  pharmacokinetics, 768-769
  uses, 763, 765, 768
Dieldrin, 814
Dienestrol, 618
Diethylcarbamazine, 787-791
Diethylpropion, 127
Diethylstilbestrol (DES):
  adverse reactions, 618, 619
  classification as an antineoplastic, 657
  history of, 7
  pharmacokinetics, 617
  structure, 615
  uses, 618, 619, 673
Difenoxin:
  adverse reactions, 570
  classification, 325
  chemistry, 335, 336
  pharmacokinetics, 336-337
  structure, 337
  uses, 337, 570

Diflorasone diacetate, 648
Diflunisal:
- adverse reactions, 354
- classification, 346, 353
- pharmacokinetics, 346, 354
- pharmacologic effects, 353-354
- structure, 353
- uses, 353

Digitalic glycosides (*see also* Digoxin and Digitoxin):
- adverse reactions, 394-395, 461
- antibodies, 396
- chemistry, 389
- contraindications, 395
- drug interactions, 394, 395, 447, 459
- history of, 3, 5
- mechanism of action, 389
- pharmacokinetics, 393
- pharmacologic effects, 391-393
- treatment of toxicity, 395-396, 807, 808
- uses, 394, 423, 459
- warnings, 395

Digitoxin:
- adverse reactions, 394-395
- chemistry, 389
- contraindications, 395
- drug interactions, 238, 298, 394, 395
- pharmacokinetics, 393
- treatment of toxicity, 395-396, 808
- uses, 394

Digoxin:
- adverse reactions, 83, 84, 394-395
- chemistry, 389
- contraindications, 395
- drug interactons, 79, 81, 136, 298, 394, 395, 412, 418, 420, 463, 566, 568, 575, 643, 750
- history of, 8, 10
- mechanism of action, 390
- pharmacokinetics, 85, 393
- pharmacologic effects, 391-393
- structure, 390
- treatment of toxicity, 395-396, 808
- uses, 350, 394, 412, 481

Digoxin-specific FAB antibodies, 396, 808
1,25-Dihydrocholecalciferol, 594
1,25-Dihydroxy vitamin D_3, *see* Calcitriol
Dihydroergotamine, 202-203
Dihydroindolones, 275, 283
Dihydrotachysterol, 594
Diloxanide furoate, 772, 782
Diltiazem:
- adverse reactions, 436
- classification, 401, 430, 478
- drug interactions, 436, 683
- history of, 10
- mechanism of action, 401, 432
- pharmacokinetics, 434, 435
- pharmacologic effects, 401, 421, 432, 434
- structure, 431
- uses, 421, 434, 435, 478

Dimaprit, 188
Dimenhydrinate, 192, 194, 196 (*see also* H_1 receptor antagonists)
Dimercaprol:
- adverse reactions, 833
- arsenic antagonist, 785
- binding properties, 832
- mechanism of action, 832
- mercury treatment, 832
- pharmacokinetics, 832-833
- route of administration and dosage, 833
- structure, 832
- uses, 808, 824, 826, 827, 828, 833

Dimetan, 815
Dimethoate, 815
2,4-Dimethoxy-4-methylamphetamine (DOM):
- classification, 262
- chemistry, 263, 265
- pharmacokinetics, 265
- structure, 265

N,N-Dimethyltriptamine (DMT):
- classification, 262
- chemistry, 262-263
- pharmacokinetics, 265
- pharmacologic effects, 381
- sources, 265

Dimetilan, 815
Dinoprostone, 214, 215
Diphenhydramine (*see also* H_1 receptor antagonists):
- adverse reactions, 76
- pharmacokinetics, 194
- pharmacologic effects, 76, 82, 188, 192, 194
- drug interactions, 81
- structure, 192
- uses, 76, 169, 193, 194, 196, 242, 316

Diphenoxylate:
- adverse reactions, 570
- classification, 325
- chemistry, 335, 336
- controlled substance schedule, 376
- drug interactions, 395
- pharmacokinetics, 336-337
- structure, 337
- uses, 337, 570

Diphenylbutylpiperidines, 275, 278, 285
Dipivefrine (dipivalyl epinephrine), 119
Dipyridamole, 351, 437, 532
Disopyramide: 83, 401, 414
Distribution, 50-52
Disulfiram:
- contraindications, 260
- drug interactions, 259, 307, 532
- mechanism of action, 74, 260
- pharmacokinetics, 260
- pharmacologic effects, 259-260
- structure, 259

Diuretics (*see also Individual Agents*):
- Classification, 455
- Carbonic anhydrase inhibitors, 465, 466

Drug interactions, 349, 394
Loop diuretics:
adverse reactions, 461-462
chemistry, 460
drug interactions, 462, 607
mechanism of action, 460, 469
pharmacokinetics, 460-462
structures, 461
uses, 462, 466
Osmotic nonelectrolytes, 466
Potassium-sparing diuretics, 455, 463-465, 466, 683
Thiazide-related compounds:
adverse reactions, 460, 469
mechanism of action, 459, 469
pharmacokinetics, 460
pharmacologic effects, 466
structures, 459-460
uses, 460
Thiazide diuretics:
adverse reactions, 458-459
drug interactions, 287, 362, 414, 447, 607
history of, 6
mechanism of action, 457, 469
pharmacologic effects, 457, 466
pharmacokinetics, 458
structures, 458
uses, 458, 459, 469, 482
DMT, *see* N,N-Dimethyltriptamine
Dobutamine:
adverse reactions, 123
pharmacokinetics, 123
pharmacologic effects, 122, 396
mechanism of action, 115
structure, 117
use, 123, 396
Docusate calcium, 573
Docusate potassium, 573
Docusate sodium, 573
DOM, *see* 2,4-Dimethoxy-4-methylamphetamine
Dopa, 105-107 (*see also* Levodopa)
Dopamine:
adverse reactions, 125
effect on lactation, 628
history of, 8
in adrenergic transmission, 106, 113
nonmicrosomal oxidative biotransformation, 70
mechanism of action, 114, 115, 125
pharmacologic effects, 125, 396
receptors, history of, 10
receptors, 110, 112
structure, 125
uses, 125, 396, 397
Dosage regimens:
multiple doses, 62-64
single dose, 61-62
Dose-response relationships, 16-20
Dose-response curves:
ceiling effect, 16
graded, 16-17
quantal, 17-18
threshold dose, 16
time-action curves, 19-20
variables, 16
Down regulation, 25, 115
Doxacurium:
history of, 30
mechanism of action, 175
pharmacokinetics, 177-178
Doxazosin:
adverse reactions, 476
classification, 130
mechanism of action, 143, 475
pharmacokinetics, 475, 476
pharmacologic effects, 398, 475
site of action, 131
structure, 475
uses, 143, 398, 475-476
Doxepin:
chemistry, 289
drug interactions, 258
mechanism of action, 291
pharmacokinetics, 294-295
pharmacologic effects, 293
structure, 290
Doxorubicin:
adverse reactions, 69, 669
classification, 657, 669
drug interactions, 550, 670
mechanism of action, 669
pharmacokinetics, 669
redox cycling mechanism, 71
uses, 663, 669
Doxycycline:
adverse reactions, 744-745
antimicrobial spectrum, 743-744
mechanism of action, 743
pharmacokinetics, 744-745
structure, 743
uses, 745, 772, 781
Doxylamine, 242
DRANO, 807
Dromostanolone propionate, 631
Dronabinol, 274
Droperidol, 283, 336
Drug:
definition, 16
interaction, 78
metabolizing microsomal system, 65, 72, 258
pharmacodynamics, 78
pharmacokinetics, 78
receptor association, 21
resistance, 24
Drug absorption, 78
Drug biotransformation:
cytochromes P-450, 66
definition, 65, 66
description, 53, 65-75
drug-drug interactions, 74
environmental factors, 74

first-order kinetics, 73
induction of the drug-metabolizing microsomal system, 73-74
pharmacogenetic variants, 75
physiologic factors, 74
reactions, 53, 65-70, 803
conjugation, 71-72
hydrolysis, 71-72
oxidation, 65-70
reduction, 69-71
zero-order kinetics, 73
Drug dependence:
controlled substances schedules, 376
depressants, 376-378
designer drugs, 383-384
hallucinogens, 381-382
marijuana, 382-383
nicotine dependence, 383
sedative dependence, 378-380
stimulants, 380-381
terms, 375-376
Drug-receptor interactions, 16-27
DTIC, *see* Dacarbazine
Dyclonine, 368
Dynorphins, 321-324
Dyphylline, 490, 491, 494

E

Echothiophate:
classification, 154
structure, 155
uses, 161
Econazole:, 758, 760, 761
ED_{50} (median effective dose), 18
Edetate calcium disodium (calcium EDTA):
adverse reactions, 832
binding properties, 831
chemistry, 831
mechanism of action, 832
pharmacokinetics, 832
routes of administration and dosage, 832
structure, 831
toxicology, 831
uses, 808, 824, 826, 832
Edrophonium:
chemistry, 158
classification, 154
mechanism of action, 154
pharmacokinetics, 158
pharmacologic effects, 158-159
structure, 155
use, 158, 159
EDTA, *see* Ethylenediaminetetraacetic acid
Eflornithine:
adverse reactions, 784
history of, 11
mechanism of action, 783-784
pharmacokinetics, 784
structure, 784
uses, 772, 784
Eicosanoids:
biosynthesis, 205-209
inhibition of biosynthesis, 209-210
mechanism of action, 210
pharmacokinetics, 211
physiologic and pharmacologic effects, 211-214, 494
terminology, 205
uses, 214-215
Elimination, 52-54
Emetine, 4
EMLA cream, 371
Enalapril:
classification, 479
history of, 3
pharmacokinetics, 481, 482
pharmacologic effects, 398
structure, 480
uses, 397, 398, 481
Enalaprilat, 481, 482
β-Endorphin, 321-323
Enflurane:
chemistry, 226
classification, 219
history of, 8
physicochemical properties, 220, 223
pharmacodynamics, 227
pharmacokinetics, 226-227
structure, 226
Enkephalins:
definition, 321
history of, 6
placebo effects, 88
Enoxacin:
adverse reactions, 727
antimicrobial spectrum, 725
chemical structure, 725
drug interactions, 727
history of, 11
mechanism of resistance, 726
mechanism of action, 724
pharmacokinetics, 726-727
uses, 727-728
Enoxaparin sodium, 528
Enprofylline, 491, 492, 494
Ephedrine:
adverse reactions, 127, 491
chemistry, 126
classification, 490
mechanism of action, 114, 115
pharmacodynamics, 126, 491
pharmacokinetics, 126-127
structure, 117
uses, 126, 490, 491
Epibatidine, 3
Epilepsy, 303-305
Epinephrine:
adverse reactions, 120-121, 491

classification, 490
drug interactions, 78, 79, 282, 296
history of, 5
in adrenergic transmission, 107
in insecticide poisoning, 814
mechanism of action, 115, 116
pharmacodynamics, 116, 118-120, 396
pharmacokinetics, 120, 491
structure, 117
uses, 121, 169, 396, 490, 491
Epoetin alfa, *see* Erythopoietin
Ergocalciferol, 543, 544, 592, 594
Ergonovine, 202, 203
Ergosterol, 757, 760
Ergot, history of, 5
Ergot alkaloids, 202
Ergotamine, 202
Erythrityl tetranitrate, 425, 428, 429
Erythromycin:
adverse reactions, 452, 732
antimicrobial spectrum, 729-730
chemical structure, 730
drug interactions, 79, 493, 683
mechanism of action, 729
mechanism of resistance, 731
pharmacodynamics, 85
pharmacokinetics, 731
uses, 351, 562, 567, 732
Erythropoietin (epoetin alfa), 12, 518-519
Esmolol (*see also* β-Adrenergic blocking agents):
classification, 130, 133, 137
pharmacolodynamic properties, 134, 137
pharmacokinetics, 135, 137
physicochemical properties, 135
structure, 132
uses, 137-138, 419
Estazolam:
chemistry, 244
mechanism of action, 238-239
pharmacokinetics, 239, 247
uses, 239, 247, 250
Estradiol (17β-estradiol):
biosynthesis, 611, 614
biotransformation, 616
chemistry, 613
pharmacokinetics, 617
physiologic effects, 613, 616, 617
secretion, 612, 630
structure, 614, 615
uses, 619, 673
Estradiol cypionate, 618
Estradiol valerate, 618
Estradiol, micronized, 617, 618
Estramustine, 657, 673
Estriol, 615, 616, 617
Estrogens:
adverse reactions, 617-618
chemistry and synthesis, 613-616
classification, 613, 657
drug interactions, 750
gender factors, 84
history of, 5, 7
mechanism of action, 616
pharmacokinetics, 87, 617, 631, 632
pharmacologic effects, 452, 616-617, 632
uses, 452, 618-619, 673
Estrogens, conjugated, 617, 618
Estrogens, esterified, 618
Estrone:
biosynthesis, 613, 614
conjugation reaction, 72
secretion, 613
structure, 614, 615
synthetic pathways, 614
Estrone sulfate, 616, 618
Estropipate, 618
Ethacrynic acid:
adverse reactions, 461
chemistry, 460
classification, 455
drug interactions, 287, 462
pharmacokinetics, 72, 461-462
structure, 461
uses, 462
Ethambutol:
adverse reactions, 751
antimicrobial activity, 750
chemistry, 750
history of, 9
mechanism of action, 750
mechanism of resistance, 750
pharmacokinetics, 750-751
structure, 750
uses, 751, 753-754
Ethanol:
adverse reactions, 86, 257-258
biotransformation, 69-72
chemistry and source, 253
dependence, 378
drug interactions, 81, 227, 237, 258-259, 282, 296, 298, 575, 607, 668
mechanism of action, 253-254
pharmacodynamics, 256
pharmacokinetics, 74, 254-256
uses, 259, 260, 808
Ethchlorvynol:
abuse, 379
adverse reactions, 241-242
controlled substance schedule, 376
drug interactions, 296
pharmacokinetics, 241
Ethinyl estradiol:
pharmacokinetics, 617
structure, 615
uses, 618, 625
Ethionamide, 752
Ethosuximide:
classification, 305
history of, 6
pharmacokinetics, 305, 311

structure, 311
uses, 305, 306, 311
Ethotoin, 305, 306, 308:
Ethyl alcohol, *see* Ethanol
Ethyl chloride, 374
Ethylene glycol:
adverse reactions, 260-261, 814
chemistry and sources, 260
pharmacokinetics, 260
treatment of poisoning, 260-261, 808
Ethylenediaminetetraacetic acid (EDTA), 831
Ethylene oxide, 816
Ethylmercury chloride, 825
Ethynodiol diacetate, 622, 623, 625
Etidocaine:
adverse reactions, 370
pharmacodynamics, 369
pharmacokinetics, 366, 368, 369, 373
structure, 366
uses, 371, 372
Etidronate sodium, 545, 594-595, 619
Etodolac:
adverse reactions, 357
classification, 346, 356
pharmacokinetics, 346, 357
structure, 356
uses, 357
Etomidate, 229-230
Etoposide (VP-16), 12, 657, 671-672
Etretinate, 543
Eucalyptus, 495
Excretion:
biliary, 53-54
mammary secretions, 54
nasal excretions, 54
renal, 53
salivary, 54
sweat, 54
tears, 54
Extended insulin zinc suspension (Ultralente insulin), 602

F

Famotidine:
adverse reactions, 198, 562
chemistry, 197
drug interactions, 199
history of, 11
mechanism of action, 197
pharmacokinetics, 198
pharmacologic effects, 188, 197-198, 562
structure, 197
uses, 561, 562
FANSIDAR (sulfadine-pyrimethamine), 772, 781
Felbamate:
adverse reactions, 311
classification, 305
drug interactions, 311
mechanism of action, 311
pharmacokinetics, 311
structure, 310
uses, 305
Felodipine:
classification, 478
pharmacokinetics, 435
pharmacologic effects, 434
uses, 434, 478
Female sex hormones (*see also Individual Categories and Agents*):
antiestrogens, 615, 619-620
estrogens, 613-619
fertility agents, 628-629
menstrual cycle, 611-613
oral contraceptives, 624-627
progestin antagonist, 624
progestins, 620-624
Fenitrothion, 815
Fenoprofen calcium:
adverse reactions, 349, 355
classification, 346, 354
pharmacokinetics, 346, 355
structure, 355
Fentanyl:
chemistry, 335
classification, 219, 325
pharmacokinetics, 327, 328, 336
structure, 336
uses, 224, 230-231, 336
Ferritin, 503, 505, 509
Ferrous fumarate, 508
Ferrous gluconate, 508
Ferrous sulfate, 508, 587
Fertility agents, 628-629 (*see also Individual Agents*)
Fibrinolytic agents, 533-534
Filgrastim:
adverse reactions, 655, 687
mechanism of action, 655, 687
pharmacokinetics, 655
uses, 655, 678, 687
Finasteride, 637
First generation cephalosporins:
pharmacokinetics, 709-710
structures, 707
Fish oils, 213, 446
FK506, 682, 683
Flavoxate, 170
Flecainide: 10, 401, 417
Fleroxacin, 724
Floxuridine, 656, 657, 662
Fluconazole, 757, 758, 762
Flucytosine:
adverse reactions, 760
history of, 11
mechanism of action, 758, 759
pharmacokinetics, 760
spectrum of activity, 759
structure, 758

uses, 760
Fludarabine phosphate, 656, 657, 659, 660
Fludrocortisone (9α-fluorohydrocortisone), 644
Flumazenil:
adverse reactions, 251
mechanism of action, 245, 251
pharmacokinetics, 251
precautions, 251
treatment in poisoning, 808
uses, 232, 251
Flunisolide, 489, 499, 808
Fluocinolone acetonide, 648
9α-Fluorohydrocortisone, *see* Fludrocortisone
Fluoroquinolones (*see also Individual Agents*):
adverse reactions, 727
antimicrobial spectrum, 725
drug interactions, 727
history of, 11
mechanism of action, 724
mechanism of resistance, 726
pharmacokinetics, 726-727
structures, 725
uses, 727-728
5-Fluorouracil:
adverse reactions, 662
classification, 656, 657
mechanism of action, 511, 662, 758, 759
pharmacokinetics, 662
structure, 658, 662
uses, 662
Fluoxetine:
adverse reactions, 298
chemistry, 297
drug interactions, 298
history of, 10
mechanism of action, 291, 297
pharmacokinetics, 295, 297-298
pharmacologic effects, 293
structure, 290
Fluoxymesterone:
adverse reactions, 634
classification, 657
pharmacokinetics, 632
relative activity, 633
structure, 631
Fluphenazine:
adverse reactions, 280
pharmacokinetics, 279
pharmacologic effects, 278
structure, 276
uses, 285
Flurandrenolide, 648
Flurazepam:
controlled substance schedule, 376
mechanism of action, 238-239
pharmacokinetics, 239, 247
structure, 238
uses, 239, 250
Flurbiprofen:
adverse reactions, 356
classification, 346, 354
history of, 10
pharmacokinetics, 346, 355-356
structure, 355
uses, 356
Flutamide, 12, 636, 657
Folic Acid:
absorption and fate, 511
chemistry and nomenclature, 511
classification, 539
diagnosis of deficiency, 514
deficiency, 514
drug interactions, 79, 447, 514
history of, 7
metabolic functions, 512-514
requirements and distribution, 514
sources, 511-512
structure, 512, 658
therapy of deficiency, 514
Folinic acid, 511, 513
Follicle-stimulating hormone (FSH):
in menstrual cycle, 611
stimulation of spermatogenesis, 630
Forcarnet:
antiviral agent, 763
mechanism of action, 764, 767
uses, 765
Formaldehyde, 804
N^5-Forminino-FH_4, 513
Formoterol, 490
Foscarnet, 11, 764, 765, 767
Fosinopril:
classification, 479
pharmacokinetics, 481, 482
structure, 480
Fumigants, 814, 816
Fungicides, 814
Furazolidone, 772, 785
Furosemide:
adverse reactions, 461-462, 804
chemistry, 460
classification, 455, 470
drug interactions, 287, 462
mechanism of action, 460
pharmacokinetics, 461-462, 470
structure, 461
uses, 462, 469, 471, 593, 594

G

G Proteins:
history of, 10
receptors and effector systems, 33-37
schematic model, 30
GABA (Gamma Aminobutyric Acid):
history of, 10
inhibition of, 181
inhibitory neurotransmitter, 233
mechanism of action, 238-239

receptor, 32-33, 254
$GABA_A$:
chloride ion influx, 234
receptors, 32-33, 233
Gabapentin, 306, 311
Gallamine:
histamine release, 177
mechanism of action, 175
pharmacokinetics, 177-178
pharmacologic effects, 176-177
structure, 174
Gallium nitrate, 594
Gamma aminobutyric acid (*see* GABA)
Ganciclovir, 764-766
Ganglionic blocking agents (*see also Individual Agents*):
antidepolarizing drugs, 171
classification, 163, 171
depolarizing drugs, 171
effects on organ systems, 171-172
mechanism of action, 170-171
pharmacologic effects, 171-172
Ganglionic transmission, 170-171
Gases and fumes, 806
Gastrointestinal drugs (*see also Individual Categories and Agents*):
acid-neutralizing compounds (antacids), 562, 567-569
antidiarrheal agents, 568-571
antiemetic drugs, 574-576
anti-infective agents, 562
antisecretory agents, 561-564
cytoprotective agents, 562, 564-567
inflammatory bowel disease, 576-579
laxatives, 571-574
peptic ulcer disease, 560-561
prokinetic drugs, 574-576
Gelatin, Absorbable, 536
Gemfibrozil
adverse reactions, 449, 452
drug interactions, 447
mechanism of action, 449
pharmacokinetics, 449
structure, 449
uses, 446, 449
Gene therapy, 498
Gentamicin:
adverse reactions, 722-723
antimicrobial spectrum, 700, 721
chemistry, 719
enhanced neuromuscular blockade, 176
mechanism of action, 719, 721
mechanism of resistance, 722
pharmacokinetics, 722
structural formula, 720
uses, 700, 723-724
Giardiasis, 772, 785
Glipizide (*see also* Sulfonylurea derivatives):
classification, 604
drug interactions, 762
pharmacokinetics, 606
structure, 605
uses, 608
Glucagon, 604, 808
Glucagon-like peptide-1 (7-36) amide, 609
Glucocorticoid inhibitors, 648-649
Glucocorticoids (*see also* Corticosteroids):
danazol receptor, 634
drug interactions, 750
effect on lactation, 628
inhibition of thyroid function, 584
Glucose:
antagonist of pentamidine, 784
transporter proteins, 599
Glutamate, 323-324
Glutamate receptors, 33, 254, 323-324
Glutethimide:
abuse, 242, 379
controlled substance schedule, 376
drug interactions, 532
pharmacokinetics, 242
treatment of toxicity, 807
uses, 242
Glyburide (*see also* Sulfonylurea derivatives):
classification, 604
drug interactions, 762
pharmacokinetics, 606
structure, 605
uses, 608
Glycerin, 573
Glycine, 33, 72
Glycopeptides (*see* also individual agents), 715-717
Glycopyrrolate, 168
GnRH Agonists, 12
Gold:
adverse reactions, 85, 821-822, 828
contraindications, 828
mechanism of action, 828
pharmacokinetics, 822, 828
poisoning, 822
treatment of poisoning, 808, 828, 833
uses, 497, 828
Gold sodium thiomalate, 828
Gonadal steroids, 616
Gonadorelin, 12
Gonadotropin releasing hormone (GnRH), 630, 636
Gonadotropin analogs, 674
Gonadotropins:
adverse reactions, 628
history of, 7
secretion 632-633
uses, 628
Goserelin, 636
Gout, 361
Granulocyte macrophage colony stimulating factor (GM-CSF), 488, 655, 686
Granulocyte-colony stimulating factor (G-CSF), 655, 687
Griseofulvin:
adverse reactions, 760

antifungal agent, 757
disulfiram-like reaction, 259
drug interactions, 532, 626
history of, 9
mechanism of action, 757, 760
pharmacokinetics, 87, 760
structure, 758
uses, 757, 760
Growth factors, 678, 686-688
Growth hormone, 12
Guaifensin, 495, 496
Guanabenz:
adverse reactions, 473
mechanism of action, 115, 122, 470, 472
pharmacokinetics, 473
pharmacologic effects, 472-473
structure, 472
uses, 473
Guanadrel:
adverse reactions, 145
classification, 130
drug interactions, 476
mechanism of action, 145
site of action, 131
structure, 145
uses, 145, 476
Guanethidine:
adverse reactions, 145,476
classification, 130
drug interactions, 81, 282, 296, 300, 476, 607
mechanism of action, 144
pharmacological effects, 144-145, 476
pharmacokinetics, 145
site of action, 131
structure, 144
uses, 145, 476
Guanfacine:
adverse reactions, 473
mechanism of action, 115, 122, 470, 472
pharmacokinetics, 473
pharmacologic effects, 472-473
structure, 472
uses, 473

H

H_1 receptor antagonists:
adverse reactions, 195
chemistry, 191
drug interactions, 258
mechanism of action, 191, 193
pharmacokinetics, 194-195
pharmacologic effects, 167, 193-194
structural classes, 192
uses, 195-196, 672, 834
H_2 receptor antagonists:
adverse reactions, 198-199, 562
chemistry, 197
drug interactions, 199, 607
history of, 8
mechanism of action, 197
pharmacokinetics, 198
pharmacologic effects, 197-198, 562
structures, 197
uses, 199, 562, 672
Halazepam:
contraindications and precautions, 250
pharmacokinetics, 246, 247, 248
structure, 245
uses, 247
Halcinonide, 648
Half-life ($t_{1/2}$), 56, 58
Hallucinogens, *see* Psychotomimetics
Halobetasol propionate, 648
Halofantrine:
adverse reactions, 778
history of, 11
mechanism of action, 777
pharmacokinetics, 777
structure, 777
uses, 772, 773, 774, 778
Haloperidol:
adverse reactions, 283
drug interaction, 282
history of, 6
mechanism of action, 277, 283
pharmacologic effects, 278, 283
pharmacokinetics, 283
structure, 283
uses, 267, 270, 283, 285
Haloprogin, 763
Halothane:
adverse reactions, 121, 225-226, 804
biotransformation, 67, 69, 72
chemistry, 224
classification, 219
drug interactions, 82, 225, 493
history of, 6
hypersensitivity reaction, 86
physicochemical properties, 220
pharmacodynamics, 224-225
pharmacokinetics, 224
structure, 224
uses, 226
Hashish, 271, 382
Hazard, definition of 803
Heavy metal antagonists, 831-834
Heavy metal poisoning, 821-834
Helminthiasis, 787
Hemp, 382
Henderson-Hasselbalch equation, 45
Heparin:
adverse reactions, 83, 527
chemistry, 526
history of, 5
mechanism of action, 526, 527
pharmacokinetics, 526-527
pharmacologic effects, 533
sources, 526

uses, 527 528
Heptachlor, 814
Herbicides, 814, 818-819
Heroin:
  chemistry, 333
  controlled substance schedule, 334, 376
  pharmacokinetics, 334
  pharmacologic effects, 334
  structure, 334
  structure-activity relationship, 326
  tolerance and physical dependence, 338-339
  withdrawal reactions, 377
Hexamethonium, 72
Histamine:
  adverse reactions, 191
  binding, 185
  biotransformation, 70, 186-187
  distribution, 185-186
  effects, 189-190
  history of, 5, 185
  in peptic ulcer disease, 560
  localization, 185-186
  mechanism of action, 188-189
  receptors, 185, 187-188, 275, 289
  release, 187, 347
  synthesis, 185, 186
  uses, 190-191
Histrelin, 636
HIV, 517
HMG-CoA reductase inhibitors *see also Individual Agents*:
  adverse reactions, 451-452
  drug interactions, 447
  mechanism of action, 450
  pharmacokinetics, 450-451
  structures, 451
  uses, 446, 447, 451
Homatropine, 169-170
Household poisons, 810
Human chorionic gonadotropin (HCG):
  in menstrual cycle, 613
  uses, 628, 629, 636
Human DNase, recombinant, 495
Human menopusal gonadotropin (HMG), 628, 629
Hydralazine:
  adverse reactions, 477
  classification, 476
  drug interaction, 553
  history of, 6
  mechanism of action, 477
  pharmacokinetics, 477
  pharmacologic effects, 398, 476, 477
  structure, 477
  uses, 397, 398, 477, 482
Hydrocarbon poisoning, 811
Hydrocarbons:
  aromatic, 814
  halogenated aliphatic, 814
  in air pollution, 811
  polyphosphorylated, 810
  sulfonated, 810
Hydrochlorothiazide:
  classification, 470
  pharmacokinetics, 458, 470
  pharmacologic effects, 457
  structure, 458
  uses, 463, 464, 469, 471
Hydrocodone, 334
Hydrocortisone (*see also* Cortisol):
  chemistry, 640
  pharmacologic effects, 644, 648
  physiologic effects, 638
  relative activity, 644
  structure, 641
  uses, 648, 759
Hydrocortisone valerate, 648
Hydrogen cyanide, 816
Hydromorphone:
  classification, 325
  controlled substance schedule, 376
  pharmacokinetics, 327, 328, 334
  structure, 334
  uses, 334
Hydroxocobalamin (Vitamin B_{12a}), 515, 818
Hydroxychloroquine, 497, 772-776
4-Hydroxycoumarin, 529
Hydroxyprogesterone, 613, 623, 641, 657
5-Hydroxytryptamine:
  agonists, 201-203
  antagonists, 203-204
  biosynthesis, 199, 200
  biotransformation, 199-200
  effects, 200-201
  physiologic function, 199
  receptors, 200, 251
  storage, 199
  uptake blockers, 289, 297
Hydroxyurea, 657, 672, 673
Hydroxyzine (*see also* H_1 receptor antagonists):
  structural class, 192
  use, 196, 252
Hyoscyamine, 163
Hyoscine, 163, 315
Hypercalcemia, 594
Hyperglycemia, 596
Hyperlipoproteinemia:
  cholesterol metabolism, 443-444
  cholesterol transport, 440-443
  classification of, 443, 444
  diagnosis of, 444-445
  hypertriglyceridemia, 444
  plasma lipid composition, 440, 442
  relationship to disease, 439-440, 443, 445
  treatment, 445
    dietary management, 445-446
    drug management, 446-453 (*see also Individual Agents*)
Hyperosmotic laxatives, 573
Hypertension:
  classification, 468, 469

definitions, 468
principles of drug therapy, 468-469
therapeutic approaches, 482-483
Hyperthyroidism, 588
Hyperuricemia, 361
Hypervitaminosis D, 593
Hypothalamic LH-releasing hormone (LHRH), 611
Hypothyroidism, 587

I

Ibuprofen:
adverse reactions, 354
classification, 346, 354
drug interactions, 355
history of, 8
pharmacokinetics, 346, 354
structure, 355
uses, 350
Idarubicin, 657, 670
Idoxuridine, 9, 764-766
Ifosfamide, 12, 656, 657, 666
Imidazole derivatives, 758, 760-761 (*see also Individual Agents*)
Imidazoline, 117, 122
Imipenem, 11, 713
Imipramine:
adverse reactions, 295
chemistry, 289
mechanism of action, 291
pharmacokinetics, 294-295
pharmacologic effects, 292-293
structure, 290
uses, 301
Immunoglobulin E (IgE), 485, 486
Immunophillins, 681
Immunopharmacologic drugs (*see also Individual Agents*):
immunostimulant agents, 684-688
immunosuppressive agents, 578, 676-684
Immunostimulating agents, 684-688
Immunosuppressive agents, 578, 676-684
Impromidine, 188
Indapamide:
adverse reactions, 460
chemistry, 460
classification, 455, 470
mechanism of action, 460
pharmacokinetics, 460, 470
structure, 460
uses, 460, 470
Indomethacin:
adverse reactions, 356-357
biotransformation, 87
classification, 346, 356
drug interactions, 349, 362, 462, 532
history of, 8
mechanism of action, 356
pharmacokinetics, 346, 356
structure, 356
uses, 215, 347, 350, 357
Inflammatory bowel disease, 576
Inotropic agents, 387 (*see also* Cardiac Glycosides)
Insecticides:
botanical, 815-816
types, 814-816
mono-carbamate, 815
organochlorine, 814
organophosphorus, 814-815
Insulin:
biologic effects, 600
chemistry and biosynthesis, 597-598
complications of insulin therapy, 603
drug interactions, 353, 607
effect on lactation, 628
history of, 5
mechanism of action, 599-600
mechanism for stimulation, 599
preparations, 601-602
secretion and degradation, 598
structure, 597
uses, 596, 603
Insulin injection (Regular insulin), 601, 602
Insulin-like growth factor 1 (IGF-1), 37, 600, 609
Insulin receptors, 37-39, 599-600
Insulin zinc suspension (Lente), 601, 602
Interferon, 12, 672-673
Interferon alpha, 678, 685
Interferon alfa-2a, 685
Interferon alfa-2b, 685
Interferon beta, 678, 685, 686
Interferon gamma, 488, 678, 685-686
Interleukin-1, 209, 347, 488
Interleukin-2, 488, 576, 686
Interleukin-3, 488
Interleukin-4, 488
Interleukin-5, 488
Interleukins, history of, 12
Iodinated glycerol, 495
Iodide:
inhibition of thyroid function, 584, 588-589
mechanism of action as a bronchomucotropic agent, 495
pharmacologic effects as a mucokinetic agent, 496
Iodine, 807
Iodoquinol, 772, 782
Ion channel receptors, 29-31
Ipecac syrup, 167, 807, 808
Ipratropium:
adverse reactions, 495
classification, 490
pharmacokinetics, 170, 495
structure, 494
uses, 170, 490, 494, 495, 500
Iron:
absorption, 505
adverse reactions, 509-510, 808, 821

complexes, 503-505
compliance, 508
deficiency, 503, 505, 507-508
drug interactions, 447
excretion, 506
pharmacokinetics, 507
preparations, 508-509
requirements, 506-507
storage, 505
treatment of toxicity, 509, 510-511, 808
transport, 505
uses, 510-511
Iron dextran, 509
Isoetharine:
adverse reactions, 491
classification, 490
mechanism of action, 115
pharmacokinetics, 124, 491
structure, 124
use, 115 490, 491
Isoflavone phytoestrogens, 620
Isoflurane:
chemistry, 227
classification, 219
physicochemical properties, 220
pharmacodynamics, 227
pharmacokinetics, 227
structure, 227
uses, 225
Isoflurophate:
classification, 154
inhibition of histamine release, 187
mechanism of action, 160, 161
structure, 155
use, 161
Isolan, 815
Isoniazid:
adverse reactions, 86, 748, 804
antimicrobial activity, 747
drug interactions, 227, 307, 553, 568, 761
history of, 9
mechanism of action, 747
mechanism of resistance, 747
pharmacokintics, 75, 87, 748
structure, 747
uses, 551, 748, 753-754
Isophane insulin suspension (NPH insulin), 601, 602, 608
Isopropyl alcohol, 261
Isoproterenol:
adverse reactions, 122, 491
cardiovascular effects, 118, 396
classification, 113, 115, 490
mechanism of action, 114, 115, 121
pharmacokinetics, 491
pharmacologic effects, 121-122
structure, 117
use, 122, 396, 490, 491
Isosorbide dinitrate, 425, 426, 429
Isosorbide mononitrate, 425, 428
Isotretinoin, 543
Isradipine:
classification, 478
pharmacokinetics, 435
pharmacologic effects, 434
uses, 434, 478
Itraconazole, 757, 758, 762
Ivermectin, 789, 798

K

Kanamycin, 719, 752, 753
Kaolin-pectin, 395
Kepone, 447
Ketamine, 8, 229
Ketanserin, 204
Ketoconazole:
adverse reactions, 649, 761
drug interactions, 683, 761
effect on steroidogenesis, 648-649
history of, 9
mechanism of action, 758
pharmacokinetics, 760-761
structure, 758
uses, 637, 649, 757, 761
Ketoprofen:
adverse reactions, 356
classification, 346, 354
pharmacokinetics, 356
structure, 355
uses, 356
Ketorolac tromethamine:
adverse reactions, 360
classification, 346, 359
history of, 10
pharmacokinetics, 346, 360
pharmacologic effects, 359-360
structure, 359
uses, 360

L

Labetalol (*see also* β-Adrenergic blocking agents):
adverse reactions, 139
classification, 130, 133, 137
mechanism of action, 138, 473
pharmacodynamic properties, 134, 138, 473, 474, 475
pharmacokinetics, 135, 138-139
physicochemical properties, 135, 474
structure, 138
uses, 138, 139, 468, 474, 482
Lactulose, 573
Laxatives (*see also Individual Agents*):
bulk laxatives, 572
classification, 571
constipation, 571

hyperosmotic laxatives, 573
lubricant laxatives, 573
miscellaneous laxatives, 573-574
saline laxatives, 573
stimulant laxatives, 572
stool softeners, 573
Lead:
adverse reactions, 808
treatment of poisoning, 808, 824
pharmacokinetics, 821-823
poisoning, 822, 823-824
sources, 821
Lead arsenate, 826
Leishmaniasis, 772, 783
Lemakalim, 497
Lente insulin, 601, 602
Leptophos, 815
Lethal concentration-50 (LCT_{50}), 803
Lethal dose-50 (LD_{50}), 803
Leu-enkephalin, 321-322, 323
Leucovorin:
adverse reactions, 662
mechanism of action, 659
growth factor, 511, 513
uses, 656, 659, 662
Leukotriene antagonists, 496
Leukotrienes (LTs):
biosynthesis, 209
in bronchospasm, 485, 496
mechanism of action, 210, 485
physiologic effects, 212
Leuprolide:
adverse reactions, 674
classification as an antineoplastic, 657
history of, 12
pharmacologic effects, 629, 636
uses, 629, 636, 674
Levamisole, 678, 687
Levarterenol, 121
LEVLEN, 625
Levo-α-acetyl methadol (LAAM), 377
Levodopa:
adverse reactions, 316
chemistry, 315
drug interactions, 282, 296, 300, 316, 568, 575
history of, 6
mechanism of action, 315
pharmacokinetics, 316, 568
uses, 169, 315, 317
Levomethadyl acetate, 338, 377
Levonorgestrel, 611, 623-625, 627
Levorphanol:
classification, 325
pharmacokinetics, 327, 328, 335
pharmacologic effects, 335
potency comparison, 327
structure, 335
Levothyroxine sodium (L-T_4), 121, 447, 587
Lidocaine:
adverse reactions, 85, 370, 415
classification, 401
drug interactions, 414, 416
history of, 6, 365
mechanism of action, 403
pharmacokinetics, 72, 83, 368, 369, 415
pharmacologic effects, 16, 83, 401, 415
structure, 366, 415
uses, 371, 372, 373, 395, 412, 415
Lindane, 814
Liothyronine sodium (L-T_3), 587
Liotrix, 587
Lipoxins, 209
5-Lipoxygenase inhibitors, 496
Lisinopril:
classification, 479
history of, 3
pharmacokinetics, 481, 482
pharmacologic effects, 398
structure, 480
uses, 397, 398, 481
Lithium carbonate:
adverse reactions, 286-287
drug interactions, 282, 287-288, 298, 436, 459, 462, 493
history of, 10
management of intoxication, 288
mechanism of action, 286
pharmacokinetics, 286
uses, 85, 286
Lobeline:
classification, 147, 171
structure, 150
pharmacologic effects, 153
use, 153
Local anesthetics, *see* Anesthetics, Local
LOESTRIN 21 1/20, 625
LOESTRIN 21 1.5/30, 625
Lomefloxacin:
adverse reactions, 727
antimicrobial spectrum, 725
drug interactions, 727
mechanism of action, 724
mechanism of resistance, 726
pharmacokinetics, 726-727
structure, 725
uses, 727-728
Lomustine (CCNU), 657, 663, 665, 666
Loop diuretics, *see* Diuretics
LO/OVRAL, 625
Loperamide:
adverse reactions, 570
classification, 325
chemistry, 335, 337
pharmacokinetics, 337
structure, 337
uses, 337, 570
Loracarbef, 710-711
Loratadine (*see also* H_1 receptor antagonists):
pharmacokintics, 195
pharmacologic properties, 194

structural class, 192
use, 196
Lorazepam:
adverse reactions, 249
contraindications and precautions, 250
controlled substance schedule, 376
pharmacodynamics, 248
pharmacokinetics, 246, 247, 248
structure, 245
uses, 219, 231-232, 247, 250, 251, 312, 314
withdrawal, 249
Lovastatin, 10, 450, 451
Loxapine, 278, 284, 297
LSD:
adverse reactions, 264, 381-382
chemistry, 262-263
classification, 262
history of, 8
mechanism of action, 263
pharmacokinetics, 263-264
pharmacologic effects, 264, 381
sensory and subjective effects, 264
structure, 263
syndrome, 263
tolerance and physical dependence, 264, 381
treatment of adverse reactions, 264
Lubricant laxatives, 573
Lugol's Solution, 589
Luteinizing hormone-releasing hormone (LHRH), 628-629
Lysergic acid diethylamide, *see* LSD
LYSOL, 807

M

Macrolides (*see also Individual Agents*):
adverse reactions, 732
antimicrobial spectrum, 729-730
mechanism of resistance, 730
mechanism of action, 729
pharmacokinetics, 731
structure, 730
uses, 732, 754
Macrophage aggregating factor (MAF), 643
Macrophage migration-inhibitory factor (MIF), 643
Magnesium aluminum trisilicate, 567, 568
Magnesium citrate, 573
Magnesium hydroxide, 567, 568, 573
Magnesium salicylate, 346, 353, 354
Magnesium salts, 414
Magnesium sulfate, 573, 808
Malaoxon, 804, 815
Malaria, 771-773
Malathion:
classification, 154, 815
pharmacokinetics, 161
structure, 155
treatment of toxicity, 807
uses, 161
Manganese, 822, 830
Mannitol:
adverse reactions, 466
classification, 455
drug interaction, 287
pharmacokinetics, 466
uses, 466, 808
MAO inhibitors *see* Monoamine oxidase inhibitors
Maprotiline:
adverse reactions, 297
drug interactions, 297
mechanism of action, 291, 297
pharmacologic effects, 293, 297
pharmacokinetics, 295, 297
Margin of safety, definition of, 804
Marijuana:
adverse reactions, 273, 382-383
chemistry, 270-271, 382
classification, 262
controlld substance schedule, 376
pharmacokinetics, 271, 382
pharmacologic effects, 273, 382
source, 270-271, 382
tolerance and dependence, 273, 382
treatment of toxicity, 273
uses, 283-274
Marine fish oils, 497
Maxindol, 376
MDMA, *see* 3,4-methylenedioxy-methamphetamine
Mebendazole:
adverse reactions, 791
chemistry, 791
contraindications and precautions, 792
mechanism of action, 791
pharmacokinetics, 791
structure, 791
uses, 788, 789, 792
Mecamylamine, 170-172
Mechlorethamine, 654, 657, 664, 665
Meclizine, *see* H_1 receptor antagonists
Meclofenamate sodium, 346, 358
Median toxic dose (TD_{50}), 18
Median effective dose (ED_{50}), 18
Medroxyprogesterone, 622, 623, 627
Mefenamic acid, 346, 358
Mefloquine, 11, 772-774, 777
Megestrol acetate, 622, 623
Meglumine antimonate, 772
Melanocyte-stimulating hormone (MSH), 321, 646
Melarsoprol, 772, 785
Melphalan:
adverse reactions, 664
classification, 657
pharmacokinetics, 666
structure, 665
uses, 656, 666
Menadiol, 779
Menadione, 70, 530, 531
Menaquinone, 529, 530
Menotropins, 636

Menthol, 495
Mepenzolate, 168
Meperidine:
  adverse reactions, 335
  chemistry, 335
  classification, 325
  controlled substance schedule, 376
  dependence, 335, 342
  drug interactions, 300, 343
  history of, 6
  pharmacokinetics, 80, 85, 327, 328, 335
  pharmacologic effects, 82, 331, 335
  potency, 327
  structure, 335
  uses, 335
Mephenytoin, 305, 306, 308
Mephobarbital:
  classification, 234, 305
  pharmacokinetics, 310
  structure, 234, 309
  uses, 238, 305
Mepivacaine:
  adverse reactions, 370, 373
  pharmacokinetics, 368, 369
  structure, 366
  uses, 371, 372, 373
Meprobamate:
  adverse reactions, 252
  controlled substance schedule, 376
  pharmacologic effects, 252
  precautions, 252
  use, 244
Mepyramine (pyrilamine), 187, 192
Mercaptopurine:
  adverse reactions, 511, 660
  classification, 656, 657
  drug interactions, 363, 660
  mechanism of action, 659, 679
  pharmacokinetics, 659-660
  structure, 658, 659, 679
  uses, 578, 660
Mercapturic acid, 72
Mercuric chloride, 807
Mercurous chloride (calomel), 824, 825
Mercury:
  chemistry, 824
  mechanism of action, 825
  pharmacokinetics, 822, 825
  poisoning, 822, 824, 825-826
  sources, 824-825
  treatment of poisoning, 808, 826, 833
Merphos, 815
Mesalamine, 577-578
Mescaline:
  chemistry, 263, 265
  classification, 262
  controlled substance schedule, 376
  mechanism of action, 263
  pharmacologic effects, 381
  structure, 265
Mesoridazine, 278, 279
Mestranol, 615, 618, 625
Metaraminol, 115, 125, 128
Met-enkephalin, 321-322, 323
Metals, 831
Metaproterenol:
  adverse reactions, 401
  clssification, 490
  mechanism of action, 115
  pharmacokinetics, 124, 491
  structure, 124
  use, 115, 124, 490, 491
Metformin, 607
Methacholine, 147-150
Methacycline, 743-745
Methadone:
  chemistry, 337
  classification, 325
  controlled substance schedule, 376
  drug interactions, 750
  history of, 6
  maintenance program, 377
  mechanism of action, 337
  pharmacokinetics, 327, 328, 337
  potency comparison, 327
  structure, 337
  uses, 338
  withdrawal reactions, 332
Methamphetamine (*see also* Amphetamine):
  classification, 127, 268
  controlled substance schedule, 376
  pharmacologic effects, 120, 126, 127
Methanol:
  adverse reactions, 260
  chemistry and sources, 260
  pharmacokinetics, 260, 804
  treatment of poisoning, 260, 808
Methcathinone, 268
Methicillin:
  adverse reactions, 700
  antimicrobial spectrum, 702
  chemistry, 702
  classification, 697
  pharmacokinetics, 699, 702
  structure, 698
  uses, 702-703
Methimazole, 584, 588
Methionine, 108, 513, 516
Methocarbamol, 181
Methohexital:
  classification, 228, 234
  pharmacodynamics, 229
  structure, 234
Methomyl, 815
Methorphan, 335
Methotrexate:
  adverse reactions, 511, 659, 680-681
  classification, 656, 657
  drug interactions, 353
  history of, 7

mechanism of action, 514, 653 654, 656
pharmacokinetics, 80, 656-657
structure, 658
uses, 497, 658-659, 677, 680
Methoxamine, 115
Methoxychlor, 814
Methoxyethylmercury chloride, 824
Methoxyflurane:
classification, 219
pharmacokinetics, 228
physicochemical properties, 220, 222, 228
structure, 228
Methscopolamine, 168
Methsuximide, 306, 311
Methyclothiazide, 470
Methyl benzethonium chloride, 810
Methyl bromide, 816
Methylcellulose, 570, 572
3-Methylcholanthrene, 72
Methyldopa:
adverse reactions, 472
drug interactions, 220, 282, 316, 436
history of, 6
mechanism of action, 122, 471-472
pharmacokinetics, 472
pharmacologic effects, 472
structure, 471
uses, 472
Methyldopate, 472
Methylene blue, 807
Methylene chloride, 811
3,4-Methylenedioxymethamphetamine (MDMA), 262, 265
Methylergonovine, 203
2-Methylhistamine, 188
4-Methylhistamine, 188
(R) α-Methylhistamine, 188
Methylmercury chloride, 825
Methylmercury dicyandiamide, 825
Methylpalmoxirate, 609
Methylphenidate:
adverse reactions, 128
classification, 115, 268
controlled substance schedule, 376
dependence, 380
drug interactions, 297
pharmacologic effects, 292
uses, 128, 380
Methylprednisolone, 642, 644
4-Methylpyrazole, 260
Methyl salicylate, 346, 350, 352
Methyltestosterone:
adverse reaction, 634
drug interactions, 683
pharmacokinetics, 632
relative activity, 633
structure, 631
uses, 633
Methylthiopurine, 67
Methylxanthines, *see* Xanthine derivatives
Methyprylon, 242, 376
Methysergide, 203
Metoclopramide:
adverse reactions, 575
drug interactions, 78-79, 575
history of, 11
mechanism of action, 574
pharmacokinetics, 575
pharmacologic effects, 574
structure, 574
uses, 575
Metocurine:
mechanism of action, 175
pharmacokinetics, 177-178
pharmacologic effects, 176-177
Metolazone:
adverse reactions, 460
classification, 455, 459, 470
mechanism of action, 459
pharmacokinetics, 460, 470
structure, 459
uses, 460
Metoprolol (*see also* β-Adrenergic blocking agents):
classification, 130, 133, 137, 473
compliance, 474
drug interactions, 79
pharmacodynamic properties, 134, 137, 473, 474
pharmacokinetics, 135, 137
physicochemical properties, 135, 474
structure, 132
uses, 137-138, 474
Metronidazole:
adverse reactions, 259, 735
antimicrobial activity, 735
disulfiram-like reaction, 259
drug interactions, 532
history of, 11
mechanism of action, 734
mechanism of resistance, 735
pharmacokinetics, 735
structure, 734
uses, 562, 567, 579, 735, 772, 781, 782, 783, 785, 789
Metyrapone, 647
Metyrosine:
adverse reactions, 145
classification, 130
mechanism of action, 145, 476
pharmacokinetics, 145
site of action, 131
uses, 145, 476
Mexiletine: 8, 401, 416
Mezlocillin:
adverse reactions, 700
antimicrobial spectrum, 704, 705
classification, 697, 704
pharmacokinetics, 697, 699, 704-705
structure, 698

uses, 705
Miconazole:
  adverse reactions, 761
  history of, 11
  mechanism of action, 758, 761
  uses, 761
MICRONOR, 625
Microsomal cytochromes P-450, 66-68
Microsomal oxidation reactions, 66-69
Microsomal ethanol oxidizing system (MEOS), 255-256
Midazolam:
  history of, 10
  pharmacokinetics, 247
  uses, 219, 231, 232, 247, 250
Mifepristone (RU 486), 624
Milrinone:
  adverse reactions, 397
  cardiovascular effects, 396
  history of, 10
  mechanism of action, 396
  pharmacokinetics, 396-397
  structure, 396
  uses, 387, 389, 396
Mineral oil, 532, 573
Minimum alveolar concentration (MAC), definition, 219-220
Minocycline, 743-745
Minoxidil, 476, 477-478, 482
Mipafox, 815
Misoprostol:
  adverse effects, 215, 565
  history, 11
  pharmacokinetics, 215, 564-565
  pharmacologic effects, 564
  structure, 564
  uses, 213, 215, 348, 565
Mithramycin, *see* Plicamycin
Mitomycin, 69, 657, 670
Mitoxantrone, 657, 670
Mivacurium:
  history of, 12
  mechanism of action, 175
  pharmacokinetics, 178, 179
  release of histamine, 177
MODICON, 625
Molindone, 278, 283-284
Monoamine oxidase inhibitors:
  adverse reactions, 296, 300, 806
  chemistry, 299
  drug interactions, 121, 298, 300, 316, 343, 607
  mechanism of action, 299
  pharmacokinetics, 295, 299-300
  structures, 290
  uses, 301
Monobactams, 714-715
Mono-carbamate insecticides, 815
N-Monomethyl-L-arsinine, 497
Moricizine: 10, 410, 418
Morphine:
  adverse reactions, 77, 331
  chemistry, 325
  classification, 325
  controlled substance schedule, 376
  histamine release, 187
  idiosyncratic reactions, 77
  mechanism of action, 324
  pharmacokinetics, 87, 326-331
  pharmacologic effects, 84, 329-330
  receptor binding, 326
  structure, 325
  structure-activity relationship, 325-326
  tolerance and physical dependence, 331-332
  treatment of toxicity, 807
  uses, 230-231, 332-333, 570
MPPP (1-methyl-4-phenylproprionoxypiperidine), 383-384
MPTP(1-methyl-4-phenyl-1,2,5,6-tetrahydropyridine, 384, 804
Mucilloid, 572
Mucokinetic agents, 495-496
Murein (peptidoglycan), 694
Muromonab-CD3, 12, 677, 684
Muscarine:
  adverse reactions, 151
  classification, 109, 147, 150-151
  mechanism of action, 88, 109-111
  pharmacodynamics, 151
  structure, 150
  treatment of toxicity, 807
Muscarinic receptors, 104, 109-111, 147-148, 275, 289

N

Nabumetone, 10, 346, 359
Nadolol (*see also* β-Adrenergic blocking agents):
  classification, 130, 133, 137
  compliance, 474
  pharmacodynamic properties, 134, 474
  pharmacokinetics, 135, 137
  physicochemical properties, 135, 474
  structure, 132
  uses, 137-138, 474
Nafarelin, 12, 636
Nafazatrom, 496, 497
Nafcillin:
  adverse reactions, 700
  classification, 697, 702-703
  pharmacokinetics, 697, 699, 702
  structure, 698
  uses, 702-703, 750
Nalbuphine:
  classification, 325
  pharmacokinetics, 327, 328
  pharmacologic effects, 339-340
  receptor binding, 326, 338
  structure, 339
  uses, 340

Nalidixic acid, 724
Nalorphine, 325, 341
Naloxone:
  chemistry, 341
  classification, 325
  history of, 6
  pharmacokinetics, 70, 342
  pharmacologic effects, 325, 341
  receptor binding, 323, 326, 341
  structure, 342
  uses, 331, 332, 339, 342, 378, 808
Naltrexone:
  adverse reactions, 343
  chemistry, 342
  classification, 325
  history of, 6
  receptor binding, 326, 341
  pharmacokinetics, 342
  pharmacologic effects, 325, 341
  structure, 342
  uses, 343, 378
Nandrolone decanoate, 631, 633
Nandrolone phenpropionate, 633
Naphazoline, 122
Naproxen:
  adverse ractions, 355
  history of, 8
  classification, 346, 354
  pharmacokinetics, 355
  structure, 355
  uses, 355
Naproxen sodium, *see* Naproxen
Narcotic analgesics, *see* Opioid analgesics
Nedocromil sodium, 489, 490, 499
NELOVA 0.5/35E, 625
NELOVA 1/35E, 625
NELOVA 1/50M, 625
NELOVA 10/11, 625
Neomycin, 176, 452, 719
Neostigmine:
  chemistry, 156
  classification, 154
  mechanism of action, 154
  pharmacokinetics, 156
  pharmacologic effects, 156-158
  structure, 155
  use, 158, 808
Netilmicin, 719-724
Neurokinin receptors, 323
Neuroleptics, 275, 297
Neuromuscular blocking agents (*see also Individual Agents*):
  adverse reactions, 180
  chemistry, 173
  classification, 163
  drug interactions, 237, 288, 416
  mechanism of action, 173-176
  pharmacologic effects, 176-178
  pharmacokinetics, 177-178
  structures, 174
  uses, 179-180
Niacin, *see* Nicotinic acid
Nicardipine:
  adverse reactions, 435, 436
  classification, 478
  pharmacokinetics, 435
  pharmacologic effects, 398, 432, 434
  structure, 431
  uses, 398, 434, 478
Niclosamide, 788, 790, 792-793
Nicotine:
  adverse reactions, 152-153, 383
  chemistry, 151
  classification, 147, 171, 815
  mechanism of action, 151-152
  pharmacodynamics, 152
  pharmacokinetics, 152
  structure, 150
  tolerance and dependence, 153, 383
  treatment of toxicity, 807
  uses, 152
  withdrawal reactions, 383
Nicotinic acid:
  adverse reactions, 447-448, 452, 552
  classification, 539
  deficiency syndrome, 551
  history of, 5
  mechanism of action, 441, 447
  pharmacologic effects, 447
  role in metabolism, 551
  structure, 447
  uses, 446, 448, 452, 540, 551
Nicotinic receptors, 31-32, 104, 108-111, 147, 173
Nifedipine:
  adverse reactions, 435-436
  classification, 430, 478
  history of, 10
  mechanism of action, 432
  pharmacokinetics, 435
  pharmacologic effects, 398, 432, 434, 497
  structure, 431
  uses, 398, 434, 478, 497
Nifurtimox, 772, 784-785
Nitrates and nitrites (*see also Individual Agents*):
  adverse reactions, 429
  classification, 425
  drug interactions, 250
  mechanism of action, 425-427
  pharmacologic effects, 427-428
  pharmacokinetics, 428
  tolerance, 429
  uses, 422, 429
Nitric oxide, 498
Nitrofurans, 87
Nitrogen dioxide, 813
Nitrogen mustard, *see* Mechlorethamine
Nitrogen oxides, 811

Nitroglycerin:
classification, 425, 476
dosage forms, 428
pharmacokinetics, 428
pharmacologic effects, 398, 476
structure, 426
tolerance, 429
uses, 397, 398, 425, 429-430, 483, 484
Nitro-imidazole, 772
Nitrous oxide:
abuse potential, 224
adverse reactions, 223
chemistry, 223
classification, 219
history of, 5
physicochemical properties, 220, 221, 222
pharmacodynamics, 223
pharmacokinetics, 223
uses, 223-224
Nizatidine:
adverse reactions, 198, 562
chemistry, 197
drug interactions, 199
history of, 11
mechanism of action, 197
pharmacokinetics, 198
pharmacologic effects, 188, 197-198, 562
structure, 197
uses, 199, 562
Nociception, *see* Pain
Nonmicrosomal oxidation reactions, 69-70
Nonsteroidal anti-inflammatory agents (NSAIDs) (*see also Individual Agents*):
adverse reactions, 213, 215, 345, 351-353, 355, 565
classification, 346
chemistry, 346
contraindications, 354
drug interactions, 258, 353, 683
history of, 8
mechanism of action, 209-210, 212, 345, 346-347
pharmacokinetics, 346, 350-351, 354
pharmacologic effects, 345, 347-350, 561
uses, 351, 353, 354, 361
Noradrenaline, *see* Norepinephrine
NORDETTE, 625
Norepinephrine:
as a neurotransmitter, 103, 105-108
biotransformation, 70, 72, 107, 108
cardiovascular effects, 118
drug interaction, 296
history of, 8
mechanism of action, 81, 114, 115, 125, 127
structure, 117, 265
NORETHIN 1/35E, 625
NORETHIN 1/50M, 625
Norethindrone, 621, 622, 625
Norethindrone acetate, 622, 623, 625
Norethynodrel, 622, 623
Norfloxacin (*see* quinolones):
adverse reaction, 727
antimicrobial spectrum 725
chemical structure, 725
drug interactions, 566, 727
history of, 11
mechanism of action, 724
spectrum, 725
uses, 727-728
Norgestimate: 623, 625
Norgestrel, 622, 623, 625
NORINYL 1 + 35, 625
NORINYL 1 + 50, 625
NOR-Q.D., 625
Nortriptyline:
adverse reactions, 295
chemistry, 289
mechanism of action, 291
pharmacokinetics, 294-295
pharmacologic effects, 292-293
structure, 290
Noscapine, 325
NPH insulin, 601, 602, 608
NSAIDs, *see* Nonsteroidal anti-inflammatory agents
Nuclear receptors, 39-40
Nystatin, 757-759

O

Octreotide, 571
Ofloxacin:
adverse reactions, 727
antimicrobial spectrum, 725, 752
drug interactions, 566, 724, 727
mechanism of action, 724
pharmacokinetics, 724-726
structure, 725
uses, 727-728, 752
Olsalazine, 577-578
Omeprazole, 11, 561, 562-563
Ondansetron, 204
Opiate, 319 (*see also* Opioid analgesics)
Opioid analgesics (*see also Individual Agents*):
agonists, 325-338
antagonists, 6, 324, 341-343
as anesthetics, 230-231
classification, 324, 325
contraindications, 343
controlled substance schedules, 376
dependence, 376-378
drug interactions, 237, 249, 258, 282, 343, 575
endogenous opioid peptides, 321-322
history of, 8
mechanism of action, 321-324
mixed agonist-antagonists, 338-341
receptor binding, 326
receptors, 322-324
sources, 319
synthetic opioid peptides, 322

tolerance, 376-377
treatment of suspected opioid-induced coma, 808
uses, 230-231, 322-323, 570
withdrawal reactions, 377
Opioid peptides, 321-322
Opium:
controlled substance schedule, 376
source of morphine, 319
treatment of toxicity, 807
uses, 570
Oral anticoagulants, *see* Anticoagulants, Oral
Oral contraceptives:
adverse reactions, 626, 628
drug interactions, 493, 532, 626, 683
effect on folate levels, 514
history of, 7, 9
pharmacologic effects, 624, 626
preparations, 625
uses, 624, 626
Oral hypoglycemic agents (*see also Individual Agents*):
Classification, 604
Biguanides, 607
Sulfonylurea derivatives:
adverse reactions, 606-607
drug interactions, 259, 350, 351, 436, 354, 447, 607, 750
mechanism of action, 599, 604
pharmacokinetics, 604-606
structures, 605
uses, 607-608
Organochlorine insecticides, 814
Organomercurial compounds, 826
Organophosphate poisoning, 161-162, 804, 807, 808
Organophosphorus insecticides, 807, 808, 814-815 (*see also* Cholinesterase inhibitors)
Orphenadrine, 169, 181, 316
ORTHO-CEPT, 625
ORTHO-CYCLEN, 625
ORTHO-NOVUM 1/35, 625
ORTHO-NOVUM 1/50, 625
ORTHO-NOVUM 7/7/7, 625
ORTHO-NOVUM 10/11, 625
ORTHO TRI-CYCLEN, 625
OVCON-35, 625
OVCON-50, 625
OVRAL, 625
OVRETTE, 625
Oxacillin:
adverse reactions, 700
classification, 697
pharmacokinetics, 697, 699, 702
structure, 698
uses, 702-703
Oxalates, 804, 807, 811
Oxalic acid, 811
Oxamniquine, 790, 793
Oxandrolone, 631, 633
Oxaprozin:
adverse reactions, 356
classification, 346, 354
history of, 10
pharmacokinetics, 356
structure, 355
uses, 356
Oxazepam:
controlled substance schedule, 376
pharmacokinetics, 246, 247, 248
structure, 245
uses, 247, 251
withdrawal, 249
Oxiconazole, 758, 761
Oxidized Cellulose, 536
Oxtriphylline, 490, 491, 494
Oxybutynin, 170
Oxycodone:
classification, 325
controlled substance schedule, 376
pharmacokinetics, 327, 328
structure, 334
uses, 334
Oxymetazoline, 122
Oxymetholone, 633
Oxymorphone:
classification, 325
controlled substance schedule, 376
pharmacokinetics, 327, 328, 334
structure, 334
uses, 334
Oxyphenbutazone:
adverse reactions, 349, 358
classification, 346, 357
pharmacokinetics, 346
uses, 358
Oxytetracycline, 743-745
Oxytocin, 214
Ozone, 813

P

PABA, *see* Para-aminobenzoic acid
Paclitaxel, 12, 657, 672
Pain: 319-321, 323
Pamidronate disodium, 594
Pancuronium:
adverse reactions, 180
mechanism of action, 175
pharmacokinetics, 177-178
pharmacologic effects, 176-177
structure, 174
Para-aminobenzoic acid (PABA), 370, 729
Para-aminosalicyclic acid, 87, 752
Papaverine, 325
Paraldehyde, 241, 376
Paramethadione:
adverse reactions, 308, 313
uses, 306, 313

Paramethasone, 642, 644
Paraoxon, 815
Paraquat, 804, 818-819
Parasympathomimetic drugs, *see* Cholinomimetic drugs
Parathion:
  adverse reactions, 801
  classification, 154, 815
  oxidation reaction, 67
  pharmacokinetics, 161
  structure, 155
  treatment of toxicity, 807
Parathion-methyl, 815
Parathyroid hormone, 590-591
Paregoric, 333, 376
Parenteral route, 48, 507-508
Parkinsonism, 314
Paromomycin:
  adverse reactions, 783
  chemistry, 719
  pharmacologic effects, 782
  uses, 772, 782, 794
Paroxetine:
  adverse reaction, 298
  chemistry, 297
  drug interactions, 298
  history of, 10
  mechanism of action, 291, 297
  pharmacokinetics, 295, 298
  pharmacologic effects, 293
  structure, 290
PAS, *see* Para-aminosalicyclic acid
PCBs, *see* Polychlorinated biphenyls
PCP, *see* Phencyclidine
Pemoline, 128
Penbutolol (*see also* β-Adrenergic blocking agents):
  classification, 130, 133, 137
  compliance, 474
  pharmacodynamic properties, 133, 134, 473, 474
  pharmacokinetics, 135, 137
  physicochemical properties, 135, 474
  uses, 137-138, 474
Penicillamine:
  adverse reactions, 834
  drug interactions, 553, 834
  mechanism of action, 833
  pharmacokinetics, 833
  route of administration and dosage, 833
  structure, 833
  uses, 808, 826, 833
Penicillin G:
  adverse reactions, 700
  antimicrobial spectrum, 700-701
  classification, 697
  drug interactions, 79, 80, 362
  history of, 697
  pharmacokinetics, 697, 699, 701, 702
  spectrum, 700-701
  structure, 698
  uses, 351, 701-702
Penicillin V:
  antimicrobial spectrum, 701
  classification, 697
  pharmacokinetics, 697, 699, 701
  structure, 698
  uses, 702
Penicillins (*see also individual Categories and Agents*):
  adverse reactions, 699-700
  allergic reactions, 804
  chemistry, 697
  classification, 697
    aminopenicillins, 703-704
    extended-spectrum penicillins, 704-705
    natural penicillins, 700-702
    penicillinase-resistant penicillins, 702-703
  pharmacokinetics, 697, 699
  structures, 698
  treatment of toxicity, 807
Pentaerythritol tetranitrate, 425, 426, 428
Pentagastrin, 190
Pentamidine, 11, 772, 783, 784
Pentazocine:
  adverse reactions, 339
  classification, 325
  pharmacokinetics, 327, 328, 339
  pharmacologic effects, 339
  receptor binding, 326, 338
  structure, 339
  tolerance and dependence, 339
  uses, 339
Pentobarbital:
  adverse effects, 237
  biotransformation, 67, 72
  classification, 234
  controlled substance schedule, 376
  pharmacokinetics, 235
  structure, 234
  uses, 238, 314
Pentostatin, 656, 657, 659, 661
Peptidoglycan, 694
Pergolide, 318
Pesticides, 814
Peyote, 376
Pharmacodynamics, definition of, 42
Pharmacokinetics (*see also individual topics*):
  absorption, 43-50
  biotransformation, 53, 65-75
  definition, 14, 20, 42, 55, 77
  distribution, 50-52
  dosage regimens, 61-64
  elimination, 52-54
  excretion, 53-54
  mathematical principles, 54-64
    apparent volume of distribution, 58-60, 803
    clearance, 60-61
    compartment models, 54-56
    kinetics, 55-58
Phenacemide, 313
Phenacetin, 349, 360

Phenanthrene methanol, 773
Phencyclidine (PCP):
adverse reactions, 381-382
binding to sigma sites, 323
chemistry, 266
classification, 262
dependence, 381
history, 8
mechanism of action, 266
pharmcokinetics, 266-267
pharmacologic effects, 267, 381
structure, 266
tolerance and dependence, 267, 381
treatment of toxicity, 267
Phendimetrazine, 127, 376
Phenelzine:
adverse reactions, 300
chemistry, 299
drug interactions, 300
mechanism of action, 299
pharmacokinetics, 295, 299
pharmacologic effects, 293
structure, 290
uses, 301
Phenformin, 607
Phenmetrazine, 268
Phenobarbital:
abuse, 379
adverse reactions, 237, 310, 804
classification, 225, 234, 305
controlled substance schedule, 376
drug interactions, 79, 225, 227, 282, 298, 307, 312, 683
mechanism of action, 309
pharmacokinetics, 235, 236, 305, 309
pharmacologic effects, 235
structure, 234, 309
uses, 238, 305, 309, 314
Phenol, 807
Phenolphthalein, 572, 807
Phenothiazines:
adverse reactions, 280-281
chemistry, 275
contraindication, 282
drug interactions, 238, 258, 282, 316, 412, 476, 575
mechanism of action, 258, 275
pharmacodynamics, 82, 167, 277, 278, 628
pharmacokinetic, 279
structure, 276
treatment of toxicity, 807
Phenoxybenzamine:
adverse reactions, 141
chemistry, 140
classification, 130
mechanism of action, 141
pharmacologic effects, 141
pharmacokinetics, 141
site of action, 131
structure, 140
uses, 141, 143
Phensuximide, 306, 311
Phenteramine, 127
Phentolamine:
adverse reactions, 140
chemistry, 139
classification, 130
drug interactions, 259
mechanism of action, 139, 140
pharmacologic effects, 139-140
pharmacokinetics, 140
site of action, 131
structure, 139
uses, 140, 471
Phenylbutazone:
adverse reactions, 86, 349, 358
classification, 346, 357
drug interactions, 79, 296, 532
hypersensitivity reaction, 86
pharmacokinetics, 67, 80, 346, 357-358
structure, 357
uses, 358
Phenylephrine:
chemistry, 116
pharmacodynamics, 119, 122
mechanism of action, 81, 114, 115
structure, 117
uses, 122, 128, 169, 371
Phenylethylamines, 116, 117
Phenylpropanolamine:
adverse reactions, 127
pharmacologic effects, 127
structure, 117
use, 122, 127
Phenytoin:
adverse reactions, 86, 308, 514
biotransformation, 65-67
classification, 305, 401
drug interactions, 136, 250, 259, 282, 298, 307, 350, 354, 412, 420, 493, 514, 566, 568, 607, 626, 683, 748
history of, 6
mechanism of action, 306-307
pharmacokinetics, 305, 307
pharmacologic effects, 401, 416
structure, 306, 416
uses, 250, 303, 305, 307-308, 314, 395, 412, 416, 545
Phosphates, 594
Phosphine, 816
Phosphonoacetic acid, 767
Phosphorous, 807
Phylloquinone, 529, 530
Physostigmine:
adverse reactions, 156
classification, 154
mechanism of action, 154
pharmacokinetics, 154-155
pharmacologic effects, 156
source, 154

structure, 155
use, 156, 167, 808
Phytonadione, 531
Plicamycin, 594, 657, 668
Pilocarpine:
adverse reactions, 151
classification, 147
pharmacodynamics, 151
pharmacokinetics, 151
structure, 150
uses, 151
Pimozide, 278, 285
Pindolol (*see* also Beta-adrenergic blocking agents):
classification, 130
compliance, 474
pharmacodynamic properties, 134, 473, 474
pharmacokinetics, 135
physicochemical properties, 135, 474
structure, 132
uses, 137-138, 474
Pioglitazone, 609
Pipecuronium, 175, 178
Piperacillin:
adverse reactions, 700
antimicrobial spectrum, 704, 705
classification, 697, 704
pharmacokinetics, 697, 699, 704-705
structure, 698
uses, 705
Pirbuterol:
classification, 490
mechanism of action, 115
structure, 124
uses, 119, 124, 490
Pirenzepine, 169, 564
Piriprost, 496, 497
Piroxicam, 346, 357
Placebo effect, 86-88
Plasminogen, 523-525
Platelet activating factor, 485, 487, 488, 497, 576
Platelet activating factor antagonists, 496, 577
Plicamycin, 594, 657
Podophyllotoxins, 671-672
Poisons (*see also* Toxicants):
classes of, 806
definition of, 803
household, 810-811
Polycarbophil, 570, 572
Polychlorinated biphenyls (PCBs), 819
Polyethylene glycol, 573-574, 810
Polyglutamate, 511-512
Polymorphism, 75
Polymyxin B, 176
Polyphenolic laxatives, 572
Polythiazide, 458, 470
Potassium:
adverse reactions, 830
arsenite, 826
treatment 807
Potassium arsenite, 826
Potassium chloride, 395
Potassium iodide, 495, 589
Potassium permanganate, 807
Potassium phosphate, 594
Potassium-sparing diuretics, 455, 463-465, 466
Pralidoxime chloride (2-PAM):
adverse reactions, 162
mechanism of action, 160, 162
pharmacokinetics, 162
uses, 161, 162, 168, 808, 815
Pramoxine, 368, 371
Pravastatin: 450, 451, 452
Prazepam:
biotransformation, 67, 248
contraindications and precautions, 250
controlled substance schedule, 376
pharmacokinetics, 246, 247, 248
structure, 245
uses, 247
Praziquantel, 788, 790, 793-794
Prazosin:
adverse reactions, 476
classification, 130
drug interactions, 436
mechanism of action, 140, 143, 475
pharmacokinetics, 475, 476
pharmacologic effects, 398, 475
site of action, 131
structure, 475
uses, 143, 398, 475-476, 482
Prednisolone:
classification, 644, 657, 677
history of, 7
pharmacologic effects, 644
relative activity, 644
structure, 642
uses, 677
Prednisone:
adverse reactions, 684
classification, 644
pharmacokinetics, 85
pharmacologic effects, 644, 646
relative activity, 644
structure, 642
uses, 500, 545, 677, 679, 682, 684
Prenalterol, 115
Prilocaine:
adverse reactions, 373
pharmacokinetics, 368, 369
structure, 366
uses, 371, 373
Primaquine:
adverse reaction, 779
chemistry, 778
mechanism of action, 778
pharmacokinetics, 87, 778
pharmacologic effects, 778
uses, 772, 774, 775, 778
Primidone:
adverse reactions, 310, 514

classification, 305
drug interactions, 514, 626
pharmacokinetics, 305, 310
structure, 310
uses, 305, 310

Probenecid:
adverse reactions, 362
chemistry, 361
drug interactions, 79, 349, 353, 362, 607, 765, 768
mechanism of action, 362
pharmacokinetics, 80, 87, 362
structure, 361
uses, 362

Probucol:
adverse reactions, 450
chemistry, 449
mechanism of action, 441, 449-450
pharmacokinetics, 450
structure, 449
uses, 446, 450

Procainamide:
adverse reactions, 413-414
chemistry, 413
classification, 401
drug interactions, 412, 414, 420
history of, 6
mechanism of action, 412-413
pharmacokinetics, 72, 75, 368, 413
pharmacologic effects, 401, 412-413
structure, 413
uses, 395, 413

Procaine:
adverse reactions, 373
drug interactions, 78-79
history of, 5, 365
mechanism of action, 413
pharmacokinetics, 72, 368, 369
structure, 366
uses, 368, 373

Procarbazine:
adverse reactions, 667-668
classification, 657
drug interactions, 259, 668
mechanism of action, 667
pharmacokinetics, 667
uses, 665, 667

Prochlorperazine, 276, 278
Procoagulant agents, 520, 534-535
Procyclidine, 169, 298, 316
Prodrug, definition of, 53, 66
Prodynorphin, 321-322
Proenkephalin, 321

Progesterone:
biological effects, 613, 616, 620, 621, 628
biosynthesis, 614, 641
chemistry, 621
pharmacodynamics, 613, 621
history of, 7
mechanism of action, 621
pharmacokinetics, 621
secretion, 612
structure, 614, 621, 641
uses, 621, 623

Progestins, 620-634 (*see also Individual Agents*)
biological effects, 621
chemistry, 621
mechanism of action, 621
pharmacokinetics, 621
physiology, 620-621
structures, 622
uses, 621, 623, 674

Proglumide, 561
Proguanil, 772
Prokinetic agents, 574-576
Prolactin, 277, 616, 621, 628
Promazine, 276, 278

Promethazine (*see also* H_1 receptor antagonists and Antipsychotic drugs):
pharmacologic effects, 194, 279
structural class, 192
structure, 276
use, 193, 194, 196

Prontosil, 69-70
Proopiomelanocortin (POMC), 321
Propafenone: 10, 401, 417-418
Propanolamine, 128
Propantheline bromide, 168-169, 395, 564
Proparacaine, 371
Propofol, 10, 230

Propoxyphene:
classification, 325
controlled substance schedule, 376
pharmacokinetics, 85, 327, 328, 338
pharmacologic effects, 338
structure, 338

Propoxur, 815

Propranolol (*see also* β-Adrenergic blocking agents):
adverse reactions, 136
classification, 133, 401
compliance, 474
drug interactions, 136, 282, 412, 493, 750
history of, 13
mechanism of action, 131, 133
pharmacokinetics, 85, 135-136
pharmacologic effects, 121, 133-135, 401, 419, 470, 474, 584
physicochemical properties, 135, 474
structures, 132
uses, 136, 252, 395, 419, 430, 471, 474, 589

Propylthiouracil, 584, 588

Prostaglandins (PGs) (*see also* Eicosanoids):
allergy and inflammation 211, 214
biosynthesis, 206-208, 347
chemistry, 205-208
classification as antiulcer drugs, 562
history of, 8
mechanism of action, 210
pharmacokinetics, 71, 211

pharmacologic effects, 213-215
physiological effects, 211-214, 485
uses, 214, 562
Protamine sulfate, 527, 601
Protein binding:
binding forces, 51
plasma protein binding, 51-52
tissue binding, 52
Protirelin, 589
Protriptyline:
chemistry, 289
mechanism of action, 291
pharmacodynamics, 293
pharmacokinetics, 295
structure, 290
uses, 301
Pseudoephedrine, 126, 568
Psilocin, 265
Psilocybin:
classification, 262
chemistry, 262-263
mechanism of action, 263
pharmacokinetics, 265
sources, 265
Psychotomimetics (Hallucinogens) (*see also Individual Agents*):
anticholinergic type, 265-266
classification, 262
LSD type, 262-265
miscellaneous type, 266-274
Psyllium husk, 573
Psyllium hydrophilic mucilloid, 572
Pyramal, 815
Pyrantel pamoate, 788, 789, 794-795
Pyrazinamide, 751, 753, 754
Pyrethrum, 815-816
Pyridostigmine:
adverse reactions, 158
classification, 154
pharmacokinetics, 158
pharmacologic effects, 158
structure, 155
use, 158, 808
Pyridoxine:
adverse reactions, 553
classification, 539
deficiency syndrome, 553
drug interactions, 316, 553, 834
role in metabolism, 552
uses, 743, 752, 552, 553
2-Pyridylethylamine, 188
Pyrilamine, *see* H_1 receptor antagonists
Pyrimethamine:
adverse reactions, 781
drug interactions, 412
mechanism of action, 514, 780
pharmacokinetics, 780
pharmacologic effects, 780
structure, 780
uses, 772, 774, 776, 780-781, 785
Pyrimethamine-sulfadiazine, 772, 781, 785
Pyrimidine, 759
Pyrolan, 815

Q

Quazepam:
mechanism of action, 238-239
pharmacokinetics, 239, 247
uses, 239, 247, 250
Quinacrine, 772, 781, 785
Quinapril:
classification, 479
pharmacokinetics, 481, 482
pharmacologic effects, 398
structure, 480
uses, 398, 481
Quinestrol, 618
Quinidine:
adverse reactions, 83, 351, 408, 411-412
chemistry, 409-410
classification, 401
drug interactions, 79, 136, 282, 395, 412, 418, 420, 532, 568, 750
history of, 5
mechanism of action, 401, 776
pharmacokinetics, 87, 411
pharmacologic effects, 401, 410-411
source, 410
structure, 410, 776
treatment of poisoning, 807-808
uses, 401, 411, 773, 776
Quinine:
adverse reactions, 351, 776-777
chemistry, 409, 410
drug interactions, 412
filler for drugs of abuse, 377
history, 4
mechanism of action, 776
pharmacokinetics, 776
pharmacologic effects, 776, 409-410
sources, 776
structure, 776
treatment of toxicity, 807
uses, 411, 772, 773, 774, 776
Quinolones, *see* Fluroquinolones
Quinone, 69-71

R

Ramipril:
classification, 479
pharmacokinetics, 481, 482
pharmacologic effects, 398
structure, 480
uses, 398, 481
Ranitidine:
adverse reactions, 198, 562

chemistry, 197
drug interactions, 199, 566, 576
mechanism of action, 197
pharmacokinetics, 198
pharmacologic effects, 188, 197-198, 562
structure, 197
uses, 199, 562
Receptor, ion selectivity, 31
Receptor-G-protein-effector system, 33-37
Receptor tyrosine kinases, 37-39
Receptor-mediated transport system, 50-51
Receptors, 20-21, 28-41
adenosine receptors, 492
adrenergic receptors, 102-103, 105, 110-112, 114, 115
benzodiazepine receptors, 246
cholinergic receptors, 31-32, 102-103, 109-112
dopaminergic receptors, 110, 112, 276-277
GABA receptors, 32-33
glutamate receptors, 33, 324
glycine receptors, 33
histamine receptors, 185, 187-188, 275, 289
5-hydroxytryptamine receptors, 200, 251
insulin receptors, 37-39, 599-600
ion channel receptors, 29-31
muscarinic receptors, 104, 109-111, 147-148, 275, 289
neurokinin receptors, 323
nicotinic acetylcholine receptors, 31-32, 104, 108-111, 147, 173
nuclear receptors, 39-40
opioid receptors, 322-324
other receptors, 40
regulation of, 112
retinoic acid receptors, 540
tyrosine kinase-associated receptors, 37-39
Receptors and intracellular signals, 28-41
Redistribution, 52
Regular insulin, 601, 602
Renal physiology, 455-457
Renin-Angiotensin system, 478-479
Reserpine:
adverse reactions, 144, 476
chemistry, 143
classification, 130
drug interactions, 316, 412
history, of, 6
mechanism of action, 143-144
pharmacologic effects, 144
site of action, 131
structure, 143
uses, 144, 470, 476
Retinoic acid receptors, 540
Retinoids, 540, 543
Retinol, *see* Vitamin A
Retinyl palmitate, 541
Ribavirin:
adverse reactions, 767
history of, 11
mechanism of action, 764
structure, 767
uses, 763, 764, 765, 767
Riboflavin, 539, 549-550
Ribosylcytosine, 658
Rifabutin, 754
Rifampin:
adverse reactions, 750
antimicrobial activity, 748-749
drug interactions, 237, 395, 493, 607, 626, 683, 761
history of, 9
mechanism of action, 748
mechanisms of resistance, 749, 753
pharmacokinetics 749-750
structure, 749
uses, 750, 753-754, 765
Rimantadine, 764
Risk, definition of, 803
Risperidone, 285
Ritodrine:
adverse reactions, 125
mechanism of action, 115
use, 120, 125
Rodenticides, 814
Rotenone, 815
RU 486, *see* Mifepristone

S

Salicylates:
adverse reactions, 85
drug interactions, 79, 362, 532, 568, 607
excretion, 80
history of, 5
treatment of toxicity, 807
Salicylic acid:
adverse reactions, 350, 352
chemistry, 345, 354
classification, 346
pharmacokinetics, 350-351, 353, 354
source, 345
structure, 346
uses, 350
Salicylism, 348, 351, 353
Saline, 495, 496, 594
Saline laxatives, 573
Salmeterol:
adverse reactions, 124
classification, 490
mechanism of action, 115, 124
pharmacokinetics, 124
pharmacologic effects, 124
uses, 115, 119, 124, 490
Salsalate, 346, 353, 354
Saralasin, 479
Sargramostim, 655-656, 678, 686-687
Sarin, 161
Scatchard plot, 23

Scopolamine:
adverse reactions, 166-167
chemistry, 163
classification as a psychotomimetic, 262
mechanism of action, 163-164, 265-266
pharmacologic effects, 164-166, 169
pharmacokinetics, 166
sources, 163
structure, 164
uses, 167-168, 169, 170, 230
Secobarbital:
adverse reactions, 237
classification, 234
controlled substance schedule, 376
pharmacokinetics, 235, 236
sedative effects, 235
structure, 234
uses, 238
Second messengers, 28-41
Second generation cephalosporins, 707, 709-711 (*see also Individual Agents*)
Sedative dependence, 379
Sedative-Hypnotic agents:
barburates, 233-238
benzodiazepines, 238-239
drug interactions, 237
miscellaneous compounds, 239-242
Sedatives, 296, 425
Selective toxicity, 691
Selegilene, 318,807
Selenium, 807
Serotonin, *see* 5-Hydroxytryptamine
Sertraline:
adverse reactions, 298
chemistry, 297
drug interactions, 298
history of, 10
mechanism of action, 291, 297
pharmacokinetics, 295, 298
pharmacologic effects, 293
structure, 290
Sevoflurane:
classification, 219
pharmcodynamics, 228
pharmacokinetics, 228
physicochemical properties, 220, 228
Silver, 807
Simvastatin, 450-451
Skeletal muscle relaxants (*see also Individual Agents*):
classification, 173
centrally-acting drugs, 173, 180-181
direct-acting muscle relaxant, 173, 180
drug interactions, 412, 414, 436
neuromuscular blocking drugs, 173-180
Slow-reacting substance (SRS), 209
Slow-reacting substance of anaphylaxis (SRS-A), 209
Soaps, 810
Sodium arsanilate, 826
Sodium bicarbonate:
as a mucokinetic agent, 495, 496
as an antacid, 567, 568
drug interactions, 79, 287, 351
uses, 495, 496, 509, 807-808
Sodium biphosphate, 573
Sodium carbonate, 810
Sodium channel, 402-404
Sodium hypochlorite, 810
Sodium iodide, radioactive ($Na^{131}I$), 588, 589
Sodium nitrate, 808, 818
Sodium nitrite, 818
Sodium nitroprusside:
adverse reactions, 484, 818
chemistry, 483
history of, 8
mechanism of action, 426, 483-484
pharmacologic effects, 398, 476
pharmacokinetics, 484
uses, 387, 397, 398, 483, 484
Sodium phosphate, 573, 810
Sodium silicate, 810
Sodium stibogluconate, 772, 783
Sodium thiosulfate, 808, 818, 827
Soman, 155, 161
Somatostatin, 323, 570
Somatotropin, 628
Sorbitan monostearate, 810
Sotalol (*see also* β-Adrenergic blocking agents):
adverse reactions, 421
classification, 130, 133, 137, 401
history of, 10
mechanism of action, 401, 421
pharmacodynamic properties, 134, 401
pharmacokinetics, 135, 137, 421
physicochemical properties, 135
uses, 138, 421, 423
Spectinomycin, 724
Spironolactone:
adverse reactions, 463
chemistry, 463
classification, 455, 470
drug interactions, 287, 395, 463
mechanism of action, 463, 649
pharmacokinetics, 463, 470
structure, 463, 649
uses, 463-464, 469, 637, 649
Standard safety margin, 19
Stanozolol, 631, 633
Steroid hormones, 654, 789
Stimulant laxatives, 572
Stimulants, 806
Stool softeners, 573
STP, *see* DOM
Stramonium, 163, 315, 807
Street drugs, 806
Streptokinase, 10, 351, 533
Streptomycin:
adverse reactions, 722-723, 752
antimicrobial spectrum, 700, 721, 752

chemistry, 719
drug interactions, 753
history of, 6
pharmacodynamics, 176
pharmacokinetics, 722
mechanism of action, 722
resistance, 752
structure, 720
uses, 700, 723-724, 751, 752, 754
Streptozocin, 657, 667
Structure-activity relationships, 13
Strychnine, 4, 804, 807
Subacute toxicity, definition of, 803
Substance P, 109, 323
Succimer, 824, 833
Succinate, 69
Succinic dihydrogenase, 505
Succinylcholine:
adverse reactions, 180, 225-226
biotransformation, 72, 87, 179
drug interactions, 82, 462
history of, 6
mechanism of action, 175-176
pharmacokinetics, 75, 84, 178, 179
pharmacologic effects, 176-177
structure, 174
uses, 179, 370
Sucralfate:
adverse reactions, 565
drug interactions, 566, 587
pharmacokinetics, 565
pharmacologic effects, 565
structure, 565
uses, 566
Sufentanil:
chemistry, 335, 336
classification, 219, 325
pharmacokinetics, 327, 328, 336
uses, 230-231, 336
Sulbactam, 705-706
Sulconazole, 758, 761
Sulfadiazine:
adverse reactions, 738
antimicrobial spectrum, 736
chemistry, 737
mechanism of action, 736
mechanism of resistance, 736
pharmacokinetics, 736-737
uses, 738-739
Sulfadoxine, 772, 781, 737-739
Sulfamerazine, 736-739
Sulfamethazine, 736-739
Sulfamethoxazole, 736-739
Sulfasalazine, 577
Sulfinpyrazone:
adverse reactions, 362
drug interactions, 349, 353, 532
pharmacokinetics, 362
pharmacologic effects, 362
structure, 362
Sulfisoxazole, 736-739
Sulfonamides (*see also Individual Agents*):
adverse reactions, 86, 779, 807, 738
antimicrobial spectrum, 736
biotransformation, 72, 87
chemistry, 607
drug interactions, 350, 354, 607
history of, 5
mechanism of action, 736
mechanism of resistance, 736
pharmacodynamics, 780
pharmacokinetics, 736-737, 80
structures, 737
treatment of toxicity, 807
uses, 738-739
Sulfonates, 810
Sulfones, 779-780
Sulfonylurea derivatives, *see* Oral hypoglycemics
Sulfur dioxide, 813
Sulfur oxides, 811
Sulindac:
adverse reactions, 357
biotransformation, 66
classification, 346, 356
pharmacokinetics, 346, 357
structure, 356
Sulmethazole:
adverse reactions, 738
antimicrobiral spectrum, 736
mechanism of action, 736
mechanism of resistance, 736
structure, 737
uses, 738-739
Sumatriptan, 201-202
Suramin, 772, 785
Sympathomimetic amines, 395
Sympathomimetic agents, *see* Adrenergic agonists

T

Tabun, 161
Tachyphylaxis, 126, 375
Tacrine:
adverse reactions, 159-160
classification, 154
mechanism of action, 159
pharmacokinetics, 159
pharmacodynamics, 159
use, 159
Tamoxifen:
adverse reactions, 619, 674
classification as an antineoplastic, 657
history of, 9
pharmacologic effects, 619
pharmacokinetics, 619
structure, 615
uses, 634, 673-674
Tazobactam, 705-706
TD_{50} (median toxic dose), 18

Teicoplanin, 717
Telenzepine, 169, 564
Temazepam:
mechanism of action, 238-239
pharmacokinetics, 239
ues, 239, 247, 250
Teniposide (VM-26), 657, 671-672
Teprotide, 479
Terazosin:
adverse reactions, 476
classification, 130
mechanism of action, 143, 475
pharmacokinetics, 475, 476
pharmacologic effects, 475
site of action, 131
structure, 475
uses, 143, 475-476
Terbutaline:
adverse reactions, 491
classification, 490
adverse reactions, 123
mechanism of action, 115
pharmacokinetics, 123, 491
pharmacologic effects, 123
structure, 123
use, 120, 123, 490, 491
Terconazole, 758, 762
Terfenadine (*see also* H_1 receptor antagonists):
adverse reactions, 195
pharmacokinetics, 194-195
pharmacologic effects, 194, 497
structural class, 192
uses, 194, 196, 496, 497
Teriparatide, 591
Terpin hydrate, 495
Testosterone:
biosynthesis, 614, 641
chemistry, 630, 633
classification, 657
gender factors, 84
history of, 5
mechanism of action, 630-631
menstrual cycle, 613
pharmacokinetics, 631-632
pharmacologic effects, 632-633
physiologic regulation, 630, 632
relative activity, 633
structure, 614, 631, 641
uses, 633-634
Testosterone cypionate, 631, 632, 633
Testosterone enanthate, 633
Testosterone propionate, 633
Tetracaine:
pharmacokinetics, 368, 369, 373
structure, 366
uses, 371, 372, 373
2,3,7,8-Tetrachlorodibenzo-p-dioxin (TCDD), 818
Tetrachlorodiphenylethane (TDE), 814
Tetrachloroethylene, 814
Tetracycline:
adverse reactions, 86, 87, 744-745, 804
antimicrobial spectrum, 743-744
drug interactions, 78, 79, 238, 566, 568, 575
history of, 6
mechanism of action, 743
mechanism of resistance, 744
neuromuscular blockade, 176
pharmacokinetics, 744-745
structure, 743
uses, 567, 776, 745, 781
Tetrahydrocannabinols:
adverse reactions, 273
chemistry, 270-271
controlled substance schedule, 376
dependence, 382
intoxication, 273
mechanism of action, 273
pharmacokinetics, 271-273
pharmacologic effects, 273
structures, 271
tolerance and dependence, 273
tratment of toxicity, 273
uses, 273-274
Tetrahydrofolic acid (FH_4), 511
Tetrahydrozoline, 117, 122
Tetraiodothyronine (T_4), 583-586 (*see also* Levothyroxine sodium)
Thallium, 437
THC, *see* Tetrahydrocannabinols
Theobromine, 491, 492
Theophylline:
adverse reactions, 225, 492-493
biotransformation, 80, 69-70
chemistry, 491
classification, 490, 491
drug interactions, 79, 493, 761
mechanism of action, 492
pharmacokinetics, 493
pharmacologic effect, 486, 492-493
structure, 492
uses, 396, 490, 491, 493-494, 498, 499, 500
Therapeutic index, 18-19, 88, 394, 804
Thiabendazole: 788, 789, 795-796
Thiamine, 539, 548-549
Thiazide diuretics, *see* Diuretics
Thiazide-related compounds, *see* Diuretics
2-Thiazoylethylamine, 188
Thiobarbiturate, 230
Thioether, 72
Thioguanine:
adverse reactions, 660
classification, 656, 657
drug interactions, 660
immunosuppressant, 680
mechanism of action, 659
pharmacokinetics, 659-660
uses, 660
Thiopental:
classification, 228, 234

distribution, 52-53
history of, 5
pharmacodynamics, 229
pharmacokinetics, 229, 235, 236
structure, 234
uses, 228
Thioperamide, 188
Thioridazine:
adverse reactions, 280-281
contraindications, 282
structure, 276
pharmacokinetics, 279
pharmacologic effects, 277, 278, 279
uses, 285
Thiotepa:
classification, 657
mechanism of action, 666
pharmacokinetics, 666
structure, 665
uses, 656, 666
Thiothixene, 278, 282, 283
2-Thiazoylethylamine, 188
Thiouracil, 72
Third generation cephalosporins, 707, 709, 711-713 (*see also Individual agents*)
Threshold limit value, definition of, 803
Thrombin, 536
Thromboxanes:
A_2 as a platelet aggregator, 212, 520, 532
biosynthesis, 206-208, 347
in bronchospasm, 485
mechanism of action, 210
physiologic effects, 212, 213
Thyroid, desiccated, 587
Thyroid hormones:
disorders of thyroid function, 586-588
effect on lactation, 628
normal thyroid function, 583-586
treatment of hyperthyroidism, 588-589
treatment of hypothyroidism, 587
Thyroxine, *see* Levothyroxine sodium
Ticarcillin:
adverse reactions, 700
antimicrobial spectrum, 704, 705
classification, 697, 704
pharmacokinetics, 699, 704-705
structure, 698
uses, 705
Ticarcillin-clavulanate, 705, 706
Ticlodipine, 12
Timolol (*see also* β-Adrenergic blocking agents):
chemistry, 131
classification, 130, 133, 137
pharmacodynamic properties, 134, 474
pharmacokinetics, 135
physicochemical properties, 135, 474
structure, 132
uses, 137-138, 474
Tin, 824
Tinidazole, 772
Tissue-type plasminogen activator (t-PA), 523-525
Tobramycin:
adverse reactions, 722-723
antimicrobial spectrum, 721
chemistry, 719
mechanism of action, 719, 721
mechanism of resistance, 722
neuromuscular blockade, 176
pharmacokinetics, 722
structure, 720
uses, 723
Tocainide:
adverse reactions, 416
classification, 401
chemistry, 416
history of, 8
mechanism of action, 401
pharmacokinetics, 416
pharmacologic effects, 401, 416
structure, 416
uses, 416, 423
α-Tocopherol, 453, 545-548
Tolazamide (*see also* Sulfonylurea derivatives):
classification, 604
disulfiram-like reaction, 259
pharmacokinetics, 605-606
structure, 605
Tolbutamide (*see also* Sulfonylurea derivatives):
classification, 604
doses, 606
disulfiram-like reaction, 259
drug interactions, 298, 762
pharmacokinetics, 605-606
structure, 605
Tolerance, definition of, 375
Tolmetin sodium, 346, 359
Tolnaftate, 757, 763
Toluene, 814
Topotecan, 657, 672
Torsemide:
adverse reactions, 461
chemistry, 460
classification, 455, 470
drug interactions, 462
pharmacokinetics, 461-462, 470
uses, 462, 469
Total body clearance, 60, 804
Toxaphene, 814
Toxicants:
Heavy metals: 821-834
Non-metallic:
air pollution, 811-813
cyanide, 816-818
herbicides, 818-819
household poisons, 810-811
pesticides, 814-816
solvents, 814
Toxicity, definition of, 803
Toxicodynamics, 804
Toxicokinetics, 803-804

Toxicology:
definitions and terms, 803
drugs used in the management of poisoning, 807-808
factors that modify toxicity, 804-805
incidence of poisoning, 805
prevention of poisoning, 805-
toxicodynamics, 804
toxicokinetics, 803-804
treatment of acute poisoning, 806-807
Toxins, definition of, 803
Toxoplasmosis, 772, 785
Tranexamic acid, 535-536
Tranycypromine:
adverse reactions, 300
chemistry, 299
drug interactions, 300
mechanism of action, 299
pharmacokinetics, 295, 300
pharmacologic effects, 292, 293
structure, 290
Trazodone:
adverse reactions, 298-299
mechanism of action, 291, 298
pharmacokinetics, 295
pharmacologic effects, 293
structure, 290
Tretinoin, 543
Triamcinolone, 642, 644
Triamcinolone acetonide, 489, 499, 648
Triamterene:
adverse reactions, 464
classification, 455, 470
drug interactions, 287
pharmacokinetics, 463, 464, 470
pharmacologic effects, 464
structure, 464
uses, 464
Triazolam:
chemistry, 244
mechanism of action, 238-239
pharmacokinetics, 239, 247
uses, 239, 247, 250
Triazole derivatives, 757, 758, 761-763 (*see also Individual Agents*)
Triazolobenzodiazepines, 244
Trichlorfon, 815
Trichlormethiazide, 470
1,1,1,-Trichloroethane, 814
Trichloroethanol, 71
Trichloroethylene, 814
2,4,5-Trichlorophenoxyacetic acid, 818
Trichomoniasis, 772, 785
Tricyclic antidepressants, *see* Antidepressants
Triethylenethiophosphoramide, *see* Thiotepa
Trifluoperazine:
adverse reactions, 280
pharmacokinetics, 279
pharmacologic effects, 277-278
structure, 276
Triflupromazine, 276
Trifluridine, 764-766
Trihexyphenidyl, 169, 316
Triiodothyronine (T_3), 583-586 (*see also* Liothyronine sodium)
TRI-LEVLEN, 625
Trimeprazine, *see* H_1 receptor antagonists
Trimethadione:
adverse reactions, 308, 313
classification, 305
uses, 305, 306, 313
Trimethaphan, 170-172
Trimethoprim:
adverse reactions, 740
antimicrobial spectrum, 739
drug interactions, 607
history of, 11
mechanism of action, 514, 739
mechanism of resistance, 739-740
pharmacokinetics, 740
structure, 739
uses, 739-740, 772, 780, 785
Trimethyl bismuth, 831
Trimipramine:
chemistry, 289
mechanism of action, 291
pharmacokinetics, 295
pharmacologic effects, 293
TRI-NORINYL, 625
Triorthocresyl phosphate (TOCP), 815
Tripelennamine, *see* H_1 receptor antagonists
TRIPHASIL, 625
Triprolidine, *see* H_1 receptor antagonists
Troleandomycin, 493
Tropicamide, 169-170
Trypanosomiasis, 772, 783
Tryptophan, 298
Tuberculosis, chemotherapy of, 753-754
Tubocurarine:
adverse reactions, 180
chemistry, 173
drug interactions, 459, 462
histamine release, 177, 187
history of, 3, 6
mechanism of action, 173-176
pharmacologic effects, 85, 176-178
pharmacokinetics, 177-178
structure, 174
uses, 179-180
Tumor necrosis factor (TNF), 643
Tyramine:
adrenergic mechanisms, 81, 114-116, 125
biotransformation, 69-70
drug interactions, 296
Tyrosine kinase-associated receptors, 37-39

U

Ultralente insulin, 602

Undecylenic acid, 757, 763
Up-regulation, 25
Uracil, 658
Urea, 287
Uricosuric agent, definition of, 349
Urokinase, 523-525, 533, 534

V

Valproic acid:
  adverse reactions, 308, 312
  classification, 305
  drug interactions, 312
  history of, 6
  mechanism of action, 312
  pharmacokinetics, 305, 312
  structure, 312
  uses, 305, 306, 312
Vancomycin:
  adverse reactions, 716-717
  antimicrobial spectrum, 716
  history of, 6
  mechanism of resistance, 716
  mechanism of action, 716
  pharmacokinetics, 716
  uses, 717, 750
Vasoactive intestinal peptide, 109, 323
Vasodilator drugs, 387, 397, 398
Vecuronium:
  mechanism of action, 175
  pharmacokinetics, 178
  structure, 174
Verapamil:
  adverse reactions, 435, 436
  classification, 401, 430, 478
  drug interactions, 136, 436
  history of, 8, 10
  mechanism of action, 401, 432
  pharmacologic effects, 401, 421, 432, 434
  pharmacokinetics, 434, 435
  structure, 431
  uses, 412, 421, 423, 434, 435, 478
Vidarabine, 9, 764-766
Vinblastine, 654, 657, 671
Vincristine, 654, 657, 671
Vitamin A:
  adverse reactions, 540, 542-543
  biochemistry, 540-541
  biotransformation, 69, 70
  deficiency syndrome, 541
  history of, 5
  mechanism of action, 540
  molecular biology, 540-541
  pharmacologic uses, 541
  pharmacology, 540-541
  role in metabolism, 541
  sources, 540
  teratogenicity, 541
Vitamin B_1, *see* Thiamine
Vitamin B_2, *see* Riboflavin
Vitamin B_6, *see* Pyridoxine
Vitamin B_{12}:
  adverse reactions, 517
  chemistry and nomenclature, 515
  classification, 539
  deficiency, 503, 513-514, 516
  diagnosis of deficiency, 516-517
  history of, 7
  mechanism of action, 515
  metabolic functions, 515-516
  pharmacokinetics, 515
  preparations, 517
  sources, 515
  structure, 515
  therapy of defiency, 517
Vitamin C, *see* Ascorbic acid
Vitamin D:
  adverse reactions, 540, 545, 593
  classification, 590, 592
  deficiency syndrome, 544
  drug interactions, 435
  history of, 5
  metabolism of, 544, 592, 593
  pharmacologic uses, 544
  role in metabolism, 544, 590
  sources, 543, 592
  uses, 543, 544-545
Vitamin D_2, 543, 592
Vitamin D_3, 543, 544, 546, 592-593
Vitamin E:
  adverse reactions, 548
  biochemistry, 545-546
  deficiency syndrome, 546
  physiology, 545
  role in metabolism, 546
  treatment of deficiency, 546
  uses, 453, 547-548
Vitamin K:
  biotransformation, 71
  drug interactions, 81, 349, 447, 531, 532
  function in blood coagulation, 529-530
Vitamins:
  classification, 539
  fat-soluble vitamins, 540-548
  federal regulations, 539-540
  water-soluble vitamins, 548-556

W

Warfarin:
  adverse reactions, 81, 531
  chemistry, 529
  drug interactions, 79, 80, 81, 298, 353, 354, 355, 412, 418, 420, 436, 531, 532, 566, 576, 607, 626, 750, 761, 762
  history of, 6
  mechanism of action, 529-530
  pharmacodynamics, 83

pharmacokinetics, 80, 530-531
structure, 529
uses, 437, 528, 531-532

X

Xanthine derivatives, 490, 491-494 (*see also* Theophylline)
Xenobiotics, 65-66, 71-74
Xylene, 814
Xylometazoline, 122

Y

Yohimbine, 130, 131, 143

Z

Zalcitabine, 763, 765, 768, 769
Zectran, 815
Zidovudine:
adverse reactions, 517, 768
antiviral agent, 763
drug interactions, 768
history of, 11
mechanism of action, 764, 768
pharmacokinetics, 768
uses, 548, 765, 766, 768
Zinc, 822, 828-829
Zolpidem, 242, 376